MOLECULAR TARGETS OF CNS TUMORS

Edited by **Miklos Garami**

Molecular Targets of CNS Tumors
Edited by Miklos Garami

Published by InTech
Janeza Trdine 9, 51000 Rijeka, Croatia

Publishing Process Manager Iva Simcic

Technical Editor Teodora Smiljanic

Cover Designer InTech Design Team

Additional hard copies can be obtained from orders@intechopen.com

Molecular Targets of CNS Tumors, Edited by Miklos Garami
p. cm.
ISBN 978-953-307-736-9

For EU product safety concerns:
IN TECH d.o.o., Prolaz Marije Krucifikse Kozulić 3, 51000 Rijeka, Croatia,
info@intechopen.com or visit our website at intechopen.com.

Meet the editor

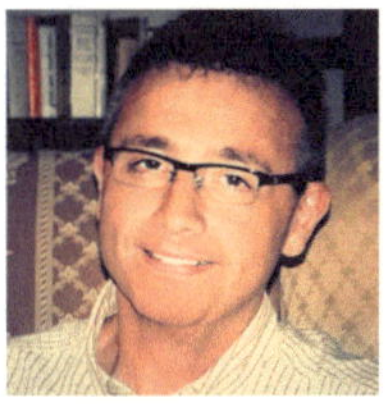

Dr. Miklós Garami, MD., MSc., PhD.; received his MD, Ph.D. and M.Sc. at Semmelweis Medical University (Budapest, Hungary) in 1991.; 2005. and 2007. He also received his Habilitation from Semmelweis Medical University (Budapest, Hungary) in 2010. Currently he is Associate Professor of Pediatrics; Head of Hungarian Pediatric Cancer Registry; Head of Unit of Pediatric Oncology and Deputy Chairman of 2nd Department of Pediatric, Semmelweis University. Dr. Miklós Garami was awarded by Hungarian Academy of Sciences (Postdoctoral Fellowship Semmelweis University (Budapest, Hungary) in 1991-1992 and by American Heart Association (Postdoctoral Fellowship University of California at San Francisco (UCSF), California, USA) in 1992-1995. Current research activities include: Pediatric oncology, investigating gene expression profiles in pediatric malignancies (CNS tumors, NBL, Ewing sc.), information systems on microcomputers. He is the author of approximately 70 scientific papers, 9 books / chapters.

Contents

Preface

Brain tumors are a various group of malignancies that remain refractory to conventional treatment approaches, including radiotherapy and cytotoxic chemotherapy. Molecular neuro-oncology has now begun to clarify the transformed phenotype of brain tumors and identify oncogenic pathways that may be amenable to targeted therapy.

Recently, there has been increasing interest in the use of targeted molecular agents for the treatment of malignant brain pediatric and adult tumors. These agents are generally well tolerated but have demonstrated only modest activity.

This book tries to cover the complexity of the rapidly developing area of targeted therapies in the field of Central Nervous System (CNS) tumors.

Brain tumors present a continuous challenge to the physicians regardless of the patients' age. The goal of this book to provide up-to-date information for physicians based description of regulatory components and effector pathways of selected CNS tumors. This book highlights some importance aspects of selected CNS tumors.

The editor would like to acknowledge the contribution of the authors and the team of the Publishing Process Management at InTech - Open Access Publisher.

Dr. med. habil. Miklos Garami, MD., MSc. PhD.
Associate Professor,
Semmelweis University,
Hungary

Part 1

CNS Tumors - Regulatory Components and Effector Pathways

1

Genetic and Immunology of Brain Tumors

Sahika Liva Cengiz and Aynur Emine Cicekcibasi
Selcuk University/Faculty of Medicine,
Turkey

1. Introduction

Tumors of the intracranial neoplasms are devastating because they frequently cause mortality or morbidity. Current studies have shown that the immune system and genetics may play a critical role in development of different kinds of brain tumors.

New insights into the causes and potential treatment of intracranial neoplasms have come from discovering connections with genes that control cell growth, differentation and development of brain cancer. Host immune response is one of key points in protection against brain tumor development.

This section will outline what is known about molecular genetics, biology and immunogenetics of brain tumors.

- We will first focus on main oncogenes which are seen in CNS tumors and try to find answer how do tumor-brain interactions contribute to development of brain tumor.
- Finally we will discuss the mechanisms of immune activation and immune escape during an anti-tumor specific response, and new concepts for immunogenetic therapeutic intervention..

Thus, the data of immunogenetic pathways that are differentially involved in tumor initiation may represent a novel approach for the treatment of malignant brain tumors.

2. Genetic and immunology of brain tumors

Brain tumors are one of the leading cause of cancer mortality and remain difficult to cure despite advances in surgery and adjuvant therapy. Recent studies are focused on the molecular and cellular analysis of the bulk tumor mass. Glioma is the most common and mortal type of brain tumors (Kleihues et al., 2002). They are typically comprised of morphologically diverse cells that express a variety of neural lineage markers. Gliomas that share similar morphology and phenotype can have a very different prognosis and response to treatment. Alterations of multiple genes in the cell cycle and regulatory pathways plays an important role in tumorigenesis and causes to formation of subtypes (Singh et al., 2003). So researches in gene therapy have been often sice 1912 because no effective therapy is achieved until now in spite of traditional treatments including surgery, radiation therapy, and chemotherapy (Culver et al., 1992). Formerly, the brain has been regarded as an immunologically privileged organ site because it possesses a distinct blood-brain barrier (BBB) and lacks discrete lymphatic structures (Yoffey & Courtice, 1970). Despite these factors minimizing central nervous system (CNS) immune function, a highly adapted system of immune surveillance presents, and effective immune responses can occur in the

CNS. Function of both the complement system (Bernheimer et al., 1988) and the antigen-antibody system, including functional B cells (Aloisi et al., 1999; Sandberg-Wollheim et al., 1986) have been found within the CNS. In the case of CNS pathologies resident antigen-presenting cells (APC) of the CNS, microglia cells, undergo activation and upregulate both major histocompatibility complex (MHC) and costimulatory molecules,and also contribute to both CD41 and CD81 specific T-cell responses (Aloisi et al., 1998; Brannan & Roberts, 2004; Hickey & Kimura, 1987; Hickey et al., 1991; Hickey, 2001; Krakowski & Owens, 2000). Actually a small number of lymphocytes are found in normal, healthy brain (Hickey & Kimura, 1987) however both resident lymphocytes and activated T cells have the capability to cross the BBB (Hickey & Kimura, 1987; Hickey et al., 1991; Hickey, 2001). Several lymphocytes also infiltrate the CNS in the presence of neoplasms (Han et al., 2010). Thus considering these factors new and more effective adjunctive treatments are needed.

3. Brain tumors and oncogenes

Oncogenes are functional mutations associated with cancer progression. They are derived from normal cellular genes called proto-oncogenes. The oncogenes that promote the tumor growth and development affecting mechanisms, such as cell proliferation, invasion, angiogenesis, and resistance to apoptosis by produced proteins are associated with the brain tumors. The protein synthesis which was gene product may increase or functional changes can be seen as a result of oncogenic mutation.

The oncogenic activation associated with nervous system tumors is in the form of gene amplification and the number of cell-specific gene increases. The most common oncogenic change is the amplification of the epidermal growth factor receptor (EGFR) gene and the mutations of the TP53 gene (Ekstrand et al., 1991; Libermann et al., 1985; Wong et al., 1987). The EGFR gene that is activated by growth factors such as EGF, TGF-α is "transmembrane tyrosine kinase" codes.

EGFR gene amplification was observed 40-50% of cases with glioblastoma multiforme, but it is rare in the anaplastic malignant astrocitoma (Brady et al., 1992; Ekstrand et al., 1991; Humphrey et al., 1990; Wong et al., 1987). This change is predictive for the malignancy degree of the astrocitomas (Ng & Lam, 1998). In malignant astrocitomas, the gene amplifications such as the MYCN, CDK4, MDM2, CCND1, and MET including the growth factors family of tyrosine kinase like EGFR were also determined (Bigner et al., 1987; .Fischer et al., 1995; He et al., 1994; Reifenberger et al., 1994).

However, these amplifications were observed lesser than EGFR. In addition, the most common amplification was 10-15% CDK4 in malignant astrocitoma and glioblastoma. Each of these genes have been associated with the malignancy degree of glial tumors. The oncogenic changes were seen less than 10% in the other CNS tumors except for malignant astrocitomas. In medulloblastoma, the CMYC and MYCN amplifications were reported. Additionally, the β-catenin and TCF mutations were also detected in rare cases (Raffel et al., 1990; Wasson et al., 1990; Zurawel et al., 1998).

4. Gene therapy

'Gene therapy' can be defined as the transfer of genetic material into a patient's tumor cells by using stereotaxic injection. Up to present,various treatment strategies utilizing gene therapy have been used, including gene transfer for modulating the immune system, enzyme prodrug ('suicide gene') therapy, oncolytic therapy, replacement/ therapeutic gene transfer, and antisense therapy (Bansal& Engelhard, 2000). Many of them have been attempted both experimentally and in clinical trials (Iwami et al., 2010; Licht et al., 1996; Lun et al., 2010; Pedersini et al., 2010; Schmidt et al., 2011; Steffens et al., 2004; Yawata et al., 2011). Mainly these approaches are based on previously established anti-neoplastic principles, like prodrug activating enzymes, inhibition of tumor neovascularization, and enhancement of the normally infirm anti-tumor immune response.

The strategies of gene therapy can be categorized as follows (Mut& Ziyal,2010).

1. Enzyme prodrug: enzyme prodrug ('suicide gene') therapy.
2. Oncolytic therapy, replacement.
3. Transfer of potentially therapeutic genes such as tumor suprosser (eg p53)
4. Antisense therapy.
5. Kemoprotection: Approaches which use the multidrug-resistance gene to protect bone marrow from myelosuppression following chemotherapy. Chemoresistance genes especially P-glycoprotein, the product of the multidrug-resistance (*MDR*1) gene, plays a major role in clinical treatment failure.
6. Gene therapy for boosting the activity of the immune system againts tumor cells

Approaches	Administered Genes
Enzyme prodrug: enzyme prodrug ('suicide gene') therapy	Suicide genes
Immuno-gene therapy	Genes of antigens and citokins
Peplasman therapy	Therapeutic genes
Kemoprotection therapy	Multi-drug resistance gene (MDR)
Antisence therapy	Antisense DNA
Oncolitic virus therapy	Oncolitic genes

Table 1. Current treatment strategies used in gene therapy. (Karaoglan &Turkmen,2010)

Immune gene therapy aims to enhance the T cell mediated immune responce againts to brain neoplasms by using genetically modified T cell therapy, vaccination therapy and cytokine therapy (Iwami et al., 2010). Cytotoxic therapy is mainly consist of either delivering of gene or virus therapy (Aboody et al., 2008; Aghi & Chiocca, 2006; Candolfi et al., 2009; Kroeger et al., 2010; Lawler et al., 2006). The most common studied conditional cytotoxic transgene is Herpes Simplex Type 1 thymidine kinase (TK), which converts the prodrug ganciclovir (or valacyclovir) into the highly toxic deoxyguanosine triphosphate causing early chain termination of nascent DNA strands (Beltinger et al., 1999). The by-stander effect of the TK approach is related to the passage of phosphorylated ganciclovir to neighboring cells through gap junctions, amplifying the cytotoxic effect of TK gene therapy (Mesnil & Yamasaki, 2000).

4.1 Vectors in gene therapy

Several viral and non-viral vectors have been engineered and used for gene transfer, both experimentally and clinically.

Virotherapy is defined delivery of conditionally replicating viral vectors that solely replicate in tumor cells and kill them (Ferguson et al., 2010; Jiang et al., 2009; Markert et al., 2009). Viruses used for glioma gene therapy can be classified into 2 categories: replicationimcompetent viruses. In the first one, the vector is derived from a virus from which all or most of its genome has been removed, so minimizing the toxicity and retaining the gene delivery efficiency. In the second, only select viral genes are deleted or mutated so that viruses can replicate in and lyse tumor cells selectively (i.e., oncolytic viral therapy) (Iwami et al., 2010).

4.1.1 Strategies in transgenic viruses (Iwami et al., 2010; Kozarsky & Wilson, 1993; Markert et al., 2009)

1. Scientists add healthy functioning genes to cells that have damage or missing genes in order to substitute the bad non-working copy of the gene with a better copy of the working gene. The extraction of reproductive are of virus was done initially. Genes have been added to and removed from the viruses so they cannot replicate on their own, but they can still break out of the tumor cells and invade nearby dividing cancer cells.
2. Injecting of the tumor cell with genes that can kill the tumor cells. For instance, suicide genes are inserted into the tumor cells. A pro-drug or an inactive form of a toxic drug is administered to the patients, and this drug will kill off any tumor cells with the suicide genes in them. This method is called enzyme prodrug ('suicide gene') therapy, Once inside the tumor cells, the viruses produce an enzyme that will turn an otherwise harmless drug into one that is toxic to the tumor cells. When the patient is treated with the drug gancyclovir, the enzyme converts it into something that is toxic to the tumor cells, and those cells die.
3. Researchers can also transfer genetic materials into cancer cells by using ex-vivo techniques. Cancer cells are taken out of the body from the patient's blood or bone marrow surgically, and the necessary genes are added to them in the laboratory.
4. Other method that is commonly used in laboratory is the in-vivo techniques. Virus or a plasmid is entirely necessary because gene cannot be directly inserted into a cell. The gene is inserted into the host's cell by using a vector. A vector acts as a bacteriophage or a plasmid (circular, small pieces of DNA) that can transfer genes from one cell to another. Vectors from the viruses adenoviruses are often used for gene therapy because viruses reproduce by inserting their genetic material into the cells they infect.

Other transferring therapeutic genes to brain tumor cells are mostly used by HSV, retrovirus and adenovirus due to following key points. Application of adenovirus mediated gene therapy was successful in liver cell and respiratory epithelium (Kozarsky & Wilson, 1993; Kramm et al., 1995). Herpes simplex virus-thymidine kinase (HSV-tk) gene, had a good tendency to neuronal cells. Retroviral vectors have long survive in target cells (Kramm et al., 1995). Oncolytic reovirus and measles viral vectors are under development for GBM virotherapy (Kroeger et al., 2010).
Gene directed prodrug therapy utilizing the herpes simplex virus thymidine kinase gene was the first gene therapy experienced clinically (Mesnil & Yamasaki, 2000; Yawata et al., 2011). The most frequent used paradigm is based on the activation of ganciclovir to a cytotoxic compound by a viral enzyme, thymidine kinase, which is expressed by tumor cells, after the gene has been introduced by a retroviral vector. This paradigm has proven to be a potent therapy with minimal side effects in several rodent brain tumor models, and has proceeded to phase 1 clinical trials (Kramm et al., 1995).
Oncolytic viral therapy: This approach uses replication-competent viruses infect and lyse the target cells. An oncolytic vector should conditionally replicate within the target tumor

cells with minimal toxicity to the surrounding normal brain tissue. Oncolytic vectors are grouped as either mesogenic (moderately pathogenic, capable of producing viable progeny and infecting adjacent cells) or lentogenic (attenuated non-pathogenic, produces defective progeny and is incapable of spreading between tissues) (Dey et al., 2010). Replicating, oncolytic viruses have been developed from several species of viruses. The most common vectors are replicating herpes simplex virus (HSV), adenovirus and replication-competent retrovirus (RCR). Replicating herpes simplex virus (HSV) vectors have been tested for the treatment of malignant glioma (Grandi et al., 2009; Granelli-Piperno et al., 2000; Parker et al., 2009). The common widely studied oncolytic HSV vector is G207, a genetically engineered HSV-1 (Markert et al., 2000).

Tumor suppressor gene therapy: Mutation or inactivation of the *p53* tumor suppressor gene is one of the early genetic alterations in the tumor progression of gliomas (Fults et al., 1992; von Deimling et al., 1992). Using a gene to encode a tumor-suppressor protein in glioma cells that is mutated or absent. Is the fundamental of this approach? TP53 is most common studied suppressor gene, whose mutations have been reported in 30-60% of malignant gliomas (Louis et al., 2001; Vousden & Lane, 2007). It is demonstrated that the replacement of wild-type p53 in tumor cells induced rapid cell death even in cells with the intact functional gene (Li et al., 1999; Roth, 2006).

Antisense therapy: Antisense oligonucleotides are single strands of DNA or RNA that are complementary to a chosen sequence. Antisense oligonucleotides specific for insulin-like growth factor-1 (IGF-1) or transforming growth factor b2 (TGF-b2) have been used in various clinical studies (Tambuyzer et al., 2009; Vauleon et al., 2010).

5. Non-viral methods

Non-viral methods provide certain advantages over viral methods, such as simple large scale production and low host immunogenicity, however small levels of transfection and expression of the gene are a disadvantage of this methods (Iwami et al., 2010).

1. Injection of naked DNA or naked PCR product,
2. Physical methods to enhance delivery
   a. Electroporation
   b. Gene gun
   c. Sonoporation
   d. Magnetofection
3. Chemical methods to enhance delivery

Synthetic oligonucleotides, lipoplexes and polyplexes, dendrimers

   a. Hybrid methods: Combination of two or more techniques. For example virosomes are combine with liposomes using an inactivated HIV or influenza virus.

Difficulties in gene therapy in brain tumors can be arranged as follows: (Mut & Ziyal, 2010).

1. Difficulties to recognize tumor cells as target for attack.
2. In order to inject gene cells into the specific region of the brain, to perform stereotactic brain surgery is mandatory.
3. After the genes are injected into the region, there is the possibility that the viral vectors that are used to transfer the genetic material into the cell might infect healthy cells as well as brain tumors.

4. The new gene might also insert into the wrong location in the DNA, thus leading to harmful mutations of the DNA and triggering unwanted reaction by the immune system.
5. The transferred genes can also be overexpressed by producing a lot of missing proteins.
6. Finally, inflammation of the lining of the brain or infection can occur after the treatment.
7. The negative side, on the other hand, is that the gene therapy will affect the development of the fetus in many unexpected ways like causing long-term illness or other side effects. The human gene pool can also be permanently affected by these gene alterations.

6. Supressive factors of gliomas on immune system

Gliomas can abstain immune system at different steps of antigen recognition and immune activation (Parney et al., 2000). Many glioma cells express low or defective levels of human leukocyte antigens (HLA) and also ave been found deficient in proper antigen presentation for cytotoxic and helper T-cell activation (Flügel et al., 1999). Inhibition of antigen presentation by microglia and macrophages in the tumor micro environment also causes to the tumors' ability to escape immune detection.

In gliomas, T cells, specifically the CD41 population, both in peripheral blood and in the tumor microenvironment, have depressed function (Roszman & Brooks, 1985; Roszman et al., 1985). Innate helper T cells (CD41) reveal weak proliferative responses and dramatically lowered synthesis of the TH1 cytokine IL-2 (Das et al., 2008).

One hypothesis sugested that these are actually resident T cells passively infiltrating the tumor across a compromised BBB caused by the tumor; alternatively, they may represent a population that once was active but has been subsequently rendered inactive by the host of immunosuppressive mechanisms found in the tumor microenvironment (Han et al., 2010).

Secretion of various immune inhibitory cytokines and molecules by glioma cells also plays an important role in glioma-associated immunosuppression. High levels of expression of TGF-b2, IL-10 and prostaglandin E2 are present in malignant gliomas (Couldwell et al., 1992; Nitta et al., 1994). TGF-b2 mRNA is found in samples of glioblastome multiforme (GBM) (Bodmer et al., 1989).

Iatrogenic factors may also cause a systemic immunosuppression in patients with glioma (Roszman & Brooks, 1985). Corticosteroids given in the treatment of tumor-associated edema may cause inhibition of cytokine production and sequestration of CD41 T cells (Barshes et al., 2004). Otherwise recent reports suggest, however, that at therapeutic doses corticosteroids may not interfere with immunotherapy (Fenstermaker & Ciesielski, 2004; Lesniak et al., 2004).

Stimulation of microglia in the existence of tumor cells reduces the secretion of proinflammatory cytokines, such as tumor necrosis factor (TNF)-a, however also increases the secretion of the inhibitory cytokine interleukin (IL)-10 (Dix et al., 1999).

7. Immunotherapy

Immunotherapy is one of the new promising therapeutic approaches that can especially target tumour cells. Adoptive and active immunotherapies using lymphokine-activated killer cells, cytotoxic T cells, tumour-infiltrating lymphocytes, autologous tumour cells, and dendritic cells are mainly used in this approach (Prasad et al., 2004).

Microglial cells constitute the first step of defense for the brain. They migrate toward inflammatory zones and, after activation, possess phagocytic properties and synthesize several types of cytokines and chemokines (Tsurushima et al., 1999). They express a number of macrophage-associated markers and major histocompatability (MHC) antigens suggesting that they may actually function as APCs in the brain thus evidence suggests that antigen presentation cells (APCs) are indeed present in the brain (Cash & Rott, 1994).
To date, it was generally suggested that immune reactions do not occur in the brain because of the blood-brain barrier (BBB) and the specific features of the brain such as the absence of conventional lymphatic vessels or the low level of circulating T cells. This hypthesiz is not true excacly. Cell based Immunotherapies are affective in brain tumors. Immune effector cells such as lymphocytes, macrophages, dendritic cells, natural killer cells (NK Cell), cytotoxic T lymphocytes (CTL), etc., work together to defend the body against tumor by targeting abnormal antigens expressed on the surface of the tumor due to mutation. An adaptive immune response implies antigen recognition (Prasad et al., 2004). A variety of immunologically based strategies, including passive immunization and adoptive cellular immunotherapy (Fujimiya et al., 1999; Inoue et al., 1996; Kruse et al., 1990; Merchant et al., 1997; Plautz et al., 1997; Plautz et al., 1998) local and systemic delivery of biological response modifiers (Dranoff et al., 1993; Färkkilä et al., 1994; Jean et al., 1998; Jean et al., 2004; Lichtor et al., 1995; Ohno et al., 2009; Thompson et al., 1996; Yu et al; 1993) and vaccination with parental and genetically modified tumor cells (Dranoff et al., 1993; Jean et al., 1998; Lichtor et al., 1995; Thompson et al., 1996; Ohno et al., 2009; Yu et al; 1993) have been attempted.

7.1 Cytokine therapy

Cytokines are a heterogeneous group of soluble small polypeptides or glycoproteins, which have either pro- or anti-inflammatory activity and immunosuppressive activity, depending on the microenvironments. The tumor microenvironment consists of a variable combination of tumor cells, endothelial cells and infiltrating leukocytes, such as macrophages, T-lymphocytes, natural killer (NK) cells, B-cells and antigen-presenting cells (APCs). Cytokine production acts as a means of communication in the tumor microenvironment (Giezeman-Smits et al., 2000). Several strategies for delivery of cytokines to the CNS have been studied, including injection/infusion of recombinant cytokines, vectors containing cytokine encoding genes, cells that secrete cytokines, or cytokines linked to toxins (Das et al., 2008).

7.2 Passive immunotherapy

Passive immunotherapy includes serotherapy and adoptive immunotherapy. Serotherapy uses monoclonal antibodies to effect an antitumor response or to achieve very specific delivery of toxins, chemotherapy, or radiotherapy to the tumor cells. An important finding of its advantage is the identification of ''tumor antigens,'' specific antigens expressed on tumor cell surfaces but not on normal brain parenchyma (Ohno et al., 2009). Targeted glioma antigens have included tenascin, EGFR and its mutated form EGFRvIII, chondroitin sulfate, vascular endothelial growth factor (VEGF) receptor, neural cell adhesion molecule (NCAM), and hepatocyte growth factor/scatter factor (Hopkins et al., 1996).
In adoptive immunotherapy, immune cells activated *ex vivo* are administrated to the tumour-bearing patient. The activated cells are either injected directly into the tumour cavity or intravenously (Han et al., 2010). The first types of cells used for gliomas were

lymphocyte-activated killer (LAK) cells (Tsuboi et al., 2003). Cytotoxic T lymphocytes (CTL) can also be used. Autologous tumour cells (ATC) are generally used as antigen source (Holladay et al., 1996; Tsuboi et al., 2003). Another approach was to collect lymphocytes from lymph nodes (Holladay et al., 1996; Plautz et al., 1998; Plautz et al., 2000; Sloan et al., 2000; Wood et al., 2000).

Active immunotherapy involves strengthing patients' immunity in vivo by vaccination against tumor antigen. Tumor vaccines for malignant glioma have been the focus of great interest currently. Successful development of glioma vaccines, however, requires proper presentation of tumor antigens and induction of effective, durable antigen-specific T cell immune response.A lot of antigen sources can be used for active immunotherapy such as intact tumour cells, tumour protein lysates, tumour-derived mRNA, peptides eluded from tumour MHC class I molecules, and synthetic peptides (Ishikawa et al., 2007; Okada et al., 2007; Sloan et al., 2000; Steiner et al., 2004).

8. Conclusion

As brain tumor neoplasms constitute a formidable therapeutic challenge, gene and immuno therapy present powerful, novel opportunities for developing adjuvant therapies in brain cancer. However, more effective researches for adjuvant treatments of malignant gliomas are needed.

9. References

Aboody, K.S.; Najbauer, J. & Dank, M.K. (2008). Stem and Progenitor Cell-Mediated Tumor Selective Gene Therapy. *Gene Therapy*, Vol.15, No.10, (May 2008), pp. 739-752, ISSN 0969-7128.

Aghi, M. & Chiocca, E.A. (2006). Gene Therapy for Glioblastoma. *Neurosurgical Focus*, Vol.20, No.4, (April 2006), E18, ISSN 1092-0684.

Aloisi, F.; Ria, F.; Columba-Cabezas, S.; Hess, H.; Penna, G. & Adorini, L. (1999). Relative Efficiency of Microglia, Astrocytes, Dendritic Cells and B Cells in Naive CD4+ T Cell Priming and Th1/Th2 Cell Restimulation. European Journal of Immunology, Vol.29, No.9, (September 1999), pp. 2705-2714, ISSN 0014-2980.

Aloisi, F.; Ria, F.; Penna, G. & Adorini, L. (1998). Microglia are more Efficient than Astrocytes in Antigen Processing and in Th1 but not Th2 Cell Activation. Journal of Immunology, Vol.160, No.10, (May 1998), pp. 4671-4680, ISSN 0022-1767.

Bansal, K. & Engelhard, H.H. (2000). Gene Therapy for Brain Tumors. *Current Oncology Reports*, Vol.2, No.5, (September 2000), pp. 463-472, ISSN 1523-3790.

Barshes, N.R.; Goodpastor, S.E. & Goss, J.A. (2004). Pharmacologic Immunosuppression. *Frontiers in Bioscience*, Vol.9, No.1, (January 2004), pp. 411-420, ISSN 1093-4715.

Beltinger, C.; Fulda, S.; Kammertoens, T.; Meyer, E.; Uckert, W. & Debatin, K.M. (1999). Herpes Simplex Virus Thymidine Kinase/Ganciclovir-Induced Apoptosis Involves Ligand-Independent Death Receptor Aggregation and Activation of Caspases. Proceedings of the National Academy of Sciences of the United States of America, Vol.96, No.15, (July 1999), pp. 8699-8704, ISSN 0027-8424.

Bernheimer, H.; Lassmann, H. & Suchanek, G. (1988). Dynamics of IgG1, IgA1, and IgM1 Plasma Cells in the Central Nervous System of Guinea Pigs with Chronic Relapsing

Experimental Allergic Encephalomyelitis. Neuropathology *and* Applied Neurobiology, Vol.14, No.2, (March-April 1988), pp. 157-167, ISSN 0305-1846.

Bigner, S.H.; Wong, A.J.; Mark, J.; Muhlbaier, L.H.; Kinzler, K.W.; Vogelstein, B. & Bigner, D.D. (1987). Relationship Between Gene Amplification and Chromosomal Deviations in Malignant Human Gliomas. *Cancer Genetics and Cytogenetics*, Vol.29, No.1, (November 1987), pp. 165-170, ISSN 0165-4608.

Bodmer, S.; Strommer, K.; Frei, K.; Siepl, C.; de Tribolet, N.; Heid, I. & Fontana, A. (1989). Immunosuppression and Transforming Growth Factor-Beta in Glioblastoma. Preferential Production of Transforming Growth Factor-Beta 2. *Journal of Immunology*, Vol.143, No.10, (November 1989), pp. 3222-3229, ISSN 0022-1767.

Brady, L.W.; Miyamoto, C.; Woo, D.V.; Rackover, M.; Emrich, J.; Bender, H.; Dadparvar, S.; Steplewski, Z.; Koprowski, H.; Black, P.; Lazzaro, B.; Nair, S.; McCormack, T.; Nieves, J.; Morabito, M. & Eshleman, J. (1992). Malignant Astrocytomas Treated with Iodine-125 Labeled Monoclonal Antibody 425 Against Epidermal Growth Factor Receptor: A Phase II Trial. *International Journal of Radiation Oncology Biology Physics*, Vol.22, No.1, (January 1992), pp. 225-230, ISSN 0360-3016.

Brannan, C.A. & Roberts, M.R. (2004). Resident Microglia from Adult Mice are Refractory to Nitric Oxide-inducing Stimuli due to Impaired NOS2 Gene Expression. *Glia*, Vol.48, No.2, (November 2004), pp. 120-131, ISSN 0894-1491.

Candolfi, M.; Kroeger, K.M.; Muhammad, A.K.; Yagiz, K.; Farrokhi, C.; Pechnick, R.N.; Lowenstein, P.R. & Castro, M.G. (2009). Gene Therapy for Brain Cancer: Combination Therapies Provide Enhanced Efficacy and Safety. *Current Gene Therapy*, Vol.9, No.5, (October 2009), pp. 409-421, ISSN 1566-5232.

Cash, E. & Rott O. (1994). Microglial Cells Qualify as the Stimulators of Unprimed CD4+ and CD8+ T Lymphocytes in the Central Nervous System. *Clinical and Experimental Immunology*, Vol.98, No.2, (November 1994), pp. 313-318, ISSN 0009-9104.

Couldwell, W.T.; Yong, V.W.; Dore-Duffy, P.; Freedman, M.S. & Antel, J.P. (1992). Production of Soluble Autocrine Inhibitory Factors by Human Glioma Cell Lines. *Journal of the Neurological Sciences*, Vol.110, No.1-2, (July 1992), pp. 178-185, ISSN 0022-510X.

Culver, K.W.; Ram, Z.; Wallbridge, S.; Ishii, H.; Oldfield, E.H. & Blaese, R.M. (1992). In Vivo Gene Transfer with Retroviral Vector-Producer Cells for Treatment of Experimental Brain Tumors. *Science*, Vol.256, No.5063, (June 1992), pp. 1550-1552, ISSN 0036-8075.

Das, S.; Raizer, J.J. & Muro, K. (2008). Immunotherapeutic Treatment Strategies for Primary Brain Tumors. *Current Treatment Options in Oncology*, Vol.9, No.1, (February 2008), pp. 32-40, ISSN 1527-2729.

Dey, M.; Ulasov, I.V. & Lesniak, M.S. (2010). Virotherapy Against Malignant Glioma Stem Cells. *Cancer Letters*, Vol.289, No.1, (March 2010), pp. 1-10, ISSN 0304-3835.

Dix, A.R.; Brooks, W.H.; Roszman, T.L. & Morford, L.A. (1999). Immune Defects Observed in Patients with Primary Malignant Brain Tumors. *Journal of Neuroimmunology*, Vol.100, No.1-2, (December 1999), pp. 216-232, ISSN 0165-5728.

Dranoff, G.; Jaffee, E.; Lazenby, A.; Golumbek, P.; Levitsky, H.; Brose, K.; Jackson, V.; Hamada, H.; Pardoll, D. & Mulligan, R.C. (1993). Vaccination with Irradiated Tumor Cells Engineered to Secrete Murine Granulocyte-Macrophage Colony-Stimulating Factor Stimulates Potent, Specific, and Long-Lasting Anti-Tumor

Immunity. Proceedings of the National Academy of Sciences of the United States of America, Vol.90, No.8, (April 1993), pp. 3539-3543, ISSN 0027-8424.

Ekstrand, A.J.; James, C.D.; Cavenee, W.K.; Seliger, B.; Pettersson, R.F. & Collins, V.P. (1991). Genes for Epidermal Growth Factor Receptor, Transforming Growth Factor Alpha, and Epidermal Growth Factor and Their Expression in Human Gliomas In Vivo. *Cancer Research*, Vol.51, No.8, (April 1991), pp. 2164-2172, ISSN 0008-5472.

Färkkilä, M.; Jääskeläinen, J.; Kallio, M.; Blomstedt, G.; Raininko, R.; Virkkunen, P.; Paetau, A.; Sarelin, H. & Mäntylä, M. (1994). Randomised, Controlled Study of Intratumoral Recombinant Gamma-Interferon Treatment in Newly Diagnosed Glioblastoma. *British Journal of Cancer*, Vol.70, No.1, (July 1994), pp. 138-141, ISSN 0007-0920.

Fenstermaker, R.A. & Ciesielski, M.J. (2004). Immunotherapeutic Strategies for Malignant Glioma. *Cancer Control*, Vol.11, No.3, (May - June 2004), pp. 181-191, ISSN 1073-2748.

Ferguson, S.D.; Ahmed, A.U.; Thaci, B.; Mercer, R.W. & Lesniak, M.S. (2010). Crossing the Boundaries: Stem Cells and Gene Therapy. *Discovery Medicine*, Vol.9, No.46, (March 2010), pp. 192-196, ISSN 1539-6509.

Fischer, U.; Müller, H.W.; Sattler, H.P.; Feiden, K.; Zang, K.D. & Meese, E. (1995). Amplification of the MET Gene in Glioma. *Genes Chromosomes & Cancer*, Vol.12, No.1, (January 1995), pp. 63-65, ISSN 1045-2257.

Flügel, A.; Labeur, M.S.; Grasbon-Frodl, E.M.; Kreutzberg, G.W. & Graeber, M.B. (1999). Microglia only Weakly Present Glioma Antigen to Cytotoxic T Cells. *International Journal of Developmental Neuroscience*, Vol.17, No.5-6, (August - October 1999), pp. 547-556, ISSN 0736-5748.

Fujimiya, Y.; Suzuki, Y.; Katakura, R. & Ohno, T. (1999). Injury to Autologous Normal Tissues and Tumors Mediated by Lymphokine-Activated Killer (LAK) Cells Generated In Vitro from Peripheral Blood Mononuclear Cells of Glioblastoma Patients. *Journal of Hematotherapy*, Vol.8, No.1, (February 1999), pp. 29-37, ISSN 1061-6128.

Fults, D.; Brockmeyer, D.; Tullous, M.W.; Pedone, C.A. & Cawthon, R.M. (1992). p53 Mutation and Loss of Heterozygosity on Chromosomes 17 and 10 During Human Astrocytoma Progression. *Cancer Research*, Vol.52, No.3, (February 1992), pp. 674-679, ISSN 0008-5472.

Giezeman-Smits, K.M.; Okada, H.; Brissette-Storkus, C.S.; Villa, L.A.; Attanucci, J.; Lotze, M.T.; Pollack, I.F.; Bozik, M.E. & Chambers, W.H. (2000). Cytokine Gene Therapy of Gliomas: Induction of Reactive CD4+ T Cells by Interleukin-4-Transfected 9L Gliosarcoma is Essential for Protective Immunity. *Cancer Research*, Vol.60, No.9, (May 2000), pp. 2449-2457, ISSN 0008-5472.

Grandi, P.; Peruzzi, P.; Reinhart, B.; Cohen, J.B.; Chiocca, E.A. & Glorioso, J.C. (2009). Design and Application of Oncolytic HSV Vectors for Glioblastoma Therapy, *Expert Review of Neurotherapeutics*, Vol.9, No.4, (April 2009), pp. 505-517, ISSN 1473-7175.

Granelli-Piperno, A.; Zhong, L.; Haslett, P.; Jacobson, J. & Steinman, R.M. (2000). Dendritic Cells, Infected with Vesicular Stomatitis Virus-Pseudotyped HIV-1, Present Viral Antigens to CD4+ and CD8+ T Cells from HIV-1-Infected Individuals. *Journal of Immunology*, Vol.165, No.11, (December 2000), pp. 6620-6626, ISSN 0022-1767.

Han, S.J.; Kaur, G.; Yang, I. & Lim, M. (2010). Biologic Principles of Immunotherapy for Malignant Gliomas. *Neurosurgery Clinics of North America*, Vol.21, No.1, (January 2010), pp. 1-16, ISSN 1042-3680.

He, J.; Allen, J.R.; Collins, V.P.; Allalunis-Turner, M.J.; Godbout, R.; Day, R.S. 3rd & James, C.D. (1994). CDK4 amplification is an alternative mechanism to p16 gene homozygous deletion in glioma cell lines. *Cancer Research*, Vol.54, No.22, (November 1994), pp. 5804-5807, ISSN 0008-5472.

Hickey, W.F. & Kimura, H. (1987). Graft-vs.-Host Disease Elicits Expression of Class I and Class II Histocompatibility Antigens and the Presence of Scattered T Lymphocytes in Rat Central Nervous System. Proceedings of the National Academy of Sciences of the United States of America, Vol.84. No.7, (April 1987), pp. 2082-2086, ISSN 0027-8424.

Hickey, W.F. (2001). Basic Principles of Immunological Surveillance of the Normal Central Nervous System. *Glia*, Vol.36, No.2, (November 2001), pp. 118-124, ISSN 0894-1491.

Hickey, W.F.; Hsu, B.L. & Kimura, H. (1991). T-lymphocyte Entry into the Central Nervous System. *Journal of Neuroscience Research*, Vol.28, No.2, (February 1991), pp. 254-260, ISSN 0360-4012.

Holladay, F.P.; Heitz-Turner, T.; Bayer, W.L. & Wood, G.W. (1996). Autologous Tumor Cell Vaccination Combined with Adoptive Cellular Immunotherapy in Patients with Grade III/IV Astrocytoma. *Journal of Neuro-Oncology*, Vol.27, No.2, (February 1996), pp. 179-189, ISSN 0167-594X.

Hopkins, K.; Papanastassiou, V. & Kemshead, J.T. (1996). The Treatment of Patients with Recurrent Malignant Gliomas with Intratumoral Radioimmunoconjugates. Recent Results *in* Cancer Research, Vol.141, pp. 159-175, ISSN 0080-0015.

Humphrey, P.A.; Wong, A.J.; Vogelstein, B.; Zalutsky, M.R.; Fuller, G.N.; Archer, G.E.; Friedman, H.S.; Kwatra, M.M.; Bigner, S.H. & Bigner, D.D. (1990). Anti-Synthetic Peptide Antibody Reacting at the Fusion Junction of Deletion-Mutant Epidermal Growth Factor Receptors in Human Glioblastoma. Proceedings of the National Academy of Sciences of the United States of America, Vol.87, No.11, (June 1990), pp. 4207-4211, ISSN 0027-8424.

Inoue, M.; Plautz, G.E. & Shu, S. (1996). Treatment of Intracranial Tumors by Systemic Transfer of Superantigen-Activated Tumor-Draining Lymph Node T Cells. *Cancer Research*, Vol.56, No.20, (October 1996), pp. 4702-4708, ISSN 0008-5472.

Ishikawa, E.; Tsuboi, K.; Yamamoto, T.; Muroi, A.; Takano, S.; Enomoto, T.; Matsumura, A. & Ohno, T. (2007). Clinical Trial of Autologous Formalin-Fixed Tumor Vaccine for Glioblastoma Multiforme Patients. *Cancer Science*, Vol.98, No.8, (August 2007), pp. 1226-1233, ISSN 1347-9032.

Iwami, K.; Natsume, A. & Wakabayashi T. (2010). Gene Therapy for High-grade Glioma. *Neurologia medico-chirurgica (Tokyo)*, Vol.50, No.9, (September 2010), pp. 727-736, ISSN 0470-8105.

Jean, W.C.; Spellman, S.R.; Wallenfriedman, M.A.; Flores, C.T.; Kurtz, B.P.; Hall, W.A. & Low, W.C. (2004). Effects of Combined Granulocyte-Macrophage Colony-Stimulating Factor (GM-CSF), Interleukin-2, and Interleukin-12 Based Immunotherapy Against Intracranial Glioma in the Rat. Journal *of* Neuro-Oncology, Vol.66, No.1-2, (January 2004), pp. 39-49, ISSN 0167-594X.

Jean, W.C.; Spellman, S.R.; Wallenfriedman, M.A.; Hall, W.A. & Low, W.C. (1998). Interleukin-12-Based Immunotherapy Against Rat 9L Glioma. *Neurosurgery*, Vol.42, No.4, (April 1998), pp. 850-856, ISSN 0148-396X.

Jiang, H.; Gomez-Manzano, C.; Lang, F.F.; Alemany, R. & Fueyo, J. (2009). Oncolytic Adenovirus: Preclinical and Clinical Studies in Patients with Human Malignant Gliomas. *Current Gene Therapy*, Vol.9, No.5, (October 2009), pp. 422-427, ISSN 1566-5232.

Karaoglan A &Turken O. Turkish Basic Neurosurgery Textbook Turkish Neurosurgical Society Textbook V2 pp:1293-1310,2010.

Kleihues, P.; Louis, D.N.; Scheithauer, B.W.; Rorke, L.B.; Reifenberger, G.; Burger, P.C. & Cavenee, W.K. (2002). The WHO Classification of Tumors of the Nervous System. Journal *of* Neuropathology *and Experimental* Neurology, Vol.61, No.3, (March 2002), pp. 215-225, ISSN 0022-3069.

Kozarsky, K.F. & Wilson, J.M. (1993). Gene Therapy: Adenovirus Vectors. *Current Opinion in Genetics & Development*, Vol.3, No.3, (June 1993), pp. 499-503, ISSN 0959-437X.

Krakowski, M.L. & Owens, T. (2000). Naive T Lymphocytes Traffic to Inflamed Central Nervous System, but Require Antigen Recognition for Activation. European Journal *of* Immunology, Vol.60, No.4, (April 2000), pp. 5731-5739, ISSN 0014-2980.

Kramm, C.M.; Sena-Esteves, M.; Barnett, F.H.; Rainov, N.G.; Schuback, D.E.; Yu, J.S.; Pechan, P.A.; Paulus, W.; Chiocca, E.A. & Breakefield, X.O. (1995). Gene Therapy for Brain Tumors. *Brain Pathology*, Vol.5, No.4, (October 1995), pp. 345-381, ISSN 1015-6305.

Kroeger, K.M.; Muhammad, A.K.; Baker, G.J.; Assi, H.; Wibowo, M.K.; Xiong, W.; Yagiz, K.; Candolfi, M.; Lowenstein, P.R. & Castro, M.G. (2010). Gene Therapy and Virotherapy: Novel Therapeutic Approaches for Brain Tumors. *Discovery Medicine*, Vol.10, No.53, (October 2010), pp. 293-304, ISSN 1539-6509.

Kruse, C.A.; Lillehei, K.O.; Mitchell, D.H.; Kleinschmidt-DeMasters, B. & Bellgrau, D. (1990). Analysis of Interleukin 2 and Various Effector Cell Populations in Adoptive Immunotherapy of 9L Rat Gliosarcoma: Allogeneic Cytotoxic T Lymphocytes Prevent Tumor Take. Proceedings of the National Academy of Sciences of the United States of America, Vol.87, No.24, (December 1990), pp. 9577-9581, ISSN 0027-8424.

Lawler, S.E.; Peruzzi, P.P. & Chiocca, E.A. (2006). Genetic Strategies for Brain Tumor Therapy. *Cancer Gene Therapy*, Vol.13, No.3, (March 2006), pp. 225-233, ISSN 0929-1903.

Lesniak, M.S.; Gabikian, P.; Tyler, B.M.; Pardoll, D.M. & Brem, H. (2004). Dexamethasone Mediated Inhibition of Local IL-2 Immunotherapy is Dose Dependent in Experimental Brain Tumors. *Journal of Neuro-Oncology*, Vol.70, No.1, (October 2004), pp. 23-28, ISSN 0167-594X.

Li, H.; Alonso-Vanegas, M.; Colicos, M.A.; Jung, S.S.; Lochmuller, H.; Sadikot, A.F.; Snipes, G.J.; Seth, P.; Karpati, G. & Nalbantoglu, J. (1999). Intracerebral Adenovirus-Mediated p53 Tumor Suppressor Gene Therapy for Experimental Human Glioma. *Clinical Cancer Research*, Vol.5, No.3, (March 1999), pp. 637-642, ISSN 1078-0432.

Libermann, T.A.; Nusbaum, H.R.; Razon, N.; Kris, R.; Lax, I.; Soreq, H.; Whittle, N.; Waterfield, M.D.; Ullrich, A. & Schlessinger, J. (1985). Amplification, Enhanced Expression and Possible Rearrangement of EGF Receptor Gene in Primary Human

Brain Tumours of Glial Origin. *Nature*, Vol.313, No.5998, (January 1985), pp. 144-147, ISSN 0028-0836.

Licht, T.; Pastan, I.; Gottesman, M.M. & Herrmann F. (1996). The Multidrug-Resistance Gene in Gene Therapy of Cancer and Hematopoietic Disorders. *Annals of Hematology*, Vol.72, No.4, (April 1996), pp. 184-193, ISSN 0939-5555.

Lichtor, T.; Glick, R.P.; Kim, T.S.; Hand, R. & Cohen, E.P. (1995). Prolonged Survival of Mice with Glioma Injected Intracerebrally with Double Cytokine-Secreting Cells. *Journal of Neurosurgery*, Vol.83, No.6, (December 1995), pp. 1038-1044, ISSN 0022-3085.

Louis, D.N.; Holland, E.C. & Cairncross, J.G. (2001). Glioma Classification: A Molecular Reappraisal. *American Journal of Pathology*, Vol.159, No.3, (September 2001), pp. 779-786, ISSN 0002-9440.

Lun, X.; Chan, J.; Zhou, H.; Sun, B.; Kelly, J.J.; Stechishin, O.O.; Bell, J.C.; Parato, K.; Hu, K.; Vaillant, D.; Wang, J.; Liu, T.C.; Breitbach, C.; Kirn, D.; Senger, D.L. & Forsyth, P.A. (2010). Efficacy and Safety/Toxicity Study of Recombinant Vaccinia Virus JX-594 in Two Immunocompetent Animal Models of Glioma. *Molecular Therapy*, Vol.18, No.11, (November 2010), pp. 1927-1936, ISSN 1525-0016.

Markert, J.M.; Liechty, P.G.; Wang, W.; Gaston, S.; Braz, E.; Karrasch, M.; Nabors, L.B.; Markiewicz, M.; Lakeman, A.D.; Palmer, C.A.; Parker, J.N.; Whitley, R.J. & Gillespie, G.Y. (2009). Phase Ib Trial of Mutant Herpes Simplex Virus G207 Inoculated Pre-and Post-Tumor Resection for Recurrent GBM. *Molecular Therapy*, Vol.17, No.1, (January 2009), pp. 199-207, ISSN 1525-0016.

Markert, J.M.; Medlock, M.D.; Rabkin, S.D.; Gillespie, G.Y.; Todo, T.; Hunter, W.D.; Palmer, C.A.; Feigenbaum, F.; Tornatore, C.; Tufaro, F. & Martuza, R.L. (2000). Conditionally Replicating Herpes Simplex Virus Mutant, G207 for the Treatment of Malignant Glioma: Results of a Phase I Trial. *Gene Therapy*, Vol.7, No.10, (May 2000), pp. 867-874, ISSN 0969-7128.

Merchant, R.E.; Baldwin, N.G.; Rice, C.D. & Bear, H.D. (1997). Adoptive Immunotherapy of Malignant Glioma Using Tumor-Sensitized T Lymphocytes. *Neurological Research*, Vol.19, No.2, (April 1997), pp. 145-152, ISSN 0161-6412.

Mesnil, M. & Yamasaki, H. (2000). Bystander Effect in Herpes Simplex Virus-Thymidine Kinase/Ganciclovir Cancer Gene Therapy: Role of Gap-Junctional Intercellular Communication. *Cancer Research*, Vol.60, No.15, (August 2000), pp. 3989-3999, ISSN 0008-5472.

Mut M,Ziyal I.(2010) V 1,975-982. Turkish Basic Neurosurgery Textbook Turkish Neurosurgical Society Textbook V1;pp975-982 V2 P:1298-1301,2010

Ng, H.K. & Lam, P.Y. (1998). The Molecular Genetics of Central Nervous System Tumors. *Pathology*, Vol.30, No.2, (May 1998), pp. 196-202, ISSN 0031-3025.

Nitta, T.; Hishii, M.; Sato, K. & Okumura, K. (1994). Selective Expression of Interleukin-10 Gene within Glioblastoma Multiforme. *Brain Research*, Vol.649, No.1-2, (June 1994), pp. 122-128, ISSN 0006-8993.

Ohno, M.; Natsume, A.; Fujii, M.; Ito, M. & Wakabayashi, T. (2009). Interferon-Beta, MCNU, and Conventional Radiotherapy for Pediatric Patients with Brainstem Glioma. *Pediatric Blood & Cancer*, Vol.53, No.1, (July 2009), pp. 37-41, 1545-5017.

Okada, H.; Lieberman, F.S.; Walter, K.A.; Lunsford, L.D.; Kondziolka, D.S.; Bejjani, G.K.; Hamilton, R.L.; Torres-Trejo, A.; Kalinski, P.; Cai, Q.; Mabold, J.L.; Edington, H.D.; Butterfield, L.H.; Whiteside, T.L.; Potter, D.M.; Schold, SC. Jr. & Pollack, I.F. (2007).

Autologous Glioma Cell Vaccine Admixed with Interleukin-4 Gene Transfected Fibroblasts in the Treatment of Patients with Malignant Gliomas. *Journal of Translational Medicine*, Vol.5, (December 2007), pp. 67, ISSN 1479-5876.

Parker, J.N.; Bauer, D.F.; Cody, J.J. & Markert, J.M. (2009). Oncolytic Viral Therapy of Malignant Glioma. *Neurotherapeutics*, Vol.6, No.3, (July 2009), pp. 558-569, ISSN 1933-7213.

Parney, I.F.; Hao, C. & Petruk, K.C. (2000). Glioma Immunology and Immunotherapy. *Neurosurgery*, Vol.46, No.4, (April 2000), pp. 778-791, ISSN 0148-396X.

Pedersini, R.; Vattemi, E. & Claudio, P.P. (2010). Adenoviral Gene Therapy in High-grade Malignant Glioma. *Drug News & Perspectives*, Vol.23, No.6, (July – August 2010), pp. 368-379, ISSN 0214-0934.

Plautz, G.E.; Barnett, G.H.; Miller, D.W.; Cohen, B.H.; Prayson, R.A.; Krauss, J.C.; Luciano, M.; Kangisser, D.B. & Shu, S. (1998). Systemic T Cell Adoptive Immunotherapy of Malignant Gliomas. Journal *of* Neurosurgery, Vol.89, No.1, (July 1998), pp. 42-51, ISSN 0022-3085.

Plautz, G.E.; Miller, D.W.; Barnett, G.H.; Stevens, G.H.; Maffett, S.; Kim, J.; Cohen, P.A. & Shu, S. (2000). T Cell Adoptive Immunotherapy of Newly Diagnosed Gliomas. *Clinical Cancer Research*, Vol.6, No.6, (June 2000), pp. 2209-2218, ISSN 1078-0432.

Plautz, G.E.; Touhalisky, J.E. & Shu, S. (1997). Treatment of Murine Gliomas by Adoptive Transfer of Ex Vivo Activated Tumor-Draining Lymph Node Cells. *Cellular Immunology*, Vol.178, No.2, (June 1997), pp. 101-107, ISSN 0008-8749.

Prasad, G.; Wang, H.; Hill, D.L. & Zhang, R. (2004). Recent Advances in Experimental Molecular Therapeutics for Malignant Gliomas. *Current Medicinal Chemistry – Anti-cancer Agents*, Vol.4, No.4, (July 2004), pp. 347-361, ISSN 1568-0118.

Raffel, C.; Gilles, F.E. & Weinberg, K.I. (1990). Reduction to Homozygosity and Gene Amplification in Central Nervous System Primitive Neuroectodermal Tumors of Childhood. *Cancer Research*, Vol.50, No.3, (February 1990), pp. 587-591, ISSN 0008-5472.

Reifenberger, G.; Reifenberger, J.; Ichimura, K.; Meltzer, P.S. & Collins, V.P. (1994). Amplification of Multiple Genes from Chromosomal Region 12q13-14 in Human Malignant Gliomas: Preliminary Mapping of the Amplicons Shows Preferential Involvement of CDK4, SAS, and MDM2. *Cancer Research*, Vol.54, No.16, (August 1994), pp. 4299-4303, ISSN 0008-5472.

Roszman, T.L. & Brooks, W.H. (1985). Neural Modulation of Immune Function. *Journal of Neuroimmunology*, Vol.10, No.1, (November 1985), pp. 59-69, ISSN 0165-5728.

Roszman, T.L.; Brooks, W.H.; Steele, C. & Elliott, L.H. (1985). Pokeweed Mitogen-Induced Immunoglobulin Secretion by Peripheral Blood Lymphocytes from Patients with Primary Intracranial Tumors. Characterization of T Helper and B Cell Function. *Journal of Immunology*, Vol.134, No.3, (March 1985), pp. 1545-1550, ISSN 0022-1767.

Roth, J.A. (2006). Adenovirus p53 Gene Therapy. Expert Opinion *on Biological* Therapy, Vol.6, No.1, (January 2006), pp. 55-61, ISSN 1471-2598.

Sandberg-Wollheim, M.; Zweiman, B.; Levinson, A.I. & Lisak, R.P. (1986). Humoral Immune Responses within the Human Central Nervous System Following Systemic Immunization. Journal *of* Neuroimmunology, Vol.11, No.3, (May 1986), pp. 205-214, ISSN 0165-5728.

Schmidt, M.; Gruensfelder, P.; Roller, J. & Hagen, R. (2011). Suicide Gene Therapy in Head and Neck Carcinoma Cells: An in Vitro Study. International Journal of *Molecular* Medicine, Vol.27, No.4, (April 2011), pp. 591-597, ISSN 1107-3756.

Singh, S.K.; Clarke, I.D.; Terasaki, M.; Bonn, V.E.; Hawkins, C.; Squire, J. & Dirks PB. (2003). Identification of a Cancer Stem Cell in Human Brain Tumors. *Cancer Research*, Vol.63, No.18, (September 2003), pp. 5821-5828, ISSN 0008-5472.

Sloan, A.E.; Dansey, R.; Zamorano, L.; Barger, G.; Hamm, C.; Diaz, F.; Baynes, R. & Wood, G. (2000). Adoptive Immunotherapy in Patients with Recurrent Malignant Glioma: Preliminary Results of Using Autologous Whole-Tumor Vaccine Plus Granulocyte-Macrophage Colony-Stimulating Factor and Adoptive Transfer of Anti-CD3-Activated Lymphocytes. *Neurosurgical Focus*, Vol.9, No.6, (December 2000), e9, ISSN 1092-0684.

Steffens, S.; Sandquist, A.; Frank, S.; Fischer, U.; Lex, C.; Rainov, N.G. & Kramm, C.M. (2004). A Neuroblastoma-Selective Suicide Gene Therapy Approach Using the Tyrosine Hydroxylase Promoter. *Pediatric Research*, Vol.56, No.2, (August 2004), pp. 268-277, ISSN 0031-3998.

Steiner, H.H.; Bonsanto, M.M.; Beckhove, P.; Brysch, M.; Geletneky, K.; Ahmadi, R.; Schuele-Freyer, R.; Kremer, P.; Ranaie, G.; Matejic, D.; Bauer, H.; Kiessling, M.; Kunze, S.; Schirrmacher, V. & Herold-Mende, C. (2004). Antitumor Vaccination of Patients with Glioblastoma Multiforme: A Pilot Study to Assess Feasibility, Safety, and Clinical Benefit. *Journal of Clinical Oncology*, Vol.22, No.21, (November 2004), pp. 4272-4281, ISSN 0732-183X.

Tambuyzer, B.R.; Ponsaerts, P. & Nouwen, E.J. (2009). Microglia: Gatekeepers of Central Nervous System Immunology. *Journal of Leukocyte Biology*, Vol.85, No.3, (March 2009), pp. 352-370, ISSN 0741-5400.

Thompson, R.C.; Pardoll, D.M.; Jaffee, E.M.; Ewend, M.G.; Thomas, M.C.; Tyler, M. & Brem, H. (1996). Systemic and Local Paracrine Cytokine Therapies Using Transduced Tumor Cells are Synergistic in Treating Intracranial Tumors. *Journal of Immunotherapy With Emphasis on Tumor Immunology*, Vol.19, No.6, (November 1996), pp. 405-413, ISSN 1067-5582.

Tsuboi, K.; Saijo, K.; Ishikawa, E.; Tsurushima, H.; Takano, S.; Morishita, Y. & Ohno, T. (2003). Effects of Local Injection of Ex Vivo Expanded Autologous Tumor-Specific T Lymphocytes in Cases with Recurrent Malignant Gliomas. *Clinical Cancer Research*, Vol.9, No.9, (August 2003), pp. 3294-3302, ISSN 1078-0432.

Tsurushima, H.; Liu, S.Q.; Tuboi, K.; Matsumura, A.; Yoshii ,Y.; Nose, T.; Saijo, K. & Ohno, T. (1999). Reduction of End-Stage Malignant Glioma by Injection with Autologous Cytotoxic T Lymphocytes. *Japanese Journal of Cancer Research*, Vol.90, No.5, (May 1999), pp. 536-545, ISSN 0910-5050.

Vauleon, E.; Avril, T.; Collet, B.; Mosser, J. & Quillien, V. (2010). Overview of Cellular Immunotherapy for Patients with Glioblastoma. *Clinical & Developmental Immunology*, pii: 689171. Epub 2010 Oct 4, ISSN 1740-2522.

von Deimling, A.; Eibl, R.H.; Ohgaki, H.; Louis, D.N.; von Ammon, K.; Petersen, I.; Kleihues, P.; Chung, R.Y.; Wiestler, O.D. & Seizinger, B.R. (1992). p53 Mutations are Associated with 17p Allelic Loss in Grade II and Grade III Astrocytoma. *Cancer Research*, Vol.52, No.10, (May 1992), pp. 2987-2990, ISSN 0008-5472.

Vousden, K.H. & Lane, D.P. (2007). p53 in Health and Disease. Nature *Reviews* Molecular Cell Biology, Vol.8, No.4, (April 2007), pp. 275-283, ISSN 1471-0072.

Wasson, J.C.; Saylors, R.L. 3rd; Zeltzer, P.; Friedman, H.S.; Bigner, S.H.; Burger, P.C.; Bigner, D.D.; Look, A.T.; Douglass, E.C. & Brodeur, G.M. (1990). Oncogene Amplification in Pediatric Brain Tumors. *Cancer Research,* Vol.50, No.10, (May 1990), pp. 2987-2990, ISSN 0008-5472.

Wong, A.J.; Bigner, S.H.; Bigner, D.D.; Kinzler, K.W.; Hamilton, S.R. & Vogelstein, B. (1987). Increased Expression of the Epidermal Growth Factor Receptor Gene in Malignant Gliomas is Invariably Associated with Gene Amplification. Proceedings of the National Academy of Sciences of the United States of America, Vol.84, No.19, (October 1987), pp. 6899-6903, ISSN 0027-8424.

Wood, G.W.; Holladay, F.P.; Turner, T.; Wang, Y.Y. & Chiga, M. (2000). A Pilot Study of Autologous Cancer Cell Vaccination and Cellular Immunotherapy Using Anti-CD3 Stimulated Lymphocytes in Patients with Recurrent Grade III/IV Astrocytoma. *Journal of Neuro-Oncology,* Vol.48, No.2, (June 2000), pp. 113-120, ISSN 0167-594X.

Yawata, T.; Maeda, Y.; Okiku, M.; Ishida, E.,; Ikenaka, K. & Shimizu, K. (2011). Identification and Functional Characterization of Glioma-specific Promoters and their Application in Suicide Gene Therapy. *Journal of Neuro-Oncology,* February 24. [Epub ahead of print]. ISSN 0167-594X.

Yoffey J.M. & Courtice FC, eds. *Lymphatics, Lymph and the Lymphomyeloid Complex.* London, New York: Academic Press; 1970. ISBN 0127720502.

Yu, J.S.; Wei, M.X.; Chiocca, E.A.; Martuza, R.L. & Tepper, R.I. (1993). Treatment of Glioma by Engineered Interleukin 4-Secreting Cells. *Cancer Research,* Vol.53, No.13, (July 1993), pp. 3125-3128, ISSN 0008-5472.

Zurawel, R.H.; Chiappa, S.A.; Allen, C. & Raffel, C. (1998). Sporadic Medulloblastomas Contain Oncogenic Beta-Catenin Mutations. *Cancer Research,* Vol.58, No.5, (March 1998), pp. 896-899, ISSN 0008-5472.

2

Genetic Instability in Paediatric and Adult Brain Tumours

Marta Viana-Pereira[1,2], Chris Jones[3] and Rui M. Reis[1,2,4]
[1]*Life and Health Sciences Research Institute (ICVS), School of Health Sciences, University of Minho, Braga,*
[2]*ICVS/3B's - PT Government Associate Laboratory, Braga/Guimarães,*
[3]*The Institute of Cancer Research, Sutton,*
[4]*Molecular Oncology Research Center, Barretos Cancer Hospital, Barretos, São Paulo,*
[1,2]*Portugal*
[3]*UK*
[4]*Brazil*

1. Introduction

1.1 Brain tumours in children and adults

Primary Central Nervous System (CNS) tumours are considered to be those that originate in the CNS and usually remain there. Primary CNS tumours, despite not leading the cancer frequency rates, rank first among cancer types for the average years of life lost (Burnet et al., 2005). By contrast with other malignancies, where research has lead to the establishment of more successful treatment options, the diagnosis of a CNS tumour, particularly the more malignant histological types, still has devastating effects on the patients and their relatives, not only due to the dismal prognosis of these tumours with extremely high rates of mortality, but also to the great morbidity that actual treatment options cause (Laughton et al., 2008; Mulhern et al., 2004; Silber et al., 1992).

The estimated annual worldwide age-standardized incidence of malignant primary CNS tumours is 3.5 per 100,000 people, which represents more than 200,000 cases. The rate is slightly higher in males (3.9 per 100,000 people per year) than in females (3.1 per 100,000 people per year) (Ferlay et al., 2008). The frequency of brain tumours is also higher in more developed countries (5.2 per 100,000 people per year) compared to less developed countries (3.0 per 100,000 people per year), probably due to diagnostic advances, as well as access to adequate health care in the developed regions (Ferlay et al., 2008; Wrensch et al., 2005). Similarly, estimated annual global age-standardized mortality of malignant primary CNS tumours is higher in males (3.0 per 100,000 people) than in females (2.2 per 100,000 people), with higher rates also in more developed countries (3.2 per 100,000 people) than in less developed regions (2.3 per 100,000 people) (Ferlay et al., 2008). The median age of diagnosis for all primary CNS tumours is 57 years, however the histology-specific median age ranges from 9 to 70 years (Central Brain Tumor Registry of the United States [CBTRUS], 2010).

In children, CNS tumours are the second most frequent malignancy after leukaemia and are therefore the most common solid tumours in childhood (Jemal et al., 2009). An estimated 3,750 new cases of childhood primary non-malignant and malignant CNS tumours are expected to be diagnosed in the United States each year. This number reflects an annual incidence rate of 4.5 cases per 100,000 people. As in adults, the rate is higher in males (4.7 cases per 100,000 people) than in females (4.3 cases per 100,000 people) (CBTRUS, 2010). Importantly, malignant brain tumours are the leading cause of cancer-related death in the childhood (Rickert & Paulus, 2001).

Pathologically, CNS tumours are generally classified according to the World Health Organization (WHO) criteria (Louis et al., 2007). There are a wide range of CNS histological entities, classified according to the cell morphology and the degree of malignant behaviour. The WHO classification (Louis et al., 2007) includes a grading scheme that is a reference for predicting the biological behaviour of the tumour. Grade I tumours generally have a low proliferative potential and the possibility of cure after surgical resection, whilst grade IV tumours are histologically malignant, mitotically active and necrotic, and are associated with rapid disease evolution contributing to the high rates of mortality and morbidity among malignant brain tumour patients. The incidence of different histological types of brain tumours varies across specific age groups (Maity et al., 2004); accordingly, the regions of the brain mostly affected in paediatric and adult tumours are also different. In adults and older children, brain tumours are mostly supratentorial (cerebrum), whereas in young children they are more commonly infratentorial (cerebellum) (Gottardo & Gajjar, 2008). This chapter will focus on malignant CNS tumours, more particularly supratentorial high-grade gliomas (WHO grades III and IV) and cerebellar medulloblastomas (grade IV), which are the most common malignant CNS tumours of adults and children, respectively.

Brain tumour aetiology is thought to be multifactorial and is likely to vary by tumour type. There is a likely connection between genetics and environment, meaning that particular genetic susceptibilities lead to increased vulnerability to environmental factors. The only proven exogenous environmental cause of brain tumours, in children or adults, is ionizing radiation, often seen in the setting of previous radiation therapy for the treatment of a former malignancy (Baldwin & Preston-Martin, 2004; Bondy et al., 2008; Ohgaki & Kleihues, 2005; Pettorini et al., 2008; Wrensch et al., 2005). Genetic susceptibility to brain tumours comes from rare syndromes and polymorphisms, specifically in pathways thought to be involved in the process of brain tumour formation. Familial tumour predisposition syndromes are associated with germline mutations, typically in tumour suppressor genes, which confer an increased susceptibility of individuals to tumour formation from childhood until their adult life (Ullrich, 2008). Some of the major syndromes associated with high-grade gliomas or medulloblastomas (with genes affected by germline mutations) are neurofibromatosis type 1 (*NF1*), Li-Fraumeni syndrome (*TP53*) and Turcot syndrome (*APC* and *MLH1*/*PMS2*/*MSH2*/*MSH6*) (complete list in **Table 1**).

1.2 High-grade glioma

The majority of CNS tumours in all age groups are gliomas. The estimated annual incidence rate of gliomas in the United States is 6.0 per 100,000 people. Overall, the broad category of gliomas accounts for 36% of all CNS tumours and 81% of malignant lesions. In young adults (20-34 years), gliomas represent 39% of all CNS tumours and 86% of malignant tumours; in adolescents (15-19 years), 45% of all CNS tumours and 81% of malignant; whereas in

Syndrome	Gene	CNS Tumour (e.g.)	Other Clinical Manifestations (e.g.)
Neurofibromatosis Type 1	*NF1*	Astrocytoma, neurofibroma, optic nerve glioma	Skin café-au-lait spots; axillary freckling; other tumours
Neurofibromatosis Type 2	*NF2*	Astrocytoma, meningioma	Posterior lens opacities, retinal hamartoma
Tuberous sclerosis	*TSC1, TSC2*	Giant cell astrocytoma	Other tumours
Li-Fraumeni syndrome	*TP53*	Astrocytoma, medulloblastoma	Other tumours
Turcot	*APC; MLH1, PMS2, MSH2, MSH6*	Medulloblastoma; glioblastoma	Skin café-au-lait spots, colorectal polyps
Gorlin	*PTCH*	Medulloblastoma	Other tumours

Table 1. Familial syndromes and genes involved causing increased risk of gliomas and medulloblastomas. *Adapted from* (Louis et al., 2007).

children less than 15 years the frequency of gliomas is higher (56%), but they only account for 74% of malignant tumours (CBTRUS, 2010). The incidence rates of gliomas by histology varies among age-specific groups; in children and adolescents grade I gliomas are the most common tumours, whereas in older patients grade IV gliomas have the highest incidence (CBTRUS, 2010). The treatment of low-grade gliomas with surgical resection alone allows in most instances the possibility of cure. High-grade gliomas by contrast remain a difficult therapeutic challenge with a poor prognosis. Conventional treatment includes surgery, radiotherapy and chemotherapy, however despite improving survival times and quality of life, current therapeutic regimens are still unable to effect a cure. In malignant histologies, tumour cells infiltrate into the surrounding brain and are generally not completely removed by surgery, which coupled with the fact that these remaining cells are often resistant to radio- and chemotherapy are the main reasons for the therapeutic failure in high-grade gliomas (Imbach, 2006). Similarly in children, surgery plays a major role in the treatment of gliomas, with the extent of tumour resection the most important prognostic factor in this age group. For the more malignant subtypes, focal radiation is used as first line adjuvant therapy, except in infants (Hargrave, 2009; Imbach, 2006). Both in adult and paediatric populations, histological type and grade of the tumour, anatomic location, extent of surgical resection, patient's age, whether radiotherapy is applied, and some chemotherapy protocols have been consistently considered prognostic factors (Stewart & Cohen, 1998; Wrensch et al., 2005).

The major subtypes of gliomas are astrocytomas, oligodendrogliomas and the mixed lineage, oligoastrocytomas.

Astrocytoma represents a highly heterogeneous histological group of neoplasms. They represent about 75% of all gliomas and can occur in most parts of the brain, and are the most frequent gliomas of childhood (CBTRUS, 2010). While malignant astrocytomas comprise only 2% of all adult tumours, their malignant nature makes them the fourth greatest cancer-related death (Davis et al., 1998). The different histological types of astrocytoma, grade I pilocytic, grade II diffuse, grade III anaplastic and grade IV glioblastoma vary in frequency, age and gender distribution, location within the brain and clinical features. The major malignant subtypes, anaplastic astrocytoma and glioblastoma, account respectively for 8%

and 51% of all gliomas, with glioblastoma representing 80% of malignant tumours (CBTRUS, 2010; Imbach, 2006; Louis et al., 2007; Reifenberger et al., 2006; Weingart et al., 2006). High-grade glioma may arise *de novo*, and are designated primary tumours, or may be considered secondary tumours developing from lower grade lesions. Whereas the great majority of adults with diffuse astrocytoma experience malignant transformation to grade III and finally to grade IV astrocytoma, the long-term risk of malignant transformation in histologically identical neoplasms in children is less than 10% (Broniscer et al., 2007). Nevertheless, the majority (about 95%) of glioblastomas are primary tumours, develop very rapidly in elderly patients (mean 62 years) after a short clinical history and present a poorer prognosis (Louis et al., 2007), whereas secondary glioblastoma mostly develop in younger patients below the age of 45 (Louis et al., 2007). Due to its invasive nature, glioblastoma cannot be completely resected and despite progress in radio- and chemotherapy, less than half of the patients survive more than a year, making glioblastoma the CNS tumour with worse prognosis, for both paediatric and adult patients (Louis et al., 2007; Reifenberger et al., 2006).

Oligodendroglioma account for a small subset of all gliomas (about 8%), being predominantly tumours of adulthood, with a peak incidence between the fourth and fifth decade of life, representing only 1-2% of all CNS tumours in children (CBTRUS, 2010). There are two grades of malignancy for oligodendrogliomas, oligodendroglioma (grade II) and anaplastic oligodendroglioma (grade III), with grading a significant predictor of survival.

Precise data on the incidence of oligoastrocytoma are not available, but reported frequencies vary from 1-20% of all gliomas, with the higher percentage thought to be overestimated due to a consultation bias. These tumours arise preferentially in the cerebral hemispheres and mainly occur in the fifth decade of life (Bromberg & van den Bent, 2009; Louis et al., 2007; Reifenberger et al., 2006; van den Bent et al., 2008). Similar to oligodendrogliomas, these tumours can also be divided in two grades of malignancy.

1.3 Medulloblastoma

Medulloblastoma represents a highly malignant, invasive embryonic tumour, and is the most common malignant CNS tumour in children, accounting together with other embryonic tumours for about 1.5% of all primary CNS tumours (CBTRUS, 2010), representing 12-25% of childhood brain tumours and only about 0,5-1% of all brain neoplasms in adults (Imbach, 2006; Sarkar et al., 2005; Taylor, 2006). The peak age incidence is 9 years, with 70% of all medulloblastomas occurring in patients less than 16 years of age. In adulthood, 80% of medulloblastomas arise before the fourth decade of life and rarely occur after the fifth decade. About 65% of patients are male (Louis et al., 2007; Reifenberger et al., 2006; Taylor, 2006). The annual incidence of medulloblastoma has been estimated at 0.5 per 100,000 children less than 15 years (CBTRUS, 2010; Reifenberger et al., 2006). Medulloblastoma presents predominantly neuronal differentiation. It is composed of densely packed small round blue cells with carrot-shaped hyperchromatic nuclei, possibly presenting neuroblastic rosettes which are associated with marked nuclear pleomorphism and high mitotic activity (Huse & Holland, 2010; Imbach, 2006; Louis et al., 2007; Taylor, 2006). The WHO classification of CNS tumours recognizes at least five different histological types of medulloblastoma: classic (70-85% of the cases); desmoplastic/nodular (15% in paediatric medulloblastoma compared to 30-40% in adults); anaplastic (about 10-22% of medulloblastomas); large cell (about 2-4% of cases) and medulloblastoma with extensive nodularity (about 3%) (Brandes et al., 2009; Imbach, 2006; Louis et al., 2007; Taylor, 2006). There is an heterogeneity among medulloblastoma histologic subtypes which exhibit a highly variable clinical behaviour, with the anaplastic and large cell subtypes being associated with worse prognosis and desmoplastic/nodular medulloblastomas portending a more favourable outcome (Gilbertson & Ellison, 2008; Huse & Holland, 2010; Imbach, 2006). About 30% of the medulloblastoma patients, particularly paediatric tumours, present metastasis via the cerebrospinal fluid pathways at diagnosis, whereas spread outside the CNS is a rare event (Carrie et al., 1994; Frost et al., 1995; Reifenberger et al., 2006). Clinical prognostic factors include tumour size, presence of metastasis, age, and amount of tumour resected (Imbach, 2006). Stratification of medulloblastoma involves distinguishing high-risk and standard-risk patients, with high-risk patients those aged less than 3 years, with incomplete surgical resection of the tumour and/or with disseminated disease (Dubuc et al., 2010; Imbach, 2006; Louis et al., 2007). Significant advances have been made in the treatment of childhood medulloblastoma, with the 5-year survival raised to 60% for high-risk disease and 80% for standard-risk tumours, however the long-term side effects of the treatment modalities applied can be severe. Actual treatment includes maximal safe surgical resection and the use of combined radio- and chemotherapy for children older than 3 years. Most therapeutic approaches for high-risk patients include relatively high doses of craniospinal radiotherapy and aggressive chemotherapeutic regimens (Hargrave, 2009; Imbach, 2006). The treatment of infants with medulloblastoma remains highly problematic as radiation therapy is especially damaging for the developing brain of very young children.

2. Genetic instability of malignant brain tumours

Cancer cells usually harbour mutations in oncogenes and tumour suppressor genes. These may play a role in key cellular processes such as proliferation, apoptosis or angiogenesis. Oncogenes are genes whose deregulated activation through mutation, translocation, amplification or over-expression promotes tumorigenesis. Tumour suppressors, on the other hand, play an inhibitory role, and can be inactivated in cancer through mutation, deletion, methylation or transcriptional repression. Genomic instability present in cancer cells occurs mainly through chromosomal instability (CIN) or microsatellite instability (MSI), together with increased frequencies of molecular alterations in cancer regulatory genes (Negrini et al., 2010; Nigg, 2005). CIN refers to the high rate by which chromosome structure and number (by gains or losses) changes over time in cancer cells compared with normal cells and MSI is characterized by the expansion or contraction of the number of oligonucleotide repeats present in microsatellite sequences (Venkatesan & Loeb, 2005).

2.1.1 Patterns of copy number change

CIN is characterised by an increased frequency of chromosomal alterations, resulting in gains, losses, deletions, insertions, translocations, amplifications, and rearrangements. Nearly all human tumours display the CIN phenotype and consequently aneuploidy. Tumours with the CIN usually harbour mutations in oncogenes and/or tumour suppressor genes, many of which are involved in the regulation of transcription (Nigg, 2005). During the last decade, the use of genome-scale profiling techniques to identify the key genetic alterations underlying different tumour types allowed fundamental findings about the drivers of oncogenesis, providing the rationale for specific targeted therapies in these malignancies. The first studies using large-scale genome profiling techniques to identify the key genetic alterations of brain tumours were only recently published (Kool et al., 2008; Parsons et al., 2008; The Cancer Genome Atlas Research Network [TCGA], 2008; Thompson et al., 2006). Nevertheless, the number of such studies have been increasing on the past few years, with the first studies in paediatric glioma patients starting to emerge (Barrow et al., 2011; Bax et al., 2010; Paugh et al., 2010; Qu et al., 2010; Schiffman et al., 2010; Zarghooni et al., 2010).

2.1.2 High-grade glioma

Comprehensive mapping of the genome of adult glioblastoma has identified common regions of chromosomal instability and gene expression signatures, identifying frequently dysregulated molecular pathways (Bredel et al., 2005; de Tayrac et al., 2009; Gardina et al., 2008; Kotliarov et al., 2006; Maher et al., 2006; Nigro et al., 2005; Parsons et al., 2008; TCGA, 2008). The number of such studies specifically addressing childhood high-grade glioma has until recently been much lower. Nevertheless, several works specifically addressing these paediatric tumours, from ours and others groups, are beginning to emerge, providing increasing evidence that the paediatric high-grade glioma genome has certain key differences from that of histologically similar adult tumours (Barrow et al., 2011; Bax et al., 2010; Paugh et al., 2010; Qu et al., 2010; Rao et al., 2010; Rickert et al., 2001; Schiffman et al., 2010; K.K. Wong et al., 2006; Zarghooni et al., 2010).

These studies have demonstrated that the retinoblastoma (RB), p53 and RTK/PI3K/MAPK pathways are commonly disrupted in adult and paediatric glioblastomas through various genetic mechanisms (TCGA, 2008; Parsons et al., 2008). Nevertheless, our data has demonstrated that paediatric tumours show deregulation of these core pathways by copy number alterations in less than half the frequency of that reported for adult tumours: 25% RTK/PI3K/MAPK, 19% p53 and 22% RB versus 59%, 70% and 66%, for adult glioblastoma (**Figure 1**) (Bax et al., 2010; TCGA, 2008). Even though isolated cases presented clear genomic events linked to activation of the sonic hedgehog (SHH) and Notch pathways activation, there is no evidence of consistently targeted pathways in paediatric high-grade gliomas. Nevertheless, low-frequency amplifications in childhood tumours included genes involved in cell cycle progression (*CCND2, CDK4, MYC,* and *MYCN*), receptor tyrosine kinases (RTKs) and ligands (*EGFR, MET, IGF1R, PDGFB,* and *NRG1*), members of the PI3K/MAPK pathway (*PIK3C2B, PIK3C2G, PIK3R5, KRAS, AKT1,* and *S6K1*), and p53 pathway regulation (*MDM4*), some of them known to be deregulated also in adult glioblastoma (**Figure 2**) (Bax et al., 2010; Paugh et al., 2010). In addition, homozygous deletions of tumour suppressor genes of known importance within the adult glioblastoma core signalling pathways included *CDKN2C, PTEN, RB1, TP53,* and *TP73* (**Figure 1**) (TCGA, 2008; Parsons et al., 2008), albeit at considerably lower frequencies in paediatric *versus* adult tumours. These numerous low-frequency amplifications and deletions identified in paediatric high-grade gliomas, such as *MYC/MYCN, CCND2, KRAS,* and *CDKN2C,* suggest that paediatric high-grade gliomas may be molecularly more similar to secondary adult glioblastomas (Beroukhim et al., 2007; Maher et al., 2006).

At the gross chromosomal level, paediatric glioblastomas can be distinguished from adult tumours by the more frequent gain of chromosome 1q and loss of 16q, and the relative scarcity of chromosome 7 gains and 10q losses. The most frequent focal amplifications are also different, with *PDGFRA* predominant in paediatric and *EGFR* adult tumours (**Table 2**). Moreover, paediatric cases without *PDGFRA* amplification seem to present overexpression of a specific *PDGFRA*-associated gene signature, which differs from that observed in adult

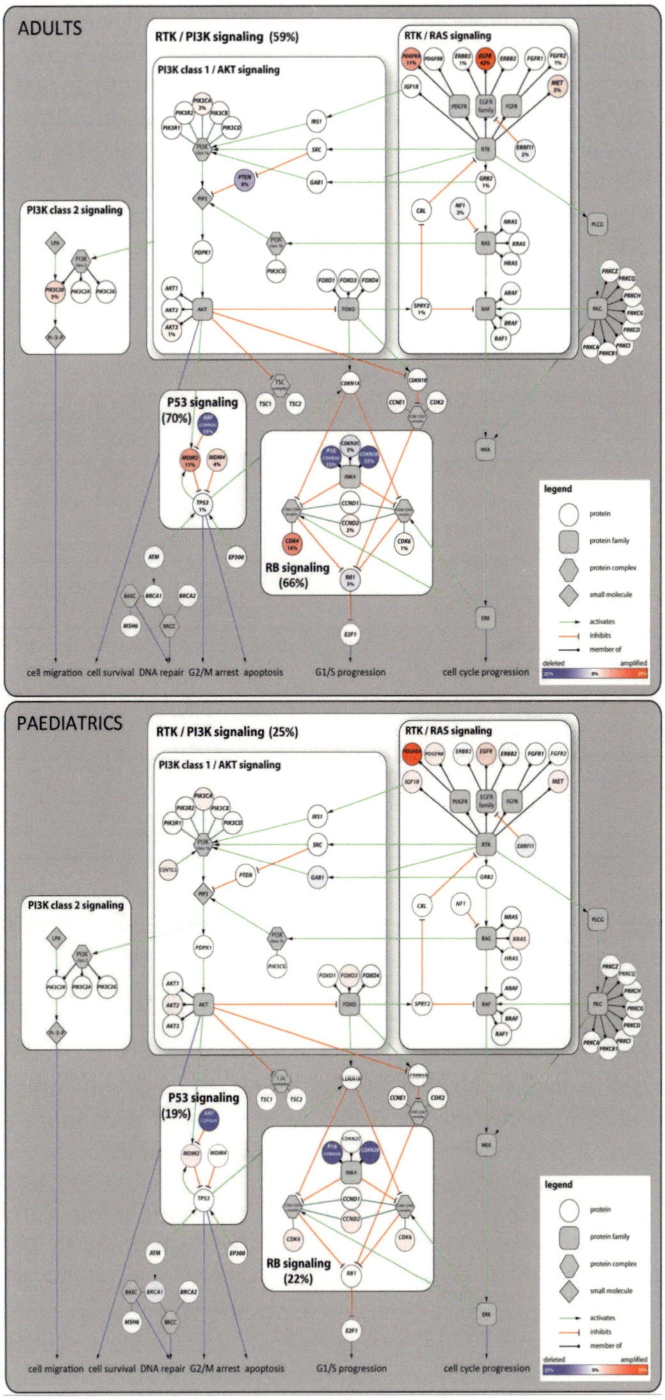

Fig. 1. Copy number alterations in core signalling Pathways in Adult and Paediatric Glioblastoma. RTK/PI3K/MAPK, p53 and RB pathways are more frequently deregulated in adult than in paediatric glioblastomas. *Adapted from* (Bax et al., 2010; TCGA, 2008).

tumours with the 4q12 amplification (Bax et al., 2010; Martinho et al., 2009; Paugh et al., 2010; Rickert et al., 2001; K.K. Wong et al., 2006). Even if *PDGFRA* amplification, 1q+ and 16q- events are more common in paediatric patients (Qu et al., 2010; Schiffman et al., 2010; Zarghooni et al., 2010), they are also present in a proportion of adult tumours. Similarly there is a small group of paediatric high-grade gliomas containing copy number alterations associated with adult tumours (*EGFR* amplification, 7+, 10q-) (Bax et al., 2010; Paugh et al., 2010). The deletion of *CDKN2A/CDKN2B* is among the most frequent focal events found in paediatric high-grade gliomas, nevertheless it is even more commonly present in adult tumours (**Table 2**) (Bax et al., 2010; TCGA, 2008; Paugh et al., 2010). In adults, secondary glioblastomas show overexpression or amplification of *PDGFRA* but rarely contain *EGFR* aberrations.

Region	Paediatric Glioblastoma (n=46)	Adult Glioblastoma (n=189)	*P*
Gains			
1q	30%	9%	0.001
7	13%	74%	<0.001
Losses			
1p	9%	2%	0.05
4q	22%	2%	<0.001
9p	17%	33%	<0.05
10q	35%	80%	<0.001
16q	24%	7%	0.003
Focal amplifications			
PDGFRA	16%	11%*	0.2
EGFR	4%	43%*	<0.001
Focal deletions			
CDKN2A	20%	55%*	<0.001

* n = 206 tumours

Table 2. Summary of copy number changes in Paediatric and Adult Glioblastoma. *Adapted from* (TCGA, 2008; Paugh et al., 2010).

Recently, missense mutations in *IDH1* were found in a significant number of adult glioblastomas that tend to occur mostly in younger patients with more protracted clinical courses (Parsons et al., 2008). These mutations were found exclusively on the R132 residue in the active site region of the protein (Parsons et al., 2008; Yan et al., 2009). Interestingly, a separate group of gliomas harbour mutations in the *IDH1* homologue *IDH2* at the analogous residue (R172). Further investigations have shown that mutations in *IDH1* and *IDH2* are present in high proportions of grade II and III astrocytic, oligodendroglial and mixed tumours (72 to 100%) along with secondary glioblastomas (up to 85%), but are largely absent in primary glioblastomas (5%) (Hartmann et al., 2009; Ichimura et al., 2009; Parsons et al., 2008; Watanabe et al., 2009; Yan et al., 2009). Additionally, *IDH* mutations are associated with other genomic abnormalities that are typically seen in gliomas, such as *TP53* mutation in low-grade astrocytoma, and 1p/19q deletion in oligodendrogliomas; they are also mutually exclusive with *EGFR* amplification and chromosome 10 loss (Sanson et al., 2009; Watanabe et al., 2009; Yan et al., 2009). These findings suggest that, although *IDH* mutations probably contribute to the early evolution of low-grade gliomas, remaining in the higher-grade lesions, they seem to have no role in the underlying biology of primary glioblastoma. Importantly, these *IDH1* hotspot mutations are not found in childhood tumours (Balss et al., 2008; Yan et al., 2009), biologically distinguishing paediatric high-grade gliomas from adult secondary glioblastoma. Nevertheless, *IDH1* mutations was recently found in 7 of the 20 high-grade gliomas from older children (14-18 years) and reported to be associated with a favourable prognosis, as observed in adults (Pollack et al., 2010a).

Oligodendrogliomas harbour specific copy number alterations related to response to therapy or prognosis, however a comparison between adult in paediatric populations is difficult, as paediatric oligodendrogliomas are extremely rare neoplasms. Still, up to 80% of adult tumours show combined loss of chromosomes 1p and 19q, associated with increased chemosensitivity to treatment and favourable clinical outcome (Smith et al., 2000, 1999), whereas deletion of these regions are rare and did not seem to anticipate a survival advantage in paediatric high-grade gliomas (Kreiger et al., 2005; Pollack et al., 2003).

Another feature of childhood high-grade gliomas that is almost entirely absent from adult tumours is the occurrence of very few or even no detectable copy number alterations in paediatric tumours (Bax et al., 2010; Paugh et al., 2010). This stable genomic profile is independent of histologic grade or type, and seems to confer an improved survival in high-grade glioma patients, in contrast to those patients with an amplifier genomic profile, who do significantly worse (Bax et al., 2010).

2.1.3 Medulloblastoma

Similarly to glial tumours, studies of genomic copy number alterations analysing large cohorts of paediatric and adult medulloblastomas have recently begun to emerge (Kool et al., 2008; Thompson et al., 2006; Korshunov et al., 2010).

The most frequent and consistent genetic event reported in medulloblastoma is the partial or complete loss of the chromosome 17p, often in association with gain of chromosome 17q (resulting in the isochromosome 17q: i(17)q), occurring in approximately 30–50% of the medulloblastomas (Biegel et al., 1997; Bigner et al., 1988; Cogen & McDonald, 1996; Lamont et al., 2004; Nicholson et al., 2000; Steichen-Gersdorf et al., 1997; Capodano et al., 1994). Although the precise mechanism by which this genomic abnormality contributes to tumorigenesis and its prognostic importance remain unclear, the common deletion region of 17p13.2-13.3 includes several confirmed and putative tumour suppressor genes, including *TP53* (Huse & Holland, 2010). Together with the deletion of 17p, *MYC* amplification is a molecular prognostic factor of medulloblastoma (Imbach, 2006). Genomic amplifications of *MYCN* and *MYC* were described as characteristics of a subset of clinically aggressive medulloblastomas that tend to exhibit large cell/anaplastic histological features (Aldosari et al., 2002; Tomlinson et al., 1994).

Recently, Korshunov and colleagues (Korshunov et al., 2010) compared a large series of adult and paediatric subsets of tumours, using array-based comparative genomic hybridization (aCGH) (34 adult and 101 paediatric patients) and validating the results in an independent series (112 adult and 303 childhood patients) by fluorescent *in situ* hybridization (FISH) analysis. Although frequencies of loss of 17p (either isolated or via i(17)q formation) were similar in both populations, isolated gains of 17q were significantly more frequent in children than adult patients, with monosomy of chromosome 17 exclusively found in adults (**Table 3**) (Korshunov et al., 2010). Additionally, amplifications of MYC/MYCN prevailed in the paediatric cohort, whereas amplification of CDK6 (at

7q21.3), was frequently present in adult tumours and absent in paediatric medulloblastomas. Of note is that both MYC/MYCN and CDK6 amplifications were associated with poor survival in paediatric and adult populations, respectively. Besides chromosome 17q, alterations on additional chromosome arms were shown to be significantly different between adult and paediatric medulloblastoma. Gains of chromosome 3q, 4 and 19 more frequently found in the adult tumours, while gains of 1q, 2 and 7 and loss of 16q was more abundant in children. The frequency of chromosome 6 deletions was similar across adult and childhood medulloblastoma, however the patterns of aberration were different, with complete loss of the chromosome and absence of concomitant aberrations frequently more present in paediatric medulloblastoma (Korshunov et al., 2010). This may explain the reason why the prognostic value of chromosome 6 deletion, a well established marker for favourable outcome in medulloblastoma (Clifford et al., 2006; Pfister et al., 2009; Thompson et al., 2006), was not found to be statistically significant for adult cases (Korshunov et al., 2010). A summary of the results from the validation cohort is presented on **Table 3**.

Region	Paediatric Medulloblastoma (n=303)	Adult Medulloblastoma (n=112)	*P*
Gains			
1q	24%	9%	<0.001
2	15%	6%	0.02
6q	11%	3%	*
7	33%	14%	<0.001
17q	17%	2%	**
Losses			
6q	12%	15%	*
17p	4%	4%	**
Focal amplifications			
CDK6	0.3%	8%	<0.001
MYC/MYCN	14%	3%	<0.001
Other Alterations			
i(17)q	39%	32%	**

* $P = 0.02$ for total Chromosome 6 aberrations; ** $P < 0.001$ for total Chromosome 17 aberrations

Table 3. Summary of copy number changes in Paediatric and Adult Medulloblastomas (validation set of adult tumours by FISH analysis). *Adapted from* (Korshunov et al., 2010).

2.2 Microsatellite Instability

DNA is continuously exposed to numerous different insults, endogenous and exogenous, that can ultimately result in DNA mutation and alteration of cell behaviour. DNA repair mechanisms are therefore essential for maintaining DNA integrity and preventing tumorigenesis (Li, 2008; Ljungman, 2010). Consequences of the failure of these molecular pathways are well illustrated in colorectal cancer, mainly HNPCC where it is present in about 90% of the tumours. In these cancers, mismatch repair (MMR)-deficient cells adopt a mutator phenotype in which there is a significant increase in cellular mutation rates (Loeb, 1991; Marra & Jiricny, 2005). The most obvious molecular signature of this mutator phenotype is the presence of microsatellite instability (MSI) (Fishel & Kolodner, 1995).

The MMR system is the major pathway responsible for repairing base-base mispairs and short insertion/deletion loops that arise during DNA replication and as intermediates of homologous recombination (Arana & Kunkel, 2010; Kunkel & Bebenek, 2000; Nigg, 2005). Such a mechanism is essential to the cells because the fidelity of replicating DNA polymerases is insufficient to generate an error-free copy of genomic DNA. Single-base substitutions are estimated to arise once in every 10^4-10^6 nucleotides incorporated, and MMR reduces the error rate to a range of 10^{-9} to 10^{-10}, which ensures that the human genome can be duplicated without mutations (Kunkel & Bebenek, 2000). Left unrepaired, these structures will give rise to base-substitution and frameshift mutations, respectively (Arana & Kunkel, 2010; Kunkel & Bebenek, 2000; Nigg, 2005). The role of the key factors of the human MMR system, the MutS homologues MSH2, MSH3 and MSH6, and the MutL homologues MLH1 and PMS2, have begun to be elucidated (Jiricny, 2006; Li, 2008; Schofield & Hsieh, 2003). MSH6 competes for binding to MSH2 with MSH3 (Boland et al., 2008), whilst MLH1 can form heterodimers with PMS2 (Li & Modrich, 1995), PMS1 (Raschle et al., 1999) or MLH3 (Lipkin et al., 2000); MLH1/PMS2 is the only complex with an essential role in mismatch correction (Nigg, 2005; Shah et al., 2010).

Microsatellites are short DNA sequence repeats that are scattered throughout the human genome (Lander et al., 2001), and whose copy number varies steadily through evolution (Ellegren, 2004). MSI is the expansion or retraction of the number of repeats within the microsatellites and it is assumed to be generated by slippage of DNA polymerases during copying of repeats, representing a hot spot for mutagenesis (Aaltonen et al., 1994; Cahill et al., 1999; Ionov et al., 1993). The classification of MSI more commonly adopted takes into account the number of markers presenting frameshift alterations. MSI tumours are therefore classified as MSI-H when, comparing to germline DNA, two or more markers present allelic shifts, or in the absence of constitutive DNA, at least three markers are altered. When one or two markers present alterations tumours are classified as MSI-L; when all markers are normal tumours are classified as microsatellite stable (MSS) (Buhard et al., 2006; Umar et al., 2004; Y.F. Wong et al., 2006). In parallel with this classification, an alternative qualitative distinction of MSI, which considers the size of the allelic shifts in the markers, has been proposed (Giunti et al., 2009; Oda et al., 2005). Samples presenting small length changes (≤6 bp) are designed Type A MSI whereas those with more extreme variations are defined as Type B MSI.

The presence and frequency of MSI in brain tumours is a controversial and poorly studied issue. Previous studies have evaluated the presence of MSI in brain tumours, particularly in gliomas, while in medulloblastomas MSI status has not been properly addressed. Reports in the literature describe the absence or rare incidence of MSI in adult patients, while in children results have been contradictory, with reported frequencies in paediatric gliomas varying between 0 and 44% (Alonso et al., 2001; Amariglio et al., 1995; Cheng et al., 1999; Dams et al., 1995; Eckert et al., 2007; Izumoto et al., 1997; Kanamori et al., 2000; Leung et al., 1998; Martinez et al., 2005; Sobrido et al., 2000; Vladimirova et al., 2007). Importantly, the methodologies for determining MSI have been highly diverse, making it difficult to draw accurate conclusions (**Table 4**). To clarify the role of MSI in paediatric *versus* adult malignant brain tumours, our group has used a highly sensitive and robust panel of MSI markers and studied series of high-grade glioma and medulloblastoma of adult and paediatric samples for the presence of MSI (Viana-Pereira et al., 2009, 2011). In our study of high-grade

Reference	Age (years)	Number of cases	MSI (%)	Markers	QMVR or comparison with germline DNA
Pollack et al., 2010b	<21	68	3 (4.4%)	Mononucleotide and Polynucleotide*	N/A
Maxwell et al, 2008	N/A	52	8 (15.4%)	Mononucleotide	QMVR
Vladimirova et al., 2007	<18	126	4 (3.2%)	Mononucleotide	-
Eckert et al., 2007	<22	71	0	Mononucleotide	N/A
	<22	553	1 (0.2%)		
Martinez et al., 2005	<18	1	0	Mononucleotide and Polynucleotide	Comparison with germline DNA
	>18	108	6 (5.6%)		
Alonso et al., 2001	<21	102	16 (15.7%)	Mononucleotide	No
	>21	104	0		
Kanamori et al., 2000	13-19	6	2 (33.3%)	Mononucleotide and Polynucleotide	Comparison with germline DNA
	20-29	8	0		
	>30	66	0		
Sobrido et al., 2000	N/A	56	10 (17.9%)	Polynucleotide	Comparison with germline DNA

*NCI recommended panel of markers (2 mononucleotide markers: BAT26 and BAT25; and 3 dinucleotide markers: D2S123, D5S346 and D17S250)

N/A - not available

Table 4. Summary of relevant studies reporting MSI analysis in brain tumours after the year 2000.

gliomas, the frequency of MSI was significantly higher in paediatric than adult tumours (Viana-Pereira et al., 2011), reflecting the bulk of the previously published data (Alonso et al., 2001; Cheng et al., 1999; Kanamori et al., 2000; Leung et al., 1998; Martinez et al., 2005). On the other hand, in medulloblastomas, no difference was observed in MSI frequency between adult and paediatric tumours, suggesting that the presence of MSI in these tumours is not age-related (Viana-Pereira et al., 2009). Overall, it seems that there are less molecular differences between adult and paediatric medulloblastomas than those reported in high-grade gliomas, in concordance with our MSI data.

One of the key considerations in the assessment of MSI is in the use of mononucleotides *versus* polynucleotides in the panel of markers used. In our studies we used a pentaplex of quasimonomorphic mononucleotide markers (NR27, NR21, NR24, BAT25 and BAT26), which is currently regarded as the most sensitive panel of markers available, with distinct advantages over the classic National Cancer Institute panel of markers (2 mononucleotide markers: BAT26 and BAT25; and 3 dinucleotide markers: D2S123, D5S346 and D17S250) to the determine MSI in populations of different ethnicities and in different types of human tumours (Buhard et al., 2004; Buhard et al., 2006; Goel et al., 2010; Y.F. Wong et al., 2006). Importantly, the use of quasimonomorphic mononucleotide markers overcomes the need for using matching germline DNA, required when using dinucleotide polymorphic markers. Despite this, still there is the need for optimization of the quasi-monomorphic variation range (QMVR) for each marker, as the allelic size estimation for these quasimonomorphic markers can be influenced by the use of specific reagents or the sequencing machine (Goel et al., 2010).

Previous studies have established MSI frequencies in gliomas using polynucleotide markers only, with frequencies ranging from 0 to 37% (Amariglio et al., 1995; Dams et al., 1995; Izumoto et al., 1997; Sobrido et al., 2000). Including both mononucleotide and polynucleotides repeat markers did not improve consistency, with contrasting results varying between 0 and 44% in paediatric gliomas cohorts or between 0 and 18% in adult tumours (Cheng et al., 1999; Kanamori et al., 2000; Leung et al., 1998; Martinez et al., 2005; Pollack et al., 2010b). Using mononucleotides only also provided contradictory results of 0 to 27% MSI in paediatric gliomas (Alonso et al., 2001; Eckert et al., 2007; Vladimirova et al., 2007). In addition to the heterogeneity of markers used to assess MSI frequency that likely accounts for the majority of variability in the data, many of the previous studies did not refer the establishment of a QMVR (for quasimonomorphic mononucleotide markers) or a direct comparison between tumour and germline DNA (for other markers).

In contrast to colorectal cancer, which presents mainly Type B MSI, we and others have shown that high-grade gliomas harbour Type A MSI (Giunti et al., 2009; Viana-Pereira et al., 2009, 2011). Moreover, we have observed that both MSI-positive medulloblastoma and high-grade glioma presented small length alterations within the microsatellites and hypothesise that this can also contribute for the high variation frequency of MSI in brain tumours reported in the literature (Alonso et al., 2001; Amariglio et al., 1995; Cheng et al., 1999; Dams et al., 1995; Eckert et al., 2007; Izumoto et al., 1997; Kanamori et al., 2000; Leung et al., 1998; Martinez et al., 2005; Sobrido et al., 2000; Vladimirova et al., 2007).

Importantly, the MSI-positive paediatric high-grade glioma mostly presented a stable genomic profile at the chromosomal level, even if microsatellite and chromosomal instability were not mutually exclusive. As mentioned above, the presence of a proportion of tumours with few or absent copy number alterations distinguishes paediatric high-grade gliomas from their adult counterparts and therefore we hypothesise that MSI might represent an alternative form of genetic instability, at least in a proportion of these paediatric tumours with no gross chromosome number alterations.

Mismatch repair deficiencies have been associated with paediatric brain tumours in a hereditary context. Case reports have described MMR germline mutations combined with NF1-like clinical features in children presenting medulloblastoma or high-grade glioma, described as a "mismatch repair-deficiency (MMR-D) syndrome" (summary in **Table 5**) (Agostini et al., 2005; De Rosa et al., 2000; Giunti et al., 2009; Hegde et al., 2005; Kruger et al., 2008; Menko et al., 2004; Ostergaard et al., 2005; Poley et al., 2007; Roy et al., 2009; Scott et al., 2007; Toledano et al., 2009; Viana-Pereira et al., submitted; Wagner et al., 2003; Wang et al., 1999). Also in our study there was a MSI-H paediatric high-grade glioma with clinical characteristics of NF1 (multiple *café-au-lait* spots). Even though there was no constitutional DNA available for evaluation of MMR germline mutations, data imply that this patient probably present a *MSH6* germline mutation, harbouring a MMR-D syndrome (de Leeuw et al., 2000).

Due to the widespread presence of microsatellites in DNA, mutations are expected to accumulate in the genome of tumour cells due to MMR deficiency, with some alterations

Family	Malignancy	Age at diagnosis	Café-au-lait spots	Affected gene	Reference
1	AML Medulloblastoma	6 7	Yes	*MLH1*	Wang et al., 1999
2	Anaplastic oligodendroglioma/ Colorectal cancer	14 / 17 18	NS	*PMS2*	De Rosa et al., 2000
	Neuroblastoma	13	NS		
3	Oligodendroglioma Rectosigmoid carcinoma	10 12	Yes	*MSH6*	Menko et al., 2004
4	Glioblastoma	8	Yes	*MSH6*	Hegde et al., 2005
5	Duodenal adenocarcinoma Colonic adenoma Glioblastoma	16 16 17	Yes	*PMS2*	Agostini et al., 2005
6	Pilocytic astrocytoma Lymphoma	9 10	Yes	*MSH6*	Ostergaard et al., 2005
	Spinal glioblastoma	2	Yes		
7	Glioblastoma Wilms tumour	4 4	Yes	*MLH1*	Wagner et al., 2003 Poley et al., 2007
8	Lymphoma Anaplastic oligodendroglioma	4 6	Yes	*MSH6?*	Poley et al., 2007
	Medulloblastoma	6	Yes		
9	Medulloblastoma AML Colon carcinomas	7 10 13	Yes	*MSH6*	Scott et al., 2007
10	Glioblastoma	6	Yes	*PMS2*	Kruger et al., 2008
	Glioblastoma Colorectal cancer Small bowel cancer Urotel carcinoma	6 15 15 15	Yes		
	Glioblastoma	9	Yes		
11	Glioblastoma	10	Yes	*PMS2*	Giunti et al., 2009
12	Glioblastoma	4	NS	*MLH1*	Giunti et al., 2009
	Glioblastoma	12	NS	*NS*	
13	Colorectal cancer Astrocytoma WHOII	14 14	Yes	*MSH2*	Toledano et al., 2009
	Anaplastic astrocytoma	13	Yes	*NS*	
14	Medulloblastoma Duodenal adenocarcinoma	16	Yes	*PMS2*	Roy et al., 2009
15	Glioblastoma	3	Yes	*MLH6?*	Viana-Pereira et al., submitted

Table 5. Cases reported in the literature with MMR-D associated with brain tumours, including the likely MMR-D cases found in our studies.

potentially contributing to tumorigenesis (Duval & Hamelin, 2002). Genes thought to harbour mutations in microsatellites due to the MSI phenotype are commonly designated MSI target genes. There are numerous MSI target genes described, however the relevance of several of them in cancer is not clear-cut (Mori et al., 2001; Woerner et al., 2003). In brain tumours, only a small number of the "classical" mutated MSI target genes have been reported: *IGFIIR* (Leung et al., 1998) and *PTEN* (Kanamori et al., 2000), each of them in a single case of MSI high-grade gliomas, and *TGFβRII,* reported in 71% of samples (Izumoto et al., 1997), although this result was never confirmed (Kanamori et al., 2000; Leung et al., 1998). We identified four additional alterations, not previously reported in brain tumours, all in genes involved in different DNA repair pathways: mutations in the *MBD4, DNAPKcs,* and *MSH6* genes and a polymorphism in *MRE11* (Viana-Pereira et al., 2009, 2011).

In summary, MSI is present in a subset of medulloblastomas and paediatric high-grade gliomas associated with molecular alterations distinctive of this phenotype, suggesting a potentially new genetic pathway correlated with the development of these tumours. As MSI is associated in other tumour types to a differential response to chemotherapy, the presence of MSI even in a small subset of brain tumours may have important translational implications in these extraordinarily treatment refractory malignancies.

3. References

Aaltonen, L.A., Peltomaki, P., Mecklin, J.P., et al. (1994). Replication errors in benign and malignant tumors from hereditary nonpolyposis colorectal cancer patients. *Cancer Research.* Vol.54, No.7, pp. 1645-1648, ISSN 0008-5472

Agostini, M., Tibiletti, M.G., Lucci-Cordisco, E., et al. (2005). Two PMS2 mutations in a Turcot syndrome family with small bowel cancers. *American Journal of Gastroenterology.* Vol.100, No.8, pp. 1886-1891, ISSN 0002-9270

Aldosari, N., Bigner, S.H., Burger, P.C., et al. (2002). MYCC and MYCN oncogene amplification in medulloblastoma. A fluorescence in situ hybridization study on paraffin sections from the Children's Oncology Group. *Archives of Pathology & Laboratory Medicine.* Vol.126, No.5, pp. 540-544, ISSN 0003-9985

Alonso, M., Hamelin, R., Kim, M., et al. (2001). Microsatellite instability occurs in distinct subtypes of pediatric but not adult central nervous system tumors. *Cancer Research.* Vol.61, No.5, pp. 2124-2128, ISSN 0008-5472

Amariglio, N., Friedman, E., Mor, O., et al. (1995). Analysis of microsatellite repeats in pediatric brain tumors. *Cancer Genetics and Cytogenetics.* Vol.84, No.1, pp. 56-59, ISSN 0165-4608

Arana, M.E. & Kunkel, T.A. (2010). Mutator phenotypes due to DNA replication infidelity. *Seminars in Cancer Biology.* Vol.20, No.5, pp. 304-311, ISSN 1044-579X

Baldwin, R.T. & Preston-Martin, S. (2004). Epidemiology of brain tumors in childhood - a review. *Toxicology and Applied Pharmacology.* Vol.199, No.2, pp. 118-131, ISSN 0041-008X

Balss, J., Meyer, J., Mueller, W., Korshunov, A., Hartmann, C., & von Deimling, A. (2008). Analysis of the IDH1 codon 132 mutation in brain tumors. *Acta Neuropathologica.* Vol.116, No.6, pp. 597-602, ISSN 0001-6322

Barrow, J., Adamowicz-Brice, M., Cartmill, M., et al. (2011). Homozygous loss of ADAM3A revealed by genome-wide analysis of pediatric high-grade glioma and diffuse intrinsic pontine gliomas. *Neuro Oncology.* Vol.13, No.2, pp. 212-222, ISSN 1522-8517

Bax, D.A., Mackay, A., Little, S.E., et al. (2010). A distinct spectrum of copy number aberrations in pediatric high grade gliomas. *Clinical Cancer Research*. Vol.16, No.13, pp. 3368-3377, ISSN 1078-0432

Beroukhim, R., Getz, G., Nghiemphu, L., et al. (2007). Assessing the significance of chromosomal aberrations in cancer: methodology and application to glioma. *Proc Natl Acad Sci U S A*. Vol.104, No.50, pp. 20007-20012, ISSN 1091-6490

Biegel, J.A., Janss, A.J., Raffel, C., et al. (1997). Prognostic significance of chromosome 17p deletions in childhood primitive neuroectodermal tumors (medulloblastomas) of the central nervous system. *Clinical Cancer Research*. Vol.3, No.3, pp. 473-478, ISSN 1078-0432

Bigner, S.H., Mark, J., Friedman, H.S., Biegel, J.A., & Bigner, D.D. (1988). Structural chromosomal abnormalities in human medulloblastoma. *Cancer Genetics and Cytogenetics*. Vol.30, No.1, pp. 91-101, ISSN 0165-4608

Boland, C.R., Koi, M., Chang, D.K., & Carethers, J.M. (2008). The biochemical basis of microsatellite instability and abnormal immunohistochemistry and clinical behavior in Lynch syndrome: from bench to bedside. *Familial Cancer*. Vol.7, No.1, pp. 41-52, ISSN 1389-9600

Bondy, M.L., Scheurer, M.E., Malmer, B., et al. (2008). Brain tumor epidemiology: Consensus from the Brain Tumor Epidemiology Consortium. *Cancer*. Vol.113, No.7, pp. 1953-1968, ISSN 0008-543X

Brandes, A.A., Franceschi, E., Tosoni, A., et al. (2009). Adult neuroectodermal tumors of posterior fossa (medulloblastoma) and of supratentorial sites (stPNET). *Critical Reviews in Oncology Hematology*. Vol.71, No.2, pp. 165-179, ISSN 1040-8428

Bredel, M., Bredel, C., Juric, D., et al. (2005). High-resolution genome-wide mapping of genetic alterations in human glial brain tumors. *Cancer Research*. Vol.65, No.10, pp. 4088-4096, ISSN 0008-5472

Bromberg, J.E.C. & van den Bent, M.J. (2009). Oligodendrogliomas: Molecular Biology and Treatment. *Oncologist*. Vol.14, No.2, pp. 155-163, ISSN 1083-7159

Broniscer, A., Baker, S.J., West, A.N., et al. (2007). Clinical and molecular characteristics of malignant transformation of low-grade glioma in children. *Journal of Clinical Oncology*. Vol.25, No.6, pp. 682-689, ISSN 0732-183X

Buhard, O., Cattaneo, F., Wong, Y.F., et al. (2006). Multipopulation analysis of polymorphisms in five mononucleotide repeats used to determine the microsatellite instability status of human tumors. *Journal of Clinical Oncology*. Vol.24, No.2, pp. 241-251, ISSN 0732-183X

Buhard, O., Suraweera, N., Lectard, A., Duval, A., & Hamelin, R. (2004). Quasimonomorphic mononucleotide repeats for high-level microsatellite instability analysis. *Disease Markers*. Vol.20, No.4-5, pp. 251-257, ISSN 0278-0240

Burnet, N.G., Jefferies, S.J., Benson, R.J., Hunt, D.P., & Treasure, F.P. (2005). Years of life lost (YLL) from cancer is an important measure of population burden--and should be considered when allocating research funds. *British Journal of Cancer*. Vol.92, No.2, pp. 241-245, ISSN 0007-0920

Cahill, D.P., Kinzler, K.W., Vogelstein, B., & Lengauer, C. (1999). Genetic instability and darwinian selection in tumours. *Trends in Cell Biology*. Vol.9, No.12, pp. pp. M57-M60, ISSN 0962-8924

Carrie, C., Lasset, C., Alapetite, C., et al. (1994). Multivariate analysis of prognostic factors in adult patients with medulloblastoma. Retrospective study of 156 patients. *Cancer*. Vol.74, No.8, pp. 2352-2360, ISSN 0008-543X

Central Brain Tumor Registry of the United States [CBTRUS]. (2010). CBTRUS Statistical Report: Primary Brain Tumors in the United States, 2004-2006. In: *Central Brain Tumor Registry of the United States*, Hinsdale, IL, Available from: www.cbtrus.org

Cheng, Y., Ng, H.K., Zhang, S.F., et al. (1999). Genetic alterations in pediatric high-grade astrocytomas. *Human Pathology*. Vol.30, No.11, pp. 1284-1290, ISSN 0046-8177

Clifford, S.C., Lusher, M.E., Lindsey, J.C., et al. (2006). Wnt/Wingless pathway activation and chromosome 6 loss characterize a distinct molecular sub-group of medulloblastomas associated with a favorable prognosis. *Cell Cycle*. Vol.5, No.22, pp. 2666-2670, ISSN 1538-4101

Cogen, P.H. & McDonald, J.D. (1996). Tumor suppressor genes and medulloblastoma. *Journal of Neurooncology*. Vol.29, No.1, pp. 103-112, ISSN 0167 -594X

Dams, E., Van de Kelft, E.J., Martin, J.J., Verlooy, J., & Willems, P.J. (1995). Instability of microsatellites in human gliomas. *Cancer Research*. Vol.55, No.7, pp. 1547-1549, ISSN 0008-5472

Davis, F.G., Freels, S., Grutsch, J., Barlas, S., & Brem, S. (1998). Survival rates in patients with primary malignant brain tumors stratified by patient age and tumor histological type: an analysis based on Surveillance, Epidemiology, and End Results (SEER) data, 1973-1991. *Journal of Neurosurgery*. Vol.88, No.1, pp. 1-10, ISSN 0022-3085

de Leeuw, W.J.F., Dierssen, J., Vasen, H.F.A., et al. (2000). Prediction of a mismatch repair gene defect by microsatellite instability and immunohistochemical analysis in endometrial tumours from HNPCC patients. *Journal of Pathology*. Vol.192, No.3, pp. 328-335, ISSN 0022-3417

de Tayrac, M., Etcheverry, A., Aurbry, M., et al. (2009). Integrative Genome-Wide Analysis Reveals a Robust Genomic Glioblastoma Signature Associated with Copy Number Driving Changes in Gene Expression. *Genes Chromosomes & Cancer*. Vol.48, No.1, pp. 55-68, ISSN 1045-2257

De Rosa, M., Fasano, C., Panariello, L., et al. (2000). Evidence for a recessive inheritance of Turcot's syndrome caused by compound heterozygous mutations within the PMS2 gene. *Oncogene*. Vol.19, No.13, pp. 1719-1723, ISSN 0950-9232

Dubuc, A.M., Northcott, P.A., Mack, S., Witt, H., Pfister, S., & Taylor, M.D. (2010). The Genetics of Pediatric Brain Tumors. *Current Neurology and Neuroscience Reports*. Vol.10, No.3, pp. 215-223, ISSN 1528-4042

Duval, A. & Hamelin, R. (2002). Genetic instability in human mismatch repair deficient cancers. *Annales de Genetique*. Vol.45, No.2, pp. 71-75, ISSN 0003-3995

Eckert, A., Kloor, M., Giersch, A., et al. (2007). Microsatellite instability in pediatric and adult high-grade gliomas. *Brain Pathology*. Vol.17, No.2, pp. 146-150, ISSN 1015-6305

Ellegren, H. (2004). Microsatellites: simple sequences with complex evolution. *Nature Reviews Genetics*. Vol.5, No.6, pp. 435-445, ISSN 1471-0056

Ferlay, J., Shin, H.R., Bray, F., Forman, D., Mathers, C., & Parkin, D.M. (2008). GLOBOCAN 2008. In: *Cancer Incidence and Mortality Worldwide: IARC Cancer Base*, Available from: http://globocan.iarc.fr

Fishel, R. & Kolodner, R.D. (1995). Identification of mismatch repair genes and their role in the development of cancer. *Current Opinion in Genetics & Development*. Vol.5, No.3, pp. 382-395, ISSN 0959-437X

Frost, P.J., Laperriere, N.J., Wong, C.S., Milosevic, M.F., Simpson, W.J., & Pintilie, M. (1995). Medulloblastoma in adults. *International Journal of Radiation Oncology Biology Physics*. Vol.32, No.4, pp. 951-957, ISSN 0360-3016

Furnari, F.B., Fenton, T., Bachoo, R.M., et al. (2007). Malignant astrocytic glioma: genetics, biology, and paths to treatment. *Genes & Development*. Vol.21, No.21, pp. 2683-2710, ISSN 0890-9369

Gardina, P.J., Lo, K.C., Lee, W., Cowell, J.K., & Turpaz, Y. (2008). Ploidy status and copy number aberrations in primary glioblastomas defined by integrated analysis of allelic ratios, signal ratios and loss of heterozygosity using 500K SNP Mapping Arrays. *Bmc Genomics*. Vol.9, ISSN 1471-2164

Gilbertson, R.J. & Ellison, D.W. (2008). The origins of medulloblastoma subtypes. *Annual Review of Pathology-Mechanisms of Disease*. Vol.3, pp. 341-365, ISSN 1553-4006

Giunti, L., Cetica, V., Ricci, U., et al. (2009). Type A microsatellite instability in pediatric gliomas as an indicator of Turcot syndrome. *European Journal of Human Genetics*. Vol.17, No.7, pp. 919-927, ISSN 1018-4813

Goel, A., Nagasaka, T., Hamelin, R., & Boland, C.R. (2010). An optimized pentaplex PCR for detecting DNA mismatch repair-deficient colorectal cancers. *PLoS ONE*. Vol.5, No.2, pp. e9393

Gottardo, N.G. & Gajjar, A. (2008). Chemotherapy for Malignant Brain Tumors of Childhood. *Journal of Child Neurology*. Vol.23, No.10, pp. 1149-1159, ISSN 0883-0738

Hargrave, D. (2009). Paediatric high and low grade glioma: the impact of tumour biology on current and future therapy. *British Journal of Neurosurgery*. Vol.23, No.4, pp. 351-363, ISSN 0268-8697

Hartmann, C., Meyer, J., Balss, J., et al. (2009). Type and frequency of IDH1 and IDH2 mutations are related to astrocytic and oligodendroglial differentiation and age: a study of 1,010 diffuse gliomas. *Acta Neuropathologica*. Vol.118, No.4, pp. 469-474, ISSN 0001-6322

Hegde, M.R., Chong, B., Blazo, M.E., et al. (2005). A homozygous mutation in MSH6 causes Turcot syndrome. *Clinical Cancer Research*. Vol.11, No.13, pp. 4689-4693, ISSN 1078-0432

Huse, J.T. & Holland, E.C. (2010). Targeting brain cancer: advances in the molecular pathology of malignant glioma and medulloblastoma. *Nature Reviews Cancer*. Vol.10, No.5, pp. 319-331, ISSN 1474-175X

Ichimura, K., Pearson, D.M., Kocialkowski, S., et al. (2009). IDH1 mutations are present in the majority of common adult gliomas but rare in primary glioblastomas. *Neuro Oncology*. Vol.11, No.4, pp. 341-347, ISSN 1522-8517

Imbach, P. (2006). Brain Tumours. In: *Pediatric Oncology: A Comprehensive Guide*, P. Imbach, T. Kühne, R. Arceci, (Eds.), pp. 95-117, Springer -Verlag Berlin, ISBN 3-540-20530-6, Heidelberg, Germany

Ionov, Y., Peinado, M.A., Malkhosyan, S., Shibata, D., & Perucho, M. (1993). Ubiquitous Somatic Mutations in Simple Repeated Sequences Reveal A New Mechanism for Colonic Carcinogenesis. *Nature*. Vol.363, No.6429, pp. 558-561, ISSN 0028-0836

Izumoto, S., Arita, N., Ohnishi, T., et al. (1997). Microsatellite instability and mutated type II transforming growth factor-beta receptor gene in gliomas. *Cancer Lett*. Vol.112, No.2, pp. 251-256,

Jemal, A., Siegel, R., Ward, E., Hao, Y.P., Xu, J.Q., & Thun, M.J. (2009). Cancer Statistics, 2009. *Ca-A Cancer Journal for Clinicians*. Vol.59, No.4, pp. 225-249, ISSN 0007-9235

Jiricny, J. (2006). The multifaceted mismatch-repair system. *Nature Reviews Molecular Cell Biology*. Vol.7, No.5, pp. 335-346, ISSN 1471-0072

Kanamori, M., Kon, H., Nobukuni, T., et al. (2000). Microsatellite instability and the PTEN1 gene mutation in a subset of early onset gliomas carrying germline mutation or promoter methylation of the hMLH1 gene. *Oncogene*. Vol.19, No.12, pp. 1564-1571, ISSN 0950-9232

Kool, M., Koster, J., Bunt, J., et al. (2008). Integrated genomics identifies five medulloblastoma subtypes with distinct genetic profiles, pathway signatures and clinicopathological features. *PLoS One*. Vol.3, No.8, pp. e3088.

Korshunov, A., Remke, M., Werft, W., et al. (2010). Adult and pediatric medulloblastomas are genetically distinct and require different algorithms for molecular risk stratification. *Journal of Clinical Oncology*. Vol.28, No.18, pp. 3054-3060, ISSN 0732-183X

Kotliarov, Y., Steed, M.E., Christopher, N., et al. (2006). High-resolution global genomic survey of 178 gliomas reveals novel regions of copy number alteration and allelic imbalances. *Cancer Research*. Vol.66, No.19, pp. 9428-9436, ISSN 0008-5472

Kreiger, P.A., Okada, Y., Simon, S., Rorke, L.B., Louis, D.N., & Golden, J.A. (2005). Losses of chromosomes 1p and 19q are rare in pediatric oligodendrogliomas. *Acta Neuropathologica*. Vol.109, No.4, pp. 387-392, ISSN 0001-6322

Kruger, S., Kinzel, M., Walldorf, C., et al. (2008). Homozygous PMS2 germline mutations in two families with early-onset haematological malignancy, brain tumours, HNPCC-associated tumours, and signs of neurofibromatosis type 1. *European Journal of Human Genetics*. Vol.16, No.1, pp. 62-72, ISSN 1018-4813

Kunkel, T.A. & Bebenek, K. (2000). DNA replication fidelity. *Annual Review of Biochemistry*. Vol.69, pp. 497-529

Lamont, J.M., McManamy, C.S., Pearson, A.D., Clifford, S.C., & Ellison, D.W. (2004). Combined histopathological and molecular cytogenetic stratification of medulloblastoma patients. *Clinical Cancer Research*. Vol.10, No.16, pp. 5482-5493, ISSN 1078-0432

Lander, E.S., Linton, L.M., Birren, B., et al. (2001). Initial sequencing and analysis of the human genome. *Nature*. Vol.409, No.6822, pp. 860-921, ISSN 0028-0836

Laughton, S.J., Merchant, T.E., Sklar, C.A., et al. (2008). Endocrine outcomes for children with embryonal brain tumors after risk-adapted craniospinal and conformal primary-site irradiation and high-dose chemotherapy with stem-cell rescue on the SJMB-96 trial. *Journal of Clinical Oncology*. Vol.26, No.7, pp. 1112-1118, ISSN 0732-183X

Leung, S.Y., Chan, T.L., Chung, L.P., et al. (1998). Microsatellite instability and mutation of DNA mismatch repair genes in gliomas. *American Journal of Pathology*. Vol.153, No.4, pp. 1181-1188

Li, G.M. & Modrich, P. (1995). Restoration of mismatch repair to nuclear extracts of H6 colorectal tumor cells by a heterodimer of human MutL homologs. *Proc Natl Acad Sci U S A*. Vol.92, No.6, pp. 1950-1954, ISSN 1091-6490

Li, G.M. (2008). Mechanisms and functions of DNA mismatch repair. *Cell Research*. Vol.18, No.1, pp. 85-98, ISSN 1001-0602

Lipkin, S.M., Wang, V., Jacoby, R., et al. (2000). MLH3: a DNA mismatch repair gene associated with mammalian microsatellite instability. *Nature Genetics*. Vol.24, No.1, pp. 27-35, ISSN 1061-4036

Ljungman, M. (2010). The DNA damage response--repair or despair? *Environmental and Molecular Mutagenesis*. Vol.51, No.8-9, pp. 879-889, ISSN 0893-6692

Loeb, L.A. (1991). Mutator phenotype may be required for multistage carcinogenesis. *Cancer Research*. Vol.51, No.12, pp. 3075-3079, ISSN 0008-5472

Louis, D.N., Ohgaki, H., Wiestler, O.D., & Cavenee, W.K. (Eds.). (2007). *WHO Classification of Tumours of the Central Nervous System*, IARC, ISBN 9283224302, Lyon, France

Maher, E.A., Brennan, C., Wen, P.Y., et al. (2006). Marked genomic differences characterize primary and secondary glioblastoma subtypes and identify two distinct molecular and clinical secondary glioblastoma entities. *Cancer Research*. Vol.66, No.23, pp. 11502-11513, ISSN 0008-5472

Maity, A., Pruitt, A.A., Judy, K.D., & Phillips, P.C. (2004). Cancer of the Central Nervous System, In: *Abeloff's Clinical Oncology*, M.D. Abeloff, J.O. Armitage, J.E. Niederhuber, M.B. Kastan, W.G. McKenzie (Eds.), pp. 1357-1362, Elsevier Churchill Livingstone, ISBN 978-0-443-06694-8, Philadelphia, US

Marra, G. & Jiricny, J. (2005). DNA Mismatch Repair and Colon Cancer. In: *Genome Instability in Cancer Development*, E.A. Nigg (Ed.), pp. 85-123, Springer Science + Business Media, Inc., ISBN 1-4020-3763-5 New York, US

Martinez, R., Schackert, H.K., Appelt, H., Plaschke, J., Baretton, G., & Schackert, G. (2005). Low-level microsatellite instability phenotype in sporadic glioblastoma multiforme. *Journal of Cancer Research and Clinical Oncology*. Vol.131, No.2, pp. 87-93, ISSN 0171-5216

Martinho, O., Longatto-Filho, A., Lambros, M.B., et al. (2009). Expression, mutation and copy number analysis of platelet-derived growth factor receptor A (PDGFRA) and its ligand PDGFA in gliomas. *British Journal of Cancer*. Vol.101, No.6, pp. 973-982, ISSN 0007-0920

Maxwell, J.A., Johnson, S.P., McLendon, R.E., et al. (2008). Mismatch repair deficiency does not mediate clinical resistance to temozolomide in malignant glioma. *Clinical Cancer Research*. Vol.14, No.15, pp. 4859-4868, ISSN 1078-0432

Menko, F.H., Kaspers, G.L., Meijer, G.A., Claes, K., van Hagen, J.M., & Gille, J.J. (2004). A homozygous MSH6 mutation in a child with cafe-au-lait spots, oligodendroglioma and rectal cancer. *Familial Cancer*. Vol.3, No.2, pp. 123-127, ISSN 1389-9600

Mori, Y., Yin, J., Rashid, A., et al. (2001). Instabilotyping: comprehensive identification of frameshift mutations caused by coding region microsatellite instability. *Cancer Research*. Vol.61, No.16, pp. 6046-6049, ISSN 0008-5472

Mulhern, R.K., Merchant, T.E., Gajjar, A., Reddick, W.E., & Kun, L.E. (2004). Late neurocognitive sequelae in survivors of brain tumours in childhood. *Lancet Oncology*. Vol.5, No.7, pp. 399-408, ISSN 1470-2045

Negrini, S., Gorgoulis, V.G., & Halazonetis, T.D. (2010). Genomic instability - an evolving hallmark of cancer. *Nature Reviews Molecular Cell Biology*. Vol.11, No.3, pp. 220-228, ISSN 1471-0072

Nicholson, J., Wickramasinghe, C., Ross, F., Crolla, J., & Ellison, D. (2000). Imbalances of chromosome 17 in medulloblastomas determined by comparative genomic hybridisation and fluorescence in situ hybridisation. *Molecular Pathology*. Vol.53, No.6, pp. 313-319

Nigg, E.A. (2005). *Genome Instability in Cancer Development*, Springer Science + Business Media, Inc., ISBN 1-4020-3763-5 New York, US

Nigro, J.M., Misra, A., Zhang, L., et al. (2005). Integrated array-comparative genomic hybridization and expression array profiles identify clinically relevant molecular subtypes of glioblastoma. *Cancer Research*. Vol.65, No.5, pp. 1678-1686, ISSN 0008-5472

Oda, S., Maehara, Y., Ikeda, Y., et al. (2005). Two modes of microsatellite instability in human cancer: differential connection of defective DNA mismatch repair to dinucleotide repeat instability. *Nucleic Acids Research*. Vol.33, No.5, pp. 1628-1636, ISSN 0305-1048

Ohgaki, H. & Kleihues, P. (2005). Epidemiology and etiology of gliomas. *Acta Neuropathologica*. Vol.109, No.1, pp. 93-108, ISSN 0001-6322

Ostergaard, J.R., Sunde, L., & Okkels, H. (2005). Neurofibromatosis von Recklinghausen type I phenotype and early onset of cancers in siblings compound heterozygous for mutations in MSH6. *American Journal of Medical Genetics Part A*. Vol.139A, No.2, pp. 96-105, ISSN 1552-4825

Parsons, D.W., Jones, S., Zhang, X., et al. (2008). An integrated genomic analysis of human glioblastoma multiforme. *Science*. Vol.321, No.5897, pp. 1807-1812, ISSN 0036-8075

Paugh, B.S., Qu, C., Jones, C., et al. (2010). Integrated molecular genetic profiling of pediatric high-grade gliomas reveals key differences with the adult disease. *Journal of Clinical Oncology*. Vol.28, No.18, pp. 3061-3068, ISSN 0732-183X

Pettorini, B.L., Park, Y.S., Caldarelli, M., Massimi, L., Tamburrini, G., & Di Rocco, C. (2008). Radiation-induced brain tumours after central nervous system irradiation in childhood: a review. *Childs Nervous System*. Vol.24, No.7, pp. 793-805, ISSN 0256-7040

Pfister, S., Remke, M., Benner, A., et al. (2009). Outcome prediction in pediatric medulloblastoma based on DNA copy-number aberrations of chromosomes 6q and 17q and the MYC and MYCN loci. *Journal of Clinical Oncology*. Vol.27, No.10, pp. 1627-1636, ISSN 0732-183X

Poley, J.W., Wagner, A., Hoogmans, M.M., et al. (2007). Biallelic germline mutations of mismatch-repair genes: a possible cause for multiple pediatric malignancies. *Cancer*. Vol.109, No.11, pp. 2349-2356, ISSN 0008-543X

Pollack, I.F., Finkelstein, S.D., Burnham, J., et al. (2003). Association between chromosome 1p and 19q loss and outcome in pediatric malignant gliomas: results from the CCG-945 cohort. *Pediatric Neurosurgery*. Vol.39, No.3, pp. 114-121, ISSN 1016-2291

Pollack, I.F., Hamilton, R.L., Sobol, R.W., et al. (2010a). IDH1 mutations are common in malignant gliomas arising in adolescents: a report from the Children's Oncology Group. *Childs Nervous System*. Vol.27, No.1, pp.87-94, ISSN 0256-7040

Pollack, I.F., Hamilton, R.L., Sobol, R.W., et al. (2010b). Mismatch repair deficiency is an uncommon mechanism of alkylator resistance in pediatric malignant gliomas: a report from the Children's Oncology Group. *Pediatric Blood & Cancer*. Vol.55, No.6, pp. 1066-1071, ISSN 1545-5009

Qu, H.Q., Jacob, K., Fatet, S., et al. (2010). Genome-wide profiling using single-nucleotide polymorphism arrays identifies novel chromosomal imbalances in pediatric glioblastomas. *Neuro Oncology*. Vol.12, No.2, pp. 153-163, ISSN 1522-8517

Rao, S.K., Edwards, J., Joshi, A.D., Siu, I.M., & Riggins, G.J. (2010). A survey of glioblastoma genomic amplifications and deletions. *Journal of Neuro-Oncology*. Vol.96, No.2, pp. 169-179, ISSN 0167-594X

Raschle, M., Marra, G., Nystrom-Lahti, M., Schar, P., & Jiricny, J. (1999). Identification of hMutLbeta, a heterodimer of hMLH1 and hPMS1. *Journal of Biological Chemistry*. Vol.274, No.45, pp. 32368-32375, ISSN 0021-9258

Reifenberger, G., Blumcke, I., Pietsch, T., & Paulus, W. (2006). Pathology Classification of Tumors of the Nervous System. In: *Neuro-Oncology of CNS Tumors*. J.C. Tonn, M. Westphal, J.T. Rutka, S.A. Grossman (Eds.), pp. 5-72, Springer-Verlag Berlin, ISBN 3-540-25833-7, Heidelberg, Germany

Rickert, C.H. & Paulus, W. (2001). Epidemiology of central nervous system tumors in childhood and adolescence based on the new WHO classification. *Child's Nervous System*. Vol.17, No.9, pp. 503-511,

Rickert, C.H., Strater, R., Kaatsch, P., et al. (2001). Pediatric high-grade astrocytomas show chromosomal imbalances distinct from adult cases. *American Journal of Pathology*. Vol.158, No.4, pp. 1525-1532

Roy, S., Raskin, L., Raymond, V.A., Thibodeau, S.N., Mody, R.J., & Gruber, S.B. (2009). Pediatric Duodenal Cancer and Biallelic Mismatch Repair Gene Mutations. *Pediatric Blood & Cancer*. Vol.53, No.1, pp. 116-120, ISSN 1545-5009

Sanson, M., Marie, Y., Paris, S., et al. (2009). Isocitrate dehydrogenase 1 codon 132 mutation is an important prognostic biomarker in gliomas. *Journal of Clinical Oncology*. Vol.27, No.25, pp. 4150-4154, ISSN 0732-183X

Sarkar, C., Deb, P., & Sharma, M.C. (2005). Recent advances in embryonal tumours of the central nervous system. *Childs Nervous System*. Vol.21, No.4, pp. 272-293, ISSN 0256-7040

Schiffman, J.D., Hodgson, J.G., VandenBerg, S.R., et al. (2010). Oncogenic BRAF mutation with CDKN2A inactivation is characteristic of a subset of pediatric malignant astrocytomas. *Cancer Research*. Vol.70, No.2, pp. 512-519, ISSN 0008-5472

Schofield, M.J. & Hsieh, P. (2003). DNA mismatch repair: molecular mechanisms and biological function. *Annual Review of Microbiology*. Vol.57, pp. 579-608

Scott, R.H., Mansour, S., Pritchard-Jones, K., Kumar, D., MacSweeney, F., & Rahman, N. (2007). Medulloblastoma, acute myelocytic leukemia and colonic carcinomas in a child with biallelic MSH6 mutations. *Nature Clinical Practice Oncology*. Vol.4, No.2, pp. 130-134, ISSN 1743-4254

Shah, S.N., Hile, S.E., & Eckert, K.A. (2010). Defective mismatch repair, microsatellite mutation bias, and variability in clinical cancer phenotypes. *Cancer Research*. Vol.70, No.2, pp. 431-435, ISSN 0008-5472

Silber, J.H., Radcliffe, J., Peckham, V., et al. (1992). Whole-brain irradiation and decline in intelligence: the influence of dose and age on IQ score. *Journal of Clinical Oncology*. Vol.10, No.9, pp. 1390-1396, ISSN 0732-183X

Smith, J.S., Alderete, B., Minn, Y., et al. (1999). Localization of common deletion regions on 1p and 19q in human gliomas and their association with histological subtype. *Oncogene*. Vol.18, No.28, pp. 4144-4152, ISSN 0950-9232

Smith, J.S., Perry, A., Borell, T.J., et al. (2000). Alterations of chromosome arms 1p and 19q as predictors of survival in oligodendrogliomas, astrocytomas, and mixed oligoastrocytomas. *Journal of Clinical Oncology*. Vol.18, No.3, pp. 636-645, ISSN 0732-183X

Sobrido, M.J., Pereira, C.R., Barros, F., Forteza, J., Carracedo, A., & Lema, M. (2000). Low frequency of replication errors in primary nervous system tumours. *Journal of Neurology, Neurosurgery & Psychiatry*. Vol.69, No.3, pp. 369-375, ISSN 1468-330X

Steichen-Gersdorf, E., Baumgartner, M., Kreczy, A., Maier, H., & Fink, F.M. (1997). Deletion mapping on chromosome 17p in medulloblastoma. *British Journal of Cancer*. Vol.76, No.10, pp. 1284-1287, ISSN 0007-0920

Stewart, E.S. & Cohen, D.G. (1998). Central nervous system tumors in children. *Seminars in Oncology Nursing*. Vol.14, No.1, pp. 34-42, ISSN 0749-2081

Taylor, M.D. (2006). Medulloblastoma, In: *Neuro-Oncology of CNS Tumors*. J.C. Tonn, M. Westphal, J.T. Rutka, S.A. Grossman (Eds.), pp. 462-469, Springer-Verlag Berlin, ISBN 3-540-25833-7, Heidelberg, Germany

The Cancer Genome Atlas Research Network [TCGA]. (2008). Comprehensive genomic characterization defines human glioblastoma genes and core pathways. *Nature*. Vol.455, No.7216, pp. 1061-1068, ISSN 0028-0836

Thompson, M.C., Fuller, C., Hogg, T.L., et al. (2006). Genomics identifies medulloblastoma subgroups that are enriched for specific genetic alterations. *Journal of Clinical Oncology*. Vol.24, No.12, pp. 1924-1931, ISSN 0732-183X

Toledano, H., Goldberg, Y., Kedar-Barnes, I., et al. (2009). Homozygosity of MSH2 c.1906G-->C germline mutation is associated with childhood colon cancer, astrocytoma and signs of Neurofibromatosis type I. *Familial Cancer*. Vol.8, No.3, pp. 187-194, ISSN 1389-9600

Tomlinson, F.H., Jenkins, R.B., Scheithauer, B.W., et al. (1994). Aggressive medulloblastoma with high-level N-*myc* amplification. *Mayo Clinic Proceedings*. Vol.69, No.4, pp. 359-365, ISSN 0025-6196

Ullrich, N.J. (2008). Inherited Disorders As A Risk Factor and Predictor of Neurodevelopmental Outcome in Pediatric Cancer. *Developmental Disabilities Research Reviews*. Vol.14, No.3, pp. 229-237, ISSN 1940-5510

Umar, A., Boland, C.R., Terdiman, J.P., et al. (2004). Revised Bethesda Guidelines for hereditary nonpolyposis colorectal cancer (Lynch syndrome) and microsatellite instability. *Journal of the National Cancer Institute*. Vol.96, No.4, pp. 261-268, ISSN 0027-8874

Vagner-Capodano, A.M., Zattara-Cannoni, H., Gambarelli, D., et al. (1994). Detection of i(17q) chromosome by fluorescent in situ hybridization (FISH) with interphase nuclei in medulloblastoma. *Cancer Genetics and Cytogenetics*. Vol.78, No.1, pp. 1-6, ISSN 0165-4608 van den Bent, M.J., Reni, M., Gatta, G., & Vecht, C. (2008). Oligodendroglioma. *Critical Reviews in Oncology/Hematology*. Vol.66, No.3, pp. 262-272, ISSN 1040-8428

Venkatesan, R.N. & Loeb, L.A. (2005). The Multiplicity of Mutations in Human Cancers. In: *Genome Instability in Cancer Development*, E.A. Nigg (Ed.), pp. 3-17, Springer Science + Business Media, Inc., ISBN 1-4020-3763-5 New York, US

Viana-Pereira, M., Almeida, I., Sousa, S., et al. (2009). Analysis of microsatellite instability in medulloblastoma. *Neuro Oncology*. Vol.11, No.5, pp. 458-467, ISSN 1522-8517

Viana-Pereira, M., Lee, A., Popov, S., et al. (2010). Microsatellite Instability in Pediatric High Grade Glioma is Associated with Genomic Profile and Differential Target Gene Inactivation. PLoS ONE. Vol.6, No.5, pp.e20588

Vladimirova, V., Denkhaus, D., Soerensen, N., Wagner, S., Wolff, J.E., & Pietsch, T. (2007). Low level of microsatellite instability in paediatric malignant astrocytomas. *Neuropathology and Applied Neurobiology*. Vol.34, No.5, pp. 547-554, ISSN 0305-1846

Wagner, A., Barrows, A., Wijnen, J.T., et al. (2003). Molecular analysis of hereditary nonpolyposis colorectal cancer in the United States: high mutation detection rate among clinically selected families and characterization of an American founder genomic deletion of the MSH2 gene. *American Journal of Human Genetics*. Vol.72, No.5, pp. 1088-1100, ISSN 0002-9297

Wang, Q., Lasset, C., Desseigne, F., et al. (1999). Neurofibromatosis and early onset of cancers in hMLH1-deficient children. *Cancer Research*. Vol.59, No.2, pp. 294-297, ISSN 0008-5472

Watanabe, T., Nobusawa, S., Kleihues, P., & Ohgaki, H. (2009). IDH1 mutations are early events in the development of astrocytomas and oligodendrogliomas. *American Journal of Pathology*. Vol.174, No.4, pp. 1149-1153

Weingart, J.D., McGirt, M.J., & Brem, H. (2006). High-Grade Astrocytoma/Glioblastoma. No.6, pp. 128-138,

Woerner, S.M., Benner, A., Sutter, C., et al. (2003). Pathogenesis of DNA repair-deficient cancers: a statistical meta-analysis of putative Real Common Target genes. *Oncogene*. Vol.22, No.15, pp. 2226-2235, ISSN 0950-9232

Wong, K.K., Tsang, Y.T.M., Chang, Y.M., et al. (2006). Genome-wide allelic imbalance analysis of pediatric gliomas by single nucleotide polymorphic allele array. *Cancer Research*. Vol.66, No.23, pp. 11172-11178, ISSN 0008-5472

Wong, Y.F., Cheung, T.H., Lo, K.W., et al. (2006). Detection of microsatellite instability in endometrial cancer: advantages of a panel of five mononucleotide repeats over the National Cancer Institute panel of markers. *Carcinogenesis*. Vol.27, No.5, pp. 951-955, ISSN 0143-3334

Wrensch, M., Fisher, J.L., Schwartzbaum, J.A., Bondy, M., Berger, M., & Aldape, K.D. (2005). The molecular epidemiology of gliomas in adults. *Neurosurgical Focus*. Vol.19, No.5, pp. E5, ISSN 1092-0684

Yan, H., Parsons, D.W., Jin, G., et al. (2009). IDH1 and IDH2 mutations in gliomas. *New England Journal of Medicine*. Vol.360, No.8, pp. 765-773, ISSN 0028-4793

Zarghooni, M., Bartels, U., Lee, E., et al. (2010). Whole-genome profiling of pediatric diffuse intrinsic pontine gliomas highlights platelet-derived growth factor receptor alpha and poly (ADP-ribose) polymerase as potential therapeutic targets. *Journal of Clinical Oncology*. Vol.28, No.8, pp. 1337-1344, ISSN 0732-183X

3

Brain Tumor Exosomes and Microvesicles: Pleiotropic Effects from Tiny Cellular Surrogates

Michael W Graner
University of Colorado Denver
Anschutz Medical Campus
Department of Neurosurgery
Aurora, Coloraodo
USA

1. Introduction

Extracellular signaling is a necessity for tissue and organ system development, maintenance, adaptation and survival. From the biologic unit of the cell to the complete organizational structure that is the organism, cell-cell, cell-tissue, tissue-organ, and organ-system communication are essential to keep the organism functioning, homeostatic, and proliferative. Cell-derived extracellular vesicles such as exosomes and microvesicles are vital players in these forms of proximal and distal messaging, acting as discrete packets of information capable of altering recipient cell phenotypes, activities, and responses. These vesicles are part of the normal biologic repertoire of the organism, but are particularly exploited by neoplasmic growths and cancers to change both the local and systemic environments to aid in tumor proliferation, invasion, and metastases, and in the defense of the tumor. This chapter will focus on exosomes and microvesicles from brain tumors, but similar stories may be told about such vesicles from almost any tumor type. Following this general introduction on exosomes and microvesicles we will discuss the experimentally determined and putative roles of exosomes in brain tumor biology, particularly in stress responses, metabolism, migration, immunology, and protection against chemotherapeutics.

2. Exosome/Microvesicle biosynthesis simplified

The interactions between cell surface components, extracellular matrix molecules, proteases and protease inhibitors, and "soluble" factors is complex (Weber, Bjerke, and Desimone ; Rozario and DeSimone ; Chirco et al. 2006; Gonzalo et al. ; Kessenbrock, Plaks, and Werb ; Stetler-Stevenson 2008; Hyytiainen, Penttinen, and Keski-Oja 2004; Tran, Griffith, and Wells 2004; Goldman 2004). However, the distinction between truly soluble factors and technically particulate forms of those factors becomes blurred in terms of exosomes and microvesicles (Peinado, Lavotshkin, and Lyden ; Camussi et al.). Exosomes and microvesicles are cell-derived, bilayer membrane-enclosed nanovesicles ranging from virus-sized entities (eg, exosomes, 30-100 nm diameter) to small bacteria-sized (eg, microvesicles, ~150 nm- 3000 nm diameter) (Johnstone 2006)—ie, "fat balls". These vesicles exist essentially anywhere there is a cell-liquid interface such as in blood, urine, semen, breast milk, bronchoalveolar lavage fluid, synovial capsule fluid, saliva, ascites, amniotic fluid, cerebrospinal fluid, and *in vitro* spent culture media (Simpson et al. 2009). The obtuse vesicular nomenclature and lack of molecular definitions for these microparticles generates confusion (Mathivanan, Ji, and Simpson); in this chapter, for these cell-derived vesicles we will refer to exosomes as extracellularly-released components of the endocytic pathway, while microvesicles will refer to "shed" vesicles released directly from cell-surface membrane budding (**Figure 1**). Please note that in this work "exosome" does not refer to the intracellular multi-subunit RNA processing complex (Mitchell et al. 1997).

Due to the directional nature of the biogenesis of the two forms of vesicle formation, exosomes and microvesicles largely retain the original topography of the cell itself, making these vesicles akin to tiny cellular surrogates (**Figure 2**). The contents include selected membrane lipids such as gangliosides GM1 and GM3, sphingomyelin, lyso-*bis*-phosphatidic acid/*bis*-monoacylglycerol phosphate (LBPA/BMP), and cholesterol. Protein contents are also strikingly conserved across exosomes and microvesicles from various cell types, including protein components of lipid raft membrane structures, tetraspanins, numerous metabolic enzymes, heat shock proteins, structural proteins, and nucleic acid binding proteins (Simpson, Jensen, and Lim 2008). Appropriately, messenger and microRNAs are also present in exosomes (Taylor and Gercel-Taylor 2008; Valadi et al. 2007) including those from high grade gliomas (Skog et al. 2008). Despite the similarities amongst the vesicles,

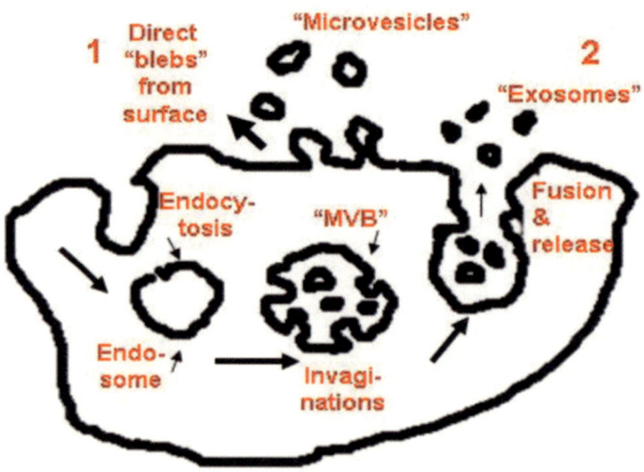

Fig. 1. Highly diagrammatic representation of the release of extracellular vesicles from a cell. Two basic mechanisms are depicted: 1) shedding or "blebbing" of vesicles directly from cell membrane surface, yielding microvesicles (sometimes called microparticles or "ectosomes"); 2) following the endocytic pathway, endosomal compartments develop invaginations that bud off into the endosomal lumen as small vesicles. The endosome is now called a multivesicular body (MVB). At this stage, the MVB may fuse with the lysosome for degradation and recycling of its contents. However, if the MVB fuses with the cell membrane, the vesicles within it are exocytically released as exosomes.

they retain sufficient cell-specific material to frequently allow identification of the cell type source of origin (Denzer et al. 2000; Bobryshev et al. 2001; Blanchard et al. 2002; Graner et al. 2009; Skog et al. 2008). Given that these durable vesicles, when released by tumors, circulate in blood and are found at particularly high levels in patients with cancer (Taylor and Gercel-Taylor 2008), exosomes and microvesicles are considered potential sources of biomarkers obtainable with minimally invasive procedures (Duijvesz et al. ; Krutovskikh and Herceg ; Simpson et al. 2009), including from urine (Dimov, Jankovic Velickovic, and Stefanovic 2009; Pisitkun, Johnstone, and Knepper 2006).

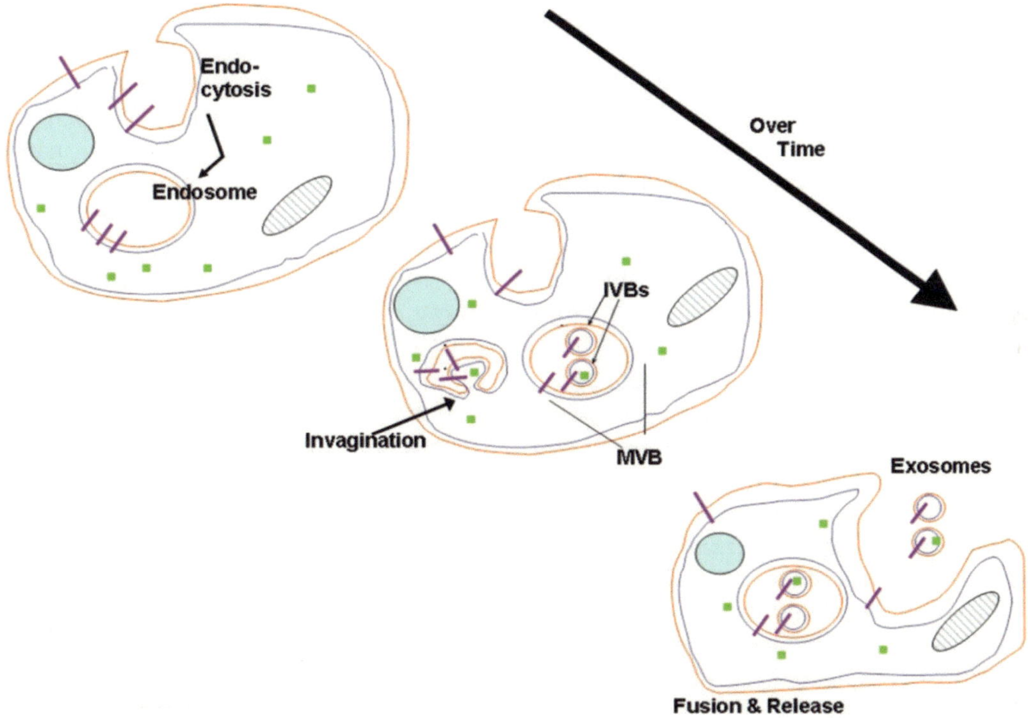

Fig. 2. The topography of exosomes mimics that of the cell of origin. Depicted is a highly diagrammatic cartoon of exosome formation showing the endocytosis of transmembrane proteins (purple lines) in the context of the outer lipid layer of the plasma membrane (shown in red) and the inner lipid layer facing the cytosol (shown in blue). During endosome formation, the cytoplasmic portion of the membrane protein remains in the cytosol; as the endosomes fuse to become more mature structures, invaginations occur, resulting in the pinching off of small vesicles into the luminal space of the endosome. These smaller vesicles may be referred to as intravesicular bodies ("IVBs") while the whole structure is denoted as a multi-vesicular body ("MVB"). The former intracellular domain of the transmembrane protein is now sequestered away from the cytosol; cytoplasmic contents also enter the IVB during formation (green dots). The typical fate of the MVB is fusion with a lysosome for content degradation and recycling. However, if the MVB instead fuses with the plasma membrane, the IVBs will be release extracellularly, and are now called "exosomes". Note that the membrane topography (red/blue positioning) and transmembrane protein orientation are the same as that of the original cell.

The mechanisms driving vesicle formation (at the level of invagination into the endosomal lumen and in the direct "blebbing" from the cell surface) have many of the same driving components, particularly the ESCRT (Endosomal Sorting Complex Required for Transport) machinery including ALIX/AIP1 (de Gassart et al. 2004) and PI3 kinase and related molecules (Stoorvogel et al. 2002). Lipid composition is also a key factor, with structure-altering, membrane-bending lipids playing key roles in the curvature-induced vesicular invaginations (Trajkovic et al. 2008; Subra et al. 2007; Laulagnier et al. 2005) . The acidic pH of the endosomal lumen also enhances lipid bending away from the limiting membrane (Subra et al. 2007) and the low pH of the tumor microenvironment likely has similar effects on microvesicle budding and extracellular activity of the vesicles (Giusti et al. 2008), including exosomes (Parolini et al. 2009). As lipid moieties such as the phosphoinositides/phosphoinositol phosphates (PIPs) and proteins such as the Rab proteins are important in intracellular vesicular identification and trafficking (Perret et al. 2005), it is not surprising that these entities also play significant roles in extracellular vesicle formation (Ostrowski et al. ; Hsu et al.) Various membrane-fusion proteins of the SNARE families are also likely involved (Thery, Zitvogel, and Amigorena 2002). Thus, the intra- and extracellular environments, various lipid players, and numerous proteins involved in intracellular vesicle identity and function all play roles in the formation , intracellular targeting, and possibly extracellular targeting, of exosomes and microvesicles.

2.1 Basics of exosome/microvesicle cargo loading: filling up the fat balls

The sorting process/cargo loading of exosomes and microvesicles is still largely a mystery; whether certain proteins are destined or chosen to become vesicle content or are "trapped" into them is not clear. However, some fundamental principles seem to hold. One of the most common protein post-translational modifications that results in a vesicular destination is ubiquitination, frequently from E3 ubiquitin ligase activities; this may be regulated to some extent by deubiquitination complexes such as signalosomes (Liu et al. 2009). Curiously, cells that are the recipients of exosomes may also activate ubiquitin ligases as part of the downstream effects of extracellular vesicle interactions (Qu et al. 2009). There are also likely ubiquitination-independent mechanisms for vesicular assimilation of proteins as well (Gauvreau et al. 2009); these may include potentially ESCRT- or Rab-driven incorporation of proteins into a "frustrated" recycling pathway where the proteins are neither returned to the cell surface nor directed toward the lysosome (de Gassart et al. 2004). Curiously, lipid sorting into such compartments is a function of the length and/or saturation of their alkyl tails (Mukherjee, Soe, and Maxfield 1999). LBPA, an unconventional negatively-charged phospholipid, is also sequestered to late endosomes/MVBs with a potential structural role (Matsuo et al. 2004). Since LBPA is mostly enriched in internal membranes, whether it plays a role in plasma membrane dynamics is unclear. Membrane partitioning such as lipid raft formation is also a key player in exosome and microvesicle biogenesis and sorting (de Gassart et al. 2003; Calzolari et al. 2006; Staubach, Razawi, and Hanisch 2009; Del Conde et al. 2005). Proteins contained within those lipid rafts are thus sorted to exosomes and microvesicles and include GPI-linked proteins such as acetylcholinesterase (Graner et al. 2009), the NKG2D ligands MICA and MICB (Hedlund et al. 2009), Gce1 and CD73 (Muller et al. 2009), and CD55 and CD59 (Rabesandratana et al. 1998), etc. As mentioned above, the gangliosides GM1 and GM3 are also present in lipid membrane microdomains (Janich and Corbeil 2007) and in exosomes (de Gassart et al. 2003; Parolini et al. 2009).

Membrane proteins that are not necessarily typical constituents of lipid raft domains may shuttle into exosomes or membrane patches of microvesicles by aggregation, such as the transferrin receptor (de Gassart et al. 2004) or by "higher-order oligomerization" induced by antibody cross-linking at the cell surface, or by artificially acylation tagging of cytosolic proteins resulting in oligomerization and trafficking to released microvesicles (Fang et al. 2007). Further studies have shown that a variety of membrane anchors can target proteins to exosomes and microvesicles, but not all with the same efficiency (Shen et al.). A number of other membrane proteins are typically found in exosomes and microvesicles and are hallmarks of them. These include members of the tetraspanin network such as CD9, CD9P-1 TSPAN8, CD63, CD81, and CO-029 (Abache et al. 2007; Gesierich et al. 2006; Pols and Klumperman 2009; Rana et al.).

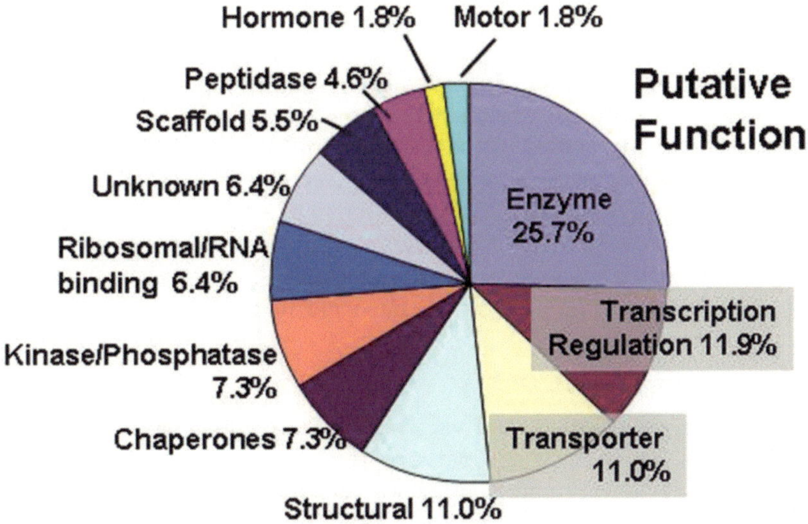

Fig. 3. Functional analysis of the proteomic content of exosomes/microvesicles derived from D283MED medulloblastoma cells. Over 130 proteins were identified by extraction of proteins from vesicles, separation of the proteins on SDS-PAGE, excision of the bands from BioSafe Coomassie Blue-stained gels, and tryptic digest of the excised bands. Peptides were separated and analyzed by LC-MS/MS, and peptides were mapped or identified by de novo sequencing using PROWL and Sequest algorithms. Proteins were categorized with Ingenuity Pathway Analysis software and by literature searches focusing on known functions; please note that many of the proteins identified were multifunctional, and this categorization represents the preponderance of evidence for function based on present literature.

Many cytosolic proteins (or at least many that are not widely recognized to have membrane associations) are exosome components; these include members of the heat shock protein (HSP) family, HSP/HSC70 and HSP90 in particular, and numerous metabolic enzymes. We have identified these proteins previously in proteomic studies of murine brain tumor exosomes and have cataloged and categorized them (Graner et al. 2009). We have performed further proteomic studies on human brain tumor exosomes (from the medulloblastoma cell line D283MED) which confirm and extend the results of the murine studies. In particular, metabolic enzymes represent the largest class of exosome proteins (**Figure 3**). While their prevalence may reflect their cellular abundance, there is a clear enrichment of these proteins in exosomes/microvesicles.

2.2 Functions and activities of tumor exosomes/microvesicles: fun with fat balls

Originally regarded as a means of cellular content disposal, particularly if cells lack lysosome activity (Johnstone et al. 1987; Johnstone, Bianchini, and Teng 1989) (ie, "garbage bags"), exosomes and microvesicles have an extensive and increasing list of activities, roles, and functions locally and systemically when released by tumors into the extracellular environment. Here we will briefly overview some of those better-characterized activities, most of which are regarded as beneficial to the tumor in terms of growth, invasion, or protection.

2.2.1 Immunologic effects: floating fat balls as stimulators or suppressants?

Exosome/microvesicle studies in tumors were originally driven by the idea that as tiny, non-replicating cellular surrogates, these vesicles could be used as cell-free anti-cancer vaccines. The premise was that exosomes and microvesicles contained tumor-specific antigens (Andre et al. 2002; Cho et al. 2005) as a source of adaptive immune cell targeting. In addition, exosomes/microvesicles contain heat shock proteins, known "danger signals" that both carry peptide antigens themselves as well as provide a potent, adjuvant-like stimulus to the innate and adaptive immune systems, particularly at the level of antigen presenting cells (Graner and Bigner 2005, 2006).

2.2.1.1 Dendritic Cell Exosomes ("DEX")

The initial works using exosome-based vaccines utilized exosomes derived from antigen-pulsed dendritic cells (DCs). DCs are perhaps the most effective "professional" antigen presenting cells known (Banchereau et al. 2000), and like all immune cells, one important means of extracellular communication for them is via the release of exosomes and microvesicles (Chaput et al. 2006). DCs process and present antigens to CD4+ and CD8+ T cells ("helper" cells and "cytotoxic or killer"/cytotoxic T lymphocyte/CTL cells, respectively), and if appropriately activated, will prime and stimulate the T cells for enhanced immune activities. From a clinical perspective, antigen-loaded and *ex vivo* activated DCs have been used in immunotherapy protocols as anti-cancer vaccines for a wide variety of tumor types and using an extraordinary range of antigen sources that are "pulsed" (applied to) the DCs (Palucka et al.). In general, *in vitro* (or *ex vivo*) DC production protocols are not standardized, require a great deal of hands-on time and effort, and the resulting cell preparations can be difficult to freeze and recover from thawing for repeated patient treatment (de Vries et al. 2005; Kalinski et al. 2009; Simon, Fonteneau, and Gregoire 2009). Exosomes and microvesicles from DCs (sometimes called "dexosomes" or "DEX") can be harvested from the culture supernatants, stored frozen, and thawed without loss of stimulating activity. They can be injected into hosts as cell-free DC-type vaccines capable of stimulating anti-tumor responses. These DEX were the first exosome-based vaccines (Zitvogel et al. 1998); DEX are capable of transferring antigen-loaded major histocompatibility class I molecules (MHC I) to recipient DCs for priming of naïve T cells in the host (Andre et al. 2004). These DC-derived vesicles were produced in a large-scale GMP setting (Lamparski et al. 2002) and were used to treat patients with metastatic melanoma in a clinical trial; the vaccines were safe, feasible, and produced one partial response with signs of specific immunity (Escudier et al. 2005). Another trial for patients with non-small cell lung cancer achieved similar results with some patients maintaining stable disease (Morse et al. 2005). As is the case for most immunotherapies, more work is needed on disabling the tumor-induced immune suppression and perhaps choosing patients with less tumor burden and lower stage, less advanced cancers to improve responses and outcomes. Nonetheless, the safety and feasibility of DEX as clinically-usable entities is evident; further advances in safe and tolerable immune stimulation, and the means to "suppression the suppression" of immunity driven by tumors are desperately needed.

2.2.1.2 Tumor-derived Exosomes ("TEX")

Tumor-derived exosomes (sometimes call "TEX") also have a history as vaccine material; as mentioned above, their antigen content and HSP-based adjuvant effects theoretically make them ideal cancer vaccines. This has proven true in a number of animal models of cancer (Altieri, Khan, and Tomasi 2004; Dai et al. 2005; Chen, Wang et al. 2006; Bu et al. 2006; Cho et al. 2009; Graner et al. 2009). One clinical trial performed in China using autologous tumor-derived (from ascites fluid of colorectal cancer patients) combined (or not) with the immune stimulant GM-CSF has been reported. One patient treated with both TEX and GM-CSF had stable disease, and another in that group had a partial response. In immune assays, delayed-type hypersensitivity (DTH) reactions were seen in patients immunized above a threshold amount, and selected patients had positive CTL assays (tetramer staining, cytotoxicity, interferon-gamma (IFNγ) release). No serious adverse events were reported (Dai et al. 2008). This trial seemed to bear out results from animal models. However, much of our current thought regarding TEX immunology is dominated by the pervading opinion that tumor-derived exosomes are purveyors of immune suppression thru increased regulatory T cell (Treg) activity, myeloid-derived suppressor cell activity, and suppression of activated T cells, natural killer (NK) cells, and inhibiting DC maturation (Taylor and Gercel-Taylor 2005; Liu et al. 2006; Valenti et al. 2007; Ichim et al. 2008; Xiang et al. 2009; Szajnik et al.). There is also evidence that TEX can prevent the binding of anti-tumor antibodies to their tumor-expressed target by essentially titrating out the antibodies, thus preventing antibody-dependent cellular cytotoxicity (ADCC) (Battke et al.). While a few of these studies have been performed in *in vivo* settings, most of the data are from human cells in *in vitro* assays. Thus, the complex interplay of *in vivo* and systemic immunity and immune suppression may be poorly represented in these assays, and our results in this area will be discussed later.

2.2.2 Coagulation and thrombosis: fat balls and clotting

Microvesicles, especially those derived from platelets, have long been known as procoagulant players in clot formation, particularly when the vesicles carry tissue factor (TF) (Freyssinet and Toti). There is an increasing awareness that microvesicles may also have roles in some of the thrombotic events that can occur in cancer (Aharon and Brenner 2009; Castellana, Kunzelmann, and Freyssinet 2009) indicating an interplay between microvesicles from other "normal" cell types such as platelets reacting with cancer cells. However, tumor-derived exosomes and microvesicles are also likely involved in this cellular cross-talk as well (Milsom et al. 2008), with the potential for coagulation to aid in delivery of growth factors or other stimuli to tumor cells. Tumor-derived microvesicles are believed to be partly responsible for Trousseau's syndrome, a coagulopathy associated with the cancerous state

(Varki 2007); the involvement of tumor vesicles likely involves the presence of TF on their surfaces (Del Conde et al. 2007). These studies further indicate the systemic roles that tumor cell-derived vesicles may play in cancer growth, progression, and generation of other co-morbidities in cancer patients.

2.2.3 Signaling capacity: influential fat balls

Exosomes and microvesicles are carriers of protein and lipid molecules with direct and indirect signaling capacities and complexes (Record et al. ; Zumaquero et al.) including members of the EGFR family (Sanderson et al. 2008) including Her2/Neu/ErbB2 (EGFR2) (Ciravolo et al.) and the tumor-specific mutant EGRFvIII (Graner et al. 2009; Al-Nedawi et al. 2008). Importantly, both EGFR and EGFRvIII may actually passage from exosomes to recipient cells, leading to activation of those pathways with phenotypic changes induced in the recipient cells (Al-Nedawi et al. 2009). In addition, tumor exosomes and microvesicles also carry active EGFR ligands such as amphiregulin (Higginbotham et al.), thus indicating that the vesicles can carry not only the signal transducer, but the signal as well.

Much of the signaling in cancer cells is devoted to proliferative drive. Exosomes and microvesicles are known to drive proliferation of tumor cells that are exposed to the vesicles (Koga et al. 2005; Skog et al. 2008); we have seen similar proliferation when pediatric and adult brain tumor cells are exposed to their endogenous exosomes (data not shown). Exosome-driven proliferation has been associated with the presence of the anti-apoptotic protein survivin in tumor exosomes (Khan et al.), and in a potential recruitment phenomenon, tumor microvesicles can enhance endothelial cell proliferation (Hong et al. 2009) which presumably may promote tumor vascularization. The mechanisms behind these proliferative responses are not clear, although we have evidence that exosomes increase overall glycolytic metabolism of recipient cells (see below) which may be either a cause for cell growth or a means to abet it. To further complicate the issue, there is at least one report in the literature of tumor exosomes/microvesicles inducing apoptosis in the recipient tumor cells (Ristorcelli et al. 2008), so it is possible that exosome effects may be cell-type or cell context specific.

2.2.4 RNA transport: fat balls as diplomatic satchels

As noted above (**Figure 3**) exosome/microvesicle proteomics revealed a relatively high percentage of RNA binding proteins typically present in exosomes. Since the biogenesis of exosomes and microvesicles intersects with some pathways of intercellular transmission of viruses, particularly at the levels of endosome (de Gassart et al. 2004; Mercer, Schelhaas, and Helenius) (also, see below), researchers began asking if exosomes and microvesicles themselves might have actual viral qualities, such as the ability to transport and transfer RNA molecules to recipient cells. This was first answered by Valadi et al (Valadi et al. 2007) when they demonstrated that exosomes did indeed possess both messenger and micro RNAs (mRNAs, miRNAs). Encapsulated in the vesicles, these RNAs were highly resistant to degradation by RNAses; furthermore, they demonstrated that mRNAs from one cell type could be passaged to another cell type, even of a different species (ie, mouse to human) resulting in translation of at least some of those messages (ie, humans cells now making mouse proteins). The numbers of mRNAs in exosomes/microvesicles and the genes represented by them are impressive (Mathivanan, Ji, and Simpson). One study involving brain tumor exosomes/microvesicles found that essentially the entire mRNA "expressome" is present in the population of collected vesicles, but there was significant enrichment for certain mRNAs in exosomes/microvesicles that did not mirror the mRNA expression distributions from cells of origin (Skog et al. 2008). This type of horizontal transmission of epigenetic materials exists with normal cell types (Ogawa et al.) and even with viable tissues in culture (Aliotta et al.) as well as with tumor cells communicating with normal cells (Hong et al. 2009).

microRNAs are recently-discovered small (22-25 nucleotide) non-coding RNAs that have potent regulatory potential (Carrington and Ambros 2003). miRNAs act as silencing RNAs, binding in an antisense fashion to regions of the 3′ untranslated regions (3′ UTRs) of mRNAs, resulting in either destabilization and degradation of the message, or prevention of translation; the net effect is translational repression of the message (Nelson et al. 2003). Following the discovery of miRNAs in exosomes (Valadi et al. 2007) there has been an explosion in the study of miRNAs in exosomes/microvesicles (for example, (Taylor and Gercel-Taylor 2008; Hunter et al. 2008; Rosell, Wei, and Taron 2009; Luo et al. 2009; Kosaka et al. ; Wang et al.)). There has been a particular emphasis on using circulating miRNAs (ie, those present in patient blood/serum) as disease biomarkers, presumably in the form of circulating exosomes/microvesicles (Rabinowits et al. 2009; Michael et al. ; De Smaele, Ferretti, and Gulino ; Kosaka, Iguchi, and Ochiya ; Wittmann and Jack ; Corcoran et al.). Thus, messenger and micro RNAs, when delivered to cells in the context of exosomes and microvesicles, have the potential to almost act virally by passaging epigenetic materials that could alter the phenotypes of the recipient cells. This represents an extraordinary form of extracellular communication, with vesicles as either mechanisms for delivery of RNAs, or perhaps as reservoirs to rapidly dispose of the RNA messages or regulatory activities. As biomarkers, the major advantage of such "circulating" RNAs over proteins or other subjects of molecular diagnostics is the ability to amplify the nucleic acid signal using PCR-based techniques, providing both increased signal and high specificity for the same biomarker, and relatively cheaply compared to some of the mass spectrometry or NMR methods needed for protein and metabolite markers.

2.2.5 Passage of pathogens / pathogenic entities: fat balls gone bad

As alluded above, the association of virus internalization, component packaging, and release in association with vesicles of the MVB and endosomal complexes or membrane lipid raft regions (Calistri et al. 2009) has prompted study of relationships between viruses and exosomes/microvesicles. For Human Immunodeficiency Virus (HIV), it has been proposed that the virus may hijack the system and egress from the cells via the plasma membrane microvesicle pathway (Booth et al. 2006) and from the exosome pathway (Nguyen et al. 2003), leading to the "Trojan exosome" hypothesis (Gould, Booth, and Hildreth 2003). However, this concept remains controversial (Coren, Shatzer, and Ott 2008). Epstein-Barr Virus (EBV) has been another well-studied virus in the exosome/microvesicle field, where it was first noticed that the EBV protein LMP1 appears in exosomes from EBV-infected cells (Flanagan, Middeldorp, and Sculley 2003; Keryer-Bibens et al. 2006). The presence of LMP1 and the immunomodulatory protein galectin-9 in exosomes derived from infected cells are implicated in immune suppression of NK and T cells, particularly affecting the inflammatory Th1-type responses (Dukers et al. 2000; Klibi et al. 2009). Hepatitis B and C viruses (HBV, HCV) are embedded in the etiology of hepatocellular carcinomas; envelope proteins from these viruses appear in exosomes from infected cells, and HBV requires MVBs for production of enveloped virons while subviral particles are released differently (Masciopinto et al. 2004; Watanabe et al. 2007). Human Herpes Virus 6 (HHV-6), an immunosuppressive, neurotropic virus, also has associations with hematologic and CNS malignancies (Ogata 2009; Saddawi-Konefka and Crawford). As with other viruses, mature virons in infected cells were found in MVB-like compartments and released in exosome-like vesicles. It is not known if these viron-containing exosomes are infectious, but the implications of infection and immune suppression aiding tumor take and progression are obvious. Finally, Cytomegalovirus (CMV) has become an increasingly interesting associate in high grade gliomas (Cobbs et al. 2002; Mitchell et al. 2008; Dziurzynski et al.). Exosomes from CMV infected cells contain CMV antigens (eg, gB) that are capable of stimulating CD4+ memory T cells (Walker, Maier, and Pober 2009), and while CMV DNA was amplified from glioblastoma (GBM) patient peripheral blood in one study (Mitchell et al. 2008), no CMV DNA was detected in another similar (but smaller) study (Lehrer et al.). However, neither of these studies used patient serum exosomes as target materials. In a proteomic study of murine SMA-560 brain tumor cell-derived exosomes, we identified the gag polyprotein pr65 and its precursor (Graner et al. 2009); these proteins originate from an endogenous murine retrovirus implicated in the progression of murine melanoma by subversion of immune surveillance (Mangeney et al. 2005). Thus, there remain many implications of viruses, virons, or viral particles/pieces in circulating tumor exosomes either as immune targets (potential antigens) or as further purveyors of immune suppression.

The roles of exosomes/microvesicles in bacterial diseases are less well studied, but there have been significant works in the mycobacter area. Exosomes from macrophage infected with *Mycobacterium avium* display antigens such as glycolipids from that pathogen. These exosomes provide pro-inflammatory signals to resting macrophage (Bhatnagar and Schorey 2007), as is true of exosomes from a number of pathogenically infected macrophage both *in vitro* and *in vivo* (Bhatnagar et al. 2007). However, while exosomes from *Mycobacterium tuberculosis*-infected macrophage contain proteomically-identified TB proteins/antigens (Giri et al.), exosomes from MTB-infected macrophage can actually suppress activation of naïve macrophage (Singh et al.). While the similarities, particularly immune relationships, between cancer and MTB infection have not gone unnoticed (Broxmeyer 2004; Schorey and Bhatnagar 2008; Cocito and Maes 1998), the roles of exosomes and microvesicles in these diseases likely remains complex.

Another intriguing (and perhaps frightening) role played by exosomes and microvesicles is in the neurodegenerative disease arena. Experimentally, prion diseases such as scrapie have been shown to be transmissible from infected cells (those with the prion protein, PrP, misfolded into the scrapie form, PrPsc) to uninfected cells by application of exosomes from the infected cells to the uninfected cells. PrPsc was found in the exosomes from the infected cells, and these cells initiated scrapie when injected into mice (Fevrier et al. 2004). PrP is a GPI-linked protein (Miesbauer et al.), and as mentioned above, membrane proteins with this lipid anchor are frequently sorted into lipid rafts that become part of the IVBs within MVBs, and eventually become exosomes. It is uncertain whether PrP converts to PrPsc in/on exosomes (Fevrier et al. 2005) but abnormal folding makes it a candidate for ubiquitination and thus sorting into MVBs/IVBs. Blood is considered the most common bodily fluid of transmission, but another study showed that at least the naturally occurring PrP protein is present in pseudo-afferent lymph fluid, and is preferentially enriched in CSF from sheep (Vella et al. 2008). Thus, there may be a neuronal reservoir for PrP (and PrPsc or other transmissible infectious prion forms) in exosomes found in CSF. For another neurodegenerative disease, Alzheimer's disease (AD), the etiology is believed to be related to the cleavage of cell surface amyloid precursor protein APP by β– and γ-secretases, resulting in formation of a peptide called Aβ. Rajendran et al (Rajendran et al. 2006) found that from cells transfected with expression vectors for APP, they could find Aβ peptides in the extracellular medium in the context of exosomes. The cells processed APP to Aβ endosomally, with Aβ ending up in MVBs and extracellularly with exosomes. In immunoelectron microscopy sections of brains from afflicted patients, AD plaques contained exosome-associated proteins (eg, ALIX), further suggesting the role of MVBs and the potential for exosome involvement in the disease. Exosomes from cells expressing APP were found to contain a number of the secretases necessary for processing of APP into its secreted form, as well as the different C-terminal forms of cleaved APP, as well as Aβ itself (Sharples et al. 2008). γ-secretase inhibition resulted in less Aβ accumulation in exosomes, suggesting a potential therapeutic approach, but also suggesting the biomarker potential of Aβ in exosomes to diagnose AD. Thus, not only can pathogenic organisms utilize the exosome/microvesicle pathways for infectious transmission, disease "particles" may utilize them as well to passage from infected or diseased cells to unaffected cells, a novel form of transmission that does not require cell-to-cell contact.

2.2.6 Drug Efflux: fat balls as HazMat crews

In our proteomic analyses of medulloblastoma exosomes, transporter molecules constituted > 10% of the proteins identified (see **Figure 3**). Thus, it may not be surprising that exosomes/microvesicles may be exit vehicles for chemotherapeutic agents applied to cancer cells as a mechanism of resistance. A cisplatin-insensitive ovarian carcinoma cell subline was found to have greatly reduced lysosome size and activity compared to its cisplatin-sensitive original line, and that insensitive line produced more exosomes than the parent line (Safaei et al. 2005). Those exosomes contained a number of lysosomal markers as well as transport molecules. When the insensitive line was treated with cisplatin, 2.5 fold more drug was effluxed from the insensitive line than the sensitive one, and at least a portion of that was found in the insoluble exosome pellet from the spent culture medium. Chen et al (Chen, Posada et al. 2006) further implicated the endosomal/MVB pathway for egress of doxorubicin, demonstrating a role for VPS4a in MVB and exosome function and packaging of drug. There may also be a role for microvesicle-based drug efflux, since the plasma membrane plays a role in resistance to doxorubicin in the K562 leukemia cell line used in these studies (Chen et al. 2007). While exosomes and microvesicles may provide drug resistance mechanisms for tumor cells, one must also consider the possibility that in normal cells, exosomes/microvesicles may perform similar cellular detoxification roles to remove noxious small molecule compounds to protect normal cells, as well.

2.3 Summary

Exosomes and microvesicles are akin to miniature versions of the cell itself, possessing lipids, proteins, and even RNAs from the originating cell; some even refer to exosomes and microvesicles as "extracellular organelles". These extracellular vesicles are intimately involved in the extracellular local and distal cross-talk between and amongst cell, tissues, and organs, and have a variety of functions associated with them. In particular, the relationships between cancer cells and associated "normal" cells, such as those of the endothelium, the microenvironment, and immune system, are all profoundly mutually influenced by these secreted vesicles in ways we are only slowly beginning to understand.

3. Brain tumor exosomes and microvesicles: fat balls on the brain

The primary literature on brain tumor extracellular vesicles is amazingly small (Graner, Cumming, and Bigner 2007; Al-Nedawi et al. 2008; Skog et al. 2008; Graner et al. 2009; Guescini, Genedani et al. ; Yang et al.), although one of the early microvesicle papers used C-6 rat glioma cells and called their vesicular entities "exosomes", but by current standards the vesicles would be called microvesicles or microparticles (Trams et al. 1981; Johnstone 2006). Our group was arguably the first to identify *bona fide* brain tumor exosomes, despite some 20 years of previous study. Brain tumor exosomes and microvesicles appear structurally and proteomically like such vesicles from other cell/tumor types in culture, and from the sera of patients with diverse tumors (Graner, Cumming, and Bigner 2007; Graner et al. 2009; Al-Nedawi et al. 2008; Skog et al. 2008). One difference has been that exosomes from both adult gliomas and pediatric medulloblastomas have proven extremely resilient to lysis and extraction (Graner et al. 2009) (M Graner, unpublished; Johan Skog, personal communication), making protein analysis in particular rather difficult. Another interesting feature is the putative presence of mitochondrial DNA contained within (and perhaps on the surface of) glioma cell line extracellular vesicles (Guescini, Genedani et al.), which has also been seen in murine myoblast vesicles as reported by the same group (Guescini, Guidolin et al.) ; this finding runs counter to other groups' findings (Valadi et al. 2007) and will likely be somewhat controversial. However, given the high glycolytic capacity of gliomas and the distressed and non-uniform appearance and activities of their mitochondria (Oudard et al. 1996; Oudard et al. 1997; Ordys et al. ; Santandreu et al. 2008), relationships between exosomes and mitochondria in cancer cells could potentially be an area of fruitful and energetic study. In the next sections we will discuss the broad range signaling abilities, metabolic effects, and immunological properties of brain tumor exosomes/microvesicles, as well as the exosome-induced migratory and protective phenotypes cells experience upon exposure to exosomes.

3.1 Brain tumor exosomes drive various activities in recipient cells: fat balls as game-changers

High grade gliomas such as glioblastomas (GBMs) are extremely heterogeneous with respect to cellular appearances and phenotypes, chromosomal abnormalities, gene and protein expression, etc, but almost universally share a lack of response to treatment (Mischel, Cloughesy, and Nelson 2004) whether the treatment is chemical, radiologic, or immunologic. Another commonality amongst GBMs is their extraordinary invasive potential that inevitably leads to tumor recurrence and patient demise (Hoelzinger, Demuth, and Berens 2007). Below we will describe mechanisms by which exosomes and microvesicles may contribute to these most nefarious features of high grade gliomas.

3.1.1 Brain tumor exosomes and EGFR signaling: fat balls carry the mail

The epidermal growth factor receptor (EGFR) has a long history as a major player and therapeutic target in brain tumors and many other tumors as well (Hatanpaa et al. ; Ye, Gao, and Cai ; Brandes et al. 2008; Vivanco and Mellinghoff ; Yarden 2001). Perhaps the most prominent mutation in EGFR in gliomas is the variant (either genomically mutated/encoded or resulting from a splice-site mutation and alternate usage) that eliminates exons 2-7 to yield "delta 2-7 EGFR" or "EGFR variant III" (EGFRvIII), reviewed in (Wikstrand et al. 1998; Pedersen et al. 2001; Sonabend, Dana, and Lesniak 2007). This mutant EGFR does not necessarily need to dimerize to signal (Chu et al. 1997) , does not bind ligand but is nonetheless constitutively active and is capable of inducing tumor growth in otherwise non-tumorigenic cells in animal models (Batra et al. 1995). EGFRvIII is expressed in 25%-67% of all GBMs (Pelloski et al. 2007; Heimberger et al. 2005) and is generally considered a marker of poorer prognosis. The receptor is heterogeneously expressed in human GBMs (generally pockets of expression) compared to the more uniform presence of the wild type EGFR (EGFRwt) (Nishikawa et al. 2004). Coupled with animal model studies, it is suspected that EGFRvIII results in both autocrine signaling loops that lead to enhance EGFRwt signaling (Ramnarain et al. 2006) and paracrine mechanisms driving increased proliferation of the bulk of the tumor mass (which expresses EGFRwt), thus maintaining tumor cell expression heterogeneity (Inda et al.). While one usually invokes soluble extracellularly-released signaling factors for these mechanisms, the work of Al-Nedawi (Al-Nedawi et al. 2008) indicates that tumor-derived microvesicles could carry and transfer EGFRvIII from cells that express the mutant receptor to cells that do not. This group transfected U373 cells to express the mutated EGFRvIII (these glioma cells normally express neither EGFR nor EGFRvIII) and collected microvesicles from the transfectants that displayed EGFRvIII. Recipient U373 [EGFRvII(-)] cells not only epigenetically "express" EGFRvIII following microvesicle receipt, but this also activates downstream signaling pathways associated with the presence of EGFRvIII including phosphorylation of ERK 1/2 and AKT, release of VEGF, increased Bcl-x expression with concurrent reduction in p27 expression, and enhanced soft agar colony formation. U373viii tumor-bearing mice also had EGFRvIII(+) microvesicles in their blood. We also found that murine glial tumor cells expressing EGFRvIII (SMA-560vIII) display the receptor on their exosome surfaces, and that patient serum exosomes/microvesicles (from 4 of 5 GBM patients) contained EGFRvIII, while all had EGFR in/on them (Graner et al. 2009). Skog et al (Skog et al. 2008) also found *EGFRvIII* mRNA transcripts in microvesicles in sera from 7 of 25 patients with GBMs; 14 of 30 patients had transcript-positive tumor biopsies (and curiously, one patient had *EGFRvIII*(+) serum microvesicles but the biopsy was negative). They also found that GBM cell line microvesicles contained angiogenic factors and could stimulate brain endothelial cells to form tubules. These cumulative results beg the question as to whether the autocrine/paracrine signaling mechanisms and resultant enhanced tumor growth and features of aggressiveness may be in part due to the passage and reception of exosomes and microvesicles from EGFRvIII-expressing cells affecting ostensibly EGFRvIII(-) cells to enhance, maintain, or extend aggressive tumorigenic phenotypes. Aside from EGFR and the vIII mutant, exosomes and microvesicles are reservoirs of other factors potentially involved in cell-cell signaling including L1-NCAM as we have shown. One of the highest scoring networks using Integrated Pathway Analysis from our proteomic efforts was "cell-to-cell signaling and interaction, cancer, hematologic system development and function" (Graner et al. 2009), implying that these vesicles have inherent signaling capacity or the ability to merge readily into signaling networks. Another important implication of the discovery of serum-borne tumor vesicles from patients with GBMs (and also, pediatric patients with medulloblastoma, data not shown) is that these vesicles escape the blood-brain barrier with potential for systemic effects, particularly involving immune function (**Section 3.2**).

3.1.2 Brain tumor exosomes and metabolomics: fat balls grease the wheels of glycolysis

Results from other brain tumor exosome/microvesicle experiments indicate that exogenously-added vesicles increase recipient tumor cell proliferation (Al-Nedawi et al. 2008; Skog et al. 2008). We have seen similar dose-dependent results in modified clonogenicity assays using U87MG cells while adding differential quantities of exosomes to those cells (**Figure 4**).

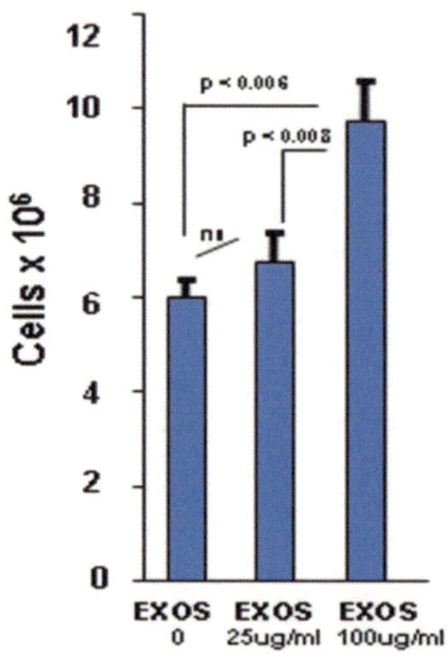

Fig. 4. Exogenous tumor exosomes increase tumor cell proliferation in a dose-dependent manner. U87 glioma cells were grown under standard conditions for 48 hrs in the presence of 0, 25, or 100 µg/ml exosomes and counted on a hemocytometer. Higher concentrations of exosomes significantly increased cell proliferation.

Proliferation assays requiring redox readouts such as MTT/MTS assays in slower-growing cell lines pulsed with exosomes suggested that the proliferative effects may involve metabolic changes in the recipient cells, and our proteomics (Graner et al. 2009) (see also **Figure 3**) strongly suggested this also. We tested this by performing metabolomics experiments on U87MG cells grown in a stem cell-like medium with serum replacement; cells were treated (or not) with 25 µg/ml exosomes for 44 hrs, and carbon flux was followed by incorporation of ^{13}C-labeled glucose as a metabolic tracer for an additional 4 hrs. Media and cells were extracted and analyzed by nuclear magnetic resonance/magnetic resonance spectroscopy (NMR/MRS), notably revealing very large increases in energy transfer compounds and glycolytic activity (**Figure 5**)

Decreased glutathione levels and increased lactate output are associated with transformation and metastasis in cell line models (Lu et al.); the lipid profile, with the exception of monounsaturated fatty acids (MUFA) and cholesterol, is remarkably stable. In a somewhat controversial finding in the literature, incubation of cells with oleic acid, a MUFA, promotes secretion of matrix metalloproteinase-9 (MMP9) and invasion of breast cancer cells (Soto-Guzman et al.). Whether there is an endogenous relationship between increased cellular MUFA production (as opposed to exogenous supplementation) and MMP activity/invasion remains to be seen, although it is possible that exosome lipid content may act in that supplementary fashion. Finally, the energy compounds and glycolysis profile, along with the soluble metabolite outputs, demonstrate that exosomes do indeed profoundly increase cellular metabolic activity in the form of glycolysis, in keeping with the Warburg effect (Ferreira). The mechanisms behind this need to be elucidated--is there increased enzymatic metabolic activity, or is there increased gene/protein expression of those enzymes, or are such enzymes actually delivered to the cells by exosomes (or any combination of these scenarios)? From our proteomic studies we have identified more than half of the enzymes in both the "preparatory" and "pay-off" phases of glycolysis (Graner et al. 2009) (and data not shown), along with a variety of other enzymes in other metabolic cycles. Thus, it is not inconceivable that exosomes themselves directly provide, or at least contribute to, some of the glycolytic enzyme repertoire that leads to enhanced glycolysis in tumor cells pulsed with exosomes. The general renewed interest in tumor metabolism (Cairns, Harris, and Mak) will hopefully prompt more research into the area of exosome metabolic effects, both downstream and perhaps even within the exosomes themselves.

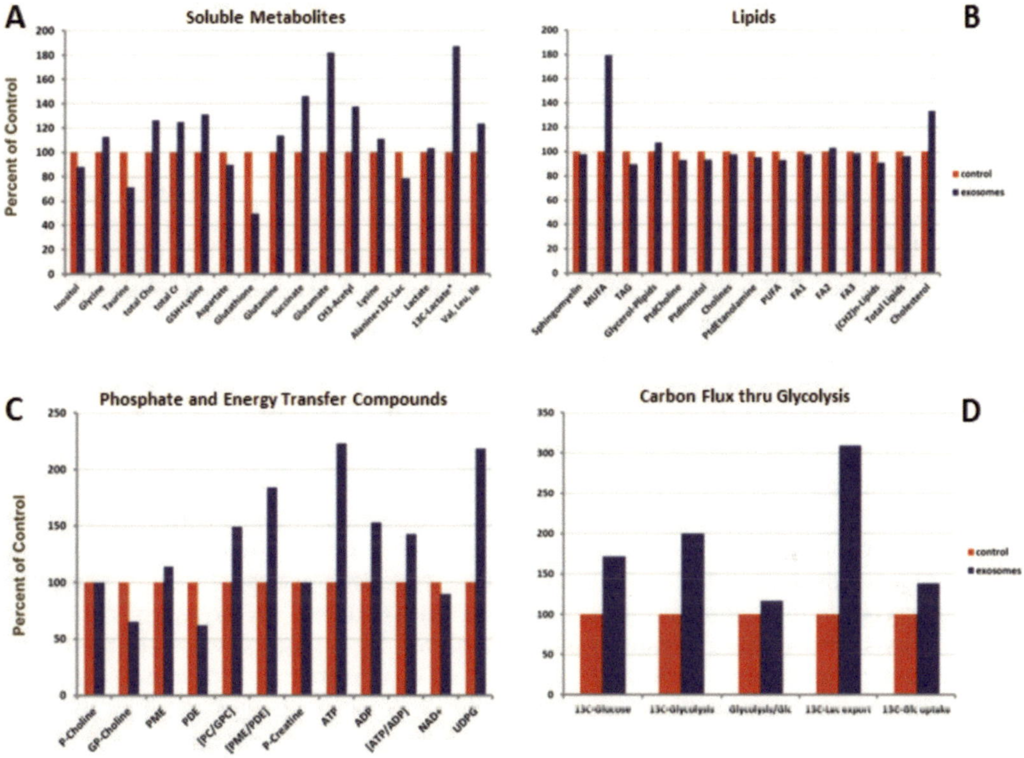

Fig. 5. U87MG exosomes applied to U87 recipient cells results in increased glycolytic activity. U87 cells were incubated with 25 µg/ml U87 exosomes for 44 hrs prior to changing the medium into medium containing ^{13}C-labeled glucose for 4 hrs (blue bars). Control cells were grown without the addition of exosomes (red bars). Cells and media were harvested and extracted for soluble and lipid-based compounds, and analyzed by NMR/MRS for quantification and determination of carbon flux. **A** shows levels of soluble metabolites compared to control (untreated) U87MG cells; **B** shows lipid profile changes following exosome pulsing; **C** shows phosphate/energy compound changes during exosome exposure, and **D** shows changes in the glycolytic profile of U87 cells following incubation with exosomes.

3.2 Brain tumor exosomes and immunology: fat balls vacillate between vaccines and vacuums

As mentioned above (**Section 2.2.1**) tumor exosomes have gone from being seen as perfect vaccine material to their current status as infamous purveyors of immune suppression. Also as mentioned, most of those immune suppression studies have been performed in tissue culture settings that may not reflect the complexity of the mammalian immune system. Aside from our previous work demonstrating that murine brain tumor exosomes were potent prophylactic vaccines and drivers of antibody production (Graner et al. 2009), there has been only one other very recent study involving brain tumor exosomes and immunology (Bu et al.). That report determined that exosomes from culture supernatant of primary gliomas effectively provided antigens to autologous dendritic cells, which in turn could generate activated CD8+ T cells with potent cytotoxicity against autologous tumors cells *in vitro*. We pointed out in our publication (Graner et al. 2009) that there are a number of putative and known antigens in or on the glioma exosomes we utilized including the aforementioned EGFRvIII and glycoprotein nmb (GPNMB, also called osteoactivin, HGFIN, and DC-HIL). GPNMB is believed to be a *bona fide* antigen target in high grade gliomas (Kuan et al. 2006; Loging et al. 2000) and possibly in breast cancer (Rose et al.) as well as in melanoma (Tse et al. 2006). The exosomes also had HSP70 on their vesicular surfaces along with HSPs 60, 90, calreticulin, and protein disulfide isomerase, all known immune stimulators or "danger signals", and capable of providing antigens to DCs. However, those exosomes also had HSP25 (human HSP27) on their surfaces, which is associated with lower immunogenicity of exosomes (Alexzander Asea, personal communication) and more aggressive tumors when cell surface localized (Bausero et al. 2004). Also we found transforming growth factor beta (TGF-β) with the exosomes, which is frequently associated with immune suppression (Flavell et al.); even the antigen GPNMB also has potential T cell inhibition activities (Tomihari et al.). Consequently, there seems to be a range of immune stimulatory and potentially immune suppressive moieties in/on the same population of exosomes. Also, quantity may be an issue. Our data suggest that tumor cell-derived exosomes at (relatively) low concentrations may inhibit interferon-gamma (IFNγ) release from mitogen-activated T cells, while at higher concentrations exosomes increase IFNγ release over control (mitogen-stimulated) T cells (**Figure 6**). Based on these data, context and quantity may be extremely relevant in the roles played by tumor exosomes in the double-edged sword of immunity. One may imagine that if peripherally activated (eg, from a draining lymph node) circulating T cells encounter low concentrations of tumor exosomes also in the periphery, circulating in blood, those T cells may face the suppressive features of the exosomes. However, if the T cells are in the vicinity of high tumor exosome concentrations (tumor under stress, or in the context of a bolus of exosomes in the form of a vaccine following a priming protocol), this may switch the T cells to an even further activated phenotype. While that ostensibly should lead to better anti-tumor immunity, it may also lead to activation induced cell death (AICD) of the T cells.

We found that tumor exosomes as antigen sources drive effective antibody production in short duration immunization protocols and with no adjuvant (Graner et al. 2009) (M Graner, unpublished) in mice. The significance of this in unclear; while antibody output is generally associated with Th2-type immune responses (ie, more regulatory than inflammatory), we nonetheless found IFNγ-producing T cells following tumor exosome vaccination concurrent with significant antibody titers against the exosomes (Graner et al. 2009). Similar enhanced simultaneous T- and B-cell immune responses have been seen when immunizing mice with

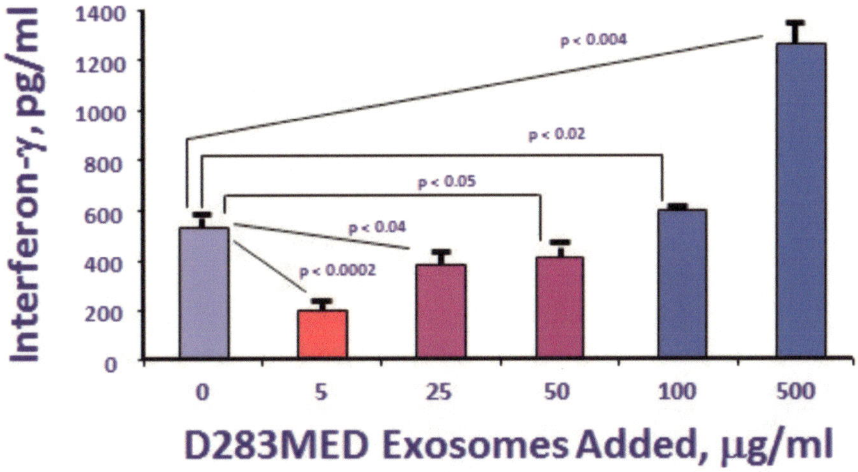

Fig. 6. Medulloblastoma exosomes differentially and dose-dependently alter interferon-gamma (IFNγ) release from mitogen activated human T cells. Peripheral blood mononuclear cells (PBMCs) were collected from a healthy donor and were stimulated with phytohemagglutinin (PHA) for 48 hrs (or not) in the presence of D283MED medulloblastoma exosomes harvested from tissue culture supernatants at the concentrations listed. After 48 hrs, media were harvested and IFNγ released from the cells was measured by specific ELISA. Statistical relationships (Student *t* tests) are shown.

heat shock protein vaccines (Li et al. 2008; Manjili et al. 2003). The relevant question here is if the antibodies have any biologic, anti-tumor activity. In the situation of true human, pre-established tumors, one may think of tumor-released exosomes acting as "auto-immunizations" against tumor antigens. However, it may be that the tumor "sheds" antigens via exosomes/microvesicles, driving futile immune responses against "decoy" circulating antigens. This may have 2 benefits for the tumor—1) driving antibody responses may serve to maintain a Th2 cytokine environment, which is suboptimal for effective cellular anti-tumor immune responses; and 2) free-floating, released exosomes may titrate out potentially "dangerous" antibodies generated against tumor antigens, thus preventing those antibodies from ever reaching the solid tumor mass. Concepts similar to this are cited above (Battke et al.). As further evidence that tumors may "offer up" exosome-bound antigens we show here that antibodies in serum from a patient with GBM show reactivity with the autologous tumor lysate on a Western blot but far more intense reactivity against the autologous serum exosomes (**Figure 7**)

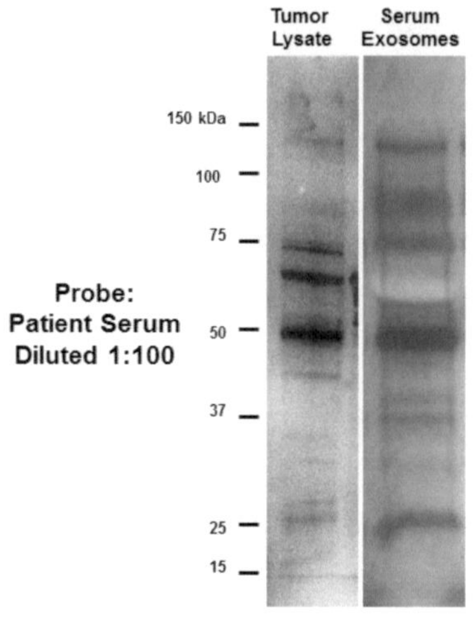

Fig. 7. Patient serum antibodies react with autologous tumor lysate and serum exosomes/microvesicles. A patient with GBM had blood drawn at the time of tumor resection. Exosomes/microvesicles were harvested from the serum; the remainder of the serum was diluted 1:100 and used to probe reducing, denaturing gels/blots of tumor lysate and lysed serum exosomes (25 µg loaded per lane). Secondary antibody was biotinylated anti-human IgA/G/M, and tertiary reagent was streptavidin HRP. ECL developing agent was used, and images captured on a FluroChem Imager. Molecular weight markers are shown to the left.

We postulate that vaccination with exosomes, particularly in relatively naïve animals, may prompt effective antibody (and T cell) generation, but in situations where the tumor has had time to "self-vaccinate" by releasing tumor exosomes, the antibody repertoire may reflect immune editing and therefore actually benefit the tumor via "ironic immunity". This concept bears further study, and such investigations are ongoing.

Thus complex interplays between stimulation, suppression, and "decoy allocation" that tie the tumor to the host immune response are further complicated by the potential roles played by exosomes. With antigens and heat shock protein danger signals, exosomes may be good vaccines; however with TGFβ content and a host of other suppressive features, tumor-released exosomes may ultimately skew the host immune response into a position that benefits the tumor by decoy antigen release and stealth regulatory cytokine environment.

3.3 Brain tumor exosomes/microvesicles and tumor migration: attractive fat balls blaze the trail

Perhaps the most distressing activity performed by high grade gliomas is their ability to migrate and invade the parenchyma with devastating consequences of bilateral presentation if the tumor crosses the corpus callosum, with the possibility of disastrous leptomeningeal dissemination. The modulation of the extracellular environment, and the ability to proximally and distally signal extracellularly are critical factors in this manifestation of the glioma phenotype (Nakada et al. 2007; Berens and Giese 1999). The cells may migrate out of the range of focused external beam radiation therapy, thus limiting its usefulness, and this migration is a clear danger in the multifocal recurrences more and more frequently seen following treatment with bevacizumab (Rahman et al. ; Iwamoto et al. 2009; de Groot et al. ;

Verhoeff et al. 2009). Obviously, glioma invasion makes truly complete surgical resections impossible. Exosomes and microvesicles, as nanovesicles released into the extracellular environment, seem like perfect vehicles for extracellular remodeling, possessing proteases such as insulin degrading enzyme (IDE) (Tamboli et al.), MMPs 1 and 14 (Medina and Ghahary ; Hakulinen et al. 2008) and ADAMs 10 and 17 (Mathews et al. ; Stoeck et al. 2006). Exosomal Rabs (Hendrix et al.), HSP90 and plasminogen (McCready et al.), and tetraspanins (Rana et al.) have been implicated in tumor cell migration/invasion as well. Recently it was shown that L1-NCAM (CD171) and its migration-inducing cleavage product were found in exosomes of brain tumor cell lines (Yang et al.), and exosomes were partially involved in an animal model of tumor metastasis by preparation of the pre-metastatic niche (Jung et al. 2009). Amidst this background we have determined that glioma exosomes (from U87MG cells, as well as D283MED cells—not shown) can promote tumor cell migration across a plastic membrane at higher levels than that promoted by FBS (**Figure 8**)

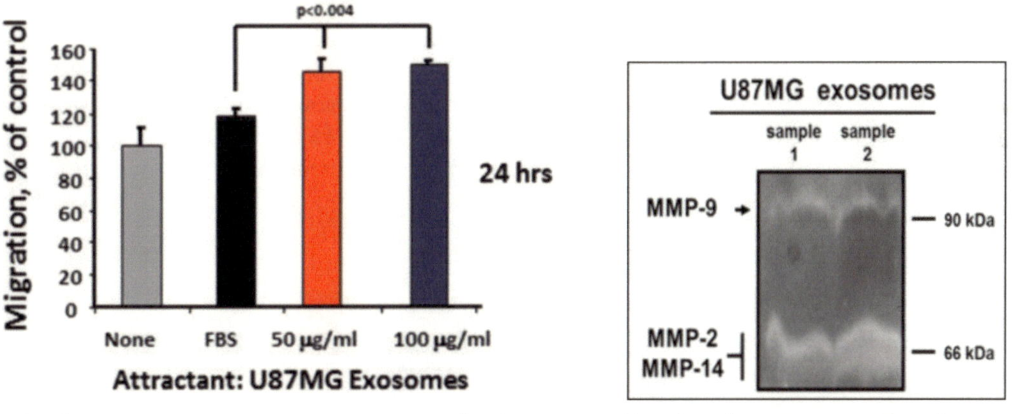

Fig. 8. Glioma exosomes promote tumor cell migration in Boyden chamber assays and possess intrinsic matrix metalloproteinase activities. **Left** U87MG cells were placed on the top chamber of an 8 µm pore-size plastic insert in wells; the lower chambers contained serum-free media, fetal bovine serum (FBS, positive control) or increasing quantities of U87 exosomes. Cells migrated for 24 hrs; the inserts were removed, the tops washed, and the bottoms were stained with crystal violet, and 5 random fields of duplicate wells were counted (avg, SD, and *t* test results shown). **Right** U87 exosomes were separated in a zymogram (gelatin) gel; MMP activation was induced, and cleared areas in the gel correspond to gelatinase activities of appropriate molecular weights for MMPs 2, 9, and 14 (confirmed by Western blotting, data not shown).

The Boyden chamber/migration assay is largely an attraction assay; the complexity of exosomes/microvesicles will make it interesting to determine what factors in or on these vesicles promote this migration and potentially could serve as attractants over a larger distance, akin to leaving "bread crumbs" of exosomes for cells to track and follow while migrating or metastasizing. The MMP activities suggest that exosomes will be able to also carve paths and remodel the extracellular matrix to allow for cells to migrate (either tumor cells out of the main mass, or even endothelial cells in for angiogenic events). These preliminary data indicate that brain tumor exosomes can both blaze paths and provide attraction for glioma migration. As this is an important area of therapeutic attention, exosome biology may play a critical role in our attempts to regain local control of high grade gliomas following surgery, thus improving recurrent-free survival.

3.4 Brain tumor exosomes/microvesicles and chemoresistance: fat balls provide protection

High grade gliomas are extremely chemoresistant (Lu and Shervington 2008; Sarkaria et al. 2008). As mentioned above (**Section 2.2.6**), exosomes have transporter molecules among their proteomic content, and we have also shown that MRP3 is in glioma exosomes (Graner et al. 2009). These may provide mechanisms for drug export, literally packaging the chemotherapeutic agent in exosomes/microvesicles. As shown above (**Section 3.1.2**), exosomes may also accelerate metabolic activity which could lead to increased breakdown or chemical modification of the drug compound. While these mechanisms are undoubtedly important in glioma chemoresistance (along with the natural protection of the blood-brain barrier), no one has ever demonstrated an impact of exosomes on cellular resistance to drugs in neuro-oncology. Since all of this discussion is currently theoretical, we have first tested this putative protective property of exogenously-added exosomes and have discovered that glioma exosomes can indeed provide protection or enhance resistance to temozolomide (**Figure 9**). In fact, even low concentrations of tumor exosomes fully complemented cell growth back to normal despite the presence of the drug (which is the chemotherapy of choice for high grade gliomas and is a component of the current standard of care for these tumors) (Stupp et al. 2005).

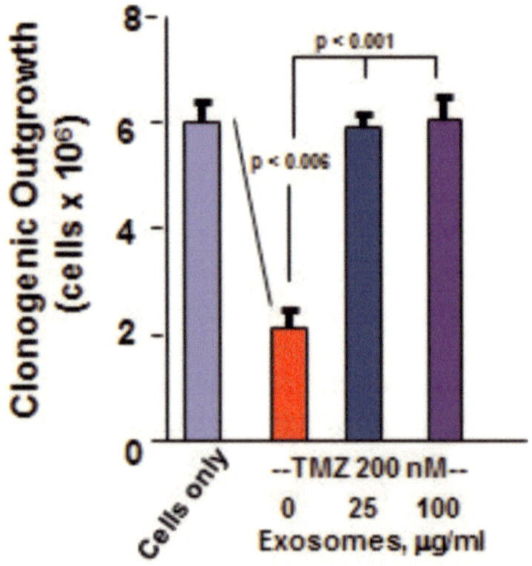

Fig. 9. Exogenously added tumor exosomes protect glioma cells from cytotoxic chemotherapy. U87MG cells were either left untreated ("Cells only") or were subjected to treatment with temozolomide/Temodar® ("TMZ") at 200 nM concentrations for 48 hrs. Exosomes at the concentrations listed were also added (or not), and cell growth was quantified in a modified clonogenicity assay as describe for **Figure 4**. Exosomes provide significant protection against the chemotherapy agent, and return cell growth to normal (+ exosomes, not significant compared to cells only).

Exosomes, by currently unknown mechanisms, provide some means of chemoresistance to the therapeutic drug of choice as the standard of care for high grade gliomas. However, this does strongly suggest that discovering this underlying mechanism may be a critical point for improving therapeutic efficacy of our drug treatments. This may go back to the cellular mechanisms for generating exosomes; however, as this is a process common apparently almost all cells, it is unclear if there are particular aspects that are tumor-specific. Iero et al (Iero et al. 2008) have suggested that a number of pharmacologic agents may be able to interfere with exosome release, but so far this does not appear to have made an impact in most of our current chemotherapy regimens.

3.5 Summary

Exosomes and microvesicles from brain tumor cells affect signaling capacities, alter metabolism, impinge on immunity, and may promote two of the most nefarious characteristics of high grade gliomas (and medulloblastomas)—their abilities to migrate and invade normal tissue, and their inherent resistance to treatment. Obviously, there is a tremendous space for research in this area as well as a great need to understand these complex vesicles and their interactions with the tumor, the tumor microenvironment, the normal tissues, and the potential systemic effects as the tumor attempts to control its surroundings locally and distally.

4. Conclusions

Exosomes and microvesicles serve as unique and profoundly important extracellular signaling vehicles both locally in the area of release, as well as at potentially great distances via the circulatory system. Despite some 20 years of research efforts devoted to these "fat balls", we are finding more and more fascinating features about them almost constantly. With intense study of the biochemical compositions of the vesicles (proteomics, ribonomics, lipidomics) we are learning more about the similarities, as well as the curious differences, between exosomes from different cellular sources. We are also developing much better understandings of the biology of vesicular formation and release—something that many viruses and pathogens have long exploited. All of this knowledge complements the ongoing work to understand our ever-increasing—and increasingly fascinating--knowledge of the biologic impacts that exosomes and microvesicles have on recipient cells, and on micro- and macroenvironments. From the perspective of neuro-oncology, there is a wealth of information waiting to be mined, particularly in the areas of immunology, proximal and distal cell signaling, microenvironment alteration for migration or protection, and how tumor cells may use the physiology of exosomes as a means of therapeutic resistance. The almost viral quality of exosomes and microvesicles as carriers of messenger and microRNAs is one example of a vastly open region ripe for progress, and it almost certainly intersects with many other areas of research. As studies of exosomes and microvesicles become accepted as legitimate science and gain mainstream appreciation, we should see further advances in the research that leads to translational applications of this knowledge. Interdisciplinary approaches will be required as expertise in genetics, proteomics, metabolomics, lipid biochemistry, and microparticle/nanovesicle technologies all have a place in these endeavors. For patients facing the dismal prognoses of brain tumors, new clinical applications resulting from more basic and translational research cannot come fast enough.

5. Acknowledgements

The author wishes to thank Dr Laura Epple, Dr Natalie Serkova, Andrea Merz, Jason White, Kamalika Nag, Ben Winston, and Matt Herring for their unpublished data, and Dr Kevin Lillehei for continued encouragement. This work was supported by a generous donation to the University of Colorado Cancer Center.

6. References

Abache, T., F. Le Naour, S. Planchon, F. Harper, C. Boucheix, and E. Rubinstein. 2007. The transferrin receptor and the tetraspanin web molecules CD9, CD81, and CD9P-1 are differentially sorted into exosomes after TPA treatment of K562 cells. *J Cell Biochem* 102 (3):650-64.

Aharon, A., and B. Brenner. 2009. Microparticles, thrombosis and cancer. *Best Pract Res Clin Haematol* 22 (1):61-9.

Al-Nedawi, K., B. Meehan, R. S. Kerbel, A. C. Allison, and J. Rak. 2009. Endothelial expression of autocrine VEGF upon the uptake of tumor-derived microvesicles containing oncogenic EGFR. *Proc Natl Acad Sci U S A* 106 (10):3794-9.

Al-Nedawi, K., B. Meehan, J. Micallef, V. Lhotak, L. May, A. Guha, and J. Rak. 2008. Intercellular transfer of the oncogenic receptor EGFRvIII by microvesicles derived from tumour cells. *Nat Cell Biol* 10 (5):619-24.

Aliotta, J. M., M. Pereira, K. W. Johnson, N. de Paz, M. S. Dooner, N. Puente, C. Ayala, K. Brilliant, D. Berz, D. Lee, B. Ramratnam, P. N. McMillan, D. C. Hixson, D. Josic, and P. J. Quesenberry. Microvesicle entry into marrow cells mediates tissue-specific changes in mRNA by direct delivery of mRNA and induction of transcription. *Exp Hematol* 38 (3):233-45.

Altieri, S. L., A. N. Khan, and T. B. Tomasi. 2004. Exosomes from plasmacytoma cells as a tumor vaccine. *J Immunother* 27 (4):282-8.

Andre, F., N. Chaput, N. E. Schartz, C. Flament, N. Aubert, J. Bernard, F. Lemonnier, G. Raposo, B. Escudier, D. H. Hsu, T. Tursz, S. Amigorena, E. Angevin, and L. Zitvogel. 2004. Exosomes as potent cell-free peptide-based vaccine. I. Dendritic cell-derived exosomes transfer functional MHC class I/peptide complexes to dendritic cells. *J Immunol* 172 (4):2126-36.

Andre, F., N. E. Schartz, N. Chaput, C. Flament, G. Raposo, S. Amigorena, E. Angevin, and L. Zitvogel. 2002. Tumor-derived exosomes: a new source of tumor rejection antigens. *Vaccine* 20 Suppl 4:A28-31.

Banchereau, J., F. Briere, C. Caux, J. Davoust, S. Lebecque, Y. J. Liu, B. Pulendran, and K. Palucka. 2000. Immunobiology of dendritic cells. *Annu Rev Immunol* 18:767-811.

Batra, S. K., S. Castelino-Prabhu, C. J. Wikstrand, X. Zhu, P. A. Humphrey, H. S. Friedman, and D. D. Bigner. 1995. Epidermal growth factor ligand-independent, unregulated, cell-transforming potential of a naturally occurring human mutant EGFRvIII gene. *Cell Growth Differ* 6 (10):1251-9.

Battke, C., R. Ruiss, U. Welsch, P. Wimberger, S. Lang, S. Jochum, and R. Zeidler. Tumour exosomes inhibit binding of tumour-reactive antibodies to tumour cells and reduce ADCC. *Cancer Immunol Immunother* 60 (5):639-48.

Bausero, M. A., D. T. Page, E. Osinaga, and A. Asea. 2004. Surface expression of Hsp25 and Hsp72 differentially regulates tumor growth and metastasis. *Tumour Biol* 25 (5-6):243-51.

Berens, M. E., and A. Giese. 1999. "...those left behind." Biology and oncology of invasive glioma cells. *Neoplasia* 1 (3):208-19.

Bhatnagar, S., and J. S. Schorey. 2007. Exosomes released from infected macrophages contain Mycobacterium avium glycopeptidolipids and are proinflammatory. *J Biol Chem* 282 (35):25779-89.

Bhatnagar, S., K. Shinagawa, F. J. Castellino, and J. S. Schorey. 2007. Exosomes released from macrophages infected with intracellular pathogens stimulate a proinflammatory response in vitro and in vivo. *Blood* 110 (9):3234-44.

Blanchard, N., D. Lankar, F. Faure, A. Regnault, C. Dumont, G. Raposo, and C. Hivroz. 2002. TCR activation of human T cells induces the production of exosomes bearing the TCR/CD3/zeta complex. *J Immunol* 168 (7):3235-41.

Bobryshev, Y. V., R. S. Lord, N. K. Golovanova, E. V. Gracheva, N. D. Zvezdina, and N. V. Prokazova. 2001. Phenotype determination of anti-GM3 positive cells in atherosclerotic lesions of the human aorta. Hypothetical role of ganglioside GM3 in foam cell formation. *Biochim Biophys Acta* 1535 (2):87-99.

Booth, A. M., Y. Fang, J. K. Fallon, J. M. Yang, J. E. Hildreth, and S. J. Gould. 2006. Exosomes and HIV Gag bud from endosome-like domains of the T cell plasma membrane. *J Cell Biol* 172 (6):923-35.

Brandes, A. A., E. Franceschi, A. Tosoni, M. E. Hegi, and R. Stupp. 2008. Epidermal growth factor receptor inhibitors in neuro-oncology: hopes and disappointments. *Clin Cancer Res* 14 (4):957-60.

Broxmeyer, L. 2004. Is cancer just an incurable infectious disease? *Med Hypotheses* 63 (6):986-96.

Bu, N., Q. L. Li, Q. Feng, and B. Z. Sun. 2006. Immune protection effect of exosomes against attack of L1210 tumor cells. *Leuk Lymphoma* 47 (5):913-8.

Bu, N., H. Wu, B. Sun, G. Zhang, S. Zhan, R. Zhang, and L. Zhou. Exosome-loaded dendritic cells elicit tumor-specific CD8(+) cytotoxic T cells in patients with glioma. *J Neurooncol.*

Cairns, R. A., I. S. Harris, and T. W. Mak. Regulation of cancer cell metabolism. *Nat Rev Cancer* 11 (2):85-95.

Calistri, A., C. Salata, C. Parolin, and G. Palu. 2009. Role of multivesicular bodies and their components in the egress of enveloped RNA viruses. *Rev Med Virol* 19 (1):31-45.

Calzolari, A., C. Raggi, S. Deaglio, N. M. Sposi, M. Stafsnes, K. Fecchi, I. Parolini, F. Malavasi, C. Peschle, M. Sargiacomo, and U. Testa. 2006. TfR2 localizes in lipid raft domains and is released in exosomes to activate signal transduction along the MAPK pathway. *J Cell Sci* 119 (Pt 21):4486-98.

Camussi, G., M. C. Deregibus, S. Bruno, V. Cantaluppi, and L. Biancone. Exosomes/microvesicles as a mechanism of cell-to-cell communication. *Kidney Int* 78 (9):838-48.

Carrington, J. C., and V. Ambros. 2003. Role of microRNAs in plant and animal development. *Science* 301 (5631):336-8.

Castellana, D., C. Kunzelmann, and J. M. Freyssinet. 2009. Pathophysiologic significance of procoagulant microvesicles in cancer disease and progression. *Hamostaseologie* 29 (1):51-7.

Chaput, N., C. Flament, S. Viaud, J. Taieb, S. Roux, A. Spatz, F. Andre, J. B. LePecq, M. Boussac, J. Garin, S. Amigorena, C. Thery, and L. Zitvogel. 2006. Dendritic cell derived-exosomes: biology and clinical implementations. *J Leukoc Biol* 80 (3):471-8.

Chen, V. Y., M. M. Posada, L. L. Blazer, T. Zhao, and G. R. Rosania. 2006. The role of the VPS4A-exosome pathway in the intrinsic egress route of a DNA-binding anticancer drug. *Pharm Res* 23 (8):1687-95.

Chen, V. Y., M. M. Posada, L. Zhao, and G. R. Rosania. 2007. Rapid doxorubicin efflux from the nucleus of drug-resistant cancer cells following extracellular drug clearance. *Pharm Res* 24 (11):2156-67.

Chen, W., J. Wang, C. Shao, S. Liu, Y. Yu, Q. Wang, and X. Cao. 2006. Efficient induction of antitumor T cell immunity by exosomes derived from heat-shocked lymphoma cells. *Eur J Immunol* 36 (6):1598-607.

Chirco, R., X. W. Liu, K. K. Jung, and H. R. Kim. 2006. Novel functions of TIMPs in cell signaling. *Cancer Metastasis Rev* 25 (1):99-113.

Cho, J. A., Y. S. Lee, S. H. Kim, J. K. Ko, and C. W. Kim. 2009. MHC independent anti-tumor immune responses induced by Hsp70-enriched exosomes generate tumor regression in murine models. *Cancer Lett* 275 (2):256-65.

Cho, J. A., D. J. Yeo, H. Y. Son, H. W. Kim, D. S. Jung, J. K. Ko, J. S. Koh, Y. N. Kim, and C. W. Kim. 2005. Exosomes: a new delivery system for tumor antigens in cancer immunotherapy. *Int J Cancer* 114 (4):613-22.

Chu, C. T., K. D. Everiss, C. J. Wikstrand, S. K. Batra, H. J. Kung, and D. D. Bigner. 1997. Receptor dimerization is not a factor in the signalling activity of a transforming variant epidermal growth factor receptor (EGFRvIII). *Biochem J* 324 (Pt 3):855-61.

Ciravolo, V., V. Huber, G. C. Ghedini, E. Venturelli, F. Bianchi, M. Campiglio, D. Morelli, A. Villa, P. D. Mina, S. Menard, P. Filipazzi, L. Rivoltini, E. Tagliabue, and S. M. Pupa. Potential role of HER2-overexpressing exosomes in countering Trastuzumab-based therapy. *J Cell Physiol.*

Cobbs, C. S., L. Harkins, M. Samanta, G. Y. Gillespie, S. Bharara, P. H. King, L. B. Nabors, C. G. Cobbs, and W. J. Britt. 2002. Human cytomegalovirus infection and expression in human malignant glioma. *Cancer Res* 62 (12):3347-50.

Cocito, C., and H. Maes. 1998. Immunological relatedness of the protective mechanisms against tuberculosis and cancer. *Eur J Clin Invest* 28 (1):1-12.

Corcoran, C., A. M. Friel, M. J. Duffy, J. Crown, and L. O'Driscoll. Intracellular and extracellular microRNAs in breast cancer. *Clin Chem* 57 (1):18-32.

Coren, L. V., T. Shatzer, and D. E. Ott. 2008. CD45 immunoaffinity depletion of vesicles from Jurkat T cells demonstrates that exosomes contain CD45: no evidence for a distinct exosome/HIV-1 budding pathway. *Retrovirology* 5:64.

Dai, S., T. Wan, B. Wang, X. Zhou, F. Xiu, T. Chen, Y. Wu, and X. Cao. 2005. More efficient induction of HLA-A*0201-restricted and carcinoembryonic antigen (CEA)-specific CTL response by immunization with exosomes prepared from heat-stressed CEA-positive tumor cells. *Clin Cancer Res* 11 (20):7554-63.

Dai, S., D. Wei, Z. Wu, X. Zhou, X. Wei, H. Huang, and G. Li. 2008. Phase I clinical trial of autologous ascites-derived exosomes combined with GM-CSF for colorectal cancer. *Mol Ther* 16 (4):782-90.

de Gassart, A., C. Geminard, B. Fevrier, G. Raposo, and M. Vidal. 2003. Lipid raft-associated protein sorting in exosomes. *Blood* 102 (13):4336-44.

de Gassart, A., C. Geminard, D. Hoekstra, and M. Vidal. 2004. Exosome secretion: the art of reutilizing nonrecycled proteins? *Traffic* 5 (11):896-903.

de Groot, J. F., G. Fuller, A. J. Kumar, Y. Piao, K. Eterovic, Y. Ji, and C. A. Conrad. Tumor invasion after treatment of glioblastoma with bevacizumab: radiographic and pathologic correlation in humans and mice. *Neuro Oncol* 12 (3):233-42.

De Smaele, E., E. Ferretti, and A. Gulino. MicroRNAs as biomarkers for CNS cancer and other disorders. *Brain Res* 1338:100-11.

de Vries, I. J., G. J. Adema, C. J. Punt, and C. G. Figdor. 2005. Phenotypical and functional characterization of clinical-grade dendritic cells. *Methods Mol Med* 109:113-26.

Del Conde, I., L. D. Bharwani, D. J. Dietzen, U. Pendurthi, P. Thiagarajan, and J. A. Lopez. 2007. Microvesicle-associated tissue factor and Trousseau's syndrome. *J Thromb Haemost* 5 (1):70-4.

Del Conde, I., C. N. Shrimpton, P. Thiagarajan, and J. A. Lopez. 2005. Tissue-factor-bearing microvesicles arise from lipid rafts and fuse with activated platelets to initiate coagulation. *Blood* 106 (5):1604-11.

Denzer, K., M. van Eijk, M. J. Kleijmeer, E. Jakobson, C. de Groot, and H. J. Geuze. 2000. Follicular dendritic cells carry MHC class II-expressing microvesicles at their surface. *J Immunol* 165 (3):1259-65.

Dimov, I., L. Jankovic Velickovic, and V. Stefanovic. 2009. Urinary exosomes. *ScientificWorldJournal* 9:1107-18.

Duijvesz, D., T. Luider, C. H. Bangma, and G. Jenster. Exosomes as biomarker treasure chests for prostate cancer. *Eur Urol* 59 (5):823-31.

Dukers, D. F., P. Meij, M. B. Vervoort, W. Vos, R. J. Scheper, C. J. Meijer, E. Bloemena, and J. M. Middeldorp. 2000. Direct immunosuppressive effects of EBV-encoded latent membrane protein 1. *J Immunol* 165 (2):663-70.

Dziurzynski, K., J. Wei, W. Qiao, M. A. Hatiboglu, L. Y. Kong, A. Wu, Y. Wang, D. Cahill, N. B. Levine, S. Prabhu, G. Rao, R. Sawaya, and A. B. Heimberger. Glioma-associated cytomegalovirus mediates subversion of the monocyte lineage to a tumor propagating phenotype. *Clin Cancer Res*.

Escudier, B., T. Dorval, N. Chaput, F. Andre, M. P. Caby, S. Novault, C. Flament, C. Leboulaire, C. Borg, S. Amigorena, C. Boccaccio, C. Bonnerot, O. Dhellin, M. Movassagh, S. Piperno, C. Robert, V. Serra, N. Valente, J. B. Le Pecq, A. Spatz, O. Lantz, T. Tursz, E. Angevin, and L. Zitvogel. 2005. Vaccination of metastatic melanoma patients with autologous dendritic cell (DC) derived-exosomes: results of thefirst phase I clinical trial. *J Transl Med* 3 (1):10.

Fang, Y., N. Wu, X. Gan, W. Yan, J. C. Morrell, and S. J. Gould. 2007. Higher-order oligomerization targets plasma membrane proteins and HIV gag to exosomes. *PLoS Biol* 5 (6):e158.

Ferreira, L. M. Cancer metabolism: the Warburg effect today. *Exp Mol Pathol* 89 (3):372-80.

Fevrier, B., D. Vilette, F. Archer, D. Loew, W. Faigle, M. Vidal, H. Laude, and G. Raposo. 2004. Cells release prions in association with exosomes. *Proc Natl Acad Sci U S A* 101 (26):9683-8.

Fevrier, B., D. Vilette, H. Laude, and G. Raposo. 2005. Exosomes: a bubble ride for prions? *Traffic* 6 (1):10-7.

Flanagan, J., J. Middeldorp, and T. Sculley. 2003. Localization of the Epstein-Barr virus protein LMP 1 to exosomes. *J Gen Virol* 84 (Pt 7):1871-9.

Flavell, R. A., S. Sanjabi, S. H. Wrzesinski, and P. Licona-Limon. The polarization of immune cells in the tumour environment by TGFbeta. *Nat Rev Immunol* 10 (8):554-67.

Freyssinet, J. M., and F. Toti. Formation of procoagulant microparticles and properties. *Thromb Res* 125 Suppl 1:S46-8.

Gauvreau, M. E., M. H. Cote, M. C. Bourgeois-Daigneault, L. D. Rivard, F. Xiu, A. Brunet, A. Shaw, V. Steimle, and J. Thibodeau. 2009. Sorting of MHC class II molecules into exosomes through a ubiquitin-independent pathway. *Traffic* 10 (10):1518-27.

Gesierich, S., I. Berezovskiy, E. Ryschich, and M. Zoller. 2006. Systemic induction of the angiogenesis switch by the tetraspanin D6.1A/CO-029. *Cancer Res* 66 (14):7083-94.

Giri, P. K., N. A. Kruh, K. M. Dobos, and J. S. Schorey. Proteomic analysis identifies highly antigenic proteins in exosomes from M. tuberculosis-infected and culture filtrate protein-treated macrophages. *Proteomics* 10 (17):3190-202.

Giusti, I., S. D'Ascenzo, D. Millimaggi, G. Taraboletti, G. Carta, N. Franceschini, A. Pavan, and V. Dolo. 2008. Cathepsin B mediates the pH-dependent proinvasive activity of tumor-shed microvesicles. *Neoplasia* 10 (5):481-8.

Goldman, R. 2004. Growth factors and chronic wound healing: past, present, and future. *Adv Skin Wound Care* 17 (1):24-35.

Gonzalo, P., V. Moreno, B. G. Galvez, and A. G. Arroyo. MT1-MMP and integrins: Hand-to-hand in cell communication. *Biofactors* 36 (4):248-54.

Gould, S. J., A. M. Booth, and J. E. Hildreth. 2003. The Trojan exosome hypothesis. *Proc Natl Acad Sci U S A* 100 (19):10592-7.

Graner, M. W., O. Alzate, A. M. Dechkovskaia, J. D. Keene, J. H. Sampson, D. A. Mitchell, and D. D. Bigner. 2009. Proteomic and immunologic analyses of brain tumor exosomes. *FASEB J* 23 (5):1541-57.

Graner, M. W., and D. D. Bigner. 2005. Chaperone proteins and brain tumors: potential targets and possible therapeutics. *Neuro-oncol* 7 (3):260-78.

———. 2006. Therapeutic aspects of chaperones/heat-shock proteins in neuro-oncology. *Expert Rev Anticancer Ther* 6 (5):679-95.

Graner, M. W., R. I. Cumming, and D. D. Bigner. 2007. The heat shock response and chaperones/heat shock proteins in brain tumors: surface expression, release, and possible immune consequences. *J Neurosci* 27 (42):11214-27.

Guescini, M., S. Genedani, V. Stocchi, and L. F. Agnati. Astrocytes and Glioblastoma cells release exosomes carrying mtDNA. *J Neural Transm* 117 (1):1-4.

Guescini, M., D. Guidolin, L. Vallorani, L. Casadei, A. M. Gioacchini, P. Tibollo, M. Battistelli, E. Falcieri, L. Battistin, L. F. Agnati, and V. Stocchi. C2C12 myoblasts release micro-vesicles containing mtDNA and proteins involved in signal transduction. *Exp Cell Res* 316 (12):1977-84.

Hakulinen, J., L. Sankkila, N. Sugiyama, K. Lehti, and J. Keski-Oja. 2008. Secretion of active membrane type 1 matrix metalloproteinase (MMP-14) into extracellular space in microvesicular exosomes. *J Cell Biochem* 105 (5):1211-8.

Hatanpaa, K. J., S. Burma, D. Zhao, and A. A. Habib. Epidermal growth factor receptor in glioma: signal transduction, neuropathology, imaging, and radioresistance. *Neoplasia* 12 (9):675-84.

Hedlund, M., A. C. Stenqvist, O. Nagaeva, L. Kjellberg, M. Wulff, V. Baranov, and L. Mincheva-Nilsson. 2009. Human placenta expresses and secretes NKG2D ligands via exosomes that down-modulate the cognate receptor expression: evidence for immunosuppressive function. *J Immunol* 183 (1):340-51.

Heimberger, A. B., D. Suki, D. Yang, W. Shi, and K. Aldape. 2005. The natural history of EGFR and EGFRvIII in glioblastoma patients. *J Transl Med* 3:38.

Hendrix, A., W. Westbroek, M. Bracke, and O. De Wever. An ex(o)citing machinery for invasive tumor growth. *Cancer Res* 70 (23):9533-7.

Higginbotham, J. N., M. Demory Beckler, J. D. Gephart, J. L. Franklin, G. Bogatcheva, G. J. Kremers, D. W. Piston, G. D. Ayers, R. E. McConnell, M. J. Tyska, and R. J. Coffey. Amphiregulin exosomes increase cancer cell invasion. *Curr Biol* 21 (9):779-86.

Hoelzinger, D. B., T. Demuth, and M. E. Berens. 2007. Autocrine factors that sustain glioma invasion and paracrine biology in the brain microenvironment. *J Natl Cancer Inst* 99 (21):1583-93.

Hong, B. S., J. H. Cho, H. Kim, E. J. Choi, S. Rho, J. Kim, J. H. Kim, D. S. Choi, Y. K. Kim, D. Hwang, and Y. S. Gho. 2009. Colorectal cancer cell-derived microvesicles are enriched in cell cycle-related mRNAs that promote proliferation of endothelial cells. *BMC Genomics* 10:556.

Hsu, C., Y. Morohashi, S. Yoshimura, N. Manrique-Hoyos, S. Jung, M. A. Lauterbach, M. Bakhti, M. Gronborg, W. Mobius, J. Rhee, F. A. Barr, and M. Simons. Regulation of exosome secretion by Rab35 and its GTPase-activating proteins TBC1D10A-C. *J Cell Biol* 189 (2):223-32.

Hunter, M. P., N. Ismail, X. Zhang, B. D. Aguda, E. J. Lee, L. Yu, T. Xiao, J. Schafer, M. L. Lee, T. D. Schmittgen, S. P. Nana-Sinkam, D. Jarjoura, and C. B. Marsh. 2008. Detection of microRNA expression in human peripheral blood microvesicles. *PLoS One* 3 (11):e3694.

Hyytiainen, M., C. Penttinen, and J. Keski-Oja. 2004. Latent TGF-beta binding proteins: extracellular matrix association and roles in TGF-beta activation. *Crit Rev Clin Lab Sci* 41 (3):233-64.

Ichim, T. E., Z. Zhong, S. Kaushal, X. Zheng, X. Ren, X. Hao, J. A. Joyce, H. H. Hanley, N. H. Riordan, J. Koropatnick, V. Bogin, B. R. Minev, W. P. Min, and R. H. Tullis. 2008. Exosomes as a tumor immune escape mechanism: possible therapeutic implications. *J Transl Med* 6:37.

Iero, M., R. Valenti, V. Huber, P. Filipazzi, G. Parmiani, S. Fais, and L. Rivoltini. 2008. Tumour-released exosomes and their implications in cancer immunity. *Cell Death Differ* 15 (1):80-8.

Inda, M. M., R. Bonavia, A. Mukasa, Y. Narita, D. W. Sah, S. Vandenberg, C. Brennan, T. G. Johns, R. Bachoo, P. Hadwiger, P. Tan, R. A. Depinho, W. Cavenee, and F. Furnari.

Tumor heterogeneity is an active process maintained by a mutant EGFR-induced cytokine circuit in glioblastoma. *Genes Dev* 24 (16):1731-45.

Iwamoto, F. M., L. E. Abrey, K. Beal, P. H. Gutin, M. K. Rosenblum, V. E. Reuter, L. M. DeAngelis, and A. B. Lassman. 2009. Patterns of relapse and prognosis after bevacizumab failure in recurrent glioblastoma. *Neurology* 73 (15):1200-6.

Janich, P., and D. Corbeil. 2007. GM1 and GM3 gangliosides highlight distinct lipid microdomains within the apical domain of epithelial cells. *FEBS Lett* 581 (9):1783-7.

Johnstone, R. M. 2006. Exosomes biological significance: A concise review. *Blood Cells Mol Dis* 36 (2):315-21.

Johnstone, R. M., M. Adam, J. R. Hammond, L. Orr, and C. Turbide. 1987. Vesicle formation during reticulocyte maturation. Association of plasma membrane activities with released vesicles (exosomes). *J Biol Chem* 262 (19):9412-20.

Johnstone, R. M., A. Bianchini, and K. Teng. 1989. Reticulocyte maturation and exosome release: transferrin receptor containing exosomes shows multiple plasma membrane functions. *Blood* 74 (5):1844-51.

Jung, T., D. Castellana, P. Klingbeil, I. Cuesta Hernandez, M. Vitacolonna, D. J. Orlicky, S. R. Roffler, P. Brodt, and M. Zoller. 2009. CD44v6 dependence of premetastatic niche preparation by exosomes. *Neoplasia* 11 (10):1093-105.

Kalinski, P., J. Urban, R. Narang, E. Berk, E. Wieckowski, and R. Muthuswamy. 2009. Dendritic cell-based therapeutic cancer vaccines: what we have and what we need. *Future Oncol* 5 (3):379-90.

Keryer-Bibens, C., C. Pioche-Durieu, C. Villemant, S. Souquere, N. Nishi, M. Hirashima, J. Middeldorp, and P. Busson. 2006. Exosomes released by EBV-infected nasopharyngeal carcinoma cells convey the viral latent membrane protein 1 and the immunomodulatory protein galectin 9. *BMC Cancer* 6:283.

Kessenbrock, K., V. Plaks, and Z. Werb. Matrix metalloproteinases: regulators of the tumor microenvironment. *Cell* 141 (1):52-67.

Khan, S., J. M. Jutzy, J. R. Aspe, D. W. McGregor, J. W. Neidigh, and N. R. Wall. Survivin is released from cancer cells via exosomes. *Apoptosis* 16 (1):1-12.

Klibi, J., T. Niki, A. Riedel, C. Pioche-Durieu, S. Souquere, E. Rubinstein, S. Le Moulec, J. Guigay, M. Hirashima, F. Guemira, D. Adhikary, J. Mautner, and P. Busson. 2009. Blood diffusion and Th1-suppressive effects of galectin-9-containing exosomes released by Epstein-Barr virus-infected nasopharyngeal carcinoma cells. *Blood* 113 (9):1957-66.

Koga, K., K. Matsumoto, T. Akiyoshi, M. Kubo, N. Yamanaka, A. Tasaki, H. Nakashima, M. Nakamura, S. Kuroki, M. Tanaka, and M. Katano. 2005. Purification, characterization and biological significance of tumor-derived exosomes. *Anticancer Res* 25 (6A):3703-7.

Kosaka, N., H. Iguchi, and T. Ochiya. Circulating microRNA in body fluid: a new potential biomarker for cancer diagnosis and prognosis. *Cancer Sci* 101 (10):2087-92.

Kosaka, N., H. Iguchi, Y. Yoshioka, F. Takeshita, Y. Matsuki, and T. Ochiya. Secretory mechanisms and intercellular transfer of microRNAs in living cells. *J Biol Chem* 285 (23):17442-52.

Krutovskikh, V. A., and Z. Herceg. Oncogenic microRNAs (OncomiRs) as a new class of cancer biomarkers. *Bioessays* 32 (10):894-904.

Kuan, C. T., K. Wakiya, J. M. Dowell, J. E. Herndon, 2nd, D. A. Reardon, M. W. Graner, G. J. Riggins, C. J. Wikstrand, and D. D. Bigner. 2006. Glycoprotein nonmetastatic melanoma protein B, a potential molecular therapeutic target in patients with glioblastoma multiforme. *Clin Cancer Res* 12 (7 Pt 1):1970-82.

Lamparski, H. G., A. Metha-Damani, J. Y. Yao, S. Patel, D. H. Hsu, C. Ruegg, and J. B. Le Pecq. 2002. Production and characterization of clinical grade exosomes derived from dendritic cells. *J Immunol Methods* 270 (2):211-26.

Laulagnier, K., H. Vincent-Schneider, S. Hamdi, C. Subra, D. Lankar, and M. Record. 2005. Characterization of exosome subpopulations from RBL-2H3 cells using fluorescent lipids. *Blood Cells Mol Dis* 35 (2):116-21.

Lehrer, S., V. Labombardi, S. Green, M. S. Pessin-Minsley, I. M. Germano, and K. E. Rosenzweig. No circulating cytomegalovirus in five patients with glioblastoma multiforme. *Anticancer Res* 31 (3):959-60.

Li, G., S. Andreansky, G. Helguera, M. Sepassi, N. Janikashvili, J. Cantrell, C. L. Lacasse, N. Larmonier, M. L. Penichet, and E. Katsanis. 2008. A chaperone protein-enriched tumor cell lysate vaccine generates protective humoral immunity in a mouse breast cancer model. *Mol Cancer Ther* 7 (3):721-9.

Liu, C., S. Yu, K. Zinn, J. Wang, L. Zhang, Y. Jia, J. C. Kappes, S. Barnes, R. P. Kimberly, W. E. Grizzle, and H. G. Zhang. 2006. Murine mammary carcinoma exosomes promote tumor growth by suppression of NK cell function. *J Immunol* 176 (3):1375-85.

Liu, Y., S. V. Shah, X. Xiang, J. Wang, Z. B. Deng, C. Liu, L. Zhang, J. Wu, T. Edmonds, C. Jambor, J. C. Kappes, and H. G. Zhang. 2009. COP9-associated CSN5 regulates exosomal protein deubiquitination and sorting. *Am J Pathol* 174 (4):1415-25.

Loging, W. T., A. Lal, I. M. Siu, T. L. Loney, C. J. Wikstrand, M. A. Marra, C. Prange, D. D. Bigner, R. L. Strausberg, and G. J. Riggins. 2000. Identifying potential tumor markers and antigens by database mining and rapid expression screening. *Genome Res* 10 (9):1393-402.

Lu, C., and A. Shervington. 2008. Chemoresistance in gliomas. *Mol Cell Biochem* 312 (1-2):71-80.

Lu, X., B. Bennet, E. Mu, J. Rabinowitz, and Y. Kang. Metabolomic changes accompanying transformation and acquisition of metastatic potential in a syngeneic mouse mammary tumor model. *J Biol Chem* 285 (13):9317-21.

Luo, S. S., O. Ishibashi, G. Ishikawa, T. Ishikawa, A. Katayama, T. Mishima, T. Takizawa, T. Shigihara, T. Goto, A. Izumi, A. Ohkuchi, S. Matsubara, and T. Takeshita. 2009. Human villous trophoblasts express and secrete placenta-specific microRNAs into maternal circulation via exosomes. *Biol Reprod* 81 (4):717-29.

Mangeney, M., J. Pothlichet, M. Renard, B. Ducos, and T. Heidmann. 2005. Endogenous retrovirus expression is required for murine melanoma tumor growth in vivo. *Cancer Res* 65 (7):2588-91.

Manjili, M. H., X. Y. Wang, X. Chen, T. Martin, E. A. Repasky, R. Henderson, and J. R. Subjeck. 2003. HSP110-HER2/neu chaperone complex vaccine induces protective immunity against spontaneous mammary tumors in HER-2/neu transgenic mice. *J Immunol* 171 (8):4054-61.

Masciopinto, F., C. Giovani, S. Campagnoli, L. Galli-Stampino, P. Colombatto, M. Brunetto, T. S. Yen, M. Houghton, P. Pileri, and S. Abrignani. 2004. Association of hepatitis C virus envelope proteins with exosomes. *Eur J Immunol* 34 (10):2834-42.

Mathews, J. A., D. R. Gibb, B. H. Chen, P. Scherle, and D. H. Conrad. CD23 Sheddase A disintegrin and metalloproteinase 10 (ADAM10) is also required for CD23 sorting into B cell-derived exosomes. *J Biol Chem* 285 (48):37531-41.

Mathivanan, S., H. Ji, and R. J. Simpson. Exosomes: extracellular organelles important in intercellular communication. *J Proteomics* 73 (10):1907-20.

Matsuo, H., J. Chevallier, N. Mayran, I. Le Blanc, C. Ferguson, J. Faure, N. S. Blanc, S. Matile, J. Dubochet, R. Sadoul, R. G. Parton, F. Vilbois, and J. Gruenberg. 2004. Role of LBPA and Alix in multivesicular liposome formation and endosome organization. *Science* 303 (5657):531-4.

McCready, J., J. D. Sims, D. Chan, and D. G. Jay. Secretion of extracellular hsp90alpha via exosomes increases cancer cell motility: a role for plasminogen activation. *BMC Cancer* 10:294.

Medina, A., and A. Ghahary. Transdifferentiated circulating monocytes release exosomes containing 14-3-3 proteins with matrix metalloproteinase-1 stimulating effect for dermal fibroblasts. *Wound Repair Regen* 18 (2):245-53.

Mercer, J., M. Schelhaas, and A. Helenius. Virus entry by endocytosis. *Annu Rev Biochem* 79:803-33.

Michael, A., S. D. Bajracharya, P. S. Yuen, H. Zhou, R. A. Star, G. G. Illei, and I. Alevizos. Exosomes from human saliva as a source of microRNA biomarkers. *Oral Dis* 16 (1):34-8.

Miesbauer, M., A. S. Rambold, K. F. Winklhofer, and J. Tatzelt. Targeting of the prion protein to the cytosol: mechanisms and consequences. *Curr Issues Mol Biol* 12 (2):109-18.

Milsom, C., J. Yu, L. May, N. Magnus, and J. Rak. 2008. Diverse roles of tissue factor-expressing cell subsets in tumor progression. *Semin Thromb Hemost* 34 (2):170-81.

Mischel, P. S., T. F. Cloughesy, and S. F. Nelson. 2004. DNA-microarray analysis of brain cancer: molecular classification for therapy. *Nat Rev Neurosci* 5 (10):782-92.

Mitchell, D. A., W. Xie, R. Schmittling, C. Learn, A. Friedman, R. E. McLendon, and J. H. Sampson. 2008. Sensitive detection of human cytomegalovirus in tumors and peripheral blood of patients diagnosed with glioblastoma. *Neuro Oncol* 10 (1):10-8.

Mitchell, P., E. Petfalski, A. Shevchenko, M. Mann, and D. Tollervey. 1997. The exosome: a conserved eukaryotic RNA processing complex containing multiple 3'-->5' exoribonucleases. *Cell* 91 (4):457-66.

Morse, M. A., J. Garst, T. Osada, S. Khan, A. Hobeika, T. M. Clay, N. Valente, R. Shreeniwas, M. A. Sutton, A. Delcayre, D. H. Hsu, J. B. Le Pecq, and H. K. Lyerly. 2005. A phase I study of dexosome immunotherapy in patients with advanced non-small cell lung cancer. *J Transl Med* 3 (1):9.

Mukherjee, S., T. T. Soe, and F. R. Maxfield. 1999. Endocytic sorting of lipid analogues differing solely in the chemistry of their hydrophobic tails. *J Cell Biol* 144 (6):1271-84.

Muller, G., C. Jung, J. Straub, S. Wied, and W. Kramer. 2009. Induced release of membrane vesicles from rat adipocytes containing glycosylphosphatidylinositol-anchored microdomain and lipid droplet signalling proteins. *Cell Signal* 21 (2):324-38.

Nakada, M., S. Nakada, T. Demuth, N. L. Tran, D. B. Hoelzinger, and M. E. Berens. 2007. Molecular targets of glioma invasion. *Cell Mol Life Sci* 64 (4):458-78.

Nelson, P., M. Kiriakidou, A. Sharma, E. Maniataki, and Z. Mourelatos. 2003. The microRNA world: small is mighty. *Trends Biochem Sci* 28 (10):534-40.

Nguyen, D. G., A. Booth, S. J. Gould, and J. E. Hildreth. 2003. Evidence that HIV budding in primary macrophages occurs through the exosome release pathway. *J Biol Chem* 278 (52):52347-54.

Nishikawa, R., T. Sugiyama, Y. Narita, F. Furnari, W. K. Cavenee, and M. Matsutani. 2004. Immunohistochemical analysis of the mutant epidermal growth factor, deltaEGFR, in glioblastoma. *Brain Tumor Pathol* 21 (2):53-6.

Ogata, M. 2009. Human herpesvirus 6 in hematological malignancies. *J Clin Exp Hematop* 49 (2):57-67.

Ogawa, R., C. Tanaka, M. Sato, H. Nagasaki, K. Sugimura, K. Okumura, Y. Nakagawa, and N. Aoki. Adipocyte-derived microvesicles contain RNA that is transported into macrophages and might be secreted into blood circulation. *Biochem Biophys Res Commun* 398 (4):723-9.

Ordys, B. B., S. Launay, R. F. Deighton, J. McCulloch, and I. R. Whittle. The role of mitochondria in glioma pathophysiology. *Mol Neurobiol* 42 (1):64-75.

Ostrowski, M., N. B. Carmo, S. Krumeich, I. Fanget, G. Raposo, A. Savina, C. F. Moita, K. Schauer, A. N. Hume, R. P. Freitas, B. Goud, P. Benaroch, N. Hacohen, M. Fukuda, C. Desnos, M. C. Seabra, F. Darchen, S. Amigorena, L. F. Moita, and C. Thery. Rab27a and Rab27b control different steps of the exosome secretion pathway. *Nat Cell Biol* 12 (1):19-30; sup pp 1-13.

Oudard, S., F. Arvelo, L. Miccoli, F. Apiou, A. M. Dutrillaux, M. Poisson, B. Dutrillaux, and M. F. Poupon. 1996. High glycolysis in gliomas despite low hexokinase transcription and activity correlated to chromosome 10 loss. *Br J Cancer* 74 (6):839-45.

Oudard, S., E. Boitier, L. Miccoli, S. Rousset, B. Dutrillaux, and M. F. Poupon. 1997. Gliomas are driven by glycolysis: putative roles of hexokinase, oxidative phosphorylation and mitochondrial ultrastructure. *Anticancer Res* 17 (3C):1903-11.

Palucka, K., H. Ueno, G. Zurawski, J. Fay, and J. Banchereau. Building on dendritic cell subsets to improve cancer vaccines. *Curr Opin Immunol* 22 (2):258-63.

Parolini, I., C. Federici, C. Raggi, L. Lugini, S. Palleschi, A. De Milito, C. Coscia, E. Iessi, M. Logozzi, A. Molinari, M. Colone, M. Tatti, M. Sargiacomo, and S. Fais. 2009. Microenvironmental pH is a key factor for exosome traffic in tumor cells. *J Biol Chem* 284 (49):34211-22.

Pedersen, M. W., M. Meltorn, L. Damstrup, and H. S. Poulsen. 2001. The type III epidermal growth factor receptor mutation. Biological significance and potential target for anti-cancer therapy. *Ann Oncol* 12 (6):745-60.

Peinado, H., S. Lavotshkin, and D. Lyden. The secreted factors responsible for pre-metastatic niche formation: old sayings and new thoughts. *Semin Cancer Biol* 21 (2):139-46.

Pelloski, C. E., K. V. Ballman, A. F. Furth, L. Zhang, E. Lin, E. P. Sulman, K. Bhat, J. M. McDonald, W. K. Yung, H. Colman, S. Y. Woo, A. B. Heimberger, D. Suki, M. D. Prados, S. M. Chang, F. G. Barker, 2nd, J. C. Buckner, C. D. James, and K. Aldape. 2007. Epidermal growth factor receptor variant III status defines clinically distinct subtypes of glioblastoma. *J Clin Oncol* 25 (16):2288-94.

Perret, E., A. Lakkaraju, S. Deborde, R. Schreiner, and E. Rodriguez-Boulan. 2005. Evolving endosomes: how many varieties and why? *Curr Opin Cell Biol* 17 (4):423-34.

Pisitkun, T., R. Johnstone, and M. A. Knepper. 2006. Discovery of urinary biomarkers. *Mol Cell Proteomics* 5 (10):1760-71.

Pols, M. S., and J. Klumperman. 2009. Trafficking and function of the tetraspanin CD63. *Exp Cell Res* 315 (9):1584-92.

Qu, J. L., X. J. Qu, M. F. Zhao, Y. E. Teng, Y. Zhang, K. Z. Hou, Y. H. Jiang, X. H. Yang, and Y. P. Liu. 2009. The role of cbl family of ubiquitin ligases in gastric cancer exosome-induced apoptosis of Jurkat T cells. *Acta Oncol* 48 (8):1173-80.

Rabesandratana, H., J. P. Toutant, H. Reggio, and M. Vidal. 1998. Decay-accelerating factor (CD55) and membrane inhibitor of reactive lysis (CD59) are released within exosomes during In vitro maturation of reticulocytes. *Blood* 91 (7):2573-80.

Rabinowits, G., C. Gercel-Taylor, J. M. Day, D. D. Taylor, and G. H. Kloecker. 2009. Exosomal microRNA: a diagnostic marker for lung cancer. *Clin Lung Cancer* 10 (1):42-6.

Rahman, R., S. Smith, C. Rahman, and R. Grundy. Antiangiogenic therapy and mechanisms of tumor resistance in malignant glioma. *J Oncol* 2010:251231.

Rajendran, L., M. Honsho, T. R. Zahn, P. Keller, K. D. Geiger, P. Verkade, and K. Simons. 2006. Alzheimer's disease beta-amyloid peptides are released in association with exosomes. *Proc Natl Acad Sci U S A* 103 (30):11172-7.

Ramnarain, D. B., S. Park, D. Y. Lee, K. J. Hatanpaa, S. O. Scoggin, H. Otu, T. A. Libermann, J. M. Raisanen, R. Ashfaq, E. T. Wong, J. Wu, R. Elliott, and A. A. Habib. 2006. Differential gene expression analysis reveals generation of an autocrine loop by a mutant epidermal growth factor receptor in glioma cells. *Cancer Res* 66 (2):867-74.

Rana, S., C. Claas, C. C. Kretz, I. Nazarenko, and M. Zoeller. Activation-induced internalization differs for the tetraspanins CD9 and Tspan8: Impact on tumor cell motility. *Int J Biochem Cell Biol* 43 (1):106-19.

Record, M., C. Subra, S. Silvente-Poirot, and M. Poirot. Exosomes as intercellular signalosomes and pharmacological effectors. *Biochem Pharmacol* 81 (10):1171-82.

Ristorcelli, E., E. Beraud, P. Verrando, C. Villard, D. Lafitte, V. Sbarra, D. Lombardo, and A. Verine. 2008. Human tumor nanoparticles induce apoptosis of pancreatic cancer cells. *FASEB J* 22 (9):3358-69.

Rose, A. A., A. A. Grosset, Z. Dong, C. Russo, P. A. Macdonald, N. R. Bertos, Y. St-Pierre, R. Simantov, M. Hallett, M. Park, L. Gaboury, and P. M. Siegel. Glycoprotein nonmetastatic B is an independent prognostic indicator of recurrence and a novel therapeutic target in breast cancer. *Clin Cancer Res* 16 (7):2147-56.

Rosell, R., J. Wei, and M. Taron. 2009. Circulating MicroRNA Signatures of Tumor-Derived Exosomes for Early Diagnosis of Non-Small-Cell Lung Cancer. *Clin Lung Cancer* 10 (1):8-9.

Rozario, T., and D. W. DeSimone. The extracellular matrix in development and morphogenesis: a dynamic view. *Dev Biol* 341 (1):126-40.

Saddawi-Konefka, R., and J. R. Crawford. Chronic viral infection and primary central nervous system malignancy. *J Neuroimmune Pharmacol* 5 (3):387-403.

Safaei, R., B. J. Larson, T. C. Cheng, M. A. Gibson, S. Otani, W. Naerdemann, and S. B. Howell. 2005. Abnormal lysosomal trafficking and enhanced exosomal export of cisplatin in drug-resistant human ovarian carcinoma cells. *Mol Cancer Ther* 4 (10):1595-604.

Sanderson, M. P., S. Keller, A. Alonso, S. Riedle, P. J. Dempsey, and P. Altevogt. 2008. Generation of novel, secreted epidermal growth factor receptor (EGFR/ErbB1) isoforms via metalloprotease-dependent ectodomain shedding and exosome secretion. *J Cell Biochem* 103 (6):1783-97.

Santandreu, F. M., M. Brell, A. H. Gene, R. Guevara, J. Oliver, M. E. Couce, and P. Roca. 2008. Differences in mitochondrial function and antioxidant systems between regions of human glioma. *Cell Physiol Biochem* 22 (5-6):757-68.

Sarkaria, J. N., G. J. Kitange, C. D. James, R. Plummer, H. Calvert, M. Weller, and W. Wick. 2008. Mechanisms of chemoresistance to alkylating agents in malignant glioma. *Clin Cancer Res* 14 (10):2900-8.

Schorey, J. S., and S. Bhatnagar. 2008. Exosome function: from tumor immunology to pathogen biology. *Traffic* 9 (6):871-81.

Sharples, R. A., L. J. Vella, R. M. Nisbet, R. Naylor, K. Perez, K. J. Barnham, C. L. Masters, and A. F. Hill. 2008. Inhibition of gamma-secretase causes increased secretion of amyloid precursor protein C-terminal fragments in association with exosomes. *FASEB J* 22 (5):1469-78.

Shen, B., N. Wu, J. M. Yang, and S. J. Gould. Protein targeting to exosomes/microvesicles by plasma membrane anchors. *J Biol Chem* 286 (16):14383-95.

Simon, T., J. F. Fonteneau, and M. Gregoire. 2009. Dendritic cell preparation for immunotherapeutic interventions. *Immunotherapy* 1 (2):289-302.

Simpson, R. J., S. S. Jensen, and J. W. Lim. 2008. Proteomic profiling of exosomes: current perspectives. *Proteomics* 8 (19):4083-99.

Simpson, R. J., J. W. Lim, R. L. Moritz, and S. Mathivanan. 2009. Exosomes: proteomic insights and diagnostic potential. *Expert Rev Proteomics* 6 (3):267-83.

Singh, P. P., C. Lemaire, J. C. Tan, E. Zeng, and J. S. Schorey. Exosomes Released from M.tuberculosis Infected Cells Can Suppress IFN-gamma Mediated Activation of Naive Macrophages. *PLoS One* 6 (4):e18564.

Skog, J., T. Wurdinger, S. van Rijn, D. H. Meijer, L. Gainche, M. Sena-Esteves, W. T. Curry, Jr., B. S. Carter, A. M. Krichevsky, and X. O. Breakefield. 2008. Glioblastoma microvesicles transport RNA and proteins that promote tumour growth and provide diagnostic biomarkers. *Nat Cell Biol* 10 (12):1470-6.

Sonabend, A. M., K. Dana, and M. S. Lesniak. 2007. Targeting epidermal growth factor receptor variant III: a novel strategy for the therapy of malignant glioma. *Expert Rev Anticancer Ther* 7 (12 Suppl):S45-50.

Soto-Guzman, A., N. Navarro-Tito, L. Castro-Sanchez, R. Martinez-Orozco, and E. P. Salazar. Oleic acid promotes MMP-9 secretion and invasion in breast cancer cells. *Clin Exp Metastasis* 27 (7):505-15.

Staubach, S., H. Razawi, and F. G. Hanisch. 2009. Proteomics of MUC1-containing lipid rafts from plasma membranes and exosomes of human breast carcinoma cells MCF-7. *Proteomics* 9 (10):2820-35.

Stetler-Stevenson, W. G. 2008. Tissue inhibitors of metalloproteinases in cell signaling: metalloproteinase-independent biological activities. *Sci Signal* 1 (27):re6.

Stoeck, A., S. Keller, S. Riedle, M. P. Sanderson, S. Runz, F. Le Naour, P. Gutwein, A. Ludwig, E. Rubinstein, and P. Altevogt. 2006. A role for exosomes in the constitutive and stimulus-induced ectodomain cleavage of L1 and CD44. *Biochem J* 393 (Pt 3):609-18.

Stoorvogel, W., M. J. Kleijmeer, H. J. Geuze, and G. Raposo. 2002. The biogenesis and functions of exosomes. *Traffic* 3 (5):321-30.

Stupp, R., W. P. Mason, M. J. van den Bent, M. Weller, B. Fisher, M. J. Taphoorn, K. Belanger, A. A. Brandes, C. Marosi, U. Bogdahn, J. Curschmann, R. C. Janzer, S. K. Ludwin, T. Gorlia, A. Allgeier, D. Lacombe, J. G. Cairncross, E. Eisenhauer, and R. O. Mirimanoff. 2005. Radiotherapy plus concomitant and adjuvant temozolomide for glioblastoma. *N Engl J Med* 352 (10):987-96.

Subra, C., K. Laulagnier, B. Perret, and M. Record. 2007. Exosome lipidomics unravels lipid sorting at the level of multivesicular bodies. *Biochimie* 89 (2):205-12.

Szajnik, M., M. Czystowska, M. J. Szczepanski, M. Mandapathil, and T. L. Whiteside. Tumor-derived microvesicles induce, expand and up-regulate biological activities of human regulatory T cells (Treg). *PLoS One* 5 (7):e11469.

Tamboli, I. Y., E. Barth, L. Christian, M. Siepmann, S. Kumar, S. Singh, K. Tolksdorf, M. T. Heneka, D. Lutjohann, P. Wunderlich, and J. Walter. Statins promote the degradation of extracellular amyloid {beta}-peptide by microglia via stimulation of exosome-associated insulin-degrading enzyme (IDE) secretion. *J Biol Chem* 285 (48):37405-14.

Taylor, D. D., and C. Gercel-Taylor. 2005. Tumour-derived exosomes and their role in cancer-associated T-cell signalling defects. *Br J Cancer* 92 (2):305-11.

———. 2008. MicroRNA signatures of tumor-derived exosomes as diagnostic biomarkers of ovarian cancer. *Gynecol Oncol* 110 (1):13-21.

Thery, C., L. Zitvogel, and S. Amigorena. 2002. Exosomes: composition, biogenesis and function. *Nat Rev Immunol* 2 (8):569-79.

Tomihari, M., J. S. Chung, H. Akiyoshi, P. D. Cruz, Jr., and K. Ariizumi. DC-HIL/glycoprotein Nmb promotes growth of melanoma in mice by inhibiting the activation of tumor-reactive T cells. *Cancer Res* 70 (14):5778-87.

Trajkovic, K., C. Hsu, S. Chiantia, L. Rajendran, D. Wenzel, F. Wieland, P. Schwille, B. Brugger, and M. Simons. 2008. Ceramide triggers budding of exosome vesicles into multivesicular endosomes. *Science* 319 (5867):1244-7.

Trams, E. G., C. J. Lauter, N. Salem, Jr., and U. Heine. 1981. Exfoliation of membrane ecto-enzymes in the form of micro-vesicles. *Biochim Biophys Acta* 645 (1):63-70.

Tran, K. T., L. Griffith, and A. Wells. 2004. Extracellular matrix signaling through growth factor receptors during wound healing. *Wound Repair Regen* 12 (3):262-8.

Tse, K. F., M. Jeffers, V. A. Pollack, D. A. McCabe, M. L. Shadish, N. V. Khramtsov, C. S. Hackett, S. G. Shenoy, B. Kuang, F. L. Boldog, J. R. MacDougall, L. Rastelli, J. Herrmann, M. Gallo, G. Gazit-Bornstein, P. D. Senter, D. L. Meyer, H. S.

Lichenstein, and W. J. LaRochelle. 2006. CR011, a fully human monoclonal antibody-auristatin E conjugate, for the treatment of melanoma. *Clin Cancer Res* 12 (4):1373-82.

Valadi, H., K. Ekstrom, A. Bossios, M. Sjostrand, J. J. Lee, and J. O. Lotvall. 2007. Exosome-mediated transfer of mRNAs and microRNAs is a novel mechanism of genetic exchange between cells. *Nat Cell Biol* 9 (6):654-9.

Valenti, R., V. Huber, M. Iero, P. Filipazzi, G. Parmiani, and L. Rivoltini. 2007. Tumor-released microvesicles as vehicles of immunosuppression. *Cancer Res* 67 (7):2912-5.

Varki, A. 2007. Trousseau's syndrome: multiple definitions and multiple mechanisms. *Blood* 110 (6):1723-9.

Vella, L. J., D. L. Greenwood, R. Cappai, J. P. Scheerlinck, and A. F. Hill. 2008. Enrichment of prion protein in exosomes derived from ovine cerebral spinal fluid. *Vet Immunol Immunopathol* 124 (3-4):385-93.

Verhoeff, J. J., O. van Tellingen, A. Claes, L. J. Stalpers, M. E. van Linde, D. J. Richel, W. P. Leenders, and W. R. van Furth. 2009. Concerns about anti-angiogenic treatment in patients with glioblastoma multiforme. *BMC Cancer* 9:444.

Vivanco, I., and I. K. Mellinghoff. Epidermal growth factor receptor inhibitors in oncology. *Curr Opin Oncol* 22 (6):573-8.

Walker, J. D., C. L. Maier, and J. S. Pober. 2009. Cytomegalovirus-infected human endothelial cells can stimulate allogeneic CD4+ memory T cells by releasing antigenic exosomes. *J Immunol* 182 (3):1548-59.

Wang, K., S. Zhang, J. Weber, D. Baxter, and D. J. Galas. Export of microRNAs and microRNA-protective protein by mammalian cells. *Nucleic Acids Res* 38 (20):7248-59.

Watanabe, T., E. M. Sorensen, A. Naito, M. Schott, S. Kim, and P. Ahlquist. 2007. Involvement of host cellular multivesicular body functions in hepatitis B virus budding. *Proc Natl Acad Sci U S A* 104 (24):10205-10.

Weber, G. F., M. A. Bjerke, and D. W. Desimone. Integrins and cadherins join forces to form adhesive networks. *J Cell Sci* 124 (Pt 8):1183-93.

Wikstrand, C. J., C. J. Reist, G. E. Archer, M. R. Zalutsky, and D. D. Bigner. 1998. The class III variant of the epidermal growth factor receptor (EGFRvIII): characterization and utilization as an immunotherapeutic target. *J Neurovirol* 4 (2):148-58.

Wittmann, J., and H. M. Jack. Serum microRNAs as powerful cancer biomarkers. *Biochim Biophys Acta* 1806 (2):200-7.

Xiang, X., A. Poliakov, C. Liu, Y. Liu, Z. B. Deng, J. Wang, Z. Cheng, S. V. Shah, G. J. Wang, L. Zhang, W. E. Grizzle, J. Mobley, and H. G. Zhang. 2009. Induction of myeloid-derived suppressor cells by tumor exosomes. *Int J Cancer* 124 (11):2621-33.

Yang, M., Y. Li, K. Chilukuri, O. A. Brady, M. I. Boulos, J. C. Kappes, and D. S. Galileo. L1 stimulation of human glioma cell motility correlates with FAK activation. *J Neurooncol.*

Yarden, Y. 2001. The EGFR family and its ligands in human cancer. signalling mechanisms and therapeutic opportunities. *Eur J Cancer* 37 Suppl 4:S3-8.

Ye, F., Q. Gao, and M. J. Cai. Therapeutic targeting of EGFR in malignant gliomas. *Expert Opin Ther Targets* 14 (3):303-16.

Zitvogel, L., A. Regnault, A. Lozier, J. Wolfers, C. Flament, D. Tenza, P. Ricciardi-Castagnoli, G. Raposo, and S. Amigorena. 1998. Eradication of established murine tumors using a novel cell-free vaccine: dendritic cell-derived exosomes. *Nat Med* 4 (5):594-600.

Zumaquero, E., P. Munoz, M. Cobo, G. Lucena, E. J. Pavon, A. Martin, P. Navarro, A. Garcia-Perez, A. Ariza-Veguillas, F. Malavasi, J. Sancho, and M. Zubiaur. Exosomes from human lymphoblastoid B cells express enzymatically active CD38 that is associated with signaling complexes containing CD81, Hsc-70 and Lyn. *Exp Cell Res* 316 (16):2692-706.

Recurrent Malignant Primary Brain Tumor: the Pathophysiology and Management

Victor Tse[1] and Harish Babu[2]
[1]*Department of Neurosurgery Kaiser Permanente Medical Center, Redwood City, CA*
[2]*Department of Neurosurgery Stanford University, Palo Alto, CA, USA*

1. Introduction

Malignant primary brain tumors exhibit high proliferation index and have the potential for local or distant dissemination. GBM is an example of this group of tumor. GBM is a World Health Organization (WHO) grade IV tumor. It represents 65% of all gliomas and 15-20% of all primary intracranial tumors (Louis et al., 2007). It is the most malignant astrocytic tumor, with histolopathological features of cellular polymorphism, high mitotic activity, microvascular proliferation, and necrosis (Louis et al., 2007). Despite advances in imaging techniques and multimodal treatment options, the overall prognosis of patients with GBM remains poor. In a large retrospective study, 2.2% of the cohort resulted in longer than 2-year survival (Scott et al., 1998). The median survival is between 12-18 months with maximal treatment. With medical advancements in the past five years, there is a slight improvement in the median survival of these patients; It is estimated that about 24% of patients who underwent gross total resection followed by adjuvant chemotherapy and radiation therapy will survive 24 months, while those without any intervention succumb rapidly from time of diagnosis (Davis et al., 1998; McLendon and Halperin, 2003). Very few cases of curative outcome or long term survival have been reported (Salvati et al., 1998; Yoshida et al., 2000). Overall, the 5-year survival rate is less than 10% with a final mortality rate of near 100% (Deen et al., 1993; Kleihues and Sobin, 2000).

GBM carries an unfavorable prognosis mainly due to its high propensity for tumor recurrence. It has been suggested that GBM recurrence is inevitable after a median survival time of 32-36 weeks (Ammirati et al., 1987; Choucair et al., 1986). The natural history of recurrent GBM (rGBM), however, is largely undefined due to the lack of uniform definition and criteria for tumor recurrence, the variability in treatment philosophy among treating physicians, and the heterogeneous nature of the disease, including distinct mechanisms believed to contribute to known subtypes of GBM. In this chapter, we have summarized the definition of recurrent GBM and provide an overview on the pathophysiology, the diagnostic pathways, and treatment algorithm of this disease. We have also included a brief synopsis on the future direction in the management and the experimental target-therapies of this disease.

2. Definition

Tumor recurrence is defined as the growth of tumor after treatment. However, the criteria used to diagnose rGBM remain ambiguous due to the variety in which new lesions present. The infiltrative nature of GBM cells makes it difficult to eliminate microscopic disease despite macroscopic gross total resection. Studies have shown that GBM recurrence most often occurs in the form of a local continuous growth within 2-3 cm from the border of the original lesion (Gaspar et al., 1992; Halperin et al., 1988; Lee et al., 1999). Choucair et al. reported that over 90% of glioma cases showed recurrence at the original tumor location, while 5% developed multiple lesions after treatment (Choucair et al., 1986). Although less common (≈10%), GBM may also recur with the development of new lesions that have little evidence of being contiguous with previous resection cavity, intraventricular spread, or dissemination along any anatomically definable subcortical white matter tracts (Loeffler et al., 1990). Bauman et al. has shown that uncommon relapse patterns are more prevalent in midline tumors and tumors that infiltrate both hemispheres (Bauman et al., 1998). Likewise, in an attempt to preserve neurological function and maintain patient quality of life, subtotal resections are sometimes performed when tumors infiltrate eloquent areas of the brain. In those circumstances, the residual tumor is treated with focal radiation in addition to conventional radiation therapy and chemotherapy. Tumor recurrence is, therefore defined by the appearance of residual tumor growth on imaging studies or the manifestation of new clinical symptoms. However, tumor recurrence is frequently used synonymously with tumor progression. Recurrent GBM is commonly referred as a change from previously documented stable tumor or an absence of tumor; it is an escape from prior tumor control. Certain authors define tumor progression from a residual tumor as a 25% increase in cross-sectional area of the tumor in the slice with the greatest amount of tumor or as a 25% increase in contrast enhancing volume (Suh and Olson, 1998), while recurrence has also been defined by a greater than 50% growth between two successive imaging studies (Barker et al., 1998). Setting aside the difference in the definition of rGBM, the "local" recurrence remains the single most striking common factor among all the patients whom have received a variety of chemotherapeutic agents, with different radiation dose and field volume, in addition to the extend of resection of the initial tumor. This suggests that the recurrence of GBM is intrinsic and independent to the choice of therapy.

3. The pathophysiology of tumor recurrence

Neural stem cell surface antigen CD133 has been used to prospectively isolate and characterize a rare population of cells within the tumor mass of GBM. This population of cells has a striking similarity to normal neural stem cells in its biology (Singh et al., 2004). Expansion of these cancer stem cells (CSC) replenishes the cells that constitute the expanding cells within the tumor. As these growing cells mature, they undergo terminal differentiation. It has been shown that there are at least two populations of cells in GBM specimens. They are the $CD133^{+}/telomerase^{High}$ which are presumed to be CSC and $CD133^{-}/telomerase^{Low}$ progenitor cells. There is general consensus that $CD133^{+}/telomerase^{High}$ CSC gives rise to $CD133^{-}/telomerase^{Low}$ progenitor cells. It is the proliferation of these progenitor cells that populate and makes up the tumor mass (Beier et al., 2011). Moreover, it has been shown that differentiated tumor cells are more susceptible to chemotherapy and radiation treatment, and are eliminated from the tumor mass. Additionally, terminally differentiated tumor cells will eventually die off by initiating cell death cascades and there is accumulation of CD133+ glioma cells following high-dose irradiation by Gamma Knife surgery (GKS) plus external beam radiation (Tamura et al., 2010). Similarly, there is an accumulation of CD133+ glioma cells, in residual tumors particularly within the necrotic areas after GKS plus EBRT treatment, whereas CD133+ cells are infrequent in tumors prior to therapy. It is postulated that the longevity of cancer stem cells and their resilience to therapies, give them the ability to serve as the reservoir for regeneration of the whole tumor, which provides a plausible explanation for the recurrence of GBM (Liu et al., 2009). Additionally, CD133+ cancer stem cells have a higher expression of BCRP1 and MGMT. The presence of anti-apoptosis protein and inhibitors of apoptosis protein families explain their ability to withstand chemotherapy (Liu et al., 2006).

An emerging hypothesis states that CSCs drive tumorigenesis by directly inducing an inflammatory phenotype within the tumor and facilitate immuno-editing. This occurs by recruiting immunocytes and promoting stromal remodeling as seen in aberrant stem cell–vascular niche that contributes to myeloproliferative diseases (Walkley et al., 2007). In response to tumor-derived cytokines, these macrophages acquire the M2 phenotype (Stout et al., 2005). Macrophages are a potent source of the mediators that perpetuate the inflammatory process, and they release reactive oxygen and nitrogen species. ROS have also been shown to modify the activity of myeloid-derived suppressor cells (MDSCs). These cells inhibit anti-tumor immunity thus promoting tumors. In combination with nitric oxide, MDSC-derived ROS contribute to the generation of peroxynitrite (Nagaraj and Gabrilovich, 2007). The latter causes the nitration of various proteins on Tyrosine, including the T-cell receptor CD8. This modification alters antigen recognition and thereby induces T-cell tolerance (Movahedi et al., 2008). Moreover, MDSCs are directly involved in tumor angiogenesis, they stimulate angiogenesis and ECM breakdown through the production of angiogenic growth factors and MMPs. Secretion of MMPs and other proteinases by macrophages enhance cancer-cell motility, dispersion and invasion. Collectively, CSCs promote expansion of tumor mass, invasion, and revival of senescence cells.

4. The clinical profile of patients with recurrent glioblastomas

The patients with rGBM tend to be male with a reasonable Karnofsky Performance Score (KPS) and in age group of 50 to 60. This skewed epidemiological profile can easily be the reflection of the variability of treatment algorithms and patients selection employed at different institutions. In a multi-center trial of 222 patients with rGBM for evaluation of intra-operative placement of biodegradable wafer, the patient cohort was predominantly male (64.5%) in the fifth decade of life (48 years old). (Brem et al., 1995). Among a cohort of 301 GBM patients, Barker et al. identified 223 patients with tumor recurrence (Barker et al., 1998). Without selection bias, 64% of patients had a KPS >70 at time of recurrence. These predominantly male patients (63%) had a mean age of 54 years. The median interval from initial diagnosis until clinical or radiographic evidence of tumor recurrence was 4.9 months.

In majority of the patients, GBM recurrence is detected during imaging surveillance or by the development of new or recurring symptoms and signs. The single most commonly reported symptom is easy fatigue. In a questionnaire-based study, patients with rGBM or anaplastic astrocytoma with a KPS >70 self-reported the following symptoms: fatigue, uncertainty about the future, motor difficulties, drowsiness, communication difficulties, and headaches (Osoba et al., 2000a). While most symptoms were likely due to tumor recurrence, the authors stated that confounding factors such as radiation necrosis and steroid treatments may have contributed to generalized fatigue, whereas headache and uncertainty of the future may have been nonspecific for brain cancer. Difficulties with motor-sensory function and vision may be directly related to mass effect or edema.

The most commonly encountered dilemma in diagnosing rGBM is the uncertainty in differentiating real tumor progression from that of pseudo-progression/radiation necrosis at and around the previously treated site. Pseudo-progression is defined as progressive contrast enhancement in imaging study within the first three months (in 58% of the cases) of finishing treatment. Patients with pseudo-progression can be symptomatic but are highly responsive to steroid therapy. They account for 28-51% of the cases, and 9-14% of these patients will eventually show stable disease or resolution. The true mechanism of pseudoprogression is unclear. It is thought to be an exacerbated response to effective therapy (Chamberlain, 2008; Chamberlain et al., 2007; de Wit et al., 2004). Conversely, radiation is toxic to both rapid dividing tumor and the surrounding endothelium and oligodendroglial cells. This will result in demyelinating and coagulopathic necrotizing reaction 4-6 months after treatment. Importantly, radiation necrosis can mimic rGBM with its contrast enhancement, progression, and edema.

Radiation necrosis versus progression of gliomas can be positively differentiated in biopsy specimens. Should a biopsy be non-feasible, imaging becomes the next best option for evaluation. Positron Emission Tomography (PET) is not used for initial diagnosis of GBM due to relatively inferior image resolution compared to MRI. Rather [^{18}F] fluorodeoxyglucose (FDG)-PET is used to demonstrate increased regional glucose metabolism, which has been shown to correlate with tumor cellularity and patient survival (Ishikawa et al., 1993). In a study evaluating surgical outcomes of rGBM, Barker et al. included four patients whose PET suggested proliferation despite an MRI indication of a <50% increase in size of residual tumor (Barker et al., 1998). It is particularly useful in the early detection of rGBM in cases with unclear MRI information. While radiation necrosis mimics tumor recurrence on MRI, it is readily detectable with PET due to its low metabolic characteristics. Therefore, PET imaging plays an important role in the management of irradiated patients who develop new lesions or symptoms (Ishikawa et al., 1993). PET imaging has a specificity of >90% in distinguishing radiation necrosis from rGBM, however, it lacks the sensitivity to make it reliable (Thompson et al., 1999). The use of amino acid tracers such as [^{11}C]methionine and [^{18}F] tyrosine is shown to improve the sensitivity especially, when MRI-PET is used (Thiel et al., 2000).

The use of serial proton magnetic resonance spectroscopy (MRS) is becoming a standard protocol in the imaging rGBMs. This imaging technique, which can append current conventional MR imaging protocols, allows serial monitoring of tumor progression. With the ability to characterize abnormal processes based on their metabolic signature, It has shown that MRS can be used to discriminate between localized radiation necrosis and recurrent tumor possessing elevated choline levels after brachytherapy (Wald et al., 1997) (See Table 1). In a recent study of 29 patients, Weybright et al. found that both tumor recurrence and radiation necrosis demonstrated increased Cho:Cr ratio, Cho/NAA ratio, and decreased NAA/Cr when compare to normal brain (Weybright et al., 1998). However, the changes appear significantly greater when comparing tumor recurrence and radiation necrosis (Cho/Cr: 2.52 vs 1.57; Cho/NAA: 3.48 vs 1.31; NAA/Cr: 0.79 vs 1.22). Similarly, Rock et. al. were able to correctly predict the histopathology of the subsequently resected specimen in the case of pure radiation necrosis or pure tumor recurrence (Rock et al., 2002). However, it was noted that in specimens with mixed necrosis and neoplasm, the spectral patterns were less definitive. Histologically, radiation injury is characterized by damage to the vascular endothelium that may result in ischemia and necrosis. In those circumstances one will expect an elevated lactate reflecting severe tissue ischemia and a severely depressed levels of NAA, choline, and creatine. In addition, radiation necrosis shows a broad peak between 0 and 2 ppm corresponding to cellular breakdown products and probably consisting of free fatty acids, and amino acids; whereas, in tumor recurrence one will find an elevated choline/NAA, elevated choline/creatine, and the presence of lactate. Unfortunately, within the same mass, there may be areas of radiation necrosis in combination with areas of viable tumor, reducing the specificity of MR spectroscopy. Thus, while MRS can be a practical noninvasive screening technique, certain limitations exist at this time.

	MRI (w/ gadolinium)	MRS	MR Perfusion	PET
Tumor	Hyperintense	↑↑ Cho / NAA ↑↑ Ch / Cr ↓↓ NAA / Cr	↑ rCBV (>2.6) ↑ Enhancement rate (dI/dt)	↑ Metabolic activity (↑ glucose uptake)
Radiation Necrosis	Hypointense	↑ Cho / NAA ↑ Ch / Cr ↓ NAA / Cr	↓ rCBV (<0.6) ↓ Enhancement rate (dI/dt)	↓ Metabolic activity (↓ glucose uptake)

Table 1. The Characteristic of Tumor and Radiation Necrosis in MRI and PET imaging studies.

Magnetic Resonance Perfusion (MRP) has recently been used to assess tissue vascular physiology and to distinguish the recurrence of tumors from radiation necrosis, especially with current interest in antiangiogenic therapy for the treatment of GBM. Contrast-enhancing T2-weighted echo-planar imaging has been evaluated for use in determining treatment response of recurrent malignant gliomas, specifically to thalidomide and carboplatin and to identify radiation necrosis (Cha et al., 2000). In general, radiation necrosis typically shows decreased relative cerebral blood volume (rCBV), whereas tumor recurrence results in high rCBV (Aronen and Perkio, 2002). For example, using gradient-echo dynamic susceptibility perfusion MR imaging, Sugahara et al found that lesions with rCBV greater than 2.6 was indicative of tumor recurrence, while rCBV of less than 0.6 was consistent with radiation necrosis (Sugahara et al., 2000). However, there was significant overlap between the groups, requiring other modalities such as PET or single photon emission computed tomography (SPECT) to allow differentiation. Using more delayed, T1-weighted MR permeability methods, Hazle et al. reliably distinguished between tumor recurrence, radiation necrosis, or a combination of both factors, using an empiric model to study the rate of contrast enhancement (Hazle et al., 1997). In this study of 95 patients, the authors found that radiation necrosis and glioma tissue enhance at different rates, with recurrent tumors having the greatest mean maximal enhancement rates, mixed radiation necrosis and tumor having intermediate rate, and pure tumor necrosis having slowest rate.

5. Treatment options

With treatment options for rGBM relatively limited, physicians, patients and the patients' families have to be realistic with their therapeutic goals. The primary goal is palliative rather than curative. The ultimate aim is to preserve or restore neurological function to allow and prolong patients' comfort, independency, dignity and improved quality of life. The Canadian GBM recommendation committee's practical guideline-2007 addresses the issue of recurrent GBM and provides a relatively clear directive for practicing physicians. It states "Selected patients with recurrent GBM may be candidates for repeat resection when the situation appears favorable based on an assessment of individual patient factors such as medical history, functional status, and location of the tumor. Entry into a clinical trial is recommended for patients with recurrent disease" (Mason et al., 2007). It essentially stating that aggressive treatment should only be entertained if there is (1) reasonable chance to prolong meaningful survival and (2) there is "follow-up" experimental or salvaging treatment. Other than that, no aggressive treatment such as surgery or radiosurgery should be considered.

Surgical intervention is essential in the initial treatment of GBM. It is well documented that the extent of surgery, ranging from biopsy to subtotal resection to gross total resection can effect overall patient survival (Black, 1991a, b; Chamberlain and Kormanik, 1998; Mahaley et al., 1989). Gross total resection can double median survival as compared to just having a biopsy, and in some study gross total resection has a significant survival advantage as compared to subtotal or partial resection (80, 48, and 44 weeks respectively) (Nitta and Sato, 1995). When faced with evidence of rGBM, surgical intervention requires clear identification of short-term goals and a diligent consideration of overall prognosis including potential treatment side effects. In patients without medical contraindications, surgery can confirm tumor recurrence, reduce intracranial pressure, improve neurological status, and possibly improve efficacy of adjunctive therapy.

In patients with low KPS score and/or other co-morbidity, stereotactic biopsy is particularly relevant in making management decisions and potentially can expand treatment options especially when imaging studies fail to differentiate between radiation necrosis and tumor recurrence. Stereotactic approach allows for the sampling of small, inaccessible, or even multiple lesions with minimal morbidity and mortality (estimated to be 2-5% and <1% respectively) (Suh and Olson, 1998). Stereotactic aspiration of tumor-associated cyst may offer short-term relief to patient symptoms secondary to mass effect. While uncommonly used, chemotherapy or radioactive agents for interstitial brachytherapy may also be introduced. Although stereotactic biopsy is frequently performed with relatively low risk, clinicians must be aware of potential complications associated with small sampling. Multiple-pass sampling may improve overall sensitivity but must be weighed against the increased risk of hemorrhage.

The efficacy and utility of re-resection alone in rGBM remains controversial due to a lack of randomized clinical trials evaluating this intervention independently. The majority of studies are confounded by the inherit selection bias to perform surgery on patients with high functional status, favorable anatomical locations, and lack of medical contraindications. The potential variability in the extent of surgical resection combined with the absence of uniform treatments for the initial disease render randomized control studies impractical. Despite these limitations, several studies in the literature provide anecdotal evidence and justification for re-resection in a select subset of patients with rGBM.

Prior redo-craniotomy studies, have showed the median survival time after surgical resection to be 14-50 weeks (Ammirati et al., 1987; Barker et al., 1998; Brem et al., 1995; Nieder et al., 2000; Sipos et al., 1997; Subach et al., 1999). The median survival from the time of initial GBM diagnosis among these patients was 13-22 months (Nieder et al., 2000). Rostomily et al. reported a prolonged progression-free survival of 7 weeks in patients undergoing combined chemotherapy plus re-resection versus chemotherapy alone (21 vs. 14 weeks) (Rostomily et al., 1994). However, the overall survival among this cohort of 51 patients was equivocal. Barker et al. performed a retrospective review of 222 patients with rGBM. In this study, the 46 patients who underwent secondary surgery and adjunctive therapy demonstrated a median survival time of 36 weeks post-resection (Barker et al., 1998). In comparison, patients who received similar chemotherapy and/or radiation had a median survival time of 23 wks. Interestingly, 28% of patients in the re-resection group had an improved KPS, while 49% had similar functional status. The authors noted that while the results were likely secondary to selection bias, subset of patients with rGBM might potentially benefit from surgical re-resection.

In addition to decreasing mass effect, redo-craniotomy allows for the potential administration of in situ delivery of chemotherapy or brachytherapy. In a randomized study evaluating the efficacy of Carmustine (BCNU) implantation during re-resection versus placebo, Brem et al. reported a 50% improvement in survival at 6 months following treatment (56% vs. 36%) (Brem et al., 1995). In this study, commonly discussed side effects such as serious intracranial infections (2.2%), post operative seizures, and steroid requirements for edema were reported to be within accepted ranges for redo surgery alone. The consensus belief that remains that the morbidity is higher in re-operation and wound dehiscence is relative common (5-18%).

Overall, surgical resection in rGBM may provide a modest benefit in survival (extends median survival by 36 weeks) and/or improvement in quality of life (10 weeks of high quality survival when the pre-operative KPS is > 70) within a subset of patients. Brem et al. showed that pre-operative performance status and age were significant prognostic factors (Brem et al., 1995). Similarly, in a multivariate analysis by Ammirati et al, performance status was found to be a significant predictor of outcome, however patient age appeared to be noncontributory (Ammirati et al., 1987). The extent of initial resection has also been shown to influence patient survival (Durmaz et al., 1997). While minor discrepancies exist among different studies, the general consensus is that surgical resection should be seriously considered in those with a high KPS (>70) and whose lesions are in a favorable location. Similarly, the time from the initial resection to clinical recurrence is also a useful prognosticator for re-operation.

6. Chemotherapy

Chemotherapy remains the main component in the salvage treatment of recurrent malignant gliomas (Chamberlain and Kormanik, 1998; Combs et al., 2005). Chemotherapeutic agents such as temozolomide (TMZ), carboplatin, procarabzine (PCB), Bevacizumab, irinotecan, and imatinib mesylate are currently been used in a variety of schema to treat rGBMs (Osoba et al., 2000b). These drugs have been administered as a single-agent, multi-agent, interstitial, intrathecal and combinatorial therapies, and are hypothesized to decrease the risk of death by approximately 15% (Stewart, 2002). In this study the 2-year survival for individuals with GBM increased from 9% to 13% when chemotherapy was used.

The treatment of rGBM tumors with TMZ is promising and with a favorable toxicity profile. One has to differentiate between treatment failure and escape. Most of the patients with rGBM are relapsed from remission. In a study by Brandes et al., patients who were treated for recurrent or progressive GBM with a TMZ chemotherapy regimen showed an overall response rate of 19% and mean time to progression of 11.7 wks (Brandes et al., 2002). Similarly, it was found that treatment of rGBM with a standard TMZ regimen (150 to 200 mg/m^2 x 5 days in 28-day cycles) produced a progression free survival of 6 months (PFS-6) of 21% vs. another chemo-agent PCB which produced an 8% PFS-6 (Yung et al., 2000). However, more recent studies have shown that a more rigorous regimen (150 mg/m^2 daily on a week on/week off cycle) may yield a PFS-6 as high as 48% with an overall PFS-12 of 81% (Wick et al., 2004). A similar study has shown that PFS-6 as high as 43.8% with an overall survival (OAS) of 8.4 months. But when TMZ is used as a five days a week cycle, the PFS-6 is noted to be 39% and the OAS is 7.8 weeks. A Various combinatorial strategies have been examined including TMZ plus marimastat, a matrix metalloproteinase inhibitor, or 13-cis-retinoic acid, resulting in a PFS-6 of 39% and 32%, respectively (Jaeckle et al., 2003).

7. Antiangiogenic treatment

Increasingly, therapy that is targeting tumor angiogenesis has proven to be effective in tumor control and stabilization. Bevacizumab targets tumor angiogenesis by neutralizing VEGF-A. In May 2009, the US food and Drug Aministration (FDA) has granted accelerated approval for Bevacizumab for use in patients with rGBM. A noticeable response (26%) with a median duration of response is 4.2 months is observed in the AV3708g trial, and a 20% response with a median duration of 3.9 months is reported in the NCI 06-C-0064E study, in which Bevacizumab is used on its own. However, it has been shown that antiangiogenic treatment in the form of monotherapy produces limited clinical effects; and its delayed onset allows tumor progression and reduces its use for end-stage disease (O'Reilly, 2006). However, the use of antiangiogenics in a combinatorial fashion may provide better results (Baumann et al., 2004). Often coupled with a chemotherapy agent, antiangiogenic therapies have been shown to be effective in primary GBM tumors producing a survival time of 16 months (Tuettenberg et al., 2005). Similarly, in determining which chemotherapeutic to use, it has been shown that PTK-787 (a VEGF receptor inhibitor) combined with TMZ produced a median time to progression of 15.1 wks vs. PTK-787 combined with CCNU which resulted in 10.4 wks (Zhang and Chakravarti, 2006). One of the most promising combinations is the use of Bevacizumab with irinotecan (CPT-11). With this regimen the PFS-6 and OSA is 50% and 8.7 months while with Bevacizumab on its own, the PFS and OAS was 42% and 9.2 months respectively (Jakobsen et al., 2011).

In our institute, the choice of salvaging chemotherapy for patients with rGBM is mainly based on their past therapeutic history and the toxicity profile. In general, we like to use

Bevacizumab, or Bevacizumab/CPT-11 as the first line therapy. It is especially preferred when Stereotactic radiosurgery is planned.

8. Stereotactic radiation and brachytherapy

Stereotactic radiosurgery (SRS) and hypofractionated radiotherapy are non-invasive methods for the delivery of localized irradiation, and have been shown to be effective in treating rGBM (Combs et al., 2005; Romanelli et al., 2009). The median survival of patients undergoing single fraction SRS therapy (median dose of 15 Gy) for rGBM tumors was 10 months (Combs et al., 2005). This finding is consistent with several other studies that report similar survival times (Mahajan et al., 2005; Shrieve et al., 1995). The risks associated with SRS treatment include the possibility of radiation induced necrosis, edema, hydrocephalus, worsening of pre-existing symptoms, and radiation toxicity. Specifically, the application of SRS to larger tumors has been avoided due to an increased risk of radiation induced toxicity and mass effect (Shaw et al., 2000). However, in a recent study hypofractionated stereotactic radiosurgery in combination with Bevacizumab resulted in a OAS of 12.5 months, PFS-6 of 65% and an over all response rate of 50%, along with relatively lower radiation toxicity profile.

The use of brachytherapy has evolved over the last decade. Primarily a treatment for rGBM, brachytherapy is associated with an increase in survival time. Interstitial brachytherapy is used to target greater radiation doses to tumor cells while limiting exposure to surrounding normal brain tissue. Latest brachytherapy techniques report a median survival time (post-brachytherapy) for rGBM of 9.1 months, a competitive figure when compared to re-resection alone, chemotherapy, or re-irradiation (Chan et al., 2005). Similarly, it has also been shown that treatment of rGBM tumors with high-activity removable iodine-125 interstitial brain implants elicits a long term (3-year) survival rate of 15% (Scharfen et al., 1992).

Unfortunately, the application of brachytherapy is limited. Only 20-30% of rGBM tumors meet the morphological and focal criteria necessary for the surgical intervention associated with brachytherapy (Salcman, 1994). In some cases, post-treatment reoperation is necessary to remove the therapeutic device or to address focal radiation necrosis. Possible complications associated with brachytherapy include the development of homonymous quadrantanopsia, focal necrosis, edema, and neurological deterioration (Shrieve et al., 1995). Nevertheless, the efficacy of brachytherapy treatment is similar to that of SRS. Comparing the outcome of patients treated with SRS vs. brachytherapy, there was an overall survival time of 10.2 months for SRS treated patients and 11.4 months for brachytherapy treated patients (Shrieve et al., 1995).

9. Novel therapies

Most of the recent developments in chemotherapy are focus on targeted molecular therapies against the epidermal growth factor receptor (EGFR), the mammalian target of rapamycin (mTOR), and other signal transduction pathway components. Small-molecule EGFR inhibitors such as gefitinib and erlotinib are well tolerated in patients with rGBM, but the results from multiple clinical trails are disappointing (Rich et al., 2004; van den Bent et al., 2009).

The use of Temsirolimus, an mTOR inhibitor, as a single agent shows marginal success. Combinations of several agents, such as EGFR inhibitors with inhibitors of mTOR and VEGF receptors (VEGFR), are now being evaluated. Agents targeting VEGF, VEGFR, and other proangiogenic signaling pathways are relatively promising. Cediranib, a small-molecule inhibitor of VEGFR, shows a response rate of 56% PFS-6 of 26% (Batchelor et al., 2007; Galanis et al., 2005). AZD2171, a pan-VEGF receptor tyrosine kinase inhibitor, normalizes tumor vasculature and alleviates edema in GBM patients (Batchelor et al., 2007). Sorafenib and sunitinib are FDA-approved TKi that target VEGFR, but they have limited activity in rGBM. Although antiangiogenic therapies are promising, the duration of response is limited. Other therapeutic approaches such as viral gene therapies, immunotherapies, and convection-enhanced delivery of targeted immunotoxins are undergoing evaluation, but their use in rGBM remains to be determined (Wen and Brandes, 2009).

10. Conclusion

Patients with GBM continue to have a poor prognosis. In patients who have completed first-line therapy, vigilant tumor surveillance with regularly scheduled imaging and clinical evaluations may enable early detection of tumor recurrence and allow for immediate treatments. With the frequent use of radiation therapy, potential radiation induced injury/necrosis remains the major nuance in differentiating patients who develop new or repeat symptoms due to tumor recurrence. Hopefully, novel imaging techniques can help to detect the activation of tumor progression at molecular and cellular levels before conventional radiographic changes are seen. But to date we still rely on MRS, MR Perfusion and diffusion studies, and PET imaging.

Limited evidence from randomized studies have shown that among patients determined to be favorable surgical candidates (high KPS, non-eloquent location, no medical contraindications), the addition of salvaging chemotherapy appears to provide progression free survival. TMZ is now the standard chemotherapy agent due to its administrative ease, minimal side effect profile and proven survival improvement. Its use is not restricted by previous administration. Re-operation should be considered in patients with high preoperative KPS or in those whose symptoms are secondary to mass effect from superficial non-eloquent regions. The benefits of SRS treatment and chemotherapy are similar and should be chosen based on their corresponding side effect profiles. In general, improved outcomes are witnessed with combinatorial radiotherapy and chemotherapy as compared to each treatment alone.

Current trends indicate that the treatment of rGBM will remain multimodal in nature. Further understanding of underlying tumor biology is essential in developing more effective strategies. Research in gene therapy, antiangiogenic antagonists, and immunotherapies, all hold great promises. With continual improvements in treatment and imaging technique it is the hope of clinicians, researchers, and patients that GBM may become a controllable disease with favorable prognosis. Nevertheless, there will be time when no further medical and surgical treatments are going to be effective in preserving the comfort and dignity of our patients. Then, as clinicians we have to have the insight to prepare our patients from the inevitable and address the end-of life issue, and introduce them to the expertise of our hospice service.

Agent	Phase	Target
2ME2	Phase II	inhibits HIF-1α
Cediranib	Phase II	VEGFR and PDGFR inhibitor
Enzastaurin	Phase II	Inhibits Protein Kinase C
Pazopanib	Phase II	VEGFR and PDGFR inhibitor
PTC299	Phase II	inhibits VEGF at the post-transcriptionally
sorafenib	Phase I/II	VEGFR, PDGFR and BRAF inhibitor
Sunitinib	Phase II	VEGFR and PDGFR inhibitor
Tandutinib	Phase II	Inhibits PDGFR
Vandetanib	Phase I/II	inhibits VEGFR and EGFR
Vatalanib	Phase I/II	VEGFR and PDGFR inhibitor
Vorinostat	Phase I	Inhibits Histone Deacetylases
ABT510	Phase II	inhibits CD36 receptor
Aflibercept	Phase I/II	decoy receptor for VEGF
ATN161	Phase II	peptide inhibits integrin a5ß1
Bevacizumab	Phase II/III	monoclonal antibody binds to VEGF
Cilengitide	Phase II/III	RGD synthetic peptide inhibits integrin avß3 and $a_v ß_5$
CT322	Phase I	Fibronectin based VEGFR inhibitor
Interferon Alfa 2b	Phase II	inhibits angiogenesis
TM601	Phase I	peptide binds to Annexin A2

The list includes use of agents as isolated or in combination with other dugs. Protein or peptide based inhibitors are shaded in grey.

Table 2. Antiangiogenic agents at various stages of clinical trial for rGBM

Neurosurgical treatment interventions are labeled in green.

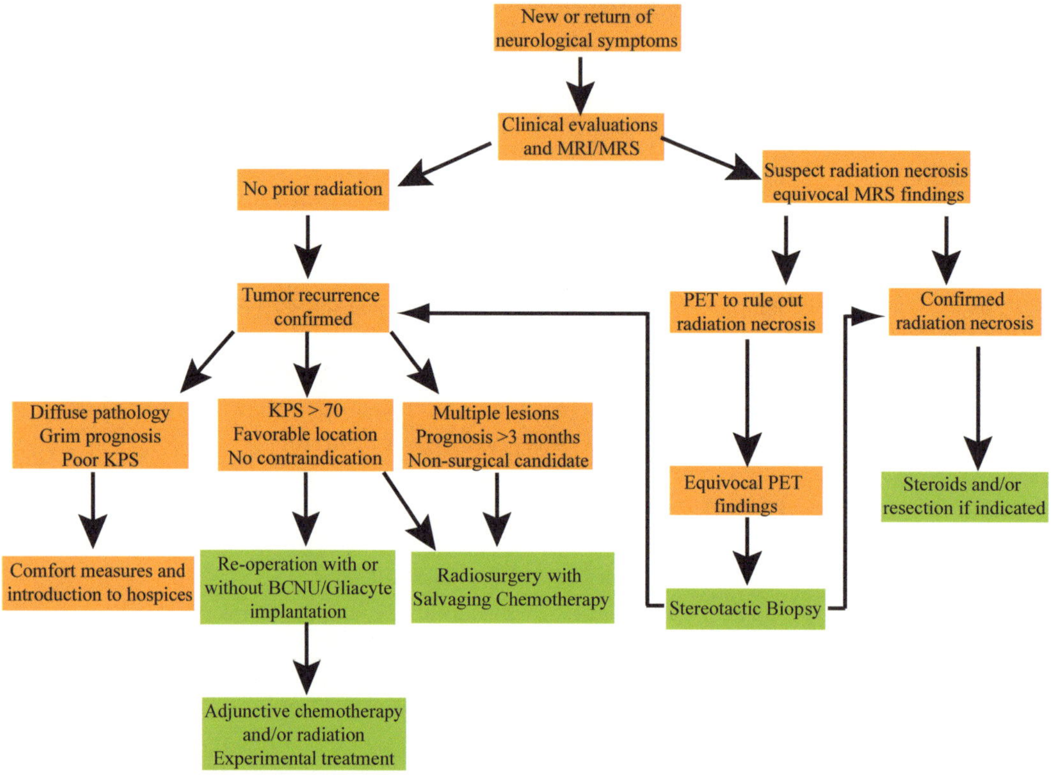

Fig. 1. Management algorithm of recurrent glioblastoma

11. References

Ammirati, M., Galicich, J.H., Arbit, E., and Liao, Y. (1987). Reoperation in the treatment of recurrent intracranial malignant gliomas. Neurosurgery *21*, 607-614.

Aronen, H.J., and Perkio, J. (2002). Dynamic susceptibility contrast MRI of gliomas. Neuroimaging Clin N Am *12*, 501-523.

Barker, F.G., 2nd, Chang, S.M., Gutin, P.H., Malec, M.K., McDermott, M.W., Prados, M.D., and Wilson, C.B. (1998). Survival and functional status after resection of recurrent glioblastoma multiforme. Neurosurgery *42*, 709-720; discussion 720-703.

Batchelor, T.T., Sorensen, A.G., di Tomaso, E., Zhang, W.T., Duda, D.G., Cohen, K.S., Kozak, K.R., Cahill, D.P., Chen, P.J., Zhu, M., *et al.* (2007). AZD2171, a pan-VEGF receptor tyrosine kinase inhibitor, normalizes tumor vasculature and alleviates edema in glioblastoma patients. Cancer cell *11*, 83-95.

Bauman, G.S., Fisher, B.J., Cairncross, J.G., and Macdonald, D. (1998). Bihemispheric malignant glioma: one size does not fit all. Journal of neuro-oncology *38*, 83-89.

Baumann, F., Bjeljac, M., Kollias, S.S., Baumert, B.G., Brandner, S., Rousson, V., Yonekawa, Y., and Bernays, R.L. (2004). Combined thalidomide and temozolomide treatment in patients with glioblastoma multiforme. Journal of neuro-oncology *67*, 191-200.

Beier, F., Beier, C.P., Aschenbrenner, I., Hildebrandt, G.C., Brummendorf, T.H., and Beier, D. (2011). Identification of CD133(-)/Telomerase (low) Progenitor Cells in Glioblastoma-Derived Cancer Stem Cell Lines. Cellular and molecular neurobiology *31*, 337-343.

Black, P.M. (1991a). Brain tumor. Part 2. N Engl J Med *324*, 1555-1564.

Black, P.M. (1991b). Brain tumors. Part 1. N Engl J Med *324*, 1471-1476.

Brandes, A.A., Ermani, M., Basso, U., Paris, M.K., Lumachi, F., Berti, F., Amista, P., Gardiman, M., Iuzzolino, P., Turazzi, S., *et al.* (2002). Temozolomide in patients with glioblastoma at second relapse after first line nitrosourea-procarbazine failure: a phase II study. Oncology *63*, 38-41.

Brem, H., Piantadosi, S., Burger, P.C., Walker, M., Selker, R., Vick, N.A., Black, K., Sisti, M., Brem, S., Mohr, G., *et al.* (1995). Placebo-controlled trial of safety and efficacy of intraoperative controlled delivery by biodegradable polymers of chemotherapy for recurrent gliomas. The Polymer-brain Tumor Treatment Group. Lancet *345*, 1008-1012.

Cha, S., Knopp, E.A., Johnson, G., Litt, A., Glass, J., Gruber, M.L., Lu, S., and Zagzag, D. (2000). Dynamic contrast-enhanced T2-weighted MR imaging of recurrent malignant gliomas treated with thalidomide and carboplatin. AJNR American journal of neuroradiology *21*, 881-890.

Chamberlain, M.C. (2008). Pseudoprogression in glioblastoma. Journal of clinical oncology : official journal of the American Society of Clinical Oncology *26*, 4359; author reply 4359-4360.

Chamberlain, M.C., Glantz, M.J., Chalmers, L., Van Horn, A., and Sloan, A.E. (2007). Early necrosis following concurrent Temodar and radiotherapy in patients with glioblastoma. Journal of neuro-oncology *82*, 81-83.

Chamberlain, M.C., and Kormanik, P.A. (1998). Practical guidelines for the treatment of malignant gliomas. The Western journal of medicine *168*, 114-120.

Chan, T.A., Weingart, J.D., Parisi, M., Hughes, M.A., Olivi, A., Borzillary, S., Alahakone, D., Detorie, N.A., Wharam, M.D., and Kleinberg, L. (2005). Treatment of recurrent glioblastoma multiforme with GliaSite brachytherapy. International journal of radiation oncology, biology, physics *62*, 1133-1139.

Choucair, A.K., Levin, V.A., Gutin, P.H., Davis, R.L., Silver, P., Edwards, M.S., and Wilson, C.B. (1986). Development of multiple lesions during radiation therapy and chemotherapy in patients with gliomas. Journal of neurosurgery *65*, 654-658.

Combs, S.E., Widmer, V., Thilmann, C., Hof, H., Debus, J., and Schulz-Ertner, D. (2005). Stereotactic radiosurgery (SRS): treatment option for recurrent glioblastoma multiforme (GBM). Cancer *104*, 2168-2173.

Davis, F.G., Freels, S., Grutsch, J., Barlas, S., and Brem, S. (1998). Survival rates in patients with primary malignant brain tumors stratified by patient age and tumor histological type: an analysis based on Surveillance, Epidemiology, and End Results (SEER) data, 1973-1991. Journal of neurosurgery *88*, 1-10.

de Wit, M.C., de Bruin, H.G., Eijkenboom, W., Sillevis Smitt, P.A., and van den Bent, M.J. (2004). Immediate post-radiotherapy changes in malignant glioma can mimic tumor progression. Neurology *63*, 535-537.

Deen, D.F., Chiarodo, A., Grimm, E.A., Fike, J.R., Israel, M.A., Kun, L.E., Levin, V.A., Marton, L.J., Packer, R.J., Pegg, A.E., *et al.* (1993). Brain Tumor Working Group Report on the 9th International Conference on Brain Tumor Research and Therapy. Organ System Program, National Cancer Institute. Journal of neuro-oncology *16*, 243-272.

Durmaz, R., Erken, S., Arslantas, A., Atasoy, M.A., Bal, C., and Tel, E. (1997). Management of glioblastoma multiforme: with special reference to recurrence. Clinical neurology and neurosurgery *99*, 117-123.

Galanis, E., Buckner, J.C., Maurer, M.J., Kreisberg, J.I., Ballman, K., Boni, J., Peralba, J.M., Jenkins, R.B., Dakhil, S.R., Morton, R.F., *et al.* (2005). Phase II trial of temsirolimus (CCI-779) in recurrent glioblastoma multiforme: a North Central Cancer Treatment Group Study. Journal of clinical oncology : official journal of the American Society of Clinical Oncology *23*, 5294-5304.

Gaspar, L.E., Fisher, B.J., Macdonald, D.R., LeBer, D.V., Halperin, E.C., Schold, S.C., Jr., and Cairncross, J.G. (1992). Supratentorial malignant glioma: patterns of recurrence and implications for external beam local treatment. International journal of radiation oncology, biology, physics *24*, 55-57.

Halperin, E.C., Burger, P.C., and Bullard, D.E. (1988). The fallacy of the localized supratentorial malignant glioma. International journal of radiation oncology, biology, physics *15*, 505-509.

Hazle, J.D., Jackson, E.F., Schomer, D.F., and Leeds, N.E. (1997). Dynamic imaging of intracranial lesions using fast spin-echo imaging: differentiation of brain tumors and treatment effects. J Magn Reson Imaging *7*, 1084-1093.

Ishikawa, M., Kikuchi, H., Miyatake, S., Oda, Y., Yonekura, Y., and Nishizawa, S. (1993). Glucose consumption in recurrent gliomas. Neurosurgery *33*, 28-33.

Jaeckle, K.A., Hess, K.R., Yung, W.K., Greenberg, H., Fine, H., Schiff, D., Pollack, I.F., Kuhn, J., Fink, K., Mehta, M., *et al.* (2003). Phase II evaluation of temozolomide and 13-cis-retinoic acid for the treatment of recurrent and progressive malignant glioma: a North American Brain Tumor Consortium study. Journal of clinical oncology : official journal of the American Society of Clinical Oncology *21*, 2305-2311.

Jakobsen, J.N., Hasselbalch, B., Stockhausen, M.T., Lassen, U., and Poulsen, H.S. (2011). Irinotecan and bevacizumab in recurrent glioblastoma multiforme. Expert opinion on pharmacotherapy *12*, 825-833.

Kleihues, P., and Sobin, L.H. (2000). World Health Organization classification of tumors. Cancer *88*, 2887.

Lee, S.W., Fraass, B.A., Marsh, L.H., Herbort, K., Gebarski, S.S., Martel, M.K., Radany, E.H., Lichter, A.S., and Sandler, H.M. (1999). Patterns of failure following high-dose 3-D conformal radiotherapy for high-grade astrocytomas: a quantitative dosimetric study. International journal of radiation oncology, biology, physics *43*, 79-88.

Liu, G., Yuan, X., Zeng, Z., Tunici, P., Ng, H., Abdulkadir, I.R., Lu, L., Irvin, D., Black, K.L., and Yu, J.S. (2006). Analysis of gene expression and chemoresistance of CD133+ cancer stem cells in glioblastoma. Molecular cancer *5*, 67.

Liu, Q., Nguyen, D.H., Dong, Q., Shitaku, P., Chung, K., Liu, O.Y., Tso, J.L., Liu, J.Y., Konkankit, V., Cloughesy, T.F., *et al.* (2009). Molecular properties of CD133+ glioblastoma stem cells derived from treatment-refractory recurrent brain tumors. Journal of neuro-oncology *94*, 1-19.

Loeffler, J.S., Alexander, E., 3rd, Hochberg, F.H., Wen, P.Y., Morris, J.H., Schoene, W.C., Siddon, R.L., Morse, R.H., and Black, P.M. (1990). Clinical patterns of failure following stereotactic interstitial irradiation for malignant gliomas. International journal of radiation oncology, biology, physics *19*, 1455-1462.

Louis, D.N., Ohgaki, H., Wiestler, O.D., Cavenee, W.K., Burger, P.C., Jouvet, A., Scheithauer, B.W., and Kleihues, P. (2007). The 2007 WHO classification of tumours of the central nervous system. Acta Neuropathol *114*, 97-109.

Mahajan, A., McCutcheon, I.E., Suki, D., Chang, E.L., Hassenbusch, S.J., Weinberg, J.S., Shiu, A., Maor, M.H., and Woo, S.Y. (2005). Case-control study of stereotactic radiosurgery for recurrent glioblastoma multiforme. Journal of neurosurgery *103*, 210-217.

Mahaley, M.S., Jr., Hipp, S.W., Dropcho, E.J., Bertsch, L., Cush, S., Tirey, T., and Gillespie, G.Y. (1989). Intracarotid cisplatin chemotherapy for recurrent gliomas. Journal of neurosurgery *70*, 371-378.

Mason, W.P., Maestro, R.D., Eisenstat, D., Forsyth, P., Fulton, D., Laperriere, N., Macdonald, D., Perry, J., and Thiessen, B. (2007). Canadian recommendations for the treatment of glioblastoma multiforme. Curr Oncol *14*, 110-117.

McLendon, R.E., and Halperin, E.C. (2003). Is the long-term survival of patients with intracranial glioblastoma multiforme overstated? Cancer *98*, 1745-1748.

Movahedi, K., Guilliams, M., Van den Bossche, J., Van den Bergh, R., Gysemans, C., Beschin, A., De Baetselier, P., and Van Ginderachter, J.A. (2008). Identification of discrete tumor-induced myeloid-derived suppressor cell subpopulations with distinct T cell-suppressive activity. Blood *111*, 4233-4244.

Nagaraj, S., and Gabrilovich, D.I. (2007). Myeloid-derived suppressor cells. Advances in experimental medicine and biology *601*, 213-223.

Nieder, C., Grosu, A.L., and Molls, M. (2000). A comparison of treatment results for recurrent malignant gliomas. Cancer treatment reviews *26*, 397-409.

Nitta, T., and Sato, K. (1995). Prognostic implications of the extent of surgical resection in patients with intracranial malignant gliomas. Cancer *75*, 2727-2731.

O'Reilly, M.S. (2006). Radiation combined with antiangiogenic and antivascular agents. Seminars in radiation oncology *16*, 45-50.

Osoba, D., Brada, M., Yung, W.K., and Prados, M. (2000a). Health-related quality of life in patients treated with temozolomide versus procarbazine for recurrent glioblastoma multiforme. J Clin Oncol *18*, 1481-1491.

Osoba, D., Brada, M., Yung, W.K., and Prados, M. (2000b). Health-related quality of life in patients treated with temozolomide versus procarbazine for recurrent glioblastoma multiforme. Journal of clinical oncology : official journal of the American Society of Clinical Oncology *18*, 1481-1491.

Rich, J.N., Reardon, D.A., Peery, T., Dowell, J.M., Quinn, J.A., Penne, K.L., Wikstrand, C.J., Van Duyn, L.B., Dancey, J.E., McLendon, R.E., *et al.* (2004). Phase II trial of gefitinib in recurrent glioblastoma. Journal of clinical oncology : official journal of the American Society of Clinical Oncology *22*, 133-142.

Rock, J.P., Hearshen, D., Scarpace, L., Croteau, D., Gutierrez, J., Fisher, J.L., Rosenblum, M.L., and Mikkelsen, T. (2002). Correlations between magnetic resonance spectroscopy and image-guided histopathology, with special attention to radiation necrosis. Neurosurgery *51*, 912-919; discussion 919-920.

Romanelli, P., Conti, A., Pontoriero, A., Ricciardi, G.K., Tomasello, F., De Renzis, C., Innocenzi, G., Esposito, V., and Cantore, G. (2009). Role of stereotactic radiosurgery and fractionated stereotactic radiotherapy for the treatment of recurrent glioblastoma multiforme. Neurosurgical focus *27*, E8.

Rostomily, R.C., Spence, A.M., Duong, D., McCormick, K., Bland, M., and Berger, M.S. (1994). Multimodality management of recurrent adult malignant gliomas: results of a phase II multiagent chemotherapy study and analysis of cytoreductive surgery. Neurosurgery *35*, 378-388; discussion 388.

Salcman, M. (1994). The value of cytoreductive surgery. Clinical neurosurgery *41*, 464-488.

Salvati, M., Cervoni, L., Artico, M., Caruso, R., and Gagliardi, F.M. (1998). Long-term survival in patients with supratentorial glioblastoma. Journal of neuro-oncology *36*, 61-64.

Scharfen, C.O., Sneed, P.K., Wara, W.M., Larson, D.A., Phillips, T.L., Prados, M.D., Weaver, K.A., Malec, M., Acord, P., Lamborn, K.R., *et al.* (1992). High activity iodine-125 interstitial implant for gliomas. International journal of radiation oncology, biology, physics *24*, 583-591.

Scott, J.N., Rewcastle, N.B., Brasher, P.M., Fulton, D., Hagen, N.A., MacKinnon, J.A., Sutherland, G., Cairncross, J.G., and Forsyth, P. (1998). Long-term glioblastoma multiforme survivors: a population-based study. Can J Neurol Sci *25*, 197-201.

Shaw, E., Scott, C., Souhami, L., Dinapoli, R., Kline, R., Loeffler, J., and Farnan, N. (2000). Single dose radiosurgical treatment of recurrent previously irradiated primary brain tumors and brain metastases: final report of RTOG protocol 90-05. International journal of radiation oncology, biology, physics *47*, 291-298.

Shrieve, D.C., Alexander, E., 3rd, Wen, P.Y., Fine, H.A., Kooy, H.M., Black, P.M., and Loeffler, J.S. (1995). Comparison of stereotactic radiosurgery and brachytherapy in the treatment of recurrent glioblastoma multiforme. Neurosurgery *36*, 275-282; discussion 282-274.

Singh, S., Hawkins, C., Clarke, I., Squire, J., Bayani, J., Hide, T., Henkelman, R., Cusimano, M., and Dirks, P. (2004). Identification of human brain tumour initiating cells. Nature *432*, 396-401.

Sipos, E.P., Tyler, B., Piantadosi, S., Burger, P.C., and Brem, H. (1997). Optimizing interstitial delivery of BCNU from controlled release polymers for the treatment of brain tumors. Cancer Chemother Pharmacol *39*, 383-389.

Stewart, L.A. (2002). Chemotherapy in adult high-grade glioma: a systematic review and meta-analysis of individual patient data from 12 randomised trials. Lancet *359*, 1011-1018.

Stout, R.D., Jiang, C., Matta, B., Tietzel, I., Watkins, S.K., and Suttles, J. (2005). Macrophages sequentially change their functional phenotype in response to changes in microenvironmental influences. J Immunol *175*, 342-349.

Subach, B.R., Witham, T.F., Kondziolka, D., Lunsford, L.D., Bozik, M., and Schiff, D. (1999). Morbidity and survival after 1,3-bis(2-chloroethyl)-1-nitrosourea wafer implantation for recurrent glioblastoma: a retrospective case-matched cohort series. Neurosurgery *45*, 17-22; discussion 22-13.

Sugahara, T., Korogi, Y., Tomiguchi, S., Shigematsu, Y., Ikushima, I., Kira, T., Liang, L., Ushio, Y., and Takahashi, M. (2000). Posttherapeutic intraaxial brain tumor: the value of perfusion-sensitive contrast-enhanced MR imaging for differentiating tumor recurrence from nonneoplastic contrast-enhancing tissue. AJNR American journal of neuroradiology *21*, 901-909.

Suh, D., and Olson, J. (1998). Management of recurrent malignant primary brain tumors. Part 1: Etiology, clinical diagnosis, and treatment options. Contemporary Neurosurgery *20*, 1–6.

Tamura, K., Aoyagi, M., Wakimoto, H., Ando, N., Nariai, T., Yamamoto, M., and Ohno, K. (2010). Accumulation of CD133-positive glioma cells after high-dose irradiation by Gamma Knife surgery plus external beam radiation. Journal of neurosurgery *113*, 310-318.

Thiel, A., Pietrzyk, U., Sturm, V., Herholz, K., Hovels, M., and Schroder, R. (2000). Enhanced accuracy in differential diagnosis of radiation necrosis by positron emission tomography-magnetic resonance imaging coregistration: technical case report. Neurosurgery *46*, 232-234.

Thompson, T.P., Lunsford, L.D., and Kondziolka, D. (1999). Distinguishing recurrent tumor and radiation necrosis with positron emission tomography versus stereotactic biopsy. Stereotactic and functional neurosurgery *73*, 9-14.

Tuettenberg, J., Grobholz, R., Korn, T., Wenz, F., Erber, R., and Vajkoczy, P. (2005). Continuous low-dose chemotherapy plus inhibition of cyclooxygenase-2 as an antiangiogenic therapy of glioblastoma multiforme. Journal of cancer research and clinical oncology *131*, 31-40.

van den Bent, M.J., Brandes, A.A., Rampling, R., Kouwenhoven, M.C., Kros, J.M., Carpentier, A.F., Clement, P.M., Frenay, M., Campone, M., Baurain, J.F., *et al.* (2009). Randomized phase II trial of erlotinib versus temozolomide or carmustine in recurrent glioblastoma: EORTC brain tumor group study 26034. Journal of clinical oncology : official journal of the American Society of Clinical Oncology *27*, 1268-1274.

Wald, L.L., Nelson, S.J., Day, M.R., Noworolski, S.E., Henry, R.G., Huhn, S.L., Chang, S., Prados, M.D., Sneed, P.K., Larson, D.A., *et al.* (1997). Serial proton magnetic resonance spectroscopy imaging of glioblastoma multiforme after brachytherapy. Journal of neurosurgery *87*, 525-534.

Walkley, C.R., Olsen, G.H., Dworkin, S., Fabb, S.A., Swann, J., McArthur, G.A., Westmoreland, S.V., Chambon, P., Scadden, D.T., and Purton, L.E. (2007). A microenvironment-induced myeloproliferative syndrome caused by retinoic acid receptor gamma deficiency. Cell *129*, 1097-1110.

Wen, P.Y., and Brandes, A.A. (2009). Treatment of recurrent high-grade gliomas. Curr Opin Neurol *22*, 657-664.

Weybright, P., Millis, K., Campbell, N., Cory, D.G., and Singer, S. (1998). Gradient, high-resolution, magic angle spinning 1H nuclear magnetic resonance spectroscopy of intact cells. Magn Reson Med *39*, 337-345.

Wick, W., Steinbach, J.P., Kuker, W.M., Dichgans, J., Bamberg, M., and Weller, M. (2004). One week on/one week off: a novel active regimen of temozolomide for recurrent glioblastoma. Neurology *62*, 2113-2115.

Yoshida, T., Kawano, N., Oka, H., Fujii, K., and Nakazato, Y. (2000). Clinical cure of glioblastoma--two case reports. Neurol Med Chir (Tokyo) *40*, 224-229.

Yung, W.K., Albright, R.E., Olson, J., Fredericks, R., Fink, K., Prados, M.D., Brada, M., Spence, A., Hohl, R.J., Shapiro, W., *et al.* (2000). A phase II study of temozolomide vs. procarbazine in patients with glioblastoma multiforme at first relapse. British journal of cancer *83*, 588-593.

Zhang, M., and Chakravarti, A. (2006). Novel radiation-enhancing agents in malignant gliomas. Seminars in radiation oncology *16*, 29-37.

Part 2

Sox Transcription Factors - CNS Tumors

5

The Role of Sox Transcription Factors in Brain Tumourigenesis

Maria Ferletta
Department of Immunology, Genetics and Pathology, Rudbeck laboratory, Uppsala University, Uppsala Sweden

1. Introduction

1.1 Brain tumours/ glioma and medulloblastoma

The total amount of brain tumours that effect humans is less than 2%. In children are brain tumours the second most common cancer type after leukaemia. Brain tumours and tumours in CNS (central nervous system) constitute 25% of all childhood tumours and is the most common cause of cancer mortality in children. Medulloblastoma is the most frequent malignant brain tumour type in children, whereas in adult glioblastoma multiforme (GBM) is the most malignant and common form. Although GBM occur in children but the diagnose is more uncommon.

Primary brain tumours are classified according to the World Health Organization (WHO) which means grading (I-IV) of the tumours based on tumour histology and pathology (Louis, et al., 2007). However, other criteria such as the age of the patient, tumour location, radiological features, surgical resection, proliferation index and genetic alterations are important when predicting a response of therapy (Louis, et al., 2007).

1.1.1 Glioma

Gliomas, tumours arise from glial cells, are the most common primary brain tumours of the central nervous system. Gliomas can be divided into astrocytomas, oligodendrogliomas, oligoastrocytomas and ependymomas based on their histological pattern (Louis, et al., 2007). Gliomas are further divided into four clinical grades based on their histology and pathology where GBM is a grade IV glioma. High grade gliomas are often biphasic tumours composed of distinct histological parts and they contain a very heterogeneous cell population (Kattar, et al., 1997). GBM develops either de novo (primary GBM), or through progression of lower grade glioma (secondary GBM). The number of genes and chromosomal changes are often correlated to glioma grade. For patients diagnosed with GBM, the mean survival time is less than 1 year. Most gliomas diffusely infiltrate the surrounding brain tissue which makes it very difficult to completely eliminate the tumour and which later makes the tumour relapse after treatment (Louis, et al., 2007). The cell-of-origin for gliomas is still not known but the origin is suggested to be a glial stem-like cell or progenitor cell.

Recently GBM is proposed to be subdivided in to four groups, classical, mesenchymal, proneural and neural, based on their specific gene-signature. The classical subgroup is primarily characterized by EGFR (Epithelial growth factor receptor) amplification and expression of stem cell and neural progenitor markers. The mesenchymal group is distinguished with deletions in *NF1* gene which results in low expression of NF1 (Neurofibromatosis type 1) and expression of mesenchymal markers such as CHI3L1 and MET. GBM of proneural origin are characterized by *PDGFR* alterations and mutations in the *IDH1* gene (isocitrate dehydrogenase 1). Further the proneural group express markers for oligodendrocytes as well as *SOX* genes. This group of GBM has somewhat longer survival. The features of the neural subgroup are expression of neural markers for instance *NEFL*, *GABRA1*, *SYT1* and *SLC12A5* (Phillips, et al., 2006; Verhaak, et al., 2010).

1.1.2 Medulloblastoma

Medulloblastoma is a highly invasive tumour located in the cerebellum, and belongs to the group of primitive neuroectodermal tumours (PNET), and generally affects children between three and nine years. Medulloblastoma is a grade IV tumour and the cell-of-origin is thought to be a pluripotent neural stem cells. Several chromosomal and genetical changes are identified in medulloblastoma. The most frequent change is isochromosome 17q. Other frequent genetical changes are affecting the Sonic hedgehog (Shh) signalling pathway, which are found in approximately 25% of medulloblastomas (Ellison, et al., 2003). Medulloblastoma is mainly divided into two subgroups, classical and desmoplastic medulloblastoma, and the tumour types differ in histology as well as in genetics (Ellison, et al., 2003). Recently medulloblastomas were subdivided into 5 different subtypes based on their characteristic gene-signature caused by genetic aberrations and mutations in specific signalling pathways as well as on their clinicopathological features (Kool, et al., 2008). The five subgroups are characterized by WNT-signalling (medulloblastoma type A), Shh-signalling (type B), neuronal differentiation (type C and D) and phosphoreceptor differentiation (type D and E) (Kool, et al., 2008).

A better insight and understanding of the molecular mechanisms behind infiltrative brain tumours and discovery of the cell-of-origin may help to generate novel ideas for treatment. Today treatment of brain tumours includes surgery if possible, radiation and chemotherapy but despite that tumours often recur and 50% of the GBM patients die within the first year (Holland, 2001). There have been many attempts to treat human gliomas but the success on the prognosis is still absent and this is mainly due to the diffuse infiltration of tumour cells into the normal brain tissue and unsuspected cell proliferation. Medulloblastomas are more sensitive to radiation and chemotherapy and about 60% are cured but many children suffer from severe side effects as motorical difficulties, learning problems and signs of fatigue (Ellison, et al., 2003).

1.2 Cancer stem cells/ progenitor cells

Current data suggest that initiation and progression of brain tumours are driven by cancer stem-like cells/progenitor cells. Cancer stem-like cells are rare tumour cells defined as cells which have the ability of unlimited self-renewal, the capacity to initiate and force tumour progression, and to differentiate into different cell lineages (Galderisi, et al., 2006). The cancer stem-like/progenitor cell has been identified in a number of studies of brain tumours (Galli, et al., 2004; Singh, et al., 2003; Yuan, et al., 2004) but exactly which cell that initially is transformed into the tumour initiating cell is still not clarified. Tumour progenitor cells have a slower division rate which could make them more resistant to treatment than the bulk tumour and which later can re-generate the tumour (Hirschmann-Jax, et al., 2004; G. Liu, et al., 2006). Cancer stem-like cells are believed to be responsible for tumour initiation, progression and for tumour relapse, which make the cancer stem-like cell become a recent and very interesting target for novel and more effective therapies. There are many mechanisms involved in regulating neural stem cells and several of these seems to be involved in brain tumour development. To identify potential tumour stem-like cells in brain tumours, different neuronal precursor markers are used and further markers are used to study their differentiation capacity. In this chapter I will discuss certain transcription factors belonging to the Sox super-family. For example Sox1-4 are involved in regulating neural precursor cells as well as the developing CNS, these transcription factors have also recently been shown to be involved in the regulation of the brain tumour stem-like cell (Gangemi, et al., 2009; Ghods, et al., 2007; Ikushima, et al., 2009). In addition, other members of the Sox super-family are suggested to be involved in the differentiation process and several of the Sox protein family members are proposed to be used as markers for different types of brain tumours.

I will discuss the new findings concerning the role of the Sox super-family in brain tumours and in brain tumour stem-like cells, as potential differentiation factors or as potential diagnostic markers of glioma but first there will be an overview of the Sox super-family and the normal expression of Sox proteins in the brain.

2. The Sox super-family

2.1 Sox structure and classification

The first identified *Sox* gene was *Sry*, the mammalian sex-determining Y-linked gene. *Sry* contains a DNA-binding motiv known as the HMG domain (high mobility group domain) (Gubbay, et al., 1992; Sinclair, et al., 1990). The HMG domain is present in a number of genes which belongs to the HMG box super-family. The HMG domain consists of 79 amino acids and some of these amino acids are conserved within the HMG box super-family, although the HMG domains can alter to a large extent. One difference with HMG domains compare to other DNA-binding domains is that the HMG domains interact with the minor groove on the DNA helix and this binding bends the DNA drastically (for review (Wegner, 1999). The Sox protein family is a group of transcription factors which all contain a highly conserved HMG domain, the domain has more than 60% similarity to the Sry HMG domain (Sox - Sry related HMG box) (Laudet, et al., 1993). To date 20 different *Sox* genes are identified in humans and mice and they are divided into eight different subgroups, A-H (Table 1). Proteins in the same subgroup share >80% of the amino acids within the HMG domain (for review (Wegner, 1999). The binding properties of the HMG domains to the DNA are similar between the Sox proteins and the DNA sequence of recognition for binding is only 6-7 base pair (for review (Kamachi, et al., 2000). Except for the HMG domain, Sox proteins contain activating and/or repressing domains, which play a part in there transcription activity (Pusch, et al., 1998; van de Wetering, et al., 1993). In addition there is evidence that Sox proteins perform their function by a complex interplay with specific partner factors to regulate gene transcription. The partner factors can be different depending on cell type, promoter and developmental stage. This enhances the specificity of the transcriptional regulation by a particular Sox protein to a large extent (for review (Kamachi, et al., 2000).

2.2 The function of Sox proteins during development and in adult

Sox proteins are involved in several developmental and adult processes in a cell specific manner. A number of Sox proteins have partial overlapping expression patterns and others not. Further, several of the Sox proteins have similar effects like Sox1, Sox2 and Sox3 are all expressed in progenitor cells during CNS development (Bylund, et al., 2003). Reduction in expression of one of Sox1-3 does not result in significant loss of function, e.g. deletion of Sox1 in mouse results in spontaneous seizures which give rise to a relatively mild CNS phenotype (Nishiguchi, et al., 1998) indicating that the similarities between Sox1-3 makes it possible for the proteins to at least some extent compensate for each other. In other cell types this may not be the case; for example Ferri et al show that neural precursors with deficient Sox2 expression in adult are dependent of correct Sox2 expression levels to generate new precursor cells and neurons (Ferri, et al., 2004). Sox2 is also essential in early embryonic development. Ablation of Sox2 in homozygous mouse case death at implantation and it is not even possible to generate Sox2 homozygous ES cells (Avilion, et al., 2003). Group C, containing Sox4, Sox11 and Sox12/22 is another group which often shows overlapping protein expression in both CNS and PNS (peripheral nervous system) (Cheung, et al., 2000; Hoser, et al., 2008).

On the other hand the same cell type can express more than one Sox protein although the proteins can have counteracting effects. One example of that is the Group B of *Sox* genes, where Sox1-3, which belong to the B1 subgroup, contains an activating domain and on the other hand Sox14 and Sox21, subgroup B2, includes a repressive domain (Uchikawa, et al., 1999). During embryogenesis and neurogenesis of the neural tube of chicken are genes of Group B1 and B2 expressed in an overlapping manner (Sandberg, et al., 2005; Uchikawa, et al., 1999). It is suggested that a proper balance between Group B1 and B2 proteins determine whether the cell stays in a progenitor/proliferating state or if the cells starts to differentiate (Sandberg, et al., 2005; Uchikawa, et al., 1999). It is shown that induced expression of Sox21 in neural cells promote differentiation by disturbing the balance between Sox1-3 and Sox21 (Sandberg, et al., 2005). Further, we have shown that an overexpression of Sox21 in glioma cells reduces glioma cell proliferation by inhibition of Sox2 (Ferletta, et al., 2011).

2.3 Expression pattern of Sox proteins in the normal CNS

The expression patterns of the different Sox proteins in brain and CNS are summarized in Table 1. Several of the Sox proteins are expressed during embryogenesis, one of the first is Sox2. Sox2 RNA is detected already at day 2.5 postcoitum (dpc) at the morula stage and Sox2 is shown to be important in the epiblast and the extra embryonic ectoderm as well as in pluripotent precursors of all embryonic and trophoblast cell types. Targed disruption of the *Sox2* gene is embryonic lethal around implantation (Avilion, et al., 2003).

Sox2 is important in early stages of the embryonic nervous system. In adult nervous system, Sox2 is mainly found in neuronal stem cells and in undifferentiated precursors (Wegner & Stolt, 2005) even though Sox2 is expressed in some differentiated neurons (Cavallaro, et al., 2008). In adult is the expression of Sox2 found in the subventricular zone (SVZ) and in the hippocampus dentate gyrus (DG) and in these regions Sox2 is found to be co-expressed with GFAP and nestin and further these cells are thought to be the adult neural stem cells (Ellis, et al., 2004; Ferri, et al., 2004; Suh, et al., 2007). All proteins of the SoxB group (Sox1-3, Sox14 and Sox21) are expressed in the developing brain to different extent during the development and many of the Sox proteins coexist throughout the CNS (Uchikawa, et al., 1999). When SoxB1 genes (*Sox1*, *Sox2* or *Sox3*) are overexpressed in chicken neural progenitor cells, the cells remain in their neural progenitor state (Bylund, et al., 2003; Graham, et al., 2003). On the other hand inhibition of SoxB1 proteins force cell-cycle exit and neuronal differentiation

(Bylund, et al., 2003). As mentioned Sox21 is able to counteract the activity of SoxB1 proteins and overexpression of Sox21 in chick embryos drives the neural progenitor cells to neuronal differentiation (Sandberg, et al., 2005). Even though all the members of the SoxB1 genes are expressed in neuronal stem cells neither the Sox1 nor the Sox3 deficient mice suffer from sever CNS defects (Nishiguchi, et al., 1998; Weiss, et al., 2003).

Sox subgroup	**Sox transcription factor**	**Expression in CNS**	**References:**
A	SRY	Midbrain and hypothalamus in adult male brain.	(Lahr, et al., 1995).
B1	SOX1	Developing CNS. Neural stem cells. Adult cerebellum: Purkinje cells, Bergman glia.	(Alcock, et al., 2009; Alcock & Sottile, 2009; Bylund, et al., 2003; Pevny, et al., 1998; Uchikawa, et al., 1999).
B1	SOX2	Developing CNS. Embryonic stem cells, neural stem cells. Adult: Neural stem cells, postmitotic neurons, pyramidal cells, Purkinje cells, Bergman glia	(Alcock, et al., 2009; Alcock & Sottile, 2009; Avilion, et al., 2003; Bylund, et al., 2003; Ferri, et al., 2004; Uchikawa, et al., 1999; Zappone, et al., 2000).
B1	SOX3	Developing CNS. Neural stem cells, mature neurons of the ventral hypothalamus	(Bylund, et al., 2003; Rizzoti, et al., 2004; Uchikawa, et al., 1999).
B2	SOX14/SOX28	Developing CNS.	(Uchikawa, et al., 1999).
B2	SOX21/SOX25	Developing CNS.	(Uchikawa, et al., 1999).
C	SOX4	Developing CNS. Oligodendrocyte precursors, neural precursors. Early differentiating cells in the CNS, neurons.	(Cheung, et al., 2000; Kuhlbrodt, Herbarth, Sock, Enderich, et al., 1998).
C	SOX11	Developing CNS. Oligodendrocyte precursors, neural precursors, mature neurons and later in differentiating brain areas as cortical plate and inferior colliculus.	(Kuhlbrodt, Herbarth, Sock, Enderich, et al., 1998; Uwanogho, et al., 1995).
C	SOX12; SOX22	Developing CNS	(Jay, et al., 1997).
D	SOX5	Developing CNS, oligodendrocyte progenitors, oligodendrocytes and neuronal subpopulations (as dorsal horn neurons). Adult: oligodendrocyte progenitors	(Stolt, et al., 2006).
D	SOX6	Developing CNS, oligodendrocyte progenitors, oligodendrocytes and neuronal subpopulations. Adult: oligodendrocyte progenitors	(Connor, et al., 1995; Stolt, et al., 2006).
D	SOX13	Developing CNS, neural progenitors and in differentiating neuronal cells.	(Y. Wang, et al., 2005).

Sox subgroup	Sox transcription factor	Expression in CNS	References:
E	SOX8	During development of CNS in neurons. Oligodendrocyte precursors, astrocytes and oligodendrocytes. Immature Bergman glia and EGL cells (external granule layer), and macroglia.	(Cheng, et al., 2001; Sock, et al., 2001; Stolt, et al., 2004).
E	SOX9	Neural stem cells, astrocytes, oligodendrocytes, Radial glia in developing CNS. Adult: neural stem cells, astrocytes and Bergman glia. Adult cerebellum: Purkinje cells	(Alcock & Sottile, 2009; Scott, et al., 2010; Stolt, et al., 2003) (Alcock, et al., 2009).
E	SOX10	Precursor and mature oligodendrocytes during development and in adult	(Kuhlbrodt, Herbarth, Sock, Hermans-Borgmeyer, et al., 1998; Stolt, et al., 2002).
F	SOX7	Abundant expressed in the brain	(Takash, et al., 2001).
F	SOX17	No expression reported.	
F	SOX18	Weak expression in brain.	(Azuma, et al., 2000).
G	SOX15/SOX20 / SOX26/SOX27	Embryonic stem cells	(H. J. Lee, et al., 2004; Maruyama, et al., 2005).
H	SOX30	Developing CNS, midbrain-hindbrain boundary (zebrafish)	(De Martino, et al., 1999).

Table 1. Sox expression in CNS.

Sox5 and Sox6, which belong to the SoxD group, are also expressed in the developing CNS and are mainly found in oligodendrocyte precursors, oligodendrocytes and different types of neurons (Stolt, et al., 2006). Sox5 and Sox6 are primarily co-expressed, as in the subventricular zone, but they can be differentially expressed as in dorsal-horn neurons where only Sox5 is found to be expressed (Stolt, et al., 2006). Further, Stolt et al showed that Sox5 and Sox6 are involved in the regulation of oligodendrocyte differentiation; the oligodendrocytes start the terminal differentiation when Sox5 and Sox6 are downregulated. Mice deficient in Sox5 and Sox6 have a higher number of oligodendrocyte precursors and the precursors are found earlier. This is the opposite to when SoxE proteins are absent (Sox8-10), which results in a reduced number or lack of oligodendrocytes (Stolt, et al., 2003; Stolt, et al., 2005). As Sox21 can counteract the function of Sox1-3 in neural stem cells, SoxD proteins are suggested to counteract the function of Sox10 in oligodendrocytes (Sandberg, et al., 2005; Stolt, et al., 2006). Sox13, also belonging to the SoxD proteins, is likewise found during the development of CNS and especially during active neurogenesis. Sox13 is primarily suggested to participate in specification and/or differentiation of neurons and Sox13 is mainly found in differentiated areas and missed in the dividing ventricular zone (Wang, et al., 2005). Sox13 starts to be expressed in neural progenitors when the differentiation program is initiated (Wang, et al., 2005). Moreover, in the developing neocortex the expression of Sox13 is very similar to the expression of Sox4 and Sox11 in the primordial plexiform layer. However later during the development only Sox13 and Sox4 are found in more differentiated neurons of the cortical plate and the expression of Sox11 is instead found in differentiating neurons of the subventricular zone (Cheung, et al., 2000; Uwanogho, et al., 1995; Wang, et al., 2005).

Sox4 and Sox11, belonging to the group of SoxC proteins, are shown to have an overlapping expression pattern during early development of the CNS particularly in differentiating areas, later the expression patterns differ to a higher extent (Cheung, et al., 2000). Both Sox4 and Sox11 are found in neural progenitors which have exited mitosis and started to differentiate even though expression are lost when the cells are full differentiated (Cheung, et al., 2000). Further, Sox4 and Sox11 are found to have comparable expression profiles in oligodendrocyte precursor cells and in neurons, both proteins are reduced during oligodendrocyte differentiation (Kuhlbrodt, Herbarth, Sock, Enderich, et al., 1998). In *Sox4*- and *Sox11*-null mice there were no signs of severe CNS defects even though they died during embryogenesis or at birth (Schilham, et al., 1996; Sock, et al., 2004). The *Sox11*-null mice die from heart defects and mutations in the *Sox11* gene are suggested to be important in human malformation syndromes (Sock, et al., 2004). Sox12 is widely expressed both during embryogenesis and adulthood, and consequently expressed in the developing CNS with sustained expression in adult (Jay, et al., 1997). Even though Sox12 has a broad expression pattern is the *Sox12*-null mice viable and fertile and since Sox12 is expressed in lower levels is the overlapping expression of Sox4 and Sox11 suggested to compensate for the loss of Sox12 (Hoser, et al., 2008).

In addition to the SoxC group, the SoxE group is expressed during the development of CNS but the expression starts just before gliogenesis. The earliest oligodendrocyte precursors in the CNS are developed from neuronal stem cells in the ventral ventricular zone and are spread from there (Pringle & Richardson, 1993). In mice, *Sox9* was deleted from neural stem cells, which resulted in defects in the specification of oligodendrocytes and astrocytes, oligodendrocyte progenitors were still detected but to a much lesser extent (Stolt, et al., 2003). Mice deficient in both *Sox8* and *Sox9* failed to generate oligodendrocytes almost completely (Stolt, et al., 2005). In the absence of only Sox8 oligodendrocytes are generated normally (Stolt, et al., 2004) suggesting that lack of Sox8 can be compensated by Sox9 and Sox10 as well as Sox8 can compensate to same extent for the lack of Sox9 and that is why there still are some oligodendrocytes generated. After specification Sox10 starts to be expressed in the developing CNS shortly after Sox8 and Sox9 in oligodendrocyte precursors but in contrast to Sox8 and Sox9, is the expression of Sox10 sustained in oligodendrocytes in adult (Kuhlbrodt, Herbarth, Sock, Hermans-Borgmeyer, et al., 1998; Stolt, et al., 2004; Stolt, et al., 2002). Sox10 is shown to be important for the terminal differentiation of oligodendrocytes (Stolt, et al., 2002) and at this stage Sox9 is downregulated and the expression of Sox8 is low which makes Sox10 crucial for the terminal differentiation and the myelination (Stolt, et al., 2004; Stolt, et al., 2002). Sox8, Sox9 and Sox10 are not essential for the neuronal stem cells but they are suggested to be important in the role of altering the neural stem cell fate to a gliogenic fate.

The only member of the G group is Sox15. In addition to Sox2, Sox15 is expressed in mouse embryonic stem cells but the mRNA is hardly detectable in the brain (Ito, 2010; H. J. Lee, et al., 2004; Maruyama, et al., 2005). In addition, when *Sox15* is targeted disrupted the mouse is viable and fertile and Sox15 is suggested to have an important role in skeletal muscle regeneration.

Sox genes are expressed in different systems and in different stages both during embryonic development and in adult. In addition to neural development and CNS, Sox proteins are reported do have important roles in lens development and in the developing PNS. Other important areas are cartilage development, chondrocyte development, haemopoiesis and sex determination (review (Wegner, 1999). Further, Sox proteins take part in several different cellular responses such as cell proliferation, survival, and differentiation in diverse cell types and tissues. Sox protein are also involved in different kinds of diseases as well as in cancer. In the next session the role of Sox proteins in brain tumourigenesis and especially the role in glioma development will be discussed.

3. The role and expression pattern of Sox proteins in brain tumourigenesis

Several of the Sox proteins have recently been identified in different kinds of brain tumours. Here I will focus on the Sox proteins which are reported to be expressed and play a role in brain tumourigenesis. I will mainly concentrate on the role in gliomagenesis but medulloblastoma and ependymoma will also be mentioned. Table 2 summaries the expression data reported in the literature and the IST (In Silico Transcriptomics) database is used to evaluate the mRNA expression of the different *Sox* genes in glioma (www.genesapiens.com) (Kilpinen, et al., 2008) and the Human protein atlas (HPA) is used to evaluate the protein expression (www.proteinatlas.org) (Berglund, et al., 2008; Uhlen, et al., 2005). Glioma is the only tumour type that is represented both in the IST and the HPA database.

3.1 The essence of Sox2 and Sox21 in brain tumours

There are surprisingly few reports about the role of Sox2 and Sox21 in brain tumour development and there are no reports about Sox1, Sox3 and Sox14, although the IST database tells us that Sox1 and Sox3 are expressed in glioma (Table 2).

Considering the recent data that the tumour-initiating cell probably is a cell of immature nature makes Sox2 extra interesting since Sox2 is reported to be expressed in ES cells, stem cells and progenitor cells (as described above), both during development and adulthood (Ferri, et al., 2004). Further Sox2 is found in the subventricular zone of the lateral ventricles and in the subgranular layer of the adult hippocampus areas where brain tumours are thought to arise (Phi, et al., 2008; Suh, et al., 2007). All ready at an early stage we showed that Sox2 was expressed in different kinds of mouse glioma induced by retroviruses containing the *PDGFB* (platelet-derived growth factor B) gene (Ferletta, et al., 2007). Further, we and others have reported that Sox2 has a broad expression pattern in human brain tumours. Sox2 is found in all sorts of glioma both high and low grade as well as in ependymoma (Ferletta, et al., 2011; Phi, et al., 2008; Schmitz, Temme, et al., 2007). Sox2 is also reported to be expressed in different kinds of paediatric brain tumours such as PNET, medulloblastoma and glioma as well as in undifferentiated and differentiated neurospheres from these tumours (Ferletta, et al., 2011; Hemmati, et al., 2003; Phi, et al., 2010). The expression data of Sox2 in medulloblastoma is a bit contradictable. In our hands the medulloblastomas are positive for Sox2 expression (Ferletta, et al., 2011) but no expression is reported by Phi et al (Phi, et al., 2010). This discrepancy can be explained if different subgroups of medulloblastoma have been used. Moreover by studying paediatric tumour-derived spheres it turned out that tumour-derived spheres were similar to normal neural stem cells, as they expressed the stem cell markers CD133, Musashi-1, melk, PSP, Bmi-1, nestin and Sox2 and the cells were able to migrate, proliferate and give rise to neurons and glia (Hemmati, et al., 2003), strengthening the idea that the brain tumours arise from a cell type of immature origin.

Up to date there is only one report about Sox21 and brain tumours. We have shown that Sox21 is expressed in gliomas of different grade, ependymoma, PNET and medulloblastoma (Ferletta, et al., 2011) (Ferletta unpublished data). In glioma, Sox2 and Sox21 are found to be co-expressed in the same cell and there is a correlation between the expression of Sox2 and Sox21, high expression of Sox2 is associated with high expression of Sox21 (Ferletta, et al., 2011). During development it is suggested that Sox2 and Sox21 have a counteracting activity (Sandberg, et al., 2005). We suggest that in brain tumour cells this fine tuning effect between Sox2 and Sox21 is disturbed and Sox21 is not able to inhibit the proliferation stimulated by Sox2. Moreover, we suggest that glioma consists of at least two cell populations: in the first population Sox21 is co-expressed with both Sox2 and GFAP and negative for fibronectin, the other cell population is instead negative for the expression of Sox2, Sox21 and GFAP but express fibronectin (Ferletta, et al., 2011). The co-expression of Sox2 and GFAP supports the idea that an adult neural stem cell in the subventricular zone could be the tumour-initiating cell of gliomagenesis. Also Phi et al report that Sox2 and GFAP are co-expressed in glial tumours of astroglial, oligodendroglial and ependymal lineages (Phi, et al., 2008). The $Sox2^{-}$/$GFAP^{-}$/$Sox21^{-}$/$fibronectin^{+}$ population could be of a more mesenchymal phenotype (Rieske, et al., 2009; Tso, et al., 2006). Further, in a study of isolation and characterization of cancer-stem-like cells from the 9L gliosarcoma cell line, they found that the expression of Sox2 was turned on when the cells were cultured as spheres compared to monolayer cultures. The cancer stem-like cells from the spheres were able to redevelop the tumour *in vivo* with a more aggressive phenotype compared to monolayer cells and sphere forming cells were less susceptible to chemotherapy, this could be a result of a slower division rate (Ghods, et al., 2007). This even more emphasizes the importance of targeting cancer stem-like cells to treat glioma.

There are a few studies where Sox2 is downregulated in glioma cells. In one investigation Sox2 expression is diminished by microRNA in GBM tumour-initiating cells which results in reduced cell proliferation and that tumour cells slowly exited the cell cycle. Reduced levels of Sox2 further result in decreased levels of Olig2 and BF1, which are transcription factors that normally are expressed in neural progenitor cells. Moreover, when tumour-initiating cells with a silenced Sox2 were orthotopically injected into NOD/SCID mice, the cells failed to recapitulate the tumour compared to tumour-initiating cells that still expressed Sox2 (Gangemi, et al., 2009). This is supported by our study showing that siRNA against Sox2 reduces the expression of Sox2 which results in decreased cell proliferation. Reduced expression levels of Sox2 additionally results in decreased expression of GFAP as well as Sox21, further supporting the correlation between Sox2, GFAP and Sox21 (Ferletta, et al., 2011). We have also investigated the correlation of Sox2 and Sox21 by using tetracycline Sox21-inducible glioma cells (by adding tetracycline Sox21 is upregulated in U-343 MGa Cl2.6 cells). The upregulation of Sox21 results in reduced expression of Sox2 and the cell proliferation was apparently decreased and this was partially a consequence of induced apoptosis (Ferletta, et al., 2011). During chicken development it is suggested that Sox2 and Sox21 must be expressed in a proper balance (Sandberg, et al., 2005; Uchikawa, et al., 1999) which supports our finding that when Sox21 is overexpressed are Sox2 and Sox21 able to act in a counteracting manner in glioma cells. From our findings we propose that Sox2 inhibitors or Sox21 activators or proteins downstream or upstream could be potential targets for novel glioma therapy.

There are a few other reports where the expression of Sox2 has been affected. Korur et al show that while Bmi1 is downregulated is the expression of Sox2 and nestin reduced and the cells become more differentiated. Bmi1 is essential for self-renewal of neural stem cells and is highly expressed in GBM. In addition, while Bmi1 is reduced is the expression of GSK3β (glycogen synthesis kinase 3 beta) also diminished and differentiation is induced while proliferation, survival, migration and clonogenicity decreases (Korur, et al., 2009). From this the authors suggest that specific inhibitors for GSK3β or LiCl could be useful to downregulate Sox2 specifically and reduce the tumourigenic role of Sox2 in glioma. Further, Sox2 is also reported to be connected to the TGF-β (transforming growth factor-β) signalling pathway, in this study Sox2 is regulated by Sox4 (Ikushima, et al., 2009), this will be further mentioned in the discussion of Sox4 below.

Yet another study shows that Sox2 is involved in self-renewal in glioma, by overexpressing Sox2 in glioma cells did the number and size of neurospheres increase. In addition there is a correlation between Sox2 expression and eIF4E (eukaryotic initiation factor 4E) in glioma tissue samples (Ge, et al., 2010). eIF4E is a mRNA 5′ cap-binding protein, which takes part in regulation of translational initiation (Richter & Sonenberg, 2005). The expression of eIF4E is upregulated in several kinds of cancer (Bjornsti & Houghton, 2004). In this study the authors suggest that eIF4E is regulating Sox2 on the protein level but not on the mRNA level and that the eIF4E-Sox2 affiliation could be a new potential therapeutic target (Ge, et al., 2010).

An immunotherapy study has been performed by Schmitz et al, who first showed that Sox2 is overexpressed in GBM. Thereafter they identified a Sox2 peptide that binds to immunogenic HLA-A*0201. The immunogenic HLA-A*0201-restricted peptide originated from Sox2 can activate tumour-directed CD8+ cytotoxic T lymphocytes (CTLs). The authors highlight the possible role of this Sox2-peptide in T-cell-based immunotherapy (Schmitz, Temme, et al., 2007).

Moreover, there is one study of the genome-wide binding pattern for Sox2 in GBM, where 4883 binding sites for Sox2 were identified. The expression of Sox2 in GBM was demolished and a microarray was performed which resulted in altered expression of 489 genes. The main groups of genes that were altered due to Sox2 knockdown were genes with signal transducer activity, transmembrane receptor genes and genes with kinase activity (Fang, et al., 2011). This study indicates that Sox2 probably is involved in several signalling pathways and cellular processes and it needs to be further investigated.

Taken together these findings strengthen the feature of Sox2 as being important for the self-renewal capacity and cell proliferation of neural stem cells as well as cancer stem-like cells and tumour cells. Several studies suggest that Sox2 or proteins up- or downstream of Sox2 could be potential targets for brain tumour therapy. The genome-wide binding screen of Sox2 stressed the difficulty of finding one solution for treating glioma or identifying one potential target that will not be involved or be to harmful to the normal adult stem cell population.

3.2 The role of Sox4 and Sox11 in glioma and medulloblastoma

3.2.1 The role of SoxC in gliomagenesis

Both Sox4 and Sox11 are reported to be expressed in glioma even though Sox4 mRNA expression was not found within the IST database (table 2). Sox11 is expressed during the development of CNS but in the adult brain is the expression of Sox11 downregulated. Compared to the adult brain Sox11 seems to be reactivated during gliomagenesis. With quantitative real-time PCR Sox11 is shown to be upregulated 5- to 600-fold in glioma (Weigle, et al., 2005). The same research group identified a ten amino-acid long peptide derived from Sox11 which has the ability to induce CD8+ cytotoxic T cells (CTLs) (Schmitz,

Wehner, et al., 2007). The Sox11 peptide was specifically expressed on glioma cells in large quantities and they suggest that this peptide could be suitable for T cell-based immunotherapy (Schmitz, Wehner, et al., 2007). Another research group confirms that Sox11 is expressed in primary GBM (Hide, et al., 2009). Further, Hide et al establish a mouse glioma cell line by overexpressing HRas in p53-deficient neural stem cells and the cell line contained both glioma-initiating cells (GICs) and non-glioma-initiating cells (non-GICs) (Hide, et al., 2009). The GICs were transformed into the mouse brain and formed glioblastoma-like tumours. They found that the GIC did not express Sox11 compared to the non-GICs which still expressed Sox11. The loss of Sox11 in GICs was also confirmed in human GIC lines. When Sox11 was overexpressed in GICs the cells lost there tumourigenic ability and the cells started to differentiate towards the direction of neurons. In addition, when Sox11 was downregulated with short hairpin RNA in non-GICs they became tumourigenic (Hide, et al., 2009). Hide et al suggest that true GICs with neural stem cell characteristics should be negative for Sox11. Sox11 is primarily found in oligodendrocytes and neuronal precursors during development which fits with the finding that the GICs are negative for Sox11 if the tumour cell-of-origin is a neural stem cell (Kuhlbrodt, Herbarth, Sock, Enderich, et al., 1998; Uwanogho, et al., 1995).

Taken together, since the expression of Sox11 seems to be high at least in primary glioma, Sox11 might be a target for T cell-based immunotherapy but if the GICs are negative for Sox11 they will escape the therapy with the risk that the relapsed tumour will be of an even more aggressive phenotype.

Sox4 has in a few reports been connected to the TGF-β cell signalling pathway in glioma. TGF-β has been shown to play several roles in glioma promoting activities such as proliferation, invasion, metastasis and angiogenesis (review (Golestaneh & Mishra, 2005). The expression of Sox2 in GICs is induced by TGF-β and while the TFG-β signalling pathway is inhibited is Sox2 downregulated and the self-renewal capacity of GICs is lost (Ikushima, et al., 2009). In this study they propose that TGF-β is not directly regulating Sox2, instead they found that Sox4 is a direct target of TGF-β signalling. Further, Sox4 overexpression is able to induce Sox2 expression and reduced expression of Sox4 in GICs results in a diminished self-renewal capacity, which suggests that Sox4 is important for maintaining the GICs (Ikushima, et al., 2009). On the contrary to Sox2, Sox4 is shown to be expressed in progenitor cells rather than in neuronal stem cells (Bylund, et al., 2003; Cheung, et al., 2000; Kuhlbrodt, Herbarth, Sock, Enderich, et al., 1998). The co-expression of Sox2 and Sox4 in glioma is supported in a DNA microarray analysis of 101 gliomas, where both Sox2 and Sox4 are identified at high levels as well as Sox11 (Tso, et al., 2006) even though there is no evidence that they are expressed in the same cell. That the TGF-β signalling pathway is mediated through Sox4 is supported by a study where the MPSS technology (massively parallel signature sequencing) was used on a pool of glioma tissue. Sox4 as well as TGFBI (transforming growth factor beta induced) were identified as alternative TGF-β mediators in addition to SMAD mediated TGF-β signalling (Lin, et al., 2010).

3.2.2 The role of Sox4 and Sox11 in medulloblastoma

The classical way to classify medulloblastomas are to divide them in to classical medulloblastoma and desmoplastic medulloblastoma (Rubinstein & Northfield, 1964). Both Sox4 and Sox11 are shown to be expressed in medulloblastoma and the expression pattern differ in the classical and the desmoplastic variants (C. J. Lee, et al., 2002). Sox4 has a strong expression in all most all classical medulloblastomas and the expression is mainly found in undifferentiated or poorly differentiated cells. In desmoplastic medulloblastoma Sox4 expression is weak and located to more differentiated cells (C. J. Lee, et al., 2002). In normal cerebellum the expression of Sox4 and Sox11 is upgregulated in granule cells that have stopped the proliferation and Sox4 and Sox11 are continued to be expressed in the deep external granular layer (EGL). As the differentiation process continues the expression of Sox11 is lost but the expression of Sox4 is sustained for some time (Cheung, et al., 2000). The expression of Sox4 in normal cerebellum fits with the expression pattern shown in medulloblastoma and since Sox4 is not expressed in more mature cells of the medulloblastoma, Sox4 is suggested to be a marker for how differentiated the tumour cells are (C. J. Lee, et al., 2002). Further, Sox4 and Sox11 are differentially expressed in medulloblastoma using microarray analysis. Sox4 was identified as a prognostic marker towards slightly better survival, in this study the medulloblastomas were not grouped in classical respectively desmoplastic medulloblastomas (de Bont, et al., 2008).

In other tissues Sox4 is suggested to take part in apoptosis, Sox4 is reported to both induce apoptosis as well as stimulate anti-apoptotic activities, which effect Sox4 has is probably cell and tissue dependent as well as depending on which extracellular signals is reaching the cell (Hur, et al., 2004; P. Liu, et al., 2006). The prognosis of a desmoplastic medulloblastoma is somewhat better compared to classical medulloblastoma (Ellison, et al., 2003).

To correctly classify the different medulloblastomas are important in the view of prognosis and better treatment. Sox4 might be a potential prognostic marker for this together with other cell specific markers. On the other hand Sox11 might be a prognostic marker in glioma connected to better survival (Hide, et al., 2009).

3.3 The feature of SoxD proteins in glioma and medulloblastoma

3.3.1 The role of Sox5 in gliomagenesis

Sox5 was first reported to be involved in gliomagenesis in our retroviral insertional mutagenesis study in mouse. We used a retrovirus containing the *PDGFB* gene to tag genes involved in the development of malignant glioma, these brain tumour lucis can mark both novel or known genes (Johansson, et al., 2004). One of the tagged genes was *Sox5*, three independent proviral insertions were found in three independent tumours. The integration sites suggest that Sox5 expression can be upregulated or truncated which can result in a truncated protein or no product at all (Johansson, et al., 2004). In the follow-up study by Tchougonova et al, *Sox5* is suggested to be a suppressor gene in PDGFB-induced gliomas predominantly in the *Ink4a*-deficient mouse background (Tchougounova, et al., 2009). In human glioma cell lines the expression of Sox5 was low and overexpression of Sox5 reduced the clone formation and the cell proliferation was inhibited. The mechanism by which Sox5 suppresses PDGFB-induced gliomas is suggested to be due to immediate cellular senescence through regulation of $p27^{Kip}$ and Akt (Tchougounova, et al., 2009). Another report confirms that Sox5 expression is lower in oligodendroglial and astrocytic tumours compared to the already low expression in normal adult brain (Schlierf, et al., 2007). Further, it is shown that *Sox5* contains a putative binding site for miR-21, which is a microRNA that functions as an anti-apoptotic factor in GBM (Chen, et al., 2008). On the contrary, another study shows that Sox5 has a higher expression in gliomas compared to normal brain and that about 25% of the glioma patients have IgG antibodies against Sox5 in there sera (Ueda, et al., 2007). The expression of IgG against Sox5 is preferably found in younger patients and the authors suggest that the presence of IgG against Sox5 is correlated to better prognosis i.e. the survival is prolonged (Ueda, et al., 2007). Taken together these data propose that Sox5 expression in glioma could have a suppressing role in gliomagenesis and the expression of Sox5 might indicate a better prognosis and in that case Sox5 could be useful as a prognostic marker.

Sox transcription factor	**Expression in brain tumour**	**Reported expression of Sox mRNA in glioma by IST database**	**Sox protein expression reported in glioma by the human protein atlas (HPA)**	**References: IST: (Kilpinen, et al., 2008) HPA: (Berglund, et al., 2008; Uhlen, et al., 2005)**
SRY	No data.	No expression.	No expression.	
SOX1	No data.	Expressed in glioma.	No data.	
SOX2	Glioma, medulloblastoma, PNET, ependymoma.	Expressed in glioma.	Expressed in all cases. Strong expression in 75% of the cases.	(Ferletta, et al., 2010; Phi, et al., 2008)
SOX3	No data.	Expressed in glioma.	No data.	
SOX14/SOX 28	No data.	No expression.	No data.	
SOX21/SOX 25	Glioma, medulloblastoma, PNET, ependymoma.	Expressed in glioma.	No data.	(Ferletta, et al., 2010)
SOX4	Glioma, medulloblastoma.	No expression.	Expressed in all cases.	(de Bont, et al., 2008; Ikushima, et al., 2009; C. J. Lee, et al., 2002; Lin, et al., 2010).
SOX11	Glioma, medulloblastoma.	Expressed in glioma.	Expressed with various intensity.	(de Bont, et al., 2008; C. J. Lee, et al., 2002; Weigle, et al., 2005).
SOX12; SOX22	No data.	No expression.	No data.	
SOX5	Glioma.	Expressed in glioma.	No data.	(Schlierf, et al., 2007).
SOX6	Glioma, central neurocytoma, medulloblastoma.	Expressed in glioma.	Expressed in 90% of the cases from high to low levels.	(Schlierf, et al., 2007; Ueda, Yoshida, et al., 2004a, 2004b).

Sox transcription factor	Expression in brain tumour	Reported expression of Sox mRNA in glioma by IST database	Sox protein expression reported in glioma by the human protein atlas (HPA)	References: IST: (Kilpinen, et al., 2008) HPA: (Berglund, et al., 2008; Uhlen, et al., 2005)
SOX13	Glioma.	No expression.	No data.	(Schlierf, et al., 2007).
SOX8	Glioma, medulloblastoma.	Expressed in glioma.	No data.	(Cheng, et al., 2001; Schlierf, et al., 2007).
SOX9	Glioma, medulloblastoma, ependymoma.	Expressed in glioma.	Expressed in all cases to varying extent.	(de Bont, et al., 2008; Kordes & Hagel, 2006; Sutter, et al., 2010)
SOX10	Glioma, ependymoma.	Expressed in glioma.	Expressed in 80% of the cases with varying intensity.	(Bannykh, et al., 2006; Ferletta, et al., 2007),
SOX7	No data.	No expression.	Expressed but with different results.	
SOX17	No data.	No expression.	Expressed in all cases, high expression in 20% of the cases.	
SOX18	No data.	No expression.	No data.	
SOX15/SOX 20/ SOX26/SOX 27	No data.	Expressed in glioma.	No data.	
SOX30	No data.	No expression.	Weak cytoplastic expression in 10% of the cases.	

Table 2. Reported expression of Sox proteins in different kinds of brain tumours, expression of Sox mRNA reported in the IST database and Sox protein expression reported in the HPA database.

3.3.2 Sox6 is expressed in both medulloblastoma and glioma

In addition to Sox5, Sox6 is reported to be expressed in glioma as well as in medulloblastoma and neurocytoma (Schlierf, et al., 2007; Ueda, Yoshida, et al., 2004a, 2004b) and the expression of Sox6 in gliomas is confirmed by the IST and HPA databases (Table 2). The presence of Sox6 in different kinds of glioma is slightly varying. Sox6 is reported to have higher mRNA expression levels in oligodendroglioma compared to astrocytomas. In GBM the expression levels are downregulated compared to normal adult brain and in astrocytomas grade II and III are the levels slightly up- or downregulated (Schlierf, et al., 2007). Another study showed that the Sox6 protein is expressed in GBM but not all cells are positive in the GBMs (Ueda, Iizuka, et al., 2004). As for Sox5 Ueda et al report that Sox6 has a higher expression in gliomas compared to normal brain and that one third of the patients develop IgG antibodies against Sox6 which is not found in the patients with other brain diseases or healthy persons (Ueda, Iizuka, et al., 2004). The same research group has continued to elucidate the possibility to vaccinate with Sox6 DNA. Glioma-bearing mice were vaccinated with a plasmid encoding the full-length Sox6 protein. The vaccinated mice developed CTLs specific for Sox6 expressing cells which resulted in a tendency of longer survival time compared to control mice (Ueda, et al., 2008). All though vaccination with Sox6 suggests an anti-tumourigenic effect, there is always a risk that the cells receiving the DNA transform (Munger, et al., 1989).

3.3.3 The expression profile of Sox13 in glioma

It is not very much known about the role of Sox13 in gliomagenesis or brain tumourigenesis. All though there is one report showing that the mRNA expression of Sox13 increased in oligodendroglioma, in astrocytomas can the expression levels be either up- or downregulated but in grade IV GBM is the expression mainly downregulated, all tumours are compared to Sox13 expression in adult brain (Schlierf, et al., 2007).

3.4 The role of SoxE proteins in tumourigenesis

3.4.1 The expression pattern of Sox8 in brain tumours

Very little is known about the role of Sox8 in brain tumourigenesis. The expression of Sox8 in gliomas is investigated by real-time RT-PCR and the expressed of Sox8 is significantly upregulated in most oligodendroglial tumours. The expression of Sox8 is increased in low-grade astrocytomas, in grade III astrocytomas the expression is more heterogeneous and in GBM is the expression of Sox8 lower than in normal brain (Schlierf, et al., 2007). The IST database supports the expression of Sox8 in glioma (table 2). Moreover Sox8 is reported to be expressed in medulloblastoma and within medulloblastoma Sox8 is found in more immature cells and not in differentiated cells which fits with the normal expression of Sox8 in microglia, oligodendrocyte progenitors as well as in EGL cells (Cheng, et al., 2001). The EGL cells have been suggested in several reports to be the cell-of-origin of medulloblastoma (Eberhart, 2007).

3.4.2 The function of Sox9 in glioma and medulloblastoma

Sox9 is found in both paediatric brain tumours as well as in adult brain tumours. In paediatric ependymoma Sox9 is predominantly overexpressed but in medulloblastoma the expression is reported to be low. Survival analysis showed that expression of Sox9 in ependymoma was associated with better overall survival (de Bont, et al., 2008). However there is another report indicating that Sox9 is expressed to a higher level in medulloblastoma (Kordes & Hagel, 2006). When studying different cell-of-origin of medulloblastoma in mice, Sox9 was identified as a stem cell marker on medulloblastomas arising from neural stem cells together with Sox2 and nestin, the expression of Sox9 or Sox2 and nestin were not found in medulloblastoma tumour cells originating from EGL cells. In human samples, a Sox2+ and nestin+ profile was identified on a subset of medulloblastoma which were more common in adult patients compared to

children and the profile was associated with poorer prognosis (Sutter, et al., 2010). In human samples the presence of Sox9 was not investigated.The conflicting data on whether Sox9 is expressed to a higher extent in medulloblastoma or not could be due to the fact that different subgroups of medulloblastoma has been studied and not mentioned and if the different medulloblastomas are raised from different cancer initiating cells as Sutter et al show then the tumours will develop in different directions. Five subgroups of medulloblastomas has been identified on the bases of their characteristic gene expressing profile (Kool, et al., 2008) maybe it is possible/necessary to subdivide them into additional and more narrowed subgroups.
The mRNA level of Sox9 in oligodendroglial tumours is lower compared to adult brain and in astrocytic tumours the expression is more varying (Schlierf, et al., 2007). On the protein level Sox9 is found in all grades of glioma with somewhat lower expression in pilocytic astrocytomas (grad I) (Kordes & Hagel, 2006). The reported expression data on Sox9 match nicely the expression data from the IST database as well as the data from the HPA database (Table 2). Moreover, we have investigated the effect of overexpressing cGKII (cyclic guanosine monophosphate (cGMP)-dependent protein kinase II) which results in reduced expression of Sox9 and PDGFRα and this is followed by dephosphorylation of Akt, suggesting a connection between Sox9, PDGFRα and the Akt signalling pathway in glioma (Swartling, et al., 2009). The Akt signalling pathway is often activated in gliomas and the PDGFRα is frequently constitutively activated (Nister, et al., 1988; Phillips, et al., 2006). Further, reduced expression of Sox9 by siRNA is decreasing the cell proliferation rate in glioma cells (Swartling, et al., 2009). In addition to gliomas, Sox9 is expressed in prostate cancers and Sox9 suppression in prostate cancer cause a downregulation of cell growth (Wang, et al., 2007) which support our findings in glioma. Further, overexpression of Sox9 in prostate cancer cells caused enhanced cell proliferation and invasion (Wang, et al., 2008). In prostate cancer Sox9 is suggested to be regulated by the Wnt/β-catenin pathway (Wang, et al., 2007). The Wnt/β-catenin signalling pathway is one of the characteristics of subgroup type A of medulloblastoma which has activated Wnt-signalling (Kool, et al., 2008). In prostate cancer the expression of Sox9 is higher in recurrent tumours suggesting that Sox9 is partially expressed by the cancer initiating cells which manage to escape the treatment (Wang, et al., 2007). Sox9 is expressed in neural stem cells and in progenitor cells in adult as well as in the embryonic CNS (Scott, et al., 2010; Stolt, et al., 2003) indicating that Sox9 could be important also for the brain tumour initiating cell, even though the type A subgroup (Wnt-signalling) of medulloblastoma has a slightly better survival rate (Kool, et al., 2008). It is also shown that Shh induces Sox9 during early generation of neural stem cells and that the expression of Sox9 is essential to keep the multipotency of the neural stem cells (Scott, et al., 2010), the Shh-signalling pathway is one of the activated pathways in subset B of medulloblastoma and is mutated in about 25% of the cases (Ellison, et al., 2003; Kool, et al., 2008). Recurrent gliomas are often of an even more aggressive and invasive phenotype compared to the primary tumour supporting the finding that Sox9 could be important for tumour cell invasion (Wang, et al., 2008).

3.4.3 The presence of Sox10 in glioma may indicate better prognosis

Sox10 was first reported to be involved in gliomagenesis in our retroviral insertional mutagenesis study as Sox5 (Johansson, et al., 2004). Five proviral integration sites were identified upstream of the transcriptional start site of *Sox10* and the positions of the proviral insertions suggests improved expression of Sox10 (Ferletta, et al., 2007; Johansson, et al., 2004).

Consistently with several other studies we have reported that Sox10 is expressed in both paediatric and adult gliomas and ependymomas with a higher expression in low grade tumours compared to high grade tumours (Addo-Yobo, et al., 2006; Bannykh, et al., 2006; Colin, et al., 2007; Ferletta, et al., 2007). On the contrary Schlierf et al found that when investigating the mRNA levels of Sox10 in glioma the expression levels were lower compared to adult brain (Schlierf, et al., 2007). The authors suggest that this could be due to the high expression of Sox10 in differentiated oligodendrocytes (Stolt, et al., 2002), meanwhile the expression in more immature oligodendrocytes are lower which is reflected in the tumour cells (Schlierf, et al., 2007). Further, Etcheverry et al has performed a whole-genome integrative analysis of methylation and gene expression profiles on GBM samples and found that the Sox10 promoter contains two hypermethylated CpG sites which are related to shorter survival. However, shorter survival time is correlated with low-expression of Sox10 in the GBM samples (Etcheverry, et al., 2010), which fits with the expression data that Sox10 is expressed to a higher extent in low grade brain tumours. We and others have not found any expression of Sox10 in medulloblastoma (Ferletta, et al., 2007; Gershon, et al., 2005). The lack of Sox10 in medulloblastomas may be explained by the theory that gliomas and medulloblastomas probably originate from different tumour-initiating cells (Marino, et al., 2000).

The expression of Sox10 by itself is not enough to characterize a subgroup of gliomas as pilocytic astrocytomas, but together with other markers it may be possible (Colin, et al., 2007; Rousseau, et al., 2006). Some researchers have tried to subgroup well-characterized gliomas depending on their expression of GFAP, vimentin, Olig2, Nkx2.2, Sox10 and nestin. They suggest that gliomas with strong expression of GFAP, vimentin, Olig2, Nkx2.2 and Sox10 can be identified as pilocytic astrocytomas, further robust expression of GFAP, vimentin and nestin can categorize GBM and oligodendrogliomas can be recognized by Olig2 expression in almost all tumour cells while Sox10 and Nkx2.2 was found in subpopulations of tumour cells, these findings are not definite but may to some degree extend the diagnostic possibilities (Colin, et al., 2007). Moreover the study indicate how heterogeneous the gliomas are and emphasize the difficulties in finding treatment that will target all different tumour cells from the bulk cells to the tumor-initiating cells.

There are very few reports about how Sox10 regulates/is regulated in brain tumours. Sox10 has in pilocytic astrocytomas been correlated with high expression of ErbB3 suggesting that Sox10 is driving the overexpression of ErbB3 which may result in induced cell proliferation (Addo-Yobo, et al., 2006). This finding is supported by the knowledge that Sox10 is regulating ErbB3 in neural crest cells during development (Britsch, et al., 2001). Further we have investigated the role of Sox10 in gliomagenesis by using the RCAS/tv-a mouse model where a gene(s) of interest can be expressed in a specific cell type as glial progenitor cells (Ntv-a mice). In this study we overexpressed *Sox10* alone or together with the oncogene *PDGFB* in the RCAS system. We found that Sox10 overexpression alone was not enough to induce any tumour formation neither in the Ntv-a wild type mice nor in the *Arf-/-* transgenic mice (Ferletta, et al., 2007). The combination of the RCAS-*Sox10* virus with the RCAS-*PDGFB* virus induced glioma and the induction was four times higher with the combination compared to RCAS-*PDGFB* alone in the *Arf-/-* null mice. Therefore we suggest that *Sox10* is not a potent oncogene by itself but in combination with other oncogenes as *PDGFB Sox10* is able to increase the gliomagenicity at least in mouse (Ferletta, et al., 2007). Autocrine stimulation of growth factors such as PDGFA are common event in human brain tumours (Nistér & Westermark, 1998). Moreover, in oligodendrocyte precursors is the expression of

Sox10 presiding the expression of PDGFRα and as soon as the expression of PDGFRα is turned on, they are co-expressed (Stolt, et al., 2002). This supports the data that a combined overexpression of Sox10 and PDGFB gives raise to glioma-like tumours and that Sox10 can increase tumour incidence. In addition, the tumours induced with RCAS-*PDGFB* alone or together with RCAS-*Sox10* both had a high expression of Sox10 suggesting that the tumour-initiating cell is of immature origin as the oligodendrocyte precursor (Ferletta, et al., 2007) and this was further supported by the expression of markers for oligodendrocyte precursors as NG2 and PDGFRα (Stallcup & Beasley, 1987) in the tumours, as well as Sox2 and nestin, markers for neural stem cells (Avilion, et al., 2003; Wiese, et al., 2004).

The wide expression pattern of Sox10 in different types of human gliomas indicates that oligodendroglioma and astrocytoma may arise from a common tumour-initiating cell. Sox10 does not appear to be an oncogene alone but when combined with other mutations Sox10 is able to increase the tumour incidence. Further, Sox10 may be used as a prognostic marker the presence of Sox10 is connected to better prognosis.

4. Conclusion

Lately there are a lot of new reports coming up about the Sox super-family and their roles in brain tumourigenesis, even though it is still a lot more to explore. Ten out of the 20 known Sox proteins are reported to be expressed in brain tumors.

There are several discussions going on in the research field as the difference between cancer stem-like cells and normal neural stem cells. Sox2, Sox9 and to some extent Sox4 are shown to be involved in the regulation of cancer stem-like cells and the presence of these proteins seems to be important for the self-renewal capacity and the cell proliferation of cancer stem-like cells. There are indications that cancer stem-like cells can escape the radiation better compared to the tumour bulk, this make the tumour able to relapse and often is the relapsed tumour even more aggressive and invasive. Specific inhibitors against Sox2, Sox9 and Sox4 or up- or downstream targets could be of therapeutic interest if it is possible to avoid too much harm on the normal stem cells and the neural progenitor cells. We also show that it is possible to inhibit the cell proliferation induced by Sox2 with Sox21.

In different studies specific peptides for T-cell-based immunotherapy have been made available for; Sox2, Sox4, Sox11, and Sox6. This needs to be further investigated, the risk with immunotherapy is that the cells receiving the DNA can transform and become tumourigenic itself. Other Sox proteins are suggested to be used as prognostic markers, as the expression of Sox5, Sox6, Sox4, Sox11 and Sox10 is associated with better survival. Unfortunately in most cases it is probably not enough with just one marker, it is a need of a combination of markers to get a prognostic overview of the tumours.

Gliomas and medulloblastomas are very heterogeneous tumour types and lately they have been divided into different subgroups depending on their genetic background, which signalling pathways are activated and common genetic mutations all this to make it a little bit easier to find a potential target for therapy.

Many of the Sox proteins are co-expressed in the same cell, some with interacting activity others with counteracting activity, but this has not been taken in to account in many of the reports about Sox proteins during brain tumourigenesis. Further, today there are several different brain tumour models in mice, both viral-induced models and transgenic models which can be used when studying the role of different Sox proteins during brain tumourigenesis to get new functional and new therapeutic ideas.

5. Acknowledgements

The work in the author's laboratory is supported by grants from the Children's Cancer Foundation, Åke Wibergs Foundation, Magnus Bergvalls Foundation and The Göran Gustafsson Foundation.

6. References

Addo-Yobo, S. O., Straessle, J., Anwar, A., Donson, A. M., Kleinschmidt-Demasters, B. K., & Foreman, N. K. (2006). Paired overexpression of ErbB3 and Sox10 in pilocytic astrocytoma. *J Neuropathol Exp Neurol, 65*(8), 769-775.

Alcock, J., Lowe, J., England, T., Bath, P., & Sottile, V. (2009). Expression of Sox1, Sox2 and Sox9 is maintained in adult human cerebellar cortex. *Neurosci Lett, 450*(2), 114-116.

Alcock, J., & Sottile, V. (2009). Dynamic distribution and stem cell characteristics of Sox1-expressing cells in the cerebellar cortex. *Cell Res, 19*(12), 1324-1333.

Avilion, A. A., Nicolis, S. K., Pevny, L. H., Perez, L., Vivian, N., & Lovell-Badge, R. (2003). Multipotent cell lineages in early mouse development depend on SOX2 function. *Genes Dev, 17*(1), 126-140.

Azuma, T., Seki, N., Yoshikawa, T., Saito, T., Masuho, Y., & Muramatsu, M. (2000). cDNA cloning, tissue expression, and chromosome mapping of human homolog of SOX18. *J Hum Genet, 45*(3), 192-195.

Bannykh, S. I., Stolt, C. C., Kim, J., Perry, A., & Wegner, M. (2006). Oligodendroglial-specific transcriptional factor SOX10 is ubiquitously expressed in human gliomas. *J Neurooncol, 76*(2), 115-127.

Berglund, L., Bjorling, E., Oksvold, P., Fagerberg, L., Asplund, A., Szigyarto, C. A., et al. (2008). A genecentric Human Protein Atlas for expression profiles based on antibodies. *Mol Cell Proteomics, 7*(10), 2019-2027.

Bjornsti, M. A., & Houghton, P. J. (2004). Lost in translation: dysregulation of cap-dependent translation and cancer. *Cancer Cell, 5*(6), 519-523.

Britsch, S., Goerich, D. E., Riethmacher, D., Peirano, R. I., Rossner, M., Nave, K. A., et al. (2001). The transcription factor Sox10 is a key regulator of peripheral glial development. *Genes Dev, 15*(1), 66-78.

Bylund, M., Andersson, E., Novitch, B. G., & Muhr, J. (2003). Vertebrate neurogenesis is counteracted by Sox1-3 activity. *Nat Neurosci, 6*(11), 1162-1168.

Cavallaro, M., Mariani, J., Lancini, C., Latorre, E., Caccia, R., Gullo, F., et al. (2008). Impaired generation of mature neurons by neural stem cells from hypomorphic Sox2 mutants. *Development, 135*(3), 541-557.

Chen, Y., Liu, W., Chao, T., Zhang, Y., Yan, X., Gong, Y., et al. (2008). MicroRNA-21 down-regulates the expression of tumor suppressor PDCD4 in human glioblastoma cell T98G. *Cancer Lett, 272*(2), 197-205.

Cheng, Y. C., Lee, C. J., Badge, R. M., Orme, A. T., & Scotting, P. J. (2001). Sox8 gene expression identifies immature glial cells in developing cerebellum and cerebellar tumours. *Brain Res Mol Brain Res, 92*(1-2), 193-200.

Cheung, M., Abu-Elmagd, M., Clevers, H., & Scotting, P. J. (2000). Roles of Sox4 in central nervous system development. *Brain Res Mol Brain Res, 79*(1-2), 180-191.

Colin, C., Virard, I., Baeza, N., Tchoghandjian, A., Fernandez, C., Bouvier, C., et al. (2007). Relevance of combinatorial profiles of intermediate filaments and transcription factors for glioma histogenesis. *Neuropathol Appl Neurobiol, 33*(4), 431-439.

Connor, F., Wright, E., Denny, P., Koopman, P., & Ashworth, A. (1995). The Sry-related HMG box-containing gene Sox6 is expressed in the adult testis and developing nervous system of the mouse. *Nucleic Acids Res, 23*(17), 3365-3372.

de Bont, J. M., Kros, J. M., Passier, M. M., Reddingius, R. E., Sillevis Smitt, P. A., Luider, T. M., et al. (2008). Differential expression and prognostic significance of SOX genes in pediatric medulloblastoma and ependymoma identified by microarray analysis. *Neuro Oncol, 10*(5), 648-660.

De Martino, S. P., Errington, F., Ashworth, A., Jowett, T., & Austin, C. A. (1999). sox30: a novel zebrafish sox gene expressed in a restricted manner at the midbrain-hindbrain boundary during neurogenesis. *Dev Genes Evol, 209*(6), 357-362.

Eberhart, C. G. (2007). In search of the medulloblast: neural stem cells and embryonal brain tumors. *Neurosurg Clin N Am, 18*(1), 59-69, viii-ix.

Ellis, P., Fagan, B. M., Magness, S. T., Hutton, S., Taranova, O., Hayashi, S., et al. (2004). SOX2, a persistent marker for multipotential neural stem cells derived from embryonic stem cells, the embryo or the adult. *Dev Neurosci, 26*(2-4), 148-165.

Ellison, D. W., Clifford, S. C., Gajjar, A., & Gilbertson, R. J. (2003). What's new in neuro-oncology? Recent advances in medulloblastoma. *Eur J Paediatr Neurol, 7*(2), 53-66.

Etcheverry, A., Aubry, M., de Tayrac, M., Vauleon, E., Boniface, R., Guenot, F., et al. (2010). DNA methylation in glioblastoma: impact on gene expression and clinical outcome. *BMC Genomics, 11*, 701.

Fang, X., Yoon, J. G., Li, L., Yu, W., Shao, J., Hua, D., et al. (2011). The SOX2 response program in glioblastoma multiforme: an integrated ChIP-seq, expression microarray, and microRNA analysis. *BMC Genomics, 12*, 11.

Ferletta, M., Caglayan, D., Mokvist, L., Jiang, Y., Kastemar, M., Uhrbom, L., et al. (2011). Forced expression of Sox21 inhibits Sox2 and induces apoptosis in human glioma cells. *Int J Cancer, 129*, 45-60.

Ferletta, M., Uhrbom, L., Olofsson, T., Ponten, F., & Westermark, B. (2007). Sox10 has a broad expression pattern in gliomas and enhances platelet-derived growth factor-B--induced gliomagenesis. *Mol Cancer Res, 5*(9), 891-897.

Ferri, A. L., Cavallaro, M., Braida, D., Di Cristofano, A., Canta, A., Vezzani, A., et al. (2004). Sox2 deficiency causes neurodegeneration and impaired neurogenesis in the adult mouse brain. *Development, 131*(15), 3805-3819.

Galderisi, U., Cipollaro, M., & Giordano, A. (2006). Stem cells and brain cancer. *Cell Death Differ, 13*(1), 5-11.

Galli, R., Binda, E., Orfanelli, U., Cipelletti, B., Gritti, A., De Vitis, S., et al. (2004). Isolation and characterization of tumorigenic, stem-like neural precursors from human glioblastoma. *Cancer Res, 64*(19), 7011-7021.

Gangemi, R. M., Griffero, F., Marubbi, D., Perera, M., Capra, M. C., Malatesta, P., et al. (2009). SOX2 silencing in glioblastoma tumor-initiating cells causes stop of proliferation and loss of tumorigenicity. . *Stem Cells, 27*, 40-48.

Ge, Y., Zhou, F., Chen, H., Cui, C., Liu, D., Li, Q., et al. (2010). Sox2 is translationally activated by eukaryotic initiation factor 4E in human glioma-initiating cells. *Biochem Biophys Res Commun, 397*(4), 711-717.

Gershon, T. R., Oppenheimer, O., Chin, S. S., & Gerald, W. L. (2005). Temporally regulated neural crest transcription factors distinguish neuroectodermal tumors of varying malignancy and differentiation. *Neoplasia, 7*(6), 575-584.

Ghods, A. J., Irvin, D., Liu, G., Yuan, X., Abdulkadir, I. R., Tunici, P., et al. (2007). Spheres isolated from 9L gliosarcoma rat cell line possess chemoresistant and aggressive cancer stem-like cells. *Stem Cells, 25*(7), 1645-1653.

Golestaneh, N., & Mishra, B. (2005). TGF-beta, neuronal stem cells and glioblastoma. *Oncogene, 24*(37), 5722-5730.

Graham, V., Khudyakov, J., Ellis, P., & Pevny, L. (2003). SOX2 functions to maintain neural progenitor identity. *Neuron, 39*(5), 749-765.

Gubbay, J., Vivian, N., Economou, A., Jackson, D., Goodfellow, P., & Lovell-Badge, R. (1992). Inverted repeat structure of the Sry locus in mice. *Proc Natl Acad Sci U S A, 89*(17), 7953-7957.

Hemmati, H. D., Nakano, I., Lazareff, J. A., Masterman-Smith, M., Geschwind, D. H., Bronner-Fraser, M., et al. (2003). Cancerous stem cells can arise from pediatric brain tumors. *Proc Natl Acad Sci U S A, 100*(25), 15178-15183.

Hide, T., Takezaki, T., Nakatani, Y., Nakamura, H., Kuratsu, J., & Kondo, T. (2009). Sox11 prevents tumorigenesis of glioma-initiating cells by inducing neuronal differentiation. *Cancer Res, 69*(20), 7953-7959.

Hirschmann-Jax, C., Foster, A. E., Wulf, G. G., Nuchtern, J. G., Jax, T. W., Gobel, U., et al. (2004). A distinct "side population" of cells with high drug efflux capacity in human tumor cells. *Proc Natl Acad Sci U S A, 101*(39), 14228-14233.

Holland, E. C. (2001). Gliomagenesis: genetic alterations and mouse models. *Nat Rev Genet, 2*(2), 120-129.

Hoser, M., Potzner, M. R., Koch, J. M., Bosl, M. R., Wegner, M., & Sock, E. (2008). Sox12 deletion in the mouse reveals nonreciprocal redundancy with the related Sox4 and Sox11 transcription factors. *Mol Cell Biol, 28*(15), 4675-4687.

Hur, E. H., Hur, W., Choi, J. Y., Kim, I. K., Kim, H. Y., Yoon, S. K., et al. (2004). Functional identification of the pro-apoptotic effector domain in human Sox4. *Biochem Biophys Res Commun, 325*(1), 59-67.

Ikushima, H., Todo, T., Ino, Y., Takahashi, M., Miyazawa, K., & Miyazono, K. (2009). Autocrine TGF-beta signaling maintains tumorigenicity of glioma-initiating cells through Sry-related HMG-box factors. *Cell Stem Cell, 5*(5), 504-514.

Ito, M. (2010). Function and molecular evolution of mammalian Sox15, a singleton in the SoxG group of transcription factors. *Int J Biochem Cell Biol, 42*(3), 449-452.

Jay, P., Sahly, I., Goze, C., Taviaux, S., Poulat, F., Couly, G., et al. (1997). SOX22 is a new member of the SOX gene family, mainly expressed in human nervous tissue. *Hum Mol Genet, 6*(7), 1069-1077.

Johansson, F. K., Brodd, J., Eklöf, C., Ferletta, M., Hesselager, G., Tiger, C. F., et al. (2004). Identification of candidate cancer-causing genes in mouse brain tumors by retroviral tagging. *PNAS, 101*(31), 11334-11337.

Kamachi, Y., Uchikawa, M., & Kondoh, H. (2000). Pairing SOX off: with partners in the regulation of embryonic development. *Trends Genet, 16*(4), 182-187.

Kattar, M. M., Kupsky, W. J., Shimoyama, R. K., Vo, T. D., Olson, M. W., Bargar, G. R., et al. (1997). Clonal analysis of gliomas. *Hum Pathol, 28*(10), 1166-1179.

Kilpinen, S., Autio, R., Ojala, K., Iljin, K., Bucher, E., Sara, H., et al. (2008). Systematic bioinformatic analysis of expression levels of 17,330 human genes across 9,783 samples from 175 types of healthy and pathological tissues. *Genome Biol, 9*(9), R139.

Kool, M., Koster, J., Bunt, J., Hasselt, N. E., Lakeman, A., van Sluis, P., et al. (2008). Integrated genomics identifies five medulloblastoma subtypes with distinct genetic profiles, pathway signatures and clinicopathological features. *PLoS One, 3*(8), e3088.

Kordes, U., & Hagel, C. (2006). Expression of SOX9 and SOX10 in central neuroepithelial tumor. *J Neurooncol, 80*(2), 151-155.

Korur, S., Huber, R. M., Sivasankaran, B., Petrich, M., Morin, P., Jr., Hemmings, B. A., et al. (2009). GSK3beta regulates differentiation and growth arrest in glioblastoma. *PLoS One, 4*(10), e7443.

Kuhlbrodt, K., Herbarth, B., Sock, E., Enderich, J., Hermans-Borgmeyer, I., & Wegner, M. (1998). Cooperative function of POU proteins and SOX proteins in glial cells. *J Biol Chem, 273*(26), 16050-16057.

Kuhlbrodt, K., Herbarth, B., Sock, E., Hermans-Borgmeyer, I., & Wegner, M. (1998). Sox10, a novel transcriptional modulator in glial cells. *J. Neuro. sci., 18*(1), 237-250.

Lahr, G., Maxson, S. C., Mayer, A., Just, W., Pilgrim, C., & Reisert, I. (1995). Transcription of the Y chromosomal gene, Sry, in adult mouse brain. *Brain Res Mol Brain Res, 33*(1), 179-182.

Laudet, V., Stehelin, D., & Clevers, H. (1993). Ancestry and diversity of the HMG box superfamily. *Nucleic Acids Res, 21*(10), 2493-2501.

Lee, C. J., Appleby, V. J., Orme, A. T., Chan, W. I., & Scotting, P. J. (2002). Differential expression of SOX4 and SOX11 in medulloblastoma. *J Neurooncol, 57*(3), 201-214.

Lee, H. J., Goring, W., Ochs, M., Muhlfeld, C., Steding, G., Paprotta, I., et al. (2004). Sox15 is required for skeletal muscle regeneration. *Mol Cell Biol, 24*(19), 8428-8436.

Lin, B., Madan, A., Yoon, J. G., Fang, X., Yan, X., Kim, T. K., et al. (2010). Massively parallel signature sequencing and bioinformatics analysis identifies up-regulation of TGFBI and SOX4 in human glioblastoma. *PLoS One, 5*(4), e10210.

Liu, G., Yuan, X., Zeng, Z., Tunici, P., Ng, H., Abdulkadir, I. R., et al. (2006). Analysis of gene expression and chemoresistance of CD133+ cancer stem cells in glioblastoma. *Mol Cancer, 5*, 67.

Liu, P., Ramachandran, S., Ali Seyed, M., Scharer, C. D., Laycock, N., Dalton, W. B., et al. (2006). Sex-determining region Y box 4 is a transforming oncogene in human prostate cancer cells. *Cancer Res, 66*(8), 4011-4019.

Louis, D. N., Ohgaki, H., Wiestler, O. D., Cavenee, W. K., Burger, P. C., Jouvet, A., et al. (2007). The 2007 WHO classification of tumours of the central nervous system. *Acta Neuropathol, 114*(2), 97-109.

Marino, S., Vooijs, M., van Der Gulden, H., Jonkers, J., & Berns, A. (2000). Induction of medulloblastomas in p53-null mutant mice by somatic inactivation of Rb in the external granular layer cells of the cerebellum. *Genes Dev, 14*(8), 994-1004.

Maruyama, M., Ichisaka, T., Nakagawa, M., & Yamanaka, S. (2005). Differential roles for Sox15 and Sox2 in transcriptional control in mouse embryonic stem cells. *J Biol Chem, 280*(26), 24371-24379.

Munger, K., Phelps, W. C., Bubb, V., Howley, P. M., & Schlegel, R. (1989). The E6 and E7 genes of the human papillomavirus type 16 together are necessary and sufficient for transformation of primary human keratinocytes. *J Virol, 63*(10), 4417-4421.

Nishiguchi, S., Wood, H., Kondoh, H., Lovell-Badge, R., & Episkopou, V. (1998). Sox1 directly regulates the gamma-crystallin genes and is essential for lens development in mice. *Genes Dev, 12*(6), 776-781.

Nister, M., Libermann, T. A., Betsholtz, C., Pettersson, M., Claesson-Welsh, L., Heldin, C. H., et al. (1988). Expression of messenger RNAs for platelet-derived growth factor and transforming growth factor-alpha and their receptors in human malignant glioma cell lines. *Cancer Res, 48*(14), 3910-3918.

Nistér, M., & Westermark, B. (1998). Mechanisms of altered growth control. *Growth factors. In: D.D. Bigner, R.E. McLendon and J.M. Bruner (eds.), Russel and Rubinstein´s pathology of tumors of the nervous system. Arnold , London., 1*, 83-116.

Pevny, L. H., Sockanathan, S., Placzek, M., & Lovell-Badge, R. (1998). A role for SOX1 in neural determination. *Development, 125*(10), 1967-1978.

Phi, J. H., Kim, J. H., Eun, K. M., Wang, K. C., Park, K. H., Choi, S. A., et al. (2010). Upregulation of SOX2, NOTCH1, and ID1 in supratentorial primitive neuroectodermal tumors: a distinct differentiation pattern from that of medulloblastomas. *J Neurosurg Pediatr, 5*(6), 608-614.

Phi, J. H., Park, S. H., Kim, S. K., Paek, S. H., Kim, J. H., Lee, Y. J., et al. (2008). Sox2 expression in brain tumors: a reflection of the neuroglial differentiation pathway. *Am J Surg Pathol, 32*(1), 103-112.

Phillips, H. S., Kharbanda, S., Chen, R., Forrest, W. F., Soriano, R. H., Wu, T. D., et al. (2006). Molecular subclasses of high-grade glioma predict prognosis, delineate a pattern of disease progression, and resemble stages in neurogenesis. *Cancer Cell, 9*(3), 157-173.

Pringle, N. P., & Richardson, W. D. (1993). A singularity of PDGF alpha-receptor expression in the dorsoventral axis of the neural tube may define the origin of the oligodendrocyte lineage. *Development, 117*(2), 525-533.

Pusch, C., Hustert, E., Pfeifer, D., Sudbeck, P., Kist, R., Roe, B., et al. (1998). The SOX10/Sox10 gene from human and mouse: sequence, expression, and transactivation by the encoded HMG domain transcription factor. *Hum Genet, 103*(2), 115-123.

Richter, J. D., & Sonenberg, N. (2005). Regulation of cap-dependent translation by eIF4E inhibitory proteins. *Nature, 433*(7025), 477-480.

Rieske, P., Golanska, E., Zakrzewska, M., Piaskowski, S., Hulas-Bigoszewska, K., Wolanczyk, M., et al. (2009). Arrested neural and advanced mesenchymal differentiation of glioblastoma cells-comparative study with neural progenitors. *BMC Cancer, 9*, 54.

Rizzoti, K., Brunelli, S., Carmignac, D., Thomas, P. Q., Robinson, I. C., & Lovell-Badge, R. (2004). SOX3 is required during the formation of the hypothalamo-pituitary axis. *Nat Genet, 36*(3), 247-255.

Rousseau, A., Nutt, C. L., Betensky, R. A., Iafrate, A. J., Han, M., Ligon, K. L., et al. (2006). Expression of oligodendroglial and astrocytic lineage markers in diffuse gliomas: use of YKL-40, ApoE, ASCL1, and NKX2-2. *J Neuropathol Exp Neurol, 65*(12), 1149-1156.

Rubinstein, L. J., & Northfield, D. W. (1964). The Medulloblastoma and the So-Called "Arachnoidal Cerebellar Sarcoma". *Brain, 87*, 379-412.

Sandberg, M., Kallstrom, M., & Muhr, J. (2005). Sox21 promotes the progression of vertebrate neurogenesis. *Nat Neurosci, 8*(8), 995-1001.

Schilham, M. W., Oosterwegel, M. A., Moerer, P., Ya, J., de Boer, P. A., van de Wetering, M., et al. (1996). Defects in cardiac outflow tract formation and pro-B-lymphocyte expansion in mice lacking Sox-4. *Nature, 380*(6576), 711-714.

Schlierf, B., Friedrich, R. P., Roerig, P., Felsberg, J., Reifenberger, G., & Wegner, M. (2007). Expression of SoxE and SoxD genes in human gliomas. *Neuropathol Appl Neurobiol, 33*(6), 621-630.

Schmitz, M., Temme, A., Senner, V., Ebner, R., Schwind, S., Stevanovic, S., et al. (2007). Identification of SOX2 as a novel glioma-associated antigen and potential target for T cell-based immunotherapy. *Br J Cancer, 96*(8), 1293-1301.

Schmitz, M., Wehner, R., Stevanovic, S., Kiessling, A., Rieger, M. A., Temme, A., et al. (2007). Identification of a naturally processed T cell epitope derived from the glioma-associated protein SOX11. *Cancer Lett, 245*(1-2), 331-336.

Scott, C. E., Wynn, S. L., Sesay, A., Cruz, C., Cheung, M., Gomez Gaviro, M. V., et al. (2010). SOX9 induces and maintains neural stem cells. *Nat Neurosci, 13*(10), 1181-1189.

Sinclair, A. H., Berta, P., Palmer, M. S., Hawkins, J. R., Griffiths, B. L., Smith, M. J., et al. (1990). A gene from the human sex-determining region encodes a protein with homology to a conserved DNA-binding motif. *Nature, 346*(6281), 240-244.

Singh, S. K., Clarke, I. D., Terasaki, M., Bonn, V. E., Hawkins, C., Squire, J., et al. (2003). Identification of a cancer stem cell in human brain tumors. *Cancer Res, 63*(18), 5821-5828.

Sock, E., Rettig, S. D., Enderich, J., Bosl, M. R., Tamm, E. R., & Wegner, M. (2004). Gene targeting reveals a widespread role for the high-mobility-group transcription factor Sox11 in tissue remodeling. *Mol Cell Biol, 24*(15), 6635-6644.

Sock, E., Schmidt, K., Hermanns-Borgmeyer, I., Bosl, M. R., & Wegner, M. (2001). Idiopathic weight reduction in mice deficient in the high-mobility-group transcription factor Sox8. *Mol Cell Biol, 21*(20), 6951-6959.

Stallcup, W. B., & Beasley, L. (1987). Bipotential glial precursor cells of the optic nerve express the NG2 proteoglycan. *J Neurosci, 7*(9), 2737-2744.

Stolt, C. C., Lommes, P., Friedrich, R. P., & Wegner, M. (2004). Transcription factors Sox8 and Sox10 perform non-equivalent roles during oligodendrocyte development despite functional redundancy. *Development, 131*(10), 2349-2358.

Stolt, C. C., Lommes, P., Sock, E., Chaboissier, M. C., Schedl, A., & Wegner, M. (2003). The Sox9 transcription factor determines glial fate choice in the developing spinal cord. *Genes Dev, 17*(13), 1677-1689.

Stolt, C. C., Rehberg, S., Ader, M., Lommes, P., Riethmacher, D., Schachner, M., et al. (2002). Terminal differentiation of myelin-forming oligodendrocytes depends on the transcription factor Sox10. *Genes Dev, 16*(2), 165-170.

Stolt, C. C., Schlierf, A., Lommes, P., Hillgartner, S., Werner, T., Kosian, T., et al. (2006). SoxD proteins influence multiple stages of oligodendrocyte development and modulate SoxE protein function. *Dev Cell, 11*(5), 697-709.

Stolt, C. C., Schmitt, S., Lommes, P., Sock, E., & Wegner, M. (2005). Impact of transcription factor Sox8 on oligodendrocyte specification in the mouse embryonic spinal cord. *Dev Biol, 281*(2), 309-317.

Suh, H., Consiglio, A., Ray, J., Sawai, T., D'Amour, K. A., & Gage, F. H. (2007). In vivo fate analysis reveals the multipotent and self-renewal capacities of Sox2+ neural stem cells in the adult hippocampus. *Cell Stem Cell, 1*(5), 515-528.

Sutter, R., Shakhova, O., Bhagat, H., Behesti, H., Sutter, C., Penkar, S., et al. (2010). Cerebellar stem cells act as medulloblastoma-initiating cells in a mouse model and a neural stem cell signature characterizes a subset of human medulloblastomas. *Oncogene, 29*(12), 1845-1856.

Swartling, F. J., Ferletta, M., Kastemar, M., Weiss, W. A., & Westermark, B. (2009). Cyclic GMP-dependent protein kinase II inhibits cell proliferation, Sox9 expression and Akt phosphorylation in human glioma cell lines. *Oncogene, 28*(35), 3121-3131.

Takash, W., Canizares, J., Bonneaud, N., Poulat, F., Mattei, M. G., Jay, P., et al. (2001). SOX7 transcription factor: sequence, chromosomal localisation, expression, transactivation and interference with Wnt signalling. *Nucleic Acids Res, 29*(21), 4274-4283.

Tchougounova, E., Jiang, Y., Brasater, D., Lindberg, N., Kastemar, M., Asplund, A., et al. (2009). Sox5 can suppress platelet-derived growth factor B-induced glioma development in Ink4a-deficient mice through induction of acute cellular senescence. *Oncogene, 28*(12), 1537-1548.

Tso, C. L., Shintaku, P., Chen, J., Liu, Q., Liu, J., Chen, Z., et al. (2006). Primary glioblastomas express mesenchymal stem-like properties. *Mol Cancer Res, 4*(9), 607-619.

Uchikawa, M., Kamachi, Y., & Kondoh, H. (1999). Two distinct subgroups of Group B Sox genes for transcriptional activators and repressors: their expression during embryonic organogenesis of the chicken. *Mech Dev, 84*(1-2), 103-120.

Ueda, R., Iizuka, Y., Yoshida, K., Kawase, T., Kawakami, Y., & Toda, M. (2004). Identification of a human glioma antigen, SOX6, recognized by patients' sera. *Oncogene, 23*(7), 1420-1427.

Ueda, R., Kinoshita, E., Ito, R., Kawase, T., Kawakami, Y., & Toda, M. (2008). Induction of protective and therapeutic antitumor immunity by a DNA vaccine with a glioma antigen, SOX6. *Int J Cancer, 122*(10), 2274-2279.

Ueda, R., Yoshida, K., Kawakami, Y., Kawase, T., & Toda, M. (2004a). Expression of a transcriptional factor, SOX6, in human gliomas. *Brain Tumor Pathol, 21*(1), 35-38.

Ueda, R., Yoshida, K., Kawakami, Y., Kawase, T., & Toda, M. (2004b). Immunohistochemical analysis of SOX6 expression in human brain tumors. *Brain Tumor Pathol, 21*(3), 117-120.

Ueda, R., Yoshida, K., Kawase, T., Kawakami, Y., & Toda, M. (2007). Preferential expression and frequent IgG responses of a tumor antigen, SOX5, in glioma patients. *Int J Cancer, 120*(8), 1704-1711.

Uhlen, M., Bjorling, E., Agaton, C., Szigyarto, C. A., Amini, B., Andersen, E., et al. (2005). A human protein atlas for normal and cancer tissues based on antibody proteomics. *Mol Cell Proteomics, 4*(12), 1920-1932.

Uwanogho, D., Rex, M., Cartwright, E. J., Pearl, G., Healy, C., Scotting, P. J., et al. (1995). Embryonic expression of the chicken Sox2, Sox3 and Sox11 genes suggests an interactive role in neuronal development. *Mech Dev, 49*(1-2), 23-36.

van de Wetering, M., Oosterwegel, M., van Norren, K., & Clevers, H. (1993). Sox-4, an Sry-like HMG box protein, is a transcriptional activator in lymphocytes. *EMBO J, 12*(10), 3847-3854.

Wang, H., Leav, I., Ibaragi, S., Wegner, M., Hu, G. F., Lu, M. L., et al. (2008). SOX9 is expressed in human fetal prostate epithelium and enhances prostate cancer invasion. *Cancer Res, 68*(6), 1625-1630.

Wang, H., McKnight, N. C., Zhang, T., Lu, M. L., Balk, S. P., & Yuan, X. (2007). SOX9 is expressed in normal prostate basal cells and regulates androgen receptor expression in prostate cancer cells. *Cancer Res, 67*(2), 528-536.

Wang, Y., Bagheri-Fam, S., & Harley, V. R. (2005). SOX13 is up-regulated in the developing mouse neuroepithelium and identifies a sub-population of differentiating neurons. *Brain Res Dev Brain Res, 157*(2), 201-208.

Wegner, M. (1999). From head to toes: the multiple facets of Sox proteins. *Nucleic Acids Res, 27*(6), 1409-1420.

Wegner, M., & Stolt, C. C. (2005). From stem cells to neurons and glia: a Soxist's view of neural development. *Trends Neurosci, 28*(11), 583-588.

Weigle, B., Ebner, R., Temme, A., Schwind, S., Schmitz, M., Kiessling, A., et al. (2005). Highly specific overexpression of the transcription factor SOX11 in human malignant gliomas. *Oncol Rep, 13*(1), 139-144.

Weiss, J., Meeks, J. J., Hurley, L., Raverot, G., Frassetto, A., & Jameson, J. L. (2003). Sox3 is required for gonadal function, but not sex determination, in males and females. *Mol Cell Biol, 23*(22), 8084-8091.

Verhaak, R. G., Hoadley, K. A., Purdom, E., Wang, V., Qi, Y., Wilkerson, M. D., et al. (2010). Integrated genomic analysis identifies clinically relevant subtypes of glioblastoma characterized by abnormalities in PDGFRA, IDH1, EGFR, and NF1. *Cancer Cell, 17*(1), 98-110.

Wiese, C., Rolletschek, A., Kania, G., Blyszczuk, P., Tarasov, K. V., Tarasova, Y., et al. (2004). Nestin expression--a property of multi-lineage progenitor cells? *Cell Mol Life Sci, 61*(19-20), 2510-2522.

Yuan, X., Curtin, J., Xiong, Y., Liu, G., Waschsmann-Hogiu, S., Farkas, D. L., et al. (2004). Isolation of cancer stem cells from adult glioblastoma multiforme. *Oncogene, 23*(58), 9392-9400.

Zappone, M. V., Galli, R., Catena, R., Meani, N., De Biasi, S., Mattei, E., et al. (2000). Sox2 regulatory sequences direct expression of a (beta)-geo transgene to telencephalic neural stem cells and precursors of the mouse embryo, revealing regionalization of gene expression in CNS stem cells. *Development, 127*(11), 2367-2382.

Part 3

Endoglin: Role of Angiogenesis - CNS Tumors

6

Angiogenesis of Primary Brain Tumors: The Role of Endoglin (CD105)

Yasuo Sugita
Department of Pathology, Kurume University School of Medicine, Japan

1. Introduction

Angiogenesis is the process by which tumors induce the blood supply crucial for growth and progression. Therefore, angiogenesis has been proposed as a prognostic marker in a variety of human neoplasms (Bellamy et al., 1999). Although the importance of angiogenesis in solid tumors is well established, its role in the clinical implication of neoangiogenesis in brain tumors is enigmatic.

Endoglin (CD105) is a receptor for transforming growth factors (TGF)-β1 and TGF-beta 3, and it modulates TGF-β signaling by interacting with the TGF-βa receptor I (TGF-βRI) and/or the TGF－β receptor II (TGF－β RII) whereas antibodies against panendothelial cells, such as anti-CD31 and anti-CD34 antibodies, have been commonly used in the evaluation of angiogenesis. These panendothelial antibodies react with not only newly forming vessels, but also with normal vessels trapped within tumor tissues (Duff et al., 2003). On the other hand, endoglin (CD105) is predominantly expressed in cellular lineages within the vascular system and is overexpressed in proliferating endothelial cells that participate in tumor angiogenesis, with weak or negative expression in the vascular endothelium of normal tissues (Balza et al., 2001). Investigators have recently shown that endoglin (CD105) is a more specific and sensitive microvessel marker than other commonly used panendothelial antibodies in malignant neoplasms of the brain, breast, colon, esophagus, urothelial bladder, and lung (Dales et al., 2004; Bodey et al., 1998; Minhajat et al., 2006; Saad et al., 2005; Santos et al., 2003; Tanaka F et al., 2010).

From this perspective, this review summarizes our current knowledge regarding the role of endoglin (CD105) in the angiogenesis of primary brain tumors and further introduces the potential role of endoglin (CD105) targeting compounds for the treatment of primary brain tumors.

2. Structure and function of endoglin (CD105)

Endoglin was designated the cluster of differentiation number 105 at the Fifth International Workshop on Human Leukocyte Differentiation Antigen. Therefore,
it was called, as an alias, CD105 (Dallas et al., 2008). Human endoglin (CD105) is a type I integral membrane protein with a large extracellular domain, a single hydrophobic transmembrane domain, and a short cytosolic domain. The expression of two alternatively spliced isoforms (L and S), long and short endoglin has been charcterized. L- endoglin and

S-endoglin are different from each other in thier cytoplasmic tails that have 47, 14 amino acids, respectively. L- endoglin is predominant and S-endoglin remains unobscure in the significance of it's function (López-Novoa & Bernabeu, 2010). Endoglin is constitutively phosphorylated on serine and threonine residues. Endoglin is an accessory protein of the TGF-β receptor family (Barbara et al., 1999; Li et al., 1999). The TGF-β receptor family of ligands contains TGF-β type 1, TGF-β type 2, and TGF-β type 3 isoforms and activins, and bone morphogenic proteins. The cytostatic domain of endoglin serves as a receptor transforming factor (TGF)-β type 1 and TGF-β type 3, and modulate TGF-β signaling through it's interaction with TGF-βRI and TGF-βRII. In endothelial cells, two TGF-β receptor type 1 pathways with opposite effects have been demonstrated: the ALK-5 that stimulates Smad 2/3 phosphorylation, and the ALK-1 that stimulates Smad 1/5 phosphorylation. Endoglin (CD105) induces TGF-β1/ALK 5 signaling that promotes endothelial proliferation and migration. On the other hand, endoglin (CD105) indirectly inhibits TGF-β1/ALK 5 signaling (Dallas et al., 2008;Fonsatti et al., 2010).

3. Endoglin (CD105) and hypoxia

Hypoxia is a major stimulus of neovascularization including tumor angiogenesis, and collateral vessel formation in ischemic cardiovascular disease. As outlined above,
endoglin (CD105), a marker of endothelial cells, is abundantly expressed in tissues undergoing angiogenesis and is a receptor for transforming growth factor β. The pivotal role of CD105 in the vascular system was demonstrated by the severe vascular defects that occur in CD105-knockout mice, but the exact mechanisms for CD105 regulation of vascular development have not been fully elucidated. In light of the function of CD105 and the importance of hypoxia in neovascularisation, Li et al. speculated that CD105 is involved in hypoxia-initiated angiogenesis, and they have investigated the effects of hypoxic stress on CD105 gene expression using tissue-cultured human microvascular endothelial cells (Li et al., 2003). As for the results, they considered that hypoxia is a potent stimulus for CD105 gene expression in vascular endothelial cells, which in turn attenuates cell apoptosis and thus contributes to angiogenesis. They also speculated that the non-TGF β-binding endoglin (CD105) in endothelial cells plays a self-protective role against apoptotic factors such as hypoxia.

Angiogenesis occurs in the human brain after a stroke, with endothelial proliferation after 3 to 4 days, a dense capillary network by 1 week, and neovascular infiltration by 2 to 4 weeks. These alternations help to sustain cerebral circulation and prevent a recurrent stroke. Therefore, to investigate the mechanisms of angiogenesis after cerebral ischemia, Zhu et al. studied the effect of hypoxia on endoglin expression in murine cerebral microvascular endothelial cells (bEND.3 cells) in vitro and the possible involvement of mitogen-activated protein kinase (MAPK) pathways (Zhu et al., 2003). The results of their investigation are as follows; namely, hypoxia increased endoglin mRNA and protein expression in bEND.3 cells, which was associated with the phosphoactivation of extracellular signal-related kinase (ERK), p38 MAPK, and Jun amino-terminal kinase (JNK). Inhibitors of p38 decreased the hypoxic induction of endoglin expression, as did dominant negative MAPK kinase 3 (MKK3), which activates p38. In contrast, constitutively active MKK3 or JNK1 potentiated the hypoxic induction of endoglin. Therefore, they considered that hypoxia induces the expression of endoglin at both the mRNA and protein levels and that induction is regulated by the p38 and perhaps also JNK pathways. In addition, Guo et al supported their theory based on the data of human strokes, although it would limit the value of the findings of Zhu et al., which were based on the use of murine endothelial cell culture and an in vivo mouse model of focal cerebral ischemia (Guo et al., 2004). Furthermore, they demonstrated that knowledge of endoglin (CD105) signaling would have practical implications for the discovery of novel therapies in a host of angiogenic disease.

Dziewulska et al. morphologically examined human brains several years after a territorial ischemic stroke to assess the development of progressing white matter damage and its pathomechanisms (Dziewulska et al., 2006). They focused on the role of TGF-β, one of the factors whose expression increases after tissue damage, and its receptor endoglin in the propagation of postischemic injury. The results of their investigation are as follows; namely, the examination of white matter adjacent to the postapoplectic cavity revealed structural changes in the capillary vessels, disturbed microcirculation, and deep endothelial cell damage with DNA fragmentation in the TUNEL reaction. Many oligodendrocytes also revealed DNA damage and an increased expression of caspase-3. In the rarefied white matter, the microvessel immune reaction to TGF-β was diminished while the expression of endoglin was heterogeneous: absent in some capillaries but increased in others in comparison to the vessels located more peripherally from the cavity and in the control material. Therefore, they considered that endoglin and TGF-β can be involved in the development of the microangiopathy responsible for the propagation of postischemic white matter injury in humans, and speculated that disturbances in endoglin expression can influence TGF-β signaling and, consequently, vessel structure and function. In addition, they considered that pronounced endoglin expression can lead to decreased vessel wall integrity while a lack of the constitutively expressed protein is probably a reflection of deep vessel damage.

Collectively, these above studies indicate that endoglin (CD105) has an important role in angiogenesis in ischemic cardiovascular disease or cerebral stroke.

4. Endoglin (CD105) and non-tumor angiogenesis

Although endoglin is expressed at low levels in normal tissue, it is highly expressed in vascular endothelial cells during embryogenesis, in inflamed tissues, and healing wounds, psoriatic skin, inflamed synovial arthritis, and vascular injury. In addition, investigators pointed out the important role of endoglin in vascular pathology. Particularly, the representative example is hereditary hemorrhagic telangiectasia (HHT), or Rendu-Osler-Weber syndrome (Fernández-L et al., 2006). This is manifested as epistaxis, mucocutaneous and gastrointestinal telangiectases, and arteriovenous malformations in the pulomanary, cerebral, or hepatic circulation. The recent isolation and characterization of circulating endothelial cells from HHT patients has revealed a decreased endoglin expression, impaired ALK1-and ALK5-dependent TGF-β signaling, disorganized cytoskelton and the failure to form cord-like structures which may lead to the fragility of small vessels with the bleeding characteristic of HHT vascular dysplasia, or to disrupted and abnormal angiogenesis after injuries and may explain the clinical symptoms associated with this disease. Furthermore, it is well known that a high incidence of arteriovenous malformations (AVMs) of central nervous system is associated with HHT type 1 and endoglin. The gene mutated in this disorder is expressed at reduced levels in the blood vessels of these patients. Since endoglin is a component of the transforming growth factor-β receptor complex critical for vascular development and homeostasis, Matsubara et al. determined its expression in sporadic cerebral AVMs and in normal brain vessels (Matsubara et al., 2011). They examined twenty cerebral AVMs and 10 normal brain samples were analyzed for endoglin, platelet endothelial cell adhesion molecule 1 (PECAM-1), alpha-smooth muscle cell actin, vimentin, and desmin by immunohistochemistry. As for the results of their investigation, in the normal brain, endoglin was found not only in the endothelium of all vessels but also in the adventitial layer of arteries and arterioles. Namely, in cerebral AVMs, the numerous vessels presented expressed endoglin in both the endothelium and adventitia. Arterialized veins, identified by lack of elastin and an uneven thickness of smooth muscle cells, revealed endoglin-positive mesenchymal cells in the adventitia and perivascular connective tissue. They found that these cells were fibroblasts since they expressed vimentin but not actin and/or desmin, and that increasing numbers of endoglin-positive endothelial and adventitial cells were seen in sporadic cerebral AVMs, but endoglin density was normal. Thus, they considered that it was not involved in the generation of these lesions. However, since the presence of endoglin in fibroblasts in the perivascular stroma, they speculated that there is an active role for this protein in vascular remodeling in response to increased blood flow and shear stress.

On the other hand, Sure et al. examined endoglin (CD105) expression of adult cavernous malformation of the central nervous system (CNS) to clarify their biological activity (Sure et al., 2005). They pointed out the histological similarities of HHT and the cavernous malformation of the CNS, and found endoglin (CD105) in the majority of cavernous malformations of the CNS. However, they considered that the role of endoglin (CD105) in cavernous malformations when compared with AVMs, since cavernous malformations are not associated with high blood flow or shear stress.

Moyamoya disease is a cerebrovascular occlusive disease characterized by progressive stenosis or occlusion at the distal ends of the bilateral internal arteries. Histological investigations on autopsy samples have demonstrated the main vascular lesion in moyamoya disease is stenosis or occlusion caused by an intimal hyperplasia. Recently, evidence has been obtained indicating that hypoxia-inducing factor-1 regulates TGF-β3.

Therefore, Takagi et al. surgically collected tiny pieces of the wall of the middle cerebral artery from patients with moyamoya disease and analyzed them using histological and immunohistochemical methods focusing on the mechanism of remodeling of the intracranial arterial walls of patients with moyamoya disease (Takagi et al., 2007). As for results of their study, middle cerebral artery specimens from moyamoya disease patients had a thicker intima than those from the control group. In moyamoya disease samples, the immunoreactivity indicating both hypoxia-inducing factor-1α and endoglin expression was higher in the endothelium and intima. No vascular endothelial growth factor immunoreactivity was detectable in the moyamoya disease samples. In addition, transforming growth factor-β3 immunoreactivity was also detected and was co-localized with that of hypoxia-inducing factor-1α and endoglin, mainly in the endothelium.

Therefore, they considered that hypoxia-inducing factor-1α and endoglin were overexpressed in the intima of the middle cerebral artery of moyamoya disease patients, and that these factors play a role in the proliferating response of moyamoya disease.

Collectively, these above studies indicate that endoglin (CD105) has an important role in the vascular remodeling of the CNS.

5. Endoglin (CD105) and tumor angiogenesis

Angiogenesis is the formation of new blood vessels from preexisting vessels or circulating endothelial progenitor cells, and it is essential for tumor growth by providing nutrients and eliminating metabolic waste products. Therefore, angiogenesis has been proposed to be a prognostic marker in a variety of human neoplasms and investigators compared the expression of endoglin with other markers in cancers from various organs.

It was reported by Saad et al. that they studied endoglin and the vascular endothelial growth factor (VEGF) expression as a possible prognostic marker in esophageal carcinoma (Saad et al., 2005). They have shown that the assesment of microvesell count using endoglin in esopageal carcinoma might be a valuable parameter for predicting patients who have a poor survival rate and higher risk of developing a metastatic disease. In addition, they reported that endoglin, by direct staining of proliferative vessels in esophageal adenocarcinoma, is a more specific and sensitive marker for tumor angiogenesis than the other commonly used panendothelial markers. Furthermore, endoglin staining also showed prognostic significance with a positive correlation with the presence of angiolymphatic invasion, tumor stage, and survival.

In breast carcinomas, as in many tumor types, marked characteristics of neoangiogenesis have been found to correlate with a high rate of metastasis. Intratumoral tumoral microvessels can be identified with panendothelial markers that stain all tumor blood vessels to the same degree. Dales et al. therefore considered that they should examine other markers more specific to activated endothelial cells that should better reflect a tumor's capability to produce new vessels, and they studied the long-term prognostic significance of neoangiogenesis in breast carcinoma by comparison of Tie-2/Tek, endoglin (CD105) and CD31 immunocytochemical expression (Dales et al., 2004). As a result, they showed that endoglin (CD105) immunoexpression in breast carcinomas is an independent prognostic indicator in node-negative patients, better in terms of overall survival than Tie-2/Tek and panendothelial marker CD31.

Information regarding the role of angiogenin and endoglin (CD105) expression in head and neck squamous cell carcinoma is extremely sparse and limited exclusively to serum protein levels. Thus, Marioni et al. investigated angiogenin expression in laryngeal squamous cell carcinoma and evaluated the relationship between angiogenin expression and endoglin (CD105), clinicopathological and prognostic parameters. As a result, they showed that angiogenin expression in laryngeal carcinoma cells and endoglin (CD105) expression in vascular endothelial cells in the de novo blood vessels can be considered potentially useful to detect laryngeal squamous cell carcinoma patients with high risk of disease recurrence who might benefit from more aggressive therapy (Marioni et al., 2004).

Most colorectal carcinomas are considered to originate from precursor lesions (adenomas). Adenomas are thought to progress to carcinoma over many years because of multiple accumulated molecular alternations, and angiogenesis is an important step in the process of colorectal carcinoma growth. Therefore, Minhajat et al. compared the expression of endoglin (CD105) in several hundred target spots with that of other endothelial markers in all tissue layers during the development of colon carcinoma using tissue microarrays and immunohistochemistry (Minhajat et al., 2006a, 2006b). As a result, they showed that endoglin (CD105) was expressed at high levels in vascular endothelial cells in the de novo blood vessels of the adenoma-carcinoma of the colon and was weakly expressed in blood vessels of the normal mucosal layers. Therefore, they considered that endoglin (CD105) was more intensely expressed in de novo microvessels. In this review, Fig. 1 shows that endoglin (CD105) was expressed at high levels in vascular endothelial cells in the de novo blood vessels of the carcinoma of the colon. Namely, although vascular endothelial expression of panendothelial marker CD 34 in normal and neoplastic layers of adenoma and adenocarcinoma from all layers did not significantly differ, endoglin (CD105) was intensely expressed in vascular endothelial cells of the neoplastic mucosal adenoma and various layers of adenocarcinoma at a level corresponding to the depth of cancer invasion.

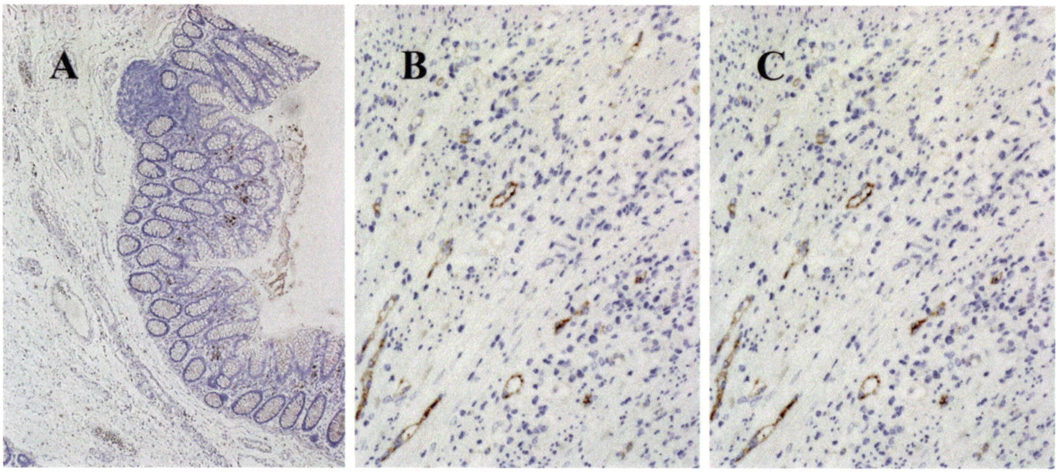

A. Endoglin (CD105)-negative endothelial cells in normal colonic tissue adjacent to colonic carcinoma. B. Vessels in colonic carcinoma at submucosal level showing endoglin (CD105)-positive endothelial cells. C. Vessels in colonic carcinoma at muscular layer level showing endoglin (CD105)-positive endothelial cells.

Fig. 1. Expression of endoglin (CD105).

Collectively, these above studies indicate that endoglin (CD105) is a better marker than panendothelial markers such as CD31, 34, etc., in the evaluation of neoangiogenesis and prediction of prognosis in various cancers.

6. Endoglin (CD105) and primary brain tumor angiogenesis

6.1 Endoglin (CD105) and glioma angiogenesis

Several investigators have shown that the degree of angiogenesis has a prognostic value in glial tumors, particularly astrocytic tumors, oligodendrogliomas. Yao et al. considered that the prognosis of glioma patients is largely determined by the histopathlogical malignacy grade, whereas within each grade, the clinical course of glioma patients is still variable because each grade tumor is not a single pathological entity but encompasses a spectrum of tumors with variable malignant potential. Also, the prediction of tumor biological behavior can thus hardly be made only by histological criteria and needs the predicting assistance of biological makers (Yao et al., 2005). Therefore, they assessed micovessel density (MVD) using an anti-105 monoclonal antibody to clarify the validity of endoglin (CD105) in the evaluation of angiogenesis in gliomas. They demonstrated that MVD expressed by endoglin (CD105) is more closely correlated the prognosis of glioma patients than MVD expressed by panendothelial marker CD 31.

The prototypic histopathology of glioblastomas is characterized by dense cellularity, striking pleomorphism, a complex form of microvascular proliferation and zones of coagulative necrosis lined by "pseudopalisading" tumor cells. It is also well known that numerous vascular changes occur at the transition of anaplastic astrocytomas to glioblastomas. Recent studies have further demonstrated that a dramatic shift in biological behavior occurs following the transition from anaplastic astrocytomas to glioblastomas. Brat and Van Meir reported that pseudopalisade formation results from the following sequence of events: i) vascular occlusion, which is related to endothelial apoptosis and associated with intravascular thrombosis; ii) hypoxia in regions surrounding vascular pathology; iii) outward migration of glioma cells away from hypoxia, creating a peripherally directed wave of cell movement; iv) death of nonmigrated cells leading to central necrosis; v) an exuberant angiogenic response creating microvascular proliferation in regions peripheral to the central hypoxia; and vi) enhanced outward expansion of infiltrating tumor cells toward a new vasculature (Brat &Van Meir, 2004). In addition, vascular glomeruli are observed in the white matter surrounding the tumor but less frequently in the cortex. The number, caliber and wall thickness mean values of the vessels are significantly higher than those of the normal brain. In this area, significant modifications in terms of vacularization and biomolecular features take place. Therefore, Sica et al. investigated that neovascularization in the tumor surrounding areas by examining endoglin (CD105) and nestin expression along with MVD while establishing their possible prognostic significance (Sica et al.,2011).. As a result, they demonstrated that a tumor neoangiogenesis occurs in glioblastoma peritumor tissue with intimate involvement of pericytes, and that endoglin (CD105)-MVD in the area located at a greater distance from the tumor margin carries prognostic significance. In this review, Fig. 2 shows that endoglin (CD105) is expressed at high levels in vascular endothelial cells in the de novo blood vessels of glioblastoma. Namely, although vascular endothelial expression of panendothelial marker CD 34 in normal and did not significantly differ normal brain, astrocytoma, and glioblastoma, endoglin (CD105) was intensely expressed in

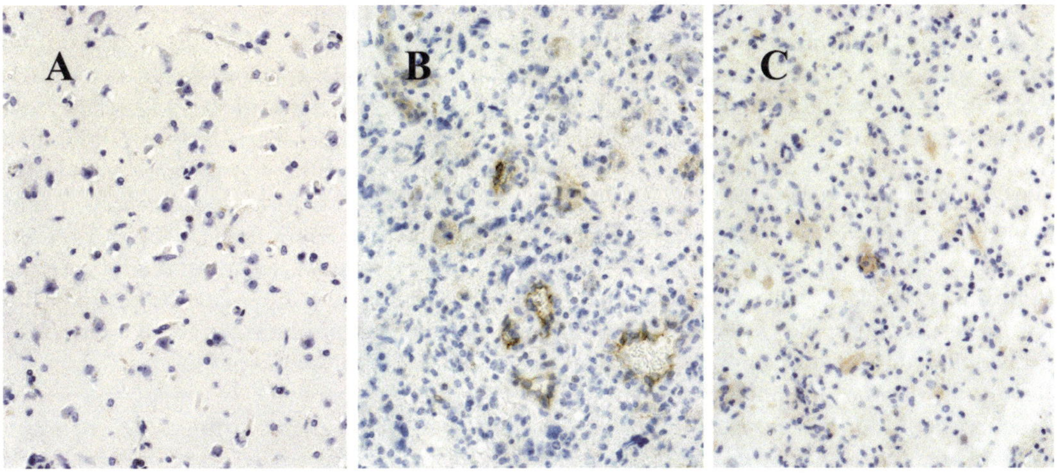

A. Endoglin (CD105)-negative endothelial cells in normal brain tissue adjacent to glioblastoma. B. Vessels in Glioblastoma(Grade IV, WHO classification) showing intensive endoglin (CD105)-expression of endothelial cells. C. Vessels in diffuse astrocytoma (Grade II, WHO classification) showing heterogenous endoglin (CD105)-expression of endothelial cells.

Fig. 2. Expression of endoglin (CD105).

vascular endothelial cells of glioblastoma, but was heterogeneous in astrocytona and negative in normal brain, respectively.
Regarding oligodendrgliomas, Netto et al. considered that oligodendrgliomas show typical vascularization with delicate and ramified blood vessels, but also the importance of angiogenesis (Netto et al., 2008). Therefore, they assessed micovessel density (MVD) using an anti-105 monoclonal antibody to clarify the validity of endoglin (CD105) in the evaluation of angiogenesis in oligodendrogliomas, and showed that endoglin (CD105)-MVD is greater in anaplastic oligodendrogliomas than oligodendrogliomas, indicating an increase in the vascular neoformation, something which must be evaluated as a possible prognostic factor in oligodendrogliomas.
Based on these collective evidences, it is indicated that endoglin (CD105) is a better marker than panendothelial markers such as CD31, 34, etc., in the evaluation of neoangiogenesis and prediction of prognosis in glial tumors, particularly glioblastomas.

6.2 Endoglin (CD105) and extraaxial tumor angiogenesis

The grading of meningiomas is geneally based on tumor subtype and histological features. Although the MIB-1 labelling index is not an included criterion in the WHO grading system, it is sometimes used to assess the prognosis of patients with meningiomas. In addition, several studies have shown that the morbidity of meniniomas is related to the degree of tumor vascularity. As mentioned above, several investigators have already shown that the degree of angiogenesis has prognostic value in primary brain tumors, particularly astrocytic tumors, oligodendrogliomas. Regarding extraaxial tumor angiogenesis, Barresi et al. investigated endoglin (CD105) in immunoexpression in meningiomas and the corresponding normal leptomeninges in order to evaluate its ability to identify newly formed neoplastic vessels as well as establish whether a correlation exists between clinicopathological parameters, so as to verify if MVD documented by endoglin (CD105) could be utilized for prognostic purposes (Barresi et al., 2008). As a result, they showed that CD 34 stained both the host entrapped vessels in menngiomas and the newly formed vessels; thus CD34 may be considered a pan-endothelial marker, while endoglin (CD105) futher appears to be a more specific marker for neo-angigenesis, and that endoglin (CD105) positive vessels were evidenced in 70% of meningiomas and atypical meningiomas were charactraized by higher endoglin (CD105) immunoexpression in general. Interestingly, they also showed that cases with higher MIB-1 labelling indexed exhibit significantly higher CD 105 counts. In this regard, they speculated that meningiomas with an intrinstically higher capability to proliferate undergo a hypoxic condition which is determined by their increased volume, and that hypoxia may be in turn responsible for the endoglin up-regulation, via the hypoxia inducible factor-1 and consequently for the higher neo-angiogenesis revealed by MVD. Furthermore, they speculated that endoglin (CD105) might be considered a target for anti-angiogenic selective immuno-therapies able to blood supply in meningiomas.
Regarding pituitary tumors, there is controversy about the behavior of angiogenesis as a function of hormonal secretion or other characteristics of pituitary tumors. Pizarro et al. studied the anti-endoglin (CD105) antibody, a glycoprotein expressed in endothelial cells and conjunctive tissue particularly associated with neovascularization, in order to determine MVD in pituitary adenomas (Pizarro et al., 2009). Their data were as follows; No significant difference was found in MVD concerning the variables of age, clinical presentation, immunohistochemical phenotype or tumor size. MVD in males was significantly higher than in females. Cell proliferation, as evaluated by the MIB-1 antibody ranged from 0% to

19.58%. No correlation was found between MIB-1 and MVD. Therefore, they speculated that the lower MVD found in pituitary adenomas in females reflects an inhibitory estrogen action on TGF-β1, a protein involved in vascular remodeling, and that, because of its role as a TGF receptor ligand, endoglin proved to be sensitive in detecting this gender difference in pituitary tumor angiogenesis.

6.3 Endoglin (CD105) and primary central nervous system lymphoma angiogenesis

Primary central nervous system lymphomas (PCNSLs) are an uncommon variant of extranodal non-Hodgkin lymphomas that involve leptomeninges, eyes or the spinal cord without evidence of systemic disease. These lymphomas do not include systemic lymphomas that have spread to the CNS. The vast majority of PCNS lymphomas are of B-cell origin (Paulus et al., 2007; Sugita et al., 2004). There have been two hypotheses to explain the pathologic processes of PCNS lymphomas. One hypothesis suggests that inflammatory lesions transform into neoplasms, such as lymphomas, in situ in the CNS. The other hypothesis suggests that a malignant B-cell clone homes to the CNS, although a putative homing signal has not been identified.

There are conflicting descriptions as to whether the degree of angiogenesis as measured by microvessel density has prognostic value in lymphomas. For example, Zhao et al. reported that vascular endothelial growth factor-A was expressed both on lymphoma cells and endothelial cells in angioimmunoblastic T-cell lymphomas, and it thus was related to lymphoma progression (Zhao et al., 2004). Salven et al. also demonstrated the simultaneous serum elevation of vascular endothelial growth factor (VEGF) and basic fibroblast growth factor (bFGF) levels to be an independent predictor of a poor prognosis in non-Hodgkin's lymphoma (Salven et al., 2000). On the other hand, Stewart et al. reported that non-Hodgkin's lymphoma may be less angiogenic than most solid tumors (Salven et al., 2002). Regarding PCNSLs, Rubenstein et al. speculated that angiotropism in PCNSLs may constitute an important paracrine growth mechanism for lymphoma progression (Rubenstein et al., 2002). However, Roser et al. commented that the lack of a correlation between apoptosis and vascularity may indicate that PCNSLs growth occurs independently of vessel formation, even though the high microvessel density in PCNSLs could play a significant role in the growth kinetics and infiltrating potential of the tumor. They also commented that this could be due to the various techniques for microvessel counting used by different laboratories rather than due to truly different results (Roser et al., 2004).

It was described by Sugita et al that CD105 staining reduced the false-positive staining of blood vessels in comparison to the commonly used panendothelial marker CD34. In addition, the survival rate of the lower-MVD patients was significantly higher than that of the higher-MVD patients when CD105 was used as a marker of angiogenesis. In contrast, when CD34 was used as a marker of angiogenesis, the survival rates did not significantly differ between these two groups. In addition, using a multivariate analysis, CD105-MVD demonstrated independent prognostic impacts in this investigation. As a result, they considered that the growth of PCNSLs was dependent on angiogenesis and that the intratumoral-MVD determined by the anti-CD105 monoclonal antibody was a reliable prognostic marker in patients with PCNSLs (Sugita et al., 2007). In general, PCNSLs are typically patchy, poorly demarcated, and angiocentric at low magnification (Russel & Rubinstein, 1989). Namely, the neoplastic transformation itself may, especially at the periphery of the tumor, remain at first relatively confined to the Virchow-Robin spaces, but thereafter may acquire a more florid expression as it infiltrates and destroys the neural parenchyma. In view of their study on the angiogenesis of PCNSLs, there may be some validity to this theory. Therefore, they demonstrated that PCNSLs may not need sufficient neoangiogenesis at the start of PCNSLs, but instead may require a higher rate of neoangiogenesis as they infiltrate and destroy the brain parenchyma at an advanced stage. In this review, Fig. 3 shows that endoglin (CD105) is expressed at high levels in vascular endothelial cells in the de novo blood vessels of PCNSL.

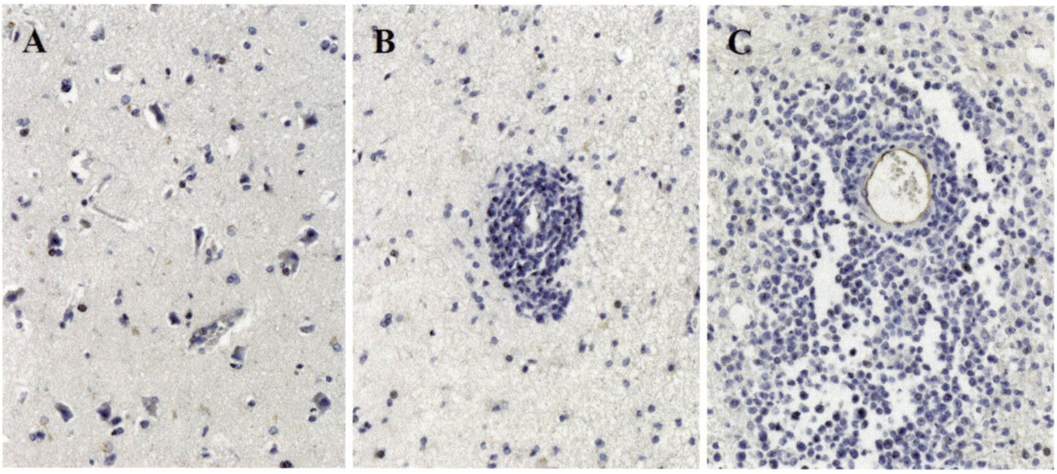

A. Endoglin (CD105)-negative endothelial cells in normal brain tissue adjacent to PCNSL. B. Endoglin (CD105)-negative endothelial cells in the periphery of PCNSL. C. Vessels in an advanced stage of PCNSL showing intensive endoglin (CD105)-expression of endothelial cells.

Fig. 3. Expression of endoglin (CD105).

7. Endoglin (CD 105) antagonists: a potential therapeutic tool for malignant brain tumors

As outlined above, endoglin (CD105) has an important role in the tumorigenesis of malignant tumors. In addition, vascular targeting agents for the treatment of cancer are designated to cause a rapid and selective shutdown of blood vessels of tumors (Thorpe F et al., 2004). Thus, endoglin (CD105) is emerging as a prime vascular target of antiangiogenetic cancer therapy. Interestingly, Takase et al. assessed cases of small cell carcinomas at autopsy using immnuohistochemistry to investigate the degree of angiogenesis status in small cell carcinoma tissue (Takase et al., 2010). As a result, they considered that small cell carcinomas are predominantly supported by newly formed vessels that are generated by endoglin (CD105)-mediated angiogenesis, and that anti-angiogenic therapy, especially endoglin (CD105)-targeting, proved an effective form of small cell carcinoma treatment.

Recent studies have shown the systemic administration of naked antihuman endoglin monoclonal antibodies to suppress established tumors, and its efficacy was markedly enhanced by combination with a chemotherapeutic drug using an antiangiogenic schedule of drug dosing. For instance, the effect of anti-endoglin (CD105) monoclonal antibodies has been investigated in several animal models. Takahashi et al. showed that antiangiogenic therapy of established tumors in human skin/severe combined immunodeficiency mouse chimeras bearing human breast cancer by anti-endoglin (CD105) monoclonal antibodies,

SN6f, SN6j, SN6k (Takahashi et al., 2001). Namely, SN6j and SN6k were effective in suppressing established tumors, whereas tumor suppression was weaker with SN6f. A combination of SN6j and SN6k that defined mutually nonoverlapping epitopes showed an addictive antitumor effect. A combination of SN6j and cyclophosphamide using an antiangiogenic schedule of drug dosing showed synergistic antitumor efficacy. They therefore considered that systemic administration of naked antihuman endoglin monoclonal antibodies can suppress established tumors, and the efficacy is markedly enhanced by combining a chemotheraputic drug using an antiangiogenic schedule of drug dosing.

Anti-metatstatic effects of an antitumor drug are extremely important. Thus, Uneda et al. investigated the anti-metatstatic activity of 3 anti-endoglin monoclonal antibodies (SN6a, SN6j, SN6k) in animal models. They showed that SN6a and SN6j effectively suppressed the formation of metastatic colonies of murine mammary carcinoma cells in the lung of metastaic models and that SN6j, SN6k and their immunoconjugates with deglycosylated ricin A-chain were effective in suppressing hepatic metastasis of murine colorectal carcinoma cells (Uneda et al., 2009). As a result, they considered that data of their investigation were clinically relevant in view of a clinical trial.

Interestingly, it was shown by Lee et al that anti-angiogenic/anti-tumor effects achieved in a prophylactic setting with an oral DNA vaccine encoding murine endoglin, carried by double attenuated Salmonella typhimurium to secondary lymphoid organ, i.e., Peyer's patches(Lee et al., 2006). Their approach was as follows; After vaccination, mice were injected with D2F2 mouse mammary carcinomas and tumor progression was evaluated. As a result, unvaccinated mice had significantly more lung metastasis, but tumors in vaccinated mice were less angiogenic. In addtion, the vaccinated mice had a longer overall survival. Regarding the effects of an oral DNA vaccine, they speculated that a $CD8^+$ T cell mediated immune response induced by this vaccine effectively suppressed dissemination of pulmonary metastasis of D2F2 breast carcinoma cells presumably by eliminating proliferating endothelial cells in the tumor vasculature. They therefore considered that the vaccine strategies can contribute to future therapies for breast carcinomas.

Regarding brain tumors, Bodey et al. investigated 62 childhood brain tumors including 34 medulloblastomas and 28 astrocytomas for the assessment of endoglin (CD105) expression (Bodey et al.,1998). Their assesment was as follows: Strong expression of endoglin (CD105) on endothelial cells was demonstrated in all 62 childhood brain tumor cases. The most striking feature of the newly formed tumor-related capillaries was the presence of a markedly enlarged perivascular space. Blood vessels in several normal human tissues (cortex, cerebellum, thymus, tonsil, spleen, lymph node, skin) used as control tissues contained significantly lower levels of endoglin (CD105), in accordance with the extremely slow turnover rate of normal endothelial cells. A close apposition between the capillaries and the adjacent parenchyma was also observed. VEGF/PF-R1 (flt-1) and VEGF/PF-R2 (flk-1) are formed de novo in a glioma progression-dependent manner. Therfore, they considered that brain tumors, especially glioblastomas, are among the most vascularized human neoplasms, and thus are candidates for antiangiogenic therapy. In addition, they further demonstrated points that substantiate the importance of endoglin (CD105) in the earliest possible detection, diagnosis and neoplasm-related angiogenesis inhibition-based treatment of mammalian solid neoplasms, especially in childhood brain tumors.

At present, a phase 1, first-in human study with the human/murine chimeric anti endoglin (CD105) monoclonal antibody TRC105 is ongoing in patients with refactory advanced or metastaic solid carcinomas (Fonsatti et al., 2010, Seon et al., 2011).

8. Conclusion

As outlined above, endoglin (CD105) has an important role in tumorigenesis of malignant tumors. In addition, based on these collective evidences, it is indicated that endoglin (CD105) is a better marker than panendothelial markers, such as CD31, 34, etc., in the evaluation of neoangiogenesis and prediction of prognosis in primary brain tumors, particularly glioblastomas. Furthermore, endoglin (CD105) is emerging as a prime vascular target of antiangiogenetic cancer therapy. Recent studies have shown the systemic administration of naked antihuman endoglin monoclonal antibodies to suppress established tumors, and that its efficacy is markedly enhanced by combination with a chemotherapeutic drug using an antiangiogenic schedule of drug dosing. Therefore, the results of endoglin expression in gliomas, PCNLs, and other primary brain tumors could thus eventually lead to better performance of therapeutic trials on antiangiogenic treatment for patients with these primary brain tumors.

9. References

Balza E, Castellani P, Zijlstra A, Neri D, Zardi L, Siri A (2001). Lack of specificity of endoglin expression for tumor blood vessels. *Int J Cancer*, 94, pp. 579-585

Barbara NP, Wrana JL, Letarte M (1999). Endoglin is an accessory protein that interacts with the signaling receptor complex of multiple members of the transforming growth factor-β superfamily. *J Biol Chem*, 274, pp. 584-594

Barresi V, Cerasoli S, Vitarelli E, Tuccari G (2007). Density of microvessels positive for CD 105(endoglin) is related to prognosis in meningiomas. *Acta Neuropathol*, 114, pp. 147-156

Bellamy WT, Richter L, Frutiger Y, Grogan TM (1999). Expression of vascular endothelial growth factor and its receptors in hematopoietic malignancies. *Cancer Res*, 59, pp.728-733

Bodey B, Bodey B Jr, Siegel SE, Kaiser HE(1998). Upregulation of endoglin (CD105) expression during childhood brain tumor-related angiogenesis. Anti-angiogenic therapy. *Anticancer Res*, 18, pp. 1485-1500

Brat DJ, and Van Meir, E.G. (2004). Vaso-occlusive and prothrombotic mechanisms associated with tumor hypoxia, necrosis, and accelerated growth in glioblastoma. *Lab Invest* 84, pp. 397-405

Dallas NA, Samuel S, Xia L, Fan F, Gray MJ, Lim SJ, Ellis LM (2008). Endoglin (CD105): A marker of tumor vasculature and potential target for therapy. Clin *Cancer Res*, 114, pp. 1931-1933

Dales JP, Garcia S, Carpentier S, Andrac L, Ramuz O, Lavaut MN, Allasia C, Bonnier P Charpin C (2004). Long-term prognostic significance of neoangiogenesis in breast carcinomas: comparison of Tie-2/Tek, CD105, and CD 31 immunocytochemical expression. *Hum Pathol*, 35, pp. 176-183

Duff SE, LI C, Garland JM, Kumar S(2003). CD105 is important for angiogenesis: evidence and potential applications. *FASEB J* 17, pp. 984-992

Dziewulska D & Rafalowska J (2006). Role of endoglin and transforming growth factor beta in progressive white matter damage after ischemic stroke. *Neuropathology*, 26, pp. 298-306

Fernández-L A, Sanz-Rodriguez F, Blanco FJ, Bernabéu C, Botella LM (2006) Hereditary hemorrhagic telangiectasia, a vascular dysplasia affecting the TGF-ß signaling pathway. *Clin Med Res*, 4, pp. 66-78

Fonsatti E, Nicolay HJM, Altomonte M, Covre A, Maio M (2010). Targeting cancervasculature via endoglin/CD105:a novel antibody-based diagnostic and therapeutic strategy in solid tumors. *Cardiovasc Res* 86, pp. 12-19

Guo B, Kumar S, Li C, Slevin M, Kumar P (2004). CD105 apotosis, and stroke. *Stroke* 35, pp. 94-95

Li C, Hampson IN, Hampson L ,Slevin M, Kumar P, Bernabeu C, Kumar S (1999). CD105 (endoglin) antagonizes the inhibitory signalng of transforming growth factor β1 on human vascular endothelial cells. *FASEB J* 14, pp. 55-64

Li C, Issa R, Kumar P, Hampson IN, Lopez-Novoa JM, Bernabeu C, Kumar S (2003). CD105 prevents apoptosis in hypoxic endothelial cells. *J Cell Sci* 116, pp. 2677-2685

Lee S-H, Mizutani N, Mizutani M, Luo Y, Zhou H, Kaplan C, Kim S-W, Xiang R, ReisfeldRA (2006). Endoglin (CD105) is a target for an oral DNA vaccine aganst breast cancer. *Cancer Immunol Immunother* 55, pp. 1565-1574

López-Novoa & Bernabeu (2010). The physological role of endoglin in the cardiovascular system. *Am J Physiol Heart Circ Physiol* 299, pp. 959-974

Marioni G, Marino F, Blandamura S, D'Alessandro E, Giacomelli L, Guzzardo V, Lionello M, Filippis C, Staffieri A (2010). Neoangiogenesis in laryngeal carcinoma:angiogenin and CD 105 expression is related to carcinoma recurrence rate and disease-free survival. *Histopathology* 57, pp. 535 -543

Matsubara S, Bourdeau A, terBrugge KG, Wallace C, Letarte M (2000). Analysis of endoglin expression in normal brain tissue and in cerebral arteriovenous malformations. *Stroke* 31, pp. 2653 -2660

Minhajat R, Mori D, Yamasaki F, Sugita Y, Satoh T, Tokunaga O (2006). Endoglin (CD 105) expression in angiogenesis of colon cancer: analysis using tissue microarrays and comparison with other endothelial markers. *Virchows Arch* 448, pp. 127-134

Minhajat R, Mori D, Yamasaki F, Sugita Y, Satoh T, Tokunaga O (2006). Organ-specific endoglin (CD 105) expression in the angiogenesis of human cancers. *Pathol Int* 12, pp. 717-723

Netto GC, Bleil CB, Hilbig A, Coutinho LM (2008). Immunohistochemical evaluation of the microvascular density through the expression of TGF-β (CD 105/endoglin) and CD34 receptors and expression of the vascular endothelial growth factor (VEGF) in oligodendrogliomas. *Neuropathology* 28, pp. 17 -23

Paulus W, Jellinger K, Morgello S, Deckert-Schluter (2007) Malignant lymphomas. In: Kleihues P and Cavenee WK (eds) *Pathology and Genetics of Tumours of the Nervous System*. International Agency for Research on Cancer Press, Lyon, pp. 198-203,

Pizarro CB, Oliveira MC, Pereira-Lima JFS, Leães CG, Kramer CK, Schuch T, Barbosa-Coutinho LM, Ferreira NP (2009). Evaluation of angiogenesis in 77 pituitary adenomas using endoglin as a marker. *Neuropathology* 29, pp. 40 -44

Roser F, Saini M, Meliss R, Ostertag H, Samii M, Bellinzona M (2004) Apoptosis, vascularity, and proliferation in primary central nervous system lymphomas: a histopathological study. *Surg Neurol* 62, pp. 393-399

Rubenstein J, Fischbein N, Aldape K, Burton E, Shuman M (2002) Hemorrhage and VEGF expression in a case of primary CNS lymphoma. *J Neurooncol* 58, pp. 53-56

Russel DS and Rubinstein LJ (1989) Primary cerebral lymphomas.In: Russel DS and Rubinstein LJ (eds) *Pathology of Tumours of the Nervous System*. Williams & Wilkins, Baltimore, pp. 592-608

Saad RS, EL-Gohary Y, Memari E, Liu YL, Silverman JF (2005): Endoglin (CD105) and vascular endothelial growth factor as prognostic markers in esophageal adenocarcinoma. *Hum Pathol* 36, pp. 955-961

Salven P, Orpana A, Teerenhovi L, Joensuu H (2000) Simultaneous elevation in the serum concentrations of the angiogenic growth factors VEGF and bFGF is an independent predictor of poor prognosis in non-Hodgkin lymphoma: a single-institution study of 200 patients. *Blood* 96, pp. 3712-3718

Santos L, Costa C, Pereira S, Koch M, Amaro T, Cardoso F, Guimaraes T, Bento MJ, Lobo F, Pinto S, Lopes C (2003): Neovascularisation is a prognostic factor of early recurrence in T1/G2 urothelial bladder tumours. *Ann Oncol* 14, pp. 1419-1424

Seon BK, Haba A, Matsuno F, Takahashi N, Tsujie M, She X, Harada N,Uneda S, Tsujie T, Toi H, Haruta Y(2011). Endoglin- targeting cancer therapy. *Curr Drug Deliv* 8, pp. 135 –143

Sica G, Lama G, Anile C, Geloso MC, La Torre G, De Bonis P, Maira G, Lauriola L, Jhanwar-Uniyal M, Mangiola A (2011). Assesment by CD105 and nestin expression in peritumor tissue of glioblastoma. *Int J Oncol* 38, pp.41-49

Sugita Y, Tokunaga O, Nakashima A, Shigemori M (2004): SHP-1 expression in primary central nervous system B-cell lymphomas in immunocompetent patients reflects maturation stage of normal B cell counterparts. *Pathol Int* 54, pp. 659-666

Sugita Y, Takase Y, Mori D, Tokunaga O, Nakashima A, Shigemori M (2007). Endoglin (CD105) is expressed on endothelial cells in the primary central nervous system lymphomas and correlates with survival. *J Neurooncol* 82, pp. 249 -256

Sure U, Freman S, Bozinov O, Benes L, Siegel AM, Bertalanffy H (2005). Endoglin- targeting cancer therapy. *J Neurosurg* 102, pp. 342–347

Takagi Y, Kikuta K, Nozaki K, Fujimoto M, Hayashi J, Imamura H, Hashimoto N (2007). Expression of hypoxia-inducing factor-1α and endoglin in intimal hyperplasia of the middle cerebral artery of patients with moyamoya disease. *J Neurosurg* 102, pp.342–347

Takahashi N, Haba A, Matsuno F, Seon BK (2001) Antiangogenic therapy of established tumors in human skin/severe combined immunodeficiency mouse chimeras by anti-endoglin (CD105) monoclonal antibodies and synergy between anti-endoglin antibody and cyclophosphamide. *Cancer Res* 61, pp7846-7854

Takase Y, Kai K, Masuda M, Akashi M, Tokunaga O (2010). Endoglin (CD 105) expression and angiogenesis status in small cell lung cancer. *Pathol Res Pract* 206, pp. 725 -730

Tanaka F, Otake Y, Yanagihara K, Kawano Y, Miyahara R, Li M, Ishikawa S, Wada H (2003). Correlation between apoptotic index and angiogenesis in non-small cell lung cancer: comparison between CD105 and CD34 as a marker of angiogenesis. *Lung Cancer* 39, pp. 289-296 Thorpe F (2004).Vascular targeting agents as cancer therapeutics. *Clin Cancer Res* 10, pp. 415 -427

Yao Y, Kubota T, Takeuchi H, Sato K (2005). Prognostic significance of microvessel density determined by an anti-CD105/endoglin monoclonal antibody in astrocytic tumors: comparison with an anti-CD31 monoclonal antibody. *Neuropathology* 25, pp.201-206

Zhao WL, Mourah S, Mounier N, Leboeuf C, Daneshpouy ME, Legrès L, Meignin V, Oksenhendler E, Maignin CL, Calvo F, Brière J, Gisselbrecht C, Janin A (2004) Vascular endothelial growth factor-A is expressed both on lymphoma cells and endothelial cells in angioimmunoblastic T-cell lymphoma and related lymphoma progression. *Lab Invest* 84, pp. 1512-1519

Zhu Y, Sun Y, Xie L, Jin K, Sheibani N, Greenberg DA (2003). Hypoxic induction of endoglin via mitogen-activated protein kinases in mouse brain microvascular endothelial cells. *Stroke* 34, pp. 2483-2488

Uneda S, Toi H, Tsujie T, Tsujie M, Harada N, Tsai H, Seon BK(2009). Anti-endoglin monoclonal antibodies are effective for suppressing metastasis and the primary tumors by targeting tumor vasculature. *Int J Cancer* 125, pp. 1446 -1453

Part 4

AQPs Proteins- CNS Tumors

7

The Role of Aquaporines in Brain Tumors

Tatsuo Sawada
Department of pathology Tokyo Women's Medical University
Japan

1. Introduction

As about 80% of the brain is water, cerebral edema, associated with various cerebral injuries is critical and crucial events as the accumulation of excessive fluids will cause fatal cerebral herniation.

Water molecular channels called aquaporines (AQP) which are small membrane-spanning proteins which are expressed at plasma membranes[1,2], There are thirteen AQPs which are divided by three groups. Recently AQPs plays roles of cell migration[3] and proliferation[4]. In central nervous system, eight AQPs (1,3,4,5,6,8,9, and 11) are expressed. AQP4 is expressed in astrocytes and AQP1 in cholloid plexus, predominantly.

Recent researches elucidated the physiological roles of AQPs expands from water channels to other function associated with tumor biology. Firstly, AQPs were found in high grade malignant tumors[5,6]. And the expression of AQPs was correlated with metastatic potentials of malignant tumors and made easier to tumor cell migrations[3].

To elucidate the characterization of the expression of AQPs especially of AQP 1 and 4, and the relation of the expression of VEGF family and their receptors, we had investigated the expression of these proteins in various tumors of the central nervous system, immunohistochemically

In this review, we survey the physiological roles of AQP 1 and 4 in central nervous system tumor, using our data and recent reports.

2. Materials and methods

Thirty-one tumors and three cerebral tissue for control were used at our study until now[7,8] Astrocytomas were reclassified according to WHO classification[9] Although we could not examine the histology of primary tumors, the histological type of metastatic carcinoma was confirmed by the charts. Non-neoplastic cerebral tissue was obtained from three patients who underwent cerebral resection for cerebral hemorrhage. No information about corticosteroid treatment including dexamemethasone, was obtained in this study.

3. Immunostainings

Tissue specimen were immuunostained by ABC methods using antihum an AQP 1, antihum an AQP4 polyclonal antibody (H80, diluted 1:50;Santa Cruz Biotechnology, Santa Cruz, CA, USA), antihuman VEGF polyclonal antibody (C-1, diluted 1:1000: Santa Cruz Biotechnology) and antihuman MIB1-LI monoclonal antibody (diluted 1:100;DAKO, Kyoto Japan)

4. Results

In glioma, immunoreaction for AQP1 and 4 were recognized in tumor cells. Negative reactions for AQP 1 and 4 in tumor cells of grade 1 meningioma, medulloblastoma, neurocytoma, and lymphoma. Some of metastatic carcinoma cells – some of metastatic carcinoma cells were negative for AQP4 but a few tumor cells were positive for AQP1. Positive reactions for AQP 1 and 4 were recognized in reactive astroglia in the surrounded cerebral area of tumor. Immunoreactions for AQP 1 were recognized only endothelial cells in neovasculature of gliomas and grade 2 meningioms but normal endothelial cells negative for AQP 1 or 4. In grade 2 meningiomas, immunoreactions for AQP1 were detected in tumor cells and endothelial cells in neovasculature. A positive correlation of distinctiveness for immunoreactions between VEGF-A and C were obtained of expression of AQPs of endothelial cells in neovasculature.

5. Discussion

Recent researches elucidated the physiological roles of AQPs expands from water channels to other functions associated with tumor biology. Firstly, AQPs were found in high grade malignant tumors. And the expression of AQPs was correlated with metastatic potentials of malignant tumors and made easier to tumor cell migrations. AQP 4 was first cloned from rat lung[10], played major roles of pathogenesis of neuromyelitis optica[11].

In cerebral tissue, metastatic carcinoma show significant cerebral edema in the surrounded area. Reactive astrocytes show positive reactions for AQP1 and 4. The mechanisem of AQPs were still unclear., but As AQP4 did not alter blood-brain barrier integry or cerebral morphology[12] but deletion increased cerebral edema. Tail et al suggested the AQP4 played the elimination of cerebral edema using rat experimental SAH models[13].

AQP4 was massively up regulated in high grade astrocytoma and the expression of VEGF families tended to show a positive relation to AQP1 and 4 in high grade astrocytoma and grade 2 meningioma. Neovasculature in high grade astrocytoma and the adjacent areas of metastatic carcinoma showed glomeruoid proliferation of neovasculaturein which the physiological blood-brain barrier impaired, showing high VEGFs expression[14]. In meningiomas, significant peritumoral edema are associated frequently(50-92%)[15]. But a few studies are available for the expression of AQPs about meningioma, Ng et al. found increased expression of AQP4 with peritumoral edema in meningioma[6]. But all cases of menigiomas Ng et al studiesd were grade 1. No grade 2 or 3 meningioma was not included. Our report showed no expression of AQP4 in tumor cells of grade 1 meningiomas[5]. Cerebral edema in high grede glioma, metastatic carcinoma and meningioma was likely the result of the relationship between cerebral blood vessels and AQP4-mediated water transport.

AQP is expressed in the apical membrane of the choroid plexus and plays a role in forming CSF[16]But Marton et al. reported over expression of AQP 1 in atypical meningioma of infancy[17]. Nagashima et al suggested the dural invasion of meningiomas facilitated

Expressions of AQP1 played some physiological roles of cystic formation of cholloid plexus tumors[18]. As we describes, Nielsen et al reported that normal cerebral endothelial cells were negative for AQP1 but highly expressed in the endothelial cells of peripheral area of injuries, and cultured endothelial cells without astrocytes are also positive for AQP1. These data suggested that astrocytes endofeet may regulates adjacent endothelial cells in the endothelial cells in normal cerebral capillaries o switch off endothelial AQP 1 expression.

Our study could obtain the positive reactions of AQP1 in high grade glioma and grade 2 meningiomas but not in benign tumors.

In tumor biology, AQP1 deletion in mice reduceds tumor growth and migration of endothelial and astroglia[19]. The migration of cells are closely related tumor malignancy, The biological roles of AQP 1 for arachnoid cell differentiation were uncertain, but our results suggested AQPs played some roles of take a malignant potentials of meningiomas..

In this study we could not take no informations about cerebral edema. Furthers studies about the relations between cerebral edema and the expressions of AQPs of meningiomas are needed.

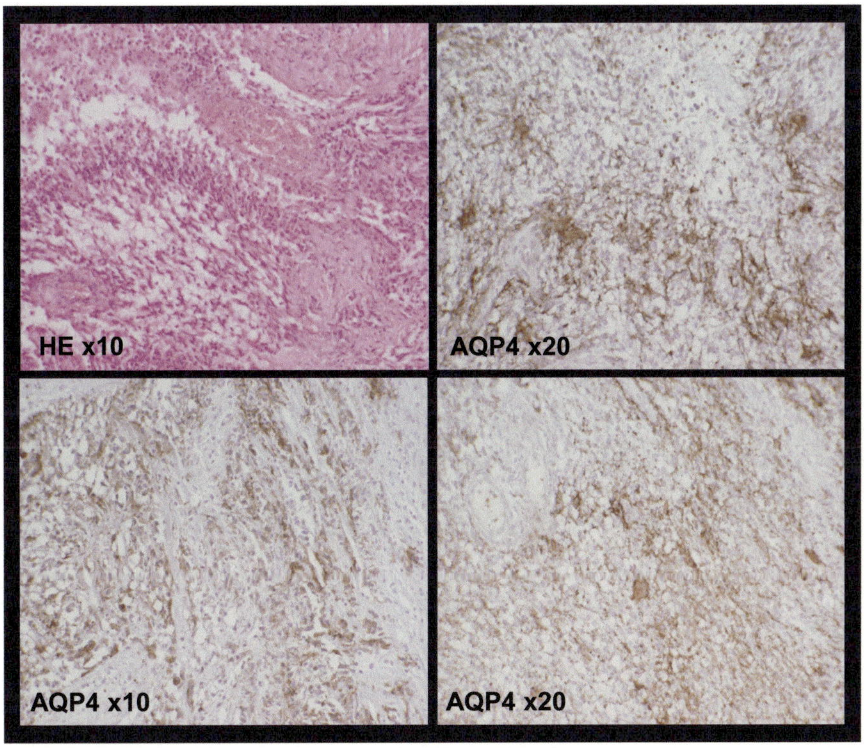

Fig. 1. Histological and immunohistochmeical findings of glioblastoma.
Histological findings (upper left) and immnunohistochemical staining for AQP4 (upper left and lower left and right). Positive findings for AQP4 are recognized in endothelial cells and tumor cells.

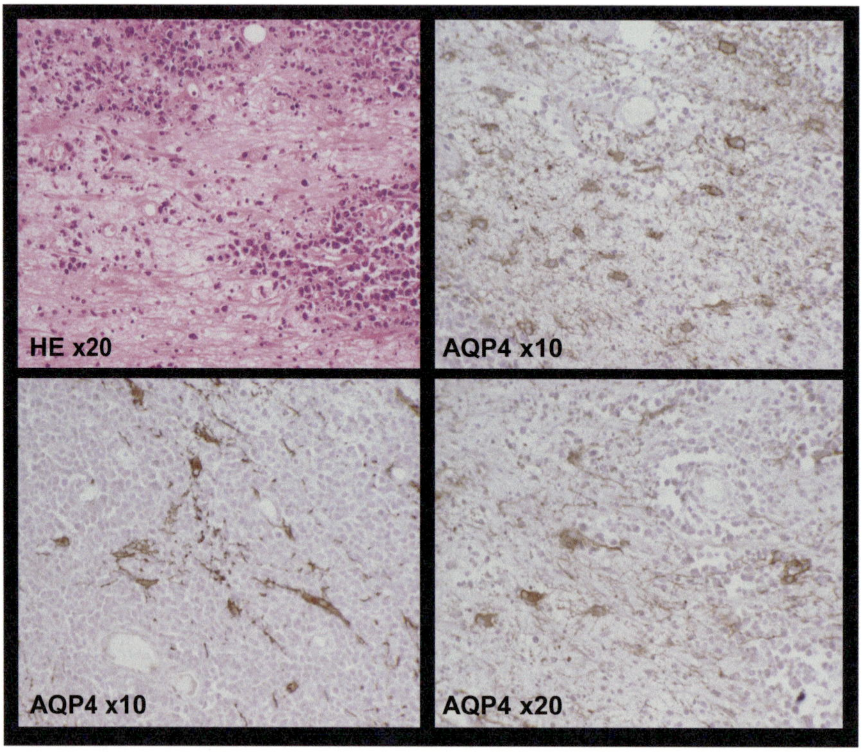

Fig. 2. Histological and immunohistochmeical findings of metastatic adenocrcinoma. Histological findings (upper left) and immnunohistochemical staining for AQP4 (upper left and lower left and right). Positive findings for AQP4 are recognized in endothelial cells and reactive astroglia.

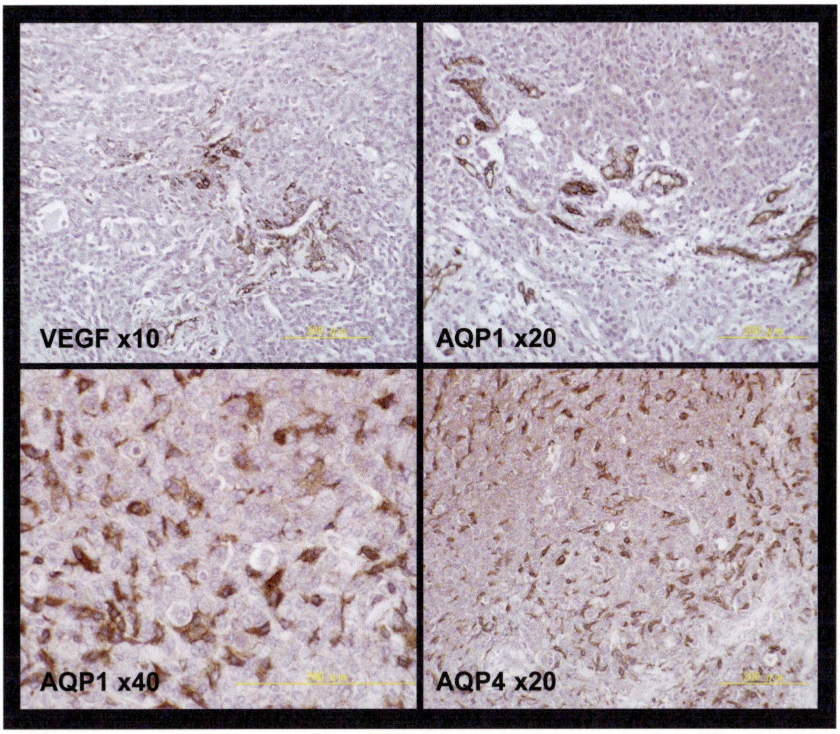

Fig. 3. Immunohistochemical findings of atypical meningioma.
Immunohistochmeical staining for VEGF (upper left), for AQP1 (upper right and lower left) and for AQP4 (lower right).
Positive findings for AQP4 in tumor cells and for AQP1 in tumor and endothelial cells are recognized.

6. References

[1] Verkman AS (1996) Water transport across mammalian membranes Am J Physiol 48:C12-C30
[2] Ishibashi K Kuwahara M Sasaki S: (2000) Molecular biology of aquaporines Rev Physiol Biochem Pharmacolol 141: 1-32
[3] Papadopuls MC, Saandoun and Verkman AS: aquaporins and cell migration Pflugers Arch-Eur J Physiol (2008)456: 693-700
[4] Hoque MO, Soria JC, Woo J et al: Aquaporin 1 is overexpressed in lung cancer and stimulates NIH-3T3 Cell proliferation and anchorage-independent growth Am J Pathology (2006) 168:1345-1353
[5] Saadoun S Papadopoulos MC, Davis DC et al: Aquaporin-4 expression is increased in oedematous human brain tumors J Neurol Neurosurg Psychiatry (2002) 72: 262-265
[6] Warth A, Kroger S, Wolburg H (2004) redistribution of aquaporin-4 in human glioblastoma correlated with loss of agrin immunoreactivity from brain capillary basal laminae. Acta Neuropathol(Berl) 107:311-318
[7] Sawada T, Kato Y,Kobayashi M: Expression of aquaporine-4 in central nervous system tumors. Brain Tumor Pathol (2007) 24:81-84
[8] Sawada T,Kato Y. Kobayashi M: Expression of aquaporine 1 and 4 in meningiomas. An immunohistochemical study Jr. Tokyo Women's Medical University(2011)81: E9-13
[9] Astrocytic tumors. WHO Classification of Tumours of the central nervous system.(2007) 13-52.WHO
[10] Hasegawa H,Sawaya R, Mohanam S et al : Molecularcloning of a mercurial-insensitive water channel expressed in selected water transporting tissue. J Biol Chem (1994) 269: 5497-5500
[11] Graber DJ, Levy M, Kerr et al : Neuromyelitis optica pathogenesis and aquaporin 4 J of Neuroinflammation (2008) 5: 22
[12] Saadoun S, Tait MJ, Reza et al: AQP4 gene deletion in mice does not alter blood-bain barrier integrity or brain morphology Neuroscience (2009) 161: 764-772
[13] Tait MJ, Saadoun S, Bell BA et al: Increased brain edema in *AQP4*-null mice in an experimental model of subarachnoid hemorrhage. Neuroscience (2010) 167: 60-67
[14] Papadopoulos MC, Saadoun, Davis et al: (2001) Emerging molecular mechanism of brain tumoe oedema Br.J neurosurg 15:101-108
[15] Kalkanis SN, Carroll RS .Zhang J et al: Correlation of vascular growth factor messengaer RNA expression with peritumoral vasogenic cerebral edemain meningiomas. J neurosurg.(1996) 85: 1095-1101
[16] Oshio K et al: Reduced cerebrospinal fluid production and intracranial pressure in mice lacking choroid plexus water channel aquapotin-1 FASEB J (2006) 19.76-78
[17] Marton E,Feletti, Basaldella L et al (2008)Atypical cystic meningioma overexpressing AQP1 in early infancy: case report with literature review Acta Paediatroca 97: 1145-1149.
[18] Longatti P, Basaldella L, Orvieto e et al:Aquaporins expression in choroid plexus tumours Pediatr Neurosurg (2006) 42: 228-33
[19] Saadoun SM, Papadopoulos MC, Watanabe H, et al: (2005) Involvement of aquaporin-4 in astroglia cell migration and glial scar formation J CellSci 118: 5691-5698

Part 5

Gliomas - Regulatory Components and Effector Pathways

8

Glioma Stem Cells

Kouichi Tabu[1], Tetsuya Taga[1] and Shinya Tanaka[2]
[1]*Department of Stem Cell Regulation, Medical Research Institute, Tokyo Medical and Dental University*
[2]*Laboratory of Cancer Research, Department of Pathology, Hokkaido University Graduate School of Medicine,*
Japan

1. Introduction

Gliomas are the most frequent primary brain tumors and are classified as grade I to IV according to their degree of malignancy (Daumas-Duport et al., 1988). Grade I and II gliomas are clinically benign or semi-benign with relatively long-term survival, while grade III and IV are malignant and lethal within several years. In particular, glioblastoma multiforme (GBM), the most malignant glioma as grade IV often relapse even after radical surgical resection and standard chemo/radiation therapies, because of their diffuse infiltration into the surrounding brain parenchyma and high degree of chemo/radioresistance. Despite extensive efforts, the overall survival of GBM patients remains still short and has not yet been dramatically improved for more than several decades.

GBMs are often composed of various types of cells with distinct morphology and clinical phenotypes. Their histological and biological multiformity has been classically explained by the stochastic clonal evolution model (Nowell, 1976). According to this model, all tumor cells should have low but inheritable ability to form tumors. However, recent evidence has suggested another concept, the cancer stem cell (CSC) hierarchy model, which shows that only a rare stem cell population has high ability to proliferate (Jordan et al., 2006). CSCs have similar characters to normal stem cells in the way of having high ability to self renew and differentiate into multiple types of progenies to organize tissue architectures. Exclusively, CSCs can proliferate uncontrollably to propagate tumor cells. CSC model have direct relevance with tumor replenishment, disease recurrence and metastatic activity, suggesting that CSCs should be the target to eradicate the tumors.

The aim of this chapter is to provide our insights into how CSCs in human glioma; i.e. glioma stem cells (GSCs) should be attacked. In the first parts, we summarize the general basis of CSC concept inclusive of the current knowledge on how a CSC is defined, how CSCs should be technically prepared and modeled, and what characteristics CSCs possess. In the following part, we highlight what abnormal signaling pathways regulate CSCs as the potential therapeutic targets. Understanding the framework of a GSC research field could help us to think of novel treatment strategy. Most importantly, however, CSCs have enhanced resistance to conventional chemotherapies. Considering this fact, we finally propose that it could be most promising strategy to disrupt the extracellular environments supporting GSCs, which is a newly emerging concept "niche therapy". We present possible cellular and molecular components of GSC niche and discuss their potentiality as innovative therapeutic targets.

2. General outlines of cancer stem cell

2.1 Heterogeniety of cancer tissue

Over the past several decades, the idea that cancer tissues are heterogeneous and composed of multiple subpopulation of cells differing in morphology, proliferation rate, metastatic potential, marker expression, and sensitivity to chemo/radiation therapies, has been highly appreciated by many investigators. This tumor heterogeneity has been classically explained by the following two models (Figure 1).

Clonal evolution (stochastic) model: Cells may acquire various combinations of genetic and epigenetic mutations asynchronously and once such mutations confer selective advantages of tumor malignancy, more aggressive and adaptive clones can dominate the whole tumor population.

In 1976, Nowell proposed the evolutionary view into tumor progression as a stochastic process of genetic instability and natural selection (Nowell, 1976). According to this model, tumor initiation occurs in the individual cells receiving multiple mutations, and cells having an advantageous mutation of growth can clonally proliferate and selectively occupy an entire tumor. During tumor progression, genetic instability yields the additional mutations by chance, resulting in a diversity of genome and cell characteristics, such as being invasive, metastatic and therapy-resistant. The adaptation to surrounding microenvironment is also a determinant of the selection. Standing on this concept, all the tumor cells should have low but inheritable ability to form tumors, therefore, the rational targets for cancer therapy is most or all of tumor cells. After this proposal, researchers have confirmed clonal expansions and genetic heterogeneity within various types of human neoplasms.

Hierarchy (cancer stem cell) model: Cells may acquire various genetic and epigenetic mutations that confer stem-like characteristics, and divide to produce its identical copy (self-renewal) and progenies terminally growth-arrested (differentiation). Such a hierarchy in a stem cell division manner results in cellular diversity of a rare stem cell and a majority of multiple types of progenies.

The CSC model is not a newly emerging concept indeed. The efforts to gain insights into tumor's malignant potential, especially their differential sensitivity to anticancer drugs were made on this concept with specimens from patients with myeloma and with ovarian cancer (Salmon et al., 1978). The technological advances of flow cytometry and discovery of stem cell surface antigens accelerated investigators to ascertain this concept, starting in human leukaemia (Bonnet and Dick, 1997) along with the subsequent identification in breast (Al-Hajj et al., 2003) and brain tumor (Singh et al., 2003).

Normal stem cells replenish normal tissues by fresh cells continuously throughout life in individual organs. Stem cells are characterized by two main hallmarks; those are multipotency and self-renewal capacity. The former is the ability to produce multiple types of functional progenies, which is associated with terminal growth-arrest. Self-renewal is the ability to produce new stem cells identical to original one with retaining the intact two main hallmarks, and thereby maintains the stem cell pool. Likewise, tumors are also organized as a hierarchy where rare CSCs stand at the top of pyramid with extensive potential to proliferate and self-renew and are responsible for maintaining the homeostasis of the tumor bulk, except that CSCs disorderly propagate tumor cells and increase cell number.

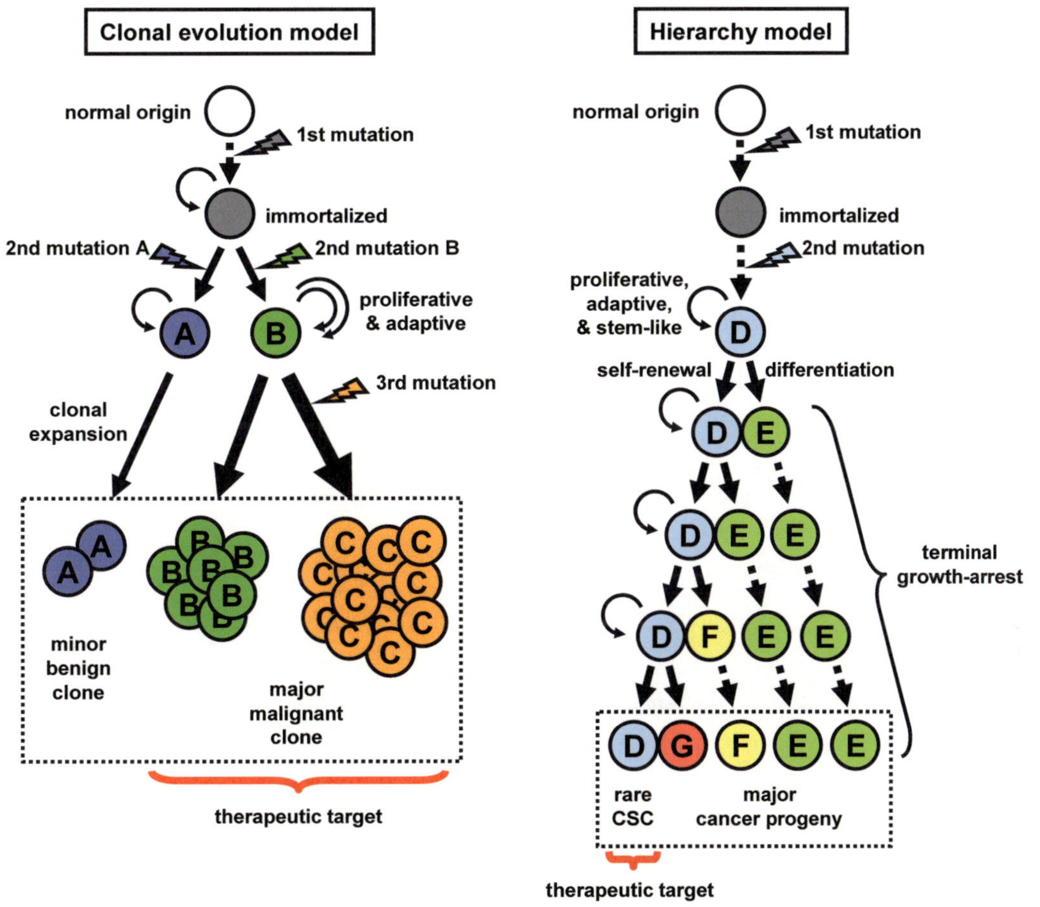

Fig. 1. The color of the arrow for 2nd mutation in Hierarchy model is changed from pale yellow to light blue.

In this concept, cancer heterogeneity means the different characteristics between CSC and differentiated cancer progenies. However, the clonal evolution model and the CSC model are not necessarily mutually exclusive. Despite types of primary cells to suffering the first set of mutations, CSCs also have genetic instability, which increases the probability of acquiring additional mutations. Potentially, CSCs might expand clonally by a symmetric division. The adaptation to surrounding microenvironment has also been recognized as important factors on normal stem cell maintenance, which is called stem cell niche. Therefore, we should consider the CSC model as a revised version by taking the idea of asymmetric division. However, we must note again that only rare CSCs are tumorigenic by definition and specific targets for cancer eradication is in a minority population within a tumor bulk.

2.2 Definition of cancer stem cell

CSCs are re-defined in the AACR Workshop 2006 on Cancer Stem Cells as "a small subset of malignant cells that constitute a pool of self-sustaining cells with the exclusive ability to maintain the tumor" (Clarke et al., 2006), and in part share the fundamental properties with normal stem cells specific to their original organs; e.g. neural stem cell for glioma.

2.3 Current methods to isolate cancer stem cell

In current studies, CSCs from cancer tissues and cell lines are firstly isolated by using diverse experimental techniques as mentioned below.

Sphere formation assay: Floating spherical cell clusters are formed *in vitro* when mitotic cells are cultured in serum-free media supplemented with mitogens (epidermal growth factor and fibroblast growth factor for neural stem cells) (Figure 2), which is originally developed to characterize the behaviour of neural stem cells (Reynolds and Weiss, 1992).

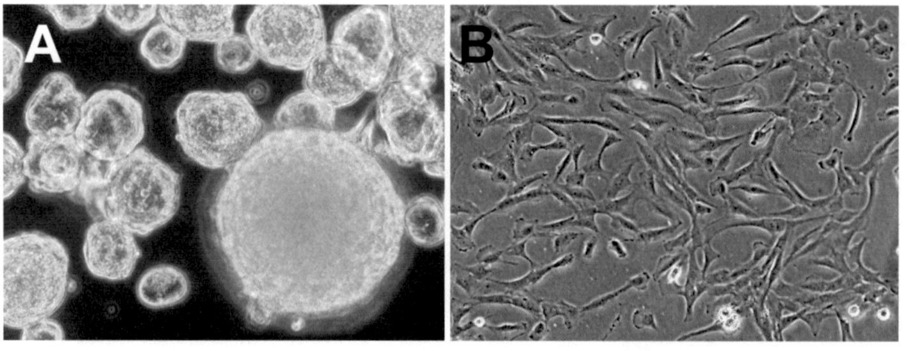

Fig. 2. Glioma spheres generated from oncogenic Ras-transformed human astrocytes (A) and differentiation of dissociated sphere cells by culturing in 10%FBS media for 1 week (B).

When cells are derived from brain, breast and others, each sphere is called neurosphere, mammosphere, and others, respectively. The number and diameter of spheres are thought to reflect the frequency of stem cells and mitotic activity of a single stem cell within the examined population, respectively. When a 1st sphere is picked up, re-dissociated into single cells, and re-cultured, the generated secondary spheres imply the sustained self-renewal potential of a true stem cell. For a while, this method has been utilized to expand cancer stem cell population by serial passage, but Bexell et al. recently showed that sphere formation is not prerequisite for enrichment of CSCs, and pointed out that glioma cells growing as monolayers are also tumorigenic (Bexell et al., 2009), like in the case of neural stem cells that can be maintained in monolayer cultures (Johe et al., 1996). In addition, it is virtually impossible to form spheres of CSC that have arisen from a tissue in which the condition of sphere assay is unestablished for normal stem cells, and even if spheres are formed, it is uncertain if they have significance for stem cell activity in the tissues. Therefore, we must note that sphere formation assay has limited utility for isolation of some types of CSCs.

Hoechst 33342 dye effluxing side population (SP): Hoechst 33342 is a fluorescent dye that binds to the AT-rich regions of DNA, and most cells are stained with this dye. In most cases, stem cells are not stained due to the high expression of ABC transporter family genes to efflux this dye. Human fetal neural stem/progenitor cells express high levels of multidrug resistance 1 (MDR1, also known as ABCB1, P-gp) gene and ATP-binding cassette sub-family G member 2 (ABCG2, also known as Bcrp), and these transporters have important roles in normal physiology on the active efflux of xenobiotics from cell body, protecting cells from cytotoxic agents. Cells with the capacity to efflux the dye were first identified in the mouse bone marrow (Goodell et al., 1996). After staining with Hoechst 33342 dye and exposure to UV laser during FACS, a population is referred to as side population (SP) cells because it appears as a "side" relative to the positively stained "main" population (MP) in FACS plots (Figure 3). Since this discovery, SP technique is applied to enrich putative stem cells and progenitors in a number of normal tissues and malignant tumors, including glioma. SP cells preferentially express high levels of stemness genes and are capable of differentiating into multiple lineages, and thus are considered to function as stem cells in the original tissues and tumors (Dean et al., 2005). Importantly, this method itself may affect the tumorigenic potential because Hoechst dye is toxic for cells. Minimally toxic concentrations of Hoechst 33342 should be also determined in the individual experiments. Rhodamine 123, which is a mitochondrial dye reflecting mitochondrial content and kinetics, has been used as a less toxic dye, by which quiescent stem cells display a low fluorescence in the flow cytometry plots. Human bone marrow hematopoietic stem cells (HSCs) have been demonstrated to be isolated by the combination of Hoechst 33342 and Rhodamine 123 (Leemhuis et al., 1996). In addition, some investigators have reported that MP cells in human GBM biopsies are also tumorigenic in mice, although transplantation of SP cells result in a shorter survival of mice than MP (Bleau et al., 2009).

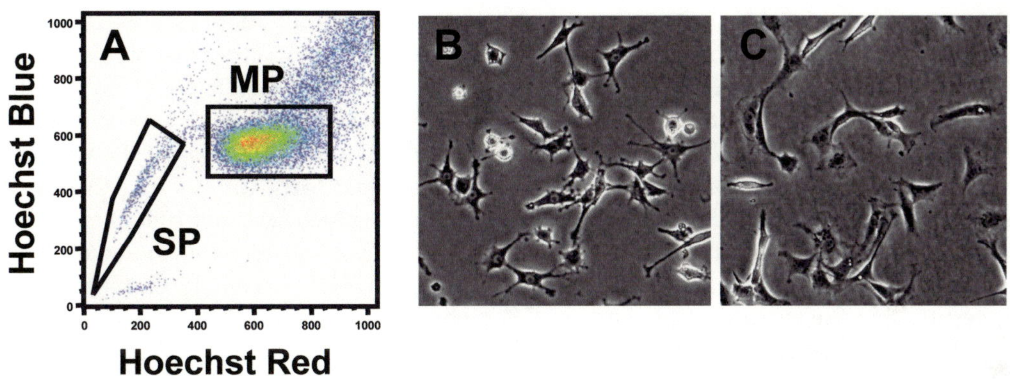

Fig. 3. FACS plots expanded by side population analysis (A) and representative images of SP (B) and MP (C) cells in the C6 glioma cell line.

Stem cell surface antigens: Potential CSCs can be identified by striking variety of cell surface markers or their combinations; e.g. CD34(+)CD38(−) for AML (Bonnet and Dick, 1997), CD44(+)CD24(−/low) for breast tumor (Al-Hajj et al., 2003) and CD133(+) for brain tumor (Singh et al., 2003). However, these methods based on the surface molecules have increased some contradiction. For instance, different stem cell markers identify distinct subpopulations of cells in one tumor, in all of which population CSC properties may sometimes confirmed. In melanoma, at least four subpopulations, CD20(+), CD133(+), BrdU label-retaining cells, and SP cells has been separately identified, all of which possess stem cell features (Zabierowski and Herlyn, 2008). This diversity of CSC markers suggests that one population isolated by certain surface molecules is still heterogeneous, and that complete enrichment of CSCs has not been achieved at least in some particular tumor types. Furthermore, the frequency of CSCs is highly variable even among the same type of tumors. In colorectal tumors, the frequency of tumor initiating cells assessed in NOD/SCID mice broadly ranges from 1.8 to 24.5% (O'Brien et al., 2007), pointing out the requirement for more refined markers (or their combinations) and assay systems. Nevertheless, it is evident that these surface markers and their roles are important keys to unveil the regulatory pathway to maintain CSCs. Actually, in many studies on human brain tumors, GSCs are isolated by the elevated expression of CD133, and the CD133(+) subpopulation has the higher ability than the other populations to regenerate the original tumors in immunodeficient mice (Singh et al., 2004).

ALDEFLUOR (aldehyde dehydrogenase activity): Measurement of ALDH activity is a recent approach for isolation of putative CSCs. The main function of ALDH enzyme is the oxidation of intracellular aldehydes. Several isoforms of ALDH family are identified in human, and ALDH1 is the primary isoform isolated from human hematopoietic progenitors. Recent studies have shown that human and murine hematopoietic progenitors can be isolated using the bodipy-aminoacetaldehyde (BAAA, commercially available in a diethyl acetate form as ALDEFLUOR), a fluorescent labeled substrate specific for ALDH activity (Ginestier et al., 2007). ALDH1 has a role in early differentiation of hematopoietic stem cells (HSCs) through conversion of retinol to retinoic acid (Chute et al., 2006). Increased ALDH activity is also found in normal neural stem cells and CSC in acute myeloid leukemia (AML) (Pearce et al., 2005) and breast carcinomas (Korkaya et al., 2008).

Xenotransplantation into immunodeficient mice: The first evidence of CSCs was obtained by transplantation experiments in the severe combined immunodeficient (SCID) mouse (Lapidot et al., 1994), and it was later re-demonstrated in the nonobese diabetic (NOD)/SCID mouse (Bonnet and Dick, 1997). However, the use of NOD/SCID mice, which T cells and B cells are lacked, has the risk to underestimate the frequency of tumorigenic human cancer cells due to the immune response of natural killer cells against the xenobiotic cells. Actually, the percentage of melanoma stem cells that form tumors in NOD/SCID/ interleukin-2 receptor γ chain (IL2Rγ)-null (NOG) mice, which lack not only T and B but natural killer cells, is higher than that in NOD/SCID mice; one in 1000 melanoma cells form tumors in NOD/SCID mice, but 1 in 4 can form tumors in NOG mice (Quintana et al, 2008), suggesting that the reported frequency of CSCs should be reevaluated in some cancers by using the more highly immunocompromised model. Thus current gold standard assay for testing whether each cell population fulfils the criteria of CSC (self-renewal, differentiation and tumorigenicity) is the orthotopic xenograft experiment where cells are transplanted at limiting dilutions into NOD/Shi-scid/IL2Rγ-null (NOG) mice and the frequency of CSCs is determined. Especially, serial transplantation into NOG mice is regarded as the best functional assay for testing the long-term self-renewal capacity. However, even the use of NOG mouse might underestimate the frequency of CSCs due to different tissue environment between mouse and human. If mouse ligands such as growth factors and adhesion molecules do not have the compatibility with human receptors, tumorigenic human cells might lose the ability to proliferate and survive in mice. Also, even being compatible, rodent normal tissues could not precisely recapitulate the patients' tumor microenvironment. Therefore, the challenges to establish humanized mouse models in which human microenvironment is recapitulated in an animal are recently highlighted.

2.4 Clinical implications of cancer stem cell

CSC model has important implications for clinical treatment of tumors, because some features of CSCs make them particularly difficult to kill. CSCs reside in relatively quiescent state on cell cycle referred as in the state of "dormancy" and this allows them to evade from typical chemotherapeutic regimens that target actively proliferating cells. Many investigators attempt to kill tumor cells independently of the cell cycle state or to selectively prompt them to enter the cycling state. Moreover, CSCs express the high level of multidrug resistant proteins and transporters associated with detoxification, and they are consequently conferred multidrug resistance by expelling chemotherapeutic reagents (Dean et al., 2005). In addition, CSCs are frequently resistant to standard radiotherapy regimens owing to their elevated expression of reactive oxygen species (ROS) scavenging (Diehn et al., 2009) and DNA damage response (Bao et al., 2006) genes. Unexpectedly, conventional chemo/radiotherapy eventuates in an increased proportion of CSC fraction and in rapid relapse of original tumor. Long-term treatment of PTEN$^{-/-}$ neurospheres isolated from PDGF-induced gliomas with temozolomide, a standard therapy for GBM patients, induces an increase in the amount of SP cells (Bleau et al., 2009). An effective therapeutic approach to CSCs enhancing the sensitivity of chemotherapeutic drugs and radiation is therefore imperative to develop.

2.5 Origin of cancer initiating cell

The revival of CSC concept triggers a debate on whether cancer origin is stem cells or terminally differentiated cells. Since 1970s, a large corpus of studies on direct introduction of viral oncogenes and mutated genes isolated from patients' tumors has demonstrated that most of normal cells are susceptible to genetic mutations leading to neoplastic transformation for the initiation and expansion of tumors. In addition to these findings, the observation that a large proportion of tumor cells retain the features of the surrounding differentiated epithelium has assured our common interpretation that oncogenic gene mutations occur in terminally differentiated cells. However, there are several controversial examples that are still difficult to explain standing on this concept for tumor cell origin. For example, malignant tumors histologically contain some degree of undifferentiated components, but differentiation of cells had been regarded as a unidirectional process under normal physiological conditions, and nuclear reprogramming had remained to be clarified until recent achievement of nuclear transfer, ES cell-fusion, or creating the induced pluripotent stem (iPS) cells (Yamanaka and Blau, 2010). In addition, terminally differentiated cells cannot normally divide to proliferate *in vivo* and thus the possibility is low that such sleeping cells have in sequence the opportunities to acquire oncogenic gene mutations, although they often undergo spontaneous immortalization *in vitro* and proliferate infinitely as cell lines. In fact, cancers prone to occur in specific tissues with the high rate of turnover in cell division, such as skin and gut but not heart. It is conceivable that this is a consequence of genetic instability during the frequent divisions of stem cells.

3. Glioma stem cell

3.1 Discovery and isolation

Subsequent to the identification in human AML and breast tumor, CSCs in human glioma i.e. glioma stem cells (GSCs) were initially identified in 2004 according to the cell surface expression of CD133 protein (Singh et al., 2004). CD133 is one of two members of pentaspan transmembrane glycoprotein prominin family and a human homolog of originally isolated mouse PROM1 selectively localizing at the apical surface of murine neuroepithelial stem cells (Weigmann et al., 1997) and HSCs from human fetal liver, bone marrow and cord blood (Yin et al., 1997). Notably, 100 CD133(+) cells recapitulated the original tumor identical to original patients' tumors in histopathological features, whereas 100,000 CD133(−) cells could not form any tumors in NOD/SCID mouse brains (Singh et al., 2004). Therefore, it was postulated that like normal neural stem-cells (NSCs), stem-like glioma cells may compose a glioma hierarchy upon differentiation and that their differentiation lineages determine tumor subtypes, i.e. astrocytomas or oligodendrogliomas. On the same year, Kondo et al. also succeeded in concentrating GSCs as stem-like SP cells from a rat C6 glioma cell line (Kondo et al., 2004). Since these discoveries, many investigators have confirmed the major utility of CD133, SP technique, and others for GSCs isolation (Table 1).

Parameters	Details of assay	Observed GSC phenotypes	References
Neurosphere culture	Culturing in serum-free media containing EGF and bFGF	self-renewal differentiation tumor formation	Singh et al. 2003
CD133 (AC133 antigen)	Magnetic sorting or flow cytometry sorting by CD133 expression	self-renewal differentiation tumor formation	Singh et al. 2004
Side population	Staining and flow cytometry sorting based on Hoechst 33342 dye efflux	self-renewal differentiation tumor formation	Kondo et al. 2004
A2B5 antigen	Flow cytometry sorting by the expression of a glial progenitor marker A2B5	tumor formation	Ogden et al. 2008
SSEA-1	Flow cytometry sorting by the expression of an embryonic marker SSEA-1 (stage-specific embryonic antigen 1)	self-renewal differentiation tumor formation	Son et al. 2009
Laminin-coated flask	Culturing in serum-free media containing EGF and bFGF on laminin-coated flask	self-renewal differentiation tumor formation	Pollard et al. 2009
Integrin alpha 6	Magnetic sorting or flow cytometry sorting by integrin alpha 6 expression alone or in combination with CD133 expression	self-renewal tumor formation	Lathia et al. 2010
Autofluorescence	Flow cytometry sorting by intrinsic autofluorescence emission around 520 nm upon laser excitation at 488 nm	self-renewal differentiation tumor formation	Clement et al. 2010

Table 1. Cell surface markers and functional assays for the isolation of glioma stem cells

However, these methods indeed produce some contradictory. First, accumulating reports have demonstrated the presence of CD133(-) GSCs (Ogden et al., 2008). Some of fresh GBM specimens and commonly used glioma cell lines do not express CD133, but nevertheless they can form tumors *in vivo* (Beier et al., 2007). Second, CD133(+) population in human gliomas are generally found at a very low frequency in flow cytometry and sometimes barely detectable, which lead to the concept that CSCs are a rare subpopulation in solid tumors, but immunohistochemical analysis by several groups and us have demonstrated that some of human GBMs contain high CD133(+) fractions (Figure 4B). This discrepancy has been thought to be partially caused by the limitation of FACS analysis; i.e. trypsin digestion during preparation of cell suspensions is predicted to cleave the 865-amino acids long-CD133 sequences at 79 different sites. And many of cleavage sites by trypsin are within the glycosylated extracellular loops containing AC133 or AC141 epitopes, although the majority of studies on CD133 have ever made use of antibodies against AC133 or AC141 glycosylated epitopes. Third, CD133 expression was found to be retained in differentiated cancer cells when a glucosylation-independent CD133 antibody was used (Florek et al., 2005). Other studies also have demonstrated that the expression of AC133 and AC141 epitopes is down-regulated independently of CD133 mRNA (Corbeil et al., 2000), and that the distribution of CD133 mRNA in adult tissues is much wider than that of immunoreactivity to the AC133 epitope (Miraglia et al., 1997). Furthermore, human CD133 transcripts have alternatively spliced variants devoid of AC133 or AC141 epitopes (Fargeas et al., 2007), and cytoplasmic localization of CD133 is also observed in human glioma sections (Sakariassen et al., 2007). In addition, we also found in human GBM sections the broadly ranged frequency of CD133(+) cells using an antibody against C-terminal intracellular region of CD133 (Figure 4A and B) and distinct discordance on the expression levels between CD133 and another neural stem cell marker Nestin (Figure 4C and D).

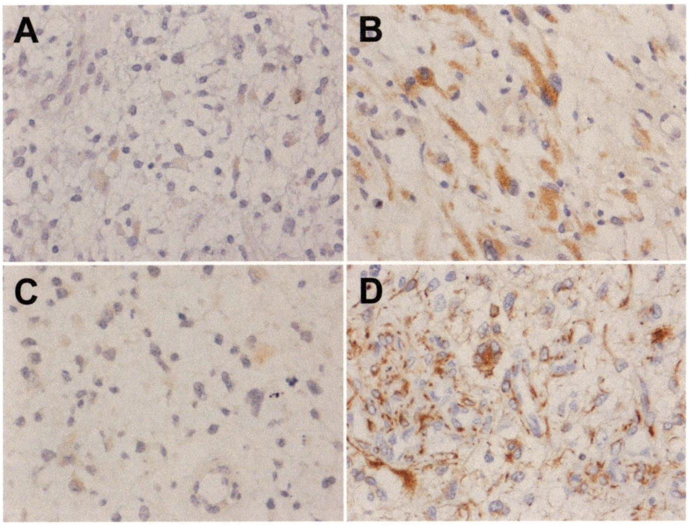

Fig. 4. (A and B) Different levels of CD133 expression in two human GBM tissues. Each tissue was stained with an anti-CD133 antibody. Relatively high frequency of CD133(+) cells are observed in B, but rarely detected in A. (C and D) The expression levels of two neural stem cell markers CD133 and Nestin does not coincide in the same GBM tissue. A GBM tissue was stained with an anti CD133 (C) and nestin (D) antibody.

Given these unresolved problems might lead to our underestimation of the size of true GSCs, it must be again deliberated whether CD133 could be utilized as a marker for GSC isolation. It may be one goal in future studies to find other markers (or their combination with CD133) to accurately define GSC population.

In contrast, SP method can compensate the disadvantage of cell surface marker-dependent isolation that fails when stem cell markers are unknown. Subsequently to the study with the C6 glioma cell line, SP cells have been detected in not only human glioma cell lines U87MG, T98G, U251 and U373, but also two primary gliomas in transgenic mouse models; Ntv-a/Ink4a$^{-/-}$Arf$^{-/-}$PTEN$^{flox/flox}$ mice (Bleau et al., 2009) and S100β-verbB:p53$^{-/-}$ mice (Harris et al., 2008), which are reported to be more self-renewable and tumorigenic than MP cells and able to reconstitute cellular heterogeneity. However, the isolation of SP cells from primary human GBMs and relevant correlation between SP and glioma malignancy have been little reported. Interestingly, Pollard and colleagues have proposed a protocol for the efficient establishment of GSC lines as culturing on laminin-coated flask, in which GSCs could be expanded in adherent culture for at least 1 year (>20 passages) with retaining stem cell properties and tumor initiation capacity (Pollard et al., 2009). They pointed out some problems on the use of the traditional neurosphere culture in GSCs isolation and highthroughput assays i.e. drug screenings. First, they claimed that the efficiency to successfully establish GSC lines from primary tumors is very low (from 1 to 30%). Second, spheroid cells tend to spontaneously undergo differentiation and apoptosis, and therefore it is complicated to identify the precise molecular targets against the true GSCs. Finally, the non-adherent aggregates make real-time observation of cellular behaviors more challenging, compared to adherent cells. Actually, they provided a proof-of-principle chemical screen using a live-cell imaging system to monitor the effects of FDA (Food and Drug Administration)-approved 450 compounds for potential anti-GSC activity, and identified 23 compounds having cytotoxic activity against all tested GSCs. This approach could greatly improve the work to probe GSC biology and to identify agents that selectively and directly target GSCs.

3.2 Signalling to regulate GSC (Therapeutic candidate)

GSC now attracts much attention with expectations that targeting GSCs could induce effective eradication of glioma. Currently, remarkable insights have been gained regarding intracellular and extracellular signalling pathways that are crucial in GSC malignancies (Figure 5), all of which are potential candidates for anti-GSC therapy.

3.2.1 Membrane-bound receptor-mediated signalling

Receptor tyrosine kinases (RTKs)

RTKs are the cell surface receptors for many growth factors, cytokines, and hormones, and have been known as not only key regulators of normal cellular processes but also critical stimuli in the development of many cancers.

The most frequent genetic alteration associated with human GBMs is amplification of EGF receptor (EGFR) gene, and its overexpression is observed in approximately 50–60% of GBM patients. The most common EGFR mutant is EGFRvIII, which is an in frame deletion variant that has a truncated extracellular domain with ligand-independent constitutive activity. The Ink4a/Arf$^{-/-}$ astrocytes dedifferentiate in response to EGF. Moreover, transduction of EGFRvIII into Ink4a/Arf$^{-/-}$ neural stem cells (NSCs)/astrocytes induces tumors displaying a common high-grade glioma phenotype (Bachoo et al., 2002). Soeda et al. (2008) have demonstrated that human GBM CSCs retain their self-renewal ability in the presence of EGF and that the tyrosine kinase inhibitors of EGF signaling, AG1478 and gefitinib suppress the proliferation and self-renewal of these cells. Mazzoleni et al. (2010) also have showed that EGFR expression is heterogenous in human GBMs and its high expression can identify tumor initiating cells. Interestingly, genomic heterogeniety of EGFR gene links to mutual communication between tumor cells, in which IL-6 and LIF proteins secreted from EGFRvIII-expressing GBM cells enhance wild-type EGFR-expressing GBM cell growth (Inda et al., 2010). From these data, targeting of EGFR seems reasonable for eradication of GSCs. However, despite several inhibitors of EGFR are now available in the glioma clinic, their efficacy is limited, suggesting that some combinatorial approach could improve clinical outcome.

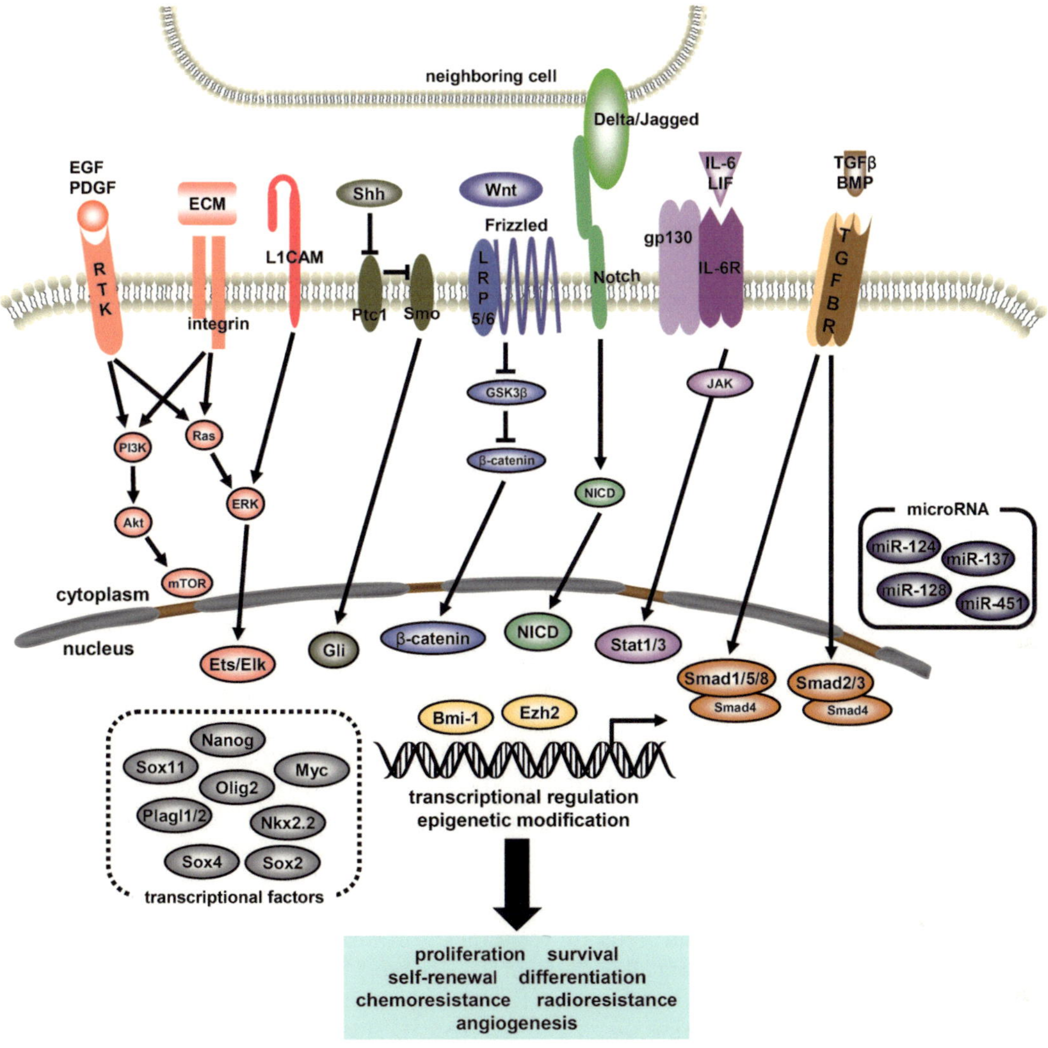

Fig. 5. Extracellular signaling and intracellular factors regulating glioma stemness.

PDGF functions in the later period in development as a potent mitogen of oligodendrocyte precursor cells (OPCs). OPCs express PDGF receptor (PDGFR), and PDGF is important for regulating OPC number and oligodendrocyte production. Additionally, PDGF signaling has been closely associated with the formation of glioma. Activation of PDGF pathway has been found in more than 80% of human oligodendrogliomas and in 50-100% of human astrocytomas. Daii et al. have reported that PDGF-B overexpression causes the proliferation of Nestin^{+} neural progenitors to form human oligodendroglioma-like tumors and also induces the dedifferentiation of GFAP(+) astrocyte into glial precursor-like cells (Dai et al., 2001). Recently, PDGFRα-expressing cells in the adult subventricular zone (SVZ) have been proposed as adult NSCs, and they are known to exhibit hyperplastic proliferation in response to excessive PDGFR activation (Jackson et al., 2006). These data suggest that PDGF/PDGFR pathway may contribute to not only glioma progression but also glioma initiation originated from immature stem-like cells.

RTK signallings are transmitted into nucleus by intracellular molecules, such as Ras/ERK and PI3K/Akt. Given that the combined activation of Ras and Akt in nestin(+) neural progenitors induces GBM in mice (Holland et al., 2000) and that the activity of drug transporter ABCG2 is regulated by PI3K/Akt pathway (Bleau et al., 2009), RTK signalling might control multiple behaviors of GSC in glioma progression and therapy-resistance.

Transforming growth factor-beta (TGF-β)

TGF-β superfamily proteins play a critical role on morphogenesis and cell lineage specification during brain development. In response to TGF-β, Smad2/3 becomes phosphorylated and forms a heterodimeric complex with Smad4, and then its complex is translocated into the nucleus to transactivate downstream target genes. Bone morphogenetic proteins (BMPs) belonging to a subset of the TGF-β superfamily is known to maintain self-renewal and multi-lineage differentiation potential of NSCs within the SVZ of the adult brain. In human GBMs, enhanced expression of the TGF-2 and TGF receptor I/II are detected. Two groups have reported that TGF-β enhances human GBM stemness and tumorigenic activity; one is through Sox4-mediated Sox2 induction (Ikushima et al., 2009) and another is through the induction of LIF secretion in an autocrine/paracrine fashion (Peñuelas et al., 2009). Consistent with these data, TGF-β receptor I inhibitor LY2109761 and SB431542 decrease the $CD44^{high}/Id1^{high}$ GBM CSCs population through the repression of Id1 and Id3 levels (Anido et al., 2010). However, TGF-β family proteins can function as both oncogenes and tumor suppressors. Lee et al. (2008) have reported that the expression of BMP receptor 1B is downregulated in human GBM CSCs through EZH2-dependent epigenetic silencing and thereby tumor stemness is maintained with impaired astroglial differentiation. Although these opposite roles of TGF-β on differentiation has remained to be resolved, these data indicate that TGF-β family proteins and their downstream targets have fundamental roles in glioma stemness and suggest that control of them could yield glioma eradication.

Interleukin-6 (IL-6)

IL-6 family of cytokines stimulate cells by forming the receptor complex composed of the each cytokine-specific receptor and the common component gp130 glycoprotein, leading to phosphorylation of signal transducers and activators of transcription (STAT3 and, to a less extent, STAT1) by gp130-associated janus kinases (JAKs). The phosphorylated STAT3 and 1 homodimerize and translocate into the nucleus where downstream target genes are transactivated. Several reports have shown that GBM tissues contain significantly higher levels of IL-6 protein, and higher IL-6 mRNA correlates with poor survival of GBM patients. In addition, phosphorylation and nuclear translocation of STAT3 positively correlate with the histopathological grade in human glioma samples (Weissenberger et al., 2004). Recent papers have demonstrated that targeting of either IL-6 receptor alpha or IL-6 by using lentiviral transduced shRNA or IL-6 antibody decrease tumor growth and survival in mice bearing intracranially xenografted human glioma (Wang et al., 2009). Likewise, STAT3 inhbitors (S3I-201 and STA-21) and RNAi-mediated knockdown of STAT3 prevent growth of human primary GBM CSCs (Sherry et al., 2009). Leukemia inhibitory factor (LIF), one of the cytokines of the IL-6 family which is known to be an essential factor for mouse embryonic stem cell self-renewal and maintenance, induces astrocytic differentiation of NSCs in cooperation with BMP2. As described above, transactivation of the LIF gene in glioma spheres by TGF-β enhances glioma stemness and then results in significantly shorter survival in mice when inoculated (Peñuelas et al., 2009). These effects of LIF on GSCs show important contrast to those on NSCs and therefore LIF inhibition might be one potential approach whose side-effects are minimized during treatment.

Sonic hedgehog (Shh), Notch, and Wnt

Because GSCs share common properties with NSCs, molecular mechanisms underlying self-renewal and differentiation are usually overlapped among them. The Shh, Notch and Wnt pathways play a major role in normal stem cell regulation and also there is much evidence that aberration of these pathways cause tumorigenesis.

Sonic hedgehog binds to the Patched-1 (Ptc1) receptor and in turn activates the transcription factors of GLI family by cancelling the Patched-mediated inactivation of Smoothened (Smo). Shh signalling regulates neural progenitor proliferation and self-renewal in adult cerebellum, and it is well known that deregulation of Shh pathway in cerebellum neural progenitors induces medulloblastoma in mouse models. In human GBMs, amplification and overexpression of Gli-1 is reported in several types of gliomas. Hsieh et al. (2011) have reported that Shh/Gli1 signaling regulates insulin-like growth factor (IGF)-1-dependent GSC proliferation and chemo/radioresistance through insulin receptor substrate 1 (IRS1) gene transactivation. Xu et al. (2008) have identified Shh-dependent CSCs in some cases of human GBMs and found that activity of Shh signaling in PTEN-positive GBMs correlates with reduced patients' survival.

Notch is a membrane-bound receptor, and its intracellular domain is proteolytically released by binding of membrane-associated ligands Delta and Jagged and in turn binds to promoters of genes encoding bHLH transcription factors. Notch activation is involved in the regulation of NSC self-renewal, but it promotes glial differentiation in some conditions. Abnormal activation of Notch signaling has been found in a wide range of human cancers, including glioma. Fan et al. (2010) have reported that a γ-secretase inhibitor GSI-18, which prevents Notch secretion, suppresses neurosphere clonogenicity *in vitro* and growth of intracranial CD133-positive GBM cells through loss of AKT and STAT3 phosphorylation. Importantly, the combination of γ-secretase inhibitors and irradiation can attenuate cell growth and clonogenic survival of GBM CSCs (Wang et al., 2010a).

Wnt signaling pathway also controls the size of the NSC population through β-catenin activation. Wnt binds to a transmembrane receptors Frizzled (Fzd), leading to the phosphorylation of the Dishevelled, which prevents glycogen synthase kinase 3β (GSK3β)-dependent degradation of β-catenin. β-catenin translocates into the nucleus where it binds to TCF/LEF and displaces corepressors to induce expression of target genes. Although Wnt is mutated in a subgroup of medulloblastomas, its role in gliomas is little known. Zheng et al. (2010) have recently proposed Wnt signaling as promising targets for GBM treatment. They identified PLAGL2 as a protooncogene amplified and/or overexpressed in human GBMs. Enhanced PLAGL2 expression promotes GSC self-renewal and contributes to gliomagenesis. They showed that PLAGL2 modulates the transcription of Wnt6 and Fzd9 and Fzd2 receptors, but in this paper transcriptome analysis is examined in only $p53^{-/-}$ NSCs, and therefore it remains still unclear whether Wnt contributes to the malignant behaviors of GSCs.

L1CAM

The neural cell adhesion molecule, L1CAM (CD171) regulates neural cell growth, survival, migration during brain development. Although the role of L1CAM in the normal adult brain is not well defined, L1CAM is overexpressed in human gliomas and associated with invasive phenotype. L1CAM is highly expressed in CD133(+) glioma cells and that its knockdown suppresses glioma growth *in vivo* and increases survival of xenografted mice with downregulation of NSC transcription factor Olig2 and upregulation of cyclin-dependent kinase inhibitor $p21^{WAF1/CIP1}$ (Bao et al., 2008). These data suggest that L1CAM is a functional marker of GSC and its inhibition might be useful as a CSC–directed therapy.

3.2.2 Nuclear transcriptional factors

Signals and stresses from outside of the cells are transduced into nucleus, where expression of downstream targets is regulated by transcriptional and/or epigenetic factors, and lead to a variety of cellular phenotypes. Some nuclear factors are currently suggested to be essential for GSC behaviors and most of them regulate the self-renewal and differentiation.

Myc

Zheng et al. (2008) have performed wide-scale transcriptome/promoter studies and found strong enrichment of Myc binding elements in human primary GBMs. They revealed that the increase of Myc expression by the defect of p53 and PTEN in GBM CSCs withstands the differentiation and then enhances tumorigenic potential. These results strongly support pro-differentiation as a potential strategy against GSCs and encourage the identification and screening of agents targeting these differentiation pathways.

Sox11

Hide et al. (2009) have identified Sox11 as a candidate to induce differentiation in GSCs. Sox11 is exclusively overexpressed in non-tumorigenic glioma cells, and overexpression of Sox11 inhibits tumorigenesis of GSCs by inducing their neuronal differentiation. Sox11 is expressed in the committed neuronal precursor cells but not in NSCs, and negatively regulates the expression of PLAGL1, which is expressed in developing neuroepithelial cells. Knockdown of PLAGL1 significantly improves overall survival of xenotransplanted mice. Considering that PLAGL2 also regulates GSC self-renewal (Zheng et al., 2010), these PLAG family genes of transcriptional factors might play essential oncogenic roles. As both PLAGL1 and PLAGL2 are known to activate IGF2 promoters, the relevance between PLAG genes, Shh, IGF, and Wnt suggest that highly complicated cross-talk of multiple signaling regulates GSC features.

Nkx2.2

Muraguchi et al. (2011) have recently identified the homeodomain transcription factor Nkx2.2 as an inducer of GSCs toward oligodendroglial differentiation by using a sophisticated mouse models developing glioma at 100% penetrance. During normal development of brain, Nkx2.2 cooperates with Olig2 to promote oligodendrocyte maturation. Overexpression of Nkx2.2 inhibits self-renewal of human GSCs by induction of oligodendroglial differentiation, and therefore reactivation of Nkx2.2 expression in glioma is suggested as a novel therapeutic strategy.

Nanog

The puluripotent protein Nanog promotes not only embryonic stem (ES) cell expansion but also GSC tumorigenicity. GBMs show ES-like stemness signature that includes the expression of Nanog, OCT4, SOX2 and c-Myc (Ben-Porath et al., 2008). Knockdown of Nanog1 or Nanog2 suppress tumor growth after orthotopic xenotransplantation of GBM spheres and this effect is mediated by a positive-feedback loop of Nanog with Gli-1, and repression of Nanog by p53, which acts in a negative-regulatory loop with Gli-1, suggesting functional crosstalk among transcriptional factors in regulating the stem cell behavior and glioma growth (Zbinden et al., 2010).

3.2.3 DNA-damage response (DDR)

The large-scale genomic analyses have revealed genomic loss of at least one allele of ATR, ATM, CHEK1, or CHEK2 in 36% of human GBM samples, which are genes encoding key components of DDR required for cell-cycle checkpoint. Approximately 50% of GBM patients with CHEK2 alterations carry defects in the p53 signaling pathway (Squatrio et al., 2010). As the defect of DNA repair factors leads cells to genomic instability, genomic loss of DDR components might contribute to glioma initiation. However, Bao et al. (2008) have reported that $CD133^+$ primary GBM cells, not $CD133^-$ cells, have high activity of DDR response and thereby can repair ionizing radiation-dependent DNA damages. Wang et al., (2010a) showed that Notch signaling promotes radioresistance through regulation of the PI3K/Akt pathway and myeloid cell leukemia 1 (Mcl-1), but it remains unelucidated why only GSCs acquire and/or retain the high activity of DDR response.

3.2.4 Epigenetic factors

The DNA-methylation and histone-modification patterns are associated with the development and progression of cancers. Hundreds of genes are subject to DNA hypermethylation at their CpG island promoters. On the contrary, DNA hypomethylation is also detected by locus-specific and genome-wide. Histone modifications are also likely important in the pathology of GBM. However, the molecular aspects of them are not yet fully determined. One important example of DNA hypermethylation is the silencing of O6-methylguanine-DNA methyltransferase (*MGMT*) gene in human GBMs (Hegi et al., 2005). *MGMT* gene encodes a DNA repair protein that removes alkyl at the O6 position of guanine, which protect glioma cells from chemotherapeutic alkylating agents, such as temozolomide. MGMT hypermethylation has been considered as a predictor of outcome after treatment, but it is unrevealed if longer patients survival is directly due to reduced MGMT expression. As epigenetic modification can alter the differentiation properties of normal stem cells, some epigenetic factors have been examined their roles in GSC maintenance and tumor development.

EZH2

Enhancer of zeste homologue 2 (EZH2) is a component of the polycomb repressive complexes (PRC) 2 that participates in transcriptional repression of specific genes by mainly trimethylation of lysine 27 of histone H3. EZH2 is upregulated in a broad range of human neoplasms and its overexpression is correlated with poor prognosis. Suvà et al. (2009) have reported that pharmacologic depletion of EZH2 by the S-adenosylhomocysteine hydrolase inhibitor 3-Deazaneplanocin A (DZNep) reduces the self-renewal and tumor-initiating properties of GBM GSCs. Interestingly, their effects are mediated by c-myc downregulation, even though EZH2 belongs to a repressive complex.

Bmi-1

B lymphoma mouse Moloney leukemia virus insertion region (Bmi)-1 is a component of PRC1 complex which allows stable silencing of gene expression. PRC1 and PRC2 cooperatively modify histone status. Abdouh et al. (2009) have reported that Bmi-1, as well as EZH2, is highly enriched in CD133(+) GBM cells and that knockdown of Bmi-1 can deplete the

CD133(+) cell population and inhibit intracranial tumor formation. Bmi-1 directly represses $p21^{Cip}$ expression. It may also directly repress FOXOA3 expression, a potent inducer of apoptosis, and thereby supports cell-cycle progression and survival (Abdouh et al. 2009). Polycomb group proteins seem to regulate important aspects of GSC biology.

3.2.5 microRNA (miRNA)

microRNAs are non-coding RNAs of 22 nucleotides in length and regulate the translation and degradation of mRNAs by base-pairing to untranslated regions (UTRs) of targets. Approximately 1000 species of microRNA are thought to exist in the human genome. One microRNA has hundreds of targets, and one gene is targeted by multiple microRNAs (Krek et al., 2005). Increasing evidence strongly suggest that microRNAs are involved in neural development. The most highly expressed microRNAs in brain are miR-124 and miR-128, both of which are preferentially expressed in neurons. Some groups have investigated the direct roles of miRNAs in GSC features. SMAD3/4-controlled miR-451 expression has been shown to increase neurosphere formation of CD133(+) GBM cells (Gal et al., 2008). Interestingly, another group has reported that miR-451 regulates the expression of MDR1, which links to chemoresistant feature in cancer cells (Zhu et al., 2008). Conversely, the expression of miR-124 and miR-137 are significantly reduced in grade III and IV malignant gliomas and overexpression of these two microRNAs promotes differentiation of human GBM stem cells, indicating their tumor suppressive roles (Silber et al., 2008). miR-128 targeting to the Bmi-1 gene expression is known to be down-regulated in human GBMs, and its restoration specifically blocks proliferation of glioma spheres (Godlewski et al., 2008).

3.3 GSC niche (Therapeutic strategy)

As well as normal NSCs, GSCs are believed to be physically situated in the specialized microenvironment called "stem cell niche". Niche cells provide extrinsic cues as described above, including soluble factors, membrane-bound ligands, and extracellular matrix (ECM) proteins. Cell-to-cell communication between stem cells and the niche regulates self-renewal, differentiation, and maintenance of proper stem cell numbers and functions. Tumor niche is thought to be composed of tumor vascular endothelial cells, stromal fibroblasts, and immune cells. Considering that CSCs display enhanced resistance to conventional chemotherapies due to their increased expression of membrane pumps, cancer treatment should be aimed at not the conventional elimination of the proliferating cancer cell population but the disruption of cellular niches to induce stem cell differentiation. The stromal components that function as niche would therefore be most promising targets to eradicate GSCs (Figure 6).

Vascular niche

Enhanced neovascularization is one of the characters of malignant gliomas and it significantly correlates with tumor aggressiveness and poor clinical prognosis. An initial report on GSC niche was proposed as a perivascular niche, where GSCs closely interact with vascular endothelium (Calabrese et al., 2007). It was verified by subsequent studies showing that glioma cells express high levels of laminin receptor integrin $\alpha6\beta1$ in the perivascular niche and CD133(+)/integrinα6 (high) glioma cells exhibit stem cell properties (Lathia et al., 2010). In addition, secreted nitric oxide (NO) from the vascular endothelium regulates adjacent Nestin(+) glioma cells (Charles et al., 2010). GSCs are themselves tightly involved in tumor angiogenesis. Folkins et al. (2009) have demonstrated that GSCs increase endothelial cell proliferation and tube formation *in vitro*. In addition, GSCs in xenografted mice increase mobilization of bone marrow-derived endothelial progenitor cells and recruit them to the tumor through amplified secretion of vascular endothelial growth factor (VEGF) and stromal-derived factor 1 (SDF-1, also known as CXCL12). Surprisingly, two groups have provided strong evidence that a proportion of the vascular endothelial cells in human GBMs are originated from the tumor cell itself, which are differentiated ones from GSCs (Wang et al., 2010b; Ricci-Vitiani et al., 2010). DAPT, a γ-secretase inhibitor that effectively inhibits Notch signalling was found to induce significant suppression of the transition from CD133(+)/CD144(−) GSCs into CD133(+)/CD144(+) endothelial progenitors. In addition, bevacizumab, a VEGFA-binding antibody, blocked further maturation from endothelial progenitors into CD105(+) endothelial cells. These data suggested again that GSCs are critical targets in glioma biology and treatment.

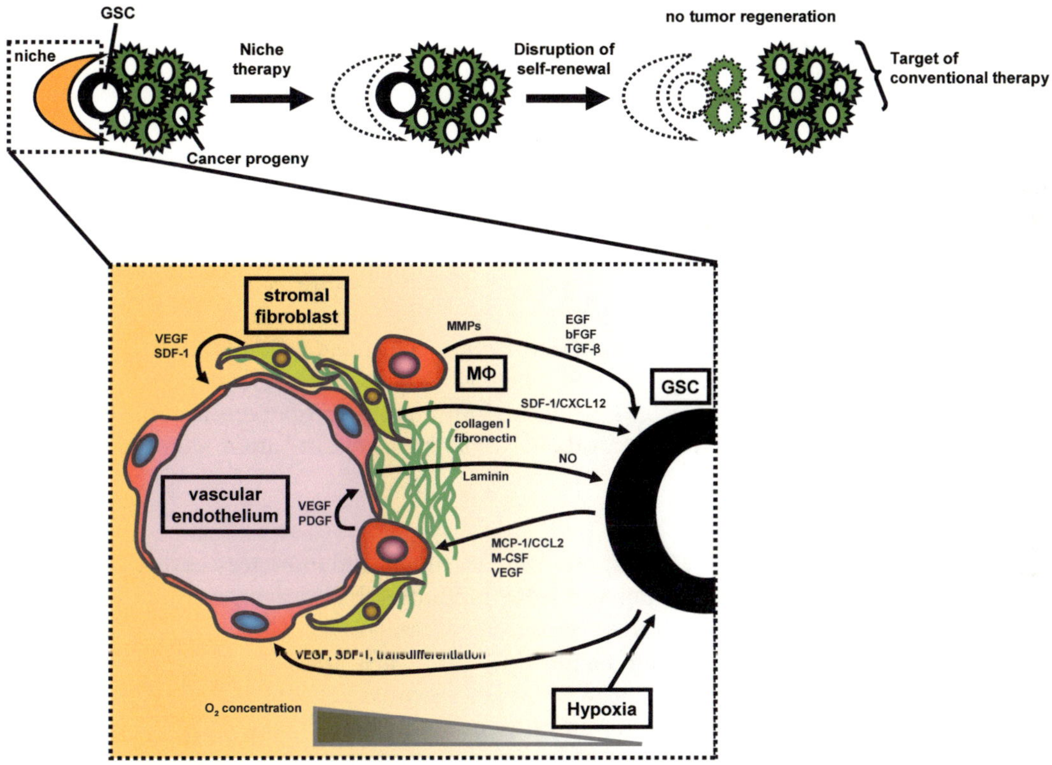

Fig. 6. The concept of niche therapy and components of GSC niche.

Hypoxic niche

Although the perivascular niche is well accepted, low oxygen areas away from tumor vessels are also recognized as secondary niches that play a role in GSC regulation. CD133 expression increases by approximately two-fold when primary glioma spheres are incubated in physiological concentrations of oxygen (7%) (McCord et al., 2009). In addition, hypoxia (1%) increases the self-renewal capacity of CD133(+) human GSCs independent of PI3K/Akt or ERK pathways (Soeda et al., 2009). The hypoxia-inducible factors (HIFs) are transcription factors that help cells to adapt to changes in oxygen concentrations. HIFs have more than 60 putative downstream genes that are involved in angiogenesis, glucose transport, glycolysis, cell survival, and metastasis. Li et al. (2009) have reported that knockdown of either HIF-1α or HIF-2α in GSCs decreases tumorigenic potential and increases the survival of xenografted mice and that elevated HIF-2α expression is correlated with poor survival of human glioma patients. Méndez et al. (2010) have also demonstrated that HIF-1α plays a role in the survival and self-renewal potential of GSCs. Some chemotherapeutic agents which target RTKs, such as gefitinib (Iressa, an inhibitor of EGFR/ERBB1) and imatinib (Glivec, an inhibitor of Bcr-Abl and PDGFRβ), have been shown to inhibit HIF-1 activity (Pore et al., 2006; Kimura et al., 2007), and further evidence has shown that hypoxia mediates resistance to chemotherapy and radiation (Teicher, 1994). The formation of necrosis, which is a resultant of increasing cellularity and poorly organized tumor vasculature, is a biologic hallmark in a highly aggressvie gliomas. Therefore, understanding of stem cell biology in hypoxic environment could also provide useful clues for glioma biology and treatment.

Cancer-associated fibroblast

Stromal fibroblasts, which are potentially originated from bone marrow-derived mesenchymal stem cells (MSCs), are observed as a cellular component in the tumor microenvironment and have important roles in the tumor progression. Especially, during tumor-induced angiogenesis, fibroblasts actively contribute to neovascularization through secretion of VEGF. They also produce ECM proteins such as fibronectin and type I collagen, both of which are involved in the initiation of tumor angiogenesis. Additionally, fibroblast-derived SDF-1 is responsible for recruiting endothelial progenitor cells into a tumor mass, thereby boosting tumor angiogenesis (Orimo et al., 2005). In parallel, the SDF-1 protein enhances tumor growth in a direct paracrine fashion via the CXCR4 receptor. Although whether stromal fibroblasts could affect GSCs behaviors is not yet so clear, it is worth noting that some MSCs are exactly detected as a tumor-stimulating component around the blood vessels and closely associated with endothelial cells/pericytes in tumor xenograft models (Spaeth et al., 2009).

Tumor-associated macrophages

Tumor-associated macrophages (TAMs) represent the major inflammatory component of the stroma in many tumors. TAMs are derived from circulating blood monocytes and recruited into the tumor region toward monocyte chemotactic protein-1 (MCP-1, also known as CCL2) and macrophage colony stimulating factor (M-CSF). TAMs display several pro-tumoral functions, including tumor growth (growth factors), neo-angiogenesis (VEGF and PDGF), matrix remodeling (MMPs), and anti-tumor immune suppression (prostaglandins, IL-10 and TGF-β) (Sica et al., 2006). There is no evidence on the exact roles of TAMs against GSCs, but ablation of TAMs might provide some therapeutic benefits against GSCs beyond disrupting vascular niche.

4. Conclusion

The existence of CSCs has altered our view on glioma biology, which prompts our re-evaluation of conventional strategies in therapies for glioma. Although some controversy is still unresolved regarding the definition, isolation methods, characteristics, and their exact roles *in vivo*, it is assured that gliomas have a cellular hierarchy and that certain subpopulation within tumors has extraordinary potential for tumor progression, therapeutic resistance, and tumor recurrence. Importantly, GSCs are highly resistant to chemo/radiotherapies, which are convinced by the currently poor record of clinical remission with conventional treatments. Therefore the development of novel therapies directed against GSCs is our urgent task. Remarkable insights into the molecular mechanisms or signaling pathways that are differentially regulated in GSCs and non-GSCs have accumulated in virtue of recent advance in this field. In this chapter, we have provided several key signaling pathways that are potentially useful for the future development of anti-GSC therapeutics, but at this point most of them are still far away from the clinical application. As an achievement, anti-vascular niche therapy with a humanized anti-VEGF-A monoclonal antibody bevacizumab, has displayed beneficial effects in phase II clinical trials, and approved for recurrent GBM patients in 2009. For relapsed or progressed GBMs, tumor responses were observed in 22 of 85 patients (26%) treated with bevacizumab alone (Friedman et al., 2009). This is the first major advance in glioma treatment over a decade. Nonetheless, our goal of glioma eradication has not been achieved. Additional basic and translational research must be carried out to exploit this promising concept for clinical advantage.

5. Acknowledgment

Our work is supported by Grants-in-Aid for Scientific Research from the Ministry of Education, Culture, Sports, Science and Technology (MEXT) of Japan to KT, TT, and ST. We wish to thank all members in Dept. of Stem Cell Regulation and Lab. of Cancer Research for their technical advice and helpful discussions.

6. References

Abdouh, M., Facchino, S., Chatoo, W., Balasingam, V., Ferreira, J. & Bernier, G. (2009). BMI1 sustains human glioblastoma multiforme stem cell renewal. *Journal of Neuroscience*, Vol.29, No.28, pp. 8884-8896

Al-Hajj, M., Wicha, M. S., Benito-Hernandez, A., Morrison, S. J. & Clarke, M. F. (2003). Prospective identification of tumorigenic breast cancer cells. *Proceedings of the National Academy of Sciences of the United States of America*, Vol.100, No.7, pp. 3983-3988

Anido, J., Saez-Borderias, A., Gonzalez-Junca, A., Rodon, L., Folch, G., Carmona, M. A., Prieto-Sanchez, R. M., Barba, I., Martinez-Saez, E., Prudkin, L., Cuartas, I., Raventos, C., Martinez-Ricarte, F., Poca, M. A., Garcia-Dorado, D., Lahn, M. M., Yingling, J. M., Rodon, J., Sahuquillo, J., Baselga, J. & Seoane, J. (2010). TGF-beta Receptor Inhibitors Target the CD44(high)/Id1(high) Glioma-Initiating Cell Population in Human Glioblastoma. *Cancer Cell*, Vol.18, No.6, pp. 655-668

Bachoo, R. M., Maher, E. A., Ligon, K. L., Sharpless, N. E., Chan, S. S., You, M. J., Tang, Y., DeFrances, J., Stover, E., Weissleder, R., Rowitch, D. H., Louis, D. N. & DePinho, R. A. (2002). Epidermal growth factor receptor and Ink4a/Arf: convergent mechanisms governing terminal differentiation and transformation along the neural stem cell to astrocyte axis. *Cancer Cell*, Vol.1, No.3, pp. 269-277

Bao, S., Wu, Q., Li, Z., Sathornsumetee, S., Wang, H., McLendon, R. E., Hjelmeland, A. B. & Rich, J. N. (2008). Targeting cancer stem cells through L1CAM suppresses glioma growth. *Cancer Research*, Vol.68, No.15, pp. 6043-6048

Bao, S., Wu, Q., McLendon, R. E., Hao, Y., Shi, Q., Hjelmeland, A. B., Dewhirst, M. W., Bigner, D. D. & Rich, J. N. (2006). Glioma stem cells promote radioresistance by preferential activation of the DNA damage response. *Nature*, Vol.444, No.7120, pp. 756-760

Beier, D., Hau, P., Proescholdt, M., Lohmeier, A., Wischhusen, J., Oefner, P. J., Aigner, L., Brawanski, A., Bogdahn, U. & Beier, C. P. (2007). CD133(+) and CD133(-) glioblastoma-derived cancer stem cells show differential growth characteristics and molecular profiles. *Cancer Research*, Vol.67, No.9, pp. 4010-4015

Ben-Porath, I., Thomson, M. W., Carey, V. J., Ge, R., Bell, G. W., Regev, A. & Weinberg, R. A. (2008). An embryonic stem cell-like gene expression signature in poorly differentiated aggressive human tumors. *Nature Genetics*, Vol.40, No.5, pp. 499-507

Bexell, D., Gunnarsson, S., Siesjo, P., Bengzon, J. & Darabi, A. (2009). CD133+ and nestin+ tumor-initiating cells dominate in N29 and N32 experimental gliomas. *International Journal of Cancer*, Vol.125, No.1, pp. 15-22

Bleau, A. M., Hambardzumyan, D., Ozawa, T., Fomchenko, E. I., Huse, J. T., Brennan, C. W. & Holland, E. C. (2009). PTEN/PI3K/Akt pathway regulates the side population phenotype and ABCG2 activity in glioma tumor stem-like cells. *Cell Stem Cell*, Vol.4, No.3, pp. 226-235

Bonnet, D. & Dick, J. E. (1997). Human acute myeloid leukemia is organized as a hierarchy that originates from a primitive hematopoietic cell. *Nature Medicine*, Vol.3, No.7, pp. 730-737

Calabrese, C., Poppleton, H., Kocak, M., Hogg, T. L., Fuller, C., Hamner, B., Oh, E. Y., Gaber, M. W., Finklestein, D., Allen, M., Frank, A., Bayazitov, I. T., Zakharenko, S. S., Gajjar, A., Davidoff, A. & Gilbertson, R. J. (2007). A perivascular niche for brain tumor stem cells. *Cancer Cell*, Vol.11, No.1, pp. 69-82

Charles, N., Ozawa, T., Squatrito, M., Bleau, A. M., Brennan, C. W., Hambardzumyan, D. & Holland, E. C. (2010). Perivascular nitric oxide activates notch signaling and promotes stem-like character in PDGF-induced glioma cells. *Cell Stem Cell*, Vol.6, No.2, pp. 141-152

Chute, J. P., Muramoto, G. G., Whitesides, J., Colvin, M., Safi, R., Chao, N. J. & McDonnell, D. P. (2006). Inhibition of aldehyde dehydrogenase and retinoid signaling induces the expansion of human hematopoietic stem cells. *Proceedings of the National Academy of Sciences of the United States of America*, Vol.103, No.31, pp. 11707-11712

Clarke, M. F., Dick, J. E., Dirks, P. B., Eaves, C. J., Jamieson, C. H., Jones, D. L., Visvader, J., Weissman, I. L. & Wahl, G. M. (2006). Cancer stem cells--perspectives on current status and future directions: AACR Workshop on cancer stem cells. *Cancer Research*, Vol.66, No.19, pp. 9339-9344

Corbeil, D., Roper, K., Hellwig, A., Tavian, M., Miraglia, S., Watt, S. M., Simmons, P. J., Peault, B., Buck, D. W. & Huttner, W. B. (2000). The human AC133 hematopoietic stem cell antigen is also expressed in epithelial cells and targeted to plasma membrane protrusions. *The Journal of Biological Chemistry*, Vol.275, No.8, pp. 5512-5520

Dai, C., Celestino, J. C., Okada, Y., Louis, D. N., Fuller, G. N. & Holland, E. C. (2001). PDGF autocrine stimulation dedifferentiates cultured astrocytes and induces oligodendrogliomas and oligoastrocytomas from neural progenitors and astrocytes in vivo. *Genes & Development*, Vol.15, No.15, pp. 1913-1925

Daumas-Duport, C., Scheithauer, B., O'Fallon, J. & Kelly, P. (1988). Grading of astrocytomas. A simple and reproducible method. *Cancer*, Vol.62, No.10, pp. 2152-2165

Dean, M., Fojo, T. & Bates, S. (2005). Tumour stem cells and drug resistance. *Nature Reviews Cancer*, Vol.5, No.4, pp. 275-284

Diehn, M., Cho, R. W., Lobo, N. A., Kalisky, T., Dorie, M. J., Kulp, A. N., Qian, D., Lam, J. S., Ailles, L. E., Wong, M., Joshua, B., Kaplan, M. J., Wapnir, I., Dirbas, F. M., Somlo, G., Garberoglio, C., Paz, B., Shen, J., Lau, S. K., Quake, S. R., Brown, J. M., Weissman, I. L. & Clarke, M. F. (2009). Association of reactive oxygen species levels and radioresistance in cancer stem cells. *Nature*, Vol.458, No.7239, pp. 780-783

Fan, X., Khaki, L., Zhu, T. S., Soules, M. E., Talsma, C. E., Gul, N., Koh, C., Zhang, J., Li, Y. M., Maciaczyk, J., Nikkhah, G., Dimeco, F., Piccirillo, S., Vescovi, A. L. & Eberhart, C. G. (2010). NOTCH pathway blockade depletes CD133-positive glioblastoma cells and inhibits growth of tumor neurospheres and xenografts. *Stem Cells*, Vol.28, No.1, pp. 5-16

Fargeas, C. A., Huttner, W. B. & Corbeil, D. (2007). Nomenclature of prominin-1 (CD133) splice variants - an update. *Tissue Antigens*, Vol.69, No.6, pp. 602-606

Florek, M., Haase, M., Marzesco, A. M., Freund, D., Ehninger, G., Huttner, W. B. & Corbeil, D. (2005). Prominin-1/CD133, a neural and hematopoietic stem cell marker, is expressed in adult human differentiated cells and certain types of kidney cancer. *Cell and Tissue Research*, Vol.319, No.1, pp. 15-26

Folkins, C., Shaked, Y., Man, S., Tang, T., Lee, C. R., Zhu, Z., Hoffman, R. M. & Kerbel, R. S. (2009). Glioma tumor stem-like cells promote tumor angiogenesis and vasculogenesis via vascular endothelial growth factor and stromal-derived factor 1. *Cancer Research*, Vol.69, No.18, pp. 7243-7251

Friedman, H. S., Prados, M. D., Wen, P. Y., Mikkelsen, T., Schiff, D., Abrey, L. E., Yung, W. K., Paleologos, N., Nicholas, M. K., Jensen, R., Vredenburgh, J., Huang, J., Zheng, M. & Cloughesy, T. (2009). Bevacizumab alone and in combination with irinotecan in recurrent glioblastoma. *Journal of Clinical Oncology*, Vol.27, No.28, pp. 4733-4740

Gal, H., Pandi, G., Kanner, A. A., Ram, Z., Lithwick-Yanai, G., Amariglio, N., Rechavi, G. & Givol, D. (2008). MIR-451 and Imatinib mesylate inhibit tumor growth of Glioblastoma stem cells. *Biochemical and Biophysical Research Communications*, Vol.376, No.1, pp. 86-90

Ginestier, C., Hur, M. H., Charafe-Jauffret, E., Monville, F., Dutcher, J., Brown, M., Jacquemier, J., Viens, P., Kleer, C. G., Liu, S., Schott, A., Hayes, D., Birnbaum, D., Wicha, M. S. & Dontu, G. (2007). ALDH1 is a marker of normal and malignant human mammary stem cells and a predictor of poor clinical outcome. *Cell Stem Cell*, Vol.1, No.5, pp. 555-567

Godlewski, J., Nowicki, M. O., Bronisz, A., Williams, S., Otsuki, A., Nuovo, G., Raychaudhury, A., Newton, H. B., Chiocca, E. A. & Lawler, S. (2008). Targeting of the Bmi-1 oncogene/stem cell renewal factor by microRNA-128 inhibits glioma proliferation and self-renewal. *Cancer Research*, Vol.68, No.22, pp. 9125-9130

Goodell, M. A., Brose, K., Paradis, G., Conner, A. S. & Mulligan, R. C. (1996). Isolation and functional properties of murine hematopoietic stem cells that are replicating in vivo. *The Journal of Experimental Medicine*, Vol.183, No.4, pp. 1797-1806

Harris, M. A., Yang, H., Low, B. E., Mukherjee, J., Guha, A., Bronson, R. T., Shultz, L. D., Israel, M. A. & Yun, K. (2008). Cancer stem cells are enriched in the side population cells in a mouse model of glioma. *Cancer Research*, Vol.68, No.24, pp. 10051-10059

Hegi, M. E., Diserens, A. C., Gorlia, T., Hamou, M. F., de Tribolet, N., Weller, M., Kros, J. M., Hainfellner, J. A., Mason, W., Mariani, L., Bromberg, J. E., Hau, P., Mirimanoff, R. O., Cairncross, J. G., Janzer, R. C. & Stupp, R. (2005). MGMT gene silencing and benefit from temozolomide in glioblastoma. *The New England Journal of Medicine*, Vol.352, No.10, pp. 997-1003

Hide, T., Takezaki, T., Nakatani, Y., Nakamura, H., Kuratsu, J. & Kondo, T. (2009). Sox11 prevents tumorigenesis of glioma-initiating cells by inducing neuronal differentiation. *Cancer Research*, Vol.69, No.20, pp. 7953-7959

Holland, E. C., Celestino, J., Dai, C., Schaefer, L., Sawaya, R. E. & Fuller, G. N. (2000). Combined activation of Ras and Akt in neural progenitors induces glioblastoma formation in mice. *Nature Genetics*, Vol.25, No.1, pp. 55-57

Hsieh, A., Ellsworth, R. & Hsieh, D. (2010). Hedgehog/GLI1 regulates IGF dependent malignant behaviors in glioma stem cells. *Journal of Cellular Physiology*, Vol.226, No.4, pp. 1118-1127

Ikushima, H., Todo, T., Ino, Y., Takahashi, M., Miyazawa, K. & Miyazono, K. (2009). Autocrine TGF-beta signaling maintains tumorigenicity of glioma-initiating cells through Sry-related HMG-box factors. *Cell Stem Cell*, Vol.5, No.5, pp. 504-514

Inda, M. M., Bonavia, R., Mukasa, A., Narita, Y., Sah, D. W., Vandenberg, S., Brennan, C., Johns, T. G., Bachoo, R., Hadwiger, P., Tan, P., Depinho, R. A., Cavenee, W. & Furnari, F. (2010). Tumor heterogeneity is an active process maintained by a mutant EGFR-induced cytokine circuit in glioblastoma. *Genes & Development*, Vol.24, No.16, pp. 1731-1745

Jackson, E. L., Garcia-Verdugo, J. M., Gil-Perotin, S., Roy, M., Quinones-Hinojosa, A., VandenBerg, S. & Alvarez-Buylla, A. (2006). PDGFR alpha-positive B cells are neural stem cells in the adult SVZ that form glioma-like growths in response to increased PDGF signaling. *Neuron*, Vol.51, No.2, pp. 187-199

Johe, K. K., Hazel, T. G., Muller, T., Dugich-Djordjevic, M. M. & McKay, R. D. (1996). Single factors direct the differentiation of stem cells from the fetal and adult central nervous system. *Genes & Development*, Vol.10, No.24, pp. 3129-3140

Jordan, C. T., Guzman, M. L. & Noble, M. (2006). Cancer stem cells. *The New England Journal of Medicine*, Vol.355, No.12, pp. 1253-1261

Kimura, Y., Inoue, K., Abe, M., Nearman, J. & Baranowska-Kortylewicz, J. (2007). PDGFRbeta and HIF-1alpha inhibition with imatinib and radioimmunotherapy of experimental prostate cancer. *Cancer Biology & Therapy*, Vol.6, No.11, pp. 1763-1772

Kondo, T., Setoguchi, T. & Taga, T. (2004). Persistence of a small subpopulation of cancer stem-like cells in the C6 glioma cell line. *Proceedings of the National Academy of Sciences of the United States of America*, Vol.101, No.3, pp. 781-786

Korkaya, H., Paulson, A., Iovino, F. & Wicha, M. S. (2008). HER2 regulates the mammary stem/progenitor cell population driving tumorigenesis and invasion. *Oncogene*, Vol.27, No.47, pp. 6120-6130

Krek, A., Grun, D., Poy, M. N., Wolf, R., Rosenberg, L., Epstein, E. J., MacMenamin, P., da Piedade, I., Gunsalus, K. C., Stoffel, M. & Rajewsky, N. (2005). Combinatorial microRNA target predictions. *Nature Genetics*, Vol.37, No.5, pp. 495-500

Lapidot, T., Sirard, C., Vormoor, J., Murdoch, B., Hoang, T., Caceres-Cortes, J., Minden, M., Paterson, B., Caligiuri, M. A. & Dick, J. E. (1994). A cell initiating human acute myeloid leukaemia after transplantation into SCID mice. *Nature*, Vol.367, No.6464, pp. 645-648

Lathia, J. D., Gallagher, J., Heddleston, J. M., Wang, J., Eyler, C. E., Macswords, J., Wu, Q., Vasanji, A., McLendon, R. E., Hjelmeland, A. B. & Rich, J. N. (2010). Integrin alpha 6 regulates glioblastoma stem cells. *Cell Stem Cell*, Vol.6, No.5, pp. 421-432

Lee, J., Son, M. J., Woolard, K., Donin, N. M., Li, A., Cheng, C. H., Kotliarova, S., Kotliarov, Y., Walling, J., Ahn, S., Kim, M., Totonchy, M., Cusack, T., Ene, C., Ma, H., Su, Q., Zenklusen, J. C., Zhang, W., Maric, D. & Fine, H. A. (2008). Epigenetic-mediated dysfunction of the bone morphogenetic protein pathway inhibits differentiation of glioblastoma-initiating cells. *Cancer Cell*, Vol.13, No.1, pp. 69-80

Leemhuis, T., Yoder, M. C., Grigsby, S., Aguero, B., Eder, P. & Srour, E. F. (1996). Isolation of primitive human bone marrow hematopoietic progenitor cells using Hoechst 33342 and Rhodamine 123. *Experimental Hematology*, Vol.24, No.10, pp. 1215-1224

Li, Z., Bao, S., Wu, Q., Wang, H., Eyler, C., Sathornsumetee, S., Shi, Q., Cao, Y., Lathia, J., McLendon, R. E., Hjelmeland, A. B. & Rich, J. N. (2009). Hypoxia-inducible factors regulate tumorigenic capacity of glioma stem cells. *Cancer Cell*, Vol.15, No.6, pp. 501-513

Mazzoleni, S., Politi, L. S., Pala, M., Cominelli, M., Franzin, A., Sergi Sergi, L., Falini, A., De Palma, M., Bulfone, A., Poliani, P. L. & Galli, R. (2010). Epidermal growth factor receptor expression identifies functionally and molecularly distinct tumor-initiating cells in human glioblastoma multiforme and is required for gliomagenesis. *Cancer Research*, Vol.70, No.19, pp. 7500-7513

McCord, A. M., Jamal, M., Shankavaram, U. T., Lang, F. F., Camphausen, K. & Tofilon, P. J. (2009). Physiologic oxygen concentration enhances the stem-like properties of CD133+ human glioblastoma cells in vitro. *Molecular Cancer Research*, Vol.7, No.4, pp. 489-497

Mendez, O., Zavadil, J., Esencay, M., Lukyanov, Y., Santovasi, D., Wang, S. C., Newcomb, E. W. & Zagzag, D. (2010). Knock down of HIF-1alpha in glioma cells reduces migration in vitro and invasion in vivo and impairs their ability to form tumor spheres. *Molecular Cancer*, Vol.9, No.pp. 133

Miraglia, S., Godfrey, W., Yin, A. H., Atkins, K., Warnke, R., Holden, J. T., Bray, R. A., Waller, E. K. & Buck, D. W. (1997). A novel five-transmembrane hematopoietic stem cell antigen: isolation, characterization, and molecular cloning. *Blood*, Vol.90, No.12, pp. 5013-5021

Muraguchi, T., Tanaka, S., Yamada, D., Tamase, A., Nakada, M., Nakamura, H., Hoshii, T., Ooshio, T., Tadokoro, Y., Naka, K., Ino, Y., Todo, T., Kuratsu, J., Saya, H., Hamada, J. & Hirao, A. (2010). NKX2.2 suppresses self-renewal of glioma-initiating cells. *Cancer Research*, Vol.71, No.3, pp. 1135-1145

Nowell, P. C. (1976). The clonal evolution of tumor cell populations. *Science*, Vol.194, No.4260, pp. 23-28

O'Brien, C. A., Pollett, A., Gallinger, S. & Dick, J. E. (2007). A human colon cancer cell capable of initiating tumour growth in immunodeficient mice. *Nature*, Vol.445, No.7123, pp. 106-110

Ogden, A. T., Waziri, A. E., Lochhead, R. A., Fusco, D., Lopez, K., Ellis, J. A., Kang, J., Assanah, M., McKhann, G. M., Sisti, M. B., McCormick, P. C., Canoll, P. & Bruce, J. N. (2008). Identification of A2B5+CD133- tumor-initiating cells in adult human gliomas. *Neurosurgery*, Vol.62, No.2, pp. 505-514; discussion 514-505

Orimo, A., Gupta, P. B., Sgroi, D. C., Arenzana-Seisdedos, F., Delaunay, T., Naeem, R., Carey, V. J., Richardson, A. L. & Weinberg, R. A. (2005). Stromal fibroblasts present in invasive human breast carcinomas promote tumor growth and angiogenesis through elevated SDF-1/CXCL12 secretion. *Cell*, Vol.121, No.3, pp. 335-348

Pearce, D. J., Taussig, D., Simpson, C., Allen, K., Rohatiner, A. Z., Lister, T. A. & Bonnet, D. (2005). Characterization of cells with a high aldehyde dehydrogenase activity from cord blood and acute myeloid leukemia samples. *Stem Cells*, Vol.23, No.6, pp. 752-760

Penuelas, S., Anido, J., Prieto-Sanchez, R. M., Folch, G., Barba, I., Cuartas, I., Garcia-Dorado, D., Poca, M. A., Sahuquillo, J., Baselga, J. & Seoane, J. (2009). TGF-beta increases glioma-initiating cell self-renewal through the induction of LIF in human glioblastoma. *Cancer Cell*, Vol.15, No.4, pp. 315-327

Pollard, S. M., Yoshikawa, K., Clarke, I. D., Danovi, D., Stricker, S., Russell, R., Bayani, J., Head, R., Lee, M., Bernstein, M., Squire, J. A., Smith, A. & Dirks, P. (2009). Glioma stem cell lines expanded in adherent culture have tumor-specific phenotypes and are suitable for chemical and genetic screens. *Cell Stem Cell*, Vol.4, No.6, pp. 568-580

Pore, N., Jiang, Z., Gupta, A., Cerniglia, G., Kao, G. D. & Maity, A. (2006). EGFR tyrosine kinase inhibitors decrease VEGF expression by both hypoxia-inducible factor (HIF)-1-independent and HIF-1-dependent mechanisms. *Cancer Research*, Vol.66, No.6, pp. 3197-3204

Quintana, E., Shackleton, M., Sabel, M. S., Fullen, D. R., Johnson, T. M. & Morrison, S. J. (2008). Efficient tumour formation by single human melanoma cells. *Nature*, Vol.456, No.7222, pp. 593-598

Reynolds, B. A. & Weiss, S. (1992). Generation of neurons and astrocytes from isolated cells of the adult mammalian central nervous system. *Science*, Vol.255, No.5052, pp. 1707-1710

Ricci-Vitiani, L., Pallini, R., Biffoni, M., Todaro, M., Invernici, G., Cenci, T., Maira, G., Parati, E. A., Stassi, G., Larocca, L. M. & De Maria, R. (2010). Tumour vascularization via endothelial differentiation of glioblastoma stem-like cells. *Nature*, Vol.468, No.7325, pp. 824-828

Sakariassen, P. O., Immervoll, H. & Chekenya, M. (2007). Cancer stem cells as mediators of treatment resistance in brain tumors: status and controversies. *Neoplasia*, Vol.9, No.11, pp. 882-892

Salmon, S. E., Hamburger, A. W., Soehnlen, B., Durie, B. G., Alberts, D. S. & Moon, T. E. (1978). Quantitation of differential sensitivity of human-tumor stem cells to anticancer drugs. *The New England Journal of Medicine*, Vol.298, No.24, pp. 1321-1327

Sherry, M. M., Reeves, A., Wu, J. K. & Cochran, B. H. (2009). STAT3 is required for proliferation and maintenance of multipotency in glioblastoma stem cells. *Stem Cells*, Vol.27, No.10, pp. 2383-2392

Sica, A., Schioppa, T., Mantovani, A. & Allavena, P. (2006). Tumour-associated macrophages are a distinct M2 polarised population promoting tumour progression: potential targets of anti-cancer therapy. *European Journal of Cancer*, Vol.42, No.6, pp. 717-727

Silber, J., Lim, D. A., Petritsch, C., Persson, A. I., Maunakea, A. K., Yu, M., Vandenberg, S. R., Ginzinger, D. G., James, C. D., Costello, J. F., Bergers, G., Weiss, W. A., Alvarez-Buylla, A. & Hodgson, J. G. (2008). miR-124 and miR-137 inhibit proliferation of glioblastoma multiforme cells and induce differentiation of brain tumor stem cells. *BMC Medicine*, Vol.6, No.pp. 14

Singh, S. K., Clarke, I. D., Terasaki, M., Bonn, V. E., Hawkins, C., Squire, J. & Dirks, P. B. (2003). Identification of a cancer stem cell in human brain tumors. *Cancer Research*, Vol.63, No.18, pp. 5821-5828

Singh, S. K., Hawkins, C., Clarke, I. D., Squire, J. A., Bayani, J., Hide, T., Henkelman, R. M., Cusimano, M. D. & Dirks, P. B. (2004). Identification of human brain tumour initiating cells. *Nature*, Vol.432, No.7015, pp. 396-401

Soeda, A., Inagaki, A., Oka, N., Ikegame, Y., Aoki, H., Yoshimura, S., Nakashima, S., Kunisada, T. & Iwama, T. (2008). Epidermal growth factor plays a crucial role in mitogenic regulation of human brain tumor stem cells. *The Journal of Biological Chemistry*, Vol.283, No.16, pp. 10958-10966

Soeda, A., Park, M., Lee, D., Mintz, A., Androutsellis-Theotokis, A., McKay, R. D., Engh, J., Iwama, T., Kunisada, T., Kassam, A. B., Pollack, I. F. & Park, D. M. (2009). Hypoxia promotes expansion of the CD133-positive glioma stem cells through activation of HIF-1alpha. *Oncogene*, Vol.28, No.45, pp. 3949-3959

Spaeth, E. L., Dembinski, J. L., Sasser, A. K., Watson, K., Klopp, A., Hall, B., Andreeff, M. & Marini, F. (2009). Mesenchymal stem cell transition to tumor-associated fibroblasts contributes to fibrovascular network expansion and tumor progression. *PLoS One*, Vol.4, No.4, pp. e4992

Squatrito, M., Brennan, C. W., Helmy, K., Huse, J. T., Petrini, J. H. & Holland, E. C. (2010). Loss of ATM/Chk2/p53 pathway components accelerates tumor development and contributes to radiation resistance in gliomas. *Cancer Cell*, Vol.18, No.6, pp. 619-629

Suva, M. L., Riggi, N., Janiszewska, M., Radovanovic, I., Provero, P., Stehle, J. C., Baumer, K., Le Bitoux, M. A., Marino, D., Cironi, L., Marquez, V. E., Clement, V. & Stamenkovic, I. (2009). EZH2 is essential for glioblastoma cancer stem cell maintenance. *Cancer Research*, Vol.69, No.24, pp. 9211-9218

Teicher, B. A. (1994). Hypoxia and drug resistance. *Cancer Metastasis Reviews*, Vol.13, No.2, pp. 139-168

Wang, H., Lathia, J. D., Wu, Q., Wang, J., Li, Z., Heddleston, J. M., Eyler, C. E., Elderbroom, J., Gallagher, J., Schuschu, J., MacSwords, J., Cao, Y., McLendon, R. E., Wang, X. F., Hjelmeland, A. B. & Rich, J. N. (2009). Targeting interleukin 6 signaling suppresses glioma stem cell survival and tumor growth. *Stem Cells*, Vol.27, No.10, pp. 2393-2404

Wang, J., Wakeman, T. P., Lathia, J. D., Hjelmeland, A. B., Wang, X. F., White, R. R., Rich, J. N. & Sullenger, B. A. (2010a). Notch promotes radioresistance of glioma stem cells. *Stem Cells*, Vol.28, No.1, pp. 17-28

Wang, R., Chadalavada, K., Wilshire, J., Kowalik, U., Hovinga, K. E., Geber, A., Fligelman, B., Leversha, M., Brennan, C. & Tabar, V. (2010b). Glioblastoma stem-like cells give rise to tumour endothelium. *Nature*, Vol.468, No.7325, pp. 829-833

Weigmann, A., Corbeil, D., Hellwig, A. & Huttner, W. B. (1997). Prominin, a novel microvilli-specific polytopic membrane protein of the apical surface of epithelial cells, is targeted to plasmalemmal protrusions of non-epithelial cells. *Proceedings of the National Academy of Sciences of the United States of America*, Vol.94, No.23, pp. 12425-12430

Weissenberger, J., Loeffler, S., Kappeler, A., Kopf, M., Lukes, A., Afanasieva, T. A., Aguzzi, A. & Weis, J. (2004). IL-6 is required for glioma development in a mouse model. *Oncogene*, Vol.23, No.19, pp. 3308-3316

Xu, Q., Yuan, X., Liu, G., Black, K. L. & Yu, J. S. (2008). Hedgehog signaling regulates brain tumor-initiating cell proliferation and portends shorter survival for patients with PTEN-coexpressing glioblastomas. *Stem Cells*, Vol.26, No.12, pp. 3018-3026

Yamanaka, S. & Blau, H. M. (2010). Nuclear reprogramming to a pluripotent state by three approaches. *Nature*, Vol.465, No.7299, pp. 704-712

Yin, A. H., Miraglia, S., Zanjani, E. D., Almeida-Porada, G., Ogawa, M., Leary, A. G., Olweus, J., Kearney, J. & Buck, D. W. (1997). AC133, a novel marker for human hematopoietic stem and progenitor cells. *Blood*, Vol.90, No.12, pp. 5002-5012

Zabierowski, S. E. & Herlyn, M. (2008). Melanoma stem cells: the dark seed of melanoma. *Journal of Clinical Oncology*, Vol.26, No.17, pp. 2890-2894

Zbinden, M., Duquet, A., Lorente-Trigos, A., Ngwabyt, S. N., Borges, I. & Ruiz i Altaba, A. (2010). NANOG regulates glioma stem cells and is essential in vivo acting in a cross-functional network with GLI1 and p53. *The EMBO Journal*, Vol.29, No.15, pp. 2659-2674

Zheng, H., Ying, H., Wiedemeyer, R., Yan, H., Quayle, S. N., Ivanova, E. V., Paik, J. H., Zhang, H., Xiao, Y., Perry, S. R., Hu, J., Vinjamoori, A., Gan, B., Sahin, E., Chheda, M. G., Brennan, C., Wang, Y. A., Hahn, W. C., Chin, L. & DePinho, R. A. (2010). PLAGL2 regulates Wnt signaling to impede differentiation in neural stem cells and gliomas. *Cancer Cell*, Vol.17, No.5, pp. 497-509

Zheng, H., Ying, H., Yan, H., Kimmelman, A. C., Hiller, D. J., Chen, A. J., Perry, S. R., Tonon, G., Chu, G. C., Ding, Z., Stommel, J. M., Dunn, K. L., Wiedemeyer, R., You, M. J., Brennan, C., Wang, Y. A., Ligon, K. L., Wong, W. H., Chin, L. & DePinho, R. A. (2008). p53 and Pten control neural and glioma stem/progenitor cell renewal and differentiation. *Nature*, Vol.455, No.7216, pp. 1129-1133

Zhu, H., Wu, H., Liu, X., Evans, B. R., Medina, D. J., Liu, C. G. & Yang, J. M. (2008). Role of MicroRNA miR-27a and miR-451 in the regulation of MDR1/P-glycoprotein expression in human cancer cells. *Biochemical Pharmacology*, Vol.76, No.5, pp. 582-588

9

Molecular Hallmarks of Gliomas

Marta Pojo and Bruno Marques Costa
Life and Health Sciences Research Institute (ICVS),
School of Health Sciences, University of Minho,
ICVS/3B's - PT Government Associate Laboratory, Braga/Guimarães
Portugal

1. Introduction

Tumors of the central nervous system (CNS) encompass a wide variety of entities, which span from benign to highly malignant. The classification of these tumors is typically based on their histopathological features or their location within the CNS. Despite these apparently simple criteria, there are a great number of independent CNS tumor types as defined by the most recent World Health Organization (WHO) classification of CNS tumors (Louis et al., 2007), which is the standard for the definition of CNS tumors worldwide. The WHO listing of CNS tumors is impressively vast and has, in fact, been surrounded by some controversy concerning the nosology of some tumor entities (e.g., the nosologic place of highly anaplastic oligoastrocytic tumors, glioblastoma with oligodendroglioma components). The age-standardized incidence rate of all primary non-malignant and malignant CNS tumors in the US is 16.5 per 100,000 person-years (9.2 per 100,000 person-years for non-malignant tumors and 7.3 per 100,000 person-years for malignant tumors) (CBTRUS, 2010). This rate is higher in females (17.2 per 100,000 person-years) than males (15.8 per 100,000 person-years). Worldwide data is available only for malignant primary CNS tumors; in this setting, the incidence rates are higher in males (approximately 3.7 per 100,000 person-years) than females (2.6 per 100,000 person-years) (Ferlay et al., 2008). In Western Europe, the male and female incidence rates of malignant CNS tumors are 6.7 per 100,000 person-years and 4.5 per 100,000 person-years, respectively. Very similar figures are observed in Northern America (6.0 and 4.5 per 100,000 person-years for males and females, respectively). Interestingly, the incidence rates are higher in more developed countries than in less developed ones, but these differences may be a consequence of differences in diagnostic practices, completeness of reporting and access to adequate health care, rather than attributable to geographic and genetic variation.

CNS tumors are considered to be primary when the tumor originally initiates in the CNS, as opposed to the far more common brain metastases derived from malignant tumors located in other organs, which are considered secondary brain tumors. Primary brain and CNS tumors account for only approximately 2% of all primary tumors (Louis et al., 2007), but they rank first among tumor types for the average years of life lost (~20 years, compared, for example, with ~6 years for prostate cancer and ~12 years for lung cancer) (Burnet et al., 2005). These tumors are the most frequent solid malignancy in children, being the leading cause of cancer-related death in children under the age of 19 (Rickert & Paulus, 2001). The impact and nature of primary brain tumors in adults is somewhat different, but they still rank second as cause of cancer death in males aged 20 to 39 years, and fifth in females of those same ages (Jemal et al., 2009). This chapter will not fully review all the types of brain and CNS malignancies, but rather focus more specifically and thoroughly in gliomas, the most common type of all primary brain tumors.

2. Classification and epidemiology of gliomas

Glioma is a broad category of tumors divided into histological subgroups based on the type of glial cell of origin or morphological similarities between tumor and normal glial cells: astrocytomas (derived from astrocytes or their precursors), oligodendrogliomas (derived from oligodendrocytes or their precursors), and oligoastrocytomas (mixed lineage) are the three major subgroups, while ependymomas (derived from ependyma or their precursors) are less common (Louis et al., 2007). They represent 36% of all primary brain and CNS tumors, and account for approximately 81% of those that are malignant, an occurrence most likely related to the fact that the number of glial cells in the CNS is an order of magnitude higher than that of neurons. In addition, glial cells retain the ability to proliferative throughout adulthood, while most neurons do not, a characteristic that may also contribute to the higher incidence of this tumor group.

The WHO classification of CNS tumors is the most commonly used classification system among the medical and research community. This system classifies gliomas according to the presumed cell of origin based on similarities of tumor cells and non-neoplastic glial cells, as determined by histological analysis. Additionally, gliomas can be graded I to IV based on their degree of differentiation and malignancy (Louis et al., 2007), which can help predict the likely behavior of the tumor. Glioma grading is typically based on tumor cells' characteristics like mitotic index, nuclear atypia, vascular proliferation and necrosis (Louis et al., 2007). Simply put, grade I tumors often present well differentiated cells, are biologically benign and can be cured; grade II gliomas are malignancies that may follow long clinical courses, but early diffuse infiltration of the surrounding brain renders them incurable by surgery; grade III tumors exhibit increased anaplasia and proliferation, being more rapidly fatal; grade IV tumors exhibit more advanced features of malignancy, such as vascular proliferation and necrosis, and are generally lethal within 12 months. In general, grades I and II tumors are considered low-grade, while grades III and IV are high-grade tumors. The cell of origin of gliomas is a matter surrounded by controversy: for a long time, gliomas were believed to arise from differentiated glial cells, but this paradigm has recently been called into question, as some evidences suggest that these tumors arise from stem cells or lineage-committed progenitor cells (Singh et al., 2004). For the purposes of this chapter, the three major histological types of glioma (astrocytomas, oligodendrogliomas, and oligoastrocytomas) are discussed with particular emphasis.

2.1 Astrocytomas

Astrocytic tumors, or astrocytomas, are the most common intracranial neoplasms, accounting for approximately 75% of all gliomas (CBTRUS, 2010). Despite sharing a same cell of origin, astrocytoma is a broad category of tumors with different characteristics that differ in their location within the CNS, age and gender distribution, morphological features, growth potential, extent of invasiveness, tendency for progression, and clinical course. These are distinctly classified into four major clinicopathological entities, mostly based on their degree of malignancy: pilocytic astrocytomas (WHO grade I), diffuse astrocytoma (WHO grade II), anaplastic astrocytoma (WHO grade III) and glioblastoma multiforme

(GBM, WHO grade IV). A brief summary of the main characteristics of these tumor types is given below, with a special emphasizes on the most common and malignant type, GBM. **Pilocytic astrocytomas** (WHO grade I) account for ~5.8% of all gliomas, with similar frequencies in both males and females. Sometimes these are also referred to as "juvenile pilocytic astrocytoma", as they occur predominantly in children and teens, being the most common CNS tumor type among people under the age of 19 (CBTRUS, 2010). **Diffuse astrocytomas** (WHO grade II), sometimes called low-grade astrocytomas, account for ~1.5% of all gliomas and occur most commonly in young adults between the ages of 20 to 40. A slight male predominance (male-to-female ratio of 1.18:1) has been reported (Louis et al., 2007). This diffusely infiltrative nature may in part contribute to the typical progression of these tumors to more malignant neoplasms like anaplastic astrocytoma and, ultimately, glioblastoma. Three histologic entities can be distinguished: fibrillary astrocytoma (the most common), gemistocytic astrocytoma, and protoplasmic astrocytoma (Louis et al., 2007). **Anaplastic astrocytomas** (WHO grade III) are high-grade gliomas which may arise from a low grade diffuse astrocytoma or may arise *de novo*, i.e., without clinical evidence of a less malignant precursor lesion. These tumors account for approximately 7.5% of all gliomas, affect males more frequently than females (reported male to female ratios range from 1.1:1 to 1.6:1) and show a peak of incidence in adults aged between 30 to 50 years (Louis et al., 2007). In most cases, these grade III malignancies will progress to glioblastoma, showing a mean time to progression of ~2 years (Louis et al., 2007). **Glioblastoma** (WHO grade IV), or glioblastoma multiforme (GBM), is the most frequent and most malignant brain tumor, accounting for approximately 51% of all primary gliomas (CBTRUS, 2010). In Europe and North America, the incidence rates are approximately 3 new cases per 100,000 people per year. The peak of incidence occurs in adults aged 45 to 70 years, but glioblastoma can develop at any age. Males are more frequently affected (male to female ratio 1.7:1), and the frequency of glioblastoma in Caucasians is two times higher than in blacks. From a clinical and biological perspective, two main subtypes of this malignancy can be distinguished: primary (or *de novo*) glioblastoma develop without the presence of any precursor neoplastic lesion and manifest after a short clinical history (usually less than 3 months); secondary glioblastoma develop from lower grade tumors (a diffuse astrocytoma or an anaplastic astrocytoma) (Ohgaki & Kleihues, 2007). Primary glioblastoma, which are by far the most common, affect primarily older patients, present a quicker tumor progression and a poorer prognosis, as compared to secondary GBM. Of note, primary and secondary glioblastomas are histologically indistinguishable, but a growing body of data has been suggesting that these two disease entities evolve through different molecular mechanisms (as further detailed later in this chapter). Two histological variants of glioblastoma include: i) giant cell glioblastoma (WHO grade IV) is a rare variant (less than 5% of glioblastomas) composed of atypic multinucleated giant tumor cells; ii) gliosarcoma (WHO grade IV) accounts for approximately 2-8% of all glioblastomas (Homma et al., 2006; Meis et al., 1991), and is characterized by a biphasic tissue pattern with alternating areas displaying glial and mesenchymal differentiation.

2.2 Oligodendrogliomas

Oligodendroglial tumors account for approximately 8.4% of all gliomas, affecting males slightly more frequent than females (male to female ratio 1.1:1) (CBTRUS, 2010). The age distribution of oligodendrogliomas shows a peak of incidence in adults aged 40 to 50 years, but they may also rarely affect children (only 2% of all brain tumors in patients younger than 14 years). Based on their degree of malignancy and other histopathological features, two histological subtypes are distinguished: oligodendroglioma (WHO grade II) and anaplastic oligodendroglioma (WHO grade III). These two entities encompass a continuum of neoplasms which range from well-differentiated to highly malignant (Louis et al., 2007). **Oligodendroglioma (WHO grade II)** account for approximately 6% of all gliomas (CBTRUS, 2010). **Anaplastic oligodendroglioma** (WHO grade III) accounts for approximately 2.4% of all gliomas (CBTRUS, 2010). Similarly to high-grade astrocytomas, anaplastic oligodendroglioma may develop *de novo* or by progression from a pre-existing low grade oligodendroglioma (WHO grade II).

2.3 Oligoastrocytomas (mixed gliomas)

Oligoastrocytomas are diffusely infiltrating gliomas that present with a mixture of two morphologically distinct tumor cell types, resembling the neoplastic cells present in astrocytomas and oligodendrogliomas (Louis et al., 2007). As such, these tumors are also often called "mixed glioma". Precise and consistent epidemiological data on oligoastrocytoma are not yet available, but they have been reported to account for approximately 2-9% of all gliomas, affecting preferentially males (male to female ratio 1.3:1). Median ages range from 35 to 45 years (CBTRUS, 2010). Oligoastrocytomas, like astrocytomas and oligodendrogliomas, are divided into low grade (WHO grade II) and high-grade (WHO grade III) oligoastrocytoma, based on the most aggressive type of neoplastic cell present in the tumor.

3. Etiology and risk factors for glioma

Typical risk factors for a variety of human tumors, including genetic and environmental factors (such as tobacco smoking, diet, excessive alcohol intake, occupational exposure to carcinogens, exposure to UV radiation, and some other personal habits), have not been consistently correlated with risk for glioma (Fisher et al., 2007). Epidemiological data suggest that approximately one third of all human cancers are related to dietary factors and lack of proper physical activity in adulthood. Additionally, a significant number of these could be prevented by vaccination (e.g., viral-related tumors) and/or behavioral changes (e.g., tobacco-related tumors and skin cancer), as their risk factors are well known. In contrast, reliable recommendations to prevent gliomas cannot be endorsed presently, as the etiology of glioma remains largely obscure. A brief summary of the most relevant potential risk factors for glioma are briefly reviewed below.

3.1 Environmental risk factors

Exposure to high-dose therapeutic radiation is the only firmly established exogenous environmental cause of glioma, which can clinically manifest only several years after the exposure (Ohgaki & Kleihues, 2005). Recent data suggest that use of high-dose chemotherapy to treat other tumors may also contribute to gliomagenesis (Edick et al., 2005). Interestingly, the degree of risk from these exposures to radiotherapy and chemotherapy may be influenced by the individual's genetic background; for example, a functional germline polymorphism in the thiopurine methyltransferase gene was shown to affect the susceptibility of children treated with cranial radiotherapy and intensive antimetabolite therapy for acute lymphocytic leukemia to further develop brain tumors (Relling et al., 1999). However, similar studies are needed to confirm these observations and extend its conclusions to adults.

Throughout life, people are exposed to a variety of endogenous and exogenous chemicals (for example, reactive oxygen and nitrogen species, *N*-nitroso compounds, several industrially used chemicals, and polycyclic aromatic hydrocarbons) through cellular metabolism, diet, occupation, and personal habits. Some of these compounds have been shown to be biologically plausible neurocarcinogens in a great number of animal and other studies; however, inconsistent or null findings have been reported for these same factors in human studies (reviewed in Wrensch et al., 2005). These inconsistent data among several association studies may result from a variety of issues, including small study sample sizes, false-positive results (due to both small sample size and lack of accurate statistical hypothesis), imprecise exposure measures (from proxy reporting and exposure history recall issues), protective exposures or conditions unaccounted for (e.g., allergies), variation in metabolic and repair pathways in the brain, differential diffusion of chemicals across the blood–brain barrier, and disease heterogeneity.

A currently hot topic is the potential association between cellular phone usage and glioma risk. While one study reported increased risk for glioma associated with long term (≥10 years) use of cellular phones (Hardell et al., 2007), other larger studies have failed to replicate this (Lahkola et al., 2007; Inskip et al., 2001; Fisher et al., 2007).

It is plausible that the failure to find strong and consistent associations between environmental risk factors and gliomas might be simply a reflection of absence of true associations (and not due to research issues). Nevertheless, considering the small number of studies examining environmental risk factors for specific well-defined glioma subtypes, it is premature to irrefutably conclude that environmental risks do not exist for glioma.

3.2 Genetic syndromes, familial aggregation, and mutagen sensitivity

Studies of genetic syndromes, familial aggregation, linkage, and mutagen sensitivity have suggested that genetics has an effect on susceptibility to glioma. Particular inherited rare genetic mutations cause a small number of genetic syndromes that have been associated with increased risk of glial tumors. Although these familial tumor syndromes account for a small proportion of cases (Ichimura et al., 2004), the elucidation of their molecular basis has greatly contributed to the understanding of gliomas, and has provided a valuable starting point for identifying candidate genes and pathways involved in gliomagenesis.

In large, carefully-designed epidemiological studies, familial glioma risks have been reported to be approximately two-fold, a magnitude that is similar to the familial association reported for other cancers for which susceptibility genes have been identified (e.g., breast cancer) (Malmer et al., 1999; Hemminki et al., 2000; Wrensch et al., 1997). The underlying causes of the pattern of familial brain tumor occurrence have been attributed to a variety of causes: one study implicates environmental factors only (Grossman et al., 1999), while others attribute multifactorial causes, polygenic causes, and autosomal recessive inheritance (de Andrade et al., 2001; Malmer et al., 2001).

Two case-control studies have suggested that peripheral lymphocytes from glioma patients are more sensitive to gamma-radiation than lymphocytes from matched controls, suggesting that increased sensitivity to radiation is an independent risk factor for gliomas (Bondy et al., 1996; 2001). The authors also propose that inherited genetic variation in the capacity to repair radiation damage may partly influence mutagen sensitivity and, ultimately, glioma risk.

3.3 Genetic polymorphisms

Since high-dose therapeutic radiation and inherited rare mutations explain only a small proportion of gliomas, neuro-oncology research has focused on genetic polymorphisms that, together with environmental risk factors, might potentially affect susceptibility to gliomas. Some of the most frequently studied polymorphisms, in the context of glioma, are in genes involved in DNA repair, carcinogen metabolism, cell cycle regulation, and immunological responses.

Because DNA repair is a mechanism of utmost importance in preserving genomic integrity, genes involved in this pathway have been extensively studied in human tumors. Glioma and some histological subtypes have been associated with specific polymorphic variants of particular DNA repair genes, such as *ERCC1* (excision repair cross-complementing 1), *ERCC2* (excision repair cross-complementing 2), *GLTSCR1* (glioma tumor suppressor candidate region gene 1), *PRKDC* (protein kinase, DNA-activated, catalytic), and *MGMT* (O^6-methylguanine-DNA methyltransferase) (Wang et al., 2004; Wiencke et al., 2005; Wrensch et al., 2005; Yang et al., 2005). However, the clear reliability of these findings is still requiring further studies to assess consistency. The DNA repair pathway is extraordinarily complex, as illustrated by the more than 130 genes known to be involved in base excision repair, direct reversal of damage, mismatch repair, nucleotide excision repair, homologous recombination, nonhomologous end joining, sanitization of nucleotide pools, activity of DNA polymerases, editing and processing of nucleases, and postreplicative repair (Wood et al., 2001). Studying genetic variants in this panoply of DNA repair genes might contribute to a better understanding of gliomagenesis, progression, and response to therapy (mostly DNA targeting agents).

Some of the most intriguing and consistent findings of the past decade of neuro-oncology research are the statistically significant inverse associations between risk of gliomas in adults and histories of allergies and/or chickenpox, IgG antibodies to varicella-zoster virus, and levels of serum IgE (Wiemels et al., 2004; Wrensch et al., 2001; 2005). A later study used germline polymorphisms in genes associated with asthma and allergies (*IL-4RA*, *IL-13* and *ADAM33*) as biomarkers for the presence of these conditions, as genetic polymorphisms could not be influenced by the presence of glioma. Remarkably, specific genotypic variants, which have been shown to increase asthma risk, were equally associated with decreased risk for glioblastoma (J. Schwartzbaum et al., 2005), further supporting the findings from self-reported case-control studies.

We have recently investigated genetic variants potentially relevant for glioma in the EGF/EGFR pathway, one of the most important growth signaling networks in human tumors, whose significance in gliomas has been well established. Previous studies have reached inconsistent conclusions regarding the relevance of a polymorphism in the *EGF* gene (*EGF*+61 A/G) as a risk factor for glioblastoma (Bhowmick et al., 2004; Vauleon et al., 2007). Later, we showed that the G allele increases the risk for gliomas, including glioblastoma and oligodendroglioma (Costa et al., 2007). Importantly, we have conclusively showed that the G variant of *EGF*+61 is associated with increased promoter activity, which may partly explain its relevance for glioma risk. In the *EGFR* gene, three polymorphisms have been described as having a transcriptional regulatory function: two single nucleotide polymorphisms in the essential promoter region, -216G/T and -191C/A, and a polymorphic $(CA)_n$ microsatellite sequence in intron 1. Preliminary studies by our group seem to indicate that the -191CA genotype is associated with higher risk for glioma, particularly oligodendroglioma, and that shorter $(CA)_n$ repeat variants are significantly associated with increased risk for glioma, particularly glioblastoma and oligodendroglioma (Costa et al., 2010c). In contrast to a study by Carpentier et al. (2006), our preliminary data does not seem to implicate the -216G/T polymorphism as a risk factor for glioblastoma.

Our understanding of cancer as a multi-factorial disease, in which several pathways contribute to various stages of tumorigenesis, warrants the need for more integrative studies to evaluate interactions among these pathways. Accordingly, the simultaneous study of DNA repair, detoxification metabolism, cell cycle, and immunological pathways will allow more proper evaluation of different molecular players in gliomagenesis.

4. Molecular pathology of glioma

During the past two decades, remarkable progress has been accomplished in the understanding of the molecular pathology of gliomas. Similarly to the multistep process of human tumorigenesis in other human tissues (Hanahan & Weinberg, 2000), malignant transformation of normal cells (either differentiated glial or stem or progenitor cells) into gliomas results from the sequential accumulation of molecular aberrations (Ohgaki & Kleihues, 2007; Furnari et al., 2007). Tumor-associated molecular dysregulation can occur at the genetic and epigenetic levels, including chromosomal gains or losses, gene mutation, amplification, deletion, DNA and histones methylation or demethylation, and transcriptional regulation (Ichimura et al., 2004); (Wen & Kesary, 2008). An overview of some important molecular pathways in the development of gliomas is summarized in **Figure 1**, and briefly discussed below.

4.1 Chromosomal aberrations

Cytogenetic studies of gliomas have identified several chromosomal regions with copy number alterations (deletions, amplifications, gains, and losses). Typically, the presence of loss of heterozygosity (LOH) and deletions in tumors might point to chromosomal regions with tumor suppressor genes (those that normally function to suppress tumor formation/progression), while amplifications and chromosomal gains might indicate regions with oncogenes (those whose function favors tumorigenesis). However, these hints may be more difficult to interpret; strikingly, some particular chromosomal regions are commonly gained or lost in glioma. To make things a little more complex, the definition of tumor suppressor genes and oncogenes is highly context-dependent (e.g., on the tumor's location and intrinsic characteristics), as some proteins play roles that, depending on the tissue and cellular context, may favor or hamper tumorigenesis (Haber & Harlow, 1997).

Combined loss of chromosome arms 1p and 19q is the most frequently detected aberration in oligodendroglial tumors (Jeuken et al., 2004). Grade II and grade III oligodendrogliomas are equally affected by these chromosomal lesions, suggesting an early role in oligodendroglial tumorigenesis. Since losses of chromosome 1p and 19q are intimately correlated (Jenkins et al., 2006), it is plausible that the corresponding putative tumor suppressor genes may be involved in biologically distinct pathways, which may act synergistically in oligodendroglial tumorigenesis. Allelic losses of chromosomes 9p and 10q, and homozygous deletion of *CDKN2A* on chromosome 9p21, are also frequent in anaplastic oligodendroglioma (WHO grade III) (Bigner et al., 1999; Ueki et al., 2002). Chromosomal aberrations are also present in the majority (~70%) of both primary and secondary glioblastoma, which present LOH of chromosome 10q (Behin et al., 2003).

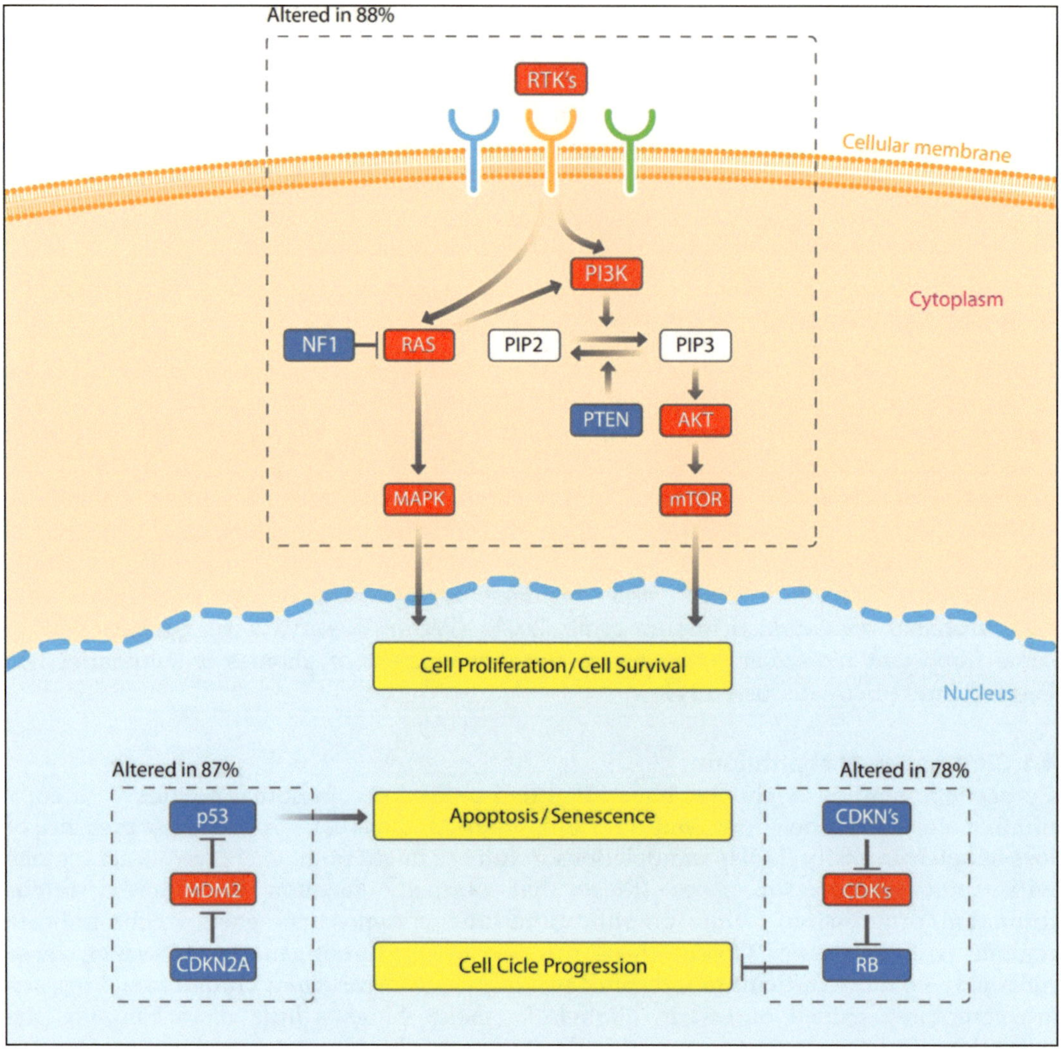

Fig. 1. Major signalling pathways commonly altered in glioblastomas: RTK/RAS/PI3K, p53, and RB. Red and blue boxes indicate proteins with activating and inactivating alterations, respectively, which can be genetic (gene amplifications or deletions, chromosomal copy number alterations and translocations, and mutations) and/or epigenetic (DNA CpG island hypermethylation, gene specific and global genome-wide DNA hypomethylation, and aberrant histone modifications). The frequency of alterations found in GBM in each pathway is indicated in the dashed boxes.

4.2 Dysregulated pathways

The histological heterogeneity of gliomas parallels with a substantial degree of molecular heterogeneity, both within and between histological subtypes of glioma (Rasheed et al., 1999; Freije et al., 2004). Several interconnected pathways are commonly altered in glioma, typically those governing cell-cycle regulation (cellular proliferation and senescence), cellular survival (apoptosis and necrosis), invasion (adhesion and migration), and angiogenesis. These molecular abnormalities result in cell's self-sufficiency with respect to growth signals, insensitivity to growth-inhibitory stimuli, evasion of programmed cell death, "limitless" replicative potential, sustained angiogenesis, tissue invasion, and metastasis.

4.2.1 Receptor tyrosine kinase (RTK) pathways

Gliomas typically present overactivation of many mitogens (growth factors) and their specific membrane receptors. In order to proliferate, normal cells require activation of mitogenic signaling pathways (upon binding of diffusible growth factors to their specific transmembrane receptors) and subsequent intracellular signal transduction, which occurs mostly through the PI3K and MAPK signaling pathways. In contrast, acquired molecular alterations in tumor cells decrease their dependence on exogenous growth stimuli, facilitating their aberrant cell division, survival, and motility. While multiple mechanisms contribute to the ability of gliomas to overcome normal impositions on the control of mitogenic signaling (MAPK and PI3K/PTEN/AKT pathways, among others), abnormal activation of receptor tyrosine kinases (RTKs) seems to be the predominant (and better studied) mechanism.

Activation of receptor tyrosine kinase pathways in gliomas occurs through a variety of mechanisms, including overexpression of both ligands and receptors (leading to autocrine activating loops), gene amplification, and/or mutation of the receptor (resulting in constitutive activation even in the absence of the ligand). In addition, particular genetic polymorphisms may influence the expression of some of the genes involved in these pathways. The two most important receptor-driven signaling pathways in both CNS development and gliomagenesis are the epidermal growth factor (EGF) and platelet-derived growth factor (PDGF) pathways.

It is well established the importance of **EGF receptor (EGFR)** in development and differentiation of normal astrocytes (Burrows et al., 1997), but this RTK also plays critical roles in glial tumors (Kapoor & O'Rourke, 2003; Rao, et al., 2003). *EGFR* gene amplification is found in a variety of solid tumors, being notably frequent in astrocytomas (up to ~40% of all glioblastomas) (Viana-Pereira et al., 2008; Wong et al., 1992). These amplified versions of *EGFR* often undergo genetic rearrangements (e.g., *EGFRvI, EGFRvII*), some of which are relevant for the oncogenic and malignant roles of EGFR (Ekstrand et al., 1992). *EGFRvIII* (also known as Δ*EGFR*, or *EGFR**), which shows an in-frame deletion of exons 2–7, is the most common *EGFR* mutant allele, occurring up to 30% of all human GBM (and in up to 60% of those that have amplified wild-type EGFR) (Frederick et al., 2000). EGFRvIII protein, which exhibit constitutive ligand-independent tyrosine kinase activity, has been found to enhance tumorigenic behavior of human glioblastoma cells by reducing apoptosis and increasing proliferation (Nagane et al., 1996) and to malignantly transform murine *Ink4a/Arf* null neural stem cells (NSCs) or astrocytes in the mouse brain (Holland et al., 1998; Bachoo et al., 2002) making it an attractive and validated therapeutic target in glioma.

PDGF receptor-α (PDGFR-α), along with its specific ligands PDGF-A and PDGF-B, are also commonly overexpressed in gliomas, particularly in high-grade tumors (Westermark et al., 1995). In contrast, strong expression of PDGFR-β occurs mostly in proliferating endothelial cells in glioblastoma. PDGF-C and PDGF-D are also frequently expressed in glioma cell lines and in glioblastoma tissues (Lokker et al., 2002). Autocrine and paracrine signaling loops may be the primary means by which the PDGFR axis exerts its effects in gliomas, as these tumors often demonstrate coexpression of both PDGF ligands and receptors. The importance of this signaling axis in gliomas has been supported by several recent studies: PDGF was shown to stimulate NSCs in the adult subventricular zone that express PDGFR-α to form glioma-like lesions in the mouse (Jackson et al., 2006); in addition, mice transgenic for neural progenitor PDGF-B expression resulted in the formation of oligodendrogliomas and forced elevation of PDGF-B levels increased overall tumor incidence (Dai et al., 2001; Shih et al., 2004). This growing body of data suggests that targeted therapy against this pathway could have therapeutic potential.

4.2.2 The PI3K-AKT pathway

Along with alterations in cell cycle regulatory pathways and RTK pathways, **intracellular signaling pathways** are also critical in glioma. Some important examples include the MAPK pathway (which plays a wide variety of cellular functions, such as regulation of cell-cell interactions, composition of extracellular matrix, and expression of genes promoting cell cycle progression (Dhanasekaran & Johnson, 2007), and the PI3K/AKT pathway (involved in an extraordinary diverse group of cellular functions, including cell growth, proliferation, differentiation, motility, survival and intracellular trafficking). Gliomas typically show increased activity of several molecular components of the MAPK and PI3K/AKT pathways, while some tumor suppressor genes that negatively regulate these pathways are often inactivated (Konopka & Bonni, 2003). For example, inactivating mutations in the tumor suppressor gene phosphatase and tensin homolog deleted on chromosome 10 (PTEN), whose protein is a negative regulator of the PI3K/AKT pathway, contribute to the abnormal activity of the pathway.

The **class IA PI3Ks** are heterodimers consisting of one regulatory subunit [one of five isoforms encoded by three genes: p85α, p55α, and p50α (*PIK3R*1); p85β (*PIK3R2*); and p55γ (*PIK3R3*)] and a catalytic isoform [p110α (*PIK3CA*), p110β (*PIK3CB*) and p110δ (*PIK3CD*)]. Activated RTKs recruit class IA PI3Ks to the membrane through their regulatory subunit. Activation of class IA PI3Ks at the membrane results in phosphorylation and conversion of the lipid phosphatidylinositol-(4,5)-bisphosphate (PIP_2) into phosphatidylinositol-(3,4,5)-triphosphate (PIP_3), which in turn recruits and activates phosphatidylinositol-dependent kinase 1 (PDK1). Activated PDK1, in turn, phosphorylates and activates protein kinase B (PKB, also known as AKT). A subsequent signaling cascade downstream of AKT ultimately results in inhibition of cell cycle arrest and apoptosis, and increased cell proliferation and survival. The tumor-suppressor phosphatase and tensin homologue (PTEN) negatively regulates PI3K signalling by dephosphorylating PIP_3, converting it back to PIP_2 (Hawkins et al., 2006).

The class IA PI3Ks are currently defined by their catalytic isoform, as the regulatory subunits appear to be functionally equivalent. Several studies have implicated class IA *PI3Ks* genes in glial tumors. Gain-of-function mutations in the *PI3KCA* gene have been found in some malignant gliomas (e.g., glioblastoma), with a reported mutation frequency up to 15% (Samuels et al., 2004; Gallia et al., 2006). Inactivation of **PTEN** by mutations or epigenetic mechanisms is a frequent event in high-grade gliomas (up to 50%), which results in uncontrolled PI3K signaling (Knobbe & Reifenberger, 2003; Ohgaki et al., 2004). Studies using elegant mouse models have recently shown that the specific inactivation of PTEN in the mouse brain caused its overgrowth and abnormal proliferation of astrocytes (Fraser et al., 2004). Also in mouse studies, inactivation of PTEN has been associated with increased angiogenesis, closely paralleling the progression from low-grade to high-grade astrocytomas in humans, which coincides with *PTEN* loss (Andrew Xiao et al., 2002; 2005).

Aberrant PI3K signaling commonly results in activation of **Akt** via phosphorylation of two key residues, T308 and S473, by PDK1 and the mammalian target of rapamycin (mTOR), respectively (Mora et al., 2004; Sarbassov et al., 2005). In fact, assessment of the phosphorylation status of these residues in Akt is often the method of choice for determining activation of the PI3K pathway in cell lines and primary tumors, including glioblastoma samples, 85% of which have been shown to exhibit activated Akt (Wang et al., 2004). Additional mechanisms by which Akt activation may become dysregulated include decreased expression of PHLPP (PH domain leucine-rich repeat protein phosphatase, which dephosphorylates S473 in Akt), decreased expression of CTMP (C-terminal modulator protein, which binds to Akt and inhibits its phosphorylation), or overexpression of PIKE-A (phosphatidylinositol-3-kinase enhancer, which binds directly to phosphorylated Akt and enhances its anti-apoptotic function) in primary glioblastoma and glioma cell lines (Ahn et al., 2004).

Despite most of the signaling pathways previously mentioned (p53, RB, RTK, MAPK, and PI3K/AKT pathways) are often considered as distinct entities, there is significant cross-talk and inter-dependence among them, which reinforces the inappropriate regulation of any single pathway perturbation. (Indeed, these pathways are sometimes referred to as genetic networks, to emphasize their highly complex relationships.) For example, since p53 enhances transcription of *PTEN* (Stambolic et al., 2001), the loss of p53 in cells with constitutively active RTK signaling can further potentiate PI3K/AKT pathway activation.

The *NF1* tumor suppressor gene encodes neurofibromin-1, which functions primarily as a RAS negative regulator, and also plays a role in adenylyl cyclase and AKT-mTOR pathways. Loss of *NF1* is a typical molecular aberration of WHO grade I pilocytic astrocytoma (Zhu & Parada, 2002), and is believed to be one of the precursor lesions in these tumors, as the absence of negative regulation of RAS oncoprotein may favor cell proliferation and, ultimately, tumor initiation.

4.2.3 Cell cycle regulators

Genes involved in **cell cycle regulation** have been frequently found mutated in glioma, highlighting the importance of such genes in cellular proliferation and senescence. The RB and p53 pathways, which regulate the cell cycle primarily by governing the G1-to-S-phase transition, are major targets of functional inactivation in glioma, through any of several molecular alterations. The inactivation of these key regulators renders tumors highly sensitive to uncontrolled cell proliferation driven by mitogenic signaling effectors, such as phosphatidylinositol 3-kinase (PI3K) and mitogen-activated protein kinase (MAPK).

The RB protein exerts its anti-proliferative effects in quiescent cells by binding and sequestering the E2F family of transcription factors, preventing the transactivation of genes essential for cell cycle progression (Sherr & McCormick, 2002). Gliomas circumvent the RB-mediated negative regulation of the cell cycle by any of the following genetic/epigenetic aberrations: mutation of the *Rb1* gene, loss of its chromosomal region (13q) when progression from low- to high-grade gliomas occurs, amplification of cyclin-dependent kinases 4 and 6 (*CDK4* and *CDK6*) genes (which encode negative regulators of RB activity), and inactivation of $p16^{Ink4a}$ (a negative regulator of CDKs) by allelic loss or DNA hypermethylation in high-grade gliomas (Louis et al., 2007). Even though the neutralization of the RB pathway alone is not sufficient to abrogate cell cycle control to the extent needed for cellular transformation (suggesting that other important cell cycle regulation pathways complement its activities in preventing gliomagenesis) (Xiao et al.

2002), the importance of its inhibition in progression from low- to higher-grade gliomas is underscored by the near-universal and mutually exclusive alterations of the molecular players of the RB pathway in both primary and secondary glioblastoma (Schmidt et al., 1994; Ueki et al., 1996).

The p53 tumor suppressor prevents the proliferation of cells with faulty genomes, mostly by halting the cell cycle in the G1 phase or by induction of an apoptotic program (Vousden & Lu, 2002). In sporadic (non-hereditary) gliomas, the p53 pathway is almost universally altered. A variety of molecular mechanisms may result in defective p53 function in glioma. Loss of p53 through either inactivating mutations in its DNA-binding domain or loss of chromosome 17p are common early events in the progression of secondary glioblastoma (Louis, 1994); in addition, germline p53 mutations in Li-Fraumeni patients, who have increased risk to develop gliomas, also underscore the importance of p53 in gliomagenesis (Malkin et al., 1990; Srivastava et al., 1990). Alternative inactivating alterations of the p53 pathway in gliomas include deletion of $p14^{ARF}$ (whose protein stabilizes p53), amplification of the chromosomal region containing *MDM2* and *MDM4* genes (which encode negative regulators of p53 activity and expression) (Riemenschneider et al., 1999), and hemizygous deletion of the tumor suppressor gene *CDH5* (whose protein plays a role in maintaining *TP53* expression) (Bagchi et al., 2007).

4.2.4 Isocitrate dehydrogenases (*IDH1* and *IDH2*) genes

Very recent studies have identified mutations in the genes encoding the cytosolic and mitochondrial isoforms of $NADP^+$-dependent isocitrate dehydrogeneses (IDH1 and IDH2, respectively) in GBMs (Balss et al., 2008; Parsons et al., 2008; Ichimura et al., 2009; Watanabe et al., 2009; Yan et al., 2009; Zhao et al., 2009; Pollack et al., 2010; Christensen et al., 2011). These enzymes catalyze the decarboxylation of isocitrate to α-ketoglutarate (α-KG), in a reaction that utilizes NADP+ and produces NADPH. This cytosolic NAPDH is essential for the regeneration of reduced glutathione, which is important in the protection of cells against oxidative damage. These mutations in *IDH1* and *IDH2* are heterozygous and of somatic origin. Until now, the mechanisms by which *IDH* mutant proteins contribute to gliomagenesis are not fully understood. The IDH1 R132H mutant variant, which is present in more than 90% of gliomas but rare in pilocytic astrocytomas, presents impaired substrate affinity, and dominantly inhibits wild-type IDH1 activity through the formation of catalytically inactive heterodimers (Zhao et al., 2009). The overexpression of mutant IDH1 was shown to reduce the formation of α-KG, and to increase the levels of HIF-1α, a critical transcription factor that promotes tumor growth under hypoxic conditions and whose stability depends on the levels of α-KG. This HIF-1α regulation by mutant IDH1 suggested that this mutation may cause oncogenic gains of function. Indeed, a later study by Dang et al., (2009) showed that mutant IDH1 converts a α-KG to 2-hydroxyglutarate (2-HG) in a NADPH-depend manner. Because mutations in *IDH1* and *IDH2* genes are restricted to a single amino acid, their detection for diagnostic purposes should be straightforward. Gliomas of astrocytic or oligodendrocytic lineage with *IDH* mutations have been shown to present distinct clinical and genetic characteristics as compared with gliomas with wild-type *IDH* genes (Yan et al., 2009), suggesting this mutation may be an early event in gliomagenesis from a stem/progenitor cell that can differentiate into both astrocytes and oligodendrocytes. Since *IDH* mutants occur in the large majority of WHO grade II or III gliomas, and in WHO grade IV secondary glioblastomas that develop from these lower-grade precursor lesions, suggests that tumors with mutated IDH's encompass a specific subgroup of glioblastomas.

4.2.5 Molecular pathways to glioblastoma

As previously mentioned, glioblastomas can be subdivided into primary or secondary GBMs, based on their clinical and biological differences. Primary GBMs are by far the most common, affect older patients, and are genetically characterized by *EGFR* amplification and mutations, LOH of chromosome 10q, and deletion of the *PTEN* and the $p16^{INK4a}$ genes (Louis et al., 2007). Secondary GBMs affect younger patients who had previously been affected by a lower grade astrocytoma, and are molecularly characterized by mutations in the *TP53* gene, overexpression of PDGFR, abnormalities in the p16 and Rb pathways, and LOH of chromosome 10q (Louis et al., 2007). Importantly, some of these molecular abnormalities are not exclusive for a specific glioblastoma subtype, but are rather present at significantly different frequencies (for example, the frequency of *TP53* mutation in secondary GBM is more than ~65%, but only ~28% in primary GBM) (Ohgaki & Kleihues, 2007). Despite being morphologically and clinically indistinguishable, as reflected by an equally poor prognosis when adjusted for patient age, primary and secondary GBMs have markedly distinct molecular features, at the levels of gene transcriptional patterns and DNA copy number aberrations (Furnari et al., 2007). Thus, these molecular distinctions strongly suggest that these GBM entities may respond differently to targeted molecular therapies, warranting the need to change the current standardize clinical management of these truly distinct diseases.

4.2.6 Epigenetic changes in glioma

In addition to genetic aberrations, gliomas also present a variety of epigenetic alterations, defined as mitotically heritable changes in gene expression that are not due to changes in the primary DNA sequence. The most well-studied epigenetic changes in gliomas occur primarily at two levels: DNA methylation at CpG dinucleotides, and post-translational modifications of histone tails. Nevertheless, other epigenetic mechanisms include noncoding RNAs (*e.g.*, microRNAs and small nucleolar RNAs), accumulation of histone variants, and chromatin remodeling, and may also be altered in brain tumors. Typical changes in DNA methylation levels observed in gliomas, as in other human tumors, include CpG island hypermethylation (associated with tumor suppressor gene silencing), gene-specific hypomethylation (resulting in aberrant oncogene activation), and genome-wide hypomethylation (potentially leading to chromosomal instability, loss of imprinting, and uncontrolled cellular proliferation). The histone modifications are quite more complex: firstly, because of the great variety of modifications that can occur in different histones (including, methylation, acetylation, phosphorylation, ubiquitylation, sumoylation, among others), and secondly, because a single histone tail residue can be mono-, di-, or tri-methylated on a single, specific lysine. In general, epigenetics is just another layer of gene expression regulation that, when altered in specific genes, may favor tumor formation and progression. While genetic and epigenetic changes in gliomas have been mostly studied independently, there is evidence that these mechanisms interact on specific genes, signaling pathways, and chromosomal domains. A summary of some of the epigenetic changes previously found in gliomas is presented in Table 1, and elegantly reviewed by Nagarajan & Costello, 2009.

<table>
<tr><th>Glioma type</th><th>Subtype (WHO grade)</th><th>Genetic Alterations</th><th>Epigenetic Alterations</th></tr>
<tr><td rowspan="4">Astrocytic tumors</td><td>Pilocytic astrocytoma (I)</td><td>NF1 loss</td><td rowspan="9">CpG island hypermethylation in tumor suppressor genes (MGMT, PCDH-gamma-A11, EMP3, THBS1, RASSF1A, CRBP1, TMS1, p16, SLC5A8, RB, PTEN, TP53, $p14^{ARF}$, TIMP3)
Genome-wide ("global") DNA hypomethylation
Aberrant levels of histone post-translational modifications (e.g., acetylation, methylation)</td></tr>
<tr><td>Diffuse astrocytoma (II)</td><td>LOH 17p; TP53 mutations; PDGFRA amplification</td></tr>
<tr><td>Anaplastic astrocytoma (III)</td><td>Gains of chromosome 7; Mutations in TP53, RB1, CDK4, CDKN2A; Deletions of 6p, 9p, 11p, 22q</td></tr>
<tr><td>Gliobastoma (IV)</td><td>Amplification of EGFR, $p14^{ARF}$, CDK4, MDM2, MDM4;
Homozygous deletion of CDKN2A, RB1;
Mutation of TP53, RB1, PTEN, IDH1, IDH2;
Allelic loss of 19q, 13q</td></tr>
<tr><td rowspan="2">Oligodendroglial tumors</td><td>Oligodendroglioma (II)</td><td>LOH 1p/19q;
TP53 mutations</td></tr>
<tr><td>Anaplastic oligodendroglioma (III)</td><td>LOH 1p/19q; 10q deletion; CDKN2A
Amplification EFGR
Mutation of IDH1</td></tr>
<tr><td rowspan="2">Oligoastrocytic tumors</td><td>Oligoastrocytoma (II)</td><td>LOH 1p/19q; TP53 mutations</td></tr>
<tr><td>Anaplastic oligoastrocytoma (III)</td><td>LOH 1p/10q;
Mutations of IDH1, TP53</td></tr>
</table>

Table 1. Common genetic and epigenetic hallmarks of gliomas

5. Molecular prognostic factors of malignant glioma

Recent studies started to identify potential biological and molecular characteristics in the tumors that may have prognostic value and help in making therapeutic decisions (Phillips et al., 2006), although such studies clearly require validation in prospectively followed and uniformly treated patients. Until now, work on the identification of prognostic markers in gliomas grants reasons for both optimism and caution with respect to improvements in the diagnosis and treatment of patients. In practice, the multitude of studies on the identification of such markers has led so far to development of only one molecular test with clinical relevance: 1p/19q testing in oligodendrogliomas. Much more effort is required for the identification of markers that truly and consistently distinguish glioma patients in ways that can assist therapeutic decisions. Below we briefly discuss the current most promising molecular prognostic factors in these tumors, which are summarized in Table 2.

Molecular Prognostic Marker	Glioma Type
Chromosome 1p/19q co-deletion	Oligodendroglioma and oligoastrocytoma
MGMT promoter methylation	GBM and anaplastic astrocytoma
Loss of chromosome 10	GBM
Activation of the PI3K/AKT pathway	GBM
Activation of MAPK members	GBM
EGFR mutation (EGFRvIII)	GBM
PTEN expression (wild-type)	GBM
Molecular signatures (proneural, proliferative and mesenchymal)	GBM
High expression of angiogenic genes	Diffusely infiltrating gliomas of all histologic types
Stem-cell like gene expression signatures	GBM
CHI3L1 (YKL-40) expression	GBM
PTEN and DLL3 expression	GBM
EGFR expression	GBM
HOXA overexpression	GBM
IDH1-2 mutations	All gliomas, but not very frequent in primary GBM

Table 2. Selected Molecular Prognostic Markers for Gliomas.

5.1 Malignant astrocytomas

O^6-methylguanine-DNA methyltransferase (MGMT, also known as AGT) is an important DNA repair enzyme that contributes to glioblastoma resistance to temozolomide. The methyl group at the O^6 position of guanine can be removed by MGMT, which is consumed by this event (Spiro et al., 2001). In a similar study to the one from the EORTC-NCIC, Hegi et al., 2005, examined the DNA methylation at the promoter region of the *MGMT* gene in tumor samples from glioblastoma patients. This epigenetic event silences *MGMT*, which decreases tumor cells' ability to repair temozolomide-induced DNA damage, resulting in increased susceptibility of the tumor cells to temozolomide. Hegi reported that glioblastoma patients with a methylated *MGMT* promoter who were treated with temozolomide had a significantly longer median overall survival (21.7 months) and a higher 2-year survival rate (46%) than patients without *MGMT* promoter methylation who were similarly treated with temozolomide (median survival of only 12.7 months and a 2-year survival rate of 13.8%), suggesting that glioblastoma patients whose tumors do not have a methylated *MGMT* promoter do not benefit from temozolomide. Despite the striking and encouraging findings supporting *MGMT* as a glioma prognostic marker and a specific predictor of temozolomide-based chemotherapy, there is a significant body of controversial data surrounding the reproducibility of such findings (summarized in Costa et al., 2010a). Much of the controversy around the prognostic value of MGMT is due in part to studies including very heterogeneous groups of patients, with different glioma histologies, grades, and treatment types often grouped together in the same analysis. Additionaly, different studies analyzed

MGMT at different levels, including methylation by methylation-specific PCR, mRNA expression by RT-PCR, and protein levels by immunohistochemistry and quantitative immunofluorescence. Due to the widely acknowledged need of replicating Hegi's findings, we investigated the potential of *MGMT* methylation as a prognostic marker of glioblastoma in a set of 90 prospectively followed patients uniformly treated with postoperative temozolomide-based chemoradiation. In line with some other reports, we found a trend for longer overall and progression-free survival in glioblastoma patients whose tumors had *MGMT* promoter methylation, but the differences failed to reach statistical significance in our data set (Costa et al., 2010a).

Recent evidences are revealing striking similarities between developmental and tumorigenic processes, suggesting that some of the molecular regulatory mechanisms necessary for normal development may be equally relevant in tumors. Homeobox (HB) genes encode transcription factors that play critical roles during normal development. These genes are broadly divided into two classes: class I includes clustered homeobox (*HOX*) genes, while class II includes divergent HB (non-*HOX*) genes that are dispersed throughout the genome (McGinnis & Krumlauf, 1992). The expression of some *HOX* genes has been shown to be altered in leukemias and several types of solid tumors. In recent years, a growing body of data has been implicating the aberrant expression of *HOXA* genes as an important mechanism in the pathophysiology of malignant astrocytomas. A study by (Abdel-Fattah et al., 2006) assessed the expression status of all *HOX* genes in primary astrocytomas and non-tumoral brain specimens, showing that a portion of these genes are aberrantly overexpressed in malignant astrocytomas. However, the relevance of these genes in glioma pathogenesis, malignancy, and prognosis was not addressed in that study. Later, Murat et al., 2008, suggested *HOX* genes may be part of a glioma stem cell signature with prognostic significance in patients treated with chemo-radiotherapy. We have recently shown that several *HOXA* genes are preferentially overexpressed in high-grade rather than in low-grade primary astrocytomas, and we have implicated the reactivation of *HOXA9* expression in GBM as a novel, independent, and negative prognostic factor in 2 independent sets of GBM patients (Costa et al., 2010b). Additionally, *HOXA9* reactivation was particularly frequent in a subgroup of GBM with aberrant chromosomal domains of transcriptional activation encompassing the *HOXA* cluster. Importantly, we demonstrated the PI3K-associated epigenetic mechanism by which this domain of activation is reversible: activation of the PI3K pathway in GBM cells decreased the levels of histone H3 lysine 27 trimethylation through inhibition of EZH2, a key histone methyltransferase. Finally, we provided functional data on the effects of *HOXA9* expression in GBM cells and immortalized astrocytes, which support its pro-proliferative and anti-apoptotic properties. Our findings revealed prognostic and therapeutic implications for oncogenic expression of the developmental transcription factor HOXA9 in malignant brain tumors, including the evaluation of PI3K inhibitors, which are being extensively tested in clinical trials. Finally, a recent study by (Gaspar et al., 2010) showed that high levels of *HOX* genes expression was a signature of resistance to temozolomide in pediatric GBM cell lines; in addition, pediatric high-grade glioma patients whose tumors expressed *HOXA* genes (particularly *HOXA9* and *HOXA10*) presented significantly shorter survival. Taken together, these recent studies point out to a very relevant role of *HOXA* genes in rendering high-grade gliomas even more malignant and resistant to therapy, resulting in particularly lethal tumors.

A genomic study by Parson and colleagues in 2008 showed that a subset of GBM patients had *IDH1* R132H mutations, and that this mutation occurred mostly in younger patients (mean age 33 years in *IDH1* mutant patients versus 53 years for patients with wild-type

IDH1). In addition, this mutation was particularly frequent in secondary GBMs (5 out of 6 secondary GBMs versus 7 out of 99 primary GBMs with IDH1 mutation), and was significantly associated with an increase in patients overall survival (Parsons et al., 2008). Yan et al. (2009) subsequently showed that *IDH1* mutation was commonly present in a variety of gliomas, including diffuse astrocytoma, anaplastic astrocytoma, and oligodendroglioma. In addition, the authors also identified a mutation affecting the analogous aminoacid residue (R172) of the *IDH2* gene, which was present in tumors without *IDH1* mutation. Importantly, the presence of either *IDH* mutation was associated with better survival of GBM and anaplastic astrocytoma patients. Christensen et al. (2011) also verified that *IDH1* mutation occurs more frequently than *IDH2* mutation in gliomas, and showed that the presence of *IDH1* or *IHD2* mutation was significantly associated with better survival of glioma patients, independently of patient age, sex, and grade-specific histology.

5.2 Malignant oligodendrogliomas and oligoastrocytomas

Tumors with 1p/19q codeletion are particularly sensitive to chemotherapy with PCV, with response rates as high as 100%, whereas patients whose tumors do not present 1p/19q codeletion show response rates of 23-31% (Ino et al., 2001; Cairncross et al., 1998). Indeed, oligodendroglioma is the first CNS neoplasm in which a molecular signature (1p and 19q codeletion) has been categorically associated with patient outcome within the context of large clinical trials (Felsberg et al., 2004). Even though the reasons for such associations are still unclear, the status of 1p and 19q, rather than classic histological analysis, is currently used as an eligibility criterion in studies involving patients with pure or mixed anaplastic oligodendrogliomas. This truly reflects a paradigm shift in the design of clinical trials for patients with these tumors, and has been regarded as a key example of the value of molecular signatures as prognostic markers of disease. Again, codeletion of 1p/19q was associated with improved survival in both studies. Although most studies of patients with pure or mixed oligodendroglioma were performed with PCV chemotherapy, temozolomide is arguably likely to have similar activity with less side effects (van den Bent, 2007; Yung et al., 1999); however, studies comparing the efficacy of these two chemotherapeutic regimens are still lacking.

6. Conclusion

Human gliomas are particularly dramatic diseases, not only because of their high lethality, but also because their etiological and prognostic factors are still not fully understood. Integrating multi-disciplinary teams to collaborate in the identification of new molecular and exogenous glioma risk factors is urgent. Possibly even more important is to rapidly improve the clinical management of glioma patients. While the current therapies used for malignant glioma and patients' outcome are not satisfactory, the recent insights on the biological and clinical features of glioma offer appealing opportunities for the development of more effective targeted therapy. The use of comprehensive genome-wide approaches to analyze genetic and epigenetic alterations, as it is the case of The Cancer Genome Atlas (TCGA, http://cancergenome.nih.gov/about/mission.asp), may foster our understanding of the complex mechanisms underlying the various layers of glioma biology (formation, progression, resistance to therapy, etc) and aid in the identification of new avenues for drug development, particularly targeted therapies. Indeed, recent developments in second generation sequencing technologies and its more widespread application hold promise to achieve these goals. Much more effort is required for the identification of molecular markers that truly and consistently distinguish glioma patients in ways that can assist therapeutic decisions. The integration of clinical and molecular data, now becoming available using recently developed tools such as gene microarrays, proteomics, and molecular imaging, will take us to an era where more targeted and effective treatments may be developed and implemented. We are cautiously optimistic that the development of a consensual molecular marker set predictive of therapy response in malignant gliomas, particularly glioblastoma, can arise in the future. Such marker set would substantially change the clinical management of these patients as it could aid the neuro-oncologist in individualizing therapy for each patient. Particularly, such marker set could allow the identification of the subset of patients who are likely to benefit from a specific therapy alone. Conversely, the ability to prospectively identify patients who are not be likely to respond to such therapy would also allow those patients to make an informed decision to participate in clinical trials with alternative novel therapies, avoiding adverse effects of specific treatments in the absence of anticipated clinical benefit. Additionally, a more in depth knowledge of the molecular determinants of treatment resistance could be the rational for designing the next generation of clinical trials for these highly malignant tumors. Finally, the identification of true molecular markers is also invaluable in the first steps of new drugs' development. Despite all the gaps in our understanding, a large amount of information is now available about the clinical and biological behavior of gliomas, and the molecular pathways that are relevant in their genesis and progression. In the quest toward individualization of glioblastoma treatment, the discovery of particular tumor molecular features, such as the status of *MGMT* methylation, *IDH1-2* mutations, and *HOXA* genes expression, may be the initial building blocks of a panel of molecular markers that truly have clinical implications. The challenge in the future will not only be to discover additional molecular markers of glioblastoma, but also to integrate all this new knowledge in an interdisciplinary manner to create an intelligible puzzle, which allows a more rational and efficient fight against this disease.

7. Acknowledgments

We wish to thank Dr. Sérgio Abreu for critical assistance in designing the figures. Bruno M. Costa is supported by grants from the Portuguese Science and Technology Foundation (FCT), Calouste Gulbenkian Foundation, and Portuguese League Against Cancer (LPCC).

8. References

Abdel-Fattah, R. et al., 2006. Differential expression of HOX genes in neoplastic and non-neoplastic human astrocytes. *The Journal of pathology*, 209(1), pp.15-24.

Ahn, J.-Y. et al., 2004. PIKE-A is amplified in human cancers and prevents apoptosis by up-regulating Akt. *Proceedings of the National Academy of Sciences of the United States of America*, 101(18), pp.6993-8.

Bachoo, R.M. et al., 2002. Epidermal growth factor receptor and Ink4a/Arf: convergent mechanisms governing terminal differentiation and transformation along the neural stem cell to astrocyte axis. *Cancer cell*, 1(3), pp.269-77.

Bagchi, A. et al., 2007. CHD5 is a tumor suppressor at human 1p36. *Cell*, 128(3), pp.459-75.

Balss, J. et al., 2008. Analysis of the IDH1 codon 132 mutation in brain tumors. *Acta Neuropathologica*, 116(1432 0533 (Electronic)), pp.597 602.

Behin, A. et al., 2003. Primary brain tumours in adults. *Lancet*, 361(9354), pp.323-331.

Bhowmick, D.A. et al., 2004. A functional polymorphism in the EGF gene is found with increased frequency in glioblastoma multiforme patients and is associated with more aggressive disease. *Cancer Research*, 64(4), pp.1220-1223.

Bigner, S.H. et al., 1999. Molecular genetic aspects of oligodendrogliomas including analysis by comparative genomic hybridization.*The American Journal of Pathology*, 155(2), pp.375-386.

Bondy, M.L. et al., 2001. Gamma-radiation sensitivity and risk of glioma. *Journal of the National Cancer Institute*, 93(20), pp.1553-7.

Bondy, M.L. et al., 1996. Mutagen Sensitivity and Risk of Gliomas: A Case-Control Analysis. *Cancer Research*, 56(7), pp.1484-1486.

Burnet, N.G. et al., 2005. Years of life lost (YLL) from cancer is an important measure of population burden--and should be considered when allocating research funds. *British Journal of Cancer*, 92(2), pp.241-245.

Burrows, R.C. et al., 1997. Response diversity and the timing of progenitor cell maturation are regulated by developmental changes in EGFR expression in the cortex. *Neuron*, 19(2), pp.251-67.

Cairncross, J. G. et al., 1998. Specific genetic predictors of chemotherapeutic response and survival in patients with anaplastic oligodendrogliomas. *Journal of the National Cancer Institute*, 90(19), pp.1473-1479.

Carpentier, C. et al., 2006. Polymorphism in Sp1 recognition site of the EGF receptor gene promoter and risk of glioblastoma. *Neurology*, 67(1526-632X (Electronic)), pp.872-874.

CBTRUS, 2010. CBTRUS - 2009-2010 Eighteen States Statistical Report Tables.

Christensen, B.C. et al., 2011. DNA methylation, isocitrate dehydrogenase mutation, and survival in glioma. *Journal of the National Cancer Institute*, 103(2), pp.143-53.

Costa, B.M. et al., 2007. Association between Functional EGF+61 Polymorphism and Glioma Risk. *Clinical Cancer Research*, 13, pp.2621-2626.

Costa, B.M. et al., 2010a. Prognostic value of MGMT promoter methylation in glioblastoma patients treated with temozolomide-based chemoradiation: a Portuguese multicentre study. *Oncology Reports*, 23, pp.1655-1662.

Costa, B.M. et al., 2010b. Reversing HOXA9 oncogene activation by PI3K inhibition: epigenetic mechanism and prognostic significance in human glioblastoma. *Cancer Research*, 70, pp.453-462.

Costa, B.M. et al., 2010c. Associations between functional EGFR polymorphisms and glioma risk. In *European Journal of Cancer Supplements*. Oslo, Norway, p. 25.

Dai, C. et al., 2001. PDGF autocrine stimulation dedifferentiates cultured astrocytes and induces oligodendrogliomas and oligoastrocytomas from neural progenitors and astrocytes in vivo. *Genes & Development*, 15(15), pp.1913-1925.

de Andrade, M. et al., 2001. Segregation analysis of cancer in families of glioma patients. *Genetic Epidemiology*, 20(2), pp.258-70.

Denning, G. et al., 2007. A short N-terminal sequence of PTEN controls cytoplasmic localization and is required for suppression of cell growth. *Oncogene*, 26(27), pp.3930-40.

Dhanasekaran, D.N. & Johnson, G.L., 2007. MAPKs: function, regulation, role in cancer and therapeutic targeting. *Oncogene*, 26(22), pp.3097-9.

Edick, M.J. et al., 2005. Lymphoid gene expression as a predictor of risk of secondary brain tumors. *Genes, Chromosomes & Cancer*, 42(2), pp.107-16.

Ekstrand, A.J. et al., 1992. Amplified and rearranged epidermal growth factor receptor genes in human glioblastomas reveal deletions of sequences encoding portions of the N- and/or C-terminal tails. *Proceedings of the National Academy of Sciences of the United States of America*, 89, pp.4309-4313.

Felsberg, J. et al., 2004. Oligodendroglial tumors: refinement of candidate regions on chromosome arm 1p and correlation of 1p/19q status with survival. *Brain Pathology*, 14, pp.121-130.

Ferlay, J. et al., 2008. *GLOBOCAN 2008* IARC, eds., Lyon: International Agency of Cancer. Available at: http://globocan.iarc.fr.

Fisher, J.L. et al., 2007. Epidemiology of brain tumors. *Neurologic clinics*, 25(4), pp.867-90, vii.

Fraser, M.M. et al., 2004. Pten loss causes hypertrophy and increased proliferation of astrocytes in vivo. *Cancer Research*, 64(21), pp.7773-9.

Frederick, L. et al., 2000. Diversity and frequency of epidermal growth factor receptor mutations in human glioblastomas. *Cancer Research*, 60(5), pp.1383-1387.

Freije, W.A. et al., 2004. Gene expression profiling of gliomas strongly predicts survival. *Cancer Research*, 64(18), pp.6503-10.

Furnari, F.B. et al., 2007. Malignant astrocytic glioma: genetics, biology, and paths to treatment. *Genes & Development*, 21, pp.2683-2710.

Gallia, G.L. et al., 2006. PIK3CA gene mutations in pediatric and adult glioblastoma multiforme. *Molecular Cancer Research*, 4, pp.709-714.

Gaspar, N. et al., 2010. MGMT-independent temozolomide resistance in pediatric glioblastoma cells associated with a PI3-kinase-mediated HOX/stem cell gene signature. *Cancer Research*, 70(22), pp.9243-52.

Grossman, S.A. et al., 1999. Central nervous system cancers in first-degree relatives and spouses. *Cancer Investigation*, 17(5), pp.299-308.

Haber, D. & Harlow, E., 1997. Tumour-suppressor genes: evolving definitions in the genomic age. *Nature Genetics*, 16(4), pp.320-2.

Hanahan, D. & Weinberg, R.A., 2000. The hallmarks of cancer. *Cell*, 100(1), pp.57-70.

Hardell, L. et al., 2007. Long-term use of cellular phones and brain tumours: increased risk associated with use for > or =10 years. *Occupational and Environmental Medicine*, 64(9), pp.626-32.

Hawkins, P.T. et al., 2006. Signalling through Class I PI3Ks in mammalian cells. *Biochemical Society Transactions*, 34(Pt 5), pp.647-62.

Hegi, M. E. et al., 2005. MGMT gene silencing and benefit from temozolomide in glioblastoma. *The New England Journal of Medicine*, 352, pp.997-1003.

Hemminki, K. et al., 2000. Cancers in the first-degree relatives of children with brain tumours. *British Journal of Cancer*, 83(3), pp.407-411.

Holland, E. C. et al., 1998. A constitutively active epidermal growth factor receptor cooperates with disruption of G1 cell-cycle arrest pathways to induce glioma-like lesions in mice. *Genes & Development*, 12(23), pp.3675-3685.

Homma, T. et al., 2006. Correlation among pathology, genotype, and patient outcomes in glioblastoma. *Journal of Neuropathology and Experimental Neurology*, 65(9), pp.846-54.

Ichimura, K. et al., 2004. Molecular pathogenesis of astrocytic tumours. *Journal of Neuro-Oncology*, 70(2), pp.137-160.

Ichimura, K. et al., 2009. IDH1 mutations are present in the majority of common adult gliomas but rare in primary glioblastomas. *Neuro-Oncology*, 11), pp.341-347.

Ino, Y. et al., 2001. Molecular subtypes of anaplastic oligodendroglioma: implications for patient management at diagnosis. *Clinical Cancer Research*, 7, pp.839-845.

Inskip, P.D. et al., 2001. Cellular-telephone use and brain tumors. *N Engl J Med*, 344(2), pp.79-86.

Jackson, E.L. et al., 2006. PDGFR alpha-positive B cells are neural stem cells in the adult SVZ that form glioma-like growths in response to increased PDGF signaling. *Neuron*, 51(2), pp.187-99.

Jemal, A. et al., 2009. Cancer Statistics, 2009. *Ca-A Cancer Journal for Clinicians*, 59(4), pp.225-249.

Jenkins, R.B. et al., 2006. A t(1;19)(q10;p10) mediates the combined deletions of 1p and 19q and predicts a better prognosis of patients with oligodendroglioma. *Cancer Research*, 66, pp.9852-9861.

Jeuken, J.W.M. et al., 2004. Molecular pathogenesis of oligodendroglial tumors. *Journal of Neuro-Oncology*, 70(2), pp.161-81.

Kapoor, G.S. & O'Rourke, D.M., 2003. Mitogenic signaling cascades in glial tumors. *Neurosurgery.*, 52(6), pp.1425-1434.

Knobbe, C.B. & Reifenberger, G., 2003. Genetic alterations and aberrant expression of genes related to the phosphatidyl-inositol-3'-kinase/protein kinase B (Akt) signal transduction pathway in glioblastomas. *Brain Pathology (Zurich, Switzerland)*, 13(4), pp.507-18.

Konopka, G. & Bonni, A., 2003. Signaling pathways regulating gliomagenesis. *Current Molecular Medicine*, 3(1), pp.73-84.

Lahkola, A. et al., 2007. Mobile phone use and risk of glioma in 5 North European countries. *International Journal of Cancer. Journal International du Cancer*, 120(8), pp.1769-75.

Lokker, N.A. et al., 2002. Platelet-derived growth factor (PDGF) autocrine signaling regulates survival and mitogenic pathways in glioblastoma cells: evidence that the novel PDGF-C and PDGF-D ligands may play a role in the development of brain tumors. *Cancer Research*, 62(13), pp.3729-3735.

Louis, D. N., 1994. The p53 gene and protein in human brain tumors. *Journal of Neuropathology & Experimental Neurology*, 53, pp.11-21.

Louis, D. N. et al., 2007. The 2007 WHO classification of tumours of the central nervous system. *Acta Neuropathologica*, 114(2), pp.97-109. Available at: ISI:000248046800001.

Malkin, D. et al., 1990. Germ line p53 mutations in a familial syndrome of breast cancer, sarcomas, and other neoplasms. *Science*, 250(4985), pp.1233-1238.

Malmer, B. et al., 1999. Familial aggregation of astrocytoma in northern Sweden: an epidemiological cohort study. *International Journal of Cancer*, 81(3), pp.366-370.

Malmer, B. et al., 2001. Genetic epidemiology of glioma. *British Journal of Cancer*, 84(3), pp.429-34.

McGinnis, W. & Krumlauf, R., 1992. Homeobox genes and axial patterning. *Cell*, 68(2), pp.283-302.

Meis, J.M. et al., 1991. Mixed glioblastoma multiforme and sarcoma. A clinicopathologic study of 26 radiation therapy oncology group cases. *Cancer*, 67, pp.2342-2349.

Mora, A. et al., 2004. PDK1, the master regulator of AGC kinase signal transduction. *Seminars in Cell & Developmental Biology*, 15(2), pp.161-70.

Murat, A. et al., 2008. Stem cell-related "self-renewal" signature and high epidermal growth factor receptor expression associated with resistance to concomitant chemoradiotherapy in glioblastoma. *Journal of clinical oncology : Official Journal of the American Society of Clinical Oncology*, 26(18), pp.3015-24.

Nagane, M. et al., 1996. A common mutant epidermal growth factor receptor confers enhanced tumorigenicity on human glioblastoma cells by increasing proliferation and reducing apoptosis. *Cancer Research*, 56, pp.5079-5086.

Nagarajan, R.P. & Costello, J.F., 2009. Epigenetic mechanisms in glioblastoma multiforme. *Seminars in Cancer Biology*, 19(3), pp.188-97.

Ohgaki, H. et al., 2004. Genetic pathways to glioblastoma: a population-based study. *Cancer Research*, 64(0008-5472 (Print)), pp.6892-6899.

Ohgaki, H. & Kleihues, P., 2005. Epidemiology and etiology of gliomas. *Acta Neuropathologica*, 109(1), pp.93-108.

Ohgaki, H. & Kleihues, P., 2007. Genetic pathways to primary and secondary glioblastoma. *The American Journal of Pathology*, 170, pp.1445-1453.

Parsons, D.W. et al., 2008. An integrated genomic analysis of human glioblastoma multiforme. *Science*, 321, pp.1807-1812.

Phillips, H.S. et al., 2006. Molecular subclasses of high-grade glioma predict prognosis, delineate a pattern of disease progression, and resemble stages in neurogenesis. *Cancer Cell*, 9, pp.157-173.

Pollack, I.F. et al., 2010. IDH1 mutations are common in malignant gliomas arising in adolescents: a report from the Children's Oncology Group. *Child's Nervous System*, pp.1433-0350.

Rao, R.D. et al., 2003. Genetic and signaling pathway alterations in glioblastoma: relevance to novel targeted therapies. *Frontiers in Bioscience*, 8, p.e270-e280.

Rasheed, B.K. et al., 1999. Molecular pathogenesis of malignant gliomas. *Current Opinion in Oncology*, 11(3), pp.162-167.

Relling, M.V. et al., 1999. High incidence of secondary brain tumours after radiotherapy and antimetabolites. *The Lancet*, 354(9172), pp.34-39.

Rickert, C.H. & Paulus, W., 2001. Epidemiology of central nervous system tumors in childhood and adolescence based on the new WHO classification. *Child's Nervous System*, 17(9), pp.503-511.

Riemenschneider, M.J. et al., 1999. Amplification and overexpression of the MDM4 (MDMX) gene from 1q32 in a subset of malignant gliomas without TP53 mutation or MDM2 amplification. *Cancer Research*, 59(24), pp.6091-6.

Samuels, Y. et al., 2004. High frequency of mutations of the PIK3CA gene in human cancers. *Science (New York, N.Y.)*, 304(5670), p.554.

Sarbassov, D.D. et al., 2005. Growing roles for the mTOR pathway. *Current Opinion in Cell Biology*, 17(6), pp.596-603.

Schmidt, E.E. et al., 1994. CDKN2 (p16/MTS1) gene deletion or CDK4 amplification occurs in the majority of glioblastomas. *Cancer Research*, 54(24), pp.6321-6324.

Schwartzbaum, J. et al., 2005. Polymorphisms associated with asthma are inversely related to glioblastoma multiforme. *Cancer Research*, 65(0008-5472 (Print)), pp.6459-6465.

Sherr, C.J. & McCormick, F., 2002. The RB and p53 pathways in cancer. *Cancer cell*, 2(2), pp.103-12.

Shih, A.H. et al., 2004. Dose-dependent effects of platelet-derived growth factor-B on glial tumorigenesis. *Cancer Research*, 64(14), pp.4783-9.

Singh, S.K. et al., 2004. Cancer stem cells in nervous system tumors. *Oncogene*, 23(43), pp.7267-7273.

Spiro, T.P. et al., 2001. Temozolomide: the effect of once- and twice-a-day dosing on tumor tissue levels of the DNA repair protein O(6)-alkylguanine-DNA-alkyltransferase. *Clinical cancer research : an official journal of the American Association for Cancer Research*, 7(8), pp.2309-17.

Srivastava, S. et al., 1990. Germ-line transmission of a mutated p53 gene in a cancer-prone family with Li-Fraumeni syndrome. *Nature*, 348, pp.747-749.

Stambolic, V. et al., 2001. Regulation of PTEN transcription by p53. *Molecular Cell*, 8(2), pp.317-25.

Trotman, L.C. et al., 2007. Ubiquitination regulates PTEN nuclear import and tumor suppression. *Cell*, 128(1), pp.141-56.

Ueki, K. et al., 1996. CDKN2/p16 or RB alterations occur in the majority of glioblastomas and are inversely correlated. *Cancer Research*, 56(1), pp.150-153.

Ueki, K. et al., 2002. Correlation of histology and molecular genetic analysis of 1p, 19q, 10q, TP53, EGFR, CDK4, and CDKN2A in 91 astrocytic and oligodendroglial tumors. *Clinical cancer research : an official journal of the American Association for Cancer Research*, 8(1), pp.196-201.

van den Bent, M.J., 2007. Anaplastic oligodendroglioma and oligoastrocytoma. *Neurologic Clinics*, 25(4), pp.1089-109, ix-x.

Vauleon, E. et al., 2007. The 61 A/G EGF polymorphism is functional but is neither a prognostic marker nor a risk factor for glioblastoma. *Cancer Genetics and Cytogenetics*, 172(1), pp.33-7.

Viana-Pereira, M. et al., 2008. Analysis of EGFR overexpression, EGFR gene amplification and the EGFRvIII mutation in Portuguese high-grade gliomas. *Antiacancer Research*, 28, pp.913-920.

Vousden, K.H. & Lu, X., 2002. Live or let die: the cell's response to p53. *Nature Reviews. Cancer*, 2(8), pp.594-604.

Wang, H. et al., 2004. Analysis of the activation status of Akt, NFkappaB, and Stat3 in human diffuse gliomas. *Lab.Invest.*, 84, pp.941-951.

Wang, L.E. et al., 2004. Polymorphisms of DNA repair genes and risk of glioma. *Cancer Research*, 64(16), pp.5560-5563.

Watanabe, T. et al., 2009. IDH1 mutations are early events in the development of astrocytomas and oligodendrogliomas. *Am.J Pathol.*, 174, pp.1149-1153.

Wen, P. & Kesary, S., 2008. Malignant gliomas in adults. *The New England Journal of Medicine*, 359(17), p.1850; author reply 1850.

Westermark, B. et al., 1995. Platelet-derived growth factor in human glioma. *Glia*, 15(3), pp.257-263.

Wiemels, J.L. et al., 2004. Reduced immunoglobulin E and allergy among adults with glioma compared with controls. *Cancer Research*, 64(22), pp.8468-73.

Wiencke, J.K. et al., 2005. Molecular features of adult glioma associated with patient race/ethnicity, age, and a polymorphism in O6-methylguanine-DNA-methyltransferase. *Cancer Epidemiology, Biomarkers & Prevention*, 14(7), pp.1774-1783.

Wong, A.J. et al., 1992. Structural alterations of the epidermal growth factor receptor gene in human gliomas. *Proceedings of the National Academy of Sciences of the United States of America*, 89, pp.2965-2969.

Wood, R.D. et al., 2001. Human DNA repair genes. *Science (New York, N.Y.)*, 291(5507), pp.1284-9.

Wrensch, M. et al., 2005. The molecular epidemiology of gliomas in adults. *Neurosurgical Prevention Focus*, 19(5), p.E5.

Wrensch, M. et al., 2005. ERCC1 and ERCC2 polymorphisms and adult glioma. *Neuro-Oncology*, 7(4), pp.495-507.

Wrensch, M. et al., 2001. Prevalence of antibodies to four herpesviruses among adults with glioma and controls. *American Journal of Epidemiology*, 154(2), pp.161-5.

Wrensch, M. et al., 1997. Familial and Personal Medical History of Cancer and Nervous System Conditions among Adults with Glioma and Controls. *The American Journal of Epidemiology*, 145(7), pp.581-593.

Xiao, A. et al., 2002. Astrocyte inactivation of the pRb pathway predisposes mice to malignant astrocytoma development that is accelerated by PTEN mutation. *Cancer Cell*, 1(2), pp.157-68.

Xiao, A. et al., 2005. Somatic induction of Pten loss in a preclinical astrocytoma model reveals major roles in disease progression and avenues for target discovery and validation. *Cancer Research*, 65(12), pp.5172-80.

Yan, H. et al., 2009. IDH1 and IDH2 mutations in gliomas. *The New England Journal of Medicine*, 360, pp.765-773.

Yang, P. et al., 2005. Polymorphisms in GLTSCR1 and ERCC2 are associated with the development of oligodendrogliomas. *Cancer.*, 103(11), pp.2363-2372.

Yung, W.K. et al., 1999. Multicenter phase II trial of temozolomide in patients with anaplastic astrocytoma or anaplastic oligoastrocytoma at first relapse. Temodal Brain Tumor Group. *Journal of clinical oncology: Official Journal of the American Society of Clinical Oncology*, 17(9), pp.2762-71.

Zhao, S. et al., 2009. Glioma-derived mutations in IDH1 dominantly inhibit IDH1 catalytic activity and induce HIF-1alpha. *Science*, 324, pp.261-265.

Zhu, Y. & Parada, L.F., 2002. The molecular and genetic basis of neurological tumours. *Nature Reviews Cancer*, 2(8), pp.616-626.

10

Integrated Network Analysis of Genetic and Epigenetic Factors in Glioblastoma Multiform

Hua Dong[1] and MomiaoXiong[2,1]

[1]*State Key Laboratory of Genetic Engineering and MOE Key Laboratory of Contemporary Anthropology, School of Life Sciences and Institutes of Biomedical Sciences, Fudan University, Shanghai,*

[2]*Human Genetics Center, University of Texas School of Public Health, Houston,TX*

[1]*China*

[2]*USA*

1. Introduction

Glioblastoma is the most common and aggressive type of primary brain tumor in humans. It is located preferentially in the cerebral hemispheres. Glioblastoma arises from complex interactions between a variety of genetic, epigenetic alterations and environmental perturbations. However, the precise mechanism of glioblastoma is unknown and its survival rate is very low. The Cancer Genome Atlas (TCGA) generates large-scale multi-dimensional genetic and epigenetic data to catalogue and identify cancer causing alterations (Kuhn, et al., 2008). Glioblastoma (GBM) is the first cancer studied by TCGA. In TCGA glioblastoma pilot project, a total of 601 genes were sequenced for detection of somatic mutations in 179 tumor and matched normal tissues pairs; expressions of 12,042 genes were measured in 243 tumor tissue samples and 10 normal tissue samples and 1 cell line; expressions of 534 miRNAs were profiled in 240 tumor tissue samples and 10 normal tissue samples and a total of 2,994 genes were examined for methylation in 239 tumor tissue samples and 1 cell line. This dataset will be used as an example for developing system biology and network approach as a general framework for integrated analysis of genetic and epigenetic alternations in cancer studies.

Biological functions and mechanisms are encoded in network properties. An important strategy for unraveling the mechanisms of initiation and progression of cancer is to conduct analysis of complex genetic and epigenetic networks and study their behaviors under genetic and epigenetic perturbations. Robustness of a biological network, ability to retain much of its functionality in the face of perturbation (Dartnell, et al., 2005), has emerged as a fundamental concept in the study of network topological properties (Demetrius and Manke, 2005). The locations of the DNA variants, mRNA, miRNA, and methylation in the genetic and epigenetic networks are likely to affect the phenotypes. We use network structural analysis as a tool to identify a set of key cancer causing genome alternations and core modules of biological networks that play an essential role in the development of cancer.

Purpose of this report is to use system biology approaches to develop novel analytic strategies for systematically integrating genetic and epigenetic data. To achieve this, we reconstruct genetic and epigenetic networks involved in tumorigenesis and study how these networks respond to perturbation such as somatic mutations and methylation. Information that defines the path from genomic variations to tumors flows from mutations and methylation through mRNA and miRNA expressions to tumor formation. Therefore, the components of complex genetic and epigenetic networks that determine cell function and response to perturbation of external stimuli include genes harboring DNA variations, mRNAs, miRNAs, and methylation connected by their co-expressions or interactions. These networks consist of three levels. The subnetworks in the first level consist of mRNA and miRNA co-expression networks, mRNA and miRNA interaction networks. The subnetworks in the second level are miRNA target gene networks. The subnetworks in the third level are eQTL networks which connect mutations to gene and miRNA expression.

Somatic mutations that are likely to cause tumorigenesis are traditionally identified by comparing differences in mutation frequencies between tumor and normal tissues individually. However, most somatic mutations are rare mutations. Due to their rarity, the frequencies of rare alleles may be compatible with sequencing errors. As a consequence, individual tests of association of rare variants with disease have little power and may not be robust. To overcome this limitation, we develop group association tests in which a group of rare genetic variants are jointly tested for assessing association of rare mutations and LOH with cancer. Multiple rare mutations, each with a minor marginal genetic effect, but collectively may make big contributions.

We reconstructed two types of networks that connect mRNAs or miRNAs. One is mRNA or miRNA co-expression networks. To take inherent sparse structure of co-expression networks, we use partial correlation method and sparse regression techniques to infer co-expression networks. Although co-expression networks are very useful for revealing transcriptional regulatory actions, they do not directly provide information on differences in regulatory effects between tumor and normal tissues. It is differences in regulatory effects that cause cancer. Therefore, we propose a new concept of a regulatory difference network that is formally referred to as mRNA or miRNA interaction networks. We detect interaction between mRNAs or miRNAs by measuring differences in their mutual information between tumor and normal tissues and develop a novel MI-based statistic to test interaction between two mRNAs or miRNAs.

miRNAs are short endogenous noncoding RNAs of 22 nt that negatively regulate gene expression through base pairing with target mRNAs (Huang, et al., 2007; Huang, et al., 2007). It is increasingly recognized that miRNAs have emerged as an important component in the regulation of gene expression, with imperfect base pairing, to target sites in the 3' UTR of messenger RNAs (Gennarino, et al., 2009). Three types of methods have been used to identify potential target genes: sequence analysis, miRNA-mRNA regression analysis, and machine learning (Huang, et al., 2007; Maziere and Enright, 2007; Yang, et al., 2008). Sequence analysis methods rely on knowledge of the base pairing between and second structure of the miRNA and the target gene. However, the sequence approach has limited specificity due to imperfect miRNA-target pairing (Huang, et al., 2007; Huang, et al., 2007). Regressing the expression of a target gene on the expression of miRNA for identifying miRNA target is based on a linear relationship between miRNA and its target mRNA. However, the relationship between miRNA and target mRNA may be nonlinear, which leads to inaccurate prediction of the miRNA target. The precision of miRNA target prediction by machine learning depends on the number of experimentally validated miRNA targets; however, the number of experimentally validated targets is limited. To improve the accuracy of target prediction, we will combine sequence analysis with regression analysis for target prediction.

2. Materials and methods

2.1 Test association of somatic mutations and LOH with glioblastoma

Cancers arise from mutations that confer growth advantage on cells (Greenman, et al., 2007).The somatic mutations in cancers can be classified either as "drivers" or "passengers" (Wood, et al., 2007). As the number of tumor tissues and normal tissues increases we can observe somatic mutations in both tumor and normal tissues. The current popular method for identifying driver mutations is to compare the difference in the mutation rates (Kuhn, et al., 2008; Parsons, et al., 2008). However, there is debate about how to assess a significant excess of mutations in tumors (Rubin and Green, 2007). We need to develop formal tests to detect differences in mutation rates between tumor and normal tissues. Most traditional statistical methods that often test the association of genetic variants individually were designed for testing association of common alleles with common diseases and are inappropriate for testing the association of rare somatic mutations. A feasible approach is to record rare sequence variants at different genome positions and to collectively test association of a set of rare variants. It has been shown that the number of rare alleles in large samples is approximately distributed as a Poisson process with its intensity depending on the total mutation rate(Joyce and Tavare, 1995). The intensity of the Poisson process within a segment of genome can be interpreted as the mutation rate. Similar to standard χ^2 test for association of SNPs which compare the difference in allele frequencies between cases and controls, the proposed statistics are to compare difference in the mutation rates between tumor and normal samples. Specifically, let $\bar{U}$ and $\bar{V}$ be the average number of rare mutations which is the intensity of the Poisson process underlying the rare variants, in the tumor and normal samples, respectively. Let S_{uv} be the pooled sample variance of the rare variants. Define the test statistic:

$$T_G = \frac{(\bar{U}-\bar{V})^2}{(\frac{1}{n_A}+\frac{1}{n_G})S_{uv}}, \tag{1}$$

where n_A and n_G are the number of sampled tumor tissues and normal tissues, respectively. Under the null hypothesis of no association of the set of rare variants with the disease, the average number of rare alleles in cases and controls should be equal and the statistic T_G is asymptotically distributed as a central $\chi^2_{(1)}$ distribution. In some cases, we may have a homozygous genotype of rare mutations. To improve the power, in this case, we can count it twice. Instead of defining statistics in terms of genotype, we can similarly define the test statistics in terms of the rare alleles, which is denoted as T_a.

$$T_a = \frac{(\bar{U}-\bar{V})^2}{(\frac{1}{2n_A}+\frac{1}{2n_G})S_{uv}}$$

To examine the validity of the test statistics, we performed a series of simulation studies. We used infinitely many allele models and software (GENOME) to generate rare variants. Suppose that the mutation rate per generation per base pair is 1.00×10^{-8}, the recombination rate between consecutive fragments is 0.0001, the migration rate per generation per individual is 0.00025, we have simulated 100 fragments with the length of each fragment equals 10k in base pair. Total of 100,000 individuals who were equally divided into cases and controls were generated in the general population. 500 to 2,000 individuals were randomly sampled from each of the cases and controls. 10,000 simulations were repeated. Table 1 summarized the type I error rates of two statistics. Table 1 showed that the estimated type I error rates of the statistics for testing association of a set of rare variants with the disease were not appreciably different from the nominal levels $\alpha = 0.05$, $\alpha = 0.01$ and $\alpha = 0.001$.

A LOH mutation was recorded when the genotype in blood or normal tissue is heterozygous, and in the tumor tissue, the reference allele loses normal function and the genotype becomes homozygous. The statistic T_G can be used to test association of LOH with glioblastoma.

Sample Sizes		T_G	T_a
2,000	α =0.001	0.0012	0.001
	α =0.01	0.0093	0.0096
	α =0.05	0.0489	0.0494
1,500	α =0.001	0.0015	0.001
	α =0.01	0.0106	0.0092
	α =0.05	0.0521	0.0500
1,000	α =0.001	0.0012	0.0007
	α =0.01	0.0106	0.0097
	α =0.05	0.0522	0.0459
500	α =0.001	0.0009	0.0008
	α =0.01	0.0102	0.0117
	α =0.05	0.0504	0.0548

Table 1. Type 1 error rates of the statistics T_G, T_a.

2.2 Lasso for co-expression networks

A co-mRNA expression or co-miRNA expression network can be constructed by joint sparse regression for estimating the concentration matrix in which off-diagonal elements represents the covariance between the corresponding variables given all other variables in the network (Peng, et al., 2009). Sparse regression for reconstruction of co-expression network is briefly introduced here. (For details, please see(Peng, et al., 2009)). Denote the mRNA or miRNA expression levels as variables $y_1,...y_q$. A variable is represented by a node. An edge connecting two nodes indicates that the connected two variables are conditionally dependent, given all other variables. Assume that the vector of q variables $Y=[y_1,...y_q]^T$ follow a normal distribution $N(0,\Sigma)$. Denote the partial correlations as $\rho^{ij}=Corr(y_i,y_j\,|\,y_{-(i,j)})$ for $1\le i<j\le q$ and $-(i,j)\equiv\{k:1\le k\ne i,j\le q\}$. If we assume the normality of the variables, then two variables y_i and y_j are conditionally dependent, given all other variables if and only $\rho^{ij}\ne 0$. Let $\Sigma^{-1}=(\sigma^{ij})$ be the concentration matrix. Then,

$$\rho^{ij}=-\frac{\sigma^{ij}}{\sqrt{\sigma^{ii}\sigma^{jj}}} \tag{2}$$

When sample size is much larger than the number of variables, the concentration matrix can be directly estimated from the inverse of the sampling covariance matrix. However, when the number of variables in the network is larger than the sample size, the inverse of sampling covariance matrix may not exist. We use sparse regression for network modeling via estimating sparse concentration matrix.

2.3 Functional module identification and gene set enrichment analysis

Co-expression networks are usually organized into functional modules that perform specific biological tasks. Genes within coexpression modules often share conserved biological functions. A dynamic tree cut procedure was used to identify modules(Langfelder, et al., 2008). A co-expression network was clustered using hierarchical clustering. Modules are defined as braches of dendrogram. One sided Fisher exact test that calculates the probability of seeing observed number of genes within a pathway or a GO category in the module by chance was used to test for enrichment of a pathway or a GO category in the module. We assembled 465 pathways from KEGG(Hashimoto, et al., 2006) and Biocarta (http://www.biocarta.com).

2.4 miRNA interaction and mRNA Interaction networks

Modern complex theory assumes that the complexity is the degree to which components engage in organized structured interactions. Intuitively, complexity can also be viewed as the degree of dependence among components. Therefore, interaction has been considered as a sensible measure of complexity of biological systems. The more interactions between components, the more complex the system is. We identify mRNA or miRNA interaction networks via detecting pair-wise interaction between mRNAs or miRNAs. We view mRNA or miRNA expressions as continuous variables. Formally, interactions can generally be defined as a stochastic dependence between two random variables. The concept of mutual information proposed by Shannon(Cover and Thomas, 1991) can serve as a general measure of interaction (dependence) between two random variables(Jakulin, et al., 2003; Matsuda, 2000; Nakahara, et al., 2003). It quantifies the stochastic dependence between two random variables. An additional asset is that mutual information measures more than linear dependence(Brillinger, 2004; McGill, 1954). Therefore, information theory will provide an unified framework for developing statistical methods to detect interaction between mRNAs or miRNAs. Similar to the detection of interaction between two SNPs where interaction between two SNPs is measured and tested as the difference in linkage disequilibrium(LD) between cases and controls(Wu, et al., 2008; Zhao, et al., 2006), we detect interaction between mRNAs or miRNAs by measuring differences in mutual information between tumor and normal tissues.

The expression of mRNAs and miRNAs are continuous variables. Usually, we assume that they follow a normal distribution. Let random variables X and Y denote the expression of a pair of mRNAs or miRNAs. Let $f(x)$, $f(y)$ and $f(x,y)$ be the distribution functions of X and Y and their joint distribution function, respectively. The mutual information between two continuous variables is defined as

$$I(X,Y) = E\left[\log \frac{f(x,y)}{f(x)f(y)}\right] \tag{3}$$

This formula shows(Cover and Thomas, 1991) that mutual information is always nonnegative and is equal to zero if and only if two random variables are independent. Therefore, mutual information can be used to measure the degree of stochastic dependence. Assuming the normal distribution of two random variables, mutual information can easily be calculated by

$$I(X,Y) = -\frac{1}{2}\log(1-\rho^2), \tag{4}$$

where ρ is a canonical correlation. Similar to using LD to test interaction between two SNPs where tests for interaction between unlinked and linked loci are developed separately, we consider two cases in testing interaction between mRNAs or miRNAs: (1) a pair of mRNAs or miRNAs in the normal tissues are independent and (2) a pair of mRNAs or miRNAs in the normal tissues are dependent.

2.4.1 A pair of mRNAs or miRNAs in the normal tissues is independent

Let $I_T(X,Y)$ and $I_N(X,Y)$ be mutual information between x_1 and x_2 in tumor and normal tissues, respectively. Let n_A and n_G be the number of tumor and normal samples, respectively. Then, $2n_A\hat{I}_T(X,Y)$ and $2n_G\hat{I}_N(X,Y)$ are asymptotically distributed as a $\chi^2_{(1)}$ distribution (Brillinger, 2004). Define the statistic:

$$T_I = 2n_A\hat{I}_T(X,Y) - 2n_G\hat{I}_N(X,Y) \tag{5}$$

It has been shown(Holm and Alouini, 2004) that under the null hypothesis of no interaction, T_I has a distribution with the following probability density function

$$f(x) = \frac{1}{2\pi}K_0(\frac{|x|}{2}) \tag{6}$$

where $K_0(\cdot)$ is the modified Bessel function of the second kind of order 0 (Jeffrey and Zwillinger, 2000).

2.4.2 A pair of mRNAs or miRNAs in the normal tissues is dependent

When a pair of mRNAs or miRNAs in the normal tissues is dependent, we can define a test statistic that has a much simpler distribution than that of test statistic T_I. Let $\hat{\rho}_A$ and $\hat{\rho}_G$ be the canonical correlation in tumor and normal tissues, respectively. We propose a novel statistic defined as

$$T_D = \frac{[I_T(X,Y) - I_N(X,Y)]^2}{(1/n_A + 1/n_G)\hat{\rho}^2} \quad (7)$$

where $I_T(X,Y) = -\frac{1}{2}\log(1-\hat{\rho}_A^2)$ and $I_N(X,Y) = -\frac{1}{2}\log(1-\hat{\rho}_G^2)$. Then T_D follows a central $\chi^2_{(1)}$ distribution under the null hypothesis of no difference in mutual information between tumor and normal tissues. To evaluate the validity of the test statistic T_D, we calculated its type 1 error rates. We simulated a population of size 1,000,000 from a bivariate normal distribution with mean $[0,0]^T$. Then, we equally sampled 100, 200 and 400 subjects as tumor and normal samples and calculated the test statistic T_D. We repeated this with 10,000 simulations. The type 1 error rates for different samples and correlation coefficients were listed in Table 2. Type I error rates for the statistics T_D to test for the interactions between two mRNAs or miRNAs were not appreciably different from the nominal levels $\alpha = 0.05$, $\alpha = 0.01$ and $\alpha = 0.001$.

ρ	Sample Sizes	Nominal Level		
		$\alpha = 0.001$	$\alpha = 0.01$	$\alpha = 0.05$
0.2	100	0.0023	0.0113	0.0552
	200	0.0010	0.0086	0.0494
	400	0.0011	0.0115	0.0529
0.5	100	0.0008	0.0103	0.0532
	200	0.0011	0.0108	0.0528
	400	0.0012	0.0104	0.0496

Table 2. Type 1 error rates of T_D for testing interaction between two continuous variables

2.5 Ranking of the nodes in the network

Biological functions and mechanisms are encoded in network properties. An important strategy for unraveling the mechanisms of initiation and progression of cancer is to conduct analysis of complex biological networks and study their behaviors under genetic and epigenetic perturbations. Robustness of a biological network, ability to retain much of its functionality in the face of perturbation(Dartnell, et al., 2005), has emerged as a fundamental concept in the study of network topological properties(Demetrius and Manke, 2005). Widely used measures of network robustness include ranking importance of the nodes in the network. One of the most efficient measures of importance in robustness analysis of the network is the damage value of a node which quantifies the effect of the removal of that particular node from the network. Formally, we define the damage value of a node as follows. Let $G = (V,E)$ be the connected component that contains node $h \ni V$, and let $\tilde{G} = (\tilde{V}, \tilde{E})$ be the largest connected component of $\tilde{G}$, after the removal of node h. Then, the value $D(h) = |V| - |\tilde{V}|$ is the damage value of node h.

2.6 Identify the genetic variants that have cis or trans regulatory effects on miRNA or mRNA expressions

Loci that are significantly associated with expression are called expression quantitative trait loci (eQTL). Somatic mutations may directly or indirectly regulate the expression of mRNAs or miRNAs. The traditional statistical methods to regress the expression levels on the individual genetic variant for identifying eQTL is inappropriate for studying the regulatory effect of somatic mutations due to their low allele frequencies. An alternative approach to current variant-by-variant regression method is groupwise regression methods in which a group of rare genetic variants are jointly analyzed. It is well known that eQTL include *cis*-eQTL in which an association exists between the expression of a specific gene (mRNA) and the genetic variants at that gene's locus, or between the expression of miRNA and the genetic variants at its host gene, and *trans*-eQTL in which there is an association between the expression of a gene or a miRNA and the genetic variants at a non-local genomic locus. Regression methods that regress the expression of a mRNA or a miRNA on the number of all mutated alleles across the region of interest to identify *cis*- or *trans*-eQTL .

2.7 miRNA target networks

miRNAs down regulate gene expressions by base-pairing with the 3′-noncoding region of the target mRNAs. It is estimated that up to 30% of genes might be regulated by miRNAs(Sassen, et al., 2008). It is hypothesized that miRNAs and their targets form complex networks to perform various biological functions. To reveal mechanisms of the GBM, we identified target genes of miRNAs and constructed miRNA target networks. Procedures for discovering the target genes consisted of two steps. The first step was to conduct sequence analysis that used sequence complementarities of miRNA and its target site to predict potential miRNA target genes. We searched the predicted potential miRNA targets in miRGen(Megraw, et al., 2007), which integrated animal miRNA targets according to combinations of four widely used target prediction programs: miRanda, PicTar, TargetScan, DIANA-microT, and experimentally supported targets from TarBase (Sethupathy, et al., 2006) and miR2Disease(Jiang, et al., 2009). Since miRNAs repress the expression of their target genes, the second step was to test the inverse relationship between the expression profile of miRNA and that of its potential targets. To achieve this, we regressed the expression of target mRNAs on the expression of miRNAs and select mRNAs with significant negative regression coefficients as miRNA targets. P-value for declaring significant evidence of miRNA target was 1.00×10^{-4} .

3. Results

3.1 Test association of somatic mutations and LOH mutations with glioblastoma

The first step for deciphering the path from somatic mutations to the GBM is to test association of somatic mutations with the GBM. The statistic T_a and T_G was applied to glioblastoma in TCGA dataset. The tumor tissues of 179 glioblastoma patients and 179 matched normal tissues were sequenced. A somatic mutation was recorded when the mutation was detected only in the tumor tissue. There were 306 genes in which at least one somatic mutation was detected. A LOH mutation was recorded when the genotype in blood or normal tissue is heterozygous, and in the tumor tissue, the reference allele loses normal function and the genotype becomes homozygous. There were 124 genes in which at least one LOH mutation was detected. We identified association of somatic mutations in 14 genes by the statistics T_a (Table 3), and association of LOH in 11 genes by the statistic T_G with glioblastoma with false discovery rate (FDR) less than 0.05 (Table 4). Genes TP53, PTEN, EGFR, NF1, RB1 and ERBB2 were reported to be associated with GBM in the previous TCGA data analysis (The Cancer Genome Atlas Research Network, 2008). The remaining 8 somatic mutated genes and 10 LOH mutated genes were newly identified by the statistics T_G or T_a. NCBI Entrez gene database (Maglott, et al., 2007) reported that : CHEK2 is

Gene	P-value	FDR	Mutation frequency
TP53	3.46E-11	5.90E-10	0.1453
PTEN	2.25E-07	1.92E-06	0.0698
EGFR	1.22E-06	6.92E-06	0.0587
FKBP9	1.38E-04	5.89E-04	0.0363
CHEK2	1.39E-03	4.73E-03	0.0475
GSTM5	2.41E-03	6.86E-03	0.0251
DST	4.28E-03	8.12E-03	0.0223
RB1	3.54E-03	8.62E-03	0.0251
NF1	4.17E-03	8.89E-03	0.0363
BCL11A	1.36E-02	2.33E-02	0.0168
ERBB2	1.57E-02	2.43E-02	0.0307
PIK3C2G	2.45E-02	3.49E-02	0.0140
FN1	3.30E-02	4.33E-02	0.0168
COL3A1	4.46E-02	4.75E-02	0.0112

Table 3. P-values for testing association of somatic mutations with the GBM

Gene	P-value	FDR	Mutation frequency
NRAP	5.71E-07	6.24E-06	0.1173
MKI67	8.19E-07	4.47E-06	0.1229
C10orf54	1.02E-04	3.70E-04	0.0391
C9orf66	1.63E-04	4.46E-04	0.0419
MYO3A	6.40E-04	1.40E-03	0.0307
PRAME	2.14E-03	3.90E-03	0.0251
EGFR	3.20E-03	4.99E-03	0.0279
IL1RL1	7.11E-03	9.71E-03	0.0196
HLA-DOA	1.30E-02	1.57E-02	0.0168
ABCA13	2.37E-02	2.59E-02	0.0140
CYP1B1	2.37E-02	2.59E-02	0.0140

Table 4. P-values for testing association of LOH with the GBM

a cell cycle checkpoint regulator and putative tumor suppressor, and associated with GBM; GSTM5 was reported to be involved in cancer, BCL11A is a proto-oncogene, and FN1 is involved in tumor metastasis and angiogenesis. Gene PRAME was reported to be associated with melanoma and acute leukemias. Association of the other 9 genes such as NRAP, MK167, C10orf54 and C9orf66 with GBM was first reported here

3.2 Network analysis of gene expressions

3.2.1 Differential expression analysis

Comparative studies of gene expression between normal and tumor tissues is one of the most widely used strategies for unraveling the molecular circuitry underlying cancer (Liang and Pardee, 2003). To uncover the mechanisms of glioblastoma, expressions of 12,042 genes were measured in 243 tumor tissue samples and 10 normal tissue samples and 1 cell line by Affymetrix HT Human Genome U133 Array Plate Set. A total of 1,697 genes were differentially expressed between tumor and normal tissues by Wilcoxon rank-sum test (P-value for declaring significance after Bonferroni correction is 4.15×10^{-6}). Of the 1,697 genes, 72 genes were cancer genes or cancer candidate genes, 25 of which were GBM related genes including *TCF12, TP53, COL4A1, COL3A1* and *COL5A2*, 11 of them were oncogenes including *CDK4* and *RAF4*; 21 of them were tumor suppressor genes including *TP53* and *RB1* (We got the oncogene and tumor suppressor gene list from database: TSGDB(Yang and Fu, 2003) and UNSW Embryology DNA Tumor Suppressor and Oncogene Database(Ackermann and Strimmer, 2009)), 242 genes were in signal transduction pathways, 908 genes were down regulated and 789 genes were up regulated. From 1,697 significantly differentially expressed genes, we identified 97 genes that were reported to be cancer related in the literatures (Table 5).

Gene	P-value	Up-down	Cancer Gene	TSG	Cancer Signaling
ICAM5	2.52E-08	Down	CAN-gene		
TCF12	2.84E-08	Up	Cancer Gene		regulation
THRB	3.2E-08	Down		oncogene	
ABR	3.2E-08	Down		TSG	
BTG1	3.28E-08	Up	Cancer Gene	TSG	
KIAA0774	3.97E-08	Down	CAN-gene		
TMEM123	3.97E-08	Up	CAN-gene		
IGFBP7	4.57E-08	Up		TSG	
MAP2K4	4.68E-08	Down	Cancer Gene	TSG	Kinase
ELK1	4.68E-08	Down		oncogene	TF
COL4A1	4.91E-08	Up	GBM		
CD93	5.14E-08	Up	CAN-gene		
CDK2AP1	6.21E-08	Up		TSG	
ITGAV	7.49E-08	Up	GBM		
EDIL3	8.81E-08	Down	GBM		
RB1	1.24E-07	Up	Cancer Gene	TSG	TF
GRM1	1.33E-07	Down	CAN-gene		
TP53	1.40E-07	Up	Cancer Gene	TSG	TF
CDH11	1.46E-07	Up	Cancer Gene		

Gene	P-value	Up-down	Cancer Gene	TSG	Cancer Signaling
CDKN2C	1.49E-07	Up	GBM		CDK inhibitors
SNAP25	1.53E-07	Down	GBM		Vesicle
LDOC1	1.67E-07	Down		TSG	
IGFBP2	1.67E-07	Up	GBM		
BCL11B	1.75E-07	Down	Cancer Gene		
FABP3	1.77E-07	Down		TSG	
RARG	1.88E-07	Down	GBM		
PTPN13	2.3E-07	Up		TSG	cytoskeleton
GABRB2	2.40E-07	Down	GBM		
EIF4A2	2.46E-07	Down	Cancer Gene		
SP110	2.69E-07	Up	CAN-gene		
GAS1	2.75E-07	Up		TSG	
RIMS2	3.59E-07	Down	CAN-gene		
VSNL1	3.83E-07	Down	GBM		Adapter
CDH12	4.01E-07	Down	Cancer Gene		
RAP1GDS1	4.38E-07	Down	CAN-gene		
LMO7	4.57E-07	Down	CAN-gene		
ATM	4.99E-07	Up	Cancer Gene	TSG	Kinase
PDE4DIP	5.21E-07	Down	Cancer Gene		
HIP1	5.69E-07	Up	Cancer Gene		cytoskeleton
PRPF4B	5.94E-07	Up	CAN-gene		
NUP214	6.34E-07	Up	Cancer Gene		Transporter
HSP90AB1	6.77E-07	Down	Cancer Gene		
LYN	7.07E-07	Up		oncogene	Kinase
COL5A2	7.54E-07	Up	GBM		
BCL10	8.04E-07	Up	Cancer Gene		apoptosis
NCKIPSD	8.04E-07	Down	Cancer Gene		
TRIM24	8.40E-07	Up	Cancer Gene		
CLTC	8.95E-07	Down	Cancer Gene		SP
RAF1	9.55E-07	Up		oncogene	Kinase
SYK	1.02E-06	Up	Cancer Gene		Kinase
PIM1	1.03E-06	Up	Cancer Gene	oncogene	
SYT1	1.04E-06	Down	CAN-gene		Vesicle
MAPK8IP2	1.08E-06	Down	CAN-gene		
CHI3L2	1.13E-06	Up	GBM		
YES1	1.21E-06	Up		oncogene	Kinase
ATP8A2	1.31E-06	Down		TSG	Molecule
GABRA1	1.31E-06	Down	GBM		Receptor
RASSF1	1.34E-06	Up		TSG	
CHIC2	1.43E-06	Up	CAN-gene		
MYT1L	1.55E-06	Down	GBM		
COL3A1	1.55E-06	Up	GBM		
NBL1	1.62E-06	Down		TSG	
NONO	1.80E-06	Up	Cancer Gene		
TPR	1.80E-06	Up	Cancer Gene		

Gene	P-value	Up-down	Cancer Gene	TSG	Cancer Signaling
NOV	1.87E-06	Down		oncogene	GF
CDK4	1.87E-06	Up	GBM	oncogene	Kinase
TCF3	1.95E-06	Up	Cancer Gene		TF
NEFM	1.95E-06	Down	GBM		Cytoskeleton
SYN2	2.08E-06	Down	GBM		
FLT3	2.17E-06	Down	Cancer Gene		Generics
CCK	2.17E-06	Down	GBM		
IDH1	2.26E-06	Up	GBM		
CDC23	2.31E-06	Up		TSG	
CHI3L1	2.31E-06	Up	GBM		
BCL6	2.35E-06	Up	Cancer Gene		
RTN1	2.40E-06	Down	GBM		
DLEU2	2.43E-06	Up		TSG	
SH3GL2	2.50E-06	Down	GBM		Vesicle
BLM	2.56E-06	Up	Cancer Gene		
SMAD4	2.56E-06	Up	Cancer Gene		TF
CACNA2D2	2.95E-06	Down		TSG	
PRRX1	2.95E-06	Up	Cancer Gene		
SV2B	2.95E-06	Down	GBM		
NEFL	3.01E-06	Down	GBM		
MCF2	3.14E-06	Down		oncogene	Cytoskeleton
CTNNA1	3.14E-06	Up		TSG	Cytoskeleton
BMPR1A	3.27E-06	Up	Cancer Gene		Receptor
MSN	3.40E-06	Up	Cancer Gene		
RPN1	3.54E-06	Up	Cancer Gene		
LPP	3.69E-06	Up	Cancer Gene		
GABRG2	3.77E-06	Down	GBM		
TRIM8	3.77E-06	Down		TSG	
COX6C	3.84E-06	Down	Cancer Gene		
FBXW7	4.00E-06	Down	Cancer Gene		Generics
ETS2	4.34E-06	Down		oncogene	TF
EWSR1	4.8E-06	Up		oncogene	
ST5	4.99E-06	Up		TSG	

*TSG: tumor suppressor gene; TF: transcription factor; SP: Structural Protein, GF: Growth Factor

Table 5. A list of 97 genes was differentially expressed.

3.2.2 Gene co-expression network analysis

To investigate the functions of the genes at the system-level and uncover the mechanism of GBM, we used partial correlation method and sparse regression techniques to infer gene co-expression networks. The largest connected coexpression network with the average shortest path 20.4 and diameter 74 had 2,115 genes and 2,276 edges (Figure 1).

To explore the relationship between co-expressions of the genes and physical interaction between their corresponding proteins, we compared the constructed co-expression gene network with the protein protein interaction (PPI) network (Chuang, et al., 2007), comprising 57, 235 interactions among 11, 203 proteins. The human PPI network was integrated from yeast two-hybrid experiments, predicted interactions based on orthology and co-citation, and curation of literature. We restricted our analysis to 3,991 genes present in both co-expression and PPI networks, consisting of 2, 131 and 12, 182 edges, respectively. The two networks shared 85 edges involving 133 genes in common. The 133 genes and their connections were shown in Figure 2. We performed functional enrichment analysis of the 133 genes using DAVID(Huang da, et al., 2009). Enriched gene functional categories include protein biosynthesis/ribosome, development processes, metabolic processes and RNA splicing. It is noticeable that the largest connected component, which consists of 29 genes, in Figure 2 corresponds to a ribosomal protein complex.

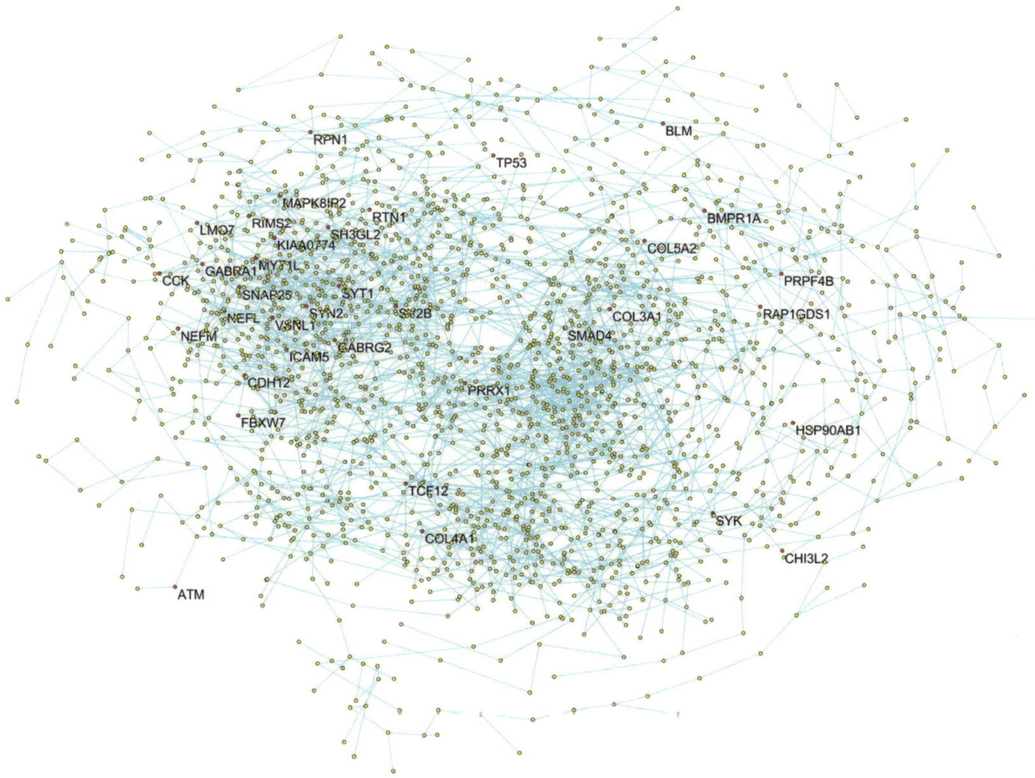

Fig. 1. The largest connected gene co-expression network. The network had 2,115 genes and 2,276 edges. Genes related to GBM were highlighted in red.

The network had 133 genes and 700 edges. This figure gives the sub-network of gene co-expressions in which a node contains both gene co-expressions and protein-protein interactions with other nodes in this sub-network.

Co-expression networks are usually organized into modules that perform specific biological process. 13 modules were significantly enriched for at least one pathway(Figure 3 and Table 6), indicating that co-expression network was organized into functional units. Enriched pathways in the modules were involved in neurodegenerative diseases, development processes, cancer related signaling pathways and metabolism. Parkinson's disease pathway was enriched in module 11 with olive green color. Genes UQCRC1, ATP5H, COX7C, NDUFA1, COX5R and COX4I1 in the module 11 are involved in mitochondria dysfunction (http://www.genome.jp/kegg/pathway/hsa/hsa05012.html). Cell cycle pathway was enriched in module 7 with yellow color. We can see that co-expressed genes CHEK2, CCNB2, CCNA2, CCNE2, MAD2L1 and BUB1 in module 7 are directly or indirectly connected in cell cycle pathway (http://www.genome.jp/dbget-bin /show_ pathway? hsa04110).

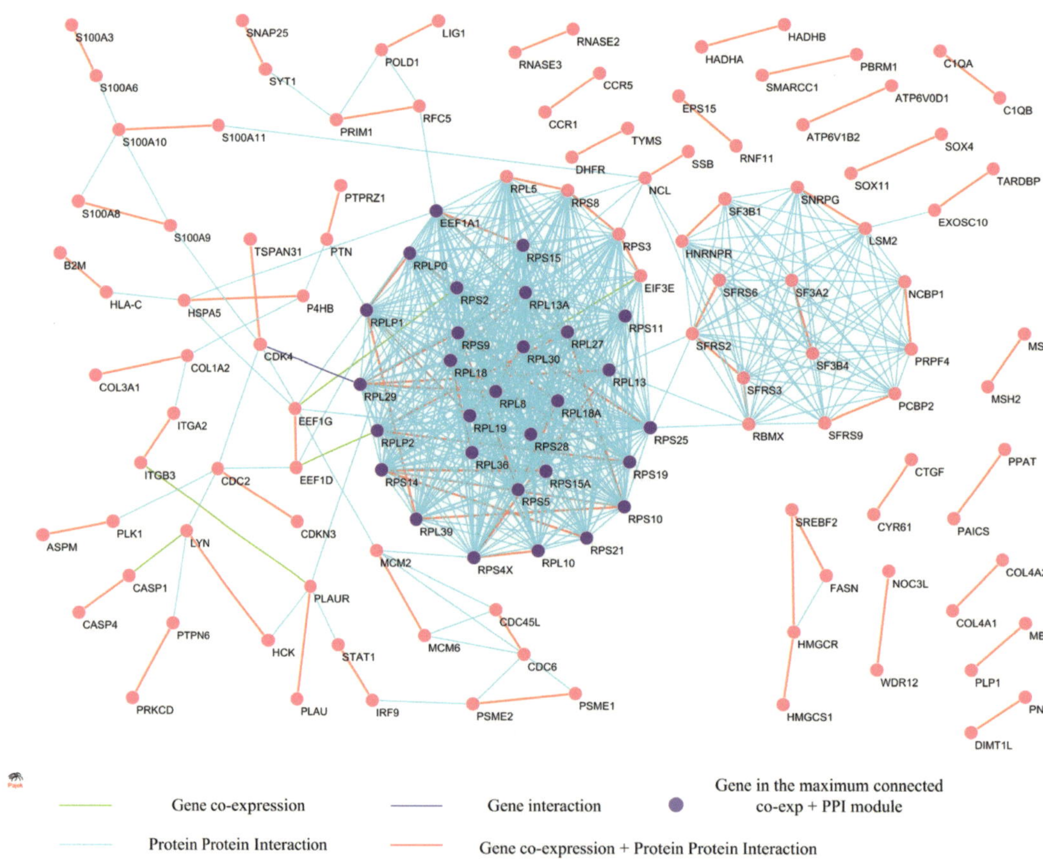

Fig. 2. Gene co-expressions and interactions supported by protein-protein interactions.

The architecture of a co-expression network is important for uncovering the genes which are involved in cancer. To identify the most important genes in the co-expression network, we used the damage value of a node as a measure to rank the importance of a node. We ranked all differentially expressed genes in the largest co-expression sub-network according to their damage values. Top 5% genes in the ranked list with the damage values greater than 15 were summarized. These genes were essential to the function of co-expression network. We suspect that these genes may be involved in the development of GBM. For example, T1A1 that had the largest damage value 38 and was over expressed in the GBM tissues plays a role in apoptosis (Forch and Valcarcel, 2001). KIAA1279 was reported to be associated with the nervous systems (Brooks, et al., 2005). It was also reported that CACYBP participates in p53-induced beta-catenin degradation and can suppress proliferation and tumorigenesis of renal cancer cells (Sun, et al., 2007). CACYBP was under expressed in gastric cancer (Ning, et al., 2007) and renal cancer (Sun, et al., 2007).

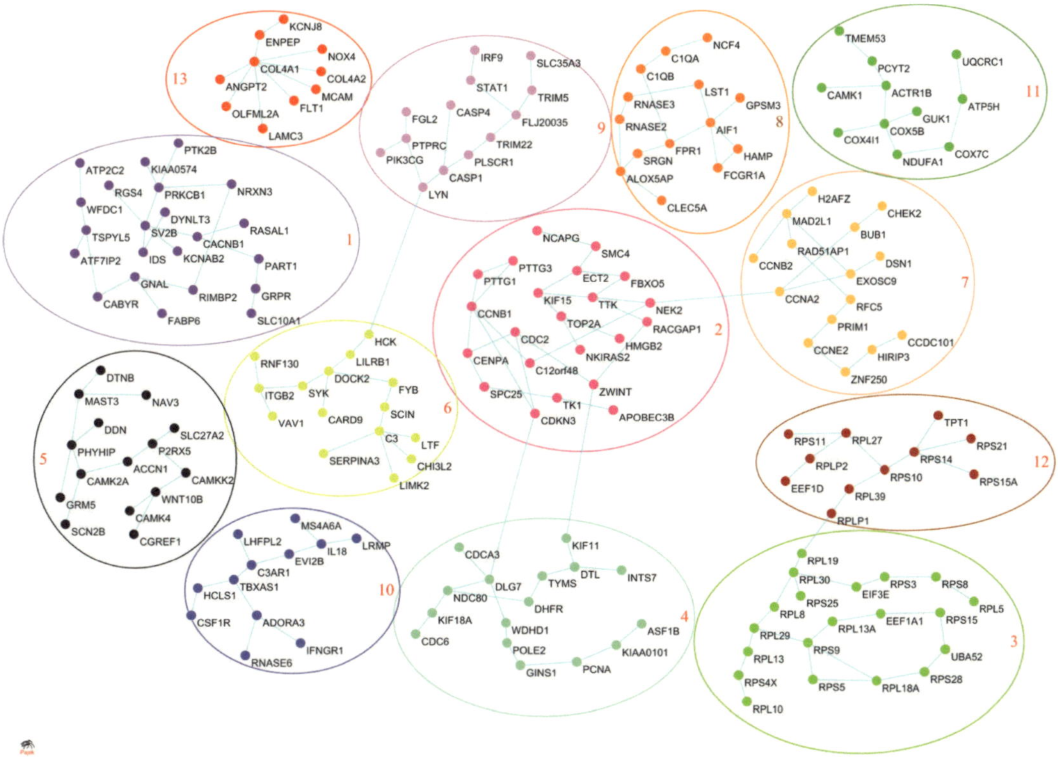

Fig. 3. 13 functional modules in the largest connected gene-coexpression network in Figure 1. The modules were indexed by the number and also represented by color. Enriched pathways in the modules were listed in Table 6.

There were three genes: TP53, COL3A1, and RAP1GDS1 whose damage values ranked the top among the cancer and cancer candidate genes (Table 5). Their removal from the network may disconnect some components in the network and hence compromise the functions of the genes in coexpression networks. TP53 and COL3A1 are GBM related genes and RAP1GDS1 is a cancer candidate gene. The p53 pathway is central to oncogenesis (El Hallani, et al., 2009). TP53, which was up regulated in GBM tissue samples, particularly, was highly over-expressed in CEREBRUM tissue samples. It was observed that TP53 had damage value 23, but was only connected with two up regulated genes: TGIF2 and EIF4A1. TGIF2 was differentially expressed (P-value$< 1.43\times10^{-7}$) and had damage value 24. TGIF2 is a novel TALE superclass homeodomain protein and a transcriptional co-repressor that interacts with Smad2 and Smad3 to negatively regulate the TGFb/Smad response in a cell, which in turn affects apoptosis and leads to cellular proliferation and differentiation. TGIF2 plays an oncogenic role through inhibition of TGFb (Imoto, et al., 2000). EIF4A1 was over expressed in tumor tissue (P-value$< 5.09 \times 10^{-6}$) and had damage value 22. EIF4A1 is ATP-dependent RNA helicase and required for mRNA binding to ribosome. EIF4A1 inhibit translation initiation and act as a tumor suppressor by forming complex with Programmed Cell Death 4 (PDCD4) (Yang, et al., 2004). COL3A1 was over expressed in GBM tissue samples (P-value$< 1.6 \times 10^{-6}$) and had damage value 21. It was also reported to be over

#	color	Category	Name	P-value
1	Purple	Cell Signaling	Ion Channel and Phorbal Esters Signaling	8.60E-03
2	Wind-Stawberry	Apoptosis	Apoptotic DNA fragmentation and tissue homeostasis	3.52E-02
		Cell Cycle Regulation	Activation of Src by Protein-tyrosine phosphatase alpha	4.23E-02
		Cell Cycle Regulation	AKAP95 role in mitosis and chromosome dynamics	4.98E-02
		Cell Cycle Regulation	Sonic Hedgehog (SHH) Receptor Ptc1 Regulates cell cycle	4.23E-02
3	Forest-Green	Translation	Ribosome	3.32E-09
4	TealBlue	Metabolism of Cofactors& Vitamins	One carbon pool by folate	4.72E-02
5	Black	Cell Signaling	Ca++/ Calmodulin-dependent Protein Kinase Activation	3.59E-03
6	Green-Yellow	Immunology	Cells and Molecules involved in local acute inflammatory response	4.68E-02
7	Yellow	Cell Growth and Death	Cell cycle	2.62E-02
8	Orange	Immunology	Classical Complement	2.85E-02
9	Lavender	Cell Signaling	IFN alpha signaling	1.03E-02
10	Blue	Cell Activation	Th1/Th2 Differentiation	3.79E-02
11	OliveGreen	Metabolism	Electron Transport Reaction in Mitochondria	1.31E-02
		Energy Metabolism	Oxidative phosphorylation	9.00E-03
		Neurodegene-rative Diseases	Parkinson's disease	8.67E-03
12	Maroon	Translation	Ribosome	1.13E-03

#	color	Category	Name	P-value
13	Red	Metabolism | Neuroscience	Vitamin C in the Brain	9.11E-03
		Cell Activation	Angiotensin-converting enzyme 2 regulates heart function	1.27E-02
		Metabolism	Intrinsic Prothrombin Activation	3.83E-02
		Metabolism	Platelet Amyloid Precursor Protein	1.47E-02
		Hematopoiesis	Regulators of Bone Mineralization	2.58E-03

Table 6. 13 Modules in gene co-expression network in Figure 3 with their enriched pathways.

expressed in ovarian cancer and breast cancer (Helleman, et al., 2006; Turashvili, et al., 2007). COL3A1 encodes a fibrillar collagen which is a major component of the extracellular matrix protein surrounding cancer cells. Presence of ECM protein prevents apoptosis of cancer cells. COL3A1 plays an important role in apoptosis, proliferation regulation and anticancer drug resistance (Sethi, et al., 1999). RAP1GDS1 was under expressed in GBM tissue samples (P-value $< 4.4\times10^{-7}$) and had damage value 18 in the co-expression network. RAP1GDS1 is a transcription factor (Cimino, et al., 2001). It was reported that translocation fusion of the *NUP98* and *RAP1GDS1* genes was recurrent in T-cell acute lymphocytic leukemia (Hussey, et al., 1999).

3.2.3 Gene interaction network analysis

To further uncover the mechanism of the GBM, the proposed MI-based statistic was applied to expressions of 12,042 genes which were measured in 243 tumor tissue samples and 10 normal tissue samples and 1 cell line to detect pair-wise mRNA interaction between the genes. We detected 967 interaction with theoretic P-values$< 1.0\times10^{-15}$ accounting for 0.1% proportion of total interactions. Pair-wise mRNA interactions were assembled into interaction networks defined by representing genes as nodes, with an edge between two nodes if an interaction was observed between the corresponding genes. The resulting largest connected mRNA interaction network consists of 187 genes and 196 edges (Figure 4) . Its average shortest path length was 5.88 and diameter was 23.

Top 10 genes with the largest damage value were SIVA1, SLC27A5, PFDN5, GBAS, COX6A1, AKR1B1, NPM3, UBE2W, CDK4 and SGCG. The gene with both the largest degree (32) and damage value (62) in the mRNA interaction network was SIVA1, an apoptosis-inducing factor. SIVA1 was over expressed in the GBM tissue samples (P-value < 0.00061). Although it was not significantly differentially expressed, regulatory relationship between SIVA1 and each one of 32 genes was significantly different between the GBM tumor tissue and normal tissue samples. This indicated that SIVA1 can act synergistically to influence the development of the GBM. SIVA1 is a pro-apoptotic protein. Function of SIVA1 is to promote DNA damage induced apoptosis and inhibit NF-κB (Barkinge, et al., 2009). SIVA1 plays an important role in cell proliferation and death (Spinicelli, et al., 2002). It was reported that SIVA1 was involved in breast cancer (Chu, et al., 2005). GBAS named as Glioblastoma-amplified sequence, was located in Chromosomal region 7p12, which contains the EGFR gene, and was reported to be co-amplified with EGFR in glioblastomas (Wang, et al., 1998). It was over expressed with p-value 1.01×10^{-5} in our expression data.CDK4 with degree (8) and damage value (13) was up regulated in the GBM tumor tissue samples and significantly differentially expressed (P-value < 1.87×10^{-8}). CDK4 was a member of the Ser/Thr protein kinase family and involved in Glioma pathway(Zhu and Parada, 2002). CDK4 was an oncogene and was reported to be associated with multiple tumors(Kim and Diehl, 2009).

3.3 Network analysis of miRNA expressions

3.3.1 Differential expression analysis

To unravel the pattern of differential regulation of miRNA, expressions of 534 microRNAs including 470 human microRNAs were profiled in 240 tumor tissue samples and 10 normal tissue samples by Agilent 8 x 15K Human microRNA-specific microarray. A total of 149 miRNAs were differentially expressed between the GBM tumor tissue and normal tissue samples which were identified by Wilcoxon rank-sum test (P-value for declaring significance after Bonferroni correction is 9.36×10^{-5}). Of 149 differentially expressed miRNAs, 73 miRNAs were up-regulated and 76 down-regulated. Among them, 21, 81 and 15 miRNAs were reported to be associated with the GBM, other cancers and other diseases, respectively, in the literatures(Jiang, et al., 2009) .

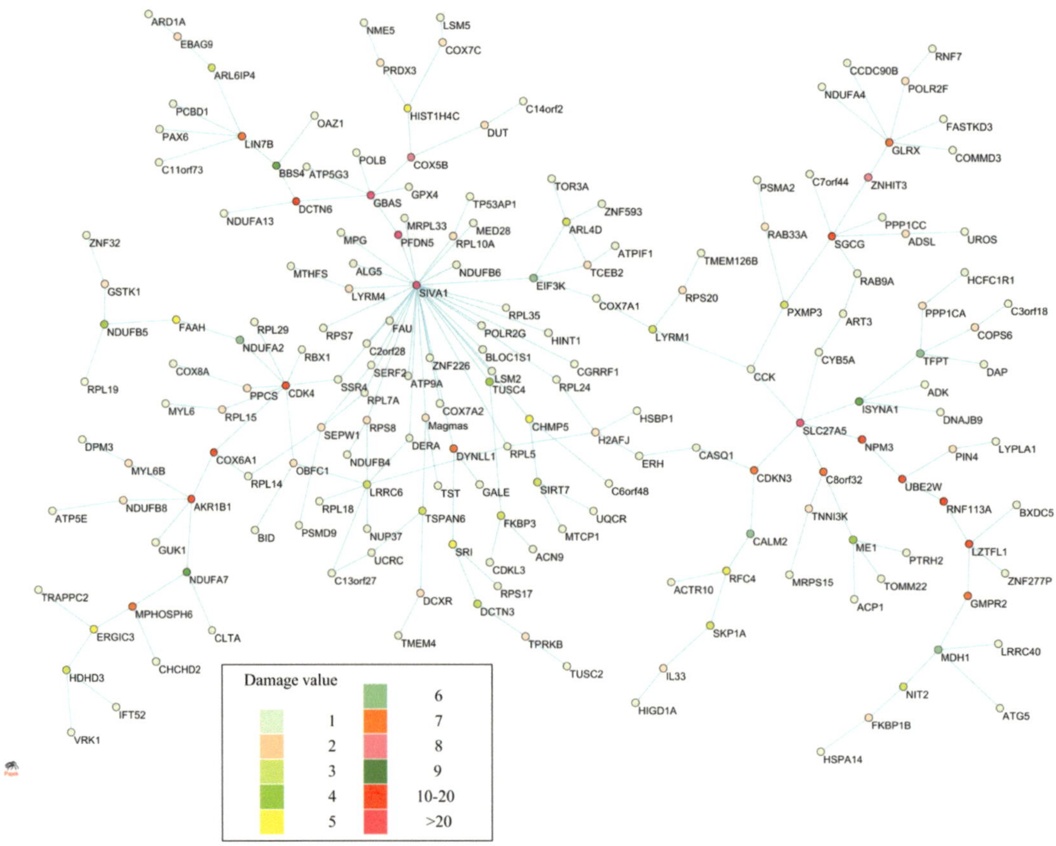

Fig. 4. Gene interaction network. The largest connected gene interaction network consists of 187 genes and 196 edges. Genes with different damage value were marked in different colors.

3.3.2 MiRNA co-expression network analysis

Similar to genes, miRNAs are not isolated, instead they act together to perform biological functions. Initiation and progression of cancer are influenced not only by individual miRNAs, but also by the coordinated effect of many miRNAs. To understand how miRNAs regulate biological processes at a system level, we reconstruct miRNA co-expression network. The largest connected miRNA coexpression network with the average shortest path 10.75 and diameter 49 had 385 miRNAs and 451 edges (Figure 5). One main feature of this miRNA coexpression network is that mir-770-5p and mir-329 divided the whole network into three subnetworks: the left, the middle and the right subnetwork. The middle subnetwork was densely connected.

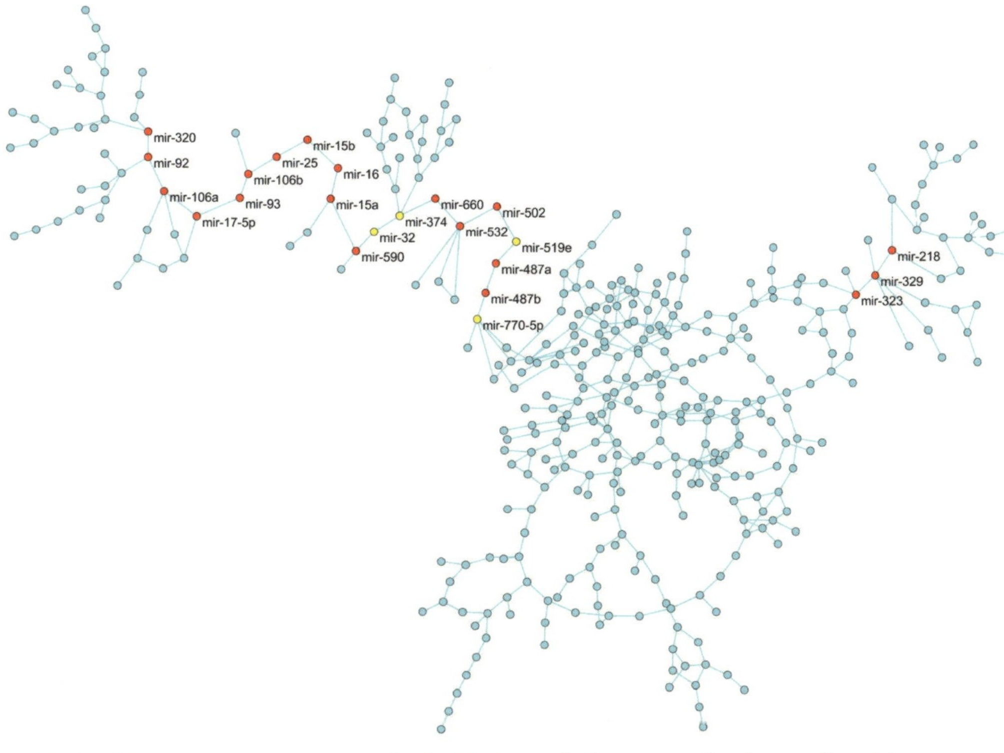

Fig. 5. MiRNAs coexpression network. MiRNAs with damage value larger than 20 were highlighted in red and yellow, where red nodes denoted significantly differentially expressed miRNAs (p-value$< 9.36 \times 10^{-5}$) and yellow nodes denoted they were not significant.

Similar to gene co-expression network, we used the damage value of a node as a robustness measure to rank the importance of a miRNA in miRNA co-expression network. We ranked all differentially expressed miRNAs in the largest miRNA co-expression network according to their damage values. There were 19 differentially expressed miRNAs with the largest damage values (>20) which we referred to as fragile miRNAs. Among the 19 fragile miRNAs, 16 miRNAs (14 miRNAs were over expressed in the GBM tissues) were in the left coexpression subnetwork, and 3 under expressed miRNAs were in the right coexpression subnetwork. The middle coexpression subnetwork contains no fragile miRNAs. Figure 5 showed that miRNAs in the middle coexpression subnetwork were densely connected. The middle coexpression network with large number of redundant miRNAs was highly robust in response to perturbation of external forces. From Figure 5, we can see that mir-487a, mir-487b, mir-502 and mir-532 were the most important components in the miRNA co-expression network. Removal of one of them would cause disconnection between the left part and right part of miRNA co-expression network and hence lead to dysfunction of the whole miRNA co-expression network. We observed that mir-487a and mi-487b were down-regulated, and mir-502 and mir-532 were up-regulated in the GBM tissues. We searched miR2disease database (Jiang, et al., 2009) and found that 7 of the 19 miRNAs were associated to GBM/glioma/ neuroblastoma (mir-15b, mir-25, mir-93, mir-17-5p, mir-323, mir-106a, mir-92), 6 others were associated with cancer and neuro-diseases(mir-487b, mir-15a, mir-16, mir-106b, mir-218, mir-320).

3.3.3 MiRNA interaction network analysis

We also used MI to quantify interaction between miRNAs and MI-based statistic to detect pair-wise interaction between miRNAs. We assembled the interacted miRNAs into miRNA interaction network. Significant P-values for declaring an interaction between miRNAs were 8.51×10^{-7} accounting for 1% proportion of total interactions. An assembled largest connected miRNA interaction network was shown in Figure 6. The network included 333 miRNAs and 563 interactions. Its average shortest path length was 5.10281 and diameter was 17.

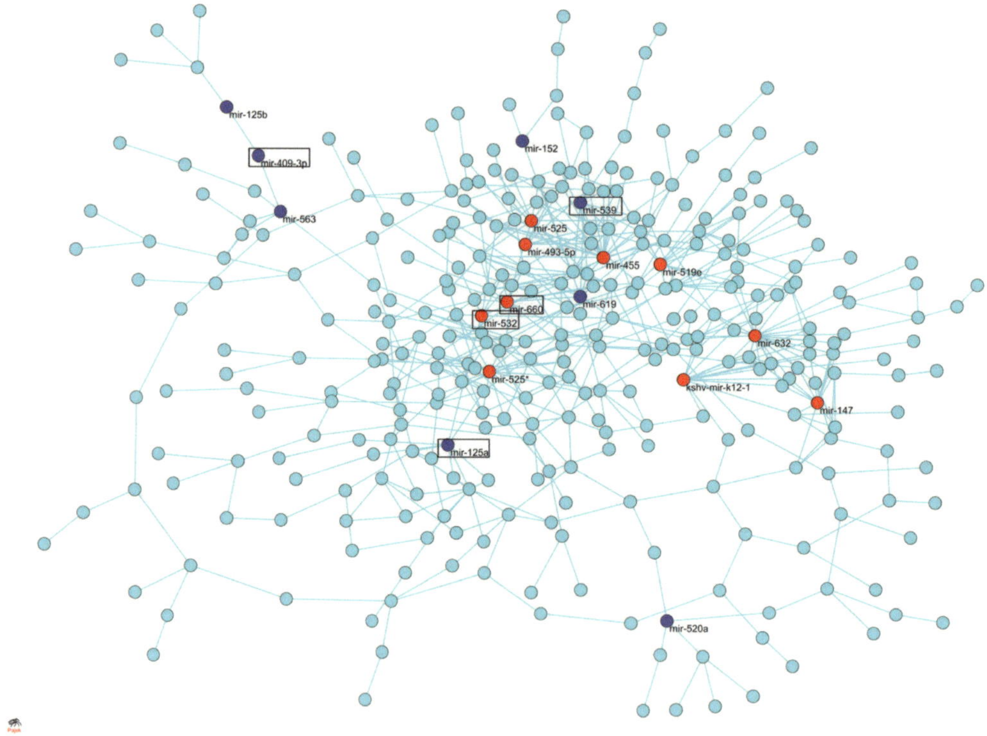

Fig. 6. MiRNA interaction network. miRNAs with damage value larger than 4 were marked in blue and miRNAs with degree larger than 9 were marked in red. Significantly differentially expressed miRNAs (p-value< 9.36×10^{-5}) were marked in black box.

To examine topological network properties of miRNA interaction networks, we also used the damage value and the degree of a node to identify cancer relevant miRNAs. Among all the miRNAs with either damage values greater than 4 or degrees greater than 9, miR-539 was associated with autism spectrum disorder (ASD), a brain development disorder(Abu-Elneel, et al., 2008). It was reported that mir-563 is involved in modulating tumors in variable microenvironments (Hebert, et al., 2007), miR-125a and miR-125b were indentified to control human neuroblastoma cell proliferation by repressing a common target gene NTRK3 (neurotrophic tyrosine kinase, receptor, type 3)(Laneve, et al., 2007). They were found to be down-modulated in primary neuroblastoma tumors and were under expressed with p-value 4.83×10^{-5} and 0.03 respectively in our dataset.

3.4 miRNA target networks

We compiled miRNA and mRNA expression data in 237 tumor tissue samples and 10 normal tissue samples for 1,697 differentially expressed mRNAs and 149 differentially expressed miRNAs. This resulted in extremely complex miRNA target networks. We found 3,953 matched miRNA-mRNA pairs for 127 differentially expressed miRNAs and 1, 089 differentially expressed genes. Of the 3,953 target-pairs, 65 down-regulated miRNAs targets 468 over expressed genes while 62 up-regulated miRNAs target 621 under expressed genes.

A total of 14 experimentally verified targets of 7 miRNAs were listed in Table 7. Of 8 miRNAs, 4 under expressed miRNAs (mir-124a, mir-29b, mir-29c and mir-33) function as tumor-suppressors and 4 over expressed miRNAs (mir-155, mir-16, mir-21 and mir-210) function as oncogenes. It has been reported that CTDSP1 was a validated target gene of mir-124a (Karginov, et al., 2007), RTN4 and SLC25A22 was validated targets of mir-16 (Selbach, et al., 2008). mir-21 was found to be over expressed in multiple cancers and down regulated tumor suppressor genes: TPM1, PTEN, PDCD4 BASP1 and RTN4 in invasion and metastasis of cancer(Yang, et al., 2009). BASP1 is a transcriptional cosuppressor for the Wilms' tumor suppressor protein WT1, thus it can regulate WT1 transcriptional activity (Carpenter, et al., 2004). Nogo-A , one protein isoforms encoded by RTN4, had turned out to be a neuronal protein involved in diverse processes that go from axonal fasciculation to apoptosis(Mingorance, et al., 2004). Mir-155 targeted a regulator of apoptosis gene: LDOC1 (Skalsky, et al., 2007). Up-regulation of miR-210 directly targeted gene EFNA3, which is crucial for endothelial cell response to hypoxia, affecting cell survival, migration, and differentiation (Fasanaro, et al., 2008). Mir-29c was reported to be under expressed in Nasopharyngeal Carcinomas and up-regulated genes COL4A1, COL4A2 and TDG (Sengupta, et al., 2008). COL4A1, COL4A2 were genes encoding extracellular matrix proteins, as we discussed previously, they played an important role in apoptosis, proliferation regulation and anticancer drug resistance (Sethi, et al., 1999) . COL4A2 was validated to be also targets of mir-29b in another research group (Li, et al., 2009). TDG was involved in DNA repair, a process frequently dysregulated in many cancers (Sengupta, et al., 2008). In mouse and human cells, miR-33 inhibits the expression of ABCA1, thereby attenuating cholesterol efflux to apolipoprotein A1 (Rayner, et al., 2010). It was also reported that the role of miR-33 controlling the hematopoietic stem cells self-renewal through p53 may lead to the prevention and treatment of hematopoietic disorders (Herrera-Merchan, et al., 2010).

The resulting miRNA target networks have several remarkable features. First, many important genes in the mRNA co-expression networks were targets of differentially expressed miRNAs. Top 17 genes with damage values greater than 19 in the gene co-expression network were negatively regulated by 34 differentially expressed miRNAs. All 17 genes and many miRNAs were crucial components in the gene and miRNA

miRNA	P-value for differential expression	Up or down regulated	Gene	P-value for differential expression	Up or down regulated	Regression coefficient	P-value for regression	Coefficient	Refer
mir-124a	8.62E-08	Down	CTDSP1	8.4E-07	Up	-17.7	2.22E-16	0.244	Karginov, et al., 2007
mir-155	1.31E-07	Up	*LDOC1	1.67E-07	Down	-197	4.00E-15	0.223	Skalsky, et al., 2007
mir-155	1.31E-07	Up	SCAMP1	3.27E-06	Down	-30.9	6.06E-10	0.145	Selbach, et al., 2008
mir-16	0.0000178	Up	*RTN4	9.44E-08	Down	-766	2.66E-08	0.119	Selbach, et al., 2008
mir-16	0.0000178	Up	SLC25A22	3.36E-08	Down	-37.8	1.97E-11	0.168	Selbach, et al., 2008
mir-16	0.0000178	Up	VTI1B	7.15E-08	Down	-122	1.03E-05	0.0765	Selbach, et al., 2008
mir-21	9.98E-08	Up	BASP1	2.98E-08	Down	-743	0.00E+00	0.349	Yang, et al., 2009
mir-21	9.98E-08	Up	RTN4	9.44E-08	Down	-246	1.16E-05	0.0756	Yang, et al., 2009
mir-210	1.48E-06	Up	EFNA3	4.67E-07	Down	-10.4	4.61E-05	0.0657	Fasanaro, et al., 2008
mir-29b	2.07E-07	Down	COL4A2	1.83E-07	Up	-164	8.92E-05	0.0609	Li, et al., 2009
mir-29c	3.66E-07	Down	COL4A2	1.83E-07	Up	-260	1.99E-07	0.105	Sengupta, et al., 2008
mir-29c	3.66E-07	Down	COL4A1	4.91E-08	Up	-389	1.35E-08	0.124	Sengupta, et al., 2008
mir-29c	3.66E-07	Down	TDG	5.21E-07	Up	-95.5	3.22E-14	0.21	Sengupta, et al., 2008
mir-33	9.6317E-06	Down	ABCA1	1.0396E-06	Up	-114.5	5.941E-12	0.176	Rayner, et al., 2010

* LDOC1 and RTN4 are tumor suppressor genes

Table 7. Experimentally verified targets.

coexpression networks. Their altered expressions played an important role in tumorigenesis. Among them, overexpressed RBBP4 (P-value 1.8×10^{-8}) with the largest damage value (37) in the table was negatively regulated by under expressed mir-29b (P-value 2.07×10^{-7} and mir-29c (P-value 3.66×10^{-7}), underexpressed TRIM8 (P-value 3.77×10^{-6}) with the damage value 29 was negatively regulated by overexpressed mir-629 (P-value 2.02×10^{-7}), overexpressed TP53 ((P-value 1.40×10^{-7}) with damage value 23 was negatively regulated by underexpressed mir-485-5p. RBBP4 has been implicated in chromatin remodeling and regulation of cell proliferation. It has been reported that RBBP4 is overexpressed in different human tumors, such as lung, liver and thyroid cancer, acute myelocytic leukemia, and acute lymphoblastic leukemia (Pacifico, et al., 2007). TRIM8 is thought of as a new tumor suppressor gene (Caligo, et al., 1997).

Second, many genes targeted by critical components in miRNA co-expression network, played important roles in regulation of neural process and tumor genesis. To study the function of the top 19 differentially expressed miRNAs with the largest damage values, we constructed mRNA target network of these 19 miRNAs with 476 nodes and 1,128 arcs and 174 edges shown in Figure 7A, where 5 underexpressed miRNAs negatively regulated 85 over expressed genes and 14 overexpressed miRNA negatively regulated 372 underexpressed genes, 1,128 arcs were miRNA-mRNA pairs, 15 edges connected co-expressed miRNAs, and remaining 159 edges linked co-expressed genes. The genes with large damage value or related to cancer in the gene co expression network were highlighted and those gene were marked in the Figure 7A. 8 genes with the damage values greater than 15 were regulated by 11 miRNAs with the damage values greater than 20. 14 of the15 cancer genes in Figure 7A were under-expressed FBXW7, GABRA1, MYT1L, NEFL, RTN1, SH3GL2, SNAP25, SV2B, SYN2, KIAA0774, VSNL1, NEFM, RIMS2, SYT1. These genes were regulated by 10 overexpressed miRNAs: mir-15b, mir-25, mir-16, mir-92, mir-15a, mir-320, mir-106b, mir-93, mir-106a, mir-17-5p, which were connected in the mRNA co-expression network (Figure 7B). They are involved in synaptic transmission process. Neuron communication occurs at the synapse via neurotransmitters. MYT1L (myelin transcription factor 1-like) regulates nervous system development. Both SYT1 and VSNL1 serve as Ca(2+) sensors in synaptic transmission(Maglott, et al., 2007). SNAP25 is a presynaptic plasma membrane protein and regulates neurotransmitter release. It is reported that SNAP25 is implicated in neuritogenesis in human neuroblastoma(Heraud, et al., 2008). GABRA1 encodes a gamma-aminobutyric acid (GABA) receptor and GABA is the major inhibitory neurotransmitter in the mammalian brain. Both NEFL and NEFM are Neurofilaments. They play a role in intracellular transport to axons and dendrites. NRGN encodes a postsynaptic protein kinase substrate that binds calmodulin in the absence of calcium and is a direct target for thyroid hormone in human brain(Maglott, et al., 2007). FBXW7 serves as a negative regulator of oncoprotein and is a general tumor suppressor. It regulates cell differentiation and proliferation. It has been reported that FBXW7 is implied in various cancers including glioblastoma(Hagedorn, et al., 2007). Remaining genes that were involved in neuron communication include SLC6A15, SYN2, SV2B and RIMS2. SLC6A15 is a neurotransmitter transporter, SYN2 is a member of the synapsin gene family, SV2B is synaptic vesicle glycoprotein and RIMS2 regulates synaptic membrane exocytosis(Maglott, et al., 2007).

Table 8 summarizes the major functions of target genes of miRNAs in Figure 7A where right-railed Fisher's exact test were used to test for significantly enriched GO categories or pathways. Table 8 shows that the target genes of these miRNAs were mainly involved in cancer related signaling pathways and nerves systems process including synapse, synaptic transmission, neurotransmitter transport, nervous system development and neurological system process. It is interesting to note that co-expressed mir-15a, mir-15b, mir-16, mir-25 and mir-92 were major miRNAs that targeted genes in both cancer related signaling pathways and nerves systems process.

Gene Ontology (GO) category or pathway	Enrichment P-values								
	mir-15b	mir-15a	mir-16	mir-25	mir-106a	mir-93	mir-106b	mir-92	mir-323
Glioma		1.9E-02							
Regulation of neurotransmitter levels		1.3E-02	1.1E-02						
Neurotransmitter transport	6.8E-03	1.5E-02	3.3E-02	3.9E-02					
Long-term potentiation	4.2E-03	3.7E-05	2.4E-03	3.1E-02		1.4E-02	5.3E-03		
Synaptic transmission	2.4E-04	4.0E-04	5.3E-04	3.0E-06		4.4E-02		1.6E-03	
Neurotransmitter secretion		1.7E-02	1.0E-02	2.9E-02					
Nervous system development	3.2E-02	1.3E-02	5.5E-03				2.7E-02		
Central nervous system development			2.5E-02						
Transmission of nerve impulse	2.3E-04	9.6E-04	4.8E-04	1.8E-06				6.0E-04	
Regulation of synaptic plasticity				4.6E-02					
Synaptic vesicle transport		2.8E-02						3.1E-02	
Regulation of synapse structure and activity				4.6E-02					
Neurological system process	7.1E-03	4.3E-03	5.1E-03	1.5E-04				3.1E-03	
Learning and/or memory	3.7E-02								
Learning	4.0E-02								
Neurofilament				2.1E-02					
Synaptic vesicle	1.1E-02		8.0E-03	2.7E-02					
Synaptosome								1.4E-02	
Synaptic vesicle membrane				3.4E-02					
Neuron projection			4.5E-02						

Synapse part				4.7E-05	1.5E-02	2.5E-03	1.6E-02	1.2E-02	
Synapse	4.9E-03	1.5E-02	2.1E-02	1.1E-07	6.2E-03	8.4E-04	5.3E-03	2.3E-04	
Axon guidance						2.1E-02			
Antigen processing and presentation									4.0E-02
Ras protein signal transduction					1.9E-02		2.3E-02		
Calcium ion transport	1.8E-03	3.6E-04	7.8E-03				4.2E-02		
Calcium signaling pathway	2.7E-04	7.5E-06	1.7E-03	1.7E-02		2.0E-04	2.2E-05		
Cell communication	1.9E-02	2.2E-02	5.6E-03	2.3E-03		1.8E-02	2.6E-02	2.5E-02	
Cell-cell signaling	1.4E-03	8.1E-04	9.5E-04	4.2E-06				7.0E-03	
Wnt signaling pathway		4.0E-02				2.9E-03	7.6E-03		
MAPK signaling pathway		1.5E-02	8.4E-03			3.8E-02	2.6E-02		
GnRH signaling pathway	1.0E-02	8.7E-05	6.6E-03						
ErbB signaling pathway		2.2E-02	3.0E-02						
B cell receptor signaling pathway						6.3E-03			
VEGF signaling pathway						8.4E-03			
T cell receptor signaling pathway						2.1E-02			
Apoptosis						2.1E-02			

Table 8. Function of target genes of 9 miRNAs.

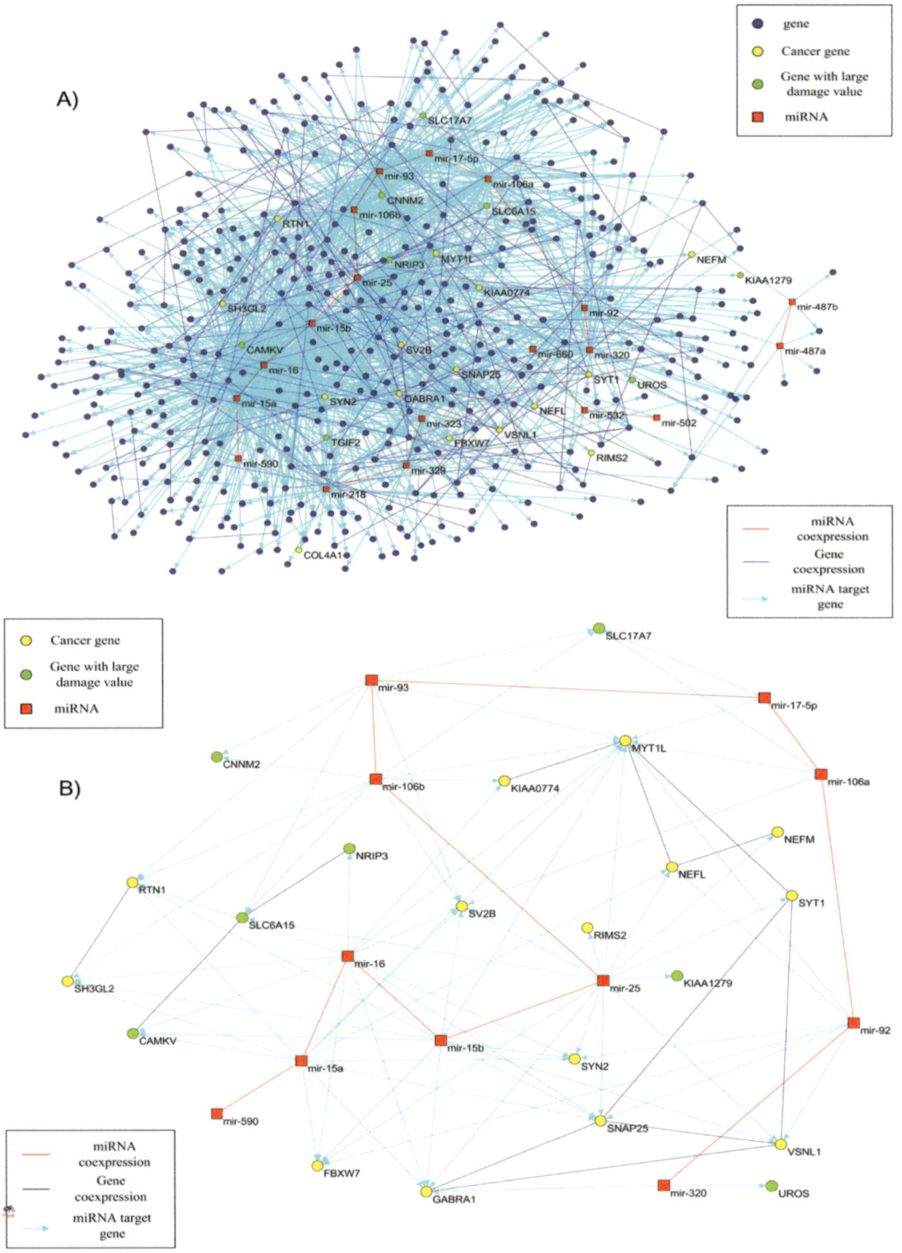

Fig. 7. MiRNA target (sub)network. (A) mRNA target networks of the 19 miRNAs with 476 nodes and 1,128 arcs and 174 edges, where 1128 arcs were miRNA-mRNA pairs, 15 edges connected coexpressed miRNAs, and remaining 159 edges linked coexpressed genes. The genes with large damage value or related to cancer in the co expression network genes were highlighted and those gene names were marked in the figure. (B) MiRNA target subnetwork. 7 genes with the damage values greater than 15 and 14 cancer related genes were regulated by 11 miRNAs with the damage values greater than 20. Those nodes and edges were extracted from Figure 7A mRNA target network.

Third, contribution of miRNAs to expression variation of some genes is very high. The proportion of expression variation of target gene explained by the linear influence of miRNA variation can be measured by the coefficient of determination (R^2). There were a total of 78 under-expressed genes with the coefficient of determination greater than 20% which were negatively regulated by 7 overexpressed miRNAs: mir-15a, mir-15b, mir-16, mir-25, mir-93, mir-106a and mir-106b. Surprisingly, up to 33% of expression variations of underexpressed gene GCC2 were explained by single overexpressed mir-25. Functional roles of GCC2 in cancer are unknown. The gene with the second largest coefficient of determination was CAMK2N1. Its 28% of expression variations were explained by overexpressed mir-106b. It was reported that CAMK2N1 is a candidate tumor suppressor (Wang, et al., 2008). Function of CAMK2N1 is to inhibit MEK/ERK activity and induce p27 accumulation which negatively regulates cell-cycle progression. Reducing expression of CAMK2N1 will accelerate tumor growth. 26% of expression variation of CPEB1 that regulates synaptic plasticity and is implied in cancer development (Hansen, et al., 2009) and GRM1 that is involved in neurotransmitter in the central nervous system and implicated in Melanoma (Namkoong, et al., 2007) was explained by overexpressed mir-25 and mir-15b, respectively. Expressions of genes SYT1, SNAP25, GABRA1, VSNL1, MYT1L, SV2B, SYN2 and SLC12A5 which were involved in synaptic transmission, were also largely regulated by miRNAs.

Fourth, we observed that one miRNA may target multiple genes (up to 179 mRNAs) directly or indirectly, and multiple miRNAs (up to 9 miRNAs) can target a given gene. More than 40% of expression variation of each of six genes (YWHAH, GABRA1, DYNC1I1, ERC2, PEX5L and CAMK2G) was explained by several miRNAs. Expressions of these genes were largely regulated by multiple differentially expressed miRNAs. YWHAH and GABRA1 are implied in neural diseases, and CAMK2G is involved in regulation of plasticity at glutamatergic synapses(Maglott, et al., 2007). Functions of other three genes are unknown.

3.5 DNA methylation analysis

To study how genes are regulated by DNA methylation in GBM, two methylation datasets: OMA-002 dataset and OMA-003 dataset were generated by TCGA project. OMA-002 dataset used the Illumina GoldenGate Methylation Cancer Panel 1 platform, which contains 1,505 CpG loci selected from 813 genes. OMA-002 dataset included 239 GBM tumor tissue samples and 1 cell line, 228 of which were shared among the miRNA expression, gene expression datasets and thus used for Methylation-miRNA regression and Methylation-gene regression analysis. OMA-003 dataset used the Custom Illumina Goldengate Methylation Cancer Panel, which contains 1,489 gene promoters. 245 GBM tumor samples and 1 cell line were used for experimented, 234 of which were shared among the miRNA expression, gene expression datasets and used for Methylation-miRNA regression and Methylation-gene regression analysis.

A total number of 341 genes were hypomethylated genes (average methylation ratio < 0.25 and fold changes <0.5) in two datasets and 113 hypermethylated genes (average methylation ratio > 0.75 and fold changes > 1.5) in glioblastomas. For OMA002 dataset we averaged the methylation ratio for several probes in one gene. To investigate the effects of aberrant methylation on gene expressions, we regressed gene expression on the methylation profile. We found that 120 hypermethylated genes negatively regulated 404 under expressed genes, and 41 hypomethylated genes negatively regulated 85 overexpressed genes. One methylated gene might influence expressions of up to 142 genes and multiple methylated genes (up to 32) might regulate a given gene. Interestingly, we found that 56.3% of expression variation of underexpressed tumor-suppressor gene BCL11B (P-value 1.75×10^{-7}) is explained by hypermethylated gene HLA-DPB1 with Average methylation 0.9631 and fold change 7.4. We also found that a total of 24 hypermethylated genes that silenced expression of BCL11B (Table 9). These hypermethylated genes include PMP22, a major component of myelin in the peripheral nervous system, GPR116, involved in neuropeptide signaling pathway, LTA, involved in apoptosis. Another gene with the largest coefficient of determination was ANXA5(P-value 3.07×10^{-6}). ANXA5 binds to phosphatidylserine, which is one of the "eat me" signals at the surface of the apoptotic cell, thus involved in apoptosis and cancers (Boersma, et al., 2005). Up to 11 hypormethylated genes were negatively correlated with overexpression of ANXA5 (Table 9).

Methylation also directly or indirectly regulates expression of miRNAs. We observed that 29 underexpressed and 26 overexpressed miRNAs were directly or indirectly regulated by 82 hypermethylated genes. One hypermethylated gene might significantly influence expressions of up to 25 miRNAs and multiple hypermethylated genes (up to 30) might influence expression of one miRNA. We also found that a total of 67 hypomethylated genes directly or indirectly induced expression variation of 38 down regulated and 23 up regulated miRNAs. One hypomethylated gene might influence expression of up to 25 miRNAs and multiple hypomethylated genes (up to 22) might influence expression of one miRNA.

A total of 542 underexpressed and 218 overexpressed genes were directly or indirectly regulated by 61 underexpressed and 62 overexpressed miRNAs, and 300 hypomethylated and 149 hypermethylated genes. In general, multiple miRNAs and methylated genes jointly contribute (in many cases, indirectly) to the variation of gene expressions. In many cases, both miRNAs and methylation repressed gene expression. However, surprisingly we observed that indirect effect of methylation on the regulation of gene expression was to increase gene expression rather than repressing gene expression. Functions of the many genes regulated by both miRNAs and methylation such as ANXA5, CACYBP, SLC17A7, SLC6A15, INA, SHANK2, PAK3, RIMS2, NBEA, VSNL1, GABRG2, PCLO, VAMP2, PLCB1, GRM7 and SNAP25 were involved in neuron communication and in nervous system. We also found that expressions of the cancer relevant genes TRIM8 (which has been tested for association with Glioblastoma), TP53, FGF13, ENC1, FBXW7, BCL2L2 were influenced by both miRNAs and methylation.

Methylated gene	Average Methylation	Fold Changes	Regu-lated	Regression coefficient	P-value	Coeffi-cient
HLA-	0.963075314	7.408272	BCL11B	-2.01E+02	0.00E+00	5.63E-01
TNF	0.954752441	5.967203	BCL11B	-1.30E+02	2.22E-16	2.59E-01
PMP22	0.912672293	40.56321	BCL11B	-5.31E+01	6.94E-13	2.06E-01
GPR116	0.945111576	7.270089	BCL11B	-7.32E+01	6.84E-11	1.72E-01

Methylated gene	Average Methylation	Fold Changes	Regu-lated	Regression coefficient	P-value	Coeffi-cient
FLJ25084	0.881295918	2.037678	BCL11B	-6.56E+01	5.84E-11	1.69E-01
EGF	0.870425384	2.451902	BCL11B	-3.42E+01	2.84E-09	1.45E-01
FCRLM1	0.819928571	46.85306	BCL11B	-2.57E+01	4.03E-09	1.39E-01
LTA	0.887046722	18.67467	BCL11B	-5.02E+01	9.74E-09	1.36E-01
TRPM5	0.84431311	2.447284	BCL11B	-4.26E+01	8.54E-08	1.19E-01
MPL	0.841936275	7.165415	BCL11B	-3.40E+01	9.62E-08	1.19E-01
BLK	0.954205021	42.40911	BCL11B	-1.01E+02	5.84E-07	1.05E-01
IL4	0.846998588	2.540996	BCL11B	-3.64E+01	8.17E-07	1.03E-01
HLA-DOB	0.886698047	39.4088	BCL11B	-4.82E+01	9.44E-07	1.01E-01
CD1D	0.955290456	3.746237	BCL11B	-6.56E+01	1.09E-06	9.92E-02
CLDN4	0.843246165	16.06183	BCL11B	-3.49E+01	1.29E-06	9.87E-02
CXCL9	0.76874477	2.520475	BCL11B	-2.14E+01	1.36E-06	9.83E-02
KISS1	0.925806122	4.571882	BCL11B	-5.68E+01	1.59E-06	9.47E-02
APOC2	0.88015625	1.614966	BCL11B	-4.65E+01	1.33E-05	9.29E-02
TNFRSF10	0.929268207	2.323171	BCL11B	-4.22E+01	4.64E-06	8.92E-02
C18orf2	0.755978723	4.142349	BCL11B	-1.77E+01	1.24E-05	8.26E-02
PLA2G2A	0.785191771	31.40767	BCL11B	-2.25E+01	1.11E-05	8.21E-02
EPHX1	0.900292887	1.809634	BCL11B	-5.92E+01	1.16E-05	8.17E-02
PLA2G2A	0.809780335	2.816627	BCL11B	-2.74E+01	2.04E-05	7.74E-02
KLK11	0.873908647	2.39427	BCL11B	-3.44E+01	2.33E-05	7.63E-02
MMP14	0.214993026	0.217165	ANXA5	-2.11E+03	0.00E+00	2.91E-01
MST150	0.230010204	0.2788	ANXA5	-1.44E+03	1.09E-13	2.12E-01
COL5A2	0.201823129	0.260417	ANXA5	-2.06E+03	1.55E-12	1.94E-01
FRZB	0.152287308	0.491249	ANXA5	-1.62E+03	2.91E-11	1.78E-01
PAX6	0.094173729	0.396521	ANXA5	-2.43E+03	3.41E-10	1.62E-01
MMP14	0.165882148	0.402139	ANXA5	-2.45E+03	3.66E-09	1.43E-01
DES	0.192259414	0.359363	ANXA5	-1.37E+03	1.66E-07	1.14E-01
LOX	0.125711297	0.177058	ANXA5	-1.69E+03	2.65E-07	1.11E-01
NEBL	0.06257483	0.161483	ANXA5	-2.18E+03	2.55E-06	9.12E-02
SPARC	0.150543933	0.174039	ANXA5	-1.99E+03	6.49E-06	8.62E-02
FGFR2	0.048397711	0.116621	ANXA5	-2.32E+03	1.94E-05	7.98E-02

Table 9. 24 hypermethylated genes negatively regulated expression of gene BCL11B and 11 hypomethylated genes regulated expression of gene ANXA5.

3.6 Deciphering the path connecting mutations to gene and miRNA expression.

To study function of somatic mutations and LOH and connect them with disease through gene expressions and miRNAs, we study their *cis* or *trans* regulatory effects on gene or miRNA expression traits. We applied the group regression method to expression profiles of 12,042 genes and expression profiles of 470 human microRNAs in 169 tumor tissue samples from glioblastomas patients, which were shared among the gene expression, miRNA expression and mutation datasets.

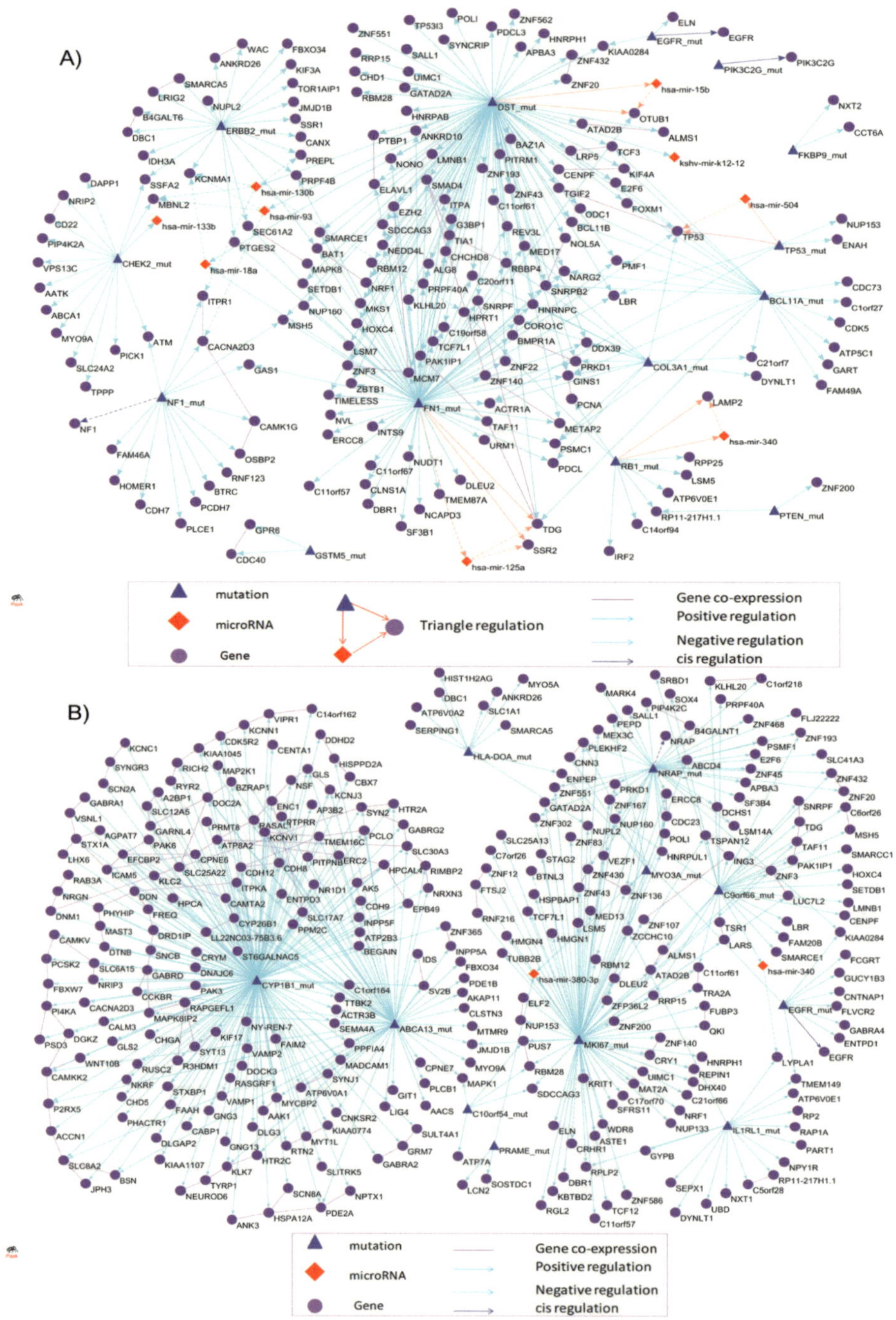

Fig. 8. Somatic and LOH mutation eQTL network. (A) Somatic mutation eQTL network. A network that connects 14 genes with somatic mutations associated with GBM, their regulated mRNAs and miRNA expressions was shown. (B) LOH mutation eQTL network. A network that connects 11 genes with LOH associated with GBM, their regulated mRNAs and miRNA expressions was shown.

Mutation	Gene expression				miRNA expression			
Gene	Gene	Damage value	P-value for gene expression	Up or down regulate	miRNA	Damage value	P-value for miRNA expression	Up or down regulated
RB1	LAMP2	0	8.22E-07	Up	hsa-mir-340	0	1.16E-06	Down
DST	OTUB1	0	5.33E-07	Down	hsa-mir-15b	45	1.30E-06	Up
FN1	SSR2	0	3.67E-07	Up	hsa-mir-125a	2	4.83E-05	Down
FN1	TDG	3	5.21E-07	Up	hsa-mir-125a	2	4.83E-05	Down
TP53	TP53	23	1.40E-07	Up	hsa-mir-504	1	1.42E-06	Down
Mutation-gene regression			miRNA-gene regression			Mutation -miRNA regression		
Regression coefficient	P-value	Coefficient of determination	Regression coefficient	P-value	Coefficient of determination	Regression coefficient	P-value	Coefficient of determination
1.03E+00	7.04E-04	6.47E-02	-2.77E+02	3.17E-06	8.50E-02	1.81E+00	4.10E-09	1.85E-01
1.23E+00	5.91E-04	6.65E-02	-2.28E+01	9.77E-07	9.34E-02	1.27E+00	3.80E-04	7.18E-02
1.54E+00	1.02E-05	1.07E-01	-2.33E+02	4.92E-05	6.52E-02	-1.18E+00	8.72E-04	6.33E-02
1.39E+00	7.60E-05	8.72E-02	-6.91E+01	4.77E-05	6.54E-02	-1.18E+00	8.72E-04	6.33E-02
2.81E-01	3.30E-02	2.62E-02	-4.14E+01	2.72E-06	8.61E-02	3.43E-01	9.10E-03	3.93E-02

Table 10. Genes with somatic mutations regulate both mRNA and miRNA expressions, and formed triangle regulation cycles.

We first studied *cis* regulatory effects of somatic and LOH mutations on mRNA or miRNA expression traits. For somatic mutation, we found four cis-eQTL: TP53, EGFR, NF1and PIK3C2G. P-values for testing association of somatic mutations in TP53 , EGFR, NF1 and PIK3C2G with their expressions were 0.033, 0.019, 0.028 and 0.006, respectively. Fold changes (defined as the ratio of their average expressions of the samples with somatic mutations over the average expressions of the samples without somatic mutations) for the 4 genes were 1.10,1.73, 0.86,1.23, respectively. Although regression analysis did not show significant association of somatic mutations in BCL11A, FN1 and COL3A1 with their expressions due to very low frequencies of mutations, the fold changes were 1.45, 0.60 and 0.20, respectively. We still observed some regulatory effects of somatic mutations on these two genes. For LOH mutation, two cis-eQTL: NRAP and EGFR were detected with P-values 0.030, 0.034 and fold change 0.90 and 2.32, respectively. Regression analysis did not show significant association of LOH mutations in gene CYP1B1 with their expressions, but the fold change were 0.48.

Next we identified *trans*-regulatory effects of somatic and LOH mutations on mRNA or miRNA expression traits. The thresholds for declaring significant association of the set of somatic mutation and LOH in the gene with mRNA and miRNA expression after Bonferroni correction for multiple tests were 1.63×10^{-4} and 4.03×10^{-4}, respectively. A network that connects 14 genes with somatic mutations associated with GBM, and their regulated mRNAs and miRNA expressions was shown in Figure 8A. Somatic mutations in these 14 genes were strongly correlated with expressions of 177 significantly differentially expressed genes, 45 of which were under-expressed and 132 were over-expressed in tumor tissue samples, a total of 262 trans gene eQTL were found. These mutations also significantly affected expressions of 23 miRNAs, 11 of which were underexpressed and 12 were overexpressed and a total of 26 trans miRNA eQTL were found. Remarkably, we found 5 paths: (1) RB1 with association of somatic mutations with GBM regulated expressions of gene LAMP2 and mir-340, and mir-340 in turn targeted gene LAMP2; (2) DST with association of somatic mutations regulated expressions of both gene OTUB1 and mir-15b and mir-15b in turn targeted gene OTUB1; (3) FN1 with association of somatic mutations regulated expressions of both SSR2 and mir-125a and mir-125a in turn targeted gene SSR2; (4) FN1 with association of somatic mutations regulated expressions of both gene TDG and mir-125a and mir-125a in turn targeted gene TDG; and (5) TP53 with association of somatic mutations regulated expressions of both gene TP53 and mir-504 and mir-504 in turn targeted TP53 (Table 10).

Similarly, Figure 8B showed a network that connects 11 genes with LOH mutations associated with GMB, their regulated mRNAs and miRNA expressions. These 11 genes with LOH as *trans*-eQTL affected 323 differentially expressed or interacted genes, 190 of which were underexpressed genes and 133 were overexpressed, a total of 409 *trans gene*-eQTL were found. The LOH also affected expressions of 19 miRNAs, 9 of which were underexpressed and 10 were overexpressed, 2 of them were differentially expressed and a total of 27 *trans miRNA*-eQTL were found.

Sources for regulating gene expressions include DNA variations, miRNAs, and methylation. To provide a comprehensive view of how DNA variations, miRNA and methylation directly or indirectly regulate gene expression, we found a total of 87 underexpressed and 48 overexpressed genes which were commonly regulated by 38 underexpressed and 28 overexpressed miRNAs, 14 hypomethylated and 107 hypemethylated genes, and 9 significant somatic mutation and 10 significant LOH mutation. Surprisingly, multiple genetic perturbations such as multiple genes with somatic mutations or LOH, multiple miRNAs and multiple methylation may directly or indirectly regulate expression of a single gene. For example, expression levels of BCL11b which is a haploinsufficient tumor suppressor gene were positively regulated by genes DST and BCL11A, with associated somatic mutations, and were negatively affected by over-expressed mir-155, mir-23a, mir-92b and mir-30a-5p, and 24 hypermethylated genes.

4. Discussion and conclusion

Genetic and epigenetic alternations that are likely to cause tumor formation are often organized into complex biological networks. Genetic and epigenetic risk factors individually cannot fully explain initiation and progression of cancer. The purpose of this report is (1) to explore the possibility of integrating altered DNA variations, mRNA and miRNA expression variation, and methylation patterns into multi-level complex genetic and epigenetic networks that contribute to tumorigenesis; (2) decipher paths from somatic mutations and LOH to tumor formation through genetic and epigenetic networks; and (3) identify key genetic and epigenetic alternations causing tumor formation by network analysis.

The approach developed here for integrating genetic and epigenetic alternations into molecular networks consists of three steps. The first step is to reconstruct single type molecular networks whose components are of the same type of molecules, either mRNAs or miRNAs. We reconstructed mRNA co-expression networks and miRNA co-expression networks for glioblastoma using partial correlation approach. The co-expression networks attempt to uncover the regulatory relationships among mRNAs or miRNAs. However, many examples show that the regulatory relationships may be changed when normal tissues become tumor tissues. To identify the alternated regulations we developed a novel mutual information-based statistic for testing interactions between mRNAs or miRNAs, which allow detecting differential regulations between tumor and normal tissues, and reconstructed mRNA and miRNA interaction networks. The second step is to identify miRNA target and reconstruct miRNA target networks that connect mRNA and miRNA co-expression networks or mRNA and miRNA interaction networks.

The third step is to decipher the paths from somatic and LOH mutations to tumor formation. The first issue is how to test association of somatic mutations or LOH with glioblastoma. We developed a group association test that is based on population genetics for assessing association of somatic mutations and LOH with cancer. We identified 14 genes harboring somatic mutations associated with glioblastoma and 11 genes harboring LOH associated with glioblastoma. The second issue is how to uncover the components of mRNA or miRNA co-expression networks and interaction networks that respond to somatic mutations and LOH associated with glioblastoma. Traditionally, when alleles are common, these components are identified by mapping *cis*-eQTL or *trans*-eQTL. However, when alleles are rare, these components are hard to find by individually mapping *cis*-eQTL or *trans*-eQTL. The approach developed here is to extend group tests for a qualitative trait to a quantitative trait. The components that respond to perturbation of rare somatic genetic variants were identified by regressing the expression of an mRNA or an miRNA on the number of all mutated alleles across the gene. We discovered large comprehensive genetic and epigenetic networks that connect genes harboring associated mutations or LOH, mRNAs and miRNAs. Interestingly, we found five triangle cycles in the networks which indicated that significantly associated somatic mutations or LOH regulated both differentially expressed mRNA and miRNA and the miRNA in turn also affected expression levels of the mRNA. The approach presented here has two remarkable features. First, it offered a powerful tool for differentiating driver mutations from passenger mutations. Second, it provides functional information on how somatic or LOH mutations lead to tumorigenesis through complex genetic and epigenetic networks. Similar to mutations, methylation is another source for causing tumorigenesis. By regressing expression levels of mRNA or miRNA on methylation level, we can incorporate methylation into network. Finally we identified large genetic and epigenetic networks including associated mutations, LOH, methylation, differentially expressed mRNAs and miRNAs to explain how mutations and methylation cause tumorigenesis through molecular networks.

Our studies support the hypothesis that cancer may be the emergent properties of large genetic and epigenetic networks that are highly interconnected. Genetic, epigenetic and environmental stimuli can be viewed as random attacks to genetic and epigenetic networks. Topological properties of the genetic and epigenetic networks are closely related to the function of cells. Cancer arises from the failure of genetic and epigenetic networks to respond to attacks. In other words, the attacked networks are unable to return to their normal states and remain functional in the face of random perturbations. We suspect that key components of network contributing to the robustness of the network also play an important role in the function of cells. We modeled over- or under-expression of mRNA and miRNA, methylation, and genetic alternation as deletion of a node in the network which will cause dynamical changes in the network and used a damage value of the node to measure its contribution to the robustness of the network. We found the several cancers related genes such as TP53 have large damage values in the genetic and epigenetic networks. These key components in the network may serve as therapeutic intervention points.

Our results are preliminary. Although network analysis may have the potential to unravel the mechanism of tumor initiation and progression, the presented network structures and their properties in this report may depend on sample size. Whether the structures of our reconstructed genetic and epigenetic network can be replicated in other samples or not is a key to the success of network analysis in cancer studies.

5. Acknowledgments

We thank the Cancer Genome Atlas Research Network for providing data and the members of TCGA's External Scientific Committee and the Glioblastoma Disease Working Group (http://cancergenome.nih.gov/components/).

6. References

Abu-Elneel, K., *et al.* (2008) Heterogeneous dysregulation of microRNAs across the autism spectrum, *Neurogenetics*, 9, 153-161.

Ackermann, M. and Strimmer, K. (2009) A general modular framework for gene set enrichment analysis, *BMC Bioinformatics*, 10, 47.

Barkinge, J.L., *et al.* (2009) The p53-induced Siva-1 plays a significant role in cisplatin-mediated apoptosis, *J Carcinog*, 8, 2.

Boersma, H.H., *et al.* (2005) Past, present, and future of annexin A5: from protein discovery to clinical applications, *J Nucl Med*, 46, 2035-2050.

Brillinger, D.R. (2004) Some data analyses using mutual information., *Brazilian J Probability Statistics*, 18, 163.

Brooks, A.S., *et al.* (2005) Homozygous nonsense mutations in KIAA1279 are associated with malformations of the central and enteric nervous systems, *Am J Hum Genet*, 77, 120-126.

Caligo, M.A., *et al.* (1997) NM23 gene expression in human breast carcinomas: loss of correlation with cell proliferation in the advanced phase of tumor progression, *Int J Cancer*, 74, 102-111.

Carpenter, B., *et al.* (2004) BASP1 is a transcriptional cosuppressor for the Wilms' tumor suppressor protein WT1, *Mol Cell Biol*, 24, 537-549.

Chu, F., *et al.* (2005) Expression of Siva-1 protein or its putative amphipathic helical region enhances cisplatin-induced apoptosis in breast cancer cells: effect of elevated levels of BCL-2, *Cancer Res*, 65, 5301-5309.

Chuang, H.Y., *et al.* (2007) Network-based classification of breast cancer metastasis, *Mol Syst Biol*, 3, 140.

Cimino, G., *et al.* (2001) Molecular evaluation of the NUP98/RAP1GDS1 gene frequency in adults with T-acute lymphoblastic leukemia, *Haematologica*, 86, 436-437.

Cover, T. and Thomas, J. (1991) *Elements of information theory.* . John Wiley and Sons Inc, New York.

Dartnell, L., *et al.* (2005) Robustness of the p53 network and biological hackers, *FEBS Lett*, 579, 3037-3042.

Demetrius, L. and Manke, T. (2005) Robustness and network evolution-an entropic principle., *Physica A: Statistical Mechanics and its Applications.* , 346, 682

El Hallani, S., *et al.* (2009) TP53 codon 72 polymorphism is associated with age at onset of glioblastoma, *Neurology*, 72, 332-336.

Fasanaro, P., *et al.* (2008) MicroRNA-210 modulates endothelial cell response to hypoxia and inhibits the receptor tyrosine kinase ligand Ephrin-A3, *J Biol Chem*, 283, 15878-15883.

Forch, P. and Valcarcel, J. (2001) Molecular mechanisms of gene expression regulation by the apoptosis-promoting protein TIA-1, *Apoptosis*, 6, 463-468.

Gennarino, V.A., *et al.* (2009) MicroRNA target prediction by expression analysis of host genes, *Genome Res*, 19, 481-490.

Greenman, C., *et al.* (2007) Patterns of somatic mutation in human cancer genomes, *Nature*, 446, 153-158.

Hagedorn, M., *et al.* (2007) FBXW7/hCDC4 controls glioma cell proliferation in vitro and is a prognostic marker for survival in glioblastoma patients, *Cell Div*, 2, 9.

Hansen, C.N., *et al.* (2009) Expression of CPEB, GAPDH and U6snRNA in cervical and ovarian tissue during cancer development, *APMIS*, 117, 53-59.

Hashimoto, K., *et al.* (2006) KEGG as a glycome informatics resource, *Glycobiology*, 16, 63R-70R.

Hebert, C., *et al.* (2007) High mobility group A2 is a target for miRNA-98 in head and neck squamous cell carcinoma, *Mol Cancer*, 6, 5.

Helleman, J., *et al.* (2006) Molecular profiling of platinum resistant ovarian cancer, *Int J Cancer*, 118, 1963-1971.

Heraud, C., *et al.* (2008) Vasoactive intestinal peptide-induced neuritogenesis in neuroblastoma SH-SY5Y cells involves SNAP-25, *Neuropeptides*, 42, 611-621.

Herrera-Merchan, A., *et al.* (2010) miR-33-mediated downregulation of p53 controls hematopoietic stem cell self-renewal, *Cell Cycle*, 9, 3277-3285.

Holm, H. and Alouini, M.-S. (2004) Sum and difference of two squared correlated Nakagami variates in connection with the McKay distribution. , *IEEE Trans. Commun.*, 52, 10.

Huang da, W., Sherman, B.T. and Lempicki, R.A. (2009) Systematic and integrative analysis of large gene lists using DAVID bioinformatics resources, *Nat Protoc*, 4, 44-57.

Huang, J.C., *et al.* (2007) Using expression profiling data to identify human microRNA targets, *Nat Methods*, 4, 1045-1049.

Huang, J.C., Morris, Q.D. and Frey, B.J. (2007) Bayesian inference of MicroRNA targets from sequence and expression data, *J Comput Biol*, 14, 550-563.

Hussey, D.J., *et al.* (1999) The (4;11)(q21;p15) translocation fuses the NUP98 and RAP1GDS1 genes and is recurrent in T-cell acute lymphocytic leukemia, *Blood*, 94, 2072-2079.

Imoto, I., *et al.* (2000) Amplification and overexpression of TGIF2, a novel homeobox gene of the TALE superclass, in ovarian cancer cell lines, *Biochem Biophys Res Commun*, 276, 264-270.

Jakulin, A., *et al.* (2003) Attribute interactions in medical data analysis., *Proceedings of the 9th Conference on Artificial Intelligence in Medicine in Europe*. Protaras, Cyprus.

Jeffrey, A. and Zwillinger, D. (2000) Table of Integrals, Series, and Products. In Gradshteyn and Ryzhik (eds). pp. 1163.

Jiang, Q., *et al.* (2009) miR2Disease: a manually curated database for microRNA deregulation in human disease, *Nucleic Acids Res*, 37, D98-104.

Joyce, P. and Tavare, S. (1995) The distribution of rare alleles, *J Math Biol*, 33, 602-618.

Karginov, F.V., *et al.* (2007) A biochemical approach to identifying microRNA targets, *Proc Natl Acad Sci U S A*, 104, 19291-19296.

Kim, J.K. and Diehl, J.A. (2009) Nuclear cyclin D1: an oncogenic driver in human cancer, *J Cell Physiol*, 220, 292-296.

Kuhn, D.E., *et al.* (2008) Experimental validation of miRNA targets, *Methods*, 44, 47-54.

Laneve, P., *et al.* (2007) The interplay between microRNAs and the neurotrophin receptor tropomyosin-related kinase C controls proliferation of human neuroblastoma cells, *Proc Natl Acad Sci U S A*, 104, 7957-7962.

Langfelder, P., Zhang, B. and Horvath, S. (2008) Defining clusters from a hierarchical cluster tree: the Dynamic Tree Cut package for R, *Bioinformatics*, 24, 719-720.

Li, Z., *et al.* (2009) Biological functions of miR-29b contribute to positive regulation of osteoblast differentiation, *J Biol Chem*, 284, 15676-15684.

Liang, P. and Pardee, A.B. (2003) Analysing differential gene expression in cancer, *Nat Rev Cancer*, 3, 869-876.

Maglott, D., *et al.* (2007) Entrez Gene: gene-centered information at NCBI, *Nucleic Acids Res*, 35, D26-31.

Matsuda, H. (2000) Physical nature of higher-order mutual information: intrinsic correlations and frustration, *Phys Rev E Stat Phys Plasmas Fluids Relat Interdiscip Topics*, 62, 3096-3102.

Maziere, P. and Enright, A.J. (2007) Prediction of microRNA targets, *Drug Discov Today*, 12, 452-458.

McGill, W. (1954) Multivariate information transmission., *Psychometrika*, 19, 97.

Megraw, M., *et al.* (2007) miRGen: a database for the study of animal microRNA genomic organization and function, *Nucleic Acids Res*, 35, D149-155.

Mingorance, A., Soriano-Garcia, E. and del Rio, J.A. (2004) [Nogo-A functions during the development of the central nervous system and in the adult], *Rev Neurol*, 39, 440-446.

Nakahara, H., *et al.* (2003) Gene interaction in DNA microarray data is decomposed by information geometric measure, *Bioinformatics*, 19, 1124-1131.

Namkoong, J., *et al.* (2007) Metabotropic glutamate receptor 1 and glutamate signaling in human melanoma, *Cancer Res*, 67, 2298-2305.

Ning, X., *et al.* (2007) Calcyclin-binding protein inhibits proliferation, tumorigenicity, and invasion of gastric cancer, *Mol Cancer Res*, 5, 1254-1262.

Pacifico, F., *et al.* (2007) RbAp48 is a target of nuclear factor-kappaB activity in thyroid cancer, *J Clin Endocrinol Metab*, 92, 1458-1466.

Parsons, D.W., *et al.* (2008) An integrated genomic analysis of human glioblastoma multiforme, *Science*, 321, 1807-1812.

Peng, J., *et al.* (2009) Partial correlation estimationby joint sparse regression model, *Journal of the American Statistical Association*, 104 735.

Rayner, K.J., *et al.* (2010) MiR-33 contributes to the regulation of cholesterol homeostasis, *Science*, 328, 1570-1573.

Rubin, A.F. and Green, P. (2007) Comment on "The consensus coding sequences of human breast and colorectal cancers", *Science*, 317, 1500.

Sassen, S., Miska, E.A. and Caldas, C. (2008) MicroRNA: implications for cancer, *Virchows Arch*, 452, 1-10.

Selbach, M., *et al.* (2008) Widespread changes in protein synthesis induced by microRNAs, *Nature*, 455, 58-63.

Sengupta, S., *et al.* (2008) MicroRNA 29c is down-regulated in nasopharyngeal carcinomas, up-regulating mRNAs encoding extracellular matrix proteins, *Proc Natl Acad Sci U S A*, 105, 5874-5878.

Sethi, T., *et al.* (1999) Extracellular matrix proteins protect small cell lung cancer cells against apoptosis: a mechanism for small cell lung cancer growth and drug resistance in vivo, *Nat Med*, 5, 662-668.

Sethupathy, P., Corda, B. and Hatzigeorgiou, A.G. (2006) TarBase: A comprehensive database of experimentally supported animal microRNA targets, *RNA*, 12, 192-197.

Skalsky, R.L., *et al.* (2007) Kaposi's sarcoma-associated herpesvirus encodes an ortholog of miR-155, *J Virol*, 81, 12836-12845.

Spinicelli, S., *et al.* (2002) GITR interacts with the pro-apoptotic protein Siva and induces apoptosis, *Cell Death Differ*, 9, 1382-1384.

Sun, S., *et al.* (2007) Overexpressed CacyBP/SIP leads to the suppression of growth in renal cell carcinoma, *Biochem Biophys Res Commun*, 356, 864-871.

The Cancer Genome Atlas Research Network, T.C.G.A.R.N. (2008) Comprehensive genomic characterization defines human glioblastoma genes and core pathways, *Nature*, 455, 1061-1068.

Turashvili, G., *et al.* (2007) Novel markers for differentiation of lobular and ductal invasive breast carcinomas by laser microdissection and microarray analysis, *BMC Cancer*, 7, 55.

Wang, C., *et al.* (2008) A novel endogenous human CaMKII inhibitory protein suppresses tumor growth by inducing cell cycle arrest via p27 stabilization, *J Biol Chem*, 283, 11565-11574.

Wang, X.Y., *et al.* (1998) GBAS, a novel gene encoding a protein with tyrosine phosphorylation sites and a transmembrane domain, is co-amplified with EGFR, *Genomics*, 49, 448-451.

Wood, L.D., *et al.* (2007) The genomic landscapes of human breast and colorectal cancers, *Science*, 318, 1108-1113.

Wu, X., Jin, L. and Xiong, M. (2008) Composite measure of linkage disequilibrium for testing interaction between unlinked loci, *Eur J Hum Genet*, 16, 644-651.

Yang, H.S., *et al.* (2004) A novel function of the MA-3 domains in transformation and translation suppressor Pdcd4 is essential for its binding to eukaryotic translation initiation factor 4A, *Mol Cell Biol*, 24, 3894-3906.

Yang, Y., *et al.* (2009) Identification of miR-21 targets in breast cancer cells using a quantitative proteomic approach, *Proteomics*, 9, 1374-1384.

Yang, Y. and Fu, L.M. (2003) TSGDB: a database system for tumor suppressor genes, *Bioinformatics*, 19, 2311-2312.

Yang, Y., Wang, Y.P. and Li, K.B. (2008) MiRTif: a support vector machine-based microRNA target interaction filter, *BMC Bioinformatics*, 9 Suppl 12, S4.

Zhao, J., Jin, L. and Xiong, M. (2006) Test for interaction between two unlinked loci, *Am J Hum Genet*, 79, 831-845.

Zhu, Y. and Parada, L.F. (2002) The molecular and genetic basis of neurological tumours, *Nat Rev Cancer*, 2, 616-626.

11

The Neural Extracellular Matrix, Cell Adhesion Molecules and Proteolysis in Glioma Invasion and Tumorigenicity

Chrissa A. Dwyer and Russell T. Matthews
SUNY Upstate Medical University, Syracuse, NY, U.S.A

1. Introduction

High-grade gliomas are the most prevalent and lethal form of primary intracranial tumors. Despite significant progress in surgical and adjuvant therapeutic treatments for gliomas, patient prognosis still remains dismal. The ability of gliomas to invade the normal surrounding brain tissue contributes to their capacity to evade therapeutic interventions, ultimately leading to tumor recurrence and subsequent disease progression (Rich & Bigner, 2004). Another major therapeutic obstacle comes from the high degree of intratumoral cellular heterogeneity. The tumor mass is comprised of both terminally differentiated cells, cells that exhibit finite capabilities of self-renewal and multipotency, and a smaller subpopulation of cells that exhibit stem cell-like qualities. These stem-like cells, termed Glioma Initiating Cells (GICs), exihibit pluripotency, self-renewal and, importantly, are capable of repopulating the original parental tumor. Therefore, more effective therapies may be derived from targeting both the infiltrative nature of gliomas and GICs (Louis, 2006; Park & Rich, 2009).

The ability of glioma tumor cells to infiltrate the normal surrounding brain tissue is a property that is restricted to intracranial tumors that are phenotypically glial within the central nervous system (CNS). As metastatic tumor cells that are highly invasive in the periphery fail to invade surrounding brain tissue once within the confines of the CNS, and invasive glioma tumors that originate in the brain rarely metastasize outside of the CNS. These findings suggest that the unique interaction between glioma tumor cells and the neural extracellular environment mediate glioma invasion (Bellail et al., 2004; Nutt et al., 2001a).

A defining attribute of the neural extracellular environment is the unique composition of the neural extracellular matrix (ECM), which unlike other peripheral matrices has low levels of fibrilliar proteins like collagens, fibronectin, and laminin (Ruoslahti, 1996). In both neural development and pathogenesis, the neural ECM regulates key biological processes including cellular migration, maturation, synapse formation, and plasticity. In the adult brain the composition of the neural ECM is largely inhibitory to cellular reorganization (Galtrey & Fawcett, 2007; Zimmermann & Dours-Zimmermann, 2008). Therefore, glioma tumor cell invasion into the normal surrounding brain tissue is derived from their ability to overcome this normally inhibitory extracellular environment. Decades of research has demonstrated that glioma tumor cells are capable of remodeling the neural extracellular space by changing the expressions of proteins involved in intercellular and extracellular interactions. Glioma tumor cells also secrete proteases that cleave the adult neural ECM and temporary produced glioma ECM to create a permissive extracellular environment supportive of tumor cell invasion (Viapiano & Matthews, 2006). In addition, recent studies have determined that the expressions of several constituents of the neural ECM are enriched in the GIC subpopulation (Gunther et al., 2008; Phillips et al., 2006), suggesting that components of the neural ECM may facilitate the stem cell-like qualities of these cells by creating a permissive extracellular niche.

Targeting either the expression of proteins that mediate intercellular or extracellular interactions or the proteases responsible for the cleavage and turnover of these proteins represent potential therapeutic avenues that require further exploration. This chapter will focus on the role of the neural ECM, proteolytic cleavage, and alterations that occur in proteins that mediate intercellular interactions to facilitate glioma tumorigenicity and invasion and their therapeutic potential.

2. The neural extracellular matrix in normal and developing brain

2.1 The neural extracellular matrix

During both neurodevelopment and in several neuropathologies, the neural ECM and molecular determinants of cell-ECM and cell-cell interactions regulate key biological processes including cellular migration, maturation, differentiation, and synapse formation (Hartmann & Maurer, 2001). The composition of the neural ECM largely dictates the permissive or inhibitory properties of the neural extracellular environment, creating a permissive environment favoring cell migration and process outgrowth during development and a notoriously inhibitory environment in the mature CNS. The neural ECM is capable of undergoing dynamic remodeling resulting from alterations in both the expression levels of ECM components and alterations in proteolytic processing (Zimmermann & Dours-Zimmermann, 2008).

2.2 The composition of the neural extracellular matrix in normal brain

The composition of the neural ECM, while most similar to cartilage, is unique and distinguishes the neural extracellular environment from that of other tissues and organs. The neural ECM is chiefly comprised of Hyaluronic Acid (HA), a repeating sugar disaccharide, proteoglycans and glycoproteins, which through their interactions organize the extracellular space of the CNS (Delpech & Delpech, 1984). The neural ECM accounts for ten to twenty percent of the total volume of the mature brain and occupies an even larger percentage in the developing brain (Ruoslahti, 1996). Unlike peripheral matrices, the neural ECM has low levels of fibrillar proteins including laminin, collagens, and fibronectin with the majority of these proteins being localized to substructures of the CNS including basement membranes, the subpial space, blood vessels, and in white matter tracts (Liesi, 1984). Instead, the backbone of the neural ECM is HA, a non-sulfated glycosaminoglycan made up of alternating glucuronic acid and N-acetylglucosamine disaccharide subunits and devoid of a protein core (Ruoslahti, 1996; Toole, 2000, 2004). HA is produced and secreted by hyaluronan synthases located at the surface of the cellular plasma membrane, recent evidence suggests that HA synthases may also play a role in tethering HA to the cellular surface to facilitate its interactions with other components of the neural ECM (DeAngelis,

1999; Itano & Kimata, 2002; Weigel et al., 1997; Spicer & McDonald, 1998; Spicer & Tien, 2004).

Since HA forms the backbone of the neural matrix, proteins that organize and bind HA to the cell surface are particularly important for defining neural ECM structure and function. In many peripheral tissues the best studied HA receptor is CD44 but it is expressed at low levels in the adult CNS. Instead, the major HA binding proteins expressed in the CNS are the lectican family members of chondroitin sulfate proteoglycans (CSPGs), also called hyalectans, which include versican, aggrecan, and brain-specific neurocan, and Brain Enriched Hyaluronan Binding protein (BEHAB)/brevican (B/b) (Bandtlow & Zimmermann, 2000; Ruoslahti, 1996; Yamaguchi, 2000). Additionally, the HA Proteoglycan binding Link Proteins (HAPLNs) work in concert with lecticans to mediate HA binding (Spicer et al., 2003). CSPGs are glycosylated proteins that are decorated with chondroitin sulfate glycosaminoglycan (CS-GAG) chains. The number and sulfation of CS-GAG chains varies for individual proteoglycans and can modulate their functions and interactions with ligands (Maeda, 2010).

The structure and molecular interactions of lecticans in the normal brain has been reviewed thoroughly in previous publications and therefore is not included here, however, the model structure of the neural matrix and the position and interactions of lecticans in this matrix is shown in Figure 1 (Ruoslahti, 1996; Viapiano & Matthews, 2006; Yamaguchi, 2000). A complete understanding of the molecular interactions and functions of lecticans in the normal brain is, however, challenging. This is due in large part to the production of several protein isoforms resulting from alternative splicing, which causes a vast and microheterogeneous array of protein products (Viapiano et al., 2003, 2005; Dours-Zimmerman & Zimmerman, 1994). Adding to this complexity, different protein isoforms from the same gene are expressed in specific temporal and regional patterns (Milev et al., 1998; Seidenbecher et al., 1998). In addition, all lecticans are cleaved by A Disintegrin And Metalloproteinase with Thrombospondin Motifs (ADAMTS) and Matrix Metalloproteinase (MMPs) family members (Westling et al., 2004; Matthews et al., 2000). Finally the glycosylation of lecticans is extremely microheterogeneous and specific glycoforms can be expressed in a very anatomically distinct and precise manner in the normal CNS (Matthews et al., 2002). The molecular heterogeneity as well as the distinct spatial and temporal expression patterns of ECM components dictates the broad functional impact the neural ECM has over the CNS in both the physiological and pathophysiological state.

2.3 The function of the neural extracellular matrix

The neural ECM regulates a diverse array of functions in both the developing and mature CNS. During neurodevelopment the ECM has been shown to play a role in cell migration, process outgrowth, cell fate decisions, synaptogenesis and regulating cortical plasticity (Bandtlow & Zimmermann, 2000; Berardi et al., 2004; Frischknecht & Seidenbecher, 2008; Maeda et al., 2010). The composition of the ECM during neurodevelopment is largely permissive and favorable for cellular migration and process outgrowth (Zimmermann & Dours-Zimmermann, 2008). The expressions of certain lectican isoforms that aid in cellular movement and process outgrowth are also elevated and undergo increased proteolytic cleavage, which enables the turnover of ECM components to facilitate cellular migration. In fact, the proteolytic activities of certain proteases have been shown to be critical for normal development to proceed (Ethell & Ethell, 2007). As the mature synaptic circuitry is established the composition of the neural ECM changes to aid in stabilizing these

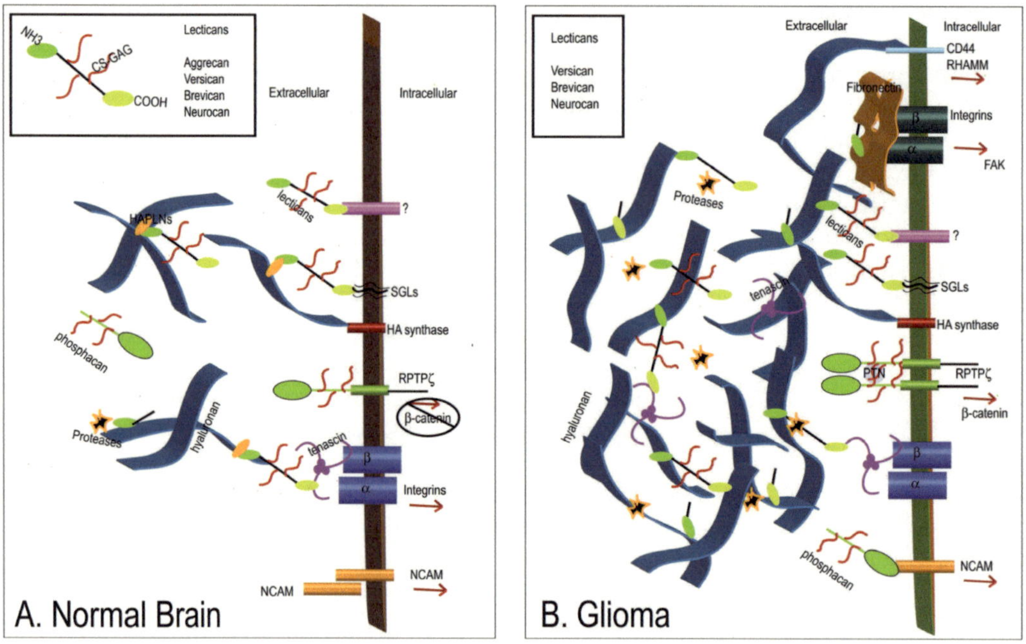

Fig. 1. Schematic Diagram of the Neural Extracellular Matrix. Diagram demonstrates the model composition of the ECM and cell-surface receptors in the normal adult brain (A) and the changes in the extracellular environment in gliomas (B). Arrows represent activation of signaling cascades.

connections, creating the notoriously inhibitory extracellular environment of the adult CNS (Galtrey & Fawcett, 2007). The expression of HA is substantially reduced and lectican family members and their specific isoforms that are inhibitory to extracellular reorganization appear (Frischknecht & Seidenbecher, 2008; Margolis et al., 1975). Often disorders and diseases that affect the CNS are accompanied by alterations in the composition of the neural ECM, which facilitates the pathophysiological condition by modifying the extracellular environment (Galtrey & Fawcett, 2007; Zimmermann & Dours-Zimmermann, 2008).

3. Extracellular matrix in brain tumors

3.1 The neural matrix facilitates glioma tumor cell invasion

While the extracellular environment of the mature CNS is notably resistant to plasticity and cellular dynamics that favor reorganization, glioma cells are capable of overcoming this inhibition to invade into the normal surrounding brain tissue. The invasive attributes of glioma cells leads to tumor cell dispersion and highly diffuse tumor-stromal boundaries, making complete surgical removal of tumor cells nearly impossible and tumor recurrence almost inevitable (Nakada et al., 2007). Brain tumor cell invasion into the normal surrounding brain tissue is a property that is restricted to tumors that are phenotypically glial and located within the CNS environment. Both non-glial tumors that originate in the CNS and tumors of non-neuroepithelial origin that metastasize to the CNS fail to invade the surrounding brain tissue, typically exhibiting well-defined brain-tumor boundaries (Bellail et al., 2004). Furthermore, gliomas rarely infiltrate the vasculature of the CNS and disseminate outside of the nervous system environment (Kleihues et al., 1993, 2002; Bellail et al., 2004). The ability of glioma cells to invade the mature CNS strongly suggests that the unique interaction between these tumors and the extracellular neural environment is critical in this invasive process. The unique composition of the neural ECM defines the extracellular environment of the CNS and, therefore, the unique ability of glioma cells to interact with the neural ECM is a critical component of their invasiveness. Consistent with this hypothesis is work from a number of labs demonstrating that glioma tumor cells synthesize and secrete a specialized composition of ECM components and cell adhesion molecules that facilitate this interaction leading to tumor cell invasion (Bellail et al., 2004; Gladson, 1999).

The composition of the ECM produced by glioma cells closely resembles that during early neurodevelopment, as both the expression levels and presence of specific protein isoforms predominately expressed during neurodevelopment are overrepresented in the ECM of gliomas. As in several invasive and metastatic tumors, the synthesis of HA is dramatically increased in glioma along with HA receptors CD44 and RHAMM which mediate aspects of glioma invasion (Delpech et al., 1993; Kuppner et al., 1992; Merzak et al., 1994; Okada et al., 1996; Park et al., 2008; Radotra & McCormick, 1997). The expression of several lectican family members and their isoforms that are predominately expressed during early nervous system development and promote cellular reorganization are also upregulated in human glioma tumors. Exemplary to this are the elevated expressions of versican (Paulus et al., 1996), B/b (Jaworski et al., 1996), neurocan (Rauch, 2004), and Receptor Protein Tyrosine Phosphatase ζ (RPTPζ, also known as RPTPβ) (Norman et al., 1998; Peles et al., 1998). A specific model of a lectican isoform that is highly expressed during neurodevelopment and reappears in glioma tumors is a variant of B/b, B/bΔg. The B/bΔg form of brevican is expressed for a short developmental window in normal human brain spanning from 16 gestational weeks to one year of age. The expression of the B/bΔg isoform reemerges in human glioma tumors causing it to be expressed in a tumor-specific manner within the adult CNS (Viapiano et al., 2005). Additionally, unlike normal adult ECM, the tumoral ECM contains traditional fibrillar matrix proteins like laminin and fibronectin, which have been shown to bind to proteoglycans to enhance tumor cell motility (Hu et al., 2008; Zheng et al., 2004). While the expressions of typical fibrillar proteins are low in the extracellular milieu of the adult brain, these common matrix elements are expressed in localized regions of the developing brain (Rutka et al., 1988; Ruoslahti, 1996). Therefore, with respect to the neural ECM, oncology recapitulates ontogeny.

While the expression of unique ECM components in glioma cells is detailed above, glioma cells also modulate the expression of cell-surface receptors, which enhances their ability to interact within the neural environment. One class of surface receptors altered in glioma tumors are cell-cell adhesion molecules, which comprise several different molecular families of receptors (Barami et al., 2006). Cell-cell adhesion molecules play important roles in regulating cell motility through interactions with ECM components and other cell adhesion molecules. Several signal transduction pathways directly regulate the cellular repertoire of adhesion molecules to dictate both extracellular and intercellular interactions. The inverse is also true, as activated cell adhesion molecules are capable of modulating intracellular signaling to influence cellular processes like adhesion, motility and even cell fate (Cavallaro & Christofori, 2004). In terms of glioma tumor pathophysiology, the activation of cell adhesion molecules are equally as important as the activation of signal transduction cascades, as signaling from both modulate tumor cell behavior.

In glioma tumors, ECM receptors like tenascin, integrins and certain cell-cell adhesion molecules mediate interactions between the extracellular environment and surface of the cell to influence cell behavior by modulating intracellular signaling. Tenascins are large molecular weight cell-surface glycoproteins that can function as receptors for proteoglycans including the lectican family members. Importantly, tenascin family members are also overexpressed in glioma specimens and have been linked to tumor cell invasion and angiogenesis (Aspberg et al., 1995; 1997; Hirata et al., 2009; Leins et al., 2003; Zagzag et al., 2002). While tenascin can function as receptors for proteoglycans, they are also secreted proteins that depend in part on interactions with cell-adhesion molecules at the cellular plasma membrane to confer their functionality. Tenascin has been shown to interact with integrins, which are integral membrane cell surface receptors involved in cell-ECM interactions (Deryugina & Bourdon, 1996; Giese et al., 1996). In addition to binding tenascin, integrins also bind fibrillar proteins like laminin and fibronectin that are expressed in the tumoral extracellular environment (Knott et al., 1998; Ohnishi et al., 1998). The interaction of integrins with both tenascin and fibrillar matrix proteins in the tumor microenvironment have been shown to enhance the motility and invasive properties of glioma tumor cells (Deryugina & Bourdon, 1996; Hirata et al., 2009). Upon binding to ECM ligands, integrins effectively transduce changes in the ECM into alterations in cellular behavior by activating signal transduction cascades that reorganize components of the cellular cytoskeleton to facilitate cell movement (D'Abaco & Kaye, 2007).

Cell-cell and cell-ECM interactions of glioma tumor cells are also critically regulated by extracellular proteases. Tumor cell invasion is strongly influenced by the proteolytic cleavage of ECM components and certain cell adhesion molecules, as proteolysis creates an extracellular environment permissive to cellular migration by facilitating the turnover of ECM components (Rao, 2003 and section 2.2). The complex interplay between HA, proteoglycans and their receptors, integrins, cell-cell adhesion molecules, and proteases present within the tumor stroma facilitate glioma invasion through the normally inhibitory extracellular environment of the mature CNS.

The restricted invasive profile of gliomas suggests that nervous system-specific proteins expressed only by neoplastic cells that are phenotypically glial may be key mediators of glioma invasion. Thus, making components of the neural ECM and adhesion molecules with expressions that are restricted or specifically enriched within the CNS appealing avenues of research for future therapeutic targets. Proteins with CNS enriched or specific expression that are overexpressed in human glioma tumors include but are not limited to B/b (Jaworski et al., 1996), specific isoforms of versican (Dours-Zimmermann & Zimmermann, 1994; Paulus et al., 1996), and RPTPζ (Muller et al., 2003). Inhibiting molecular mechanisms leading to glioma tumor cell invasion is critical to effectively curing these deadly tumors. Furthermore, the identification of pro-invasive mediators that are both nervous system and tumor-specific would create molecular targets for novel therapies with reduced off-target effects, thus limiting the potential of inducing broad systemic toxicity.

3.2 Proteolytic degradation of the neural extracellular matrix is critically involved in tumor cell invasion

In order for glioma tumor cells to invade the normal surrounding brain tissue, tumor cells must both interact with the ECM of the adult CNS, which is accomplished through the synthesis of tumor-produced ECM, altered receptor expression, and proteolytic cleavage.

Several different families of proteases are overexpressed in gliomas including MMPs, ADAMTS, serine, cysteine, and asparate and play important roles in mediating glioma tumor invasion and progression (Levicar et al., 2003). Proteases expressed by glioma tumor cells degrade the mature inhibitory ECM of the adult CNS and the glioma-expressed matrix elements. Proteolytic activity allows for turnover of ECM components and facilitates invasion by dynamically remodeling the extracellular environment to become more permissive to cellular reorganization (Yamamoto et al., 2002). Therefore, glioma tumor cell invasion is dependent on both the overproduction and proteolytic cleavage of ECM components. The importance of ECM cleavage is highlighted by previous work on B/b that showed both its overexpression and proteolytic processing are required for increased glioma cell invasion, as a mutated non-cleavable form of B/b did not enhance cell invasion (Viapiano et al., 2008). In addition to mediating aspects of invasion, proteases belonging to these families have also been linked to increases in glioma tumor cell proliferation and angiogenesis (Lakka et al., 2005). The regulation of proteolytic activity in gliomas is complex with each level of regulation representing a facet for potential therapeutic intervention.

Proteolytic activity can be regulated at different levels resulting from either an increase in transcription or activation, as most proteases require cleavage of an inactive pro-peptide form for enzymatic activity. The proteolytic activity of both ADAMTS and MMP family members are naturally inhibited by endogenously occurring proteins belonging to the Tissue Inhibitor of Metalloproteinases (TIMP) family (Brew & Nagase, 2010). In several disease pathologies including gliomas, an imbalance between protease activity and TIMP expression accounts for elevated levels of proteolysis in the pathogenic state (Kachra et al., 1999). Therefore, both the overexpression and activation of ADAMTS and MMP proteases along with the TIMP family of endogenous protease inhibitors are attractive therapeutic targets for their role as molecular determinants of glioma tumor cell invasion.

The functional role of proteases in glioma tumor pathology is exemplified by the MMP family members, which have important roles in the progression of most neoplasms and happen to be the most well characterized protease family in glioma tumors (Levicar et al., 2003). The MMPs comprise a large family of matrix peptidases that are classified on the basis of their preferred substrate, for which there is considerable overlap between family members (Rao, 2003). MMPs are produced both by glioma tumor cells and endothelial cells that comprise the tumor vasculature (Raithatha et al., 2000). Two of the most well documented MMPs in glioma are MMP-2 and MMP-9, also known as gelatinase-A and gelatinase-B, respectively. Their expressions are increased in glioma tumors and have been correlated with increased glioma tumor cell invasiveness (Nakagawa et al., 1996; Wild-Bode et al., 2001; Levicar et al., 2003). Additionally, the expression of these proteases correlated with the degree of glioma tumor malignancy, as increased levels of MMP-2 and MMP-9 were observed in high-grade glioma tumors relative to low-grade (Wang et al., 2003). Knocking down the expression of MMP-9 in an invasive glioma cell line resulted in decreased tumor cell infiltration into the surrounding brain tissue and decreased cell motility and invasion in vitro (Zhao et al., 2010). Upstream signaling molecules that regulate the expressions of MMP-2 and MMP-9 are also potential therapeutic targets of interest. Previous studies have shown that JNK and ERK signaling positively regulate the expression of MMP-9, and interfering with either of these pathways reduced the invasiveness of a glioma cell line (Lakka et al., 2000).

Based on elevated MMP expression, activation, and function in glioma tumor invasion and progression, a considerable amount of investigation into using chemical inhibitors of MMPs as therapeutic agents to reduce the pathogenesis of glioma tumors has ensued. Clinical trials using a broad MMP inhibitor failed to improve patient prognosis and caused systemic toxicity in patients, in the form of joint pain (Groves et al., 2006; Levin et al., 2006). The expression of MMPs in cartilage and their role in maintaining normal cartilage and joint physiology presumably accounted for these deleterious affects (Itoh et al., 2002). Findings from these studies suggest that the function of MMPs in both the pathogenesis of glioma tumors and its role in normal physiology are more complex than is currently understood. Additionally, these findings suggest that other proteases that play less of a role in maintaining normal physiology while still mediating aspects of glioma tumor invasion may be better candidates for therapeutic intervention.

Specific ADAMTS family members exemplify proteases that are attractive therapeutic candidates on the basis of their contribution to glioma tumor invasion and disease progression and seemingly less critical role in maintaining normal physiology (Majumdar et al., 2007; Nakada et al., 2005). Interestingly, the expression and activity of ADAMTS-4 and 5 are enriched in human glioma tumors relative to normal adult brain (Held-Feindt et al., 2006), with the expression of ADAMTS-5 being the most significantly upregulated in glioma (Nakada et al., 2005). Their expression has been shown to contribute significantly to glioma invasion and disease progression, which is mediated by their ability to cleave components of the extracellular matrix such as B/b (Matthews et al., 2000; Nakada et al., 2005) and versican (Sandy et al., 2001). Therefore, the preferred substrates of ADAMTS-4 and 5 in the CNS are presumably more restricted than other proteases, favoring extracellular matrix components that are enriched in glioma tumors with CNS-specific expression. Importantly, ADAMTS-4 and 5 are seemingly dispensable for normal physiology, as double knockout animals exhibited no deleterious affects and were indistinguishable from controls (Majumdar et al., 2007). Thus suggesting that targeting the systemic expression of ADAMTS-4 and 5 would have fewer off-target effects.

The pro-invasive contribution of ADAMTS-4 and 5 to proteolytic cleavage is further enhanced by recent work that described a novel molecular mechanism between these proteases and glioma produced ECM to facilitate glioma cell invasion. Importantly, the proteolytic cleavage of B/b by ADAMTS-4 and 5 was found to reveal cryptic binding sites on B/b to promote its motogenic effects (Hu et al., 2008). The proteolytic cleavage fragments of B/b were shown to effectively bind to fibronectin, which caused the polymerization of fibronectin microfibrils surrounding the surface of the cell and increased glioma tumor cell adhesion and motility. The interaction between B/b and fibronectin was only observed for the N-terminal proteolytic cleavage fragment of B/b and not for the full-length form of the protein. B/b mediated increases in cell adhesion and motility were found to be dependent on both its proteolytic processing and interaction with fibronectin, as a forced reduction in fibronectin expression attenuated the motogenic effects of B/b (Hu et al., 2008). In the adult brain the proposed mechanisms would be inconceivable given the lack of fibronectin expression, however the tumor-specific expression of it by glioma cells enables mechanisms of B/b-mediated cell motility to proceed in a nervous system specific manner that is critically dependent on proteolysis.

4. Tumoral cellular interactions within the extracellular space of the CNS

4.1 Extracellular interactions mediate tumor cell invasion

Dispersion of cells within the brain requires direct interactions of the tumor cells with the surrounding environment and ultimately activation of signaling pathways downstream of these interactions. In gliomas, cellular interactions within the environment are mediated by a number of key receptor systems.

The most well-studied matrix receptors are the **Integrins**. Integrins are a family of cell surface receptors that communicate changes in the extracellular environment to intracellular mediators by activating several signal transduction cascades. Integrins are comprised of a large family of heterodimeric transmembrane glycoproteins, the dimerization of different integrin subunits dictates the specificity and preference of these receptors for particular ECM components (Akiyama, 1996). In gliomas the tumor-specific overexpression of integrins $\alpha V\beta 3$ and $\alpha V\beta 5$ have been described along with their localization along blood vessels and on the surface of glioma tumor cells, suggesting they play a role in angiogenesis and cell motility (Bello et al., 2001; D'Abaco & Kaye, 2007; Gladson, 1996; Schnell et al., 2008). Cilengitide, a synthetic RGD pentapeptide that acts as an inhibitor of integrins $\alpha V\beta 3$ and $\alpha V\beta 5$, has shown promising clinical results and is now being evaluated in Phase III clinical trials (Nabors et al., 2007, Tabatabai et al., 2010).

In addition to integrins, HA binding proteins like the lecticans mediate the interaction between the extracellular environment and glioma tumor cells. **BEHAB/ brevican (B/b),** a nervous-system specific lectican family member, is significantly upregulated in human glioma specimens relative to normal brain (Jaworski et al., 1996). The expression of B/b is limited to invasive tumors of glial phenotype within the intracranial environment, thus mirroring the restricted invasive profile of gliomas (Jaworski et al., 1996). Of importance, previous studies have shown that increased B/b expression led to elevated tumor cell invasion and tumor aggressiveness in animal models (Nutt et al., 2001b). Likewise, RNAi mediated knockdown of B/b decreased tumor cell invasion and reduces tumor aggressiveness leading to prolonged survival of animal models (RTM, unpublished findings). It has been determined that the upregulation of B/b expression in gliomas occurs at both the level of transcription and translation, suggesting that a glioma-specific signaling pathway is responsible for regulating increased B/b expression (Gary et al., 2000; Viapiano et al., 2005). These unknown regulatory mechanisms represent potentially valuable therapeutic candidates, as they presumably would be regulators of glioma cell motility with nervous system and tumor specific expression.

Understanding the function of B/b overexpression is challenging due to the presence of several post-translationally modified protein isoforms, all of which are present in glioma specimens at levels far greater than normal brain. These include the full-length secreted protein, proteolytic cleavage fragments, and tumor-specific isoforms B/bsia and B/bΔg (Viapiano et al., 2003, 2005). B/bsia is an over sialidated form of B/b, exhibiting typical post-translational increases in sialic acid modifications observed in many neoplasms (Viapiano et al., 2005). B/bΔg is a hypoglycosylated full-length protein isoform resulting from decreased decoration of the full-length core protein with O-linked oligosaccharides. Interestingly, B/bΔg is bound to the cellular plasma membrane by unknown mechansisms that are distinct from those tethering other B/b isoforms to the cellular surface. While the exact contribution of the B/bΔg isoform to B/b-mediated increases in cell motility and invasion is undetermined, B/bΔg is the most highly upregulated isoform of B/b present in human and rodent glioma tumor specimens and its localization to the cellular plasma membrane is suggestive of an important pathogenic function (Viapiano et al., 2003, 2005). Both the tumor-specific expression and cellular localization of B/bΔg make it an attractive therapeutic target for either its participation in B/b-mediated motogenic effects or for targeted drug delivery methods.

B/b also undergoes proteolytic processing by the ADAMTS-4 and 5 family members resulting in cleavage of the 150kDa full-length protein into a 50kDa and 100kDa N and C-terminal cleavage fragments, respectively (Matthews et al., 2000, Viapiano, 2005). The proteolytic processing of B/b is required for B/b-mediated increases in tumor cell motility as discussed previously (Viapiano et al., 2008; Hu et al., 2008). The overexpression and proteolytic processing of B/b was found to activate Epidermal Growth Factor Receptor (EGFR) signaling resulting in elevated levels of fibronectin expression which was assembled into microfibrils at the cells surface in a B/b-dependent manner. Increased expression of integrin β3 and N-cadherin were also observed in response to B/b overexpression and these affects were found to be specific to glioma cells cultured in the presence of fibronectin (Hu et al., 2008). The summation of findings on B/b expression and function in glioma suggests that targeting B/b at the levels of transcriptional regulation, post-translational modifications, and proteolytic processing all represent novel avenues that could potentially reduce glioma tumor cell invasion.

Versican, another member of the lectican family of CSPGs, is also highly expressed in glioma specimens along with other systemic cancer types like breast cancer. In human glioma specimens and cell lines many different spice variants of versican are overxpressed including both the nervous system-specific V2 isoform and the more broadly expressed V0/V1 isoforms (Arslan et al., 2007; Dours-Zimmerman & Zimmerman, 1994; Paulus et al., 1996). The expression of versican in glioma has been linked to increased tumor size, angiogenesis and glioma cell motility (Zheng et al., 2004). Protein isoforms containing the G3 domain of versican, which consists of the C-terminal domains common to lectican family members, has been shown to be abundantly expressed in glioma specimens and play a role in regulating tumor growth and angiogenesis. Overexpression of the versican G3 domain in glioma cells resulted in tumors of increased size and enhanced vasculature in animal xenographs compared to controls. Versican G3 conditioned media was found to enhance endothelial cell adhesion, proliferation and migration. Furthermore, the overexpression of versican G3 was found to increase the expression of fibronectin and Vascular Endothelial Growth Factor (VEGF). The elevated expression levels of fibronectin and VEGF formed a complex with versican G3 that could be co-immunoprecipitated, the additive effects of all three components of the complex - versican, fibronectin and VEGF to endothelial cells exacerbated the effect that either component alone or in pairs had on the adhesion, proliferation and migration of endothelial cells, substantially increasing it (Zheng et al., 2004). More recently, the ability of transforming growth factor β- 2 (TGFβ- 2) was shown to have an enhancing effect on the expression of versican V0/V1 isoforms. Furthermore, the addition of TGFβ- 2 exerted a motogenic effect on glioma cells that was partially mediated by increased V0/V1 expression (Arslan et al., 2007).

The overexpression of versican VI was found to induce neuronal differentiation of PC12 cells, an immortal cell line used to model neural precursor cells, through an integrin-dependent mechanism resulting from activation of EGFR and downstream signaling through ERK (Wu et al., 2004). While a versican-mediated affect on EGFR signaling in glioma tumor cells remains unexplored, mechanisms leading to B/b-mediated increases in cell invasion closely resemble those described for versican (Hu et al., 2008). Therefore it is interesting to speculate that overexpression of certain lecticans (B/b or versican or perhaps neurocan) by glioma tumor cells may be sufficient to mediate tumor cell motility by utilizing similar pathomechanisms stemming from increased fibronectin expression, EGFR activation, and integrin expression. Versican also undergoes proteolytic processing in glioma, however the function of this cleavage in the pathogenesis of glioma remains unexplored (Westling et al., 2004). Versican represents an attractive therapeutic target for its functional role in glioma tumor growth, angiogenesis and cell motility.

The pro-invasive function of proteoglycans like B/b and versican may be, in-part, mediated by their interaction with cell-surface receptors, like **tenascins**. Tenascins are large secreted extracellular glycoproteins that bind to the cell surface through interactions with integrins (Bourdon & Ruoslahti, 1989). Tenascin-C and tenasin-R have been shown to bind to proteoglycans with high affinity to bridge the molecular gap between secreted proteoglycans in the extracellular space and the cellular plasma membrane (Aspberg et al., 1995, 1997; Barnea et al., 1994; Milev et al., 1997). Pioneering studies demonstrated that tenascin proteins are expressed by glioma cell lines in vitro and are present at higher levels in glioma specimens relative to normal brain tissue (Ventimiglia et al., 1992; Zagzag et al., 1995). Additionally, the use of tenascin as an immobilized protein substrate was found to enhance human glioma cell migration through an $\alpha 2\beta 1$ integrin-dependent mechanism (Deryugina and Bourdon, 1996).

Subsequent to these studies, four tenascin family members were identified including tenascin-C, R, W, and X, all of which have been implemented in several physiological and pathophysiological functions including embryonic development, wound healing and are present in several solid tumor types. Tenascin-R expression is restricted to the CNS, while other tenascin family members are ubiquitously expressed (Hirata et al., 2009). The expressions of both tenascin-C and W have been identified surrounding tumor vasculature in glioma specimens, however tenascin-C is the best studied in glioma for its role in enhancing tumor cell invasion. In GBM patients, increased expression of tenascin-C is correlated with an adverse prognosis. Moreover, the endogenous expression of tenascin-C in GBM tumor cells was found to enhance cell invasion and correlated with reactive changes in the normal brain tissue surrounding GBM tumors in patients (Hirata et al., 2009). Like several ECM components, tenascin-C-mediated increases in glioma cell invasion are dependent on proteolytic processing. In glioma tumor cells tenascin-C is cleaved predominantly by MMP-12, and the inhibition of MMP-12 activity attenuated tenascin-C mediated glioma cell invasion (Sarkar et al., 2006). The tumor-specific upregulation of tenascin-C along with its pro-invasive function make it an attractive therapeutic target for anti-invasive therapies and it has shown some promise in clinical trials (Riva et al., 1999a ,b).

Another proteoglycan that has also been shown to interact with tenascins and is upregulated in glioma specimens is **(RPTPζ)/ Phosphacan** (Adamsky et al., 2001; Muller et al., 2003). RPTPζ is a transmembrane receptor tyrosine kinase phosphatase, which like the lecticans is also a CSPG bearing extensive decoration with CS-GAG chains. However unlike the lecticans, RPTPζ lacks an HA binding domain and does not interact directly with the HA scaffold of the neural extracellular space. The N-terminal protein domains of RPTPζ, are comprised of a carbonic anhydrase-like domain and a fibronectin type III-like domain. The central domain, which contains the transmembrane domain bears CS-GAG moieties that modulate the interaction of RPTPζ with several of its ligands, and the C-terminal protein domains are made up of two intracellular phosphatase domains (Peles et al., 1998).

While the protein structures of RPTPζ and lectican CSPGs are highly divergent, both RPTPζ, neurocan and versican have several common ligands including tenascins, NCAM, L1-CAM, contactin, and Transient Axonal Glycoprotein 1 (TAG-1/ axonin-1) (Peles et al., 1998; Rauch et al., 2001). RPTPζ is encoded from the PTPRZ1 gene and has four known isoforms resulting from alternative splicing. These include the full-length receptor form RPTPζ, a short-receptor form, a secreted form, phosphacan, which lacks the transmembrane regions and intracellular phosphatase domains, and a truncated secreted form, PSI (Phosphacan Short Isoform) (Garwood et al., 2003). RPTPζ expression is enriched in the CNS and is upregulated in human glioma tumors along with its soluble ligand pleiotrophin (PTN)/ HB-GAM relative to normal brain (Muller et al., 2003). Upon binding to PTN, RPTPζ receptors cluster resulting in the inactivation of endogenous phosphatase activity, which leads to increased phosphorylation of downstream effector molecules like β-catenin. Phosphorylation of β-catenin stabilizes the protein and facilitates canonical β-catenin/cadherin and WNT pathway signaling, which have implications in cell motility, proliferation and cell fate decisions (Meng et al., 2000). In glioma tumor cells, RNAi mediated knockdown of RPTPζ in a human glioma cell line reduced the size of engrafted tumors in rodent models and decreased the proliferation rate of tumor cells in vitro. The reduction in RPTPζ expression also decreased PTN-mediated increases in cell proliferation and motility (Ulbricht et al., 2006). A similar study also found that RPTPζ knockdown cells had reduced motility on a PTN-immobilized substrate but did not see any affects on cell proliferation (Muller et al., 2003). Given that RPTPζ is upregulated in human glioma tumors, localized to the cellular surface and regulates complex cellular behaviors that contribute to glioma pathogenesis, RPTPζ is a prime candidate target for future glioma therapies. Both cell-ECM and cell-cell adhesion molecules play critical roles in translating changes in the extracellular environment to alterations in the cellular cytoskeleton

4.2 Intercellular interactions mediate tumor cell invasion

While interactions with the ECM mediate aspects of glioma invasion, this process also involves interactions between both adjacent tumor cells and tumor cells with normal cells within the CNS, which are typically mediated by cell adhesion molecules.

Cell-cell adhesion molecules typically exhibit homophilic binding to mediate intercellular interactions with adjacent cells expressing the same cell-adhesion molecule but have also been shown to interact with constituents of the ECM through heterophilic binding (Hinsby et al., 2004). In addition to mediating intercellular adhesion, molecules like the Immunoglobulin (Ig) superfamily of Cell Adhesion Molecules (CAMs) and cadherins also modulate signal transduction cascades to translate extracellular interactions into intracellular changes by impinging on the activation of receptor tyrosine kinases, molecular components of the WNT signaling cascade, and RhoGTPases (Cavallaro & Christofori, 2004). The functional roles of cell-cell adhesion molecules in glioma invasion are complex, as either their ability to enhance or inhibit glioma cell motility is dependent on both post-translational modifications and interactions with specific ligands. Neuronal- cadherin (N-cadherin) provides an exemplary model of this, as the degree of organization and maturation of N-cadherin cell-cell junctions impacts the migratory capacity of glioma cells, wherein more organized cell-cell junctions inhibit cell motility. However, the organization and maturation of cell-cell junctions depends critically on the presence or absence of specific ECM ligands (Perego et al., 2002). As a result of these complex biochemical underpinnings, the expressions and functions of specific cell-cell adhesion molecules have been differentially reported, most likely resulting from context-specific interactions that have yet to be fully understood.

The Ig-CAMs play important roles in cell migration and invasion in several physiological and pathophysiological functions including development, wound healing and cancer metastasis. The Neural Cell Adhesion Molecule (NCAM) has a complex role in mediating aspects of glioma tumor cell adhesion, migration and invasion. The overexpression of NCAM was found to decrease glioma tumor cell motility through non-homophilic interactions by blocking binding of glioma tumor cells to extracellular substrates. Both the intracellular and extracellular portions of the NCAM receptor independently were found to block glioma cell motility, for which the extracellular Ig domains were determined to be critical. Therefore the attenuation of motility by the overexpression of the NCAM extracellular domain was believed to be due to the heterophilic interaction of the Ig domains with a constituent of the ECM thereby competing off endogenous motogenic receptors (Prag et al., 2002). More recently, a loss of NCAM expression in gliomas of increasing WHO grade was determined, suggesting that the negative regulation of NCAM is involved in glioma progression. The loss of NCAM expression was also correlated with more diffuse brain-tumor interfaces (Duenisch et al. 2011).

Interestingly, NCAM is the major substrate for Poly Sialic Acid (PSA) modifications resulting in PSA-NCAM. The overexpression of enzymes that attach the PSA moiety resulted in increased invasion of intracranial grafts compared to PSA negative NCAM alone. Furthermore, increased tumor cell invasion was observed for both PSA positive and negative NCAM glioma tumor cells in NCAM knockout mice, lacking NCAM expression in the nervous system environment, suggesting that the PSA modification serves to attenuate NCAM homophilic interactions to mediate increased glioma cell invasion (Suzuki et al., 2005). Furthermore, the expression of PSA-NCAM was found to correlate with an adverse progonisis for GBM patients (Amoureux et al. 2010). Therefore the negative regulation of NCAM homophilic binding resulting from either a decrease in NCAM expression or the glycosylation of NCAM to yield PSA-NCAM enhances glioma tumor cell motility and invasion.

The **cadherin** family members are calcium dependent cell-cell adhesion molecules that interact with catenins to signal changes in the actin cyctoskleton. Studies have demonstrated that N-cadherin is expressed by glioma cells, however conflicting evidence exists as to the function of this expression (Barami et al., 2006). Regardless of these conflicting reports, it has been determined that N-cadherin proteolytic cleavage by the ADAMTS-related protease ADAM-10 is a key mediator of GBM cell motility (Kohutek et al., 2009). Both epithelial-cadherin (E-cadherin) and N-cadherin have been found to play important roles in mediating glioma tumor cell motility with the CNS, but recent studies suggest that elevated E-cadherin levels at the expense of N-cadherin in glioma cell lines has been associated with increased tumor aggressiveness (Lewis-Tuffin et al. 2010). Further investigation into the complex pathomechanisms of cell-cell adhesion molecules and their heterophilic interactions with ligands of the ECM in the context of glioma cell dissemination is important to understanding the macroscopic contribution of the neural extracellular environment to glioma invasion and progression.

5. Glioma tumor initiating cells and the neural ECM

In addition to the ability of glioma tumor cells to invade the normal surrounding brain tissue, another major therapeutic obstacle is the presence of a tumor stem cell-like population of cells that reside within the solid tumor mass. This small cellular subpopulation is resistant to radiotherapy and capable of repopulating the original parental tumor leading to tumor recurrence and disease progression (Chalmers, 2007). Interestingly, constituents of the neural ECM and cell-cell adhesion molecules are also implicated in the pathomechanisms of this small but lethal cellular subpopulation.

5.1 Cancer initiating cells are present in human glioma tumors

Cancer initiating cells (CICs) also called "cancer stem cells" were initially identified in human leukemia, and have since been described in several solid tumor types including gliomas (Galli et al., 2004; Singh et al., 2003, 2004). CICs were first isolated from human glioma tumors by culturing tumor cells in a media composition that closely resembles neural stem cell media, comprised of a serum-free base with Epidermal Growth Factor (EGF) and basic Fibroblast Growth Factor (bFGF). The resulting GIC population exhibited several distinct phenotypic characteristics from other glioma tumor cells, which serve as criterion to operationally define GICs and are: 1. the ability to self-renew, 2. multipotency – the ability to differentiate into every cellular subclass present within the CNS, and 3. the ability to phenotypically recapitulate the original parental tumor upon orthotopic transplantation (Galli et al., 2004; Singh et al., 2004). The presence of a GIC subpopulation within human glioma tumors suggests a complex intratumoral heterogeneity, wherein GICs are molecularly and phenotypically distinguishable from other glioma tumor cells. Recent evidence suggests that GICs are highly refractory to current adjuvant therapeutic treatments resulting from their slow progression through the cell cycle and upregulation of DNA repair mechanisms (Bao et al., 2006). According to the controversial "cancer stem cell hypothesis", CICs maintain stem-like characteristics that fuel the growth of the tumor by giving rise to all other tumor cell types through a process that closely resembles normal cellular differentiation and effective eradication of tumors requires the ablation of the CIC population.

While a significant amount of research supports the role of GICs in the pathophysiology of gliomas and the resemblance of GICs to their glial and neural stem cells counterparts, the utility of GICs as a model for primary glioma tumors is unparalleled. Initial evidence suggested that glioma tumor cells cultured in serum free media with EGF and bFGF more closely resembled original parental tumors both molecularly and phenotypically than serum cultured cell lines (Lee et al., 2006). These findings were seminal as they suggested, regardless of the controversy surrounding "cancer stem cells", that GICs are likely a more representative model of primary glioma tumors than traditional serum cultured cell lines.

GICs are highly tumorigenic and a significant amount of research has gone into identifying molecular markers of the most highly tumorigenic subpopulation. Although controversial, CD133 expression has been correlated to increased GIC tumorigenicity (Campos & Herold-Mende, 2011). While both CD133+ and CD133- GIC cells have been found to be highly tumorigenic, recent evidence suggests that two subpopulations of CD133- cells are present within glioma tumors; one which is tumorigenic and gives rise to CD133+ cells and another that is not (Chen et al., 2010). Thus offering a solution to the long-standing conundrum surrounding the correlation between CD133 expression and tumorigenicity.

5.2 Neural extracellular matrix expression denotes subtypes of gliomas and glioma initiating cells

High-grade gliomas, glioblastoma muliforme, were so named for the considerable intra as well as intertumoral heterogeneity observed across individual glioma tumors. In efforts to better characterize glioma subtypes and begin an investigation into the value of individualized patient-tailored therapies, molecular subclasses of hundreds of primary glioma tumors were evaluated on the basis of their gene expression profile signatures. In this seminal study by Phillips and colleagues, three molecular subpopulations of glioma tumors were identified proneural, proliferative, and mesenchymal (Phillips et al., 2006). The identification of different molecular subclasses of glioma tumors set the stage for an investigation into the presence of distinct molecular subtypes of GICs. Gunther and colleagues created GIC cell lines from nine human GBM tumors and their molecular gene profile signatures determined (Gunther et al., 2008). Interestingly, two distinct molecular subpopulations of GICs emerged as separate clusters, cluster-1 and cluster-2. GIC cell-lines belonging to cluster-1 cells grew as spheres, had increased multipotency, expressed high levels of CD133, and created highly invasive intracranial tumors. In contrast, cluster-2 GICs grew as adherent or semi-adherent cultures, were restricted in cell fate, had little or no expression of CD133 expression, and exhibited low tumorigenicity and resulted in poorly invasive tumors in vivo (Gunther et al., 2008).

Lottaz and colleagues determined that cluster-1 GICs were most similar to proneural GBM tumors, while cluster-2 GICs were closely related to the mesenchymal GBM subtype (Lottaz et al., 2010). In accordance with these findings, the expression of BCAN was specifically enriched in the proneural GBM subtype and cluster-1 GICs which were found to be more highly tumorigenic than cluster-2 GICs and correlated with increased CD133 expression (Gunther et al., 2008). Work from our own lab has replicated these findings demonstrating that B/b is highly expressed by GICs with a phenotype similar to that described for cluster-1 cells. While the exact function of B/b expression by GICs is currently under investigation, the unique pathophysiological properties of GICs suggest that B/b may have broader functionality than observed in terminally differentiated glioma tumor cells. Likewise the restricted expression of CD44 was also identified in cluster-2 GICs along with integrins β1 and β5 (Gunther et al., 2008), again suggesting that differential expression of neural ECM components may contribute to differences in the pathophysiology of distinct molecular subclasses of GICs. The identification of neural ECM expression by GICs suggests that molecular constituents of the neural ECM could be employed as therapeutic targets that also impinge on the highly tumorigenic GIC subpopulation to reduce tumor recurrence and improve patient prognosis. Further research is needed to characterize the function of neural ECM components and cell adhesion molecules in the GIC population to fully evaluate the efficacy of targeting their expression to improve the prognosis of patients with GBM tumors.

5.3 The neural extracellular matrix and glioma initiating cells

While the function of neural ECM expression by GICs remains largely unknown, GICs are phenotypically and molecularly similar to normal neural stem cells (NSCs) (Rebetz et al., 2008). Suggesting that the microenvironment, or stem cell-like niche, surrounding GICs may share several parallels with the composition and function of the microenvironment surrounding NSCs during neurodevelopment and in the adult brain (Denysenko et al., 2010). In support of this hypothesis, the stem-cell niche that comprises the normal NSC microenvironment contains elevated levels of several ECM components whose expressions are enriched in GICs and gliomas including but not limited to laminin (Shen et al., 2008) and tenascin-C (Garcion et al., 2004). Moreover, NSCs themselves have been shown to express the same neural ECM constituents expressed by GICs including the lectican family members (Kabos et al., 2004), phosphacan/ RPTPζ (Abaskharoun et al., 2010b, a), tenascin-C (Abaskharoun et al., 2010a), integrin α6β1 (Shen et al., 2008).

Of importance, both GICs and NSCs reside in highly vascularized niches and are often localized surrounding blood vessels (Gilbertson and Rich, 2007; Shen et al., 2008). Normal NSCs reside in the subventricular zone (SVZ) of the developing brain, which is inherently highly vascularized (Shen et al., 2008). In the adult SVZ, the association between endothelial cells comprising the vasculature of the stem cell microenvironment and NSCs are mediated by an interaction between laminin on endothelial cells and a major laminin binding integrin, α6β1. The inhibition of integrin α6 was found to disrupt the association between endothelial cells and NSCs and caused a significant decline in NSC proliferation. These findings highlight the functional significance of a close association between vascular endothelial cells and stem cells in maintaining their stem cell-like properties (Shen et al., 2008). Similar findings have also been reported for GICs, which further supports the hypothesis that the composition of the microenvironment surrounding GICs closely mirrors that for NSCs and as a result may have common functions in maintaining the stem cell-like state.

In gliomas the vasculature that comprises the GIC microenvironment typically arises de novo as part of tumorigenesis, or as recent evidence suggests from the differentiation of GICs into endothelial cells (Ricci-Vitiani et al., 2010). The close association between tumor vasculature endothelial cells and GICs was found to be imperative for maintaining the stem cell-like phenotype of this cellular population (Williams et al., 2010). Moreover, the expression of integrin α6 was identified as a marker of GICs residing within the perivascular niche. The inhibition of this cell adhesion molecule was found to block the interaction between laminin on vascular endothelial cells and GICs, which subsequently impeded GIC self-renewal, proliferation, and tumorigenic capacity (Lathia et al., 2010). These studies suggest that targeting the microenvironment, or stem cell-like niche, surrounding GICs may be a therapeutically advantageous approach to force the GIC subpopulation out of its stem cell-like state and to become subsequently more responsive to adjuvant therapies. Therefore, the components that comprise this unique stem cell-like microenvironment surrounding GICs represent attractive therapeutic candidates to inhibit tumor recurrence.

6. Conclusion

The ability of glioma cells to interact with and invade into the extracellular environment within the CNS is a critical contributor to the pathogenesis of these tumors and poor patient prognosis. Gliomas modulate their surrounding environment through the expression of unique matrix elements and cleavage of the normal matrix. In addition, they alter expression of cell surface receptors to mediate unique interactions within this neural environment. Recently, work suggests that GICs also employ a similar strategy to surround themselves with a neurogenic microenvironment. Therefore, therapeutic interventions that interfere with the expressions of neural ECM constituents, cell surface receptors, and cell adhesion molecules may represent ideal targets both to impede glioma invasion and also the tumorigenic qualities of GICs, thus targeting two major contributors to tumor recurrence and disease progression. Further work understanding the role of the ECM in glioma tumor pathogenesis is critical to develop better strategies for treatment of patients with gliomas.

7. References

Abaskharoun M, Bellemare M, Lau E, Margolis RU (2010a) Glypican-1, phosphacan/receptor protein-tyrosine phosphatase-zeta/beta and its ligand, tenascin-C, are expressed by neural stem cells and neural cells derived from embryonic stem cells. ASN Neuro 2:e00039.

Abaskharoun M, Bellemare M, Lau E, Margolis RU (2010b) Expression of hyaluronan and the hyaluronan-binding proteoglycans neurocan, aggrecan, and versican by neural stem cells and neural cells derived from embryonic stem cells. Brain Res 1327:6-15.

Adamsky K, Schilling J, Garwood J, Faissner A, Peles E (2001) Glial tumor cell adhesion is mediated by binding of the FNIII domain of receptor protein tyrosine phosphatase beta (RPTPbeta) to tenascin C. Oncogene 20:609-618.

Akiyama SK (1996) Integrins in cell adhesion and signaling. Hum Cell 9:181-186.

Amoureux MC, Coulibaly B, Chinot O, Loundou A, Metellus P, Rougon G, Figarella-Branger D (2010) Polysialic acid neural cell adhesion molecule (PSA-NCAM) is an adverse prognosis factor in glioblastoma, and regulates olig2 expression in glioma cell lines. BMC Cancer 10:91.

Arslan F, Bosserhoff AK, Nickl-Jockschat T, Doerfelt A, Bogdahn U, Hau P (2007) The role of versican isoforms V0/V1 in glioma migration mediated by transforming growth factor-beta2. Br J Cancer 96:1560-1568.

Aspberg A, Binkert C, Ruoslahti E (1995) The versican C-type lectin domain recognizes the adhesion protein tenascin-R. Proc Natl Acad Sci U S A 92:10590-10594.

Aspberg A, Miura R, Bourdoulous S, Shimonaka M, Heinegard D, Schachner M, Ruoslahti E, Yamaguchi Y (1997) The C-type lectin domains of lecticans, a family of aggregating chondroitin sulfate proteoglycans, bind tenascin-R by protein-protein interactions independent of carbohydrate moiety. Proc Natl Acad Sci U S A 94:10116-10121.

Bandtlow CE, Zimmermann DR (2000) Proteoglycans in the developing brain: new conceptual insights for old proteins. Physiol Rev 80:1267-1290.

Bao S, Wu Q, McLendon RE, Hao Y, Shi Q, Hjelmeland AB, Dewhirst MW, Bigner DD, Rich JN (2006) Glioma stem cells promote radioresistance by preferential activation of the DNA damage response. Nature 444:756-760.

Barami K, Lewis-Tuffin L, Anastasiadis PZ (2006) The role of cadherins and catenins in gliomagenesis. Neurosurg Focus 21:E13.

Barnea G, Grumet M, Milev P, Silvennoinen O, Levy JB, Sap J, Schlessinger J (1994) Receptor tyrosine phosphatase beta is expressed in the form of proteoglycan and binds to the extracellular matrix protein tenascin. J Biol Chem 269:14349-14352.

Bellail AC, Hunter SB, Brat DJ, Tan C, Van Meir EG (2004) Microregional extracellular matrix heterogeneity in brain modulates glioma cell invasion. Int J Biochem Cell Biol 36:1046-1069.

Bello L, Francolini M, Marthyn P, Zhang J, Carroll RS, Nikas DC, Strasser JF, Villani R, Cheresh DA, Black PM (2001) Alpha(v)beta3 and alpha(v)beta5 integrin expression in glioma periphery. Neurosurgery 49:380-389; discussion 390.

Berardi N, Pizzorusso T, Maffei L (2004) Extracellular matrix and visual cortical plasticity: freeing the synapse. Neuron 44:905-908.

Bourdon MA, Ruoslahti E (1989) Tenascin mediates cell attachment through an RGD-dependent receptor. J Cell Biol 108:1149-1155.

Brew K, Nagase H (2010) The tissue inhibitors of metalloproteinases (TIMPs): an ancient family with structural and functional diversity. Biochim Biophys Acta 1803:55-71.

Campos B, Herold-Mende CC (2011) Insight into the complex regulation of CD133 in glioma. Int J Cancer 128:501-510.

Cavallaro U, Christofori G (2004) Cell adhesion and signalling by cadherins and Ig-CAMs in cancer. Nat Rev Cancer 4:118-132.

Chalmers AJ (2007) Radioresistant glioma stem cells--therapeutic obstacle or promising target? DNA Repair (Amst) 6:1391-1394.

Chen R, Nishimura MC, Bumbaca SM, Kharbanda S, Forrest WF, Kasman IM, Greve JM, Soriano RH, Gilmour LL, Rivers CS, Modrusan Z, Nacu S, Guerrero S, Edgar KA, Wallin JJ, Lamszus K, Westphal M, Heim S, James CD, VandenBerg SR, Costello JF, Moorefield S, Cowdrey CJ, Prados M, Phillips HS (2010) A hierarchy of self-renewing tumor-initiating cell types in glioblastoma. Cancer Cell 17:362-375.

D'Abaco GM, Kaye AH (2007) Integrins: molecular determinants of glioma invasion. J Clin Neurosci 14:1041-1048.

DeAngelis PL (1999) Hyaluronan synthases: fascinating glycosyltransferases from vertebrates, bacterial pathogens, and algal viruses. Cell Mol Life Sci 56:670-682.

Delpech A, Delpech B (1984) Expression of hyaluronic acid-binding glycoprotein, hyaluronectin, in the developing rat embryo. Dev Biol 101:391-400.

Delpech B, Maingonnat C, Girard N, Chauzy C, Maunoury R, Olivier A, Tayot J, Creissard P (1993) Hyaluronan and hyaluronectin in the extracellular matrix of human brain tumour stroma. Eur J Cancer 29A:1012-1017.

Denysenko T, Gennero L, Roos MA, Melcarne A, Juenemann C, Faccani G, Morra I, Cavallo G, Reguzzi S, Pescarmona G, Ponzetto A (2010) Glioblastoma cancer stem cells: heterogeneity, microenvironment and related therapeutic strategies. Cell Biochem Funct 28:343-351.

Deryugina EI, Bourdon MA (1996) Tenascin mediates human glioma cell migration and modulates cell migration on fibronectin. J Cell Sci 109 (Pt 3):643-652.

Dours-Zimmermann MT, Zimmermann DR (1994) A novel glycosaminoglycan attachment domain identified in two alternative splice variants of human versican. J Biol Chem 269:32992-32998.

Duenisch P, Reichart R, Mueller U, Brodhun M, Bjerkvig R, Romeike B, Walter J, Herbold C, Regenbrecht CR, Kalff R, Kuhn SA (2011) Neural cell adhesion molecule isoform 140 declines with rise of WHO grade in human gliomas and serves as indicator for the invasion zone of multiform glioblastomas and brain metastases. J Cancer Res Clin Oncol 137:399-414.

Ethell IM, Ethell DW (2007) Matrix metalloproteinases in brain development and remodeling: synaptic functions and targets. J Neurosci Res 85:2813-2823.

Frischknecht R, Seidenbecher CI (2008) The crosstalk of hyaluronan-based extracellular matrix and synapses. Neuron Glia Biol 4:249-257.

Galli R, Binda E, Orfanelli U, Cipelletti B, Gritti A, De Vitis S, Fiocco R, Foroni C, Dimeco F, Vescovi A (2004) Isolation and characterization of tumorigenic, stem-like neural precursors from human glioblastoma. Cancer Res 64:7011-7021.

Galtrey CM, Fawcett JW (2007) The role of chondroitin sulfate proteoglycans in regeneration and plasticity in the central nervous system. Brain Res Rev 54:1-18.

Garcion E, Halilagic A, Faissner A, ffrench-Constant C (2004) Generation of an environmental niche for neural stem cell development by the extracellular matrix molecule tenascin C. Development 131:3423-3432.

Garwood J, Heck N, Reichardt F, Faissner A (2003) Phosphacan short isoform, a novel non-proteoglycan variant of phosphacan/receptor protein tyrosine phosphatase-beta, interacts with neuronal receptors and promotes neurite outgrowth. J Biol Chem 278:24164-24173.

Gary SC, Zerillo CA, Chiang VL, Gaw JU, Gray G, Hockfield S (2000) cDNA cloning, chromosomal localization, and expression analysis of human BEHAB/brevican, a brain specific proteoglycan regulated during cortical development and in glioma. Gene 256:139-147.

Giese A, Loo MA, Norman SA, Treasurywala S, Berens ME (1996) Contrasting migratory response of astrocytoma cells to tenascin mediated by different integrins. J Cell Sci 109 (Pt 8):2161-2168.

Gilbertson RJ, Rich JN (2007) Making a tumour's bed: glioblastoma stem cells and the vascular niche. Nat Rev Cancer 7:733-736.

Gladson CL (1996) Expression of integrin alpha v beta 3 in small blood vessels of glioblastoma tumors. J Neuropathol Exp Neurol 55:1143-1149.

Gladson CL (1999) The extracellular matrix of gliomas: modulation of cell function. J Neuropathol Exp Neurol 58:1029-1040.

Groves MD, Puduvalli VK, Conrad CA, Gilbert MR, Yung WK, Jaeckle K, Liu V, Hess KR, Aldape KD, Levin VA (2006) Phase II trial of temozolomide plus marimastat for recurrent anaplastic gliomas: a relationship among efficacy, joint toxicity and anticonvulsant status. J Neurooncol 80:83-90.

Gunther HS, Schmidt NO, Phillips HS, Kemming D, Kharbanda S, Soriano R, Modrusan Z, Meissner H, Westphal M, Lamszus K (2008) Glioblastoma-derived stem cell-enriched cultures form distinct subgroups according to molecular and phenotypic criteria. Oncogene 27:2897-2909.

Hartmann U, Maurer P (2001) Proteoglycans in the nervous system--the quest for functional roles in vivo. Matrix Biol 20:23-35.

Held-Feindt J, Paredes EB, Blomer U, Seidenbecher C, Stark AM, Mehdorn HM, Mentlein R (2006) Matrix-degrading proteases ADAMTS4 and ADAMTS5 (disintegrins and metalloproteinases with thrombospondin motifs 4 and 5) are expressed in human glioblastomas. Int J Cancer 118:55-61.

Hinsby AM, Berezin V, Bock E (2004) Molecular mechanisms of NCAM function. Front Biosci 9:2227-2244.

Hirata E, Arakawa Y, Shirahata M, Yamaguchi M, Kishi Y, Okada T, Takahashi JA, Matsuda M, Hashimoto N (2009) Endogenous tenascin-C enhances glioblastoma invasion with reactive change of surrounding brain tissue. Cancer Sci 100:1451-1459.

Hu B, Kong LL, Matthews RT, Viapiano MS (2008) The proteoglycan brevican binds to fibronectin after proteolytic cleavage and promotes glioma cell motility. J Biol Chem 283:24848-24859.

Itano N, Kimata K (2002) Mammalian hyaluronan synthases. IUBMB Life 54:195-199.

Itoh T, Matsuda H, Tanioka M, Kuwabara K, Itohara S, Suzuki R (2002) The role of matrix metalloproteinase-2 and matrix metalloproteinase-9 in antibody-induced arthritis. J Immunol 169:2643-2647.

Jaworski DM, Kelly GM, Hockfield S (1995) The CNS-specific hyaluronan-binding protein BEHAB is expressed in ventricular zones coincident with gliogenesis. J Neurosci 15:1352-1362.

Jaworski DM, Kelly GM, Piepmeier JM, Hockfield S (1996) BEHAB (brain enriched hyaluronan binding) is expressed in surgical samples of glioma and in intracranial grafts of invasive glioma cell lines. Cancer Res 56:2293-2298.

Kabos P, Matundan H, Zandian M, Bertolotto C, Robinson ML, Davy BE, Yu JS, Krueger RC, Jr. (2004) Neural precursors express multiple chondroitin sulfate proteoglycans, including the lectican family. Biochem Biophys Res Commun 318:955-963.

Kachra Z, Beaulieu E, Delbecchi L, Mousseau N, Berthelet F, Moumdjian R, Del Maestro R, Beliveau R (1999) Expression of matrix metalloproteinases and their inhibitors in human brain tumors. Clin Exp Metastasis 17:555-566.

Kleihues P, Burger PC, Scheithauer BW (1993) The new WHO classification of brain tumours. Brain Pathol 3:255-268.

Kleihues P, Louis DN, Scheithauer BW, Rorke LB, Reifenberger G, Burger PC, Cavenee WK (2002) The WHO classification of tumors of the nervous system. J Neuropathol Exp Neurol 61:215-225; discussion 226-219.

Knott JC, Mahesparan R, Garcia-Cabrera I, Bolge Tysnes B, Edvardsen K, Ness GO, Mork S, Lund-Johansen M, Bjerkvig R (1998) Stimulation of extracellular matrix components in the normal brain by invading glioma cells. Int J Cancer 75:864-872.

Kohutek ZA, diPierro CG, Redpath GT, Hussaini IM (2009) ADAM-10-mediated N-cadherin cleavage is protein kinase C-alpha dependent and promotes glioblastoma cell migration. J Neurosci 29:4605-4615.

Kuppner MC, Van Meir E, Gauthier T, Hamou MF, de Tribolet N (1992) Differential expression of the CD44 molecule in human brain tumours. Int J Cancer 50:572-577.

Lakka SS, Gondi CS, Rao JS (2005) Proteases and glioma angiogenesis. Brain Pathol 15:327-341.

Lakka SS, Jasti SL, Kyritsis AP, Yung WK, Ali-Osman F, Nicolson GL, Rao JS (2000) Regulation of MMP-9 (type IV collagenase) production and invasiveness in gliomas by the extracellular signal-regulated kinase and jun amino-terminal kinase signaling cascades. Clin Exp Metastasis 18:245-252.

Lathia JD, Gallagher J, Heddleston JM, Wang J, Eyler CE, Macswords J, Wu Q, Vasanji A, McLendon RE, Hjelmeland AB, Rich JN (2010) Integrin alpha 6 regulates glioblastoma stem cells. Cell Stem Cell 6:421-432.

Lee J, Kotliarova S, Kotliarov Y, Li A, Su Q, Donin NM, Pastorino S, Purow BW, Christopher N, Zhang W, Park JK, Fine HA (2006) Tumor stem cells derived from glioblastomas cultured in bFGF and EGF more closely mirror the phenotype and genotype of primary tumors than do serum-cultured cell lines. Cancer Cell 9:391-403.

Leins A, Riva P, Lindstedt R, Davidoff MS, Mehraein P, Weis S (2003) Expression of tenascin-C in various human brain tumors and its relevance for survival in patients with astrocytoma. Cancer 98:2430-2439.

Levicar N, Nuttall RK, Lah TT (2003) Proteases in brain tumour progression. Acta Neurochir (Wien) 145:825-838.

Levin VA, Phuphanich S, Yung WK, Forsyth PA, Maestro RD, Perry JR, Fuller GN, Baillet M (2006) Randomized, double-blind, placebo-controlled trial of marimastat in glioblastoma multiforme patients following surgery and irradiation. J Neurooncol 78:295-302.

Lewis-Tuffin LJ, Rodriguez F, Giannini C, Scheithauer B, Necela BM, Sarkaria JN, Anastasiadis PZ (2010) Misregulated E-cadherin expression associated with an aggressive brain tumor phenotype. PLoS One 5:e13665.

Liesi P (1984) Laminin and fibronectin in normal and malignant neuroectodermal cells. Med Biol 62:163-180.

Lottaz C, Beier D, Meyer K, Kumar P, Hermann A, Schwarz J, Junker M, Oefner PJ, Bogdahn U, Wischhusen J, Spang R, Storch A, Beier CP (2010) Transcriptional profiles of CD133+ and CD133- glioblastoma-derived cancer stem cell lines suggest different cells of origin. Cancer Res 70:2030-2040.

Louis DN (2006) Molecular pathology of malignant gliomas. Annu Rev Pathol 1:97-117.

Lundell A, Olin AI, Morgelin M, al-Karadaghi S, Aspberg A, Logan DT (2004) Structural basis for interactions between tenascins and lectican C-type lectin domains: evidence for a crosslinking role for tenascins. Structure 12:1495-1506.

Maeda N, Fukazawa N, Ishii M (2010) Chondroitin sulfate proteoglycans in neural development and plasticity. Front Biosci 15:626-644.

Majumdar MK, Askew R, Schelling S, Stedman N, Blanchet T, Hopkins B, Morris EA, Glasson SS (2007) Double-knockout of ADAMTS-4 and ADAMTS-5 in mice results in physiologically normal animals and prevents the progression of osteoarthritis. Arthritis Rheum 56:3670-3674.

Margolis RU, Margolis RK, Chang LB, Preti C (1975) Glycosaminoglycans of brain during development. Biochemistry 14:85-88.

Matthews RT, Gary SC, Zerillo C, Pratta M, Solomon K, Arner EC, Hockfield S (2000) Brain-enriched hyaluronan binding (BEHAB)/brevican cleavage in a glioma cell line is mediated by a disintegrin and metalloproteinase with thrombospondin motifs (ADAMTS) family member. J Biol Chem 275:22695-22703.

Matthews RT, Kelly GM, Zerillo CA, Gray G, Tiemeyer M, Hockfield S (2002) Aggrecan glycoforms contribute to the molecular heterogeneity of perineuronal nets. J Neurosci 22:7536-7547.

Meng K, Rodriguez-Pena A, Dimitrov T, Chen W, Yamin M, Noda M, Deuel TF (2000) Pleiotrophin signals increased tyrosine phosphorylation of beta beta-catenin through inactivation of the intrinsic catalytic activity of the receptor-type protein tyrosine phosphatase beta/zeta. Proc Natl Acad Sci U S A 97:2603-2608.

Merzak A, Koocheckpour S, Pilkington GJ (1994) CD44 mediates human glioma cell adhesion and invasion in vitro. Cancer Res 54:3988-3992.

Milev P, Fischer D, Haring M, Schulthess T, Margolis RK, Chiquet-Ehrismann R, Margolis RU (1997) The fibrinogen-like globe of tenascin-C mediates its interactions with neurocan and phosphacan/protein-tyrosine phosphatase-zeta/beta. J Biol Chem 272:15501-15509.

Milev P, Maurel P, Chiba A, Mevissen M, Popp S, Yamaguchi Y, Margolis RK, Margolis RU (1998) Differential regulation of expression of hyaluronan-binding proteoglycans in developing brain: aggrecan, versican, neurocan, and brevican. Biochem Biophys Res Commun 247:207-212.

Miura R, Aspberg A, Ethell IM, Hagihara K, Schnaar RL, Ruoslahti E, Yamaguchi Y (1999) The proteoglycan lectin domain binds sulfated cell surface glycolipids and promotes cell adhesion. J Biol Chem 274:11431-11438.

Morgenstern DA, Asher RA, Fawcett JW (2002) Chondroitin sulphate proteoglycans in the CNS injury response. Prog Brain Res 137:313-332.

Muller S, Kunkel P, Lamszus K, Ulbricht U, Lorente GA, Nelson AM, von Schack D, Chin DJ, Lohr SC, Westphal M, Melcher T (2003) A role for receptor tyrosine phosphatase zeta in glioma cell migration. Oncogene 22:6661-6668.

Nabors LB, Mikkelsen T, Rosenfeld SS, Hochberg F, Akella NS, Fisher JD, Cloud GA, Zhang Y, Carson K, Wittemer SM, Colevas AD, Grossman SA (2007) Phase I and correlative biology study of cilengitide in patients with recurrent malignant glioma. J Clin Oncol 25:1651-1657.

Nakada M, Nakada S, Demuth T, Tran NL, Hoelzinger DB, Berens ME (2007) Molecular targets of glioma invasion. Cell Mol Life Sci 64:458-478.

Nakada M, Miyamori H, Kita D, Takahashi T, Yamashita J, Sato H, Miura R, Yamaguchi Y, Okada Y (2005) Human glioblastomas overexpress ADAMTS-5 that degrades brevican. Acta Neuropathol 110:239-246.

Nakagawa T, Kubota T, Kabuto M, Fujimoto N, Okada Y (1996) Secretion of matrix metalloproteinase-2 (72 kD gelatinase/type IV collagenase = gelatinase A) by malignant human glioma cell lines: implications for the growth and cellular invasion of the extracellular matrix. J Neurooncol 28:13-24.

Norman SA, Golfinos JG, Scheck AC (1998) Expression of a receptor protein tyrosine phosphatase in human glial tumors. J Neurooncol 36:209-217.

Nutt CL, Matthews RT, Hockfield S (2001a) Glial tumor invasion: a role for the upregulation and cleavage of BEHAB/brevican. Neuroscientist 7:113-122.

Nutt CL, Zerillo CA, Kelly GM, Hockfield S (2001b) Brain enriched hyaluronan binding (BEHAB)/brevican increases aggressiveness of CNS-1 gliomas in Lewis rats. Cancer Res 61:7056-7059.

Ohnishi T, Hiraga S, Izumoto S, Matsumura H, Kanemura Y, Arita N, Hayakawa T (1998) Role of fibronectin-stimulated tumor cell migration in glioma invasion in vivo: clinical significance of fibronectin and fibronectin receptor expressed in human glioma tissues. Clin Exp Metastasis 16:729-741.

Okada H, Yoshida J, Sokabe M, Wakabayashi T, Hagiwara M (1996) Suppression of CD44 expression decreases migration and invasion of human glioma cells. Int J Cancer 66:255-260.

Oohira A, Matsui F, Tokita Y, Yamauchi S, Aono S (2000) Molecular interactions of neural chondroitin sulfate proteoglycans in the brain development. Arch Biochem Biophys 374:24-34.

Park DM, Rich JN (2009) Biology of glioma cancer stem cells. Mol Cells 28:7-12.

Park JB, Kwak HJ, Lee SH (2008) Role of hyaluronan in glioma invasion. Cell Adh Migr 2:202-207.

Paulus W, Baur I, Dours-Zimmermann MT, Zimmermann DR (1996) Differential expression of versican isoforms in brain tumors. J Neuropathol Exp Neurol 55:528-533.

Peles E, Schlessinger J, Grumet M (1998) Multi-ligand interactions with receptor-like protein tyrosine phosphatase beta: implications for intercellular signaling. Trends Biochem Sci 23:121-124.

Perego C, Vanoni C, Massari S, Raimondi A, Pola S, Cattaneo MG, Francolini M, Vicentini LM, Pietrini G (2002) Invasive behaviour of glioblastoma cell lines is associated with altered organisation of the cadherin-catenin adhesion system. J Cell Sci 115:3331-3340.

Phillips HS, Kharbanda S, Chen R, Forrest WF, Soriano RH, Wu TD, Misra A, Nigro JM, Colman H, Soroceanu L, Williams PM, Modrusan Z, Feuerstein BG, Aldape K (2006) Molecular subclasses of high-grade glioma predict prognosis, delineate a pattern of disease progression, and resemble stages in neurogenesis. Cancer Cell 9:157-173.

Prag S, Lepekhin EA, Kolkova K, Hartmann-Petersen R, Kawa A, Walmod PS, Belman V, Gallagher HC, Berezin V, Bock E, Pedersen N (2002) NCAM regulates cell motility. J Cell Sci 115:283-292.

Properzi F, Fawcett JW (2004) Proteoglycans and brain repair. News Physiol Sci 19:33-38.

Radotra B, McCormick D (1997) Glioma invasion in vitro is mediated by CD44-hyaluronan interactions. J Pathol 181:434-438.

Raithatha SA, Muzik H, Muzik H, Rewcastle NB, Johnston RN, Edwards DR, Forsyth PA (2000) Localization of gelatinase-A and gelatinase-B mRNA and protein in human gliomas. Neuro Oncol 2:145-150.

Rao JS (2003) Molecular mechanisms of glioma invasiveness: the role of proteases. Nat Rev Cancer 3:489-501.

Rauch U (2004) Extracellular matrix components associated with remodeling processes in brain. Cell Mol Life Sci 61:2031-2045.

Rauch U, Feng K, Zhou XH (2001) Neurocan: a brain chondroitin sulfate proteoglycan. Cell Mol Life Sci 58:1842-1856.

Reardon DA, Neyns B, Weller M, Tonn JC, Nabors LB, Stupp R (2011) Cilengitide: an RGD pentapeptide alphanubeta3 and alphanubeta5 integrin inhibitor in development for glioblastoma and other malignancies. Future Oncol 7:339-354.

Rebetz J, Tian D, Persson A, Widegren B, Salford LG, Englund E, Gisselsson D, Fan X (2008) Glial progenitor-like phenotype in low-grade glioma and enhanced CD133-expression and neuronal lineage differentiation potential in high-grade glioma. PLoS One 3:e1936.

Ricci-Vitiani L, Pallini R, Biffoni M, Todaro M, Invernici G, Cenci T, Maira G, Parati EA, Stassi G, Larocca LM, De Maria R (2010) Tumour vascularization via endothelial differentiation of glioblastoma stem-like cells. Nature 468:824-828.

Rich JN, Bigner DD (2004) Development of novel targeted therapies in the treatment of malignant glioma. Nat Rev Drug Discov 3:430-446.

Riva P, Franceschi G, Frattarelli M, Riva N, Guiducci G, Cremonini AM, Giuliani G, Casi M, Gentile R, Jekunen AA, Kairemo KJ (1999a) 131I radioconjugated antibodies for the locoregional radioimmunotherapy of high-grade malignant glioma--phase I and II study. Acta Oncol 38:351-359.

Riva P, Franceschi G, Frattarelli M, Lazzari S, Riva N, Giuliani G, Casi M, Sarti G, Guiducci G, Giorgetti G, Gentile R, Santimaria M, Jermann E, Maeke HR (1999b) Loco-regional radioimmunotherapy of high-grade malignant gliomas using specific monoclonal antibodies labeled with 90Y: a phase I study. Clin Cancer Res 5:3275s-3280s.

Ruoslahti E (1996) Brain extracellular matrix. Glycobiology 6:489-492.

Rutka JT, Apodaca G, Stern R, Rosenblum M (1988) The extracellular matrix of the central and peripheral nervous systems: structure and function. J Neurosurg 69:155-170.

Sandy JD, Westling J, Kenagy RD, Iruela-Arispe ML, Verscharen C, Rodriguez-Mazaneque JC, Zimmermann DR, Lemire JM, Fischer JW, Wight TN, Clowes AW (2001) Versican V1 proteolysis in human aorta in vivo occurs at the Glu441-Ala442 bond, a site that is cleaved by recombinant ADAMTS-1 and ADAMTS-4. J Biol Chem 276:13372-13378.

Sarkar S, Nuttall RK, Liu S, Edwards DR, Yong VW (2006) Tenascin-C stimulates glioma cell invasion through matrix metalloproteinase-12. Cancer Res 66:11771-11780.

Schnell O, Krebs B, Wagner E, Romagna A, Beer AJ, Grau SJ, Thon N, Goetz C, Kretzschmar HA, Tonn JC, Goldbrunner RH (2008) Expression of integrin alphavbeta3 in gliomas correlates with tumor grade and is not restricted to tumor vasculature. Brain Pathol 18:378-386.

Seidenbecher CI, Gundelfinger ED, Bockers TM, Trotter J, Kreutz MR (1998) Transcripts for secreted and GPI-anchored brevican are differentially distributed in rat brain. Eur J Neurosci 10:1621-1630.

Shen Q, Wang Y, Kokovay E, Lin G, Chuang SM, Goderie SK, Roysam B, Temple S (2008) Adult SVZ stem cells lie in a vascular niche: a quantitative analysis of niche cell-cell interactions. Cell Stem Cell 3:289-300.

Singh SK, Clarke ID, Terasaki M, Bonn VE, Hawkins C, Squire J, Dirks PB (2003) Identification of a cancer stem cell in human brain tumors. Cancer Res 63:5821-5828.

Singh SK, Hawkins C, Clarke ID, Squire JA, Bayani J, Hide T, Henkelman RM, Cusimano MD, Dirks PB (2004) Identification of human brain tumour initiating cells. Nature 432:396-401.

Spicer AP, McDonald JA (1998) Characterization and molecular evolution of a vertebrate hyaluronan synthase gene family. J Biol Chem 273:1923-1932.

Spicer AP, Tien JY (2004) Hyaluronan and morphogenesis. Birth Defects Res C Embryo Today 72:89-108.

Spicer AP, Joo A, Bowling RA, Jr. (2003) A hyaluronan binding link protein gene family whose members are physically linked adjacent to chondroitin sulfate proteoglycan core protein genes: the missing links. J Biol Chem 278:21083-21091.

Suzuki M, Suzuki M, Nakayama J, Suzuki A, Angata K, Chen S, Sakai K, Hagihara K, Yamaguchi Y, Fukuda M (2005) Polysialic acid facilitates tumor invasion by glioma cells. Glycobiology 15:887-894.

Tabatabai G, Weller M, Nabors B, Picard M, Reardon D, Mikkelsen T, Ruegg C, Stupp R (2010) Targeting integrins in malignant glioma. Target Oncol 5:175-181.

Tonn JC, Kerkau S, Hanke A, Bouterfa H, Mueller JG, Wagner S, Vince GH, Roosen K (1999) Effect of synthetic matrix-metalloproteinase inhibitors on invasive capacity and proliferation of human malignant gliomas in vitro. Int J Cancer 80:764-772.

Toole BP (2000) Hyaluronan is not just a goo! J Clin Invest 106:335-336.

Toole BP (2004) Hyaluronan: from extracellular glue to pericellular cue. Nat Rev Cancer 4:528-539.

Ulbricht U, Eckerich C, Fillbrandt R, Westphal M, Lamszus K (2006) RNA interference targeting protein tyrosine phosphatase zeta/receptor-type protein tyrosine phosphatase beta suppresses glioblastoma growth in vitro and in vivo. J Neurochem 98:1497-1506.

Ventimiglia JB, Wikstrand CJ, Ostrowski LE, Bourdon MA, Lightner VA, Bigner DD (1992) Tenascin expression in human glioma cell lines and normal tissues. J Neuroimmunol 36:41-55.

Viapiano MS, Matthews RT (2006) From barriers to bridges: chondroitin sulfate proteoglycans in neuropathology. Trends Mol Med 12:488-496.

Viapiano MS, Matthews RT, Hockfield S (2003) A novel membrane-associated glycovariant of BEHAB/brevican is up-regulated during rat brain development and in a rat model of invasive glioma. J Biol Chem 278:33239-33247.

Viapiano MS, Hockfield S, Matthews RT (2008) BEHAB/brevican requires ADAMTS-mediated proteolytic cleavage to promote glioma invasion. J Neurooncol 88:261-272.

Viapiano MS, Bi WL, Piepmeier J, Hockfield S, Matthews RT (2005) Novel tumor-specific isoforms of BEHAB/brevican identified in human malignant gliomas. Cancer Res 65:6726-6733.

Wang M, Wang T, Liu S, Yoshida D, Teramoto A (2003) The expression of matrix metalloproteinase-2 and -9 in human gliomas of different pathological grades. Brain Tumor Pathol 20:65-72.

Weigel PH, Hascall VC, Tammi M (1997) Hyaluronan synthases. J Biol Chem 272:13997-14000.

Westling J, Gottschall PE, Thompson VP, Cockburn A, Perides G, Zimmermann DR, Sandy JD (2004) ADAMTS4 (aggrecanase-1) cleaves human brain versican V2 at Glu405-Gln406 to generate glial hyaluronate binding protein. Biochem J 377:787-795.

Wild-Bode C, Weller M, Wick W (2001) Molecular determinants of glioma cell migration and invasion. J Neurosurg 94:978-984.

Williams RF, Sims TL, Tracey L, Myers AL, Ng CY, Poppleton H, Nathwani AC, Davidoff AM (2010) Maturation of tumor vasculature by interferon-beta disrupts the vascular niche of glioma stem cells. Anticancer Res 30:3301-3308.

Wu Y, Sheng W, Chen L, Dong H, Lee V, Lu F, Wong CS, Lu WY, Yang BB (2004) Versican V1 isoform induces neuronal differentiation and promotes neurite outgrowth. Mol Biol Cell 15:2093-2104.

Yamada H, Watanabe K, Shimonaka M, Yamaguchi Y (1994) Molecular cloning of brevican, a novel brain proteoglycan of the aggrecan/versican family. J Biol Chem 269:10119-10126.

Yamada S, Bu XY, Khankaldyyan V, Gonzales-Gomez I, McComb JG, Laug WE (2006) Effect of the angiogenesis inhibitor Cilengitide (EMD 121974) on glioblastoma growth in nude mice. Neurosurgery 59:1304-1312; discussion 1312.

Yamaguchi Y (2000) Lecticans: organizers of the brain extracellular matrix. Cell Mol Life Sci 57:276-289.

Yamamoto M, Ueno Y, Hayashi S, Fukushima T (2002) The role of proteolysis in tumor invasiveness in glioblastoma and metastatic brain tumors. Anticancer Res 22:4265-4268.

Zagzag D, Friedlander DR, Miller DC, Dosik J, Cangiarella J, Kostianovsky M, Cohen H, Grumet M, Greco MA (1995) Tenascin expression in astrocytomas correlates with angiogenesis. Cancer Res 55:907-914.

Zagzag D, Shiff B, Jallo GI, Greco MA, Blanco C, Cohen H, Hukin J, Allen JC, Friedlander DR (2002) Tenascin-C promotes microvascular cell migration and phosphorylation of focal adhesion kinase. Cancer Res 62:2660-2668.

Zhao Y, Xiao A, diPierro CG, Carpenter JE, Abdel-Fattah R, Redpath GT, Lopes MB, Hussaini IM (2010) An extensive invasive intracranial human glioblastoma xenograft model: role of high level matrix metalloproteinase 9. Am J Pathol 176:3032-3049.

Zheng PS, Wen J, Ang LC, Sheng W, Viloria-Petit A, Wang Y, Wu Y, Kerbel RS, Yang BB (2004) Versican/PG-M G3 domain promotes tumor growth and angiogenesis. Faseb J 18:754-756.

Zimmermann DR, Dours-Zimmermann MT (2008) Extracellular matrix of the central nervous system: from neglect to challenge. Histochem Cell Biol 130:635-653.

12

Portrait of Transcriptional Expression Profiles Displayed by Different Glioblastoma Cell Lines

Paulo R. D. V. Godoy et al.[1]
University of São Paulo,
Brazil

1. Introduction

Glioblastoma multiforme (GBM) is among the most lethal of all human tumors, with the average survival of approximately 1 year from diagnosis (Avgeropoulos and Batchelor, 1999). In glioblastomas, LOH 10q is the most frequent genetic alteration (69%), followed by *EGFR* amplification (34%), *TP53* mutations (31%), *p16INK4a* deletion (31%), and *PTEN* mutations (24%)(Ohgaki and Kleihues, 2005).
Treatments of patients with GBM include surgery, radiotherapy and parallel adjuvant chemotherapy (Stupp et al., 2005). While radiotherapy has been found to significantly prolong survival rates for GBM patients, a poor prognosis and radioresistance are typical characteristics of this disease (Stupp et al., 2007).
The antitumoral drug Temozolomide (TMZ) constitutes, in combination with radiotherapy, the current standard of care for glioblastoma (Stupp et al., 2005). However, the action of TMZ may be counteracted in tumors by the expression of the DNA repair enzyme MGMT, which repairs TMZ-induced DNA lesions (Hegi et al., 2005). MGMT activity and resistance to TMZ were highly correlated, indicating that MGMT is a major predictor of response to TMZ in glioma cells (Hermisson et al., 2006). According to the authors, collectively, MGMT expression and *TP53* status may become valuable parameters to predict cell responses to TMZ treatment in patients with GBM. Modulation of *MSH6*, *PARP1* and *NTL1*, DNA repair genes involved in mismatch repair and base excision repair (BER), were found at transcription and protein levels in GBM cells resistant to TMZ (Zhang et al., 2010).
Other genotoxic agents exert different effects in GBM cells with different *TP53* status. UV light (UV-C) (Batista et al., 2009) and chloroethylating agents (ACNU and BCNU) (Batista et al., 2007), significantly induce apoptosis in *TP53*-mutated glioma cells, while WT *TP53* cells are more sensitive to methylating agents, including TMZ (Hermisson et al., 2006; Roos et al., 2007).
Efforts have been made to overcome drug and radio-resistance of GBM cells, but the heterogeneity of these tumors seems to be critical, and molecular analysis is an important tool to elucidate the mechanisms underlying cellular responses to antitumoral agents. Recently, application of genome-scale methodologies has opened the opportunity to study

---

[1] Stephano S. Mello, Daniele A. Magalhães, Flavia S. Donaires, Ana P. Lima-Montaldi, Patricia Nicolucci, Eduardo A. Donadi, Geraldo A. S. Passos and Elza T. Sakamoto-Hojo

transcript profiles for thousands of genes simultaneously, thus providing a picture on how different biological processes can be modulated under irradiation, drug treatment or even between different cell types, on the basis of the lists of differentially expressed genes (either induced or repressed genes) provided by the microarray experiments. This approach allows comparisons between different biological situations (Tusher et al., 2001; Sakamoto-Hojo et al., 2003; Fachin et al., 2007; Fachin et al., 2009). In a previous work, several stress response/DNA repair genes, such as *HSPA9B*, *INPP5A*, *PIP5K1A*, *FANCG*, and *TPP2* were found up-regulated in U343MG-a GBM cells analyzed at 6 h following irradiation with 1 Gy, reflecting the radio-resistance of these cells; at this condition, the survival rate was 61%, and a broad spectrum of other biological processes was found associated to the list of differentially expressed genes in irradiated cells (Bassi et al., 2008).

TP53 gene plays a role in drug and radioresistance mechanisms, but the complex network of signaling pathways involving this gene is not well elucidated. TP53 is a multifunctional protein that acts in cell cycle blockage and signaling pathways towards DNA repair, contributing to the maintenance of genome integrity in response to a variety of genotoxic stresses (Bartussek et al., 1999). Alternatively, TP53 protein triggers a cascade of signaling pathways culminating in apoptosis, depending on the extent of DNA damage (Prise et al., 2005). The TP53 protein is also a transcription factor that regulates the expression of a large number of target genes (Vogelstein et al., 2000). Many TP53 target genes have been described (el-Deiry, 1998; Horn and Vousden, 2007; Laptenko and Prives, 2006; Sbisa et al., 2007), and some other targets have been computationally predicted by the analysis of their binding sites (Hoh et al., 2002; Smeenk et al., 2008; Veprintsev and Fersht, 2008).

According to the literature data, there are controversial findings about the outcome of patients in relation to the *TP53* status of tumors; this gene may positive or negatively influences the cell radioresistance, as well as it can exert no influence in cellular responses to therapies (McIlwrath et al., 1994; Slichenmyer et al., 1993; Smith et al., 1995).

2. Objective

In the present work, we aim to compare gene expression profiles displayed by four GBM cell lines in the absence of any kind of treatment, using the microarray method, looking for molecular signatures that can provide new clues towards the understanding of GBM biology and radioresistance mechanisms. The results on the transcriptional profiles presented by a number of genes with different biological functions are discussed on the light of literature data regarding GBM cell responses to ionizing radiation and antitumor drugs, generally provided by survival assays.

3. Materials and methods

3.1 GBM cell lines

Human GBM U343 MG-a cell line was kindly donated by Dr. James T. Rutka (The Arthur and Sonia Labatt Brain Tumour Research Center, Canada), while T98G, U251MG, and U87MG were supplied by the American Type Culture Collection (ATCC) (Rockville, Maryland, USA). T98G and U251MG cell lines harbor three mutations (*TP53, CDKN2A*, and *PTEN*) while U343MG-a and U87MG cells are wild-type (WT) for *TP53*, and mutant (MT) for *CDKN2A* and *PTEN* genes (Ishii et al., 1999).

3.2 Cell culture and total RNA extraction

For gene expression analysis, cells were thawed from the nitrogen and sub-cultured for four passages in the presence of HAM F10 + DEM medium plus 15% fetal bovine serum and kept at 37°C and 5% CO_2. After the fourth sub-culturing, they were incubated for two days, and total RNA extraction was performed in replicate at 48 h, by using the Trizol reagent (Invitrogen, Carlsbad, CA, USA) according to the manufacturer's instructions. The quality of RNA samples was evaluated by denaturing agarose gel electrophoresis under standard conditions. To remove the contaminating DNA, RNA samples used in cDNA microarrays were treated with the Deoxyribonuclease I (Amplification Grade kit, Invitrogen), according to manufacturer's instructions.

3.3 cDNA microarray method

Four experiments in duplicate using GBM cells were carried out using a glass slide microarray containing 4500 clones of cDNA probe (in duplicates) from the human IMAGE Consortium cDNA library [http://image.llnl.gov/image/; kindly provided by Dr. Catherine Nguyen (INSERM-CNRS, Marseille, France)], and prepared according to the protocol described by Hegde et al (2000).

Microarrays were spotted onto glass slides (Corning) using a Generation III Array Spotter Amersham-Molecular Dynamics according to the manufacturer's instructions. Each cDNA sample was spotted twice on the slide (duplicate spots). The cDNA complex probes were prepared using the CyScribe Post Labelling Kit (Amersham Biosciences, England) (Fachin et al., 2009). Hybridizations were carried out using an automatic system (Automatic Slide Processor, Amersham Biosciences, England) and signals were immediately captured after the final wash procedure, using a Generation III laser scanner (Amersham Biosciences, England).

In an attempt to characterize the clones present in the array slide, the gene set was submitted to the NIH-DAVID bioinformatic tool, in order to obtain biological functions associated with the gene sequences present in the arrays, as well as the number of genes associated with each biological process. Among all clones, 2334 were identified by official gene symbol (HUGO), distributed in classes according to biological processes (Table 1).

3.3.1 Data acquisition and gene expression analysis

The image quantification was performed using the Spot software, (http://spot.cmis.csiro.au/spot/, CSIRO, Australia). Filtering, normalization and data analysis were done using the R statistical environment (Ihaka and Gentleman, 1996), in addition to Limma (Smyth et al., 2005), Bioconductor (Ihaka and Gentleman, 1996), Aroma (Bengtsson, 2004) and KTH (Wirta, 2004). The background to each feature was subtracted from the foreground value. Furthermore, the spots were evaluated by their circularity and calculations on the median versus mean deviation, so that those presenting irregular circularity, or with large differences between mean and median values, were considered unreliable. The raw data (red – R and green – G) was transformed into MA format before normalization, where $M = \log2(R/G)$ and $A = 1/2 \times \log2(R \times G)$. These procedures were followed by the application of the Print-tip Lowess normalization for each slide. Following the normalization procedure, microarray data were exported to tab-delimited tables in MEV format and analyzed in MEV (v. 3.1) software (Saeed et al., 2003). The microarrays data analysis involved the application of the statistical method SAM - Significance Analysis of

GOTERM-BIOLOGICAL PROCESS - FAT	%	PValue
GO:0007242~intracellular signaling cascade	10.28	3.90E-09
GO:0006793~phosphorus metabolic process	9.43	8.50E-16
GO:0006468~protein amino acid phosphorylation	6.73	6.81E-13
GO:0008104~protein localization	6.68	2.00E-04
GO:0042981~regulation of apoptosis	6.47	1.20E-05
GO:0007049~cell cycle	5.96	2.63E-04
GO:0033554~cellular response to stress	5.78	1.27E-11
GO:0006259~DNA metabolic process	4.50	4.42E-06
GO:0006974~Response to DNA damage stimulus	4.07	5.32E-10
GO:0006281~DNA repair	3.43	8.95E-11
GO:0007243~protein kinase cascade	3.43	1.53E-05
GO:0007167~enzyme linked receptor protein signaling pathway	3.08	1.04E-04
GO:0009314~response to radiation	1.93	5.82E-04
GO:0000165~MAPKKK cascade	1.89	1.69E-04
GO:0022604~regulation of cell morphogenesis	1.41	4.85E-04
GO:0006310~DNA recombination	1.29	9.19E-05
GO:0031344~regulation of cell projection organization	1.11	2.05E-04
GO:0006302~double-strand break repair	0.94	3.35E-05
GO:0006289~nucleotide-excision repair	0.86	5.76E-05
GO:0050770~regulation of axonogenesis	0.81	3.26E-04
GO:0051291~protein heterooligomerization	0.77	2.99E-04
GO:0050772~positive regulation of axonogenesis	0.51	1.85E-04
GO:0000723~telomere maintenance	0.51	6.05E-04
GO:0032925~regulation of activin receptor signaling pathway	0.30	7.62E-04

Table 1. Percentage of genes for each biological process analyzed for a total of 2334 genes present in a glass slide microarray. The array gene set (containing 4300 image clones) was submitted to NIH-DAVID (Dennis et al. 2003).

Microarray (Tusher et al., 2001), with the objective to compare MT versus WT *TP53* cell lines in terms of expression profiles. We used FDR< 0.68% to select only highly significant differentially expressed genes.

Information regarding biological functions were obtained at S.O.U.R.C.E. (http://genome-www5.stanford.edu/cgi-bin/SMD/source/source), and NCBI (http://www.ncbi.nlm.nih.gov/). Gene functional groups were given by DAVID tool (Dunne et al., 2003), choosing *Homo sapiens* as the current background, Gene Ontology: GOTERM_BP_FAT as parameters, and Functional Annotation Chart as the analyzing tool. The main biological functions associated to the list of differentially expressed genes were selected.

Every modulated gene was compared to a list of previously identified genes with TP53 binding sites using genome-wide tiling Chromatin immunoprecipitation (ChIP)-on-chip approach (Smeenk et al., 2008) or (ChIP) with the paired-end ditag (PET) (Wei et al., 2006) in order to point out genes that could be modulated by TP53 transactivation.

4. Results

4.1 Transcript profiles displayed by GBM cell lines

4.1.1 Hierarchical cluster analysis

Gene expression profiles studied by the cDNA microarray method generated interesting results about the transcriptional profiles exhibited by each cell line. Analysis of gene cluster uses standard statistical algorithms in order to arrange genes according to similarity of expression patterns, and the results can be graphically represented (Eisen et al., 1998). The analysis of hierarchical clustering was performed to compare MT and WT *TP53* cells regarding transcript profiles by using a set of genes previously selected by the SAM analysis. The results of the hierarchical clustering showed that MT *TP53* cells were grouped apart from the WT *TP53* cells. The mutant cell lines (T98G and U251) were not separated within a gene cluster, indicating more similarity in the basal transcription levels between cell lines; in contrast, the proficient cell lines (U87 and U343) were clustered apart from each other (**Fig.1**).

4.1.2 Differentially expressed genes indicated by Significant Analysis of Microarrays (SAM)

The statistical analysis performed by SAM indicated that MT *TP53* cell lines showed 29 down-regulated and 68 up-regulated genes, compared with WT *TP53* cells, for FDR ≤ 0.68%. For this small list of highly significant differentially expressed genes, the magnitude of fold-changes ranged from -1.68 to +1.93 by comparing MT *versus* WT *TP53* (Supp. Table 1).

For the list of differentially expressed genes, biological gene functions were studied by the DAVID-NIH bioinformatic tool (Dennis et al., 2003; Huang da et al., 2009). Out of 97 modulated genes, 73 were suitable for functional grouping procedure, since 10 genes were not grouped and 14 I.D. clones were still unknown. The most relevant categories (represented by a variable number of genes) were related to neurological system process (11%), regulation of apoptosis (10%), cellular response to stress (8%), regulation of cell proliferation (8%), cell-cell adhesion (5%), DNA repair (5%), response to ionizing radiation (4%), histone modification (4%), cell division (4%), etc. (**Fig.2.**). For discussion, we selected 36 genes on the basis of biological functions that can be possibly related to responses to genotoxic agents (**Table-2**), in order to find out clues for understanding the mechanisms underlying the sensitivity or resistance to anticancer therapies. Some of candidate genes that may participate in chemo- and/or radioresistance are involved in stress responses (*RUVBL2, ASNS, RNF8, LIG4* and *CAV1*) and cell adhesion (*CDH8, CDH13, CD93* and *ITGA5*), and other important cathegories, such as regulation of cell proliferation (*IGF1R, CDH13, CAV1, DUSP22, ADAMTS1, LIG4*) and apoptosis (*IGF1R, CDH13, IFT57, CRH, HSPB1, ASNS* and *LIG4*.

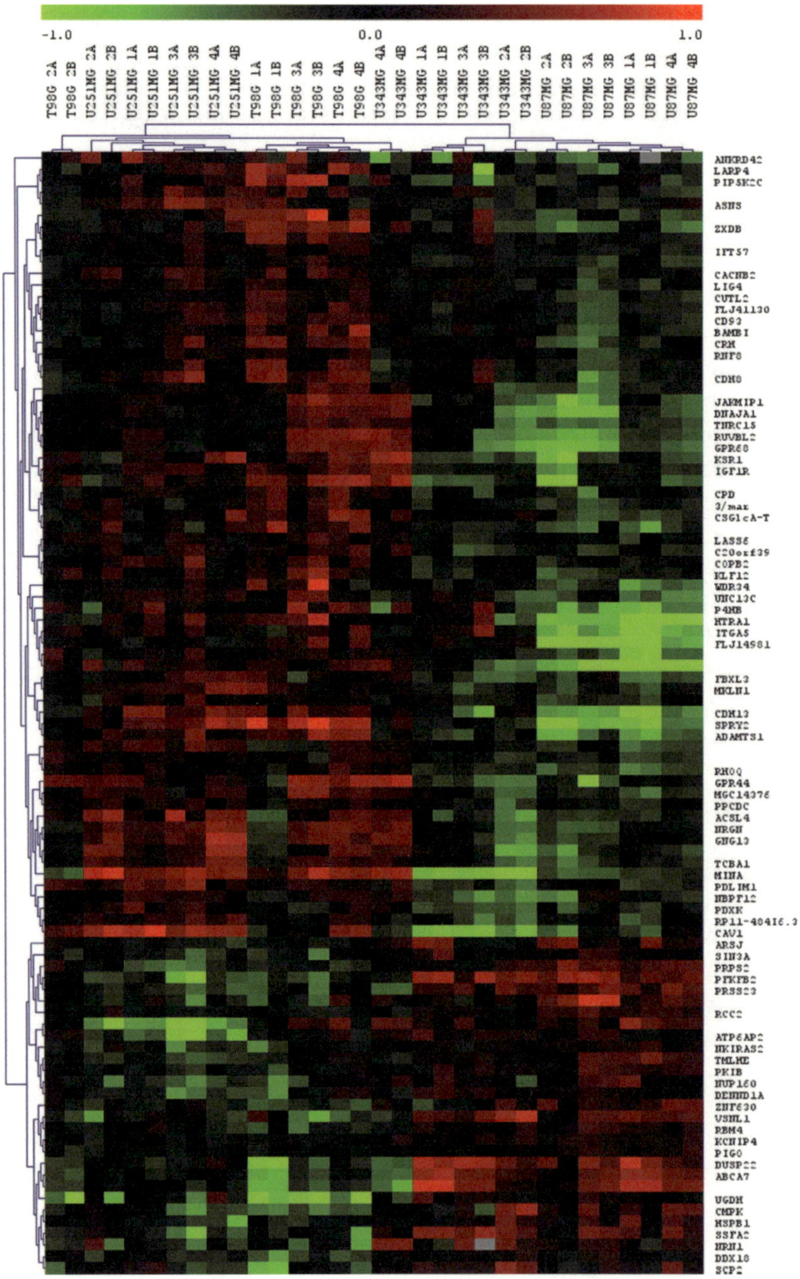

Fig. 1. Hierarchical clustering obtained for a gene set previously selected by the SAM method (FDR≤0.68%) for the results displayed by four GBM cell lines (T98G, U251MG, U343MG-a e U87MG), under normal proliferation in culture. The data set was provided by 4 experiments in duplicate. Experiments are represented by numbers (1-4) and the replicates are represented by letters (A and B). The expression level of each gene is represented according to the scale at the top (red indicates induction; green means repression; grey color represents data loss).

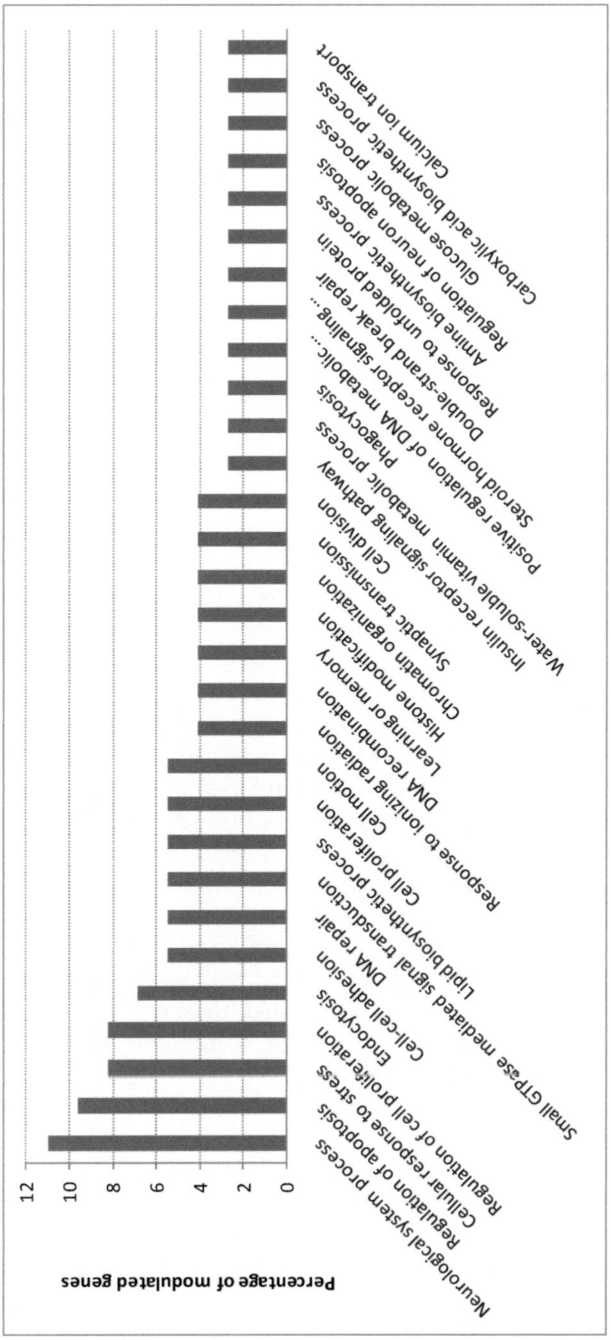

Fig. 2. Main Biological functions associated to the list of differentially expressed genes (out of 97 genes, 73 genes were recognized by the system) when comparing MT and WT *TP53* GBM cell lines. The results were analyzed by DAVID-NIH (Dennis et al., 2003; Huang da et al., 2009) as a bioinformatic tool to group differentially expressed genes according to their functions.

A comparative analysis of differentially expressed genes (obtained by SAM) was carried out with previously identified genes with *TP53* binding sites using ChIP-PET and ChIP-on-chip analysis (Smeenk et al., 2008; Wei et al., 2006). When comparing with ChIP- PET gene lists, we observed only one common gene (*LASS6*), while the comparison involving the gene list of our work with the ChIP-on-chip list, we found five common genes (*ARSJ, RCC2, CDH8, CDH13* and *HTRA1*).

5. Discussion

Expression profiles displayed by GBM cells provided results to compare these cells with other tumor types (Castells et al., 2010; Castells et al., 2009; Dreyfuss et al., 2009; Marucci et al., 2008; Reddy et al., 2008), normal tissues (Sallinen et al., 2000), or even regions in the same tumor (Mehrian Shai et al., 2005). However, there is no data in the literature comparing transcript profiles of GBM cell lines presenting similar genetic background. While T98G and U251MG harbor mutations for *TP53, CDKN2A*, and *PTEN*, U343MG-a and U87MG cell lines differ from others by the presence of a known WT *TP53* (Ishii et al., 1999). Expression profiles displayed by GBM cell lines were studied in the absence of any treatment. The hierarchical clustering analysis compared WT and MT *TP53* GBM cells regarding transcript profiles using a set of highly significant differentially expressed genes previously selected by SAM (FDR $\leq$ 0.68%). The results showed distinct expression profiles for WT *TP53* and MT *TP53* cells, whose patterns separate the mutant from WT cells. The mutant cell lines (T98G and U251MG) were not completely separated from each other within the cluster, indicating similarity of transcript patterns between the two cell lines. In contrast, *TP53* proficient cell lines (U87MG and U343MG-a) were clustered apart from each other. These results indicate the potential of the DNA microarray analysis to discriminate molecular profiles displayed by GBM cell lines presenting similar mutational background for *CDKN2A* and *PTEN* genes, but with different *TP53* status.
The statistical analysis performed by SAM (FDR $\leq$ 0.68%) indicated that MT *TP53* cell lines showed 28 down-regulated and 66 up-regulated genes, when compared to WT *TP53* cells (Table. 2). For the list of differentially expressed genes, biological gene functions were studied by the DAVID-NIH bioinformatic tool (Dennis et al., 2003; Huang da et al., 2009), and several biological processes were associated to the list of significant differentially expressed genes, such as: metabolism, response to ionizing radiation, cell adhesion, cell motion, apoptosis, DNA repair and transcription.
In addition, metabolic process was directly related with several biological functions as follow: insulin receptor signalling, water soluble vitamin metabolic process, steroid hormone receptor signalling, cellular response to nutrient levels, amine biosynthetic process, lipid biosynthetic process, calcium ion transport, lipid transport, glucose metabolic process, carboxylic acid biosynthetic process, and cellular amino acid derivative metabolic process. Other gene functions related to learning/memory, regulation of neuron apoptosis, synaptic transmission, and neurological system processes are intrinsic to the neural nature of GBM cells. DNA and RNA metabolism/regulation were also associated to several differentially expressed genes (Table. 2).
Three genes (*RNF8, CAV1* and *LIG4*) playing roles in ionizing radiation responses were found up-regulated in MT *TP53* cells, and this feature may influence the responsiveness to radiotherapy. It is already known that ionizing radiation causes DNA double-strand breaks (DSBs) that are highly cytotoxic lesions. Cells have a complex DNA-damage response that

Symbol	CloneID	Biological Process	Fold change	q-value (%)
SPRY2	40262	cell-cell signaling, development, organogenesis, regulation of signal transduction	1.93	0.00
CAV1	24651	cellular calcium ion homeostasis, cholesterol efflux, response to gamma radiation, regulation of apoptosis,	1.86	0.00
CDH13	31093	cell adhesion, homophilic cell adhesion	1.61	0.00
HTRA1	132044	proteolysis and peptidolysis, regulation of cell growth	1.55	0.00
ADAMTS1	34684	integrin-mediated signaling pathway, negative regulation of cell proliferation, heart trabecula formation, kidney development, ovulation from ovarian follicle, proteolysis	1.54	0.00
ITGA5	135671	cell-matrix adhesion, integrin-mediated signaling pathway	1.35	0.75
GPR68	22652	G-protein coupled receptor protein signaling pathway, inflammatory response, signal transduction	1.34	0.00
GPR44	25625	G-protein coupled receptor protein signaling pathway, immune response, calcium-mediated signaling, chemotaxis	1.34	0.75
RUVBL2	22267	chromatin modification, DNA recombination, DNA repair, regulation of growth, regulation of transcription	1.33	0.00
MKLN1	33715	cell motility, cell-matrix adhesion, signal transduction	1.31	0.00
KSR1	220655	Ras protein signal transduction, intracellular signaling cascade, protein amino acid phosphorylation	1.31	0.75
GNG13	178213	G-protein coupled receptor protein signaling pathway, signal transduction	1.30	0.75
CDH8	38939	cell adhesion, homophilic cell adhesion	1.30	0.00
DNAJA1	24473	protein folding, response to unfolded protein	1.28	0.75
RHOQ	131061	small GTPase mediated signal transduction	1.26	0.00
FBXL3	25778	protein ubiquitination	1.26	0.00
CRH	34671	immune response, learning and/or memory, pregnancy, signal transduction, synaptic transmission	1.24	0.00
IGF1R	21519	axonogenesis, brain development, exocrine pancreas development, male sex determination, regulation of apoptosis	1.24	0.00
ASNS	27208	amino acid biosynthesis	1.23	0.90
CD93	35503	cell-cell adhesion, macrophage activation, phagocytosis	1.19	0.00
COPB2	24627	intracellular protein transport, vesicle-mediated transport	1.18	0.00
CACNB2	34651	Synaptic transmission, ion transport	1.16	0.71
LASS6	35147	lipid biosynthetic process, regulation of transcription, DNA-dependent	1.15	0.75
LIG4	39274	single strand break repair	1.14	0.75
RNF8	39161	protein ubiquitination	1.14	0.00

Symbol	CloneID	Biological Process	Fold change	q-value (%)
KCNIP4	21478	ion transport	-1.13	0.00
RCC2	136887	cell cycle, cell division, mitosis	-1.14	0.90
RBM4	141446	DNA recombination, DNA repair, DNA replication, estrogen receptor signaling pathway, glucocorticoid receptor signaling pathway, mRNA splicing	-1.19	0.00
DENND1A	21467	synaptic vesicle endocytosis	-1.21	0.74
HSPB1	23827	cell death, response to heat	-1.23	0.00
ARSJ	32854	Unknown	-1.24	0.00
ATP6AP2	131821	angiotensin maturation, positive regulation of transforming growth factor-beta1 production, regulation of MAPKKK cascade	-1.29	0.00
UGDH	139835	UDP-glucose metabolism, electron transport	-1.41	0.00
DUSP22	182999	apoptosis, cell proliferation, development, inactivation of MAPK, protein amino acid dephosphorylation	-1.55	0.00
PFKFB2	53158	glucose catabolic process, positive regulation of insulin secretion, pyruvate metabolic process	-1.68	0.00

Table 2. List of highly significant differentially expressed genes provided by SAM (FDR ≤0.68%), comparing MT and WT TP53 GBM cell lines. Positive fold-change value means up-regulation, while negative fold-change value means down-regulation in MT *TP53* cells, compared to WT TP53 cells.

includes the spatial reorganization of DSB repair and signalling proteins into subnuclear structures surrounding DSB sites (Bartek and Lukas, 2007; Maser et al., 1997). In this context, RNF8 protein is an important component of the DNA damage response; it can be recruited to the DNA damage sites, thus triggering the formation of ubiquitin conjugates, promoting the recruitment of important proteins to DSB sites, thereby enhancing DNA-damage checkpoint events (G2/M) and guaranting cell survival (Kolas et al., 2007). There is also evidence that RNF8 participates in histone ubiquitylation and protects the genome integrity by licensing the DSB-flanking chromatin to concentrate repair factors near the DNA lesions (Mailand et al., 2007). LIG4 is also a key protein playing role in DSB repair by non-homologous end joining (NHEJ) pathway (Helleday et al., 2007), while *CAV1* presents a tumor suppressor function in non-neoplastic tissue, being down-regulated upon transformation, but re-expressed upon progression in metastatic and multidrug-resistant tumors (Burgermeister et al., 2008). *CAV1* was also associated with multidrug resistance (Belanger et al., 2004; Belanger et al., 2003), and radioresistance (Barzan et al., 2010; Cordes et al., 2007; Li et al., 2005).

In MT *TP53* cells, other stress response genes (*RUVBL2* and *ASNS*) were up-regulated, while *RBM4* was down-regulated. *RUVBL2* participates in chromatin-remodelling (Lee et al., 2010), which could also let the lesion available to DNA repair genes. *ASNS* is a gene whose response elements function as an enhancer to mediate the transcriptional activation of the gene, either by the amino acid response (AAR) or the unfolded protein response (UPR pathway), triggered by amino acid limitation or endoplasmic reticulum stress (Siu et al.,

2002), respectively. These pathways initiate a wide array of adaptive mechanisms and ultimately, if necessary, programmed cell death (Harding et al., 2003; Zinszner et al., 1998); The role of *RBM4* in response to stress stimulus is the activation of internal ribosome entry site (IRES)-mediated translation, promoting the expression of stress-response genes; therefore, the down-regulation of *RBM4* in MT *TP53* cells might compromise the translational regulation of stress-associated mRNAs (Markus and Morris, 2009).

Several genes playing roles in cell adhesion were also differentially expressed in GBM cell lines, and this result is in accordance with the association of these genes in acquired chemo- and radioresistance (Kraus et al., 2002). In the present work, three cadherins (*CDH8, CDH13* and *CD93*), and one integrin *ITGA5* were found up-regulated in MT *TP53* cells, relatively to WT counterparts. Cadherins are integral membrane proteins that mediate calcium-dependent cell-cell adhesion. They may play an important role in the development and maintenance of tissues, and possibly are involved in the invasion and metastasis of malignant tumors. While *CDH8* participates in neural circuitry, *CD93* is involved in phagocytosis (Bohlson et al., 2005), *CDH13* play a role in apoptosis (Chan et al., 2008), and *ITGA5* in cell spreading (Fang et al., 2010).

A comparative analysis of differentially expressed genes (provided by SAM) was performed with previously identified genes with TP53 binding sites; this comparison was possible by using ChIP-PET and ChIP-on-chip analyses (Smeenk et al., 2008; Wei et al., 2006). For the ChIP- PET gene lists, we observed only one common gene (*LASS6*), which was up-regulated in MT *TP53* cells. *LASS6* is a ceramide sintase, producing ceramides that have antiproliferative and pro-apoptotic effects (Ruvolo, 2003). This gene plays a role in apoptosis induction in colon cancer cells (Schiffmann et al., 2010), and enhanced tumor development and growth *in vivo* in human head and neck squamous cell carcinomas (HNSCCs) (Senkal et al., 2010).

In addition, the comparison involving our modulated gene list, comparing MT and WT *TP53* GBM cells, using the ChIP-on-chip list, provided five common genes: *ARSJ, RCC2, CDH8, CDH13* and *HTRA1*). While *CDH8, CDH13* and *HTRA1* were up-regulated, *ARSJ* and *RCC2* were down-regulated in MT *TP53* cells. *CDH8* and *CDH13* are cadherins and were already discussed as possible targets to chemo- and radioresistance (Kraus et al., 2002). *HTRA1* is a tumor suppressor-like factor when overexpressed in cancer cell lines. (Baldi et al., 2002; Chien et al., 2004). This gene was also associated to cisplatin therapy responses in various cancer types (Catalano et al., 2011; Chien et al., 2006; Komatsu et al., 2006). These genes cannot be transactivated by TP53, according to the *TP53* status in T98G and U251MG cells. However, the majority of the genome-wide TP53 target sites can also be bounded by overexpressed p63 and p73 in vivo, suggesting that they may possibly play an important role at TP53 binding sites (Smeenk et al., 2008). *ARSJ* and *RCC2* genes were not described to be related with stress responses or cancer, and were up-regulated in WT *TP53* GBM cells, compared to MT, and probably, they can be associated to transactivation properties of TP53.

Thus, in the present work, most genes involved in stress responses (*RUVBL2, ASNS, RNF8, LIG4* and *CAV1*), cell adhesion (*CDH8, CDH13, CD93* and *ITGA5*), and genes associated to p63 and p73 binding sites (*LASS6* and *HTRA1*) were up-regulated in MT *TP53* cells. At least some of them may have the potential to be directly involved in radio- or chemoresistance. Therefore, the loss of *TP53* function may compromise cellular responses to anticancer agents.

It is already known that mechanisms underlying the cellular radiosensitivity seem to vary among different cell lineages, but at what extent the radiosensitivity depends on *TP53* function is a matter of investigation since long time ago. Several authors demonstrated that the loss of *TP53* function decreases the sensitivity of GBM cells to irradiation (Bartussek et al., 1999; McIlwrath et al., 1994; Roy et al., 2006; Yount et al., 1996), and the same was observed for other tumor types (Fan et al., 1994; Komarova et al., 1997; Merritt et al., 1994). However, in primary gliomas, the *TP53* mutation confers an improved prognosis in adult glioma patients due to a better response to radiation therapy (Tada et al., 1998). This is consistent with the results obtained in *in vitro* studies, in which glioma cells lacking WT *TP53* function were more susceptible to radiation-induced apoptosis than their isogenic counterparts expressing WT *TP53* (Hara et al., 2004).

It is important to emphasize that all these articles in the literature took into account the *TP53* status, but not other mutations inherent to GBM. In the present work, we studied four GBM cell lines with different *TP53* status; T98G and U251MG are mutated and U343MG-a and U87MG are wild-type for *TP53* gene, but they are similar regarding the fact that they harbor mutations for *CDKN2A* and *PTEN*, according to Ishi et al. (1999). In experiments on cell survival performed by the clonogenic survival assay, the results provided by several authors indicated that MT *TP53* cells were, in general, more radioresistant than WT *TP53* cells (Bassi et al., 2008; Chautard et al., 2010; de la Pena et al., 2006; Lee et al., 2006; Roy et al., 2006).

As described above, several differentially expressed genes provided by the comparison between MT *versus* WT *TP53* GBM cells are involved in the mechanism of resistance to ionizing radiation and/or multidrug resistance. In general, cytotoxicity of DNA damaging agents correlates with the induction of DSB, which can be produced directly or indirectly into the DNA molecule. Whereas ionizing radiation induces DSB directly, the drug TMZ generates DSB only after two or more cycles of DNA replication, as a secondary effect (Caporali et al., 2004). Therefore, *TP53* mutation has the potential to change the sensitivity of GBM cells to anticancer agents currently used in therapy, and probably, the changes in the expression profiles exhibited by several genes acting down-stream in the signalling cascade of damage responses may compromise the outcome of drug- and radio- therapies. In order to understand these alterations in terms of transcript profiles, we are currently studying at what extent *TP53* status influences gene expression profiles in irradiated GBM cells (*manuscript in preparation*); we found several differentially expressed genes in irradiated MT *TP53* cells that are probably implicated in tumor resistance; among them, we can mention *CLSTN2*, *ROBO2*, and *BMPR1B* (with role in cell-cell adhesion), *BTRC*, *CYP26B1*, and *ANLN* (cell cycle regulators).

However, the data in the literature regarding the role of *TP53* in mediating sensitivity to anticancer agents still present controversies. It has been reported that the absence of a functional *TP53* increases TMZ sensitivity in glioma cell lines, an effect that is independent of MGMT status (Blough et al., 2011). Glioma cell lines that did not express a functional *TP53* were significantly more sensitive to TMZ than cell lines that were functionally intact for *TP53* expression (Blough et al., 2011). An example of this inconsistency comes from the results obtained with T98G cell line (MT *TP53*), in with the role of MGMT in mediating TMZ resistance was confirmed by the co-exposure to the MGMT inhibitor O6-BG, causing a reduction in the EC50, as evaluated by the clonogenic survival assay (Hermisson et al.,

2006). Nevertheless, the roles of *TP53* in terms of its influence on drug sensitivity are difficult to elucidate, since the dependence on the cell type, and the kind of antitumor agent used(Fukushima et al., 2009). In addition, the genetic background is also critical, since GBM cells often harbor other mutations for cell cycle regulator genes, and other tumor suppressor genes, as already mentioned for the four GBM cell lines studied in the present work, which carry two other mutations (*CDKN2A* and *PTEN*).

The control of cell proliferation is very critical in the tumor development, and may also be influenced by the *TP53* status (Facoetti et al., 2008). Several genes playing roles in the regulation of cell proliferation were found differentially expressed in MT *TP53* cells, relatively to WT: *IGFR1, CDH13, DUSP22, ADAMTS1, CAV1,* and *LIG4*. These last two genes also play a role in stress responses, as mentioned before.

Tumor growth also depends on the rate of apoptosis (Amirlak and Couldwell, 2003), and apoptosis is directly involved in gliomagenesis and resistance towards classical genotoxic approaches in cancer therapy. It has been reported that GBM cells are virtually resistant to different apoptotic stimuli (Adamson et al., 2009; Eisele and Weller, 2011), but the mechanisms underlying these responses are still unclear, and may depend on several treatment conditions and type of genotoxic agent. In the present work, the list of differentially expressed genes also indicated several genes implicated in apoptosis. Those genes, such as *IGF1R, CDH13, IFT57, CRH, HSPB1* and *ASNS*, were up-regulated in MT *TP53* GBM cells, relatively to WT cells. *IGF1R* participates in cell proliferation and protection of cell death (Trojan et al., 2007), while *CDH13, ITF57, CRH* and *ASNS* participates in apoptosis induction (Andreeva and Kutuzov, 2010; Chan et al., 2008; Gdynia et al., 2008; Gervais et al., 2002; Minas et al., 2007; Siu et al., 2002). Considering that the ability of cells to undergo apoptosis is dependent of a complex signaling cascade involving pro- and anti-apoptotic genes, among other gene classes, the up-regulation of several apoptosis related genes in MT *TP53* cells might influence responses of GBM cells submitted to anticancer agents.

In this work, we showed some distinct transcript profiles for MT and WT *TP53* GBM cells, pointing out several genes that might influence cell sensitivity to chemo- and/or radiotherapy.

6. Conclusions

The present data comparing transcript profiles displayed by GBM cell lines with different *TP53* status showed that several biological processes were associated to the list of highly significant differentially expressed genes. Gene classes associated with those genes (stress response, DNA repair, proliferation, cell division, cell adhesion, apoptosis, etc) provided a picture on transcript profiles under normal conditions of cell proliferation in cultured GBM cell lines. However, these gene classes reflect wide amplitude of cellular processes that might be involved in cellular defense mechanisms under conditions of cell injury provoked by irradiation or drug treatment. These results support the hypothesis that MT *TP53* cells might be more resistant than WT *TP53* cells to some genotoxic stresses, such as ionizing radiation and TMZ. While this hypothesis still should be tested, altogether, the information obtained in this work provides a relevant basic contribution towards the understanding of GBM responses to therapies, and for designing novel therapeutic strategies for patients with GBM, based on their *TP53* status, but also considering other gene mutations.

7. Supplementary data

Symbol	Gene Name	CloneID	Fold change	q-value (%)
SPRY2	Sprouty homolog 2 (Drosophila)	40262	1.93	0.00
CAV1	Caveolin 1, caveolae protein, 22kDa	24651	1.86	0.00
MINA	MYC induced nuclear antigen	139217	1.79	0.00
	Clone 25220 mRNA sequence	25220	1.63	0.00
CDH13	Cadherin 13, H-cadherin (heart)	31093	1.61	0.00
HTRA1	HtrA serine peptidase 1	132044	1.55	0.00
ADAMTS1	ADAM metallopeptidase with thrombospondin type 1 motif, 1	34684	1.54	0.00
MPND	MPN domain containing	24532	1.39	0.00
ARRB1	Arrestin, beta 1	21814	1.38	0.00
ACSL4	Acyl-CoA synthetase long-chain family member 4	133988	1.36	0.00
ITGA5	Integrin, alpha 5 (fibronectin receptor, alpha polypeptide)	135671	1.35	0.75
P4HB	Prolyl 4-hydroxylase, beta polypeptide	132702	1.34	0.00
GPR68	G protein-coupled receptor 68	22652	1.34	0.00
GPR44	G protein-coupled receptor 44	25625	1.34	0.75
PDLIM1	PDZ and LIM domain 1	135689	1.33	0.00
RUVBL2	RuvB-like 2 (E. coli)	22267	1.33	0.00
	In multiple ClusterIDs	261714	1.32	0.00
	Unknown	134004	1.32	0.00
ZXDB	Zinc finger, X-linked, duplicated B	38972	1.31	0.90
MKLN1	Muskelin 1, intracellular mediator containing kelch motifs	33715	1.31	0.00
LARP4	La ribonucleoprotein domain family, member 4	41347	1.31	0.71
KSR1	Kinase suppressor of ras 1	220655	1.31	0.75
JAKMIP1	Janus kinase and microtubule interacting protein 1	32109	1.30	0.00

GNG13	Guanine nucleotide binding protein (G protein), gamma 13	178213	1.30	0.75
ANKRD42	MRNA; cDNA DKFZp761C0524 (from clone DKFZp761C0524)	30094	1.30	0.00
CDH8	cadherin 8, type 2	38939	1.30	0.00
NRGN	Neurogranin (protein kinase C substrate, RC3)	178825	1.30	0.75
USP53	Ubiquitin specific peptidase 53	142468	1.30	0.69
PIP5K2C	Phosphatidylinositol-5-phosphate 4-kinase, type II, gamma	133173	1.30	0.75
WDR34	WD repeat domain 34	133474	1.29	0.00
TCBA1	Na+/K+ transporting ATPase interacting 2	41427	1.29	0.00
MGC14376	Chromosome 17 open reading frame 91	24659	1.28	0.00
DNAJA1	DnaJ (Hsp40) homolog, subfamily A, member 1	24473	1.28	0.75
KLF12	Kruppel-like factor 12	34367	1.28	0.00
UNC13C	unc-13 homolog C (C. elegans)	22137	1.27	0.00
RHOQ	Ras homolog gene family, member Q	131061	1.26	0.00
FBXL3	F-box and leucine-rich repeat protein 3	25778	1.26	0.00
RP11-484I6.3	Chromosome 13 open reading frame 27	24463	1.25	0.00
	Unknown	132487	1.25	0.75
CRH	Corticotropin releasing hormone	34671	1.24	0.00
IGF1R	insulin-like growth factor 1 receptor	21519	1.24	0.00
ASNS	Asparagine synthetase (glutamine-hydrolyzing)	27208	1.23	0.90
CSGlcA-T	Chondroitin polymerizing factor 2	39955	1.23	0.75
NBPF12	Neuroblastoma breakpoint family, member 1	24976	1.23	0.90
BAMBI	BMP and activin membrane-bound inhibitor homolog (Xenopus laevis)	41406	1.22	0.00
PDXK	Pyridoxal (pyridoxine, vitamin B6) kinase	25360	1.22	0.00
	Transcribed locus	136399	1.21	0.75
TNRC15	Transcribed locus	37482	1.21	0.75

	Calneuron 1	39092	1.20	0.75
3-Mar	Membrane-associated ring finger (C3HC4) 3	24707	1.20	0.00
	Unknown	39306	1.19	0.69
CD93	CD93 molecule	35503	1.19	0.00
C20orf39	Transmembrane protein 90B	35704	1.19	0.00
	In multiple ClusterIDs	41186	1.19	0.71
	CXXC finger protein 5	136782	1.18	0.00
PPCDC	Phosphopantothenoylcysteine decarboxylase	135984	1.18	0.00
COPB2	Clone 24627 mRNA sequence	24627	1.18	0.00
	CDNA FLJ34038 fis, clone FCBBF2005645	38618	1.18	0.00
FLJ41130	hypothetical LOC401113	40009	1.18	0.00
CPD	Carboxypeptidase D	40521	1.18	0.75
	Unknown	34967	1.16	0.90
CACNB2	calcium channel, voltage-dependent, beta 2 subunit	34651	1.16	0.71
CUTL2	Cut-like homeobox 2	41354	1.16	0.90
	Unknown	34966	1.15	0.00
LASS6	LAG1 homolog, ceramide synthase 6	35147	1.15	0.75
LIG4	Ligase IV, DNA, ATP-dependent	39274	1.14	0.75
RNF8	Ring finger protein 8	39161	1.14	0.00
IFT57	Intraflagellar transport 57 homolog (Chlamydomonas)	34942	1.12	0.00
PIGO	Phosphatidylinositol glycan anchor biosynthesis, class O	21678	-1.12	0.71
KCNIP4	Kv channel interacting protein 4	21478	-1.13	0.00
RCC2	Regulator of chromosome condensation 2	136887	-1.16	0.90
PKIB	Protein kinase (cAMP-dependent, catalytic) inhibitor beta	152289	-1.17	0.00
DDX18	DEAD (Asp-Glu-Ala-Asp) box polypeptide 18	149416	-1.17	0.00
SIN3A	SIN3 homolog A, transcription regulator (yeast)	26455	-1.18	0.00

RBM4	RNA binding motif protein 4	141446	-1.19	0.00
NKIRAS2	NFKB inhibitor interacting Ras-like 2	137971	-1.20	0.00
DENND1A	DENN/MADD domain containing 1A	21467	-1.21	0.74
TMLHE	Trimethyllysine hydroxylase, epsilon	21457	-1.22	0.00
HSPB1	heat shock 27kDa protein 1	23827	-1.23	0.00
ZNF630	Zinc finger protein 630	141069	-1.24	0.00
ARSJ	Arylsulfatase family, member J	32854	-1.24	0.00
NUP160	Nucleoporin 160kDa	33299	-1.25	0.00
SCP2	Sterol carrier protein 2	137004	-1.26	0.68
NRN1	Neuritin 1	140197	-1.28	0.00
ATP6AP2	ATPase, H+ transporting, lysosomal accessory protein 2	131821	-1.29	0.00
PRPS2	Phosphoribosyl pyrophosphate synthetase 2	146194	-1.32	0.00
	Transcribed locus, weakly similar to XP_933787.2 PREDICTED: hypothetical protein [Homo sapiens]	53331	-1.34	0.00
PRSS23	Protease, serine, 23	143887	-1.35	0.00
CMPK	Cytidine monophosphate (UMP-CMP) kinase 1, cytosolic	140570	-1.36	0.00
UGDH	UDP-glucose 6-dehydrogenase	139835	-1.41	0.00
VSNL1	Visinin-like 1	26570	-1.42	0.00
	Transcribed locus	139645	-1.44	0.00
SSFA2	Sperm specific antigen 2	140589	-1.45	0.00
ABCA7	ATP-binding cassette, sub-family A (ABC1), member 7	182933	-1.45	0.00
	Unknown	181796	-1.54	0.00
DUSP22	Dual specificity phosphatase 22	182999	-1.55	0.00
PFKFB2	6-phosphofructo-2-kinase/fructose-2,6-biphosphatase 2	53158	-1.68	0.00

Table 1. List of significantly modulated genes provided by the statistical analysis by SAM (FDR ≤0.68%), comparing MT versus WT *TP53* GBM cell lines.

8. Acknowledgment

This study was supported by FAPESP (Fundação de Amparo à pesquisa de São Paulo), proc. nº: 04/15611-6, 06/01947-8 and 01953-8/06; CNPq (Conselho Nacional de Desenvolvimento Científico e Tecnológico); CAPES (Coordenação de Aperfeiçoamento de Pessoal de nível Superior); and FAEPA - HC FMRP/USP (Fundação de Apoio ao Ensino, Pesquisa e Assistência).

9. References

Adamson, C., Kanu, O. O., Mehta, A. I., Di, C., Lin, N., Mattox, A. K., and Bigner, D. D. (2009). Glioblastoma multiforme: a review of where we have been and where we are going. Expert Opin Investig Drugs *18*, 1061-1083.

Amirlak, B., and Couldwell, W. T. (2003). Apoptosis in glioma cells: review and analysis of techniques used for study with focus on the laser scanning cytometer. J Neurooncol *63*, 129-145.

Andreeva, A. V., and Kutuzov, M. A. (2010). Cadherin 13 in cancer. Genes Chromosomes Cancer *49*, 775-790.

Avgeropoulos, N. G., and Batchelor, T. T. (1999). New treatment strategies for malignant gliomas. Oncologist *4*, 209-224.

Baldi, A., De Luca, A., Morini, M., Battista, T., Felsani, A., Baldi, F., Catricala, C., Amantea, A., Noonan, D. M., Albini, A., *et al.* (2002). The HtrA1 serine protease is down-regulated during human melanoma progression and represses growth of metastatic melanoma cells. Oncogene *21*, 6684-6688.

Bartek, J., and Lukas, J. (2007). DNA damage checkpoints: from initiation to recovery or adaptation. Curr Opin Cell Biol *19*, 238-245.

Bartussek, C., Naumann, U., and Weller, M. (1999). Accumulation of mutant p53(V143A) modulates the growth, clonogenicity, and radiochemosensitivity of malignant glioma cells independent of endogenous p53 status. Exp Cell Res *253*, 432-439.

Barzan, D., Maier, P., Zeller, W. J., Wenz, F., and Herskind, C. (2010). Overexpression of caveolin-1 in lymphoblastoid TK6 cells enhances proliferation after irradiation with clinically relevant doses. Strahlenther Onkol *186*, 99-106.

Bassi, C., Mello, S., Cardoso, R., Godoy, P., Fachin, A., Junta, C., Sandrin-Garcia, P., Carlotti, C., Falcao, R., Donadi, E., *et al.* (2008). Transcriptional changes in U343 MG-a glioblastoma cell line exposed to ionizing radiation. Hum Exp Toxicol *27*, 919-929.

Batista, L. F., Roos, W. P., Christmann, M., Menck, C. F., and Kaina, B. (2007). Differential sensitivity of malignant glioma cells to methylating and chloroethylating anticancer drugs: p53 determines the switch by regulating xpc, ddb2, and DNA double-strand breaks. Cancer Res *67*, 11886-11895.

Batista, L. F., Roos, W. P., Kaina, B., and Menck, C. F. (2009). p53 mutant human glioma cells are sensitive to UV-C-induced apoptosis due to impaired cyclobutane pyrimidine dimer removal. Mol Cancer Res *7*, 237-246.

Belanger, M. M., Gaudreau, M., Roussel, E., and Couet, J. (2004). Role of caveolin-1 in etoposide resistance development in A549 lung cancer cells. Cancer Biol Ther *3*, 954-959.

Belanger, M. M., Roussel, E., and Couet, J. (2003). Up-regulation of caveolin expression by cytotoxic agents in drug-sensitive cancer cells. Anticancer Drugs *14*, 281-287.

Blough, M. D., Beauchamp, D. C., Westgate, M. R., Kelly, J. J., and Cairncross, J. G. (2011). Effect of aberrant p53 function on temozolomide sensitivity of glioma cell lines and brain tumor initiating cells from glioblastoma. J Neurooncol *102*, 1-7.

Bohlson, S. S., Zhang, M., Ortiz, C. E., and Tenner, A. J. (2005). CD93 interacts with the PDZ domain-containing adaptor protein GIPC: implications in the modulation of phagocytosis. J Leukoc Biol *77*, 80-89.

Burgermeister, E., Liscovitch, M., Rocken, C., Schmid, R. M., and Ebert, M. P. (2008). Caveats of caveolin-1 in cancer progression. Cancer Lett *268*, 187-201.

Caporali, S., Falcinelli, S., Starace, G., Russo, M. T., Bonmassar, E., Jiricny, J., and D'Atri, S. (2004). DNA damage induced by temozolomide signals to both ATM and ATR: role of the mismatch repair system. Mol Pharmacol *66*, 478-491.

Castells, X., Acebes, J. J., Boluda, S., Moreno-Torres, A., Pujol, J., Julia-Sape, M., Candiota, A. P., Arino, J., Barcelo, A., and Arus, C. (2010). Development of a predictor for human brain tumors based on gene expression values obtained from two types of microarray technologies. OMICS *14*, 157-164.

Castells, X., Garcia-Gomez, J. M., Navarro, A., Acebes, J. J., Godino, O., Boluda, S., Barcelo, A., Robles, M., Arino, J., and Arus, C. (2009). Automated brain tumor biopsy prediction using single-labeling cDNA microarrays-based gene expression profiling. Diagn Mol Pathol *18*, 206-218.

Catalano, V., Mellone, P., d'Avino, A., Shridhar, V., Staccioli, M. P., Graziano, F., Giordani, P., Rossi, D., Baldelli, A. M., Alessandroni, P., *et al.* (2011). HtrA1, a potential predictor of response to cisplatin-based combination chemotherapy in gastric cancer. Histopathology.

Chan, D. W., Lee, J. M., Chan, P. C., and Ng, I. O. (2008). Genetic and epigenetic inactivation of T-cadherin in human hepatocellular carcinoma cells. Int J Cancer *123*, 1043-1052.

Chautard, E., Loubeau, G., Tchirkov, A., Chassagne, J., Vermot-Desroches, C., Morel, L., and Verrelle, P. (2010). Akt signaling pathway: a target for radiosensitizing human malignant glioma. Neuro Oncol *12*, 434-443.

Chien, J., Aletti, G., Baldi, A., Catalano, V., Muretto, P., Keeney, G. L., Kalli, K. R., Staub, J., Ehrmann, M., Cliby, W. A., *et al.* (2006). Serine protease HtrA1 modulates chemotherapy-induced cytotoxicity. J Clin Invest *116*, 1994-2004.

Chien, J., Staub, J., Hu, S. I., Erickson-Johnson, M. R., Couch, F. J., Smith, D. I., Crowl, R. M., Kaufmann, S. H., and Shridhar, V. (2004). A candidate tumor suppressor HtrA1 is downregulated in ovarian cancer. Oncogene *23*, 1636-1644.

Cordes, N., Frick, S., Brunner, T. B., Pilarsky, C., Grutzmann, R., Sipos, B., Kloppel, G., McKenna, W. G., and Bernhard, E. J. (2007). Human pancreatic tumor cells are sensitized to ionizing radiation by knockdown of caveolin-1. Oncogene *26*, 6851-6862.

de la Pena, L., Burgan, W. E., Carter, D. J., Hollingshead, M. G., Satyamitra, M., Camphausen, K., and Tofilon, P. J. (2006). Inhibition of Akt by the alkylphospholipid perifosine does not enhance the radiosensitivity of human glioma cells. Mol Cancer Ther *5*, 1504-1510.

Dreyfuss, J. M., Johnson, M. D., and Park, P. J. (2009). Meta-analysis of glioblastoma multiforme versus anaplastic astrocytoma identifies robust gene markers. Mol Cancer *8*, 71.

Eisele, G., and Weller, M. (2011). Targeting apoptosis pathways in glioblastoma. Cancer Lett.

Eisen, M. B., Spellman, P. T., Brown, P. O., and Botstein, D. (1998). Cluster analysis and display of genome wide expression patterns. Proc Natl Acad Sci U S A *95*, 14863-14868.

el-Deiry, W. S. (1998). Regulation of p53 downstream genes. Semin Cancer Biol *8*, 345-357.

Facoetti, A., Ranza, E., and Nano, R. (2008). Proliferation and programmed cell death: role of p53 protein in high and low grade astrocytoma. Anticancer Res *28*, 15-19.

Fan, S., el-Deiry, W. S., Bae, I., Freeman, J., Jondle, D., Bhatia, K., Fornace, A. J., Jr., Magrath, I., Kohn, K. W., and O'Connor, P. M. (1994). p53 gene mutations are associated with decreased sensitivity of human lymphoma cells to DNA damaging agents. Cancer Res *54*, 5824-5830.

Fang, Z., Yao, W., Xiong, Y., Zhang, J., Liu, L., Li, J., Zhang, C., and Wan, J. (2010). Functional elucidation and methylation-mediated downregulation of ITGA5 gene in breast cancer cell line MDA-MB-468. J Cell Biochem *110*, 1130-1141.

Fukushima, T., Takeshima, H., and Kataoka, H. (2009). Anti-glioma therapy with temozolomide and status of the DNA-repair gene MGMT. Anticancer Res *29*, 4845-4854.

Gdynia, G., Lehmann-Koch, J., Sieber, S., Tagscherer, K. E., Fassl, A., Zentgraf, H., Matsuzawa, S., Reed, J. C., and Roth, W. (2008). BLOC1S2 interacts with the HIPPI protein and sensitizes NCH89 glioblastoma cells to apoptosis. Apoptosis *13*, 437-447.

Gervais, F. G., Singaraja, R., Xanthoudakis, S., Gutekunst, C. A., Leavitt, B. R., Metzler, M., Hackam, A. S., Tam, J., Vaillancourt, J. P., Houtzager, V., *et al.* (2002). Recruitment and activation of caspase-8 by the Huntingtin-interacting protein Hip-1 and a novel partner Hippi. Nat Cell Biol *4*, 95-105.

Hara, S., Nakashima, S., Kiyono, T., Sawada, M., Yoshimura, S., Iwama, T., Banno, Y., Shinoda, J., and Sakai, N. (2004). p53-Independent ceramide formation in human glioma cells during gamma-radiation-induced apoptosis. Cell Death Differ *11*, 853-861.

Harding, H. P., Zhang, Y., Zeng, H., Novoa, I., Lu, P. D., Calfon, M., Sadri, N., Yun, C., Popko, B., Paules, R., *et al.* (2003). An integrated stress response regulates amino acid metabolism and resistance to oxidative stress. Mol Cell *11*, 619-633.

Hegi, M. E., Diserens, A. C., Gorlia, T., Hamou, M. F., de Tribolet, N., Weller, M., Kros, J. M., Hainfellner, J. A., Mason, W., Mariani, L., *et al.* (2005). MGMT gene silencing and benefit from temozolomide in glioblastoma. N Engl J Med *352*, 997-1003.

Helleday, T., Lo, J., van Gent, D. C., and Engelward, B. P. (2007). DNA double-strand break repair: from mechanistic understanding to cancer treatment. DNA Repair (Amst) *6*, 923-935.

Hermisson, M., Klumpp, A., Wick, W., Wischhusen, J., Nagel, G., Roos, W., Kaina, B., and Weller, M. (2006). O6-methylguanine DNA methyltransferase and p53 status predict temozolomide sensitivity in human malignant glioma cells. J Neurochem *96*, 766-776.

Hoh, J., Jin, S., Parrado, T., Edington, J., Levine, A. J., and Ott, J. (2002). The p53MH algorithm and its application in detecting p53-responsive genes. Proc Natl Acad Sci U S A *99*, 8467-8472.

Horn, H. F., and Vousden, K. H. (2007). Coping with stress: multiple ways to activate p53. Oncogene *26*, 1306-1316.

Kolas, N. K., Chapman, J. R., Nakada, S., Ylanko, J., Chahwan, R., Sweeney, F. D., Panier, S., Mendez, M., Wildenhain, J., Thomson, T. M., *et al.* (2007). Orchestration of the DNA-damage response by the RNF8 ubiquitin ligase. Science *318*, 1637-1640.

Komarova, E. A., Chernov, M. V., Franks, R., Wang, K., Armin, G., Zelnick, C. R., Chin, D. M., Bacus, S. S., Stark, G. R., and Gudkov, A. V. (1997). Transgenic mice with p53-responsive lacZ: p53 activity varies dramatically during normal development and determines radiation and drug sensitivity in vivo. Embo J *16*, 1391-1400.

Komatsu, M., Hiyama, K., Tanimoto, K., Yunokawa, M., Otani, K., Ohtaki, M., Hiyama, E., Kigawa, J., Ohwada, M., Suzuki, M., *et al.* (2006). Prediction of individual response to platinum/paclitaxel combination using novel marker genes in ovarian cancers. Mol Cancer Ther *5*, 767-775.

Kraus, A. C., Ferber, I., Bachmann, S. O., Specht, H., Wimmel, A., Gross, M. W., Schlegel, J., Suske, G., and Schuermann, M. (2002). In vitro chemo- and radio-resistance in small cell lung cancer correlates with cell adhesion and constitutive activation of AKT and MAP kinase pathways. Oncogene *21*, 8683-8695.

Laptenko, O., and Prives, C. (2006). Transcriptional regulation by p53: one protein, many possibilities. Cell Death Differ *13*, 951-961.

Lee, J. S., Kim, Y., Kim, I. S., Kim, B., Choi, H. J., Lee, J. M., Shin, H. J., Kim, J. H., Kim, J. Y., Seo, S. B., *et al.* (2010). Negative regulation of hypoxic responses via induced Reptin methylation. Mol Cell *39*, 71-85.

Lee, Y. J., Chung, D. Y., Lee, S. J., Ja Jhon, G., and Lee, Y. S. (2006). Enhanced radiosensitization of p53 mutant cells by oleamide. Int J Radiat Oncol Biol Phys *64*, 1466-1474.

Li, J., Hassan, G. S., Williams, T. M., Minetti, C., Pestell, R. G., Tanowitz, H. B., Frank, P. G., Sotgia, F., and Lisanti, M. P. (2005). Loss of caveolin-1 causes the hyper-proliferation of intestinal crypt stem cells, with increased sensitivity to whole body gamma-radiation. Cell Cycle *4*, 1817-1825.

Mailand, N., Bekker-Jensen, S., Faustrup, H., Melander, F., Bartek, J., Lukas, C., and Lukas, J. (2007). RNF8 ubiquitylates histones at DNA double-strand breaks and promotes assembly of repair proteins. Cell *131*, 887-900.

Markus, M. A., and Morris, B. J. (2009). RBM4: a multifunctional RNA-binding protein. Int J Biochem Cell Biol *41*, 740-743.

Marucci, G., Morandi, L., Magrini, E., Farnedi, A., Franceschi, E., Miglio, R., Calo, D., Pession, A., Foschini, M. P., and Eusebi, V. (2008). Gene expression profiling in glioblastoma and immunohistochemical evaluation of IGFBP-2 and CDC20. Virchows Arch *453*, 599-609.

Maser, R. S., Monsen, K. J., Nelms, B. E., and Petrini, J. H. (1997). hMre11 and hRad50 nuclear foci are induced during the normal cellular response to DNA double strand breaks. Mol Cell Biol *17*, 6087-6096.

McIlwrath, A. J., Vasey, P. A., Ross, G. M., and Brown, R. (1994). Cell cycle arrests and radiosensitivity of human tumor cell lines: dependence on wild-type p53 for radiosensitivity. Cancer Res *54*, 3718-3722.

Mehrian Shai, R., Reichardt, J. K., Ya-Hsuan, H., Kremen, T. J., Liau, L. M., Cloughesy, T. F., Mischel, P. S., and Nelson, S. F. (2005). Robustness of gene expression profiling in glioma specimen samplings and derived cell lines. Brain Res Mol Brain Res *136*, 99-103.

Merritt, A. J., Potten, C. S., Kemp, C. J., Hickman, J. A., Balmain, A., Lane, D. P., and Hall, P. A. (1994). The role of p53 in spontaneous and radiation-induced apoptosis in the gastrointestinal tract of normal and p53-deficient mice. Cancer Res *54*, 614-617.

Minas, V., Rolaki, A., Kalantaridou, S. N., Sidiropoulos, J., Mitrou, S., Petsas, G., Jeschke, U., Paraskevaidis, E. A., Fountzilas, G., Chrousos, G. P., *et al.* (2007). Intratumoral CRH modulates immuno-escape of ovarian cancer cells through FasL regulation. Br J Cancer *97*, 637-645.

Ohgaki, H., and Kleihues, P. (2005). Population-based studies on incidence, survival rates, and genetic alterations in astrocytic and oligodendroglial gliomas. J Neuropathol Exp Neurol *64*, 479-489.

Prise, K. M., Schettino, G., Folkard, M., and Held, K. D. (2005). New insights on cell death from radiation exposure. Lancet Oncol *6*, 520-528.

Reddy, S. P., Britto, R., Vinnakota, K., Aparna, H., Sreepathi, H. K., Thota, B., Kumari, A., Shilpa, B. M., Vrinda, M., Umesh, S., *et al.* (2008). Novel glioblastoma markers with diagnostic and prognostic value identified through transcriptome analysis. Clin Cancer Res *14*, 2978-2987.

Roos, W. P., Batista, L. F., Naumann, S. C., Wick, W., Weller, M., Menck, C. F., and Kaina, B. (2007). Apoptosis in malignant glioma cells triggered by the temozolomide-induced DNA lesion O6-methylguanine. Oncogene *26*, 186-197.

Roy, K., Wang, L., Makrigiorgos, G. M., and Price, B. D. (2006). Methylation of the ATM promoter in glioma cells alters ionizing radiation sensitivity. Biochem Biophys Res Commun *344*, 821-826.

Ruvolo, P. P. (2003). Intracellular signal transduction pathways activated by ceramide and its metabolites. Pharmacol Res *47*, 383-392.

Sallinen, S. L., Sallinen, P. K., Haapasalo, H. K., Helin, H. J., Helen, P. T., Schraml, P., Kallioniemi, O. P., and Kononen, J. (2000). Identification of differentially expressed genes in human gliomas by DNA microarray and tissue chip techniques. Cancer Res *60*, 6617-6622.

Sbisa, E., Catalano, D., Grillo, G., Licciulli, F., Turi, A., Liuni, S., Pesole, G., De Grassi, A., Caratozzolo, M. F., D'Erchia, A. M., *et al.* (2007). p53FamTaG: a database resource of human p53, p63 and p73 direct target genes combining in silico prediction and microarray data. BMC Bioinformatics *8 Suppl 1*, S20.

Schiffmann, S., Ziebell, S., Sandner, J., Birod, K., Deckmann, K., Hartmann, D., Rode, S., Schmidt, H., Angioni, C., Geisslinger, G., and Grosch, S. (2010). Activation of ceramide synthase 6 by celecoxib leads to a selective induction of C16:0-ceramide. Biochem Pharmacol *80*, 1632-1640.

Senkal, C. E., Ponnusamy, S., Bielawski, J., Hannun, Y. A., and Ogretmen, B. (2010). Antiapoptotic roles of ceramide-synthase-6-generated C16-ceramide via selective regulation of the ATF6/CHOP arm of ER-stress-response pathways. FASEB J *24*, 296-308.

Siu, F., Bain, P. J., LeBlanc-Chaffin, R., Chen, H., and Kilberg, M. S. (2002). ATF4 is a mediator of the nutrient-sensing response pathway that activates the human asparagine synthetase gene. J Biol Chem *277*, 24120-24127.

Slichenmyer, W. J., Nelson, W. G., Slebos, R. J., and Kastan, M. B. (1993). Loss of a p53-associated G1 checkpoint does not decrease cell survival following DNA damage. Cancer Res *53*, 4164-4168.

Smeenk, L., van Heeringen, S. J., Koeppel, M., van Driel, M. A., Bartels, S. J., Akkers, R. C., Denissov, S., Stunnenberg, H. G., and Lohrum, M. (2008). Characterization of genome-wide p53-binding sites upon stress response. Nucleic Acids Res *36*, 3639-3654.

Smith, M. L., Chen, I. T., Zhan, Q., O'Connor, P. M., and Fornace, A. J., Jr. (1995). Involvement of the p53 tumor suppressor in repair of u.v.-type DNA damage. Oncogene *10*, 1053-1059.

Stupp, R., Hegi, M. E., Gilbert, M. R., and Chakravarti, A. (2007). Chemoradiotherapy in malignant glioma: standard of care and future directions. J Clin Oncol *25*, 4127-4136.

Stupp, R., Mason, W. P., van den Bent, M. J., Weller, M., Fisher, B., Taphoorn, M. J., Belanger, K., Brandes, A. A., Marosi, C., Bogdahn, U., *et al.* (2005). Radiotherapy plus concomitant and adjuvant temozolomide for glioblastoma. N Engl J Med *352*, 987-996.

Tada, M., Matsumoto, R., Iggo, R. D., Onimaru, R., Shirato, H., Sawamura, Y., and Shinohe, Y. (1998). Selective sensitivity to radiation of cerebral glioblastomas harboring p53 mutations. Cancer Res *58*, 1793-1797.

Trojan, J., Cloix, J. F., Ardourel, M. Y., Chatel, M., and Anthony, D. D. (2007). Insulin-like growth factor type I biology and targeting in malignant gliomas. Neuroscience *145*, 795-811.

Veprintsev, D. B., and Fersht, A. R. (2008). Algorithm for prediction of tumour suppressor p53 affinity for binding sites in DNA. Nucleic Acids Res *36*, 1589-1598.

Vogelstein, B., Lane, D., and Levine, A. J. (2000). Surfing the p53 network. Nature *408*, 307-310.

Wei, C. L., Wu, Q., Vega, V. B., Chiu, K. P., Ng, P., Zhang, T., Shahab, A., Yong, H. C., Fu, Y., Weng, Z., *et al.* (2006). A global map of p53 transcription-factor binding sites in the human genome. Cell *124*, 207-219.

Yount, G. L., Haas-Kogan, D. A., Vidair, C. A., Haas, M., Dewey, W. C., and Israel, M. A. (1996). Cell cycle synchrony unmasks the influence of p53 function on radiosensitivity of human glioblastoma cells. Cancer Res *56*, 500-506.

Zhang, J., Stevens, M. F., Laughton, C. A., Madhusudan, S., and Bradshaw, T. D. (2010). Acquired resistance to temozolomide in glioma cell lines: molecular mechanisms and potential translational applications. Oncology *78*, 103-114.

Zinszner, H., Kuroda, M., Wang, X., Batchvarova, N., Lightfoot, R. T., Remotti, H., Stevens, J. L., and Ron, D. (1998). CHOP is implicated in programmed cell death in response to impaired function of the endoplasmic reticulum. Genes Dev *12*, 982-995.

13

Genetics and Biology of Glioblastoma Multiforme

Anália Carmo[1], Inês Crespo[1,2] and Maria Celeste Lopes[1,2]
[1]*Center for Neuroscience and Cell Biology, University of Coimbra*
[2]*Faculty of Pharmacy, University of Coimbra*
Portugal

1. Introduction

Glioblastoma multiforme (GBM), the most common and biologically aggressive type of glioma is characterized by intra and intertumoral heterogeneity on the cytopathological, transcriptional, and genomic levels. GBMs account for 17.1% of brain and central nervous system (CNS) tumors and constitute 60-70% of all gliomas (The Central Brain Tumor Registry of the United States (CBTRUS) Statistical Report: NPCR/SEER, 2004-2006). Glial tumors can arise anywhere in the brain, but usually localize in the cerebral hemispheres and very rarely metastasize outside the CNS. In general, GBM affects individuals of both sexes and all age groups, but are usually more frequent in male patients (Bondy, et al., 2008) and the peak age at onset is between the fifth and the seventh decades of life (Wen, & Kesari, S., 2008).

Due to this complexity, and to the existence of a cancer stem cell (CSC) subpopulation, GBM presents an uncontrolled cellular proliferation, diffuse infiltration, propensity for necrosis, angiogenesis, resistance to apoptosis, and genomic instability (Louis, 2006) that makes this cancer one of the most difficult to treat. Despite multimodal aggressive treatment that includes surgical resection, followed by local radiotherapy and systemic chemotherapy (Furnari, et al., 2007), the median survival of GBM patients is 12-14 months. Unfortunately, only a small fraction of GBM patients (< 3%) survive for more than 36 months (Sonoda, et al., 2009). The existence of the blood-brain barrier and the diffuse infiltration into the surrounding brain limits the delivery of therapeutic agents, and increases the possibility of therapeutic toxicity. On the other hand, GBM tumors seem to overcome the effect of these therapies, through the ability to repair radiation-induced injury accomplished by aberrant or amplified growth and survival signaling pathways (Noda, et al., 2009), and ultimately becoming resistant to treatment.

Molecular therapeutic strategies targeting altered signaling pathways have successfully improved patient outcome, however, it is still not possible to distinguish, in advance, which patients are the most likely to effectively benefit from specific drugs. Favorable prognostic factors associated with longer survival include young age at the time of diagnosis, absent or minimal neurological damage signs and a good initial Karnofsky performance score (KPS) (Bussiere, et al., 2005). Recent data have reported that hypermethylation of the O6-methylguanine-DNA methyltransferase (*MGMT*) gene promoter is associated with prolonged progression-free survival in GBM patients treated with alkylating agents (Hegi, et al., 2005), and the extent of tumor resection is also found to enhance the chances for a favorable outcome (Stummer, et al., 2006). Additionally, recent large-scale studies integrating genetic and gene expression datasets, have identified molecular subtypes within GBM that seem to have relevance to predict patient outcome and response to treatment (Freije, et al., 2004; Phillips, et al., 2006).

2. Histological characterization of GBM

Histological classification and grading criteria for glial neoplasms are well established, basing on morphologic evidences of cellular differentiation and on the presence or absence of histopathological features, such as cellularity, nuclear pleomorphism, mitotic activity, endothelial cell proliferation and necrosis (Furnari, et al., 2007).

Although the specific cell type of glioma origin is currently unknown, these brain tumors are probably originated from glial cells (or their precursors), the generic name of the non-neuronal cells that provide nutrients to neuronal cells, regulate metabolism and synaptic transmission. There are three main types of glial cells: astrocytes, oligodendrocytes and ependymal cells. Gliomas are classified as astrocytomas, oligodendrogliomas, oligoastocytomas (tumors presenting morphological features of both astrocytes and oligodendrocytes), or ependymomas, according to their presumable line of differentiation, that is, whether they resemble to these three types of glial cells. In the most widely accepted histological classification system of the CNS tumors, proposed by the World Health Organization (WHO) and recently revised (Louis, et al., 2007), each glioma type is further subdivided based on an increasing malignancy scale from grade I to IV, using a combination of criteria with predictive value in determining clinical outcome. Grade I tumors are biologically benign, displaying low proliferative potential and the possibility of cure following surgical resection alone. Grade II (diffuse) tumors are low-grade malignancies that may follow long clinical courses, with 5 to 8-years median survival, and some of these neoplasms tend to progress to higher grades of malignancy. Despite low-level proliferative activity, early diffuse infiltration of the surrounding brain renders them incurable by surgery. Grade III (anaplastic) tumors exhibit histological evidence of malignancy, including increased focal or dispersed anaplasia, cell proliferation, nuclear atypia and mitotic activity, and are more rapidly fatal, with survival times often less than 3 years. Grade IV designation is assigned to tumors exhibiting advanced cytologically malignant features, such as microvascular proliferation and necrosis, and as they are resistant to radio/chemotherapy they are generally lethal. Therefore, the type and grade of the tumor, as well as its localization, are currently recognized as the major factors determining patient prognosis.

GBM is classified as WHO grade IV astrocytomas due to the resemblance of the tumor cells to astrocytes, to the existence of microvascular proliferation and areas of necrosis (Brat, & Van Meir, 2004). This is a highly cellular tumor with pleomorphic, basophilic nuclei and either indistinct cytoplasmic borders or plump, pink cytoplasm with fibrillary backgrounds. Yet, even within a single tumor, the cellular composition can vary widely and mixed histologic features are typical. Most frequently, these tumors arise *de novo* as an aggressive highly invasive tumor, usually with no evidence of prior symptoms, antecedent or lower grade pathology - primary GBMs. Two-thirds of patients with this GBM subtype have a clinical history of <3 months (Ohgaki, et al., 2004), presenting a very rapid development of clinical symptoms. In contrast, secondary GBMs derive from the progressive transformation of lower grade astrocytomas, with ~70% of grade II gliomas transforming into grade III/IV within 5-10 years of diagnosis (Maher, et al., 2001; Ohgaki, & Kleihues, 2009). True secondary GBMs are uncommon, accounting for ≤ 10% of all GBM cases (Ohgaki, et al., 2004). These two GBM types also affect patients at different ages: primary GBM constitute the great majority of GBM cases in older patients, while secondary GBM are quite rare and tend to occur in patients below the age of 45 years (Ohgaki, & Kleihues, 2007). Regardless of their distinct clinical histories or likely differences in prognosis and response to therapy, primary and secondary GBMs are usually histologically indistinguishable. Though both GBM subtypes achieve a common phenotypic endpoint, recent genomic profiles have revealed different transcriptional patterns and different DNA alterations, suggesting that these tumors arise through two different genetic pathways (Ohgaki, & Kleihues, 2007).

In addition to those subtypes, there are two other uncommon GBM variants, recognized as distinct clinico-pathological entities in the current WHO classification: i) gliosarcoma (GS) represents about 2% of GBMs and contains a biphasic growth pattern with clearly identifiable of both glial and sarcomatous components, the latter of which is associated with aberrant mesenchymal differentiation and is absent in all other glioma subtypes; ii) giant cell GBM (GC-GBM) constitutes approximately 5% of GBMs and is characterized by well-circumscribed masses of enlarged and bizarre tumor cells, often appearing multinucleated. This histological variant has been associated with longer survival (Shinojima, et al., 2004). In addition, other GBM subtypes with divergent patterns of differentiation have been described: i) small-cell GBM (SC-GBM), which can morphologically resemble anaplastic oligodendroglioma (AO), displays a monomorphic cell population characterized by small, round to slightly elongated, densely packed cells with mildly hyperchromatic nuclei and minimal discernible cytoplasm; ii) GBM with oligodendroglioma component (GBM-O), containing variable oligodendroglial foci, have a significantly better prognosis than other variants of GBMs (Klink, et al., 2010).

As these GBM subtypes/variants share similar morphologic features, precise GBMs subclassification is becoming increasingly important. Conventional histological analysis is still the primary methodology to determine diagnosis and treatment. Despite its current utility, it still relies on a subjective interpretation which has an impact on its reproducibility between different observers (Figarella-Branger, & Bouvier, 2005). Moreover, tumors sharing a common morphology can behave differently, even within the same tumor type and grading subgroup, which renders the histological classification of limited value in determining optimal therapy or response to treatment. Taken together, these evidences suggest that underlying genetic and molecular abnormalities, other than the histological parameters alone, may account for tumoral variability and could be predictive of clinical behavior and survival (Gravendeel, et al., 2009).

3. Cells of origin of GBM

GBMs display a rather heterogeneous cellular composition and, to date, the specific cells of origin for the formation of these malignant gliomas remain unknown. Traditional neuro-oncology postulated that tumors with an astrocytic phenotype arise from astrocytes. However, to undergo oncogenic events, mature glial cells would have to be proliferative and it is currently accepted that most brain cells do not undergo division, during adult life. Additionally, no epidemiological evidence indubitably relates processes likely to evoke reactive proliferation or astrogliosis, such as trauma, with the development of glial tumors (Bondy, et al., 2008; Fisher, et al., 2007). On the other hand, gliomas mostly occur in adults, suggesting that their cells of origin must be present in the adult brain. It is now known that in addition to glial progenitor cells, neural stem cells (NSCs) also reside in the subventricular zone (SVZ) of adult human brain (Gil-Perotin, et al., 2009; Sanai, et al., 2005). During human development, the one important source of NSCs is the SVZ, and this region is widely viewed as the source of cells that can initiate primary brain tumors (Sanai, et al., 2005). Indeed, many gliomas are either periventricular or contiguous with the SVZ (Lim, et al., 2007).

The "neural-stem cell hypothesis" proposes that a rare subset of cells within GBM tumors may have significant expansion capacity and the ability to generate new tumors. The remainder of tumor cells, which predominantly constitutes GBM tumors, may represent partially differentiated cells with limited progenitor capacity or terminally differentiated cells that cannot form new tumors. Evidences sustain the observation that transformation of NSCs and their progenitors, through a sequence of genetic and/or epigenetic alterations, may lead to the formation of tumor-initiating cells (TICs) also in gliomas (Dietrich, et al., 2008; Singh, et al., 2004), rather than from a differentiated cell type. In fact, TICs are identified in the early stages of tumor development and may not yet have acquired the full tumorigenic potential of other premalignant cells with additional genetic mutations, referred to as cancer stem cells (CSCs). It was demonstrated that GBM-CSCs share some characteristics with normal NSCs, including the ability to self-renew and proliferate, as well as the capacity to engraft and migrate (Galli, et al., 2004; Sanai, et al., 2005; Singh, et al., 2003). The self-renewal ability of both NSCs and CSCs is provided by either symmetric cell division, which produces two daughter stem cells, or by asymmetric cell division, which produces a stem cell and a progenitor cell. The progenitor cell will then differentiate and migrate, while the stem cell retains the capacity of self-renewal and remains in the germinal zone (Berger, et al., 2004), maintaining intact the core population of stem cells. CSCs can also express stem cell markers typical of normal NSCs such as the cluster of differentiation 133 (CD133), also known as prominin-1 (originally described in mouse neuroepithelium and hematopoietic stem and progenitor cells), and the intermediate filament protein nestin (NES) (Galli, et al., 2004; Sanai, et al., 2005; Singh, et al., 2003). Several studies reported that CD133+ cells isolated from human brain tumor, when implanted into the brain of immunodeficient mice, were capable to generate a new and highly invasive tumor at low inoculation numbers, whereas CD133- GBM cells failed to have a tumor-initiating activity (Marumoto, et al., 2009; Singh, et al., 2004). However, recent studies indicate that CD133- cell subpopulation can also form orthotopic tumors, thus acting as brain tumor stem cells (Chen, et al., 2010). These evidences may partially reflect the presence of other types of GBM-CSCs devoid of CD133, which are not entirely defined by the expression of typical NSCs markers. Thus, the CD133 marker used to identify GBM-CSCs is likely only one of a variety of cell specific markers, still unknown to this point. Although the clinical value of CD133-expression in GBM tumors remains unclear, some groups have reported that the increased expression of CD133 was correlated with the poor prognosis and the decreased survival of glioma patient (Pallini, et al., 2008; Zeppernick, et al., 2008). Moreover, the frequency of CD133+ cells was shown to increase with tumor grade, suggesting that CD133 expression could serve as a prognostic factor for malignant progression and tumor regrowth. In this sense, several studies have provided evidence that GMB-CSCs may contribute to resistance to radiotherapy and chemotherapy in GBM (Eramo, et al., 2006;

Kang, & Kang, 2007). In CD133+ cells, the overexpression of drug resistance genes such as *BCRP1*, DNA-mismatch repair genes, such as *MGMT*, as well as genes related to the inhibition of the apoptosis (Juillerat-Jeanneret, et al., 2008), seems to contribute to the tumor's resistance to chemotherapy.

Like normal NSCs, brain CSCs are thought to reside in the perivascular area of the tumor, called "the vascular niche", where they are sheltered from apoptotic stimuli and maintain a proper balance between self-renewal and differentiation (Calabrese, et al., 2007; Gilbertson, & Rich, 2007). Evidences of reciprocal relationship between GBM-CSCs and their microenvironment demonstrated that CSCs not only receive the signals from surrounding niche, but are also capable of modulating it. It was also demonstrated that CSCs stimulated angiogenesis by secreting vascular endothelial growth factor (VEGF) but these cells also depended on the factors brought by vasculature (Calabrese, et al., 2007). Thus, GMB-CSCs and vascular niche may give positive feed-back to each other in order to promote tumor maintenance and expansion. Moreover, it was also hinted that vascular microenvironment might protect CSCs from chemo- and radiotherapies, enabling these cells to reform an initial clinical response (Dick, & Lapidot, 2005). The influence of the tumor microenvironment may also be reflected on the phenotypic endpoint of gliomas. In this way, the occurrence of specific genetic events on precursor cells or mature cells, in combination with the local environment, possibly alters the activity of particular cellular control pathways. Accordingly, progenitor cells that undergo *TP53* mutations generally activate pathways that induce astrocytic differentiation, whereas similar cells that undergo chromosomal loss of 1p and 19q most often become committed to an oligodendroglial phenotype (Alcantara Llaguno, et al., 2009). Several lines of evidence in the literature indicate that loss of *TP53* affects the properties of adult neural stem cells by providing a proliferative advantage (Armesilla-Diaz, et al., 2009; Gil-Perotin, et al., 2006). Regarding the effect of different tumorigenic events, more evidences come from targeting oncogenic stimuli to specific cell types. For instance, whereas overexpressing oncogenic Ras and Akt in progenitor cells results in mouse brain tumors that are histologically similar to human GBMs (Holland, et al., 2000), overexpression of platelet-derived growth factor-B (PDGF-B) in the same cells produces tumors histologically similar to oligodendrogliomas (Dai, et al., 2001). Taken together, these evidences point at the involvement of immature precursor cells in the development of tumor malignant phenotype. On the contrary, the existence of cells in the adult brain capable to revert to a less mature state, in response to certain stimuli (Canoll, & Goldman, 2008), supports the hypothesis that mature glial cells may be the target of transformation in gliomagenesis. In fact, these cells may be induced to dedifferentiate into transformed glia with stem cell–like properties, as observed in mice models, through retroviral transfection of EGF receptor (EGFR) in association with Ink4a/Arf (Bachoo, et al., 2002), or by generating pluripotent stem cells from mouse embryonic and adult differentiated fibroblast (Takahashi, & Yamanaka, 2006). However, the concept of dedifferentiation of mature glia is questionable and fails to explain adequately the origin of some gliomas, such as mixed oligoastrocytomas and gliosarcomas. These types are composed by a biphasic tissue pattern with areas of astrocytic and oligodendroglial differentiation or gliomatous and mesenchymal differentiation, respectively (Louis, et al., 2007). The presence of two morphologically distinct cell types within a tumor suggests either independent transformation events in two terminally differentiated cells or, more likely, the transformation of a single, bipotential progenitor cell (Chekenya, & Pilkington, 2002) that retains the capacity to differentiate into both cell types. If malignant transformation occurs in the progenitor cell, one would expect a similar genetic profile in both cell types, especially on the level of chromosomal changes. Indeed, loss of heterozygosity (LOH) on chromosomes 1p and 19q was observed in both the astrocytic and oligodendrocytic components of mixed oligoastrocytomas, strongly suggesting a common cell of origin for both cells types (Kraus, et al., 1995).

Despite all the evidences already mentioned, GBM may develop from cells with different origins or via different molecular steps, which accounts for their heterogeneity. In this sense, the availability of more reliable and precise approaches for the classification of gliomas based on tumorigenic mechanisms would be extremely useful. Recently, integrated molecular genetic analysis has assumed an increasing part in the improvement of classification and therapeutic strategies for GBM patients.

4. Molecular characterization of GBM

It is recognized that morphologic changes observed during the process of malignant transformation, reflect the sequential acquisition of genetic alterations. So far, several studies have identified DNA copy number (CN) alterations, such as chromosomal and gene deletions, amplifications and gains, LOH and mutations as recurrent events in gliomagenesis, suggesting the involvement of tumor suppressor genes and oncogenes in tumor initiation or progression (Dahlback, et al., 2009; Furnari, et al., 2007a; Kotliarov, et al., 2006; Ohgaki, & Kleihues, 2009; Parsons, et al., 2008). CN changes are thought to affect genes expression either through overexpression of large amplification regions or inactivation of genes in deleted regions (Bralten, et al., 2010; Rao, et al., 2010). Ultimately, these genetic alterations seem to modify crucial cellular processes and often result in deregulation of metabolic key pathways affecting growth signaling and cell cycle control (Kanu, et al., 2009), as will be further discussed in the following section.

Over the past years, specific alterations associated with abnormal GBM features were identified, using classical cytogenetics and molecular methodologies, including interphase fluorescence *in situ* hybridization (iFISH) and comparative genomic hybridization (CGH). Given the large heterogeneity within GBMs, particular genetic changes may occur in some tumors and not in others, pointing out to distinct molecular subtypes of histologically defined GBM (Liang, et al., 2005). In fact, GBM profiling has identified differences in the molecular abnormalities observed between primary and secondary GBM. Specifically, primary GBMs typically harbor amplification and/or a high rate of *EGFR* mutation, cyclin-dependent kinase inhibitor 2A (*CDKN2A/p16*), deletion in chromosome 9p, and phosphatase and tensin homologue (*PTEN*) deletion in chromosome 10. The most common EGFR mutant type -variant 3 (EGFRvIII)- is due to an in-frame deletion of exons 2–7, and it is constitutively active in EGFR-mediated signal-transduction pathway, what confers cell proliferation and survival advantages (Ohgaki, & Kleihues, 2007; Van Meir, et al., 2010). The deletion in *PTEN* results in increased protein kinase B /mammalian target of rapamycin (AKT/mTOR) activity, which promotes cell survival, proliferation, and invasion (Louis, 2006; Sathornsumetee, & Rich, 2008). Recently, *ERBB2* mutations have also been identified as a recurrent event in primary GBMs. In contrast, secondary GBM are characterized by the occurrence of early detected mutations in the tumor suppressor gene *TP53* on chromosome 17p, especially those involving codons 248 and 273 or G:C→A:T mutations at CpG sites (Ohgaki, et al., 2004), abnormalities in the p16 and retinoblastoma (RB) pathways, and loss of heterozygosity of chromosome 10q. Isocitrate dehydrogenase 1 (*IDH1*) mutations have been recently identified as a very early and frequent genetic alteration in the pathway to secondary GBMs, but rarely occurring in primary GBMs (Ichimura, et al., 2009).

Similarly, primary and secondary GBMs show significantly different mRNA and protein expression profiles, reflecting their significant differences in genetic alterations (Ohgaki, & Kleihues, 2007). Genes typically expressed in primary GBMs include *Fas* (Tohma, et al., 1998), *VEGF* (Karcher, et al., 2006), and *VEGF* fms-related tyrosine kinase 1, probably reflecting large ischemic necrosis (Tohma, et al., 1998). The insulin-like growth factor binding protein-2 (IGFBP-2), a modulator of the action of insulin-like growth factors, is also typically expressed at a high level in primary GBMs (Godard, et al., 2003). Primary GBMs also preferentially express genes characteristic of a stromal response, suggesting the importance of extracellular signaling (Tso, et al., 2006). The adipocyte lipid binding protein 1 (AEBP1), a transcriptional repressor that has been shown to interact with PTEN inhibiting its function (Reddy, S. P. et al., 2008), is up-regulated in the majority of primary GBMs. Proteins expressed uniquely in primary GBMs include tenascin-X precursor (TN-X), enolase 1 (ENO1), centrosome-associated protein 350 (CAP350), and EGFR.

On the other hand, achaete-scute complex homolog 1 (ASCL1), a protein that activates transcription and plays a role in the neuronal commitment and differentiation, is found to be highly overexpressed in secondary GBMs, which is accompanied by inhibition of Notch signaling (Somasundaram, et al., 2005). Other proteins typically expressed in secondary GBMs include excision repair cross-complementing 6 (ERCC6), dual oxidase 2 (DUOX2), heterogeneous nuclear ribonucleoprotein A3 (HNRPA3), WNT-11 protein precursor, cadherin-related tumor suppressor homolog precursor, ADAMTS-19 (Furuta, et al., 2004), platelet–derived growth factor-AB (PDGF-AB) (Karcher, et al., 2006), and PDGF receptor (PDGFR).

From the different genetic profiles recognized within GBM, it became clear that the underlying molecular characteristics of the tumor are essential to understand its variability and to identify potential therapeutic targets, however, do not allow by themselves to predict patient's outcome or response to treatment. Thus, in the past few years, efforts have been made to further characterize GBM into specific molecular subclasses, defined by combinations of over- or underexpressed genes with potential impact on survival. Recently, the availability of large-scale microarray-based genomic/expression profiling, together with advances in bioinformatics methods provided a comprehensive view of the genome-wide aberrations in malignant gliomas. Emerging studies integrating DNA CN alterations and gene expression data allowed refining GBM's classification (Liang, et al., 2005; Marko, et al., 2008; Mischel, et al., 2003; Tso, et al., 2006), and revealed a significant correlation between tumor subsets and survival (Freije, et al., 2004; Nutt, et al., 2003; Phillips, et al., 2006). Promising findings from whole-genome analysis came also from The Cancer Genome Atlas (TCGA) Research Network (The Cancer Genome Atlas (TCGA) Research Network, 2008; Verhaak, et al., 2010). In a recent multidimensional study expanding previous GBM classification, patterns of somatic mutations, DNA CN, and gene expression were assessed in a large cohort, to perform an integrated molecular classification of GBM (Verhaak, et al., 2010). Consequently, on the basis of prior naming and considering the expression profiles observed, four subtypes of tumors with a common morphologic diagnosis of GBMs were identified into Classical, Mesenchymal, Proneural and Neural. The first GBM subtype was labeled "Classical" since tumors of this subtype have a characteristic profile of highly proliferative cells and common gains on chromosome 7, paired with losses on chromosome

10 and frequent focal losses on chromosome 9p21.3. High-level amplification of the *EGFR* gene or gene rearrangements (point or vIII EGFR mutation) are frequently observed in this subtype and uncommon in other subtypes. Homozygous 9p21.3 deletion, targeting *CDKN2A*, is almost mutually exclusive with aberrations of other RB pathway components, such as *Rb1*, *CDK4*, and *CCDN2*, suggesting that the RB pathway is almost exclusively affected through *CDKN2A* deletion, in samples with focal *EGFR* amplification. Alterations in the *TP53*, neurofibromin 1*(NF1)*, *PDGFRA*, or *IDH1* genes are nearly absent. Classical GBMs are responsiveness to the radiation and chemotherapies. At the gene expression level, the Classical subtype demonstrates elevated expression of the neural precursor and stem cell marker *NES*, and both Notch (*NOTCH3*, *JAG1*, and *LFNG*) and Sonic hedgehog (*SMO*, *GAS1*, and *GLI2*) signaling pathways.

The second GBM subtype was labeled as "Mesenchymal" since tumors display overexpression of mesenchymal markers, such as *CHI3L1/YKL40* and *MET* genes, as well as the astrocytic markers *CD44* and *MERTK*. Mesenchymal GBMs have frequent inactivation of the *NF1*, *TP53*, and *PTEN* genes. Comutations of *NF1* and *PTEN*, both intersecting with the AKT pathway, are also observed in the Mesenchymal subtype. Genes in the tumor necrosis factor (TNF) super family and NF-kB pathways are highly expressed in this subtype, potentially as a consequence of higher overall necrosis and associated inflammatory infiltrates. These tumors are responsive to aggressive chemotherapy and radiation therapies and might in addition be responsive to Ras, phosphoinositide 3-kinase (PI3K), and angiogenesis inhibitors.

The third GBM subtype was called "Proneural," and these tumors are characterized by an expression profile reminiscent of gene activation in neuronal development. Thus, they present activation of oligodendrocytic (*PDGFRA*, *OLIG2*, *TCF3*, and *NKX2-2*) and proneural (*SOX*, *DCX*, *DLL3*, *ASCL1*, and *TCF4*) development genes. These tumors are also characterized by *TP53* gene mutations and LOH, and mutations in *PDGFRA*, *IDH1*, and *PIK3CA/PIK3R1* genes are also observed. Focal amplification of the *PDGFRA* locus, associated with high levels of *PDGFRA* expression, is seen almost exclusively in this tumor type. Interestingly, *PIK3CA/PIK3R1* mutations in the Proneural subtype is mostly observed in samples with no *PDGFRA* abnormalities. Amplification of chromosome 7 and loss on chromosome 10 are significant, but less frequent findings than in the Classical subtype. This GBM subtype may be responsive to inhibitors of the hypoxia-inducible factor (HIF), PI3K, and PDGFRA pathways. In this group, patients are younger and survival is slightly better than in the other 3 tumor subtypes.

The fourth GBM subtype called "Neural" is less well defined and has gene expression signatures similar to those found in normal brain tissue, with activation of neuron markers such as *NEFL*, *GABRA1*, *SYT1*, and *SLC12A5*. These tumors demonstrate a low degree of infiltration by normal cells; nevertheless, their expression signature is suggestive of cells with a differentiated phenotype.

Despite the existence of well defined differences in the genetic profile of the four subtypes, all tumor subgroups present inactivation of the p53 and RB tumor suppressor pathways, and activation of the receptor tyrosine kinase pathway. These observations suggest rather strongly that although molecular genetic profiling may eventually guide therapeutic decisions for patients with specific GBM subtypes, further studies linking the genetic alterations and the consequent affected signaling pathways, may be the key to better understand the occurrence and progression of these tumors.

5. Signaling pathways altered in GBM

5.1 EGFR/Akt/PTEN pathway

EGFR is a member of the erbB family receptor tyrosine kinase proteins, which comprises EGFR itself (ErbB1) (EGFR/HER1), ErbB2 (HER2/neu), ErbB3 (HER3), and ErbB4 (HER4) (Mellinghoff, et al., 2005; Ranson, 2004). These receptors are composed of an extracellular ligand-binding domain, a transmembrane lipophilic domain, and an intracellular tyrosine kinase domain. The binding of a specific set of ligands [EGF; transforming growth factor-α (TGF-α)] to the receptor promotes EGFR dimerization and the autophosphorylation of the receptors on tyrosine residues (Arora, & Scholar, 2005; Baselga, 2006). Upon autophosphorylation, several signal transduction pathways downstream of EGFR become activated such as the Ras/Raf/mitogen-activated protein kinase pathway, the PI3K/Akt pathway, protein kinase C (PKC), the signal transduction and activator of transcription (STAT), an the VEGF among others (Arora, & Scholar, 2005; Baselga, 2006). Taking in consideration that these signaling pathways control cell growth, regulate cell survival and apoptosis and that it was reported and overexpression of EGFR in several epithelial tumors, the EGFR/Akt/PTEN pathway is considered a potential target for cancer therapy (Arora, & Scholar, 2005; Baselga, 2006).

Regarding the activation of PI3K by EGFR it is known that there is a recruitment of PI3K to the cell membrane and phosphorylation of phosphatidynositol-4,5-bisphosphate to the respective 3-phosphate (PIP3), which in turns activates downstream effectors molecules such as Akt (Hirose, et al., 2005; Furnari, et al., 2007). Activated Akt regulates the function of downstream signaling proteins involved in cell cycle, proliferation, apoptosis and invasion, therefore, once deregulated, Akt may contribute to tumorigenesis. Activated Akt deregulates cell growth by stabilization of cyclin D and promotion of the nuclear entry of the mouse double minute protein 2 (MDM2), leading to the degradation of p53 (Han, et al., 2010). Akt might also inhibit p21 expression through its phosphorylation and activation of MDM2 (Zhou, et al., 2001). On the other hand, activated Akt exerts anti-apoptotic activity by phosphorylating and inactivating pro-apoptotic signaling proteins, such as BAD and caspase 9 (Dasari, et al., 2010). The involvement of Akt in diverse tumorigenic activities suggests that Akt activation alone might be sufficient to induce cancer (Testa, & Bellacosa, 2001). Moreover, Akt activation may contribute to tumor invasion/metastasis by stimulating secretion of matrix metalloproteinases (Dasari, et al., 2010). The action of PI3K enzyme is directly antagonized by a phosphatase encoded by the *PTEN* gene located at 10q23.3.

PTEN is a tumor suppressor gene that encodes a central domain with homology to the catalytic region of protein tyrosine phosphatases. For that reason, PTEN is a negative regulator of the PI3K pathway by removing the third phosphate from the inositol ring of the second messenger PIP3 (Mellinghoff, et al., 2005). Therefore, PTEN inactivation results in accumulation of PIP3 levels and persistent signaling through the serine/threonine kinase Akt. In addition, the amino terminal domain of PTEN, with homology to tensin and auxilin, is important in regulating cell migration and invasion by directly dephosphorylating focal adhesion kinase (FAK) (Furnari, et al., 2007; Ohgaki, & Kleihues, 2007). There are also some reports indicating that PTEN plays a significant role in inducing G1 cell cycle arrest and apoptosis, along with regulating cell differentiation (Di Cristofano, & Pandolfi, 2000).

As it is referred, *EGFR* mutation was detected in several tumor types. In GBMs, amplification of the *EGFR* gene occurs in 40% of primary GBMs but rarely in secondary

GBMs. EGFR overexpression is also more common in primary GBMs (60%) than in secondary GBMs (10%). All primary GBMs with amplification of the *EGFR* gene, also show EGFR overexpression (Ohgaki, & Kleihues, 2007; Van Meir, et al., 2010). EGFR amplicons are often mutated, being the most frequent type the variant 3 (EGFRvIII) with an in-frame deletion of exons 2 to 7 within the extracellular ligand-binding domain. This in-frame deletion is associated with constitutive activation of the receptor and failure to attenuate signaling by receptor down-regulation (Ohgaki, & Kleihues, 2007; Van Meir, et al., 2010). The constitutively active EGFRvIII can enhance cell proliferation through activation of the PI3K/Akt pathway and therefore may play a very important role in gliomagenesis (Mellinghoff, et al., 2005; Mizoguchi, et al., 2006).

For this reason, EGFR has been a prime target for therapeutic intervention in GBM with small molecule kinase inhibitors, antibody-based immunotherapy and, more recently, with small interfering RNA (siRNA)-directed neutralization of either wild-type EGFR or the EGFRvIII allele (Van Meir, et al., 2010). In fact, several small-molecule EGFR-inhibitors such as gefitinib and erlotinib have been used in clinical trials but progression-free survival was not prolonged (van den Bent, et al., 2009). The inability to increase survival of GBM patients was also observed with lapatanib (EGFR/HER-2 inhibitor) (Neyns, et al., 2009; Thiessen, et al., 2009), and with the cetuximab, the monoclonal antibody against EGFR (Neyns, et al., 2009).

The unsuccess of EGFR inhibitors in GBM treatment seems to be associated to the inactivation of PTEN and to the activation of the PI3K/Akt. Mutations in *PTEN* were detected in 15 to 40% of GBMs and almost exclusively in primary GBMs (Ohgaki, & Kleihues, P., 2007; Zhou, et al., 1999). PTEN loss could thus promote resistance to EGFR kinase inhibitors by dissociating EGFR/EGFRvIII inhibition from downstream inhibition of the PI3K signaling pathway.

The activation of PI3K/Akt pathway could also be due to the occurrence of mutations. In fact, it was reported that in up to 10% of GBMs, Akt activation is due to mutations that amplify or activate the catalytic and regulatory subunits of PI3K (Stommel, et al., 2007; The Cancer Genome Atlas (TCGA) Research Network, 2008). It was also reported that PI3K could be activated by c-MET and PDGFR alpha, which could be co-activated in EGFR-amplified tumors (Furnari, et al., 2007).

Taken together, these results indicate that PI3K activation plays a central role in the resistance of GBM to EGFR inhibitors, since there are several mechanisms that may provide alternative routes for maintaining PI3K activation. Haas-Kogan et al. demonstrated *in vitro* and in glioma patients that high levels of EGFR coupled with low levels of activated Akt were associated with a favorable response to EGFR inhibitors (Haas-Kogan, et al., 2005). Therefore, a possible therapeutic strategy in GBM should control the activation of EGFR and the activation of PI3K or key mediators of PI3K. However, since PI3K upon activation may potentially phosphorylate several proteins involved in cell proliferation, apoptosis and migration, it remains to be determined which downstream effectors of Akt are most critical for gliomagenesis. One of those downstream effectors, associated with increased cell proliferation, is the serine/threonine kinase mTOR which forms the catalytic core of at least two functionally distinct complexes (mTORC1 and mTORC2). mTOR integrates growth-inhibitory signals such as deprivation of glucose and amino acids, ATP depletion, hypoxia and lack of growth factors, in order to generate adaptive cellular responses (Wullschleger, et al., 2006). Deregulated mTOR signaling sustains proliferation of malignant cells by antagonizing these physiological starvation signals (Wullschleger, et al., 2006). Therefore, it seems plausible that the commonly observed activation of mTOR signaling in GBM contributes to the typical pattern of GBM pathology, with necrotic cores and aggressive growth at the tumor margins (Masri, et al., 2007).

Once activated, the mechanism of mTOR action could occur through different mechanisms depending on the activated complex: mTOR complex 1 or complex 2. The mTORC2 is composed by rictor (rapamycin-insensitive regulator of mTOR), mSIN1, protor and mLST8. This complex is activated by PI3K, phosphorylates Akt on serine 473 (Ser473) of its C-terminal hydrophobic motif, promoting maximal Akt activity and acting as an upstream activator of Akt (Foster, & Fingar, 2010). mTORC2 also activates additional kinases, including serum glucocorticoid-induced protein kinase and PKCα, all of which may play important roles in regulating cellular proliferation and growth (Foster, & Fingar, 2010). mTORC2 activity is elevated in glioma cell lines and seems to enhance motility and to promote glioma cell proliferation *in vitro* (Akhavan, et al., 2010). Further, in a recent drosophila model of gliomagenesis promoted by constitutive coactivation of EGFR-Ras-Akt, mTORC2 activity was required for glial proliferation suggesting that mTORC2 signaling is essential for growth in the context of enhanced signal flux through the PI3K pathway (Akhavan, et al., 2010; Read, et al., 2009). However, the mechanism of mTORC2 is not clearly understood and future studies will be needed to determine the role of mTORC2 in gliomagenesis.

The mTOR complex 1 (mTORC1 or the mTOR-raptor complex which is rapamycin-sensitive) is regulated by both nutrients and growth factor signaling. mTORC1 acts as a downstream effector of PI3K/Akt signaling, regulates the translation initiation and ribosome biogenesis and plays a role in cell growth, proliferation and survival (Akhavan, et al., 2010; Foster, & Fingar, 2010; Manning, & Cantley, 2007). The translational effects of mTOR1 signaling are mediated by phosphorylation of its two direct target molecules, eukaryotic translation initiation factor 4E binding protein 1 (4E-BP1) and ribosomal protein S6 kinase 1 (S6K1), at specific sites. In a serial cell line transformation model, mTORC1 signaling through S6K1 was required for glioma formation, highlighting its functional importance (Akhavan, et al., 2010; Foster, & Fingar, 2010; Manning, & Cantley, 2007).

In the preclinical studies, mTOR inhibitors, specially rapamycin, were very promising since it was reported an increase in apoptotic and non-apoptotic cell death (Rao, et al., 2005), cell cycle arrest (Tanaka, et al., 2007) and decreased angiogenesis (Del Bufalo, et al., 2006). However, the results from phase I and II single-agent clinical trials of rapamycin conducted in glioma were disappointing (Heimberger, et al., 2005). The unsuccess could be related to the fact that mTORC1 plays a dual role as a positive and negative regulator of PI3K/Akt signaling and to the inability of rapamycin and its derivatives to target mTORC2. Recently, it was suggested a different interpretation of the clinical failure of rapamycin in GBM patients, namely, that the lack of efficacy is a consequence of incomplete inhibition rather than an injudicious choice of molecular target (Cloughesy, & Mischel, 2011). Cloughesy and Mischel hypothesize that since mTORC1 is both a positive and a negative regulator of the PI3K/Akt signaling pathway, the treatment with rapamycin causes derepression of mTORC1-mediated feedback and may paradoxically induce a more rapid clinical progression by promoting PI3K activity in GBM patients treated with rapamycin. To test this possibility, rapamycin treatment was reinstituted in patients after surgery and patients were monitored for progression. The results showed that rapamycin treatment led to Akt activation in seven of 14 patients, presumably due to loss of negative feedback, which was associated with a significantly shorter time to progression, during postsurgical maintenance of rapamycin therapy (Guertin, & Sabatini, 2009). These results highlight the importance of pathway cross-talk in determining response to targeted therapy and put in evidence the importance of combined therapy (Cloughesy, & Mischel, 2011).

In fact, in the last years, several clinical trials used dual PI3K/mTOR inhibitors. Some of those inhibitors showed efficacy against a panel of GBM cell lines but, surprisingly, in preclinical GBM models, dual PI3K/mTOR inhibitors have failed to promote tumor cell apoptosis (Maira, et al., 2008). The remarkable plasticity of tumor cells was recently demonstrated in studies showing that mTORC1 inhibition leads to MAPK pathway activation through a PI3K-dependent mechanism (Carracedo, et al., 2008; Cloughesy, et al., 2008).

Mitogen-activated protein kinases (MAPKs) are serine/threonine protein kinases that transmit signals from the membrane to the nucleus in response to growth factors and cellular stress. Three principal isoforms of MAPKs exist: extracellular signal regulated kinase (ERK), c-jun NH2-terminal kinase (JNK) and p38 MAPK (p38). Activation of MAPKs occurs through phosphorylation of threonine and tyrosine residues of the Thr-X-Tyr motif by MAPK kinases (MEKs). In GBM, the existence of mutations affecting the expression or the activity of these serine/threonine protein kinases was not reported. However, since MAPKs may contribute to cellular proliferation and could be activated in response to the inhibition of PI3K/mTOR, its role in gliomagnesisis is under investigation.

In spite of the unsuccess of the mTOR inhibitors, the mTOR signaling pathway remains one of the most important therapeutic targets and several studies are being carried on, in order to evaluate the role of mTORC2 and of mTORC1, the interaction between PI3K/mTOR, and the interaction between mTOR, EGFR and MAPK.

5.2 p53 and cell cycle progression

The tumor suppressor p53 encoded by *TP53* gene was discovered in 1979 (DeLeo, et al., 1979; Lane, & Crawford, 1979; Linzer, & Levine, 1979). At the beginning, p53 was considered a tumor antigen but today it is known that the wild-type gene product functions as a tumor suppressor that regulates cell cycle progression and apoptosis in response to a wide variety of stress signals, including DNA damage (Baker, et al., 1989). When cells are exposed to various genotoxic agents, p53 is stabilized, accumulates in the nucleus, binds and transcriptionally regulates the promoters of >2500 potential effectors genes (Levine, et al., 2006). This leads to the expression of cell cycle checkpoint proteins and prevents the propagation of cells with unstable genomes, predominantly by halting the cell cycle in the G1 phase, or by initiating a program of apoptosis or proliferative arrest (Van Meir, et al., 2010). The best characterized of these effectors is the *p21* gene, which once transcriptionally activated blocks cell cycle progression in the G1 phase by inhibiting the function of the cyclin D family of proteins (Van Meir, et al., 2010). The cyclin D family is constituted by the regulatory subunits of the cyclin/cyclin–dependent kinase complexes that regulate cell cycle entry and progression by inducing the phosphorylation and inactivation of RB (Van Meir, et al., 2010). Due to the ability to coordinate the cellular responses to cellular stress factors, p53 was called "cellular gatekeeper" (Levine, 1997) or "the guardian of the genome" (Lane, 1992).

Since p53 function is critical for normal cell growth and development, its activity is tightly regulated by phosphorylation, which is the first step to induce stabilization of p53, and also through its interaction with MDM2, the endogenous E3-ligase that targets p53 for proteasome degradation (Michael, & Oren, 2003). MDM2 itself is transcriptionally activated by p53, thus creating a negative feedback loop that maintains p53 at very low levels in the absence of cellular damage. Upon stress, particularly DNA damage, Ser15 and Ser20 within the p53 N-terminal are phosphorylated by a broad range of kinases, including ATM, ATR, DNA-PK, Chk1, and Chk2 in a manner that prevents MDM2 from interacting with p53, thus resulting in p53 stabilization (Soussi, & Wiman, 2007; Wade, et al., 2010). Another mechanism to stabilize p53 is by direct inhibition of the MDM2 ubiquitin ligase activity through its association with Arf, the alternative transcript of the Ink4a tumor suppressor locus, which may induce G1- and G2-phase arrest (Matheu, et al., 2008).

In 50% of the human tumors, the p53 pathway is inactivated via indirect mechanisms such as MDM2 amplification, viral infection or loss of Arf, leading to p53 destabilization (Brooks, & Gu, 2006). The other 50% of the tumors present missense mutations that originate a subset of p53 mutant proteins with oncogenic properties that may contribute to the neoplastic transformation (Soussi, & Wiman, 2007; Wade, et al., 2010).

In GBM, *TP53* is the most frequently mutated gene, and the majority of its mutations occur in "Proneural" subtype of GBM samples (The Cancer Genome Atlas (TCGA) Research Network, 2008; Verhaak, et al., 2010). In addition, the TCGA reported that mutations are clustered in the DNA binding domain, a hotspot for *p53* mutations in human cancers (The Cancer Genome Atlas (TCGA) Research Network, 2008). In secondary GBM, loss of p53 is detectable in two thirds of the tumors and may occur through either point mutations that prevent DNA binding, or loss of chromosome 17p. In primary GBM, *TP53* inactivation is now considered a common event which may occur via amplification or overexpression of the p53 negative regulators MDM2 and MDM4, which suppresses p53's transcriptional activity (Foster, & Fingar, 2010; Ohgaki, et al., 2004; Zheng, et al., 2008).

According to the TCGA, in GBM the inactivation of the p53 pathway occurs in the form of *Arf* deletions (55%), amplifications of *MDM2* (11%) and *MDM4* (4%), in addition to mutations of p53 itself (The Cancer Genome Atlas (TCGA) Research Network, 2008). Among the 91 samples sequenced by this Network, genetic lesions in *TP53* were mutually exclusive of those in *MDM2* or *MDM4* but not of those in ARF (encoded by *CDKN2A*).

Since MDM2 is considered the main regulator of p53, the inhibition of p53-MDM2 interaction is regarded as having therapeutic potential. A number of different strategies have been employed to develop small molecules that bind specifically to the N-terminal region of MDM2, that interacts with p53 (Shangary, & Wang, 2009). The most promising candidate described so far has been nutlin-3A (Vassilev, et al., 2004). In fact, glioma C6 cells were quite sensitive to nutlin-3A treatment but further studies will be needed to understand the real potential of this strategy (Merkel, et al., 2010).

5.3 Retinoblastoma signaling pathway

The RB pathway consists of several proteins: the cyclin-dependent kinase inhibitor (CDKN), the cyclin D-dependent protein kinases (cdk4, cdk6), the E2F-family of transcription factors (heterodimers of E2F1-8 with DP1-2) and the RB-family (RB, p107, p130) (Knudsen, & Wang, 2010; Scambia, et al., 2006; Van Meir, et al., 2010). The *Rb* gene is localized on the 13q14 chromosome and was the first known human suppressor of tumors (Huang, et al., 1988). The RB family consists of pRb/p105, p107 and pRb2/p130 which have an homologous functional domain known as the pocket region. This region allows the interaction of RB proteins with multiple peptides and the assembly of nuclear protein-complexes that regulate transcription factor activities, G1-phase cell cycle arrest, cell proliferation and differentiation

(Weinberg, 1995). Since RB is phosphorylated and dephosphorylated during the cell cycle, its activity depends on the phosphorylation status: the hyperphosphorylated (inactive) form predominates in proliferating cells, whereas the hypophosphorylated (active) form is generally more abundant in quiescent or differentiating cells (Harbour, & Dean, 2000). In quiescent cells, hypophosphorylated RB blocks proliferation by binding and sequestering the E2F family of transcription factors, which prevents the activation of genes essential for cell cycle progression, ensuring that transcription factors remain inactive during M and G0 phases (Furnari, et al., 2007). In proliferating cells, growth factors lead to the induction of cyclin D1, as well as to the degradation of the Cdk2/cyclin E inhibitor, p27Kip1 (White, et al., 2005). These activated Cdk complexes trigger the phosphorylation of RB in late G1-phase, which is maintained in S-, G2-, and M-phases. The pRB enables E2F release leading to transcriptional activation of growth promoting genes which are required for transcription of cellular genes that participate in growth control and DNA synthesis (Furnari, et al., 2007; Harbour, & Dean, 2000; Malumbres, & Barbacid, 2001). Among the E2F-regulated genes are cyclin E, cyclin A2 and Emi1, which are key effectors of the G1/S transition in normal cells (Furnari, et al., 2007; Knudsen, & Wang, 2010).

One of the negative regulators of the RB signaling pathway is the Ink4-family of proteins, p16Ink4a, p15Ink4b, p18Ink4c, and p19Ink4d which are small heat-stable proteins containing the AKN (ankyrin repeat) domain (Knudsen, & Wang, 2010). Each of the Ink4 proteins can bind to and inhibit the activity of Cdk4 and Cdk6. The Ink4 proteins compete with the D-cyclins for Cdk4/6 to prevent the formation of the active kinase complex that phosphorylates pRB (Knudsen, & Wang, 2010).

In the comprehensive analysis of the genome and transcriptome of 206 primary GBM tumors performed by the TCGA project, the sequence of 601 genes in 91 of the 206 tumor samples was analyzed. The results have shown that the RB pathway was altered in 78% of the primary GBM tumor samples, directly by mutations, deletions or promoter methylations at *Rb* loci, as well as indirectly by alterations on the positive or negative regulators (The Cancer Genome Atlas (TCGA) Research Network, 2008). *Rb* promoter methylation and gene silencing were more frequently found in secondary GBMs (43%) than in primary GBMs (14%) (Grzmil, & Hemmings, 2010; Xiao, et al., 2002). The alterations in the RB-pathway included homozygous deletion and mutation of *CDKN2A* (p16Ink4a) and *Rb1* (RB) in 52% and 11% of the samples, respectively, and homozygous deletion of *CDKN2B* (p15Ink4b) and *CDKN2C* (p18Ink4c) in 47% and 2% of the tumor samples, respectively. On the other hand, the *CDK4*, *CDK6*, and *CCND2* (cyclin D2) genes were amplified in 18%, 1%, and 2% of the GBM tumors examined (The Cancer Genome Atlas (TCGA) Research Network, 2008).

In spite of the importance of RB pathway, several *in vitro* and *in vivo* studies demonstrated that the neutralization of this pathway alone is insufficient to abrogate cell cycle control, suggesting that cell cycle is also regulated by other signaling pathways (Furnari, et al., 2007).

In the last years, several studies have been performed in order to establish a therapeutic strategy based on the manipulation of the cyclin–RB–E2F pathway. The development of small molecules that specifically inhibit certain cyclin/CDK complexes, or that could affect E2F-dependent transcription, as well as peptides that can mimic the functional regions of RB proteins inactivated in specific tumors, is currently under investigation (Scambia, et al., 2006).

5.4 Vascular endothelial growth factors

Vascular endothelial growth factors (VEGFs) were originally described as vascular permeability factors (VPF), since they were released by tumor cells that promote vascular leakage (Keck, et al., 1989). VEGFs are predominantly produced by endothelial, hematopoietic and stromal cells in response to hypoxia, and upon stimulation with growth factors such as transforming growth factors, interleukins or PDGF.

VEGFs are dimeric cysteine-linked secreted glycoproteins with a molecular weight of approximately 40 kDa. In mammals, VEGFs are encoded by a family of genes that includes *VEGF-A, -B, -C, -D* and *PlGF* (Cebe-Suarez, et al., 2006; Van Meir, et al., 2010).

VEGFs bind to three variants of type III receptor tyrosine kinases, VEGF receptor 1, 2 and 3 (Cebe-Suarez, et al., 2006). The binding of VEGF to its cognate receptors induces dimerization and subsequent phosphorylation of the receptors, leading to the activation of several intracellular signaling molecules such as PI3K, phospholipase Cg (PLCg), PKC, nitric oxide synthase (NOS), MAPKs and focal adhesion kinases (FAKs) (Karkkainen, & Petrova, 2000).

VEGF has been demonstrated to be one of the dominant drivers of angiogenesis contributing to tumor growth and progression (Criscuolo, G. R. et al., 1990). Due to this role, inhibitors of VEGF are widely used in cancer therapy in order to reduce angiogenesis (Ferrara, & Kerbel, 2005; Huang, et al., 2003), to cause regression of tumor vessels, and to reduce tumor growth (Huang, et al., 2003).

Extensive experimental data support the concept that angiogenesis is required for GBM growth (Jain, et al., 2007; Schmidt, et al., 1999; Van Meir, et al., 2010). The process is driven primarily by tumor secreted VEGF-A, but there are a large number of alternative secreted proangiogenic factors, including basic FGF (bFGF), angiopoietins, PDGF, interleukin-8 (IL-8), and hepatocyte growth factor/scatter factor (HGF/SF). Endothelial cells in the vicinity of the tumor express VEGFR2, which establishes a paracrine signaling loop that stimulates endothelial cell growth and proliferation. The level of VEGF production in a tumor increases with the degree of malignancy. In a study of surgical glioma specimens, high-grade tumors produced greater than 10-fold more VEGF compared with low-grade tumors (Schmidt, et al., 1999). It was also demonstrated that EGFR activation transcriptionally upregulates VEGF expression in GBM cells (Mischel, et al., 2003).

A targeted molecular therapy for GBM included agents that interfere with angiogenesis. The early trials with the first generation of anti-angiogenic agents (for example, thalidomide), conducted in GBM patients, had disappointing results (Jain, et al., 2007). The new generation of antiangiogenic drugs evaluated in clinical trials uses the anti-VEGF antibody bevacizumab, which neutralizes VEGF, and the VEGF-receptor tyrosine kinase inhibitors (TKIs) (sorafinib and sunitinib) (Jain, et al., 2007). Bevacizumab, a humanized anti-VEGF antibody, has shown promising results in exploratory phase II trials of recurrent GBM. However, these results are based on small patient cohorts and, because anti-angiogenic agents directly affect vessel permeability, the imaging response assessment based on contrast enhancement (CE) is highly ambiguous (Vredenburgh, et al., 2007). However, there is increasing interest in targeting proangiogenic molecules that function by alternative mechanisms (Van Meir, et al., 2010). For example, the neuropilins are nontyrosine kinase receptors that are activated by VEGF binding and potentiate VEGFR signaling. The angiopoietins (Ang-1 and Ang-2) are involved in the stability and maintenance of the tumor vasculature. Binding of Ang-2 to its cognate receptor, Tie-2 destabilizes vessels, which is a requirement for angiogenesis to proceed (Holash, et al., 1999). Inhibitors of specific chemotactic signaling may also have therapeutic value, since tumor cells secrete chemokines that serve to recruit proangiogenic myeloid cells to the tumor (Van Meir, et al., 2010). However, it must be noted that antibodies and many of these low-molecular weight compounds may not cross the blood-brain barrier.

6. Conclusion

Despite all the evidences already mentioned, the mechanism of gliomagenesis and the cells of origin for GBM remain unknown. Several studies suggest that different cells of origin give rise to distinct types of GBM-CSC. Thus, GBM may also develop differently from different cells of origin or via different molecular steps, which accounts for their heterogeneity. From the therapeutic point of view, the inter- and intratumoral heterogeneity presents a unique challenge for GBM treatment.

In the last years, many progresses were done in order to identify the molecular signature of GBM, and these recent studies confirmed that each GBM is characterized by alterations in several signaling pathways that control cellular proliferation and apoptosis such as EGFR/mTOR/Akt/PTEN, p53, RB, VEGF, which contribute to the unsuccess of monotherapies and put in evidence the need to perform combined therapy, adjusted to the genetic and molecular alterations of each patient.

In addition, these studies reinforced the remarkable plasticity of GBM cells that allow cells to switch from one signaling pathway to another, according to the difficulties imposed by the therapeutic agents.

Thus, combined therapeutic strategies, targeting both the brain tumor stem cells and the molecular alterations that characterize the brain tumor of each patient, could turn out to be the most effective approach to increase the survival of GBM patients.

7. References

Akhavan, D.; Cloughesy, T. F. & Mischel, P. S. (2010). mTOR signaling in glioblastoma: lessons learned from bench to bedside. *Neuro Oncol,* Vol.12, No 8, (Aug,2010), pp. 882-9, ISSN 1523-5866

Alcantara Llaguno, S.; Chen, J.; Kwon, C. H. (2009). Malignant astrocytomas originate from neural stem/progenitor cells in a somatic tumor suppressor mouse model. *Cancer Cell,* Vol.15, No 1, (Jan 6,2009), pp. 45-56, ISSN 1878-3686

Armesilla-Diaz, A.; Bragado, P.; Del Valle, I. (2009). p53 regulates the self-renewal and differentiation of neural precursors. *Neuroscience,* Vol.158, No 4, (Feb 18,2009), pp. 1378-89, ISSN 0306-4522

Arora, A. & Scholar, E. M.(2005). Role of tyrosine kinase inhibitors in cancer therapy. *J Pharmacol Exp Ther,* Vol.315, No 3, (Dec,2005), pp. 971-9, ISSN 0022-3565

Bachoo, R. M.; Maher, E. A.; Ligon, K. L. (2002). Epidermal growth factor receptor and Ink4a/Arf: convergent mechanisms governing terminal differentiation and transformation along the neural stem cell to astrocyte axis. *Cancer Cell,* Vol.1, No 3, (Apr,2002), pp. 269-77, ISSN 1535-6108

Baker, S. J.; Fearon, E. R.; Nigro, J. M. (1989). Chromosome 17 deletions and p53 gene mutations in colorectal carcinomas. *Science,* Vol.244, No 4901, (Apr 14,1989), pp. 217-21, ISSN 0036-8075

Baselga, J. (2006). Targeting tyrosine kinases in cancer: the second wave. *Science,* Vol.312, No 5777, (May 26,2006), pp. 1175-8, ISSN 1095-9203

Berger, F.; Gay, E.; Pelletier, L. (2004). Development of gliomas: potential role of asymmetrical cell division of neural stem cells. *Lancet Oncol,* Vol.5, No 8, (Aug,2004), pp. 511-4, ISSN 1470-2045

Bondy, M. L.; Scheurer, M. E.; Malmer, B. (2008). Brain tumor epidemiology: consensus from the Brain Tumor Epidemiology Consortium. *Cancer,* Vol.113, No 7 Suppl, (Oct 1,2008), pp. 1953-68, ISSN 0008-543X

Bralten, L. B.; Kloosterhof, N. K.; Gravendeel, L. A. (2010). Integrated genomic profiling identifies candidate genes implicated in glioma-genesis and a novel LEO1-SLC12A1 fusion gene. *Genes Chromosomes Cancer,* Vol.49, No 6, (Jun,2010), pp. 509-17, ISSN 1098-2264

Brat, D. J. & Van Meir, E. G. (2004). Vaso-occlusive and prothrombotic mechanisms associated with tumor hypoxia, necrosis, and accelerated growth in glioblastoma. *Lab Invest,* Vol.84, No 4, (Apr,2004), pp. 397-405, ISSN 0023-6837

Brooks, C. L. & Gu, W. (2006). p53 ubiquitination: Mdm2 and beyond. *Mol Cell,* Vol.21, No 3, (Feb 3,2006), pp. 307-15, ISSN 1097-2765

Bussiere, M.; Hopman, W.; Day, A. (2005). Indicators of functional status for primary malignant brain tumour patients. *Can J Neurol Sci,* Vol.32, No 1, (Feb,2005), pp. 50-6, ISSN 0317-1671

Calabrese, C.; Poppleton, H.; Kocak, M. (2007). A perivascular niche for brain tumor stem cells. *Cancer Cell,* Vol.11, No 1, (Jan,2007), pp. 69-82, 1535-6108 (Print)

Canoll, P. & Goldman, J. E. (2008). The interface between glial progenitors and gliomas. *Acta Neuropathol,* Vol.116, No 5, (Nov,2008), pp. 465-77, ISSN 1432-0533

Carracedo, A.; Ma, L.; Teruya-Feldstein, J. (2008). Inhibition of mTORC1 leads to MAPK pathway activation through a PI3K-dependent feedback loop in human cancer. *J Clin Invest,* Vol.118, No 9, (Sep,2008), pp. 3065-74, ISSN 0021-9738

Cebe-Suarez, S.; Zehnder-Fjallman, A. & Ballmer-Hofer, K. (2006). The role of VEGF receptors in angiogenesis; complex partnerships. *Cell Mol Life Sci,* Vol.63, No 5, (Mar,2006), pp. 601-15, ISSN 1420-682X

Chekenya, M. & Pilkington, G. J. (2002). NG2 precursor cells in neoplasia: functional, histogenesis and therapeutic implications for malignant brain tumours. *J Neurocytol,* Vol.31, No 6-7, (Jul-Aug,2002), pp. 507-21, ISSN 0300-4864

Chen, R.; Nishimura, M. C.; Bumbaca, S. M. (2010). A hierarchy of self-renewing tumor-initiating cell types in glioblastoma. *Cancer Cell,* Vol.17, No 4, (Apr 13,2010), pp. 362-75, ISSN 1878-3686

Cloughesy, T. F. & Mischel, P. S. (2011). New strategies in the molecular targeting of glioblastoma: how do you hit a moving target? *Clin Cancer Res,* Vol.17, No 1, (Jan 1,2011), pp. 6-11, ISSN 1078-0432

Cloughesy, T. F.; Yoshimoto, K.; Nghiemphu, P. (2008). Antitumor activity of rapamycin in a Phase I trial for patients with recurrent PTEN-deficient glioblastoma. *PLoS Med,* Vol.5, No 1, (Jan 22,2008), pp. e8, ISSN 1549-1676

Criscuolo, G. R.; Merrill, M. J. & Oldfield, E. H. (1990). Characterization of a protein product of human malignant glial tumors that induces microvascular permeability. *Adv Neurol,* Vol.52, No 1990), pp. 469-74, ISSN 0091-3952

Dahlback, H. S.; Brandal, P.; Meling, T. R. (2009). Genomic aberrations in 80 cases of primary glioblastoma multiforme: Pathogenetic heterogeneity and putative cytogenetic pathways. *Genes Chromosomes Cancer,* Vol.48, No 10, (Oct,2009), pp. 908-24, ISSN 1098-2264

Dai, C.; Celestino, J. C.; Okada, Y. (2001). PDGF autocrine stimulation dedifferentiates cultured astrocytes and induces oligodendrogliomas and oligoastrocytomas from neural progenitors and astrocytes in vivo. *Genes Dev,* Vol.15, No 15, (Aug 1,2001), pp. 1913-25, ISSN 0890-9369

Dasari, V. R.; Kaur, K.; Velpula, K. K. (2010). Upregulation of PTEN in glioma cells by cord blood mesenchymal stem cells inhibits migration via downregulation of the PI3K/Akt pathway. *PLoS One,* Vol.5, No 4, 2010), pp. e10350, ISSN 1932-6203

Del Bufalo, D.; Ciuffreda, L.; Trisciuoglio, D. (2006). Antiangiogenic potential of the Mammalian target of rapamycin inhibitor temsirolimus. *Cancer Res,* Vol.66, No 11, (Jun 1,2006), pp. 5549-54, ISSN 0008-5472

DeLeo, A. B.; Jay, G.; Appella, E. (1979). Detection of a transformation-related antigen in chemically induced sarcomas and other transformed cells of the mouse. *Proc Natl Acad Sci U S A,* Vol.76, No 5, (May,1979), pp. 2420-4, ISSN 0027-8424

Di Cristofano, A. & Pandolfi, P. P. (2000). The multiple roles of PTEN in tumor suppression. *Cell,* Vol.100, No 4, (Feb 18,2000), pp. 387-90, ISSN 0092-8674

Dick, J. E. & Lapidot, T. (2005). Biology of normal and acute myeloid leukemia stem cells. *Int J Hematol,* Vol.82, No 5, (Dec,2005), pp. 389-96, ISSN 0925-5710

Dietrich, J.; Imitola, J. & Kesari, S. (2008). Mechanisms of Disease: the role of stem cells in the biology and treatment of gliomas. *Nat Clin Pract Oncol,* Vol.5, No 7, (Jul,2008), pp. 393-404, ISSN 1743-4262

Eramo, A.; Ricci-Vitiani, L.; Zeuner, A. (2006). Chemotherapy resistance of glioblastoma stem cells. *Cell Death Differ,* Vol.13, No 7, (Jul,2006), pp. 1238-41, ISSN 1350-9047

Ferrara, N. & Kerbel, R. S. (2005). Angiogenesis as a therapeutic target. *Nature,* Vol.438, No 7070, (Dec 15,2005), pp. 967-74, ISSN 1476-4687

Figarella-Branger, D. & Bouvier, C. (2005). [Histological classification of human gliomas: state of art and controversies]. *Bull Cancer,* Vol.92, No 4, (Apr,2005), pp. 301-9, ISSN 1769-6917

Fisher, J. L.; Schwartzbaum, J. A.; Wrensch, M. (2007). Epidemiology of brain tumors. *Neurol Clin,* Vol.25, No 4, (Nov,2007), pp. 867-90, vii, ISSN 0733-8619

Foster, K. G. & Fingar, D. C. (2010). Mammalian target of rapamycin (mTOR): conducting the cellular signaling symphony. *J Biol Chem,* Vol.285, No 19, (May 7,2010), pp. 14071-7, ISSN 1083-351X

Freije, W. A.; Castro-Vargas, F. E.; Fang, Z. (2004). Gene expression profiling of gliomas strongly predicts survival. *Cancer Res,* Vol.64, No 18, (Sep 15,2004), pp. 6503-10, ISSN 0008-5472

Furnari, F. B.; Fenton, T.; Bachoo, R. M. (2007). Malignant astrocytic glioma: genetics, biology, and paths to treatment. *Genes Dev,* Vol.21, No 21, (Nov 1,2007), pp. 2683-710, ISSN 0890-9369

Furuta, M.; Weil, R. J.; Vortmeyer, A. O. (2004). Protein patterns and proteins that identify subtypes of glioblastoma multiforme. *Oncogene,* Vol.23, No 40, (Sep 2,2004), pp. 6806-14, ISSN 0950-9232

Galli, R.; Binda, E.; Orfanelli, U. (2004). Isolation and characterization of tumorigenic, stem-like neural precursors from human glioblastoma. *Cancer Res,* Vol.64, No 19, (Oct 1,2004), pp. 7011-21, ISSN 0008-5472

Gil-Perotin, S.; Alvarez-Buylla, A. & Garcia-Verdugo, J. M. (2009). Identification and characterization of neural progenitor cells in the adult mammalian brain. *Adv Anat Embryol Cell Biol,* Vol.203, No 2009), pp. 1-101, ix, ISSN 0301-5556

Gil-Perotin, S.; Marin-Husstege, M.; Li, J. (2006). Loss of p53 induces changes in the behavior of subventricular zone cells: implication for the genesis of glial tumors. *J Neurosci,* Vol.26, No 4, (Jan 25,2006), pp. 1107-16, ISSN 1529-2401

Gilbertson, R. J. & Rich, J. N. (2007). Making a tumour's bed: glioblastoma stem cells and the vascular niche. *Nat Rev Cancer,* Vol.7, No 10, (Oct,2007), pp. 733-6, ISSN 1474-1768

Godard, S.; Getz, G.; Delorenzi, M. (2003). Classification of human astrocytic gliomas on the basis of gene expression: a correlated group of genes with angiogenic activity emerges as a strong predictor of subtypes. *Cancer Res,* Vol.63, No 20, (Oct 15,2003), pp. 6613-25, ISSN 0008-5472

Gravendeel, L. A.; Kouwenhoven, M. C.; Gevaert, O. (2009). Intrinsic gene expression profiles of gliomas are a better predictor of survival than histology. *Cancer Res,* Vol.69, No 23, (Dec 1, 2009), pp. 9065-72, ISSN 1538-7445

Grzmil, M. & Hemmings, B. A. (2010). Deregulated signalling networks in human brain tumours. *Biochim Biophys Acta,* Vol.1804, No 3, (Mar,2010), pp. 476-83, ISSN 0006-3002

Guertin, D. A. & Sabatini, D. M. (2009). The pharmacology of mTOR inhibition. *Sci Signal,* Vol.2, No 67, 2009), pp. pe24, ISSN 1937-9145

Haas-Kogan, D. A.; Prados, M. D.; Tihan, T. (2005). Epidermal growth factor receptor, protein kinase B/Akt, and glioma response to erlotinib. *J Natl Cancer Inst,* Vol.97, No 12, (Jun 15,2005), pp. 880 7, ISSN 1460 2105

Han, L.; Zhang, A. L.; Xu, P. (2010). Combination gene therapy with PTEN and EGFR siRNA suppresses U251 malignant glioma cell growth in vitro and in vivo. *Med Oncol,* Vol.27, No 3, (Sep,2010), pp. 843-52, ISSN 1559-131X

Harbour, J. W. & Dean, D. C. (2000). The Rb/E2F pathway: expanding roles and emerging paradigms. *Genes Dev,* Vol.14, No 19, (Oct 1,2000), pp. 2393-409, ISSN 0890-9369

Hegi, M. E.; Diserens, A. C.; Gorlia, T. (2005). MGMT gene silencing and benefit from temozolomide in glioblastoma. *N Engl J Med,* Vol.352, No 10, (Mar 10,2005), pp. 997-1003, ISSN 1533-4406

Heimberger, A. B.; Wang, E.; McGary, E. C. (2005). Mechanisms of action of rapamycin in gliomas. *Neuro Oncol,* Vol.7, No 1, (Jan,2005), pp. 1-11, ISSN 1522-8517

Hirose, Y.; Katayama, M.; Mirzoeva, O. K. (2005). Akt activation suppresses Chk2-mediated, methylating agent-induced G2 arrest and protects from temozolomide-induced mitotic catastrophe and cellular senescence. *Cancer Res,* Vol.65, No 11, (Jun 1,2005), pp. 4861-9, ISSN 0008-5472

Holash, J.; Maisonpierre, P. C.; Compton, D. (1999). Vessel cooption, regression, and growth in tumors mediated by angiopoietins and VEGF. *Science,* Vol.284, No 5422, (Jun 18,1999), pp. 1994-8, ISSN 0036-8075

Holland, E. C.; Celestino, J.; Dai, C. (2000). Combined activation of Ras and Akt in neural progenitors induces glioblastoma formation in mice. *Nat Genet,* Vol.25, No 1, (May,2000), pp. 55-7, ISSN 1061-4036

Hu, B.; Guo, P.; Bar-Joseph, I. (2007). Neuropilin-1 promotes human glioma progression through potentiating the activity of the HGF/SF autocrine pathway. *Oncogene,* Vol.26, No 38, (Aug 16,2007), pp. 5577-86, ISSN 0950-9232

Huang, H. J.; Yee, J. K.; Shew, J. Y. (1988). Suppression of the neoplastic phenotype by replacement of the RB gene in human cancer cells. *Science,* Vol.242, No 4885, (Dec 16,1988), pp. 1563-6, ISSN 0036-8075

Huang, J.; Frischer, J. S.; Serur, A. (2003). Regression of established tumors and metastases by potent vascular endothelial growth factor blockade. *Proc Natl Acad Sci U S A,* Vol.100, No 13, (Jun 24,2003), pp. 7785-90, ISSN 0027-8424

Ichimura, K.; Pearson, D. M.; Kocialkowski, S. (2009). IDH1 mutations are present in the majority of common adult gliomas but rare in primary glioblastomas. *Neuro Oncol,* Vol.11, No 4, (Aug,2009), pp. 341-7, ISSN 1522-8517

Jain, R. K.; di Tomaso, E.; Duda, D. G. (2007). Angiogenesis in brain tumours. *Nat Rev Neurosci,* Vol.8, No 8, (Aug,2007), pp. 610-22, ISSN 1471-003X

Juillerat-Jeanneret, L.; Bernasconi, C. C.; Bricod, C. (2008). Heterogeneity of human glioblastoma: glutathione-S-transferase and methylguanine-methyltransferase. *Cancer Invest,* Vol.26, No 6, (Jul,2008), pp. 597-609, ISSN 1532-4192

Kang, M. K. & Kang, S. K. (2007). Tumorigenesis of chemotherapeutic drug-resistant cancer stem-like cells in brain glioma. *Stem Cells Dev,* Vol.16, No 5, (Oct,2007), pp. 837-47, ISSN 1547-3287

Kanu, O. O.; Hughes, B.; Di, C. (2009). Glioblastoma Multiforme Oncogenomics and Signaling Pathways. *Clin Med Oncol,* Vol.3, No (Apr 8,2009), pp. 39-52, ISSN 1177-9314

Karcher, S.; Steiner, H. H.; Ahmadi, R. (2006). Different angiogenic phenotypes in primary and secondary glioblastomas. *Int J Cancer,* Vol.118, No 9, (May 1,2006), pp. 2182-9, ISSN 0020-7136

Karkkainen, M. J. & Petrova, T. V. (2000). Vascular endothelial growth factor receptors in the regulation of angiogenesis and lymphangiogenesis. *Oncogene,* Vol.19, No 49, (Nov 20,2000), pp. 5598-605, ISSN 0950-9232

Keck, P. J.; Hauser, S. D.; Krivi, G. (1989). Vascular permeability factor, an endothelial cell mitogen related to PDGF. *Science,* Vol.246, No 4935, (Dec 8,1989), pp. 1309-12, ISSN 0036-8075

Klink, B.; Schlingelhof, B.; Klink, M. (2010). Glioblastomas with oligodendroglial component - common origin of the different histological parts and genetic subclassification. *Anal Cell Pathol (Amst),* Vol.33, No 1, 2010), pp. 37-54, ISSN 2210-7185

Knudsen, E. S. & Wang, J. Y. (2010). Targeting the RB-pathway in cancer therapy. *Clin Cancer Res,* Vol.16, No 4, (Feb 15,2010), pp. 1094-9, ISSN 1078-0432

Kotliarov, Y.; Steed, M. E.; Christopher, N. (2006). High-resolution global genomic survey of 178 gliomas reveals novel regions of copy number alteration and allelic imbalances. *Cancer Res,* Vol.66, No 19, (Oct 1,2006), pp. 9428-36, ISSN 1538-7445

Kraus, J. A.; Koopmann, J.; Kaskel, P. (1995). Shared allelic losses on chromosomes 1p and 19q suggest a common origin of oligodendroglioma and oligoastrocytoma. *J Neuropathol Exp Neurol,* Vol.54, No 1, (Jan,1995), pp. 91-5, ISSN 0022-3069

Lane, D. P. (1992). Cancer. p53, guardian of the genome. *Nature,* Vol.358, No 6381, (Jul 2,1992), pp. 15-6, ISSN 0028-0836

Lane, D. P. & Crawford, L. V. (1979). T antigen is bound to a host protein in SV40-transformed cells. *Nature,* Vol.278, No 5701, (Mar 15,1979), pp. 261-3, ISSN 0028-0836

Levine, A. J. (1997). p53, the cellular gatekeeper for growth and division. *Cell,* Vol.88, No 3, (Feb 7,1997), pp. 323-31, ISSN 0092-8674

Levine, A. J.; Hu, W. & Feng, Z. (2006). The P53 pathway: what questions remain to be explored? *Cell Death Differ,* Vol.13, No 6, (Jun,2006), pp. 1027-36, ISSN 1350-9047

Liang, Y.; Diehn, M.; Watson, N. (2005). Gene expression profiling reveals molecularly and clinically distinct subtypes of glioblastoma multiforme. *Proc Natl Acad Sci U S A,* Vol.102, No 16, (Apr 19,2005), pp. 5814-9, ISSN 0027-8424

Lim, D. A.; Cha, S.; Mayo, M. C. (2007). Relationship of glioblastoma multiforme to neural stem cell regions predicts invasive and multifocal tumor phenotype. *Neuro Oncol,* Vol.9, No 4, (Oct,2007), pp. 424-9, ISSN 1522-8517

Linzer, D. I. & Levine, A. J. (1979). Characterization of a 54K dalton cellular SV40 tumor antigen present in SV40-transformed cells and uninfected embryonal carcinoma cells. *Cell,* Vol.17, No 1, (May,1979), pp. 43-52, ISSN 0092-8674

Louis, D. N. (2006). Molecular pathology of malignant gliomas. *Annu Rev Pathol,* Vol.1, No 2006), pp. 97-117, ISSN 1553-4006

Louis, D. N.; Ohgaki, H.; Wiestler, O. D. (2007). The 2007 WHO classification of tumours of the central nervous system. *Acta Neuropathol,* Vol.114, No 2, (Aug,2007), pp. 97-109, ISSN 0001-6322

Maher, E. A.; Furnari, F. B.; Bachoo, R. M. (2001). Malignant glioma: genetics and biology of a grave matter. *Genes Dev,* Vol.15, No 11, (Jun 1,2001), pp. 1311-33, ISSN 0890-9369

Maira, S. M.; Stauffer, F.; Brueggen, J. (2008). Identification and characterization of NVP-BEZ235, a new orally available dual phosphatidylinositol 3-kinase/mammalian target of rapamycin inhibitor with potent in vivo antitumor activity. *Mol Cancer Ther,* Vol.7, No 7, (Jul,2008), pp. 1851-63, ISSN 1535-7163

Malmer, B.; Adatto, P.; Armstrong, G. (2007). GLIOGENE an International Consortium to Understand Familial Glioma. *Cancer Epidemiol Biomarkers Prev,* Vol.16, No 9, (Sep,2007), pp. 1730-4, ISSN 1055-9965

Malumbres, M. & Barbacid, M. (2001). To cycle or not to cycle: a critical decision in cancer. *Nat Rev Cancer,* Vol.1, No 3, (Dec,2001), pp. 222-31, ISSN 1474-175X

Manning, B. D. & Cantley, L. C. (2007). AKT/PKB signaling: navigating downstream. *Cell,* Vol.129, No 7, (Jun 29,2007), pp. 1261-74, ISSN 0092-8674

Marko, N. F.; Toms, S. A.; Barnett, G. H. (2008). Genomic expression patterns distinguish long-term from short-term glioblastoma survivors: a preliminary feasibility study. *Genomics,* Vol.91, No 5, (May,2008), pp. 395-406, ISSN 1089-8646

Marumoto, T.; Tashiro, A.; Friedmann-Morvinski, D. (2009). Development of a novel mouse glioma model using lentiviral vectors. *Nat Med,* Vol.15, No 1, (Jan,2009), pp. 110-6, ISSN 1546-170X

Masri, J.; Bernath, A.; Martin, J. (2007). mTORC2 activity is elevated in gliomas and promotes growth and cell motility via overexpression of rictor. *Cancer Res,* Vol.67, No 24, (Dec 15,2007), pp. 11712-20, ISSN 1538-7445

Matheu, A.; Maraver, A. & Serrano, M. (2008). The Arf/p53 pathway in cancer and aging. *Cancer Res,* Vol.68, No 15, (Aug 1,2008), pp. 6031-4, ISSN 1538-7445

Mellinghoff, I. K.; Wang, M. Y.; Vivanco, I. (2005). Molecular determinants of the response of glioblastomas to EGFR kinase inhibitors. *N Engl J Med,* Vol.353, No 19, (Nov 10,2005), pp. 2012-24, ISSN 1533-4406

Merkel, C. A.; da Silva Soares, R. B.; de Carvalho, A. C. (2010). Activation of endogenous p53 by combined p19Arf gene transfer and nutlin-3 drug treatment modalities in the murine cell lines B16 and C6. *BMC Cancer,* Vol.10, No 2010), pp. 316, ISSN 1471-2407

Michael, D. & Oren, M. (2003). The p53-Mdm2 module and the ubiquitin system. *Semin Cancer Biol,* Vol.13, No 1, (Feb,2003), pp. 49-58, ISSN 1044-579X

Mischel, P. S.; Shai, R.; Shi, T. (2003). Identification of molecular subtypes of glioblastoma by gene expression profiling. *Oncogene,* Vol.22, No 15, (Apr 17,2003), pp. 2361-73, ISSN 0950-9232

Mizoguchi, M.; Betensky, R. A.; Batchelor, T. T. (2006). Activation of STAT3, MAPK, and AKT in malignant astrocytic gliomas: correlation with EGFR status, tumor grade, and survival. *J Neuropathol Exp Neurol,* Vol.65, No 12, (Dec,2006), pp. 1181-8, ISSN 0022-3069

Neyns, B.; Sadones, J.; Joosens, E. (2009). Stratified phase II trial of cetuximab in patients with recurrent high-grade glioma. *Ann Oncol,* Vol.20, No 9, (Sep,2009), pp. 1596-603, ISSN 1569-8041

Noda, S. E.; El-Jawahri, A.; Patel, D. (2009). Molecular advances of brain tumors in radiation oncology. *Semin Radiat Oncol,* Vol.19, No 3, (Jul,2009), pp. 171-8, ISSN 1532-9461

Nutt, C. L.; Mani, D. R.; Betensky, R. A. (2003). Gene expression-based classification of malignant gliomas correlates better with survival than histological classification. *Cancer Res,* Vol.63, No 7, (Apr 1,2003), pp. 1602-7, ISSN 0008-5472

Ohgaki, H.; Dessen, P.; Jourde, B. (2004). Genetic pathways to glioblastoma: a population-based study. *Cancer Res,* Vol.64, No 19, (Oct 1,2004), pp. 6892-9, ISSN 0008-5472

Ohgaki, H. & Kleihues, P. (2007). Genetic pathways to primary and secondary glioblastoma. *Am J Pathol,* Vol.170, No 5, (May,2007), pp. 1445-53, ISSN 0002-9440

Ohgaki, H. & Kleihues, P. (2009). Genetic alterations and signaling pathways in the evolution of gliomas. *Cancer Sci,* Vol.100, No 12, (Dec,2009), pp. 2235-41, ISSN 1349-7006

Pallini, R.; Ricci-Vitiani, L.; Banna, G. L. (2008). Cancer stem cell analysis and clinical outcome in patients with glioblastoma multiforme. *Clin Cancer Res,* Vol.14, No 24, (Dec 15, 2008), pp. 8205-12, ISSN 1078-0432

Parsons, D. W.; Jones, S.; Zhang, X. (2008). An integrated genomic analysis of human glioblastoma multiforme. *Science,* Vol.321, No 5897, (Sep 26,2008), pp. 1807-12, ISSN 1095-9203

Phillips, H. S.; Kharbanda, S.; Chen, R. (2006). Molecular subclasses of high-grade glioma predict prognosis, delineate a pattern of disease progression, and resemble stages in neurogenesis. *Cancer Cell,* Vol.9, No 3, (Mar,2006), pp. 157-73, ISSN 1535-6108

Ranson, M. (2004). Epidermal growth factor receptor tyrosine kinase inhibitors. *Br J Cancer,* Vol.90, No 12, (Jun 14,2004), pp. 2250-5, ISSN 0007-0920

Rao, R. D.; Mladek, A. C.; Lamont, J. D. (2005). Disruption of parallel and converging signaling pathways contributes to the synergistic antitumor effects of simultaneous mTOR and EGFR inhibition in GBM cells. *Neoplasia,* Vol.7, No 10, (Oct,2005), pp. 921-9, ISSN 1522-8002

Rao, S. K.; Edwards, J.; Joshi, A. D. (2010). A survey of glioblastoma genomic amplifications and deletions. *J Neurooncol,* Vol.96, No 2, (Jan,2010), pp. 169-79, ISSN 1573-7373

Read, R. D.; Cavenee, W. K.; Furnari, F. B. (2009). A drosophila model for EGFR-Ras and PI3K-dependent human glioma. *PLoS Genet,* Vol.5, No 2, (Feb,2009), pp. e1000374, ISSN 1553-7404

Reddy, S. P.; Britto, R.; Vinnakota, K. (2008). Novel glioblastoma markers with diagnostic and prognostic value identified through transcriptome analysis. *Clin Cancer Res,* Vol.14, No 10, (May 15,2008), pp. 2978-87, ISSN 1078-0432

Sanai, N.; Alvarez-Buylla, A. & Berger, M. S. (2005). Neural stem cells and the origin of gliomas. *N Engl J Med,* Vol.353, No 8, (Aug 25,2005), pp. 811-22, ISSN 1533-4406

Sathornsumetee, S. & Rich, J. N. (2008). Designer therapies for glioblastoma multiforme. *Ann N Y Acad Sci,* Vol.1142, No (Oct,2008), pp. 108-32, ISSN 1749-6632

Scambia, G.; Lovergine, S. & Masciullo, V. (2006). RB family members as predictive and prognostic factors in human cancer. *oncogene,* Vol.25, No 38, 2006), pp. 5302-5308, ISSN 0950-9232

Schmidt, N. O.; Westphal, M.; Hagel, C. (1999). Levels of vascular endothelial growth factor, hepatocyte growth factor/scatter factor and basic fibroblast growth factor in human gliomas and their relation to angiogenesis. *Int J Cancer,* Vol.84, No 1, (Feb 19,1999), pp. 10-8, ISSN 0020-7136

Schwartzbaum, J.; Jonsson, F.; Ahlbom, A. (2003). Cohort studies of association between self-reported allergic conditions, immune-related diagnoses and glioma and meningioma risk. *Int J Cancer,* Vol.106, No 3, (Sep 1,2003), pp. 423-8, ISSN 0020-7136

Shangary, S. & Wang, S. (2009). Small-molecule inhibitors of the MDM2-p53 protein-protein interaction to reactivate p53 function: a novel approach for cancer therapy. *Annu Rev Pharmacol Toxicol,* Vol.49, No 2009), pp. 223-41, ISSN 0362-1642

Shinojima, N.; Kochi, M.; Hamada, J. (2004). The influence of sex and the presence of giant cells on postoperative long-term survival in adult patients with supratentorial glioblastoma multiforme. *J Neurosurg,* Vol.101, No 2, (Aug,2004), pp. 219-26, ISSN 0022-3085

Singh, S. K.; Clarke, I. D.; Terasaki, M. (2003). Identification of a cancer stem cell in human brain tumors. *Cancer Res,* Vol.63, No 18, (Sep 15,2003), pp. 5821-8, ISSN 0008-5472

Singh, S. K.; Hawkins, C.; Clarke, I. D. (2004). Identification of human brain tumour initiating cells. *Nature,* Vol.432, No 7015, (Nov 18,2004), pp. 396-401, ISSN 1476-4687

Somasundaram, K.; Reddy, S. P.; Vinnakota, K. (2005). Upregulation of ASCL1 and inhibition of Notch signaling pathway characterize progressive astrocytoma. *Oncogene,* Vol.24, No 47, (Oct 27,2005), pp. 7073-83, ISSN 0950-9232

Sonoda, Y.; Kumabe, T.; Watanabe, M. (2009). Long-term survivors of glioblastoma: clinical features and molecular analysis. *Acta Neurochir (Wien),* Vol.151, No 11, (Nov,2009), pp. 1349-58, ISSN 0942-0940

Soussi, T. & Wiman, K. G. (2007). Shaping genetic alterations in human cancer: the p53 mutation paradigm. *Cancer Cell,* Vol.12, No 4, (Oct,2007), pp. 303-12, ISSN 1535-6108

Stommel, J. M.; Kimmelman, A. C.; Ying, H. (2007). Coactivation of receptor tyrosine kinases affects the response of tumor cells to targeted therapies. *Science,* Vol.318, No 5848, (Oct 12,2007), pp. 287-90, ISSN 1095-9203

Stummer, W.; Pichlmeier, U.; Meinel, T. (2006). Fluorescence-guided surgery with 5-aminolevulinic acid for resection of malignant glioma: a randomised controlled multicentre phase III trial. *Lancet Oncol,* Vol.7, No 5, (May,2006), pp. 392-401, ISSN 1470-2045

Takahashi, K. & Yamanaka, S. (2006). Induction of pluripotent stem cells from mouse embryonic and adult fibroblast cultures by defined factors. *Cell,* Vol.126, No 4, (Aug 25,2006), pp. 663-76, ISSN 0092-8674

Tanaka, K.; Sasayama, T.; Mizukawa, K. (2007). Specific mTOR inhibitor rapamycin enhances cytotoxicity induced by alkylating agent 1-(4-amino-2-methyl-5-pyrimidinyl)methyl-3-(2-chloroethyl)-3-nitrosourea (ACNU) in human U251 malignant glioma cells. *J Neurooncol,* Vol.84, No 3, (Sep,2007), pp. 233-44, ISSN 0167-594X

Testa, J. R. & Bellacosa, A. (2001). AKT plays a central role in tumorigenesis. *Proc Natl Acad Sci U S A,* Vol.98, No 20, (Sep 25,2001), pp. 10983-5, ISSN 0027-8424

The Cancer Genome Atlas (TCGA) Research Network. (2008). Comprehensive genomic characterization defines human glioblastoma genes and core pathways. *Nature,* Vol.455, No 7216, (Oct 23,2008), pp. 1061-8, ISSN 1476-4687

Thiessen, B.; Stewart, C.; Tsao, M. (2009). A phase I/II trial of GW572016 (lapatinib) in recurrent glioblastoma multiforme: clinical outcomes, pharmacokinetics and molecular correlation. *Cancer Chemother Pharmacol,* No (Jun 5,2009), pp. 353-361, ISSN 1432-0843

Tohma, Y.; Gratas, C.; Van Meir, E. G. (1998). Necrogenesis and Fas/APO-1 (CD95) expression in primary (de novo) and secondary glioblastomas. *J Neuropathol Exp Neurol,* Vol.57, No 3, (Mar,1998), pp. 239-45, ISSN 0022-3069

Tso, C. L.; Freije, W. A.; Day, A. (2006). Distinct transcription profiles of primary and secondary glioblastoma subgroups. *Cancer Res,* Vol.66, No 1, (Jan 1,2006), pp. 159-67, ISSN 0008-5472

van den Bent, M. J.; Brandes, A. A.; Rampling, R. (2009). Randomized phase II trial of erlotinib versus temozolomide or carmustine in recurrent glioblastoma: EORTC brain tumor group study 26034. *J Clin Oncol,* Vol.27, No 8, (Mar 10,2009), pp. 1268-74, ISSN 1527-7755

Van Meir, E. G.; Hadjipanayis, C. G.; Norden, A. D. (2010). Exciting new advances in neuro-oncology: the avenue to a cure for malignant glioma. *CA Cancer J Clin,* Vol.60, No 3, (May-Jun,2010), pp. 166-93, ISSN 1542-4863

Vassilev, L. T.; Vu, B. T.; Graves, B. (2004). In vivo activation of the p53 pathway by small-molecule antagonists of MDM2. *Science,* Vol.303, No 5659, (Feb 6,2004), pp. 844-8, ISSN 1095-9203

Verhaak, R. G.; Hoadley, K. A.; Purdom, E. (2010). Integrated genomic analysis identifies clinically relevant subtypes of glioblastoma characterized by abnormalities in PDGFRA, IDH1, EGFR, and NF1. *Cancer Cell,* Vol.17, No 1, (Jan 19,2010), pp. 98-110, ISSN 1878-3686

Vredenburgh, J. J.; Desjardins, A.; Herndon, J. E., 2nd. (2007). Phase II trial of bevacizumab and irinotecan in recurrent malignant glioma. *Clin Cancer Res,* Vol.13, No 4, (Feb 15,2007), pp. 1253-9, ISSN 1078-0432

Wade, M.; Wang, Y. V. & Wahl, G. M. (2010). The p53 orchestra: Mdm2 and Mdmx set the tone. *Trends Cell Biol,* Vol.20, No 5, (May,2010), pp. 299-309, ISSN 1879-3088

Weinberg, R. A. (1995). The retinoblastoma protein and cell cycle control. *Cell,* Vol.81, No 3, (May 5,1995), pp. 323-30, ISSN 0092-8674

Wen, P. Y. & Kesari, S. (2008). Malignant gliomas in adults. *N Engl J Med,* Vol.359, No 5, (Jul 31,2008), pp. 492-507, ISSN 1533-4406

White, J.; Stead, E.; Faast, R. (2005). Developmental Activation of the Rb-E2F Pathway and Establishment of Cell Cycle-regulated Cyclin-dependent Kinase Activity during Embryonic Stem Cell Differentiation. *Mol. Biol. Cell,* Vol.16, No 4, (April 1, 2005,2005), pp. 2018-2027

Wullschleger, S.; Loewith, R. & Hall, M. N. (2006). TOR signaling in growth and metabolism. *Cell,* Vol.124, No 3, (Feb 10,2006), pp. 471-84, ISSN 0092-8674

Xiao, A.; Wu, H.; Pandolfi, P. P. (2002). Astrocyte inactivation of the pRb pathway predisposes mice to malignant astrocytoma development that is accelerated by PTEN mutation. *Cancer Cell,* Vol.1, No 2, (Mar,2002), pp. 157-68, ISSN 1535-6108

Zeppernick, F.; Ahmadi, R.; Campos, B. (2008). Stem cell marker CD133 affects clinical outcome in glioma patients. *Clin Cancer Res,* Vol.14, No 1, (Jan 1,2008), pp. 123-9, ISSN 1078-0432

Zheng, H.;Ying, H.; Yan, H. (2008). p53 and Pten control neural and glioma stem/progenitor cell renewal and differentiation. *Nature,* Vol.455, No 7216, (Oct 23,2008), pp. 1129-33, ISSN 1476-4687

Zhou, B. P.; Liao, Y.; Xia, W. (2001). HER-2/neu induces p53 ubiquitination via Akt-mediated MDM2 phosphorylation. *Nat Cell Biol,* Vol.3, No 11, (Nov,2001), pp. 973-82, ISSN 1465-7392

Zhou, X. P.; Li, Y. J.; Hoang-Xuan, K. (1999). Mutational analysis of the PTEN gene in gliomas: molecular and pathological correlations. *Int J Cancer,* Vol.84, No 2, (Apr 20,1999), pp. 150-4, ISSN 0020-7136

14

Chemokines in Glioma Progression

Marco Locatelli and Alberto Mantovani
Neurosurgery, Fondazione IRCCS Ca' Granda Ospedale Maggiore Policlinico Milano
Istituto Clinico Humanitas IRCCS, Department of Translation Medicine
Università degli Studi di Milano
Italy

1. Introduction

Gliomas represent a formidable challenge in terms of pathophysiologic and clinical behaviour.

The frequently used term "glioma" applies to neoplasms derived from components of neuroglia: astrocytes, oligodendrocytes and ependima cells with the corrisponding tumors, astrocytomas, oligodendrogliomas and ependymomas (Louis et al 2007, Graham et al 2006). They represent the most common primary intra-axial brain tumor (40% of intracranial tumors with an estimated incidence of 12.000 new cases /year in the U.S.). Importantly, when discussing gliomas, the terms benign and malign have little meaning; the WHO classification provides a grading system to subdivide gliomas. Grading is based on cellularity, presence of giant cells, anaplasia, mitotic activity, microvascular proliferation with or without endothelial proliferation, necrosis and pseudopalisading. Astrocytomas and oligodendrogliomas are usually defined as grade II (III in the anaplastic form) while glioblastomas are grade IV. So a simpler classification describes these tumors as being of low or high grade.

From a clinical point of view the grading system has an inverse correlation to patient survival and it is important in taking decisions as to the therapeutic strategies.

With the exception of one or two entities (e.g. pilocytic astrocytoma-grade I), a low grade glioma will continue to acquire genetic mutations and eventually will transform into a high grade neoplasm. This process is defined dedifferentiation and represents the major cause of morbidity with low-grade astrocytomas. Genetic markers that correlate with a higher degree of malignant degeneration include loss of heterozygosity at chromosomes 10 & 17, alteration in tumor suppressor genes 9p, 13q, 19q & 22q, changes in epidermal growth factor receptor (EGRF) and platelet derived growth factor (PDGF) and mutation of the p53 suppressor gene.

To underline the importance of this behaviour, the gliomas that developed in the adult are frequently defined as "diffuse" because of their ability to profoundly infiltrate the brain parenchyma (Louis et al 2007).

Glioblastomas (the most malignant form of glial tumors) are characterized by extensive dissemination of tumor cells within the brain that are hallmarked histologically by the presence of vascular endothelial proliferation and wide areas of necrosis often presenting hemorrhagic components. Besides invasion, enhanced proliferation, angiogenesis and

---

All authors contributed equally to the chapter.

resistance to apoptosis are all involved in the progression and maintenance of this malignancy.
As mentioned above gliomas still represent a formidable clinical challenge. In spite of optimal and multidisciplinary treatment (in high grade forms, surgery followed by chemotherapy and radiotherapy) the prognosis of patients affected with gliomas is poor and it becomes dramatic in patients with glioblastomas. As a matter of fact patients with glioblastomas survive less than 1 year and prognosis has not consistently changed over the last two decades. Again, the reason of this defeat can be found in the rapidly expanding nature of these tumors and their capability of invading the normal brain by active cell migration.
Inflammatory cells are a key component of the tumor microenvironment (Mantovani et al 2008; Hanahan and Weinberg 2011). Chemokines play an important role in orchestrating leukocytes recruitment in tumors including gliomas. Moreover, these molecules affect various aspects of tumor cell function (Balkwill et al 2004, Mantovani et al 2006-2008, Lazennec and Richmond 2010). Here we will review available information on the expression and role of chemokines in gliomas.

2. The chemokine universe

Chemokines are a large family of small chemoattractant cytochines. They comprise approximately 50 ligands and 20 receptors in humans. The number and position of conserved cysteine residues divide this family of related molecules into two major (CXC and CC) and two minor (C and CX3C) chemokine classes (Mantovani et al 2006, Charo and Ransohoff 2006).
Chemokine receptors are G-protein coupled, seven transmembrane receptors. Based on the chemokine class they bind, the receptors have been named CXCR1-7 (bind to CXC chemokines); CCR1 through CCR10 (bound to CC chemokines), XCR1 (bound to the C chemokine, lymphotactin/XCL1) and CX3CR1 (bound to the CX3C chemokine, fractalkine/CXCL1) (Zlotnik 2006). Another classification is between homeostic and inflammatory molecules according to the chemokine constitutive (e.g. SDF1/CXCL12) or inflammatory-induced (e.g. CCL2) production, respectively Importantly, if this classification is useful it can be criticized because it does not take into account chemokines classified as inflammatory that are locally but constitutively expressed by tumor cells or in a tissue specific manner (e.g. CX3CL1 in brain).
The most important targets of chemokines are leukocytes. Their ability to orchestrate leucocyte trafficking under basal and inflammatory conditions is generally named as chemotaxis, but chemokine control is also exerted on cell adhesion, proliferation, survival and gene transcription (Campbell and Butcher 2000).
Moreover, chemokine action is not only limited to white cells but it extends to many other cell populations. In particular, chemokine and chemokine receptors are widely expressed into the central nervous system both by neurons and glial cells. The chemokine network in the central nervous system is involved in several brain processes such as cell migration, regulation of neuronal survival, neurotransmission and cell-cell communication (Ambrosini and Aloisi 2004). For this reason chemokine and chemokine receptors can be considered the third major transmitter system in the brain (Adler et al 2005). Interestingly, the chemokine universe seems to be altered in neurodegenerative disorders such as Alzheimer like dementia, multiple sclerosis and brain tumors (Ransohoff et al 2009, Sciumè et al 2010-2011, Marchesi et al 2010, Trettel et al 2010).

3. Chemokines in gliomas

3.1 Glioma cell expression of chemokine and chemokine receptors

The migratory ability of gliomas has been investigated by electron microscopy and it was shown that neoplastic cells easily adjust their shape and size to slip through the narrow brain spaces, a process that requires Cl channels (Mc Coy and Sontheimer 2007).

It is now established that migrating malignant cells exploit chemokine receptors to invade surrounding tissues thus leading to distant metastasis (Balkwill 2004, Zlotnik 2006, Mantovani et al 2010).

The expression of chemokines and chemokine receptors is considered to play a role in tumor cell proliferation, invasion, migration and ability to metastasize. This expression can be activated or amplified by both stromal cells and tumor cells themselves (Mantovani et al 2010).

Moreover the immune cell infiltration in the neoplastic area largely depends on the chemokine expression.

Since 1990 the production of chemokines by cell lines of glioma has been described (IL-8/CXCL8; MCP1/CCL2 etc). In particular, CCL2 was described to be expressed in low and high grade glioma cells both "in vitro" and "in vivo" (Jiang et al 1990, Kasahara et al 1991, Nitta et al 1992, Kuratsu et al 1993). In 1997 Desbaillets and colleagues demonstrated high levels of expression of CXCL8 and its receptors CXCR1 and CXCR2 within the necrotic areas surrounding brain tumor cells. Significantly, the presence of these two receptors was described in endothelial cells of new blood vessels, suggesting they may be implicated in neoangiogenesis.

At the early 2000s an important role of the CXCR4/CXCL12 axis has been identified for the regulation of different aspects of glioma tumor progression. High levels of this complex expression were demonstrated in areas nearby tumor necrosis (Rempel et al 2000). CXCR4 as well as CXCL8 were also demonstrated to be expressed both in glioma cells lines and primary glioblastomas. Interestingly, CXCL8 and CXCL12 "in vivo" secretion can also arise from other cellular populations such as endothelial cells and macrophage/microglial cells, and these populations are implied in gliomagenesis (Hong et al 2009). The expression of CXCL10, CXCL8 and CCL2 is increased by CXCL12-induced CXCR4 stimulation in gliomas thus creating a sort of amplification loop which influence tumor growth, angiogenesis and immune cells infiltration.

The increased expression of IP10/CXCL10 and of CCL3L1 and their receptors found in glioma cells compared to "normal" astrocytes lead to hypothesize an autocrine role for these axes in glioma control (Maru et al 2008). The high expression of CX3CL1 (or fractalkine) in the brain has suggested that also CX3CL1/CX3CR1 axis may play a role in malignancies of the central nervous system (Locatelli et al 2010, Marchesi et al 2010, Sciumè et al 2010). Indeed, neurons and astrocytes are major producers of the ligand and microglia express the receptor CX3CR1 expression has been detected both in glial cells and in neurons. Experimental evidence established that this axis play a major role in the neuron/microglia cross-talk and in neuroprotection under conditions of inflammation (Cardona et al 2006, Gunther et al 2005, Miller et al 2008).

Using a murine model a positive in situ hybridization for CX3CR1 corresponding with the localisation of CD11b-positive microglia was described (Liu et al 2008). As for human glioblastomas CX3CR1 immunopositivity was found in neoplastic cells (Ludwig et al 2005, Locatelli et al 2010).

Moreover, Sciumè and colleagues in 2010 described that glioblastomas cells express both the membrane-bound and the secreted form of CX3CL1 and its receptor CX3CR1. Marked expression of CX3CR1 was similar across low and high grade tumor though it was highest in glioblastomas. The presence of receptor expression in low grade tumor suggests that its upregulation is an early event during malignant transformation. In a recent paper (Erreni et al 2010) CX3CR1 was similarly detected in low and high grade tumors while the uppermost score of CX3CL1 were found in grades II and IV. Accordingly, the expression of fractlakine was inversely correlated to the patient survival.

Notably, constitutive expression of CX3CL1 in CX3CR1 positive glioblastomas negatively regulates tumor cell invasiveness by promoting their aggregation (Sciumè et al 2010). CX3CL1 is induced by TNF α and TNF β in neurons (Chen et al 2002, Sciumè et al 2010). These mediators are frequently present in tumors including gliomas and may be involved in the modulation of CX3CL1/CX3CR1 axis in neoplastic conditions (Mantovani et al 2008, Balkwill et al 2009).

In 2005 Ludwig and colleagues demonstrated that another membrane-bound chemokine, CXCL16 is upregulated in human glioma being this chemokine expression low in normal brain and substantially limited to brain endothelial cells.

Expression of chemokines and their receptors is modulated by factors produced by gliomas or by the tumor microenvironment. Examples are CXCL8, CXCL12 anCXCR4 which are up regulated in hypoxic conditions or upon stimulation with VEGF, an angiogenetic growth factor expressed in glioma tissues (Desbaillets et al 1997, Zagzag et al 2008).

3.2 Chemokines in glioma invasion

The peculiar adhesive function of fractalkine in the nervous system suggests that this chemokine/receptor complex plays a role in the neurotropism of cancer cells to peripheral nerves. This is a distinct and largely underestimated way of metastasis compared to blood and lymphatic routes; many human carcinomas such as bladder, prostate and pancreas take advantage of this route (Marchesi et al 2010).

The invasive process of glioma cells requires the detachment of invading cells from the primary mass of the tumor, attachment to extracellular matrix components and degradation of this matrix. At this point tumor cell migration into brain structures can take place. CX3CL1 would have a negative role in this process, as suggested by the increase in glioma cell invasion properties by the blockade induced by CX3CR1-CX3CL1 axis. Moreover, the reduced CX3CR1 expression consequent to TGF-beta 1 activation can favour glioma invasiveness (Sciumè et al 2010).

Another axis which is acquiring an increasing consideration in this complex process is the CXCL12/CXCR4 axis. This axis has been linked to glioma progression both "in vitro" and "in vivo" (Zhou et al 2002, Zhang et al 2005, Ehtesham et al 2006, Bajetto et al 2006) because of its ability to activate metalloproteinases, including the membrane type-2-MMP. Accordingly, invasive human glioma cell overexpress CXCR4 while noninvasive glioma cell do not. These data were confirmed "in vivo" in neoplastic cells from a rat C6 glioma cell line (Ehtesham et al 2006).

Co-expression of CXCL12 and its receptors is mainly localized to the pseudopalisade zones that surround necrotic foci (Rempel et al 2000). These regions are believed to represent tumor cells which are leaving necrotic regions because of their low or absent oxygen levels. In hypoxic condition, tumor cells release an angiogentic growth factor (VEGF) which promotes the over-expression of CXCL12 and consequently tumor invasion outside the hypoxic area (Zagzag et al 2008).

Promotion of glioma cell invasion is also mediated by Gro-alpha/CXCL1 that is expressed by oligodendroglioma and anaplastic astrocytomas (Zhou et al 2005). Interestingly CXCL1 overexpression conferred increased tumorigenicity to U251 cells following implantation into the brain of nude mice (Zhou et al 2005).

3.3 Chemokine role in glioma proliferation

In addition to CXCL12, also CXCL8, CXCL10 and CCL3L1 have been described to promote glioma cell proliferation in vitro (Kouno et al 2004, Maru et al 2008). Notably, a correlation between CXCL8 expression levels in cells surrounding necrotic areas and histologic grade in glioma has been demonstrated (Desbaillets et al 1997).

Chemokines also contribute to create a proangiogenic microenvironment by promoting attraction of endothelial cells and leukocytes to the tumor. The chemokine receptor panel of human microvascular endothelial cells includes CXCR2, CXCR3B, CXCR4 and CX3CR1 (Bernardini et al 2003).

As mentioned above, CXCR4 is expressed by both tumor cells and vascular endothelial cells in different grades of gliomas; this is associated with CXCL12 production in the tumor microenvironment, which is capable to modulate migration, proliferation and survival of endothelial and tumor cells (Salmaggi et 2004). It was demonstrated that CXCR4 is expressed by both tumor cells and vascular endothelial cells in all grades of gliomas. The administration of AMD-3100, a CXCR4 antagonist, inhibits the growth of glioblastoma xenografts in mouses, demonstrating the dependence of tumor cells proliferation on CXCR4 (Rubin et al 2003).

3.4 Chemokine network and leukocyte infiltration

Besides its direct effects on tumor growth, the network of chemokines implicated in human astrcytomas can influence the degree and phenotype of immune cell infiltration. However, it is well accepted that glioma cells can be recognized by both innate and adaptive immunity (Mantovani et al 2008, Friese et al 2004, Dunn et al 2007). T-cell infiltration has been described to be present in neuroephitelial tumors, on the contrary NK cells are poorly included in the glioma lymphocyte infiltrate (Vaquero et al 1989).

To date, data regarding the specificity and function of tumor -infiltrating lynphocytes such as the involvement of the chemokine network in the recruitment of these cells or tumor infiltrating microglia/macrophages are lacking. Glia derived CCL2 might be implicated in the process leading to the abundant tumor infiltration by macrophages/microglia and T cells (Jordan et al 2008). CCL2 expression by glioma cells would be advantageous for tumor progression thanks to the attraction of T regulatory cells that suppress lymphocyte anti tumor effector functions and of microglia cells with reduce anti-tumor functions. Another effect would be the secretion of metalloproteinases. The corresponding receptors were the CCR2 on microglia and CCR4 on T regulatory cells (Hussain et al 2006). The role of the CX3CL1/CX3CR1 chemokine/receptor pair in microglial and lymphocyte infiltration remains to be defined.(Liu et al 2008, Rodero et al 2008)

3.5 Concluding remarks

Available information strongly suggest that chemokines play an important role in gliomas. In particular, evidence suggests that they are orchestrators of leukocyte recruitment in the glioma microenvironment. Moreover, glioma cells express a defined repertoire of chemokine receptors including CXCR4/CXCL12, CX3CL1/CX3CR1 axis.

On the basis of available information and extrapolation from other tumors, chemokine receptors expressed on gliomas may have a broad impact on biological and clinical behaviour of the tumor, affecting different functions including invasion, cell survival and proliferation.

Despite increasing evidence on this complexity, further investigations of this network will allow a better understanding of tumor specificities, biological behaviour and therapeutic failures.

These data and considerations raise the possibility of targeting components of the chemokine system to complement available therapeutic strategies against gliomas.

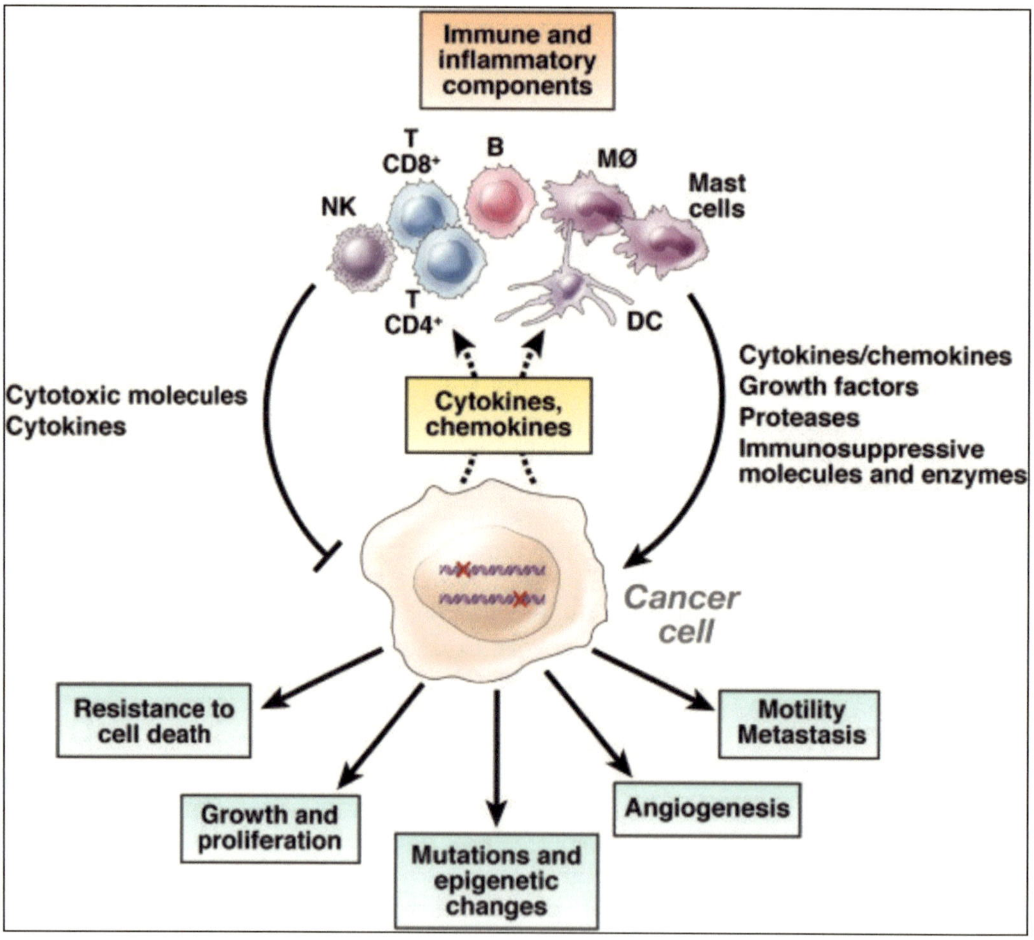

Fig. 1. Inflammatory mediators in gliomas. Innate and adaptive immune cells together with inflammatory molecules and cancer cells are part of an inflammatory microenvironment which may have an impact on biological and clinical behaviour of gliomas.

4. References

Adler M.W., Geller E.B., Chen X., Rogers T.J. 2005 Viewing chemokines as a third major system of communication in the brain. AAPS J. 7, E865-E870.

Ambrosini E., Aloisi F. 2004 Chemokines and glial cells: a complex network in the central nervous system. Neurochem. Res. 29, 1017-1038.

Bajetto A., Barbieri F., Dorcaratto A., Barbero S., Daga A., Porcile C., Ravetti J.L., Zona G., Spaziante R., Corte G., Schettini G., Florio T. 2006 Expression of CXC chemokine receptor 1-5 and their liigands in human glioma tissues role of CXCR4 and SDF1 in glioma cell proliferation and migration. Nurochem. Int. 49, 540-550.

Balkwill F. 2004 Cancer and the cytokine network. Nat. Rev. Cancer 4: 540.

Bernardini G., Ribatti D., Spinetti G., Morbidelli L., Ziche M., Santoni A., Capogrossi M.C., Napolitano M. 2003 Analysis of the role of chemokine in angiogenesis. J. Immunol. Meth. 273, 83-101.

Campbell J.J., Butcher E.C. 2000 Chemokines in tissue-specific and microenvironments-specific lymphocyte homing. Curr. Opin. Immunol. 12, 336-341.

Cardona A.E., Piorro E.P., Sasse M.E., Kostenko V., Cardona S.M., Dijkstra I.M., Huang D., Kidd G., Dombrowski S., Dutta R., Lee J.C., Cook D.N., Jung S., Lira S.A., Littman D.R., Ransohoff R.M., 2006 Control of microglial neurotoxicity by the fractalkine receptor. Nat. Neurosci. 9, 917-924.

Chen S., Luo D.,Streit W.J., Harrsion J.K., 2002 TGF-beta 1 upregulates CX3CR1 expression and inhibits fractalkine-stimulated signaling in rat microglia. J. Neuroimmunol. 133, 46-55.

Charo IF, Ransohoff RM. 2006 The many roles of chemokines and chemokine receptors in inflammation. N Engl J Med. Feb 9;354(6):610-21

Desbaillets I., Tada M., de Tribolet N., Diserens A.C., Hamou M.F., Van Meir E.G. 1997 Upregulation of interleukin 8 by oxygen-deprived cells in glioblastomas suggests a role in leukocyte activation, chemotaxis, and angiogenesis. J.Exp. Med.186, 1201-1212.

Dunn GP., Dunn IF, Curry WT. 2007 Focus on TILs: prognostic significance of tumor infiltrating lymphocytes in human glioma. Cancer Immun. 7, 12.

Erreni M, SolinasG., Brescia P., Osti D., Zunino F., Colombo P., Destro A., Roncalli M., Mantovani A., Draghi R., Levi D., Rodriguez Y Baena R., Gaetani P., Pelicci G., Allavena P. 2010 Human glioblastoma tumours and neural cancer stem cells express the chemokine CX3CL1 and its receptor CX3CR1. Eur. J. Cancer 46(18) 3383-3392.

Ehtesham M., Winston J.A., Kabos P., Thompson R.C. 2006 CXCR4 expression mediates glioma cell invasiveness. Oncogene 25, 2801-2806.

Friese MA, Steinle A., Weller M. 2004 The innate immune response in the central nervous system and its role in glioma immune surveillance. Onkologie 27, 487-491.

Graham D.I., Nicoll J.A.R, Bone I. Adams-Graham'S Introduction to Neuropathology 2006 Hodder Arnold.

Gunther K., Leier J., Henning G., Dimmler A., Weissbach R., Hohenberger W., Forster R. 2005 Prediction of lymph node metastasis in colorectal carcinoma by expression of chemokine receptor CCR7. Int. J. Cancer 116, 726-733.

Hanahan D, Weinberg RA. 2011 Hallmarks of cancer: the next generation. Cell. Mar 4;144(5):646-74.

HongT.M., Teng L.J., Shun C.T., Peng M.C., Tsai J.C. 2009 Induced interleukin-8 expression in goliomas by tumor-associated macrophages. J. Neurooncol. 93, 289-301.

Hussain S.F., Yang D., Suki D., Aldape K., Grimm E., Heimberger A.B. 2006 The role of human glioma infiltrating microglia/macrophages in mediating antitumor immune responses. Neuro-Oncology 8, 261-279.

Jiang Y., Valente A.J., Williamson M.J., Zhang L., Graves D.T. 1990 Post-translational modification of a monocyte-specific chemoattractant synthesized by glioma, osteosarcoma and vascular smooth muscle cells. J. Biol. Chem. 265, 18318-18321.

Jordan J.T., Sun W., Hussain S.F., DeAngulo G., Prabhu S.S., Heimberger A.B., 2008 Preferential migration of regulatory T cells mediated by glioma-secretd chemokines can be blocked with chemotherapy. Cancer Immunol. Immunother. 57, 123-131.

Kasahara T., Mukaida N., Yamashita K., Yagisawa H., Akahoshi T., Matshushima K., 1991 IL-1 and TNF-alpha induction of IL-8 and monocyte chemotactic and activating factor (MCAF) mRNA expression in a human astrocytoma cell line. Immunology 74, 60-67.

Kouno J., Nagai H., Nagahata T., Onda M., Yamaguchi H., Adachi K., Takahashi H., Teramoto A., Erni M. 2004 Up-regulation of CC chemokine, CCL3L1, and receptors, CCR3, CCR5 in human glioblastomas that promotes cell growth. J. Neurooncol. 70, 301-307.

Kuratsu J., Yoshizato K., Yoshimura T., Leonard E.J., Takeshima H., Ushio Y., 1993 Quantitative study of monocyte chemoattractant protein-1 (MCP-1) in cerebrospinal fluid and cyst fluid from patients with malignant glioma. J. Nattl. Cancer Inst. 85, 1836-1839.

Lazennec G, Richmond A 2010. Chemokines and chemokine receptors: new insights into cancer-related inflammation. Trends Mol Med. Mar;16(3):133-44.

Liu C., Luo D., Streit W.J., Harrison J.K., 2008 CX3CL1 and CX3CR1 in the GL261 murine model of glioma: CX3CR1 deficicnecy does not impact tumor growth or infiltration of microglia and lymphocytes. J. Neuroimmunol. 198, 98-105.

Ludwig A., Schulte A., Schnack C., Hundhausen C., Reiss K., Broadway N., Held-Feindt J., Mentlein R. 2005 Enhanced expression and shedding of the transmembrane chemokine CXCL16 by reactive astrocytes and glioma cells. J. Neurochem. 93, 1293-1303.

Locatelli M., Boiocchi L., Ferrero S., Martinelli Boneschi F., Zavanone M., Pesce S., Allavena P., Gaini S.M., Bello L., Mantovani A. 2010 Human glioma tumors express high levels of the chemokine receptor CX3CR1. Eur. Cytokine Netw. 21, 27-31.

Louis D.N., Ohgaki H., Wiestler O.D., Cavenee W.K., Burger P.C., Jouvet A., Scheithauer B.W., Kleihues P. 2007 The 2007 WHO classification of tumours of the central nervous system . Acta neuropathol. 114, 97-114.

Mantovani A, Savino B, Locati M, Zammataro L, Allavena P, Bonecchi R. The chemokine system in cancer biology and therapy. Cytokine Growth Factor Rev. 2010 Feb;21(1):27-39.

Mantovani A., Allavena P., Sica A., Balkwill F. 2008 Cancer-related inflammation. Nature 454 436-444.

Mantovani A., Bonecchi R., Locati M. 2006 Tuning inflammation and immunity by chemokine sequestration: decoys and more. Nat. Rev. Immunol. 6, 907-918.

Marchesi F., Locatelli M., Erreni M., Allavena P., Mantovani A. 2010 Role of CX3CR1/CX3CL1 axis in primary and secondary involvement of the nervous system by cancer. J. Neuroimmunol. 224, 39-44.

Maru S.V., Holloway K.A., Flynn G., Lancashire C.L., Loughlin A.J., Male D.K., Romero I.A., 2008 Chemokine production and chemokine receptor expression by human glioma cells: role of CXCL10 in tumor cell proliferation. J. Neuroimmunol. 199, 35-45. Marchesi F., Locatelli M., Erreni M., Allavena P., Mantovani A. 2010 Role of CX3CR1/CX3CL1 axis in primary and secondary involvement of the nervous system by cancer. J. Neuroimmunol. 224, 39-44.

McCoy E., Sontheimer H. 2007 Expression and function of water channels (aquaprins) in migrating malignant astrocytes. Glia 55:1034.

Miller R.J., Rostene W., Apartis E., Banisadr G., Biber K., Milligan E.D., White F.A., Zhang J. 2008 Chemokine action in the nervous system. J. Neurosci. 28, 11792-11795. McCoy E., Sontheimer H. 2007 Expression and function of water channels (aquaprins) in migrating malignant astrocytes. Glia 55:1034.

Nitta T., Allegretta M., Okumura K., Sato K., Steinman L. 1992 Neoplastic and reactive human astrocytes express interleukin-8 gene. Neurosurg. Rev. 15, 203-207.

Ransohoff RM. 2009 Chemokines and chemokine receptors: standing at the crossroads of immunobiology and neurobiology. Immunity. Nov 20;31(5):711-21.

Ransohoff RM. 2009 Immunology: In the beginning. Nature. Nov 5;462(7269):41-2.

Rempel S.A., Dudas S., Ge S., Gutierrez J.A. 2000 Identification and localization of the cytochine SDF1 and its receptor, CXC chemokine receptor 4, to regions of necrosis and angiogenesis in human glioblastoma. Clin. Cancer Res. 6, 102-111.

Rodero M., Marie Y., Coudert M., Blondet E., Mokhtari K., Rousseau A., Raoul W., Carpentier C., Sennlaub F., Deterre P., Delattre J.Y., Debre P., Sanson M., Combadiere V., 2008. Polymorphism in the microglial cell-mobilizing CX3CR1 gene is associated with serviva in patients with glioblastomas. J. Clin. Oncol. 26, 5957-5964.

Rubin J.B., Kung A.L., Klein R.S., Chan J.A., Sun Y., Schmidt K., Kieran M.W., Luster A.D., Segal R.A., 2003 A small –molecule antagonist of CXCR4 inhibits intracranial growth of primary brain tumors. Proc. Natl. Acad. Sci. U.S.A. 100, 13513-13518.

Salmaggi A., Gelati M., Pollo B., Frigerio S., Eoli M., silavni A., Broggi G., Ciusani E., Croci D., Boiardi A., de Rossi M. 2004 CXCL12 in malignant glial tumors: a possible role in angiogenesis and cross-talk between endothelial and tumoral cells. J. Neurooncol. 67, 305-317.

Sciumè G., Soriani A., Piccoli M., Frati L., Santoni A., Bernardini G. 2010 CX3CR1/CXCL1 axis negatively controls glioma cell invasion and is modulated by transforming growth factor-beta 1. Neuro-Oncology. Doi:10,1093/neuonc/nop076.

Sciumè G., Santoni A., Bernardini G. 2011 Chemokines and glioma: invasion and more. J. Neuroimmunol. 224 8-12.

Trettel F, Di Angelantonio S, Limatola C, Ransohoff RM. Chemokines and chemokine receptors in the nervous system. Rome, 24/25 October, 2009, 2nd workshop. J Neuroimmunol. 2010 Jul 27;224(1-2):1-7.

Vaquero J., Coca S., Oya S., Martinez R., Ramiro J., Salazar F.G. 1989 Presence and significance of NK cells in glioblastomas. J. Neurosurg. 70, 728-731.

Zagzag D., Esencay M., Mendez O., Yee H., Smirnova I., Huang Y., Chiriboga L., Lukyanov E., Liu M., Newcomb E.W., 2008 Hypoxia- and vascular endothelial growth factor-induced stromal cell-derived factor-1 alpha/CXCR4 expression in glioblastomas: one plausible explanation of Scherer's structures Am. J. Pathol. 173, 545-560.

Zhang J., Sarkar S., Yong V.W. 2005 The chemokine stromal cell derived factor-1 (CXCL12) promotes glioma invasiveness through MT"-matrix metalloproteinase. Carcinogenesis 26, 2069-2077.

Zhou Y., Larsen P.H. Hao C., Yong V.W. 2002 CXCR4 is a major chemokine receptor on glioma cells and mediates their survival. J. Biol. Chem. 227, 49481-49487.

Zlotnik A., Yoshie O., Nomiyama H. 2006 The chemokine and chemokine receptor superfamilies and their molecular evolution. Genome Biol. 7, 243.

15

Biomarkers of Glioma

Shufang Liang and Guobo Shen
State Key Laboratory of Biotherapy and Cancer Center, West China Hospital,
West China Medical School, Sichuan University
P.R. China

1. Introduction

According to the analysis of American Brain Tumor Association, the brain tumors are common with an incidence of 12.8 per 100,000 people. Glioma is the most common subgroup of brain tumors. It is a type of tumor that origins in the brain or spine. It is called a "glioma" because it arises from glial cells. According to the specific type of cells from which they originate, gliomas are categorized as glioblastoma (WHO grade IV), astrocytoma (WHO grades I–III), oligodendro -glioma (WHO grades II and III), and mixed glioma (WHO grades II and III) (McCarthy et al, 2011). It is reported that about 50% gliomas are glioblastomas, which are the most common and malignant phenotypic astrocytoma. They are most common in adults from ages 45-55, and affect more men than women. About 9% of brain tumors in childhood are glioblastomas.

Gliomas are difficult to treat. Usually the prognosis for patients with high-grade gliomas (especially for glioblastomas) is very poor, which has a mean survival only from 10 to 12 months (Reddy, et al, 2008). It is found that about 10,000 Americans are diagnosed annually with malignant gliomas, about half of these patients are survival 1 year after diagnosis, and 25% after two years. The traditional approach to treat the glioma contains surgery, radidtion therapy and chemotherapy. Although with these treatments or combined approaches, the tumor will be suppressed at some means, the survival rate of the patients is still very low.

Biomarker is a characteristic that is objectively measured as an indicator of normal biological processes, pathogenic processes or a pharmacological response to a therapeutic intervention (Atkinson et al., 2001; Marrer & Dieterle, 2007). And tumor/cancer biomarkers are involved in tumors which contain a wide variety of objects, including DNA, mRNA, secreted proteins, cell surface receptors, transcription factors, and metabolites, or processes such as apoptosis, angiogenesis or proliferation. The markers are produced either by the tumor itself or by other tissues or cells, in response to the presence of tumors or other associated irritation, like inflammation (Kulasingam & Diamandis, 2008). They can be found in the tumor tissues, tumor cell lines, secreted molecules and in the serum or other body fluid, and so on. The tumor/cancer biomarkers can help doctors to profile the cancer predisposition, state of cancerous development, early diagnosis, prognosis after tretment, and decide which drugs and at what does it might be most effective to the patients with tumors. They are also benefit to screen the targeted drug for the tumor treatment.

Recent years, the tumor/cancer biomarkers have played important roles in the diagnosis, therapy and prognosis in tumors. For example, prostate-specific antigen (PSA), as a best-known cancer biomarker, is widely used to screen and diagnosis the prostate cancer (Barry, 2001). In the United States (US), most prostate cancers are diagnosed through measurement of serum PSA. The serum PSA level correlates directly with prostate cancer risk and aggressiveness, as well as the outcomes after treatment. PSA testing is also useful in monitoring patients for tumor recurrence after treatment (Loeb & Catalona, 2007). The *HER2/neu* gene or protein has been found over-expression in 10% to 34% of breast cancers. It has been used as a diagnostic biomarker and also a treatment target in breast cancer. The clinical trial presented that systemic administration of anti-HER2 antibodies trastuzumab (Herceptin), alone and in combination with chemotherapy in patients with HER-2/*neu* overexpressing primary tumors, can increase the time to recurrence and overall response rates in metastatic breast cancer (Ross & Fletcher, 1998).

Gliomas are difficult to remove due to several reasons. Firstly, some drugs can not get into gliomas directly because of the blood-brain barrier. Secondly, the gliomas can infiltrate the tissues around them, the traditional approaches, including surgery, radidtion therapy and chemo-therapy, can not get rid of them completely. Finally, gliomas may have more than one kind of tumor cells in them, so chemotherapy drug, which is only directed at one kind of tumor cells, can not kill the all tumor cells. Therefore, the investigations of glioma biomarkers for diagnosis, prognosis and therapy are an urgent mission for the scientist in future.

2. The research progress of glioma biomarkers

As far as we known, glioma biomarkers can be identified from the serum, cerebrospinal fluid, glioma cell lines or directly from glioma tissues. These biomarkers will help us to diagnose the gliomas in the earlier period, treat the glioma against the specific target and monitor the prognosis after treatment.

2.1 Diagnostic biomarkers for glioma

Currently, the examinations used in clinical diagnosis for glioma include computed tomography (CT) scan, magnetic resonance imaging (MRI) scan, angiogram, skull x-ray, spinal tap, myelogram and biopsy. But it is still difficult to diagnose in the earlier period of gliomas, until if we can find some specific biomarkers associated with the eraly development of gliomas, the diagnosis will be easy to decide. Diagnostic (or screening) biomarkers are used to detect and identify a given type of cancer in an individual. These markers are expected to have high specificity and sensitivity (Kulasingam & Diamandis, 2008).

(1) YKL-40

YKL-40, also known as CHI3L1 or human cartilage glycoprotein-39, is a secreted glycoprotein. High levels of YKL-40 in serum have been implicated as a serum marker in a number of cancers including breast (Johansen et al, 1995; Jensen et al, 2003), colorectal (Cintin et al, 1999), and ovarian cancer (Dehn et al, 2003; Hogdall et al, 2003). Although the function of YKL-40 is not well elucidated, it is often over-expressed in epithelial cancers and gliomas. Previous studies suggested that YKL-40 was a marker associated with a poorer clinical outcome and a genetically defined histological subgroup of high-grade gliomas (Nutt et al, 2005).TheYKL-40 was also implicated as an important marker of radiation therapeutic response and overall survival in glioblastoma (Pelloski et al, 2005).

Later, Hormigo et al. found that except for YKL-40, matrix metalloproteinase-9 (MMP-9) protein was also highly differentially expressed in malignant gliomas (Hormigo et al, 2006). YKL-40 and MMP-9 were determined by ELISA using serum samples from patients with gliomas, and the results indicated that the values correlated with the patient's radiographic status and survival. So , YKL-40 and MMP-9 may be used as a biomarker in glioma patients' serum and help confirm the absence of active disease in glioblastoma multiforme.

(2) GFAP

Another protein, glial fibrillary acidic protein (GFAP), first reported by Eng et al. in 1971, is a member of the cytoskeletal protein family and is widely detected in astroglial cells and neural stem cells (Eng et al, 1971, 2000; Doetsch, 2003; Jung et al, 2007). It is also expressed in astrocytoma and glioblastoma multiforme (Jacque et al, 1978; Hamaya et al, 1985; Abaza et al, 1998). A serum marker for malignant gliomas may improve both differential diagnoses with different histological subtypes and clinical management of glioma tumor patients. Jung et al. investigated GFAP levels in the serum of glioblastoma multiforme patients and various control groups. Their studies showed that the serum GFAP levels of these patients were significantly higher than those of patients with WHO grade II or III astrocytomas or of patients with brain metastases. And the serum GFAP concentration was closely linked with the glioblastoma volume and tumor necrosis volume imaged from magnetic resonance imaging scans. Therefore, the serum GFAP may be used as a diagnostic biomarker for glioblastoma multiforme. But it is necessary to evaluate whether the serum GFAP could be used to monitor therapeutic effects or have a prognostic value in future studies (Jung et al, 2007). Furthermore, it is reported that GFAP does not provide a better staining for distinguishing histologic subtypes of high-grade glioma by immunohistochemistry. Compared with GFAP, YKL-40 staining, is a stronger marker, provided a better class distinction. In addition, using a combination of YKL-40 and GFAP staining could afford even greater diagnostic accuracy (Nutt et al, 2005).

(3) Other potential biomarkers

Cerebrospinal fluid (CSF) was usually used to screen glioma biomarkers because of its closer relation with glioma and its relative ease of collection (Maurer et al, 2003). Furthermore, CSF has about 1000 proteins, which is 100~400 fold lower than in serum, and this will be facilitated to screen the specific protein biomarkers (Omenn, 2005). In the past decades, many markers have been found in CSF of glioma patients, such as S100, neuron-specific enolase (NSE), recoverin (protein A) and vascular endothelial growth factor (VEGF) (Gronowitz et al, 1984; Cochran & Wen, 1985; Taomoto et al., 1987; Sampath et al., 2004; Khwaja et al, 2007). However, these biomarkers could not be widespread used due to the limitation of repetition in CSF examinations.

Recently, new candidate biomarkers have been identified by proteomics analysis for CSF samples. For example, Khwaja et al. used two-dimensional gel electrophoresis (2-DE) and cleavable Isotope-Coded Affinity Tag (cICAT) to analyze CSF proteome to detect specific biomarkers in brain tumors with differing histologies and grades (Khwaja et al, 2007). Finally, 20 potential tumor-specific markers were specially identified in high-grade astrocytoma. These potential markers may also play important role in the development and malignant progression of human astrocytoma and will be the treatment targets in glioma.

Furthermore, exosome is now becoming a hot spot to look for cancer biomarkers. Exosomes are 50-90 nm vesicles-like objects secreted by various mammalian cells. An exosome is formed intracellularly when a segment of cell membrane spontaneously invaginates and is endocytosed (Keller et al, 2006). It is reported that dendritic cells and B cells could secrete exosomes, which indicated that exosomes may play a functional role in mediating adaptive immune responses to pathogens and tumors (Li et al, 2006). Exosomes can also be detected in urine and they might serve as a diagnosis and treatment response marker in prostate cancer (Pisitkun et al, 2004; Nilsson et al, 2009). Therefore, exosomes, which are released from tumors into the blood, can also be used for diagnosis. The released exosomes by glioblastoma tumor cells contain mRNA, microRNA and angiogenic proteins (Balaj et al, 2011). Furthermore, the glioblastoma-derived exosomes serve as a vehicle to deliver genetic information and proteins in the tumor environment. Tumor mutations in glioma can be detected in exosomes from serum, which is also facilitating a blood-based biomarker detection for solid tumors (Skog et al, 2008). Thus, tumor-derived exosomes may be used as a diagnostic biomarker and aid in therapeutic decisions for glioma patients.

Although the histopathologic methods are often used to classify the pathologic grade of gliomas in clinical diagnosis, the results are usually subjective and less accurate. To overcome the limitations, cDNA microarray has been performed to screen diagnostic and prognostic markers for glioblastoma. The growth arrest and DNA-damage-inducible α (GADD45α) and follistatin-like 1 (FSTL1) were over-expressed in most primary and secondary glioblastomas, whereas superoxide dismutase 2 and adipocyte enhancer binding protein 1 were up-regulated in the majority of primary glioblastomas (Reddy et al, 2008). All the results were validated by real-time reverse transcription quantitative PCR and immunohistochemical analysis. These findings suggested that GADD45α and FSTLI are glioblastoma-specific whereas superoxide dismutase 2 and adipocyte enhancer binding protein1 are primary glioblastoma-specific diagnostic markers. It is interesting to found that the diffusion parameters could also be evaluated as early biomarkers of disease progression in glioblastoma multiforme (Khayal et al, 2010).

2.2 Prognostic biomarkers for glioma

Tumor prognostic biomarkers are used once the tumor status has been confirmed. These biomarkers are expected to predict the probable course of the tumors including its recurrence, and they therefore have important influences on the aggressiveness of therapy (Kulasingam & Diamandis, 2008).

It is known that O(6)-methylguanine-DNA methyltransferase (MGMT) can recover the carcinogenic lesion in DNA induced by alkylating mutagens. What's more, it has been showed that methylation of the MGMT's promoter plays a significant role in carcinogenesis (Hegi et al, 2005). The hypermethylation in MGMT promoter has been detected in other various of human cancers, such as colon cancer, nonsmall-cell lung cancer, head and neck carcinoma, lymphomas, Leukemias, pancreatic carcinoma , melanoma, renal carcinoma and bladder carcinoma (Esteller et al, 1999). The hypermethylation frequency of MGMT promoter varies widely in different subtype glioma. It has ranged from 35% to 73% in glioblastoma, about 50%~84% in diffusely infiltrating anaplastic gliomas (World Health Organization grade III), as well as about 43%~93% in the WHO grade II counterparts (Deimling et al, 2011). Although the methylation of MGMT status appears to be a useful prognostic marker in the elderly patients with newly diagnosed glioblastoma (Gerstner et al, 2009). In fact, MGMT immunohistochemistry analysis had some lacks for routine diagnostic purposes due to the observer variability as well as lack of association with the MGMT promoter methylation status (Preusser et al, 2008).

As is known to all, the ras GTPase-activating-like protein IQGAP1 functions as a scaffold protein which is involved in cellular motility and morphogenesis (Mateer et al, 2003). It is participated in many signaling pathways to regulate cell adhesion, polarization and migration. For example, IQGAP1 was played as a VEGFR2-associated scaffold protein to organize ROS-dependent VEGF signaling, which could promote the migration and proliferation of endothelial cell to repair the injured vessels (Yamaoka-Tojo et al, 2004). It is also identified as a core component of neuronal motility signal transduction and it is involved in epithelial carcinogenesis and metastasis (Briggs & Sacks, 2003; Kholmanskikh et al, 2006; Balenci et al, 2006). But, one recent study found that IQGAP1 may be used as a marker to discriminate the human glioblastoma from oligodendroglioma (Balenci et al, 2006)

Another known protein, the insulin-like growth factor-binding protein 2 (IGFBP2) is usually detected in many human tumors, including malignancies of the lung, colon, adrenal glands, ovary, prostate, CNS and lymphoid tumors (Dunlap et al, 2007). Its overexpression is often linked with an increasingly malignant status of the tumor, indicating a potential oncogene function of IGFBP-2 in tumorigenesis (Hoeflich et al, 2001). IGFBP2 was also identified as a specific marker for central nervous system (CNS) tumors and might serve as a marker of tumor differentiation (Muller et al, 1994; Akmal et al, 1995). Furthermore, the plasma IGFBP2 levels are obviously higher in high-grade glioma patients than in low-grade glioma patients and healthy subjects. All these data indicate the plasma IGFBP2 has a biomarker's role in glioma (Lin et al, 2009).

The coexpression of IQGAP1 and IGFBP2 is strongly associated with poor prognosis in astrocytoma and oligodendroglioma. These findings might complement the WHO classification system to permit more precise classification for glioma subtypes. Besides, in glioblastoma patients who had shown long-term survival of >3 years after initial diagnosis, the expression of IQGAP1 and IGFBP2 were not be detected. Thus, the absence of IQGAP1 and IGFBP2 may be a good prognostic marker in glioblastoma patients. However, the relationship between IQGAP1 and IGFBP2 and their roles in glioma biology are still need to be elucidated in future (McDonald et al, 2007).

Matrix-assisted laser desorption ionization- mass spectrometry (MALDI-MS) is a high-throughput and accurate tool in proteomics research. It has been used to profile the glioma-specific protein patterns which can provide clinically relevant information on tumor malignancy. The glioma-specific protein patterns could accurately classify glioma subtypes and discriminate patient survival patterns. Still, there are several discriminatory proteins were identified, including calcyclin, dynein light chain 2 (DLD2), calpactin I light chain, astrocytic phosphoprotein (PEA-15), fatty acid-binding protein 5 (FABP5) and tubulin - specific chaperone A. These proteins were reported to be involved in various aspects of tumorigenesis. These differential expression proteins in gliomas may provide as diagnostic and prognostic markers (Schwartz et al, 2005).

Tumor is a disease coupled with multiple gene alterations. The gene expression pattern may predict the survival time in patients with high-grade gliomas independently of other factors (Czernicki et al, 2007). Proteins are the true executors that directly perform functions regulated by genes. Therefore, the protein changes would be more attractive in cancer biomarker discovery (Liang et al, 2011). Khalil used the two-dimensional difference gel electrophoresis (2D-DIGE) compared protein patterns between glioma tissues and non-tumor brain tissues. About 20 unique differential proteins were identified, and these proteins with diagnostic or prognostic value are still needed to be validated in future

research (Khalil, 2007). In addition, the gelsolin protein is significantly lower expressed in the increscent glioma histopathologic grade. And in astrocytoma, the overall survival in the low-expression group was significantly poorer than in the high expression group. Therefore, gelsolin may be a prognostic marker for astrocytoma patients (Ohnishi et al, 2009). Besides, the B-chain of α_2 -heremans-schmid glycoprotein in serum can be used as a potential biomarker for glioma prognosis (Petrik et al, 2008).
DNA microarray is usually used to measure gene expression levels, single nucleotide polymorphisms or genotype. It is one of the fastest-growing new technologies in cancer research. By DNA microarray, it was found that metalloproteinase-4 (TIMP-4) and its putative partner CD63 were coexpressed in glioblastomas and pilocytic astrocytomas. High TIMP-4 /CD63 co-expression level has been found to be an independent prognostic marker associated with progression and shorter survival in glioblastomas. On the contrary,the higher co-expression indicted adverse outcomes in diffuse astrocytoma and oligoastrocytoma patients (Rorive et al, 2010). Similarly, a high level of osteopontin protein in serum indicates a poor prognosis in glioblastoma patients, and it may be a poor prognostic biomarker in glioblastoma patients (Sreekanthreddy et al, 2010).
Gene mutation is another factor in carcinogenesis. Recently, the isocitrate dehydrogenase 1 (IDH1) was analyzed by direct sequencing in a series of 404 glioma patients with different grade. It is found that the mutation rates in the codon 132 of IDH1 were obviously decreased with increscent glioma grade, which indicated that the codon 132 mutations of IDH1 could be an important prognostic marker in grade 2 to 4 gliomas (Sanson et al, 2009). The codon 132 mutation of IDH1was detected in more than 70% of WHO grade II - III astrocytomas , oligodendrogliomas, as well as in glioblastomas which are developed from those lower-grade gliomas. Gliomas, without mutations in IDH1 codon 132, often had mutations in codon 172 of the IDH2 gene. The results showed that patients with such mutations in IDH usually had a better prognosis than those with wild-type IDH genes (Yan et al, 2009).

2.3 Therapeutic targets for glioma

Recent developments in the field of tumor biology have elucidated signalling pathways and genes involved in the development of gliomas, which represent new potential therapeutic targets, and many targeted therapies are currently being tested in clinical trials (Sanson, 2008).

(1) Receptor tyrosine kinases (RTKs)-mediated signaling

The antiangiogenesis strategy has been widely used in molecularly targeted therapy for malignant glioma. Angiogenesis in tumors is caused by a number of factors involved in many signaling pathways, in which the VEGF-VEGFR2 is a major and more attractive pathway. Currently, many angiogenesis inhibitors or antibodies have been applied in clinical studies. These inhibitors or antibodies were usually design to anti-specific factors, including VEGF itself, VEGFR, and other upstream /downstream factors regulated the VEGF signaling pathway, such as Cox-2, HIF-1α, and so on(Chi et al, 2009).
Gliomas are highly heterogeneous in terms of biological alterations. Mutations in *EGFR* and genes for other receptor tyrosine kinases (RTKs), namely platelet-derived growth factor (*PDGFR*), *HER2/neu* and *MET*, lead to activation of downstream PI3K-AKT and ERK-MEK pathways in gliomas. Therefore, several antiangiogenic inhibitors, which downregulate EGFR-mediated signaling, have recently been developed and tested as therapeutic agents, including cediranib (Recentin, AstraZeneca), vatalanib (Novartis Pharmaceuticals, Basel,

Switzerland), sunitinib (Sutent, Pfizer), sorafenib (Nexavar, Bayer Pharmaceuticals, Leverkusen, Germany), vandetanib (Zactima, AstraZeneca) and VEGF trap (Aflibercept, Regeneron Pharmaceuticals, NY,USA) (Lukas et al,2009; *Roesler* et al, 2010). Besides small-molecule inhibitors, therapies can be targeted to tumor cells (e.g., EGFR inhibitors) or tumor blood vessels with the monoclonal antibody against VEGF, bevacizumab (Avastin; Genentech, CA, USA).

However, followed by the antiangiogenesis therapy at long time, the patients will have a high resistance to anti-VEGF therapies. Soda et al. investigated the resistance mechanism of anti-VEGF therapy to glioma in the transduction of p53+/− heterozygous mice containing oncogenes and in the GFAP-Cre recombinase (Cre) mice. It was found that mouse glioblastoma cells could be transdifferented into vascular endothelial cells (tumor -derived endothelial cells, TDECs) in the hypoxia situation, and this process was independent of VEGF. A further study has showed that the formation of TDECs are also presented in the xenograft model of human glioblastoma spheres directly from the patients with glioblastoma (Sodaa et al, 2011). These studies show that the TDECs may have an important role in the resistance to anti-VEGF therapy, and hence they could be a candidate target for glioblastoma therapy. But there are still many questions need to be answered. For example, what are the signaling molecules that participate in the production of TDECs? Is this mechanism of VEGF-A resistance uniform to all glioblastoma or are there alternate pathways used for different subsets of glioblastoma? (Sodaa et al, 2011; Hormigo et al, 2011).

(2) PI3K/AKT/mTOR pathways

PI3K pathways regulate several malignant phenotypes including antiapoptosis, cell growth, and proliferation. Activation of PI3K pathway is associated with poor prognosis in glioma patients (Sathornsumetee et al, 2007). Activated PI3K phosphorylates several downstream effectors including AKT. AKT is a serine/threonine kinase that regulates cell growth, proliferation, and apoptosis. The mTOR is a serine/threonine kinase downstream from AKT.

Several mTOR inhibitors have been studied in the treatment of malignant glioma. These include sirolimus (Rapamune; Wyeth Pharmaceuticals,Madison, NJ) FDA-approved for the prophylaxis of solid organ transplant rejection, and temsirolimus (CCI-779, Torisel; Wyeth Pharmaceuticals) FDA-approved for use in renal cancer (Lukas et al, 2009). And everolimus (RAD001; Novartis Oncology, East Hanover, NJ) and deferolimus (AP23573; ARIAD/Merck), still experimental, have all been evaluated in clinical trials alone or in combination with other therapies in gliomas. Although data strongly support the view of the PI3K-AKT-mTOR pathway as an important target, current clinical results on the use of mTOR inhibitors remain disappointing. For example, the Phase II studies using temsirolimus as monotherapy found only limited activity in recurrent glioblastoma multiforme. Because pathways are complex interactive networks characterized by cross-talk and homeostatic feedback loops that can greatly influence response to therapy.

(3) Histone deacetlyase (HDAC)

Histone deacetylases (HDACs), regulating histone acetylation, are now considered to be a promising target for gliomas. The epigenetic therapies, particularly HDAC inhibitors (HDACis), have been proposed as potential novel drugs. Suberoylanilide hydroxamic acid (SAHA, vorinostat, Zolinza; Merck), FDA-approved for cutaneous T-celllymphoma, is being evaluated in clinical trials of multiple cancers, including malignant gliomas (Sathornsumetee *et al, 2007; Roesler* et al, 2010).

(4) Other targets and therapeutic approaches

Advances in the understanding of cellular and molecular alterations in gliomas have led to the emergence of experimental molecularly targeted therapies. The targeted therapies for glioma include small molecules and antibodies targeted at growth factor pathways, intracellular signaling cascades and epigenetic molecular targets, as well as RNAi, gene therapy and neural stem cells as therapeutic tools (*Roesler* et al, 2010).
The receptor protein tyrosine phosphatase β (RPTPβ) have a role to facilitate tumor cell adhesion and migration by interactions with extracellular matrix components and the growth factor pleiotrophin. Over-expression of RPTPβ was found in several types of solid tumor, but with low expression in normal tissue (Foehr et al, 2006). It is reported that RPTPβ was displayed strong staining in oligodendrogliomas, and may be a novel oligodendroglioma marker (Hägerstrand et al, 2008). Therefore, RPTPβ may perform a role of potential therapy target in gliomas and other tumors. The monoclonal antibodies of RPTPβ obtained from immunizing mice could kill glioma cells in vitro and significantly suppress the growth of human glioma tumors in a xenograft mouse model (Foehr et al, 2006).
The PBEF1 (Pre-B-cell colony enhancing factor 1) gene may be a potential malignant astrocytoma serum marker and prognostic indicator in glioblastoma (Reddy et al, 2008). PBEF1 gene encodes nicotinamide phosphoribosyltransferase (NMPRTase), which has an important role in the salvage pathway of NAD^+ biosynthesis. The inhibitor of NMPRTase, such as FK866, can reduce cellular NAD^+ levels and induce apoptosis in tumors (Khan et al, 2006). Therefore, the novel inhibitor of NMPRTase may be used as an anti-tumor drug in glioma therapy (Chandra et al, 2011).
However, targeting a single component of cell signaling, or a single signaling pathway, is not likely to effectively reduce tumor growth in glioma patients. Preclinical studies should characterize the effects of multi-targeted inhibitors, combining several targeted inhibitors, and combining targeted therapies with cytotoxic chemotherapy.
Tumor stem cells are a kind of specific tumor cells which have the stem cell like properties. It is reported that glioma stem cells display self-renewal and proliferation properties, unlimited life span, a high migration rate and resistance to chemotherapy, and they are capable of replenishing the whole tumor cell population (Singh et al, 2003; 2004). The glioma stem cells have been involved in many signaling pathways, including Notch, Hedgehog, Wnt, Myc, PI3K and MAPK cascades, and so on (Das et al, 2008; Li et al, 2009; Roesler et al, 2010). According to the important roles of glioma stem cells, the drugs that directly and specifically kill the glioma stem cells will be more effective than other ways in glioma therapy. Some studies have proposed the possible strategies to target the glioma stem cells. One way is using differentiating agents (like bone morphogenetic proteins, BMPs)to induce the glioma stem cells into mature, astrocytic cells, and another way is regulating the expression of targeting genes involved in glioma stem cell proliferation (Piccirillo et al, 2006; Horvath et al, 2006).

3. Discussion and outlook

It is clear that more and more high-throughput, accurate technologies or strategies have been used in identification of glioma biomarkers (shown in Figure 1). These techniques include ELISA (Hormigo et al, 2006; Lin et al, 2009; Sreekanthreddy et al, 2010), 2-DE (Khwaja et al, 2007; Khalil, 2007; Ohnishi et al, 2009), DNA microarray (Reddy et al, 2008),

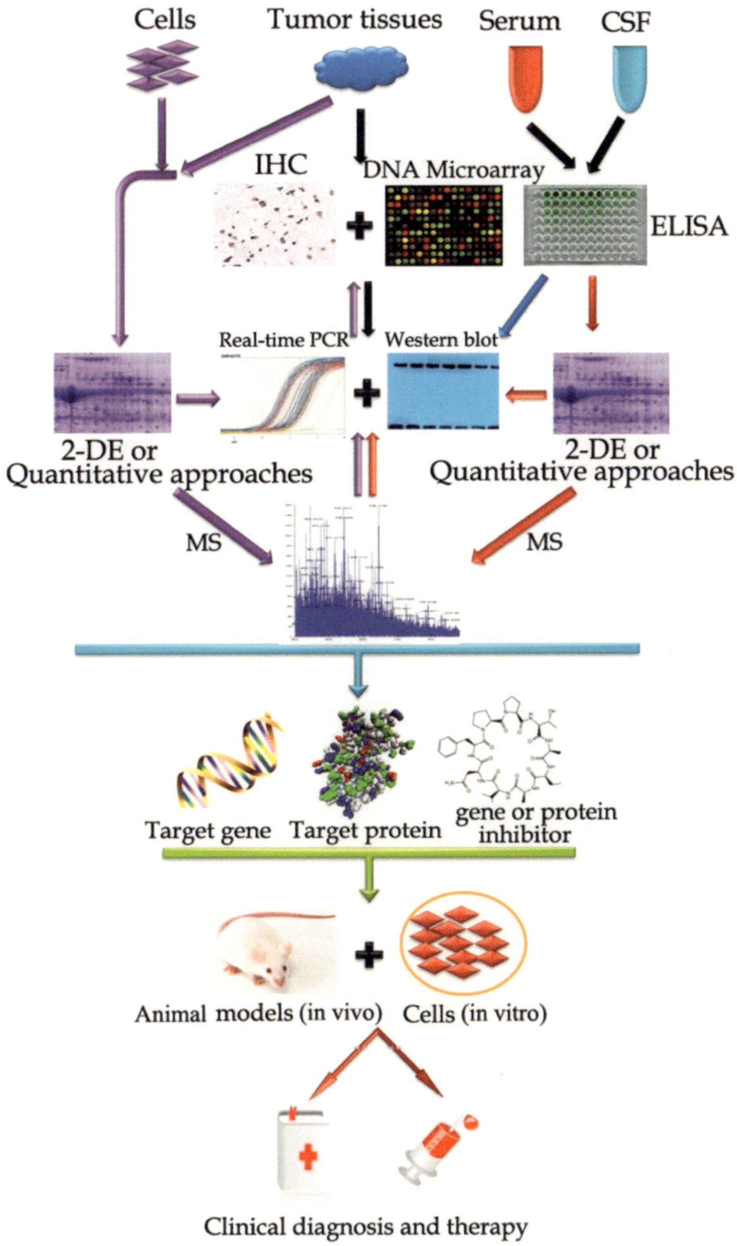

Fig. 1. Current different techniques are used in the glioma biomarker discovery.
a. CSF: Cerebrospinal fluid; IHC: immunohistochemistry; ELISA: enzyme linked immunosorbent assay; 2-DE: two-dimensional electrophoresis; MS: mass spectrometry.
b. The quantitative approaches here contain the isotope-coded affinity tag (ICAT), stable isotope labeling with amino acids in cell culture (SILAC), isobaric tagging for relative and absolute quantitation (iTRAQ).

MALDI-MS or SELDI-TOF -MS (Petrik et al, 2008; Schwartz et al, 2005),direct sequencing (Sanson et al, 2009), ICAT (Khwaja et al, 2007), and transgenic mouse etc (Sodaa et al, 2011). A number of quantitative approaches summarized in Figure 1, with different technical advantages and challenges, have been developed for glioma biomarker discovery. However, many complementary technologies are being developed and either alone or in combination will undoubtedly allow their potential in biomedical research and translation into clinical practice.

Recently, we have investigated the protein prfiling in low-grade gliomas by a quantative SILAC (stable isotope labeling with amino acids in cell culture) –based protemoics strategy in order to screen novel glioma-specific proteins (Liang et al, 2009a; Shen et al, 2010). Besides, the quantative protemoics strategy also contains the isotope-coded affinity tag (ICAT), isobaric tagging for relative and absolute quantitation (iTRAQ), and so on. With these high-throughput and sensitive approaches, more specific glioma biomarkers will be identified (Liang et al, 2009b).

In conclusion, the glioma biomarkers primarily can be classed into three kinds, including diagnostic biomarkers, prognostic markers and therapeutic targets. In fact, only few biomarkers could be used in clinical applications, such as o (6)-methylguanine-DNA methyltransferase (MGMT) (Gerstner et al, 2009; Deimling et al, 2011), VEGF and VEGFR (Chi et al, 2009), and so on (shown in Table 1). The other potential biomarkers for glioma are

Target gene/protein	Clinical Application	Phase	Drug
MGMT (Methylguanine methyl transferase)	diagnosis and prognosis	---	---
EGFR (Epidermal growth factor receptor)	therapy	Phase II	MAb-425
		---	Erlotinib
		Phase III	Nimotuzimab
		Phase I/II	Gefitinib
		Phase I/II	Cetuximab
VEGF (Vascular endothelial growth factor)	therapy	Phase II	Bevacizumab / Irinotecan
VEGFR (Vascular endothelial growth factor receptor)	therapy	Phase I/II	Vatalanib
PDGFR (Platelet-derived growth factor receptor)	therapy	Phase II	Crenolanib (CP-868,596)
		Phase II	Nilotinib
		Phase I/II	Imatinib
mTOR (mammalian target of rapamycin)	therapy	Phase III	Everolimus
		Phase II	Temsirolimus
		Phase I	Sirolimus+Gefitinib
HDAC (histone deacetlyase)	therapy	Phase I/II	SAHA
COX-2 (cyclooxegenase-2)	therapy	Phase I/II	Celecoxib

Table 1. Glioma biomarkers in clinical applications

Target gene/ protein (or other object)	Candidate Applications	Localization (a)	References
YKL-40	Diagnosis & prognosis	Serum or tumor tissues	Nutt et al, 2005; Hormigo et al, 2006
MMP-9	Diagnosis & prognosis	Serum	Hormigo et al, 2006
GFAP	Diagnosis & prognosis	Serum or tumor tissues	Nutt et al, 2005; Jung et al, 2007
Exosomes	Diagnosis	Serum or tumor tissues	Skog et al, 2008; Balaj et al, 2011
GADD45α and FSTL1	Diagnosis	Tumor tissues	Reddy et al, 2008
Diffusion parameters	Diagnosis	Tumor tissues	Khayal et al, 2010
MGMT	Diagnosis & prognosis	Tumor tissues	Gerstner et al, 2009
IQGAP1	Diagnosis & prognosis	Tumor tissues	Balenci et al, 2006; McDonald et al, 2007
IGFBP2	Diagnosis & prognosis	Serum or tumor tissues	McDonald et al, 2007; Lin et al, 2009
***Calcyclin,*DLC2 , *CalpactinI light chain, *PEA-15, *FABP5, *Tubulin-specific chaperone A**	Diagnosis & prognosis	Tumor tissues	# Schwartz et al, 2005 (b)
AHSG	Prognosis	Serum	Petrik et al, 2008
Gelsolin	Prognosis	Tumor tissues	Ohnishi et al, 2009
IDH1/IDH2 mutation	Prognosis	Tumor tissues	Sanson et al, 2009, Yan et al, 2009
TIMP-4/CD63	Prognosis	Tumor tissues	Rorive et al, 2010
Osteopontin protein	Prognosis	Serum	Sreekanthreddy et al, 2010
FoxM1	Therapy	Tumor tissues	Liu et al, 2006
RPTPβ	Diagnosis & therapy	Tumor tissues	Foehr et al, 2006, Hägerstrand et al, 2008
PBEF1(NMPRTase)	Prognosis & therapy	Serum or tumor tissues	Reddy et al, 2008, Chandra et al, 201
Glioma stem cells	Therapy	Tumor tissues	Piccirillo et al, 2006; Horvath et al, 2006
TDECs (tumor -derived endothelial cells)	Therapy	Tumor tissues	Sodaa et al, 2011; Hormigo et al, 2011

a. The sample pool where the biomarkers were identified.
b. The biomarkers with * tag were identified in the same study with # tag.

Table 2. Some novel potential glioma biomarkers

promised to need a further validation and confirmation (shown in Table 2). There have some limitations for application of glioma biomarkers in the clinical trial. Firstly, the specification of biomarkers is always not certainly. Because of the biomarkers are usually detected in both normal and tumor samples, and other diseases can also cause the changes of biomarkers. And then, the investigation strategy of biomarkers are significantly various. Even if used the same type samples, the results will be remarkably difference. Finally, the patients with tumors are usually difference from each other, also called the individual difference. Besides, the overall samples used in biomarker identification are still limited due to various gaps. In spite of this, the studies of glioma biomarker identification still have a bright future by the continuous efforts of biologists.

4. Acknowledgments

This work was financially supported by the grants from National Key Basic Program of China (2011CB910703), National Natural Sciences Foundation of China (30970654, 31071235), Program for New Century Excellent Talents in University (NCET-10-0595) and Sichuan Science Research Program for Young Scholars (2010JQ0016).

5. References

Abaza, MS.; Shaban, F.; Narayan, R. & Atassi, M. (1998). Human glioma associated intermediate filament proteins: over-expression, co-localization and cross-reactivity. *Anticancer Res.*, Vol.18, pp.1333–1340.

Akmal, S., Yun, K., MacLay, J., Higami, Y., & Ikeda, T. (1995). Insulin-like growth factor 2 and insulin-like growth factor binding protein 2 expression in hepatoblastoma. *Hum. Pathol*, Vol.26, pp.846–851.

Atkinson, A.; Colburn, W.; DeGruttola,V.; DeMets, D.; Downing, G.; Hoth, D.; Oates, J.;Peck, C.; Schooley R.; Spilker B.; Woodcock, J. & Zeger, S. (2001). Biomarkers and surrogate endpoints: preferred definitions and conceptual framework. *Clin Pharmacol Ther*, Vol.69, pp.89-95.

Balaj, L.; Lessard, R.; Dai, L.; Cho,Y.; Pomeroy, S.; Breakefield, X. & Skog, Johan. (2011).Tumour microvesicles contain retrotransposon elements and amplified oncogene sequences. *Nature Communications*, Vol.2, doi:10.1038 /ncomms1180.

Balenci, L.; Clarke, I.; Dirks, P.; Assard, N.; Ducray, F.; Jouvet, A.; Belin, M.; Honnorat, J. & Baudier, J. (2006). IQGAP1 Protein Specifies Amplifying Cancer Cells in Glioblastoma Multiforme. *Cancer Res*, Vol.66, No.18, pp.9074-9082.

Barry, M. Clinical practice. (2001). Prostate-specific-antigen testing for early diagnosis of prostate cancer. *N. Engl. J. Med.*, Vol.344, No.18, pp.1373-1377.

Briggs, M. & Sacks, D. (2003). IQGAP proteins are integral components of cytoskeletal regulation. *EMBO Rep*, Vol.4, pp.571–574.

Chandra, N.; Bhagavat, R.; Sharma, E.; Sreekanthreddy, P. & Somasundaram, K. (2011). Virtual screening, identification and experimental testing of novel inhibitors of PBEF1/Visfatin/ NMPRTase for glioma therapy. Journal of Clinical Bioinformatics, Vol.1, pp.5

Chi, A.; Sorensen, A.; Jain, R. & Batchelor, T. (2009). Angiogenesis as a Therapeutic Target in Malignant Gliomas. The Oncologist 2009;14:621–636

Cintin, C.; Johansen, J.; Christensen, I.; Price, P.; Sorensen, S. & Nielsen, H. (1999). Serum YKL-40 and colorectal cancer. *Br J Cancer,* Vol.79, pp.1494–1499.

Czernicki, T.; Zegarska, J.; Paczek, L.; Cukrowska,B.; Grajkowska, W.; Zajaczkowska, A.; Brudzewski, K.; Ulaczyk, J. & Marchel, A. (2007). Gene expression profile as a prognostic factor in high-grade gliomas. *Int J Oncol,* Vol.30, pp. 55-64.Das, S.; Srikanth, M.; Kessler, J. (2008). Cancer stem cells and glioma. *Nat. Clin. Pract.Neurol.*, Vol. 4, No.8, pp.427-435.

Dehn, H.; Høgdall, E.; Johansen J.; Price, J.; Jørgensen, M.; Engelholm, S. & Høgdall, C. (2003). Plasma YKL-40, as a prognostic tumor marker in recurrent ovarian cancer. *Acta Obstet Gynecol Scand*, Vol.82, pp.287–293.

Doetsch, F. (2003).The glial identity of neural stem cells. *Nat Neurosci.,* Vol.6, pp.1127–1134.

Dunlap, S.; Celestino, J.; Wang, H.; Jiang, R. & Hollan, E. (2007).Insulin-like growth factor binding protein 2 promotes glioma development and progression. *PNAS,* 2007 vol. 104, no. 28, 11736–11741

Eng, L.; Vanderhaeghen, J.; Bignami, A. & Gerstl, B. (1971). An acidic protein isolatedfrom fibrous astrocytes. *Brain Res.*, Vol.28, pp.351–354.

Eng, L.; Ghirnikar, R. & Lee, Y. (2000). Glial fibrillary acidic protein: GFAP-thirty-one years (1969-2000). *Neurochem Res.*, Vol. 25, pp. 1439–1451.

Esteller, M.; Hamilton, S.; Burger, P.; Baylin, S. & Herman, J. (1999). Inactivation of the DNA repair gene O6-methylguanine-DNA methyltransferase by promoter hypermethylation is a common event in primary human neoplasia. *Cancer Res,* Vol.59, pp.793–797.

Foehr, E.; Lorente, G.; Kuo, J.; Ram, R.; Nikolich, K. & Urfer, R. (2006). Targeting of the Receptor Protein Tyrosine Phosphatase B with a Monoclonal Antibody Delays Tumor Growth in a Glioblastoma Model. *Cancer Res,* Vol.66, pp.2271-2278.

Gerstner, E.; Yip, S.; Wang, D.; Louis, D.; Iafrate, A. & Batchelor,T. (2009). MGMT methylation is a prognostic biomarker in elderly patients with newly diagnosed glioblastoma. *Neurology,* Vol.73, pp.1509-1510.

Hägerstrand, D.; Smits, A.; Eriksson, A.; Sigurdardottir, S.; Olofsson,T.; Hartman,M.; Nistér, M.; Kalimo, H. & Östman, A. (2008). Gene expression analyses of grade II gliomas and identification of rPTPβ/ζ as a candidate oligodendroglioma marker. *Neuro-Oncology,* Vol.10, pp. 2-9.

Hamaya, K.; Doi, K.; Tanaka, T. & Nishimoto, A. (1985).The determination of glial fibrillary acidic protein for the diagnosis and histogenetic study of central nervous system tumors: a study of 152 cases. *Acta Med Okayama,* Vol.39, pp. 453–462.

Hegi, M.; Diserens, A.; Gorlia, T, Hamou, M.; de Tribolet, N.; Weller, M.; Kros, J.; Hainfellner, J.; Mason, W.; Mariani, L.; Bromberg, J.; Hau, P.; Mirimanoff, R.; Cairncross, J.; Janzer,R. & Stupp R. (2005). MGMT gene silencing and benefit from temozolomide in glioblastoma. *N. Engl. J. Med.,* Vol.352, No.10, pp.997–1003.

Hoeflich, A.; Reisinger, R.; Lahm, H.; Kiess, W.; Blum, W.; Kolb, H.; Weber, M. & Wolf, E. (2001). Insulin-like growth factor-binding protein 2 in tumorigenesis : protector or promoter? *Cancer Res,* Vol.61, pp.8601-8610.

Hogdall, E.; Johansen, J.; Kjaer, S.; Price, P.; Christensen, L.; Blaakaer, J.; Bock, J.; Glud, E. & Hogdall, C. (2003). High plasmaYKL-40 level in patients with ovarian cancer stage III is related to shorter survival. *Oncol. Rep.*, Vol.10, pp.1535-1538.

Hormigo, A.; Gu, B.; Karimi, S.; Riedel, E.; Panageas, K.; Edgar, M.; Tanwar, M.; Rao, J.; Fleisher, M.; DeAngelis, L. & Holland, E. (2006). YKL-40 and Matrix Metalloproteinase-9 as potential serum biomarkers for patients with high-grade gliomas. *Clin Cancer Res*, Vol.12, No.19, pp.5698-5704.

Hormigo, A.; Ding, B. & Rafiia, S. (2011). A target for antiangiogenic therapy: vascular endothelium derived from glioblastoma. *PNAS*, Vol. 108, No. 11,pp. 4271–4272.

Horvath, S.; Zhang, B.; Carlson, M.; Lud, K.; Zhu, S.; Felciano, R.; Laurance, M.; Zhao, W.; Qi, S.; Chen, Z.; Lee, Y.; Scheck, A.; Liau, L.; Wu, H.; Geschwind, D.; Febbo, P.; Kornblum, H.; Cloughesy, T.; Nelsona, S.; Mischel, P. (2006). Analysis of oncogenic signaling networks in glioblastoma identifies ASPM as a molecular target. *PNAS*, Vol.103, pp.17402-17407.

Jacque, C.; Vinner, C.; Kujas, M.; Raoul, M.; Racadot, J. & Baumann, N. (1978). Determination of glial fibrillary acidic protein (GFAP) in human brain tumors. *J Neurol Sci.*, Vol.35, pp.147–155.

Jensen, B.; Johansen, J. & Price, P. (2003). High levels of serum HER-2/neu and YKL-40 independently reflect aggressiveness of metastatic breast cancer. *Clin Cancer Res*, Vol.9, pp.4423-4434.

Johansen, J.; Cintin C.; Jorgensen, M.; Kamby, C. & Price, P. (1995). Serum YKL-40: a new potential marker of prognosis and location of metastases of patients with recurrent breast cancer. *Eur J Cancer*, Vol.31, pp.1437- 1442.

Jung, C.; Foerch, C.; Schänzer, A.; Heck, A.; Plate, K.; Seifert, V.; Steinmetz, H.; Raabe, A. &Sitzer, M. (2007). Serum GFAP is a diagnostic marker for glioblastoma multiforme. *Brain*, Vol.130, pp.3336-3341.

Keller, S.; Sanderson, M.; Stoeck, A. & Altevogt, P. (2006). Exosomes: from biogenesis and secretion to biological function. *Immunol. Lett.*, Vol.107, No.2, pp.102–108.

Khalil, A. (2007). Biomarker discovery: a proteomic approach for brain cancer profiling. *Cancer Sci*, Vol.98, pp.201-213.

Khan, J.; Tao, X. & Tong, L. (2006). Molecular basis for the inhibition of human NMPRTase, a novel target for anticancer agents. *Nature Struct. Mol. Biol.*, Vol.13,pp. 582-588.

Khayal, I.; Polley, M.; Jalbert, L.; Elkhaled, A.; Chang, S.; Cha, S.; Butowski, N. & Nelson S. (2010). Evaluation of diffusion parameters as early biomarkers of disease progression in glioblastoma multiforme. *Neuro-oncology*, Vol.12, No.9, pp.908-916.

Kholmanskikh, S.; Koeller, H.; Wynshaw-Boris, A.; Gomez, T.; Letourneau, P. & Ross, M. (2006). Calcium-dependent interaction of Lis1 with IQGAP1 and Cdc42 promotesneuronal motility. *Nat Neurosci*, Vol.9, pp.50–57.

Khwaja, F.; Reed, M.; Olson, J.; Schmotzer, B.; Gillespie, G.; Guha, A.; Groves, M.; Kesari, S.; Pohl, J. & Meir, E. (2007). Proteomic identification of biomarkers in the cerebrospinal fluid (CSF) of astrocytoma patients. *J Proteome Res.*, Vol.6, pp.559-570.

Kulasingam, V. & Diamandis, E. (2008). Strategies for discovering novel cancer biomarkers through utilization of emerging technologies. *Nat Clin Prac Oncol*, Vol.5, No.10, pp.588-599.

Li, X.; Zhang, Z.; Schluesener, H. & Xu, S. (2006). Role of exosomes in immune regulation. *J. Cell. Mol. Med,* Vol.10, No.2, pp. 364–375.

Li, Z.; Wang, H.; Eyler, C.; Hjelmeland, A.; Rich, J. (2009). Turning cancer stem cells insideout: an exploration of glioma stem cell signaling pathways. *J. Biol. Chem.,* Vol.284, No.25, pp.16705-16709.

Liang, S.; Shen, G.; Liu, Q.; Xu, Y.; Zhou, L.; Xiao, S.; Xu, Z.; Gong, F.; You, C. & Wei, Y. (2009a). Isoform-specific expression and characterization of 14-3-3 proteins in human glioma tissues discovered by SILAC-based Proteomic analysis. *Proteomics Clin. Appl.,* Vol. 3, pp. 743-753.

Liang, S.; Shen, G.; Xu, X.; Xu, X.; Wei, Y. (2009b) Affinity purification combined with mass spectrometry-based proteomics to study mammalian protein complex and protein-protein interactions. *Current Proteomics,* Vol.6(1), pp.25-31

Liang, S.; Xu, Z.; Xu, X.; Zhao, X.; Huang, C.; Wei, Y. (2011). Quantitative proteomics for cancer biomarker discovery. *Comb Chem High T Scr,* in press.

Lin,Y.; Jiang,T.; Zhou, K.; Xu, L.; Chen, B.; Li, G.; Qiu, X.; Jiang, T.; Zhang, W. & Song, S. (2009). Plasma IGFBP-2 levels predict clinical outcomes of patients with high-grade gliomas. *Neuro-Oncology,* Vol.11, pp. 468–476.

Liu, Mi.; Dai, B.; Kang, S.; Ban, K.; Huang, F.; Lang, F.; Aldape, K.; Xie, T.; Pelloski, C.;

Xie, K.; Sawaya, R. & Huang, S. (2006). FoxM1B is overexpressed in human glioblastomas and critically regulates the tumorigenicity of glioma cells. *Cancer Res.,* Vol. 66, No.7, pp. 3593-3602.

Loeb, S. & Catalona, W. (2007). Prostate-specific antigen in clinical practice. *Cancer Lett.,* Vol.249, pp.30–39.

Lukas, R.; Boire, A.; Nicholas, M. (2009). Targeted therapy in the treatment of malignant gliomas. *OncoTargets & Therapy,* Vol.2, pp. 115-133.

Marrer, E. & Dieterle, F. (2007). Promises of biomarkers in drug development –a reality check. *Chem Biol Drug Des.,* Vol.69: 381-394.

Mateer, S.; Wang, N. & Bloom, G. (2003). IQGAPs: integrators of the cytoskeleton, cell adhesion machinery, and signaling networks. *Cell Motil Cytoskeleton,* Vol.55, pp. 147–155.

Maurer, M.; Berger, C.; Wolf, M.; Futterer, C.; Feldmann,R., Jr.; Schwab, S. & Kuschinsky, W.(2003). The proteome of human brain microdialysate. *Proteome Sci.,* Vol.1, pp.7-15.

McCarthy, B.; Rankin, K.; Il'yasova, D.; Erdal, S.; Vick, N.; Ali-Osman, F.; Bigner, D. & Davis, F. (2011). Assessment of type of allergy and antihistamine use in the development of glioma. *Cancer Epidemiol Biomarkers Prev,* Vol.20, pp.370-378.

McDonald, K.; O'Sullivan, M.; Parkinson, J.; Shaw, J.; Payne, C.; Brewer, J.; Young, L.; Reader, D.; Wheeler, H.; Cook, R.; Biggs, M.; Little, N.; Teo, C.; Stone, G. & Robinson, B. (2007). IQGAP1 and IGFBP2: valuable biomarkers for determining prognosis in glioma patients. *J Neuropathol Exp Neurol,* Vol. 66, No. 5, pp.405-417.

Muller, H., Oh, Y., Lehrnbecher, T., Blum, W., & Rosenfeld, R. (1994). Insulin-like growth factor-binding protein-2 concentrations in cerebrospinal fluid and serum of children with malignant solid tumors or acute leukemia. *J. Clin. Endocrinol. Metab,* Vol.79, pp. 428–434.

Nilsson, J.; Skog, J.; Nordstrand, A.; Baranov, V.; Mincheva-Nilsson, L.; Breakefield, X. & Widmark, A. (2009). Prostate cancer-derived urine exosomes: a novel approach to biomarkers for prostate cancer. *Br J Cancer,* Vol.100, Noo.10, pp. 1603–1607.

Nutt, C.; Betensky, R.; Brower, M.; Batchelor, T.; Louis, D. & Stemmer-Rachamimov, A. (2005). YKL-40 is a differential diagnostic marker for histologic subtypes of high-grade gliomas.*Clin Cancer Res,* Vol.11, pp.2258-2264.

Ohnishi, M.; Matsumoto,T.; Nagashio, R.; Kageyama, T.; Utsuki, S.; Oka, H.; Okayasu, I. & Sato, Y. (2009). Proteomics of tumor-specific proteins in cerebrospinal fluid of patients with astrocytoma: usefulness of gelsolin protein. *Pathol Int,* Vol. 59, pp. 797–803.

Omenn, G. (2005). Exploring the human plasma proteome. *Proteomics,* Vol.5, pp.3223- 3225.

Pelloski, C.; Mahajan, A.; Maor, M.; Chang, E.; Woo, S.; Gilbert, M.; Colman, H.; Yang, H.; Ledoux, A.; Blair, Hi.; Passe, S.; Jenkins, R. & Aldape, K. (2005). YKL-40 Expression is associated with poorer response to radiation and shorter overall survival in glioblastoma. *Clin Cancer Res,* Vol.11, pp.3326-3334.

Petrik, V.; Saadoun, S.; Loosemore, A.; Hobbs, J.; Opstad, K.; Sheldon, J.; Tarelli, E.; Howe,F.; Bell, B. & Papadopoulos, M. (2008). Serum α_2-HS glycoprotein predicts survival in patients with glioblastoma. *Clinical Chemistry,* Vol.54, pp.4 713-4722.

Piccirillo, S.; Reynolds, B.; Zanetti, N.; Lamorte, G.; Binda, E.; Broggi, G.; Brem, H.; Olivi, A.; Dimeco, F.;Vescovi, A. (2006). Bone morphogenetic proteins inhibit the tumorigenic potential of human brain tumour-initiating cells. *Nature,* Vol.444, pp.761-765.

Pisitkun, T.; Shen, R. & Knepper, M. (2004). Identification and proteomic profiling of exosomes in human urine. *PNAS,* Vol.101, No.36, pp.13368–13373.

Preusser, M.; Janzer, R.; Felsberg, J.; Reifenberger, G.; Hamou, M.; Diserens, A.; Stupp, R.; Gorlia, T.; Marosi, C.; Heinzl, H.; Hainfellner, J. & Hegi, M. (2008). Anti-O6 -Methylguanine-Methyltransferase (MGMT) immunohistochemistry in gioblastoma multiforme: observer variability and lack of association with patient survival impede its use as clinical biomarker. *Brain Pathology,* Vol.18, pp. 520-532.

Reddy, P.; Umesh, S.; Thota, B.; Tandon, A.; Pandey, P.; Hegde, A.; Balasubramaniam, A.; Chandramouli, B.; Santosh,V.; Rao, M.; Kondaiah, P. & Somasundaram, K. (2008). PBEF1/NAmPRTase /Visfatin .a potential malignant astrocytoma/glioblastoma serum marker with prognostic value. *Cancer Biol. Ther.,* Vol.7, No.5, 665-670.

Reddy, S.; Britto, R.; Vinnakota, K.; Aparna, H.; Sreepathi, H.; Thota, B.; Kumari, A.; Shilpa, B.; Vrinda, M.; Umesh, S.; Samuel,C.; Shetty, M.; Tandon, A.; Pandey, P.; Hegde,S.; Hegde, A.; Balasubramaniam, A.; Chandramouli, B.; antosh, V.; Kondaiah, P.; Somasundaram, K. & Rao, M. (2008). Novel glioblastoma markers with diagnostic and prognostic value identified through transcriptome analysis. *Clin Cancer Res,* Vol.14, No.10, pp.2978-2987.

Roesler, R.; Brunetto, A.; Abujamra, A.; de Farias, C.; Brunetto, A.; Schwartsmann, G. (2010).Current and emerging molecular targets in glioma. *Expert Rev. Anticancer Ther.* Vol.10, No.11, 1735-1751.

Rorive, S.; Lopez, X.; Maris, C.; Trepant, A.; Sauvage, S.; Sadeghi, N.; Roland, I.; Decaestecker, C. & Salmon, I. (2010). TIMP-4 and CD63: new prognostic biomarkers in human astrocytomas. *Mod pathol,* Vol.23, pp.1418-1428.

Ross, J. & Fletcher, J. (1998). The HER-2/*neu* oncogene in breast cancer: prognostic factor, predictive factor, and target for therapy. *The Oncologist,* Vol.3, pp.237-252.

Sanson, M.; Marie, Y.; Paris, S.; Idbaih, A.; Laffaire, J.; Ducray, F.; Hallani, S.; Boisselier, B.; Mokhtari, K.; Hoang-Xuan, K. & Delattre, J. (2009). Isocitrate dehydrogenase 1 codon 132 mutation is an important prognostic biomarker in gliomas. *J Clin Oncol.* , Vol. 27, No.25, pp.4150-4154.

Sanson M. (2008). Targets for glioma treatment: from bench to bedside. *Curr Opin Oncol.* ,Vol.20(6),pp.650-651.

Schwartz, S.; Weil, R.; Thompson, R.; Shyr, Y.; Moore, J.; Toms, S.; Johnson, M & Caprioli1, R. (2005). Proteomic-based prognosis of brain tumor patients using direct-tissue matrix -assisted laser desorption ionization mass spectrometry. *Cancer Res,* Vol.65, No.17, pp. 7674-81.

Shen, G.; Liang, S.; Xu, Z.; Zhou, L.; Xiao, S.; Xia, X.; Li, R.; Liao, Y.; You, C. & Wei, Y. (2010).Downregulated expression of HSP27 in human low-grade glioma tissue discovered by a quantitative proteomic analysis. *Proteome Sci.,* Vol.8, pp.17-28.

Singh, S.; Clarke, I.; Terasaki, M.;, Bonn,V.; Hawkins, C.; Squire, J.; Dirks, P. (2003). Identification of a cancer stem cell in human brain tumors. *Cancer Res.,* Vol.63, No.18, pp.5821-5828.

Singh, S.; Hawkins, C.; Clarke, I.; Squire, J.; Bayani, J.; Hide, T.; Henkelman, R.; Cusimano, M.; Dirks, P. (2004). Identification of human brain tumour initiating cells. *Nature,* Vol. 432, No.7015, pp.396-401.

Skog, J.;, Würdinger, T.; van Rijn, S.; Meijer, D.; Gainche, L.; Sena-Esteves, M.; Curry, W., Jr.;Carter, B.; Krichevsky, A. & Breakefield, X. (2008). Glioblastoma microvesicles transport RNA and proteins that promote tumour growth and provide diagnostic biomarkers. *Nat Cell Biol.,* Vol.10, No.12, pp.1470–1476.

Sodaa,Y.; Marumotoa, T.; Friedmann-Morvinskia, D.; Sodaa, M.; Liua, F.; Michiuec, H.; Pastorinod, S.; Yange, M.; Hoffmane, R.; Kesarid, S. & Vermaa, I. (2011). Transdifferentiation of glioblastoma cells into vascular endothelial cells. *PNAS,* Vol.108, No. 11, PP. 4274–4280.

Sreekanthreddy, P.; Srinivasan, H.; Kumar, D.; Nijaguna, M.; Sridevi, S.; Vrinda, M.; Arivazhagan, A.; Balasubramaniam, A.; Hegde, A.; Chandramouli, B.; Santosh, V.;

Rao, M.; Kondaiah, P. & Somasundaram, K. Identification of potential serum biomarkers of glioblastoma: serum osteopontin levels correlate with poor prognosis. *Cancer Epidemiol Biomarkers Prev,* Vol.19, No.6, pp.1409–1422.

von Deimling, A.; Korshunov, Andrey. & Hartmann, C. (2011). The next generation of glioma biomarkers: MGMT methylation, BRAF fusions and IDH1 mutations. *Brain Pathology,* Vol.21, pp.74–87.

Yamaoka-Tojo, M.; Ushio-Fukai, M.; Hilenski, L.; Dikalov, S.; Chen, Y.; Tojo, T.; Fukai, T.; Fujimoto, M.; Patrushev, N.; Wang, N.; Kontos, C.; Bloom, G. & Alexander, R. (2004). IQGAP1, a novel vascular endothelial growth factor receptor binding protein, is involved in reactive oxygen species–dependent endothelial migration and proliferation. *Circ. Res.,* Vol.95, pp.276-283.

Yan, H.; Parsons, D.; Jin, G.; McLendon, R.; Rasheed, B.; Yuan, W.; Kos, I.; Batinic-Haberle, I.; Jones, S.; Riggins, G.; Friedman, H.; Friedman, A.; Reardon, D.; Herndon, J.;

Kinzler, K.; Velculescu, V.; Vogelstein, B. & Bigner, D. (2009). IDH1 and IDH2 mutations in gliomas. *N. Eng. J. Med.*, Vol.360, pp.765-773.

http://en.wikipedia.org/wiki/Glioma

16

MicroRNA (miRNA) Regulation in Glioma: Implications in Development, Progression, Grading, Prognosis and Therapy

Kumaravel Somasundaram*, Soumya Alige Mahabala Rao and Zahid Nawaz

Department of Microbiology and Cell Biology, Indian Institute of Science, Bangalore India

1. Introduction

Neoplasms, which arise in cells originating from central nervous system (CNS) or peripheral nervous system (PNS) result in a class of tumours called neuroectodermal tumours. Generally after development ceases, neurons become post-mitotic and only the glial cells retain the capacity to divide and proliferate. So it is quite appreciable that most of the brain tumours are of glial origin and are referred as gliomas. Based on the cell type involved in malignancy, gliomas can be astrocytomas (astrocytes), oligodendrogliomas (oligodendrocytes), oligoastrocytomas (mixture of astrocytes and oligodendrocytes) and ependymomas (ependymal cells). Astrocytomas account for more than 60% of all primary brain tumours hence forming the majority of neoplasms of the CNS. On the other hand, neurofibroma and schwannoma are the two most common glial tumours of the PNS.

According to WHO (2007) classification, astrocytomas are classified into grades I–IV based on the intensity of malignancy as determined by histopathological criteria. Grade I (Pilocytic astrocytoma; PA) gliomas are generally benign and often circumscribed, whereas grade II (Diffuse astrocytoma; DA), III (Anaplastic astrocytoma; AA) and IV (Glioblastoma; GBM) gliomas are malignant and they diffusely infiltrate the brain. The most malignant and common form of infiltrating astrocytic tumours is glioblastoma with a median survival of less than one year. GBM can be further divided into two subtypes based on certain genetic and clinical features: primary and secondary GBM. Primary GBM arises as a *de novo* process, without any antecedent history of low grade lesions, whereas secondary GBM develops progressively from lower grades, generally over a period of 5–10 years.

Like any other neoplasm, the underlying cause of gliomagenesis is the genomic alterations like deletions, amplifications, mutations, aberrant DNA methylation and chromosomal rearrangements, which result in the activation of oncogenes and inactivation of tumour suppressors. With the discovery of hundreds of miRNA genes in the past few years that produce non-coding RNA transcripts with no significant open reading frame, it has become evident that the genomic complexity of the cancer cell is far greater than expected.

miRNAs are single-stranded non coding RNAs of 19–25 nucleotides in length, generated from endogenous transcripts that contain a local hairpin structure. They function as guide

* Corresponding author

molecules in post-transcriptional gene silencing by base pairing with target mRNAs, leading either to the cleavage of the target mRNA or its translational repression. miRNAs are one of the largest gene families, accounting for ~1% of the genome (Kim, 2005). According to recent studies, miRNAs play key roles in diverse regulatory pathways which control development, differentiation, apoptosis, cell proliferation and organogenesis. miRNAs and their targets seem to form intricate regulatory networks, as a single miRNA can bind to and regulate different mRNA targets and conversely, a single mRNA can be synergistically controlled by multiple miRNAs. Recently, the work by the Bartel and Burge laboratories predicted that over one third of the human genes are regulated by miRNAs (Lewis *et al.*, 2005).

The location of miRNA genes in fragile sites of the genome provides a circumstantial evidence of an etiological role of miRNAs in tumour formation. Because miRNAs are generally negative regulators of gene expression, changes in the amounts of these RNAs can be tumorigenic if they target a tumour suppressor or an oncogene. For example, over accumulation of an miRNA that targets a tumour suppressor would result in less of that protective factor. In contrast, reduced accumulation of an miRNA that targets a proto-oncogene could lead to excessive amounts of the oncogenic protein. Either way, the net outcome is an imbalance in the activities of tumour suppressor genes and oncogenes, hence resulting in malignancy.

We review here the discovery and biology of miRNAs including their structure, regulation and biogenesis along with different methods available today to assay miRNA expression. A detailed account of the literature on differential miRNA expression and their functional characterization in glioma is provided. In addition, the potential utility of miRNAs in glioma diagnosis, classification, prognosis and targeted therapy is also discussed.

2. Discovery and biology of miRNAs

miRNAs were initially discovered as small temporal RNAs (stRNAs) that played a role in the developmental transitions in *Caenorhabditis elegans*. The first miRNA to be discovered was lin-4 in *C. elegans* in the year 1993 (Lee *et al.*, 1993). The discovery of lin-4 and its target specific translational repression pointed to a new way of gene regulation. In the year 2000, the second miRNA, let-7 was discovered in the same organism and since then a huge number of miRNAs have been discovered. A total of 15172 miRNA entries have been recorded so far from various organisms (Release 16, miRBase) which also include 1048 miRNAs from *Homo sapiens* (http://www.mirbase.org/).

A small RNA must fulfill the following criteria to be classified as an miRNA. Its expression should be authenticated by hybridization to a size-fractionated RNA sample by employing northern blotting. It should be detected by methods like PCR after reverse transcription of RNA (RT-PCR), primer extension analysis, RNase protection assay and microarray. However, northern blotting remains the method of choice for the confirmation of miRNAs, as the blot generally detects both the mature form (a ~22-nucleotide band) and the hairpin precursor (a ~70-nucleotide band) of the predicted miRNA. The small RNA sequence must exist in the stem portion of the hairpin precursor. The precursors are ~60–80 nucleotides in animals, but the lengths are more variable in plants. In addition, the small RNA sequences should be conserved phylogenetically. Lastly, the evidence can be consolidated if the precursor of the predicted miRNA accumulates in ablated Dicer background. However, this criterion is not in vogue, because of the technical challenges that are involved in depleting Dicer in different cells.

2.1 miRNA gene structure

Most of the miRNA genes are transcribed as independent transcription units. The transcripts thus synthesized are referred as primary miRNAs and are equipped with a 7-methyl guanosine cap in the 5' end as well as a poly A tail in the 3' end which are the unique features of class II gene transcripts. This evidence supports the fact that majority of miRNAs, if not all, are transcribed by RNA polymerase II (Lee *et al.*, 2004). Treatment of human cells with α-amanitin at levels which inhibit RNA polymerase II activity, also brings down the global levels of primary miRNAs. Furthermore, chromatin immunoprecipitation (ChIP) experiments have also revealed the physical association of RNA polymerase II with miRNA promoters and thereby establishing the fact that miRNAs are RNA polymerase II transcribed.

miRNAs can be transcribed either individually i.e. a single primary transcript gives rise to a single mature miRNA or they can be transcribed in a polycistronic fashion, in which case distinct miRNAs are produced from a single primary transcript. The miRNAs arising from a single gene cluster can be related to each other, suggesting that the miRNAs might have assembled as a result of gene duplication and may be playing a synergistic role in the production of a particular phenotype.

Based on the genomic location of the transcription units of miRNAs, they can be grouped broadly as: intergenic miRNAs and intragenic miRNAs. Intergenic miRNAs exist as independent genetic elements, their transcription being driven by their own promoter. The intragenic class can be either intronic or exonic in nature owing to the fact whether the stem loop sequence of the precursor miRNA comes from the intron or exon of the protein coding gene or sometimes a non-protein coding gene. In both types, the miRNA gene can be mono or polycistronic. The expression of intragenic miRNAs can be either controlled by their own independent promoter or the miRNAs would be co-transcribed with the parent gene, in which case the pre-miRNA would be processed subsequent to intron splicing. Some miRNAs derive their stem loop sequence from rather short introns and hence bypass the processing action of Drosha and are called Mirtrons (Ruby *et al.*, 2007).

2.2 miRNA gene regulation

The expression of miRNAs can be modulated at a number of levels, which broadly include the transcription of the primary transcript and the multiple steps of the miRNA biogenesis. But it continues to remain a dilemma that which step is regulated and how the regulation is achieved. Regulation at the level of transcription seems more likely to be the major control mechanism. A number of RNA polymearse II associated transcription factors regulate the expression of miRNA genes, for instance TP53, a tumour suppressor, transactivates the miR-34 family of miRNAs (He *et al.*, 2007). Overall, the expression of a particular miRNA seems to be under the control of developmental and tissue specific signalling. Apart from this, there are reports that miRNAs are also modulated post transcriptionally. Post transcriptional regulation is attributed to differential Drosha processing. An example of post transcriptional regulation involves the induction of miR-21 in response to bone morphogenetic protein (BMP) / transforming growth factor beta (TGF-β) signalling without actual transcriptional activation (Davis *et al.*, 2008). TGF-β and BMP signalling activates the Smad mediated Drosha processing of the pri-miR-21.

Majority of miRNA genes being transcribed by the same RNA polymerase as protein coding genes, the mechanisms of epigenetic control known for protein coding genes are likely to be applicable to miRNA loci as well. Aberrant DNA methylation of tumour suppressor genes is a common occurrence in cancer; accordingly several miRNA loci including miR-9-1, miR-193a, miR-137, miR-342, miR-203 and miR-34b/c, are found to be hypermethylated in multiple human cancers (Lujambio *et al.*, 2008). Conversely, the let-7a-3 locus is hypomethylated in lung adenocarcinoma and elevated expression of this locus results in enhanced oncogenic gene transcription (Brueckner *et al.*, 2007;). miRNA promoters are also regulated by histone modifications during development and pathogenesis (Davis and Hata, 2009).

2.3 Biogenesis of miRNAs

miRNA biogenesis involves initial transcription as a largely unstructured precursor, termed as primary miRNA (pri-miRNA), which is subsequently processed in the nucleus to give rise to a 70-nucleotide precursor miRNA hairpin intermediate (pre-miRNA). The pre-miRNA gets transported to the cytoplasm where it undergoes further processing to give rise to a mature miRNA (**Figure.1**).

Most of the miRNA genes are transcribed by RNA polymerase II to generate a stem-loop containing primary miRNA (pri-miRNA), which can range in size from hundreds of nucleotides to tens of kilobases (Lee *et al.*, 2004). Like mRNAs, RNA polymerase II transcribed pri-miRNAs contain 5' cap structures, are polyadenylated, and may be spliced (Cai *et al.*, 2004). The pri-miRNA is processed within the nucleus by a multiprotein complex called the microprocessor. The microprocessor is a 650 kDa complex in humans and is constituted by two key components: Drosha, an RNase III enzyme and DiGeorge syndrome critical region 8 gene (DGCR8), a double-stranded RNA-binding domain (dsRBD) protein (Gregory *et al.*, 2004; Landthaler *et al.*, 2004). DGCR8 is also known as Pasha in *D. melanogaster* and *C. elegans*. The activity of Drosha and DGCR8 results in the production of a ~70 nucleotide hairpin structure known as the precursor miRNA (pre-miRNA). The 2-nucleotide 3' overhang, characteristic of RNase III mediated cleavage, is recognized by exportin-5, which transports the pre-miRNA into the cytoplasm via a Ran-GTP-dependent mechanism (Bohnsack *et al.*, 2004; Lund *et al.*, 2004; Yi *et al.*, 2003). The pre-miRNA is finally cleaved off the loop to produce the mature miRNA duplex about 22 nucleotide in length by Dicer, yet another member of RNase III superfamily of bidentate nucleases.

Dicer is accompanied by dsRBD proteins like TRBP (TAR-RNA binding protein) (Chendrimada *et al.*, 2005; Lee *et al.*, 2006). Dicer and TRBP recruit members of the Argonaute family and the trimeric complex thus formed is referred to as RNA Induced Silencing Complex (RISC) (Gregory *et al.*, 2005; Maniataki and Mourelatos, 2005). Argonaute proteins form the catalytic component of the RISC complex as they aid in strand selection of the miRNA duplex in addition to the possession of slicer activity by virtue of which they slice the target mRNA. In mammals, Ago2 is the sole enzyme equipped with endonucleolytic activity (Liu *et al.*, 2004; Meister *et al.*, 2004). One of the miRNA strands which has relatively less stability at the 5' end is incorporated into the RISC complex while as the other miRNA strand is generally degraded (Du and Zamore, 2005). It is often possible that both strands of the miRNA duplex could function as mature miRNAs but their abundance may be drastically different (Ruby *et al.*, 2006).

The miRNA then guides the RISC to specific mRNA targets, the basis of which is sequence complementarity generally in the 3' UTR of the target mRNA. In cases of perfect or near perfect complementarity to the mRNA, the target mRNA can be cleaved and degraded and if there is less complementarity, it results in translational repression (Hutvagner and

Zamore, 2002). Most animal miRNAs bind imperfectly to their targets and promote translational repression, rather than cleavage and degradation. However, the seed sequence representing 2-8 nucleotides from the 5′ end of miRNA requires a perfect complementarity. The mechanism of translational repression is somewhat vague with some evidences suggesting that miRNAs block translational initiation while as others suggest a block in elongation.

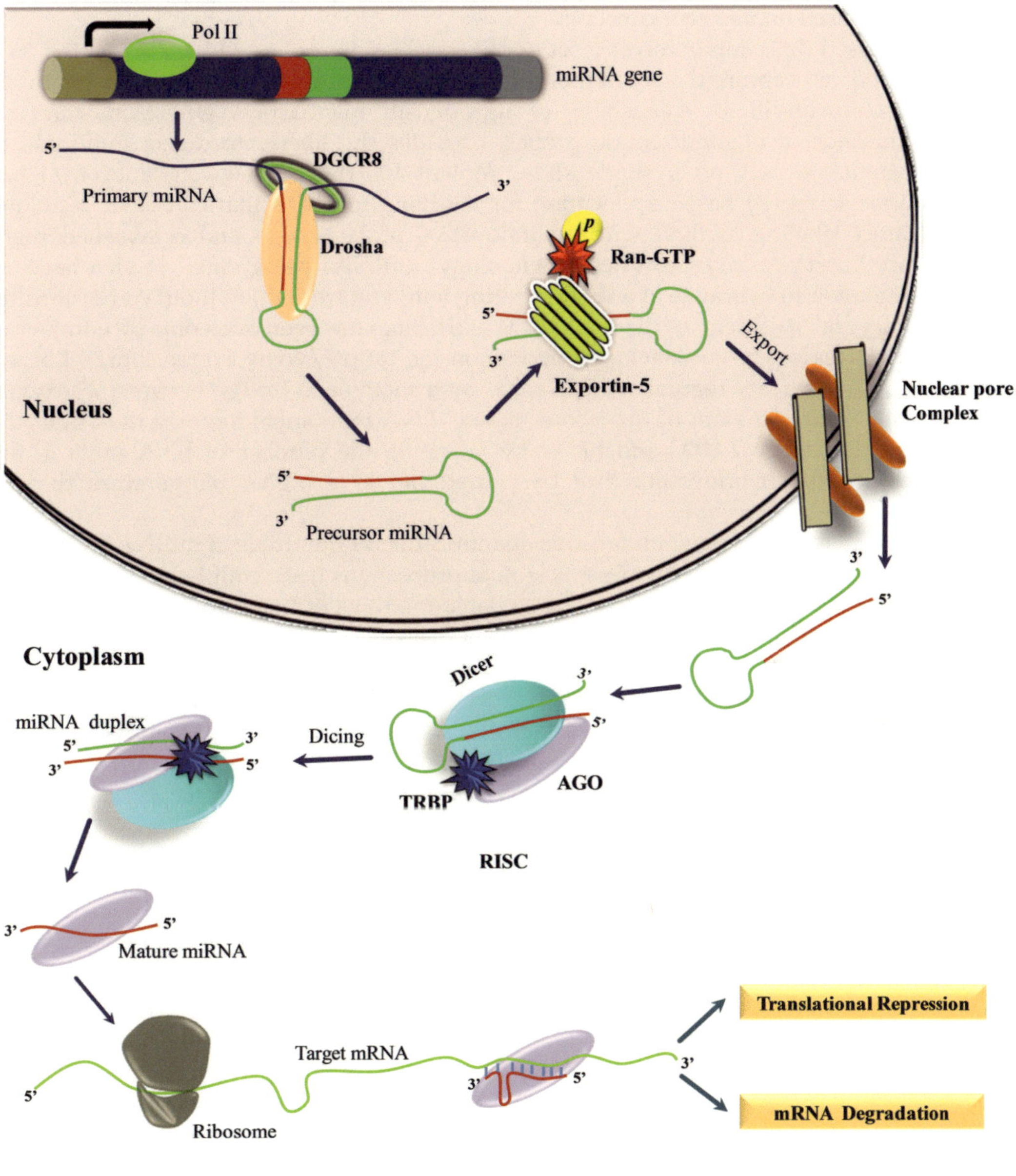

Fig. 1. Schematic representation of miRNA biogenesis pathway.

3. Methods to quantitate miRNA levels

An array of techniques and methodologies can be employed to quantify the levels of miRNAs both absolutely and relatively. These include northern blotting, microarrays, bead based arrays and quantitative real-time RT-PCR. Northern blotting is a low throughput technique as well as less sensitive requiring more input RNA but it can be used to detect both mature and pre-miRNA molecules. Genome wide miRNA expression studies are chiefly carried out by employing various microarray platforms provided by different private firms and are based on different concepts.

Microarray based detection involves a set of oligonucleotide probes which are spotted on a glass slide and can capture the small molecule RNAs like miRNAs, if allowed to hybridize under optimum conditions. Availability of high density microarrays, where one can spot several thousands of oligonucleotide probes, provides the liberty to detect hundreds of miRNAs simultaneously on a single slide. Agilent Inc (http://www.agilent.com/) has developed a microarray based application for studying miRNAs that combines a unique miRNA direct labeling method with an innovative probe design and established high-performance SurePrint inkjet synthesis technology. miRNAs being small in size have an inherent limitation to hybridize at a single melting temperature (Tm) without compromising the sensitivity and specificity of the method. This problem has been overcome by employing locked nucleic acids (LNAs) developed by Exiqon Inc (http://www.exiqon.com/). Locked nucleic acids differ from regular nucleic acids by a methylene bridge between 2′ oxygen atom and the 4′ carbon atom of the ribose moiety. LNA monomers increase the Tm of the nucleic acid duplex by 2-10°C and hence by adjusting the number of LNA units in the oligonucleotide, the hybridization can be carried out at a higher temperature thereby increasing the specificity.

Bead-based arrays also allow simultaneous quantification of hundreds of miRNAs (Luminex Inc). This methodology also uses oligonucleotide probes which are coupled to carboxylated polystyrene microspheres that incorporate variable mixtures of two fluorescent dyes hence allows the detection of each microsphere with a distinct color by a flow cytometer. Each microsphere is coupled with oligonucleotide molecules that are specific for a particular miRNA. The method involves RNA extraction, followed by biotinylation and finally hybridization. The microspheres are washed, incubated with streptavidin–phycoerythrin, and analyzed on a Luminex analyzer. The analyzer identifies the fluorescent microsphere as well as quantitates the intensity of the streptavidin–phycoerythrin fluorescence, resulting in the identification of miRNAs present in the sample.

Expression analysis is more commonly performed by quantitative real-time RT-PCR. Quantification of mature miRNAs usually involves reverse transcription of the miRNA with a stem–loop primer. miRNA specific cDNA is then used in the real-time PCR reaction. A mixture of forward and reverse primers and a dual-labeled probe (TaqMan®) are used to amplify and detect the specific cDNA (Life Technologies Corp.). The probe has a reporter dye on the 5′ end and a quencher on the 3′ end. If the target sequence is present during the PCR, the probe binds to the target sequence. During the extension stage of the PCR cycle, the reporter dye is released by the 5′ exonuclease activity of *Taq* polymerase, and because the reporter and quencher have been separated, the fluorescence from the reporter dye is detected. A variation of quantitative real time RT-PCR using SybrGreen based chemistry has also been employed (System Biosciences, Qiagen etc.). The technique involves cDNA synthesis for the miRNA pool followed by real time PCR using a miRNA specific forward primer and a reverse primer essentially derived from RT primer.

4. miRNA regulation in glioma

Since the initial reports by Ciafre *et al* and Chan *et al,* there is an increasing body of literature accumulated on the role of miRNAs in glioma development (**Table. 1**) (Chan *et al.*, 2005; Ciafre *et al.*, 2005). Various miRNA profiling studies carried out in glioma tissue samples identified differentially regulated miRNAs in gliomas. Several studies also reported the in-depth investigation of specific miRNAs in glioma cells including functional characterization to understand the effects of regulation of miRNA in glioma cells with respect to various transformation related phenotypes like cell proliferation, cell death, migration and invasion. Many of these studies also included the prediction and experimental validation of targets of miRNA by using various accepted techniques.

4.1 Large scale expression profiling of miRNAs in glioma

The first report of expression profiling of large number of miRNAs in glioma was almost simultaneously reported by two groups (Chan *et al.*, 2005; Ciafre *et al.*, 2005). Ciafre *et al* used a microarray chip to profile the expression of 245 miRNAs in GBM tissue samples (Ciafre *et al.*, 2005). The samples included nine GBM tissue samples, matched adjacent peripheral region as normal brain tissue and glioma cell lines. With the additional validation by northern blotting, this study identified miR-221 as GBM upregulated and miR-128, miR-181a, miR-181b and miR-181c as GBM downregulated miRNAs. Chan *et al* analyzed the expression of 180 mammalian miRNAs using a nylon membrane based oligonucleotide array in three primary high-grade gliomas and eight non-neoplastic fetal and adult brain tissues. They found miR-21 as the most upregulated miRNA in high grade gliomas among a total eight miRNAs (Chan *et al.*, 2005). Silber *et al* analyzed the expression of 192 miRNAs by quantitative RT-qPCR with four AAs, four GBMs and four Glioses (as normal brain tissues) and found that 35 miRNAs were significantly deregulated in AA or GBM tumours (Silber *et al.*, 2008). Thirteen (37%) of these miRNAs were differentially expressed in both AA and GBM in comparison to glioses, 16 (45%) were differentially expressed only in GBM tumours and 6 (17%) were differentially expressed only in AA tumours. Another study carried out microarray based expression profiling of 245 miRNAs and found that eleven miRNAs were downregulated and eight miRNAs were upregulated in GBM (Godlewski *et al.*, 2008). Malzkorn *et al* analyzed the expression of 157 miRNAs in four glioma patients who had the progression of grade II to grade IV by real time RT-PCR (Malzkorn *et al.*). This revealed the differential expression of 14 miRNAs - of which, 12 miRNAs (miR-9, miR-15a, miR-16, miR-17, miR-19a, miR-20a, miR-21, miR-25, miR-28, miR-130b, miR-140 and miR-210) were upregulated during progression whereas 2 (miR-184 and miR-328) of them were downregulated (Malzkorn *et al.*). The authors validated the expression of selected miRNAs (miR-16, miR-17, miR-19a, miR-20a, miR-140 and miR-184) in an independent set of low grade and secondary GBM samples thus confirming the grade associated regulation of these miRNAs. Modulation of miR-17 and miR-328 in glioma cell lines revealed an important role of these miRNAs in glioma cell proliferation, apoptosis and cell invasion phenotypes (Malzkorn *et al.*).

While the above studies were relatively small, investigating couple of hundred miRNAs and used fewer tissue samples, Rao *et al* recently profiled the expression of 756 human miRNAs in malignant astrocytoma- AA (n=13) and GBM (n=26), along with the normal brain samples (n=7) and found that 55 miRNAs were upregulated and 29 miRNAs were downregulated in malignant astrocytomas in comparison to normal brain samples

Serial No.	miRNA	Function*	Target/s **	miRNA site confirmation ***	Phenotype/s affected	References
1	miR-7	Tumour suppressor	EGFR, IRS-1, IRS-2	Yes	Cell proliferation, cell cycle, apoptosis, invasion	(Kefas *et al.*, 2008)
2	miR-15b	Tumour suppressor	CCNE1	Yes	Cell proliferation, cell cycle	(Xia *et al.*, 2009a)
3	miR-21	Oncogenic	-	-	Cell proliferation	(Chan *et al.*, 2005)
			PDCD4	-	Apoptosis	(Chen *et al.*, 2008)
			-	-	Chemosensitivity of cells to S-TRAIL, *In vivo* tumour growth	(Corsten *et al.*, 2007)
			RECK	Yes	Migration, invasion	(Gabriely *et al.*, 2008)
			TIMP3	No	Migration, invasion	(Gabriely *et al.*, 2008)
			SPRY2	Yes	Migration, invasion	(Kwak *et al.*)
			LRRFIP1	Yes	Chemosensitivity of cells to VM-26	(Li *et al.*, 2009b)
			p53, Bax, DAXX, APAF1, p21, TAp63, TGFBR2	No	Apoptosis, cell growth, cell cycle	(Papagiannakopoulos *et al.*, 2008)
			-	-	Chemosensitivity of cells to taxol	(Ren *et al.*)
			-	-	Chemosensitivity of cells to temozolomide	(Shi *et al.*)
4	miR-26a	Oncogenic	PTEN	Yes	*In vivo* tumour growth	(Huse *et al.*, 2009)
			PTEN, Rb1, MAP3K2/MEKK2	Yes	*In vivo* transformation of NIH3T3 cells	(Kim *et al.*)
5	miR-34a	Tumour suppressor	c-Met, Notch 1, Notch 2	Yes	Cell proliferation , cell cycle, apoptosis, invasion	(Li *et al.*, 2009a)
6	miR-124, miR-137	Tumour suppressor	CDK6	Yes	Cell cycle, induction of differentiation	(Silber *et al.*, 2008)

Serial No.	miRNA	Function*	Target/s **	miRNA site confirmation ***	Phenotype/s affected	References
7	miR-125b	Tumour suppressor	CDK6 and CDC25	No	Proliferation, cell cycle	(Shi *et al.*)
		Oncogenic	BMF1	No	Cell viability, apoptosis	(Xia *et al.*, 2009c)
8	miR-146b	Tumour suppressor	EGFR	Yes	Invasion, migration	(Xia *et al.*, 2009b)
9	miR-128	Tumour suppressor	Bmi1	Yes	*In vivo* tumour growth, Neurosphere formation, cell proliferation	(Godlewski *et al.*, 2008)
			E2F3a	Yes	Cell proliferation	(Zhang *et al.*, 2009)
10	miR-181a/b	Tumour suppressor	-	-	Proliferation, apoptosis, invasion, anchorage independent growth	(Shi *et al.*, 2008)
11	miR-218	Tumour suppressor	IKK-B	Yes	Migration, invasion	(Song *et al.*)
12	miR-221/222	Oncogenic	p27, p57	Yes	Cell cycle	(Medina *et al.*, 2008)
			PUMA	Yes	Apoptosis	(Zhang *et al.*)
13	miR-296	Oncogenic	HGS	Yes	Endothelial tubule formation, migration, *in vivo* tumour neovascularization	(Wurdinger *et al.*, 2008)
14	miR-451	Tumour suppressor	-	-	Cell proliferation , cell cycle, apoptosis, invasion	(Nan *et al.*)

* miRNAs are classified to have 'oncogenic' or 'tumour suppressor' function based on their pro-tumorigenic or anti-tumorigenic property respectively.
** miRNA targets are identified based on the reduction in the protein level with miRNA overexpression along with the reduction in the reporter activity of the 3′-UTR reporter.
*** miRNA site confirmation indicates whether the predicted miRNA binding site is confirmed by site directed mutagenesis that abolishes the effects of miRNA overexpression on the reporter activity.

Table 1. Characterization of the role of miRNAs in glioma

(Rao *et al.*). Besides the validation of several deregulated miRNAs, this study also developed a 23 miRNA expression signature that could distinguish between AA and GBM with high accuracy.

4.2 Specific miRNAs in glioma development

4.2.1 miR-21

miR-21 is found to be upregulated in different kinds of human cancers including glioma. miR-21, being one of the well studied miRNAs in cancer, is shown to have oncogenic roles by targeting multiple tumour suppressors in human cancers. The expression profiling of miRNAs in glioblastoma tissues as well as in glioma cell lines identified miR-21 as an upregulated miRNA in glioma (Chan *et al.*, 2005). Subsequently, the over expression of miR-21 in gliomas was confirmed by several studies (Ciafre *et al.*, 2005; Conti *et al.*, 2009; Gabriely *et al.*, 2008); (Papagiannakopoulos *et al.*, 2008; Rao *et al.*, ; Silber *et al.*, 2008).

Modulation of miRNA levels in glioma cell lines indicated that miR-21 had pro-proliferative (Chan *et al.*, 2005; Papagiannakopoulos *et al.*, 2008; Zhou *et al.*) and anti-apoptotic effects (Chan *et al.*, 2005; Papagiannakopoulos *et al.*, 2008). miR-21 also affected cell cycle progression (Papagiannakopoulos *et al.*, 2008) and the tumour growth *in vivo* (Corsten *et al.*, 2007; Zhou *et al.*). miR-21 was also shown to modulate the chemosensitivity of glioma cells to many chemotherapeutic agents like doxorubicin, secretable tumour necrosis factor related apoptosis inducing ligand (S-TRAIL), taxol, VM-26 and temozolomide (Corsten *et al.*, 2007; Li *et al.*, 2009b; Papagiannakopoulos *et al.*, 2008; Ren *et al.*, ; Shi *et al.*). Papagiannakopoulos *et al* undertook systems biology approach to understand the role of miR-21 in glioblastoma development. The network analysis of bioinformatically predicted targets of miR-21 showed that the over expressed miRNA was linked to three major cancer pathways - p53, TGF beta and mitochondrial apoptosis pathways. The knock down of miR-21 in glioma cell line upregulated many tumour suppressor proteins like p53, Bax, DAXX, APAF1, p21, TAp63 and TGFBR2 (Papagiannakopoulos *et al.*, 2008).

Since miR-21 is one of the most upregulated miRNAs, efforts are being made to identify its direct targets. While the tumour suppressor proteins like PTEN (phosphatase and tensin homolog), TPM1 (Tropomyosin 1) and maspin were well characterized as direct targets of miR-21 in other cancers, they were not validated in glioblastoma (Novakova *et al.*, 2009). Nevertheless, it was shown that the anti-apoptotic nature of the miR-21 can be partly attributed to its target PDCD4 (programmed cell death 4), as the over-expression of miR-21 inhibited PDCD4-dependent apoptosis (Chen *et al.*, 2008). In addition to its effects on growth, miR-21 also affected the property of invasion that causes infiltrating pattern of glioma growth *in vivo* (Gabriely *et al.*, 2008). Using the target prediction algorithms and the transcript profiling, the matrix metalloprotease inhibitors, RECK and TIMP3 were identified as miR-21 targets thus substantiating a pro-invasion and -migration role for miR-21 (Gabriely *et al.*, 2008). The promotion of invasion was also attributed to another target of miR-21, *sprouty*, the negative regulator of Ras/MAPK pathways (Kwak *et al.*).

4.2.2 miR-26a

The upregulation of miR-26a and its consequence on cellular pathways leading to the pro-tumorigenic effects are well studied in glioblastoma. In GBM, PTEN expression was found to be directly regulated by miR-26a (Huse *et al.*, 2009). The miR-26a locus was found to be amplified and it was often associated with the monoallelic loss of PTEN suggesting that the residual PTEN transcript made in PTEN +/- cases was nullified by miR-26a, analogous to loss of heterozygosity. Using The Cancer Genome Atlas (TCGA) data, authors demonstrated that, in patients with monoallelic PTEN deletion, amplification of miR-26a locus served as another mechanism to inactivate PTEN. In the mouse glioma model, miR-26a mediated PTEN repression enhanced tumour formation and substituted the loss of heterozygosity of PTEN locus. Further studies carried out by Kim *et al* demonstrated that hsa-miR-26a is a cooperating component of a frequently occurring oncogenic amplicon containing CDK4 and CENTG1 which regulate the RB1 and PI3 kinase/AKT pathways (Kim *et al.*). By integrating the TCGA data for copy number, mRNA, miRNA, and DNA methylation, they identified PTEN, RB1, and MAP3K2/MEKK2 to be the functional targets of miR-26a in GBM. They also demonstrated that miR-26a alone could transform NIH3T3 cells and promote the growth of glioma cells *in vivo* by directly regulating the expressions of PTEN, RB1, and MAP3K2/MEKK2. This led to the increased AKT activation and decreased c-JUN N-terminal kinase-dependent apoptosis resulting in increased proliferation. In both PTEN-positive and PTEN-deficient glioma cells, the over expression of miR-26a induced the tumour growth *in vivo,* and it was further increased if the cells were over expressing CDK4 or CENTG1. GBM patients with the amplification of miR-26a-CDK4 locus had markedly decreased survival. Thus, the amplification of hsa-miR-26a, CDK4, and CENTG1 increased the aggressiveness of the tumour by cooperately regulating RB1, PI3K/AKT, and JNK pathways (Kim *et al.*).

4.2.3 miR-221 and miR-222

The comprehensive analysis of miRNA expression during serum stimulation of quiescent T98 glioblastoma cells revealed that miR-221 and miR-222 were upregulated as cells progressed beyond the G1-S phase transition (Medina *et al.,* 2008). miR-221 and miR-222 were found to target CDK inhibitors- p27 and p57 and prevent quiescence when elevated during growth factor deprivation and induced cell death by causing precocious S-phase entry. Further, the inhibition of the expression of these miRNAs in glioma cell lines led to the increased apoptosis (Zhang *et al.*). The effect of the miRNA on apoptosis was also attributed to its ability to target pro-apoptotic gene PUMA. The over expression of PUMA reversed the phenotypes caused by the over expression of the miRNAs. In tumour xenograft model, inhibition of miR-221/222 reduced the tumour volume compared to the scramble control along with increased apoptosis, reduced Ki-67 staining, increased PUMA and Bax and reduced Bcl-2 expression. In human glioma tissue samples, the down regulation of PUMA negatively correlated with the upregulation of miR-221/222 suggesting the importance of the regulation in the clinical samples.

4.2.4 miR-296

The profiling of miRNAs upon co-culturing human brain endothelial cells (HBMVECs) with human glioma cell line U87 identified that miR-296 is the only upregulated miRNA (Wurdinger *et al.,* 2008). The miR-296 expression also increased in HBMVECs upon treatment with angiogenic factors like EGM, VEGF and EGF. Treatment of HBMVECs with VEGF resulted in the tubule formation, increased the migration distance and also increased the miR-296 level in dose dependent manner. Treatment of cells with miR-296 inhibitors led to decreased tubule formation and migration distance. On the other hand, the overexpression of the miRNA led to increased tubule formation. The target prediction algorithms and subsequently, experimental evidences suggested that HGS, hepatocyte growth factor regulated receptor kinase substrate, to be the target of the miR-296. HGS was previously known to regulate the levels of VEGFR2 and PDGFRβ receptors. These studies suggested that the miR-296 in HBMVECs target HGS with the resultant upregulation of VEGFR2 and PDGFRβ receptors thereby promoting angiogenesis. To understand the *in vivo* role of miR-296 in tumour angiogenesis, nude mice-bearing subcutaneous U87 xenografts were injected with cholesterol-conjugated miR-296 antisense oligonucleotide. The quantification of tumour neovascularization revealed that the mice injected with antisense miR-296 showed reduced tumour neovascularization as compared to the mice injected with the mismatch control. The endothelial cells derived from human glioma showed upregulation of miR-296 compared to the normal brain with concomitant downregulation of HGS and the upregulation of the receptors-VEGFR2 and PDGFRβ. These observations demonstrate the importance of miR-296 in the angiogenesis of malignant glioma.

4.2.5 miR-7

miR-7 was found to be a tumour suppressor miRNA and was downregulated in glioma compared to the normal brain. The *in vivo* experiments suggested that re-expression of miR-7 into glioma cells decreased the cell count, invasion and increased apoptosis (Kefas *et al.*, 2008). Oncogenic proteins, EGFR, IRS-1 and IRS-2 were identified as the targets of miR-7. The miR-7 inhibited the Akt pathway but this inhibition could not be rescued by the over expression of wild type or the mutant EGFR. Further investigation revealed that the impaired processing as the mechanism of downregulation of miR-7 in glioma. This study unraveled the tumour suppressor property of the miR-7 by targeting the receptors-EGFR, IRS1 and IRS2, thereby counteracting the pro-proliferative effect of the pathway.

4.2.6 miR-34a

miR-34a was found to act as a tumour suppressor in glioma by targeting multiple oncogenes like c-Met, Notch1, Notch2 and CDK6 (Li *et al.*, 2009a). The miR-34a expression in glioma tissues was downregulated compared to the normal brain. As the earlier reports suggested that miR-34a is a target of p53, authors analyzed the expression of the miRNA in cell lines with wild type p53 and with mutant p53 and found that the expression of miR-34a in mutant p53 is lower compared to that in those cell lines bearing wild type p53. In the glioma tissues, the c-Met and the miR-34a expression negatively correlated suggesting the miRNA mediated regulation of c-Met in glioma. To assess the effect of the miRNA on cell proliferation, cell cycle and apoptosis, the miR-34a was over expressed in different cell lines, along with human astrocytes. The miR-34a over expression reduced the proliferation, the increased G1/G0 population only in cancer cell lines, but not in normal human astrocytes. The invasion of the cells also decreased with miR-34a over expression. The over expression of c-met partially but significantly rescued the effect of miR-34a over expression on cell cycle where as the over expression of Notch1 and Notch2 rescued miR-34a effect on apoptosis. *In vivo* studies suggested that the miR-34a over expression in U87 cells led to the development of much smaller tumours compared to the control U87 cells.

4.2.7 miR-124 and miR-137

Expression profiling revealed that the levels of miR-124 and miR-137 were significantly decreased in AA and GBM relative to non-neoplastic brain tissue (Silber *et al.*, 2008). During the differentiation of cultured mouse neural stem cells following growth factor withdrawal, the levels of these miRNAs were increased. The re-expression of these miRNAs with the DNA methylation inhibitor treatment suggested a possible regulation of these miRNAs by epigenetic phenomenon like methylation. The over expression of miR-124 or miR-137 induced morphological changes and also induced differentiation marker profile. Further studies identified that miR-124 and miR-137 target CDK6 resulting in reduced phosphorylated RB and G1 cell cycle arrest.

4.2.8 miR-128

The expression analysis revealed that miR-128 was downregulated miRNAs in glioma (Godlewski *et al.*, 2008; Zhang *et al.*, 2009). Over expression of the miRNA led to the decreased cell proliferation and tumour growth *in vivo* (Godlewski *et al.*, 2008) suggesting the tumour suppressor nature of the miRNA. miR-128 was shown to target Bmi1 (B lymphoma mouse Moloney leukemia virus insertion region) oncogene. In the GBM tumours, the downregulation of miR-128 correlated with the corresponding upregulation of Bmi1 oncogene. The miR-128 over expression caused the reduction of H3K trimethylation and pAkt and also increased p21 suggesting that the cellular pathways regulated by Bmi1 were altered with miRNA over expression leading to the decreased neurosphere formation. miR-128 was also shown to directly target E2F3a transcription factor generally upregulated in glioma. The over expression of E2F3a rescued the cell growth inhibition caused by the over expression of the miR-128 (Zhang *et al.*, 2009).

4.2.9 miR-218

miR-218 had reduced expression in glioma cell lines compared to the normal brain (Song *et al.*). The over expression of the miRNA in glioma cell lines resulted in the decreased migration and invasion of the glioma cells with concomitant decreased MMP-9 activity. The over expression of miR-218 in glioma cell lines also resulted in the downregulation of the targets of NF-kB pathway suggesting the role of the miRNA in regulating the pathway. Using the target prediction algorithms, authors identified that miR-218 targeted IKK-β thereby regulating NF-κB pathway (Song *et al.*).

4.2.10 miR-125b

The expression of miR-125, a previously identified brain-specific miRNA, was found to be reduced when glioma cells were treated with *a*ll *t*rans *r*etinoic *a*cid (ATRA) (Xia *et al.*, 2009c). The over expression of miR-125b increased the cell viability in the presence or in the absence of ATRA along with the decrease in the apoptosis. The authors identified Bmf (Bcl-2 modifying factor) as the direct target of miR-125b. In contrast to this report, another study reported that the over expression of miR-125b in glioma cells led to the decreased cell growth and caused the reduced progression of the cells through cell cycle by downregulating the levels of CDK6 and CDC25 (Shi *et al.*). The study also reported that miR-125b was expressed at a higher level in CD133 positive glioma stem cells compared to the CD133 negative non-stem cell population.

4.2.11 miR-451

miR-451 is one of the significantly downregulated miRNA in glioma compared to the normal brain (Nan *et al.*). The over expression of miR-451 in glioma cell lines led to decreased proliferation and invasion, in addition to Go/G1 arrest and apoptosis induction. The over expression of miR-451 reduced Akt, cyclinD1, MMP2, MMP9 and Bcl-2 also increased p27/kip levels suggesting the tumour suppressor nature of the miRNA. However, the above identified miR-451 targets have not been experimentally validated (Nan *et al.*).

4.2.12 miR-15b

The modulation of miR-15b in U87 and U118 glioma cell lines demonstrated that miR-15b affects the cell growth and the cell cycle progression (Xia *et al.*, 2009a). The bioinformatics prediction identified cyclins- cyclin E1 and cyclin D to be the targets of miR-15b. The authors further demonstrated that cyclin E1 was indeed a direct target of miR-15b.

4.2.13 miR-181a and miR-181b

The miRNAs- miR-181a and miR-181b were found to be downregulated in glioma by multiple studies (Ciafre *et al.*, 2005; Conti *et al.*, 2009; Malzkorn *et al.*). The overexpression of these miRNAs in glioma cell lines resulted in the reduction of cell growth *in vivo*, anchorage independent growth, invasion and apoptosis (Shi *et al.*, 2008).

4.2.14 miR-146b

The modulation of miR-146b in glioma cell line revealed that the migration and invasion were inhibited by miR-146b (Katakowski *et al.*, ; Xia *et al.*, 2009b). miR-146 was found to target MMP-16 which could potentially mediate the reduced migration and invasion seen upon miR-146b overexpression (Xia *et al.*, 2009b). miR-146b was also shown to directly target EGFR (Katakowski *et al*).

5. Applications of miRNA in glioma: accurate grading, better prognosis and novel therapeutic approaches

The rationale for using miRNAs in glioma diagnosis and therapeutic modalities is as follows. The identification of differences in the genetic alterations in miRNA genes and miRNA transcript levels in tumour samples compared to normal tissues provides an automatic basis for their utility for glioma diagnosis, classification and prognosis. In fact, classification of multiple cancers based on the expression pattern of couple of hundred miRNAs was found to be more accurate than using expression of approximately 16,000 protein coding genes (Lu *et al.*, 2005). Even though several miRNAs have been shown to be regulated in different grades of glioma, variation in the expression of individual miRNAs within a glioma grade suggests that distinct subgroups within each grade of glioma could be identified. It is likely that these subgroups may have different prognosis. miRNAs also appear to be an attractive target for therapeutic intervention because the aberrantly expressed miRNAs seem to play key role in the development of cancer and that correcting the miRNA deficiencies either by antagonizing or restoring miRNA function may offer a therapeutic gain (Bader *et al.*).

Although several miRNAs have been identified to be either upregulated or down regulated in glioblastoma, there were only few studies which particularly investigated the differential regulation of miRNAs between different grades of glioma. Real time RT-PCR analysis of several miRNAs in WHO grade II and grade IV samples which spontaneously progressed from the same set of patients identified twelve miRNAs (miR-9, miR-15a, miR-16, miR-17, miR-19a, miR-20a, miR-21, miR-25, miR-28, miR-130b, miR-140 and miR-210) to be upregulated and two miRNAs (miR-184 and miR-328) to be downregulated in grade IV tumours thus characterizing their role in progression (Malzkorn *et al.*). Analysis of miRNA microarray data by prediction analysis of microarrays (PAM), a 23 miRNA expression signature was identified that could distinguish GBM (grade IV) from AA (grade III) with an accuracy of 95% (Rao *et al.*).

While many studies identifying an individual miRNA or miRNA expression signatures predicting patient survival in several cancers like lung cancer, lymphocytic leukemia; lung adenocarcinoma, breast and pancreas cancers have been published, there are only a few reports with respect to glioblastoma. Expression profiling of 84 astrocytoma samples belonging to different grades and 20 normal adjacent tissue samples and subsequent multivariate Cox proportional hazard regression analysis and Kaplan-Meier survival analysis identified low expression of miR-181b or miR-106a or high expression of miR-21 to be associated with poor patient survival (Zhi *et al.*). Another recent study analysed the miRNA (n=304) expression data from a total of 222 GBM patients derived from The Cancer Genome Atlas (TCGA) data set using Cox proportional hazard regression analysis and identified a 10 miRNA expression signature that predicted survival (Srinivasan *et al.*). More importantly, using multivariate analysis along with patient age, the 10 miRNA expression signature was found to be an independent predictor of patient survival. In addition, the authors developed a risk score for each patient based on the expression of each of these ten miRNAs and subsequently showed that the risk score could segregate the patients into high and low risk groups with significantly different survival times. It was also interesting to note that the miRNA set included three miRNAs (miR-20a, miR-106a and miR-17-5p) that were protective and seven miRNAs (hsa-miR-31, hsa-miR-222, hsa-miR-148a, hsa-miR-221, hsa-miR-146b, hsa-miR-200b and hsa-miR-193a) that were risky with respect to their association between their expression and patient survival. The protective miRNAs were expressed at an elevated level in the low risk group compared to the high risk group and the risky miRNAs were expressed at a higher level in the high risk group than in the low risk group. It was suggested that the protective and risky nature of these miRNAs is indicative of their functions being either inhibitory or promoting, respectively, of various properties of cancer cells like proliferation, migration, invasion etc.

The use of miRNAs in cancer therapy involves two approaches. The first approach, which is rather more commonly followed, is to inhibit oncogenic miRNAs with a gain of function using miRNA antagonists. The second approach involves reintroduction of a tumour suppressor miRNA with the resultant restoration of loss of function. An interesting view of the potential use of miRNA based cancer therapy is that targets that are considered to be undruggable could be targeted using miRNA approach. It was estimated that approximately only 20% of all human proteins are targetable by small molecules and inhibitory antibodies with the remaining 80% of genes coming under the category that are currently considered undruggable (Verdine, 2006). Since the RNA interference based approach using miRNAs can essentially target any human gene, this approach opens up a large number of potential targets.

Several reports have shown the potential use of miRNA-based approach in glioma therapy as a proof-of-principle. miR-21 being one of the most upregulated miRNAs in gliomas, with anti-apoptotic and pro-invasive functions, appears to be an automatic choice for therapeutic interventions. Corsten *et al* studied the combined effect of inhibiting miR-21 and neural precursor cells (NPC)-mediated secretable variant of the cytotoxic agent tumour necrosis factor–related apoptosis inducing ligand (S-TRAIL) on glioma (U87) tumour growth using an intra-cranial glioma model using athymic mice (Corsten *et al.*, 2007). The ability of U87 glioma cells to form tumour reduced significantly upon introduction of locked nucleic acid (LNA) antimiR-21 oligonucleotides. Further, simultaneous injection of NPCs expressing S-TRAIL along with miR-21 anti-miR treated U87 cells led to synergistic cytotoxicity with the complete elimination of tumour growth. In another study involving a tumour suppressor miRNA - miR-34a, its reintroduction into U87 glioma cells led to strong inhibition of tumour growth in xenograft models (Li *et al.*, 2009a). miR-296, which belongs to the new family of angiomirs, which are proangiogenic, was found to be elevated in human primary brain microvascular endothelial cells upon co-culturing with U87 glioma cells (Wurdinger *et al.*, 2008). Intravenous administration of miR-296 antagomirs into mice bearing subcutaneous U87 tumours resulted in significant reduction of angiogenesis in tumour xenografts suggesting the potential utility in glioma therapy.

6. Conclusions

miRNAs have generated a huge excitement in the field of cancer biology. During the last six years, several studies have established the regulation of miRNAs in glioma development, identified their targets and demonstrated their role in cell proliferation, apoptosis, cell cycle regulation, migration, invasion and angiogenesis. This indicates that defects in miRNA regulatory network appear to play a key role in glioblastoma pathogenesis. Many of these studies have clearly showed as a proof-of-concept, the utility of miRNA based approach in glioma diagnosis, grading, prognosis and therapy. However, additional studies are needed to confirm these findings for the eventual application in clinics. With total number of known human miRNAs is 1040 (Release 16, miRBase), one of important needs is to carry out more comprehensive analysis of all known miRNAs in large number of tumour tissue samples. Efforts towards identifying targets, their experimental validation and establishing the relationships with various altered molecular pathways in cancer are also very important. In addition to improved understanding of biology of glioma development and progression, miRNA study appears to provide newer improved methods useful for variety of purposes in clinical medicine. Like with other biomarkers, the use of miRNAs in glioma classification and prognosis requires more studies in large cohorts at independent laboratories. The use of miRNA based glioma therapy appears to be very highly promising. The development of better methods of *in vivo* delivery of miRNAs is likely to harness the utility of miRNA in glioma therapy.

7. Acknowledgements

This study was supported by a grant from DBT, Government of India. Infrastructural support by funding from ICMR, DBT, DST and UGC to MCB is acknowledged. SAR and ZN gratefully acknowledge SRF from CSIR.

8. References

Bader AG, Brown D, Winkler M The promise of microRNA replacement therapy. *Cancer Res* 70: 7027-30.

Bohnsack MT, Czaplinski K, Gorlich D (2004). Exportin 5 is a RanGTP-dependent dsRNA-binding protein that mediates nuclear export of pre-miRNAs. *RNA* 10: 185-91.

Brueckner B, Stresemann C, Kuner R, Mund C, Musch T, Meister M *et al* (2007). The human let-7a-3 locus contains an epigenetically regulated microRNA gene with oncogenic function. *Cancer Res* 67: 1419-23.

Cai X, Hagedorn CH, Cullen BR (2004). Human microRNAs are processed from capped, polyadenylated transcripts that can also function as mRNAs. *RNA* 10: 1957-66.

Chan JA, Krichevsky AM, Kosik KS (2005). MicroRNA-21 is an antiapoptotic factor in human glioblastoma cells. *Cancer Res* 65: 6029-33.

Chen Y, Liu W, Chao T, Zhang Y, Yan X, Gong Y *et al* (2008). MicroRNA-21 down-regulates the expression of tumor suppressor PDCD4 in human glioblastoma cell T98G. *Cancer Lett* 272: 197-205.

Chendrimada TP, Gregory RI, Kumaraswamy E, Norman J, Cooch N, Nishikura K *et al* (2005). TRBP recruits the Dicer complex to Ago2 for microRNA processing and gene silencing. *Nature* 436: 740-4.

Ciafre SA, Galardi S, Mangiola A, Ferracin M, Liu CG, Sabatino G *et al* (2005). Extensive modulation of a set of microRNAs in primary glioblastoma. *Biochem Biophys Res Commun* 334: 1351-8.

Conti A, Aguennouz M, La Torre D, Tomasello C, Cardali S, Angileri FF *et al* (2009). miR-21 and 221 upregulation and miR-181b downregulation in human grade II-IV astrocytic tumors. *J Neurooncol* 93: 325-32.

Corsten MF, Miranda R, Kasmieh R, Krichevsky AM, Weissleder R, Shah K (2007). MicroRNA-21 knockdown disrupts glioma growth in vivo and displays synergistic cytotoxicity with neural precursor cell delivered S-TRAIL in human gliomas. *Cancer Res* 67: 8994-9000.

Davis BN, Hata A (2009). Regulation of MicroRNA Biogenesis: A miRiad of mechanisms. *Cell Commun Signal* 7: 18.

Davis BN, Hilyard AC, Lagna G, Hata A (2008). SMAD proteins control DROSHA-mediated microRNA maturation. *Nature* 454: 56-61.

Du T, Zamore PD (2005). microPrimer: the biogenesis and function of microRNA. *Development* 132: 4645-52.

Gabriely G, Wurdinger T, Kesari S, Esau CC, Burchard J, Linsley PS *et al* (2008). MicroRNA 21 promotes glioma invasion by targeting matrix metalloproteinase regulators. *Mol Cell Biol* 28: 5369-80.

Godlewski J, Nowicki MO, Bronisz A, Williams S, Otsuki A, Nuovo G *et al* (2008). Targeting of the Bmi-1 oncogene/stem cell renewal factor by microRNA-128 inhibits glioma proliferation and self-renewal. *Cancer Res* 68: 9125-30.

Gregory RI, Chendrimada TP, Cooch N, Shiekhattar R (2005). Human RISC couples microRNA biogenesis and posttranscriptional gene silencing. *Cell* 123: 631-40.

Gregory RI, Yan KP, Amuthan G, Chendrimada T, Doratotaj B, Cooch N *et al* (2004). The Microprocessor complex mediates the genesis of microRNAs. *Nature* 432: 235-40.

He L, He X, Lowe SW, Hannon GJ (2007). microRNAs join the p53 network--another piece in the tumour-suppression puzzle. *Nat Rev Cancer* 7: 819-22.

Huse JT, Brennan C, Hambardzumyan D, Wee B, Pena J, Rouhanifard SH *et al* (2009). The PTEN-regulating microRNA miR-26a is amplified in high-grade glioma and facilitates gliomagenesis in vivo. *Genes Dev* 23: 1327-37.

Hutvagner G, Zamore PD (2002). A microRNA in a multiple-turnover RNAi enzyme complex. *Science* 297: 2056-60.

Katakowski M, Zheng X, Jiang F, Rogers T, Szalad A, Chopp M MiR-146b-5p suppresses EGFR expression and reduces in vitro migration and invasion of glioma. *Cancer Invest* 28: 1024-30.

Kefas B, Godlewski J, Comeau L, Li Y, Abounader R, Hawkinson M *et al* (2008). microRNA-7 inhibits the epidermal growth factor receptor and the Akt pathway and is down-regulated in glioblastoma. *Cancer Res* 68: 3566-72.

Kim H, Huang W, Jiang X, Pennicooke B, Park PJ, Johnson MD Integrative genome analysis reveals an oncomir/oncogene cluster regulating glioblastoma survivorship. *Proc Natl Acad Sci U S A* 107: 2183-8.

Kim VN (2005). MicroRNA biogenesis: coordinated cropping and dicing. *Nat Rev Mol Cell Biol* 6: 376-85.

Kwak HJ, Kim YJ, Chun KR, Woo YM, Park SJ, Jeong JA *et al* Downregulation of Spry2 by miR-21 triggers malignancy in human gliomas. *Oncogene*.

Landthaler M, Yalcin A, Tuschl T (2004). The human DiGeorge syndrome critical region gene 8 and Its D. melanogaster homolog are required for miRNA biogenesis. *Curr Biol* 14: 2162-7.

Lee RC, Feinbaum RL, Ambros V (1993). The C. elegans heterochronic gene lin-4 encodes small RNAs with antisense complementarity to lin-14. *Cell* 75: 843-54.

Lee Y, Hur I, Park SY, Kim YK, Suh MR, Kim VN (2006). The role of PACT in the RNA silencing pathway. *EMBO J* 25: 522-32.

Lee Y, Kim M, Han J, Yeom KH, Lee S, Baek SH *et al* (2004). MicroRNA genes are transcribed by RNA polymerase II. *EMBO J* 23: 4051-60.

Lewis BP, Burge CB, Bartel DP (2005). Conserved seed pairing, often flanked by adenosines, indicates that thousands of human genes are microRNA targets. *Cell* 120: 15-20.

Li Y, Guessous F, Zhang Y, Dipierro C, Kefas B, Johnson E *et al* (2009a). MicroRNA-34a inhibits glioblastoma growth by targeting multiple oncogenes. *Cancer Res* 69: 7569-76.

Li Y, Li W, Yang Y, Lu Y, He C, Hu G *et al* (2009b). MicroRNA-21 targets LRRFIP1 and contributes to VM-26 resistance in glioblastoma multiforme. *Brain Res* 1286: 13-8.

Liu J, Carmell MA, Rivas FV, Marsden CG, Thomson JM, Song JJ *et al* (2004). Argonaute2 is the catalytic engine of mammalian RNAi. *Science* 305: 1437-41.

Lu J, Getz G, Miska EA, Alvarez-Saavedra E, Lamb J, Peck D *et al* (2005). MicroRNA expression profiles classify human cancers. *Nature* 435: 834-8.

Lujambio A, Calin GA, Villanueva A, Ropero S, Sanchez-Cespedes M, Blanco D *et al* (2008). A microRNA DNA methylation signature for human cancer metastasis. *Proc Natl Acad Sci U S A* 105: 13556-61.

Lund E, Guttinger S, Calado A, Dahlberg JE, Kutay U (2004). Nuclear export of microRNA precursors. *Science* 303: 95-8.

Malzkorn B, Wolter M, Liesenberg F, Grzendowski M, Stuhler K, Meyer HE *et al* Identification and functional characterization of microRNAs involved in the malignant progression of gliomas. *Brain Pathol* 20: 539-50.

Maniataki E, Mourelatos Z (2005). A human, ATP-independent, RISC assembly machine fueled by pre-miRNA. *Genes Dev* 19: 2979-90.

Medina R, Zaidi SK, Liu CG, Stein JL, van Wijnen AJ, Croce CM *et al* (2008). MicroRNAs 221 and 222 bypass quiescence and compromise cell survival. *Cancer Res* 68: 2773-80.

Meister G, Landthaler M, Patkaniowska A, Dorsett Y, Teng G, Tuschl T (2004). Human Argonaute2 mediates RNA cleavage targeted by miRNAs and siRNAs. *Mol Cell* 15: 185-97.

Nan Y, Han L, Zhang A, Wang G, Jia Z, Yang Y *et al* MiRNA-451 plays a role as tumor suppressor in human glioma cells. *Brain Res* 1359: 14-21.

Novakova J, Slaby O, Vyzula R, Michalek J (2009). MicroRNA involvement in glioblastoma pathogenesis. *Biochem Biophys Res Commun* 386: 1-5.

Papagiannakopoulos T, Shapiro A, Kosik KS (2008). MicroRNA-21 targets a network of key tumor-suppressive pathways in glioblastoma cells. *Cancer Res* 68: 8164-72.

Rao SA, Santosh V, Somasundaram K Genome-wide expression profiling identifies deregulated miRNAs in malignant astrocytoma. *Mod Pathol* 23: 1404-17.

Ren Y, Zhou X, Mei M, Yuan XB, Han L, Wang GX *et al* MicroRNA-21 inhibitor sensitizes human glioblastoma cells U251 (PTEN-mutant) and LN229 (PTEN-wild type) to taxol. *BMC Cancer* 10: 27.

Ruby JG, Jan C, Player C, Axtell MJ, Lee W, Nusbaum C *et al* (2006). Large-scale sequencing reveals 21U-RNAs and additional microRNAs and endogenous siRNAs in C. elegans. *Cell* 127: 1193-207.

Ruby JG, Jan CH, Bartel DP (2007). Intronic microRNA precursors that bypass Drosha processing. *Nature* 448: 83-6.

Shi L, Chen J, Yang J, Pan T, Zhang S, Wang Z MiR-21 protected human glioblastoma U87MG cells from chemotherapeutic drug temozolomide induced apoptosis by decreasing Bax/Bcl-2 ratio and caspase-3 activity. *Brain Res* 1352: 255-64.

Shi L, Cheng Z, Zhang J, Li R, Zhao P, Fu Z *et al* (2008). hsa-mir-181a and hsa-mir-181b function as tumor suppressors in human glioma cells. *Brain Res* 1236: 185-93.

Shi L, Zhang J, Pan T, Zhou J, Gong W, Liu N *et al* MiR-125b is critical for the suppression of human U251 glioma stem cell proliferation. *Brain Res* 1312: 120-6.

Silber J, Lim DA, Petritsch C, Persson AI, Maunakea AK, Yu M *et al* (2008). miR-124 and miR-137 inhibit proliferation of glioblastoma multiforme cells and induce differentiation of brain tumor stem cells. *BMC Med* 6: 14.

Song L, Huang Q, Chen K, Liu L, Lin C, Dai T *et al* miR-218 inhibits the invasive ability of glioma cells by direct downregulation of IKK-beta. *Biochem Biophys Res Commun* 402: 135-40.

Srinivasan S, Patric IR, Somasundaram K A Ten-microRNA Expression Signature Predicts Survival in Glioblastoma. *PLoS One* 6: e17438.

Verdine GL (2006). Drugging the "undruggable". *Harvey Lect* 102: 1-15.

Wurdinger T, Tannous BA, Saydam O, Skog J, Grau S, Soutschek J *et al* (2008). miR-296 regulates growth factor receptor overexpression in angiogenic endothelial cells. *Cancer Cell* 14: 382-93.

Xia H, Qi Y, Ng SS, Chen X, Chen S, Fang M *et al* (2009a). MicroRNA-15b regulates cell cycle progression by targeting cyclins in glioma cells. *Biochem Biophys Res Commun* 380: 205-10.

Xia H, Qi Y, Ng SS, Chen X, Li D, Chen S *et al* (2009b). microRNA-146b inhibits glioma cell migration and invasion by targeting MMPs. *Brain Res* 1269: 158-65.

Xia HF, He TZ, Liu CM, Cui Y, Song PP, Jin XH *et al* (2009c). MiR-125b expression affects the proliferation and apoptosis of human glioma cells by targeting Bmf. *Cell Physiol Biochem* 23: 347-58.

Yi R, Qin Y, Macara IG, Cullen BR (2003). Exportin-5 mediates the nuclear export of pre-microRNAs and short hairpin RNAs. *Genes Dev* 17: 3011-6.

Zhang CZ, Zhang JX, Zhang AL, Shi ZD, Han L, Jia ZF *et al* MiR-221 and miR-222 target PUMA to induce cell survival in glioblastoma. *Mol Cancer* 9: 229.

Zhang Y, Chao T, Li R, Liu W, Chen Y, Yan X *et al* (2009). MicroRNA-128 inhibits glioma cells proliferation by targeting transcription factor E2F3a. *J Mol Med* 87: 43-51.

Zhi F, Chen X, Wang S, Xia X, Shi Y, Guan W *et al* The use of hsa-miR-21, hsa-miR-181b and hsa-miR-106a as prognostic indicators of astrocytoma. *Eur J Cancer* 46: 1640-9.

Zhou X, Ren Y, Moore L, Mei M, You Y, Xu P *et al* Downregulation of miR-21 inhibits EGFR pathway and suppresses the growth of human glioblastoma cells independent of PTEN status. *Lab Invest* 90: 144-55.

17

MicroRNA in Human Gliomas

Alfredo Conti, Lucia Merlo, Domenico La Torre
and M'Hammed Aguennouz
Department of Neuroscience, University of Messina
Italy

1. Introduction

Glioblastoma multiforme (GBM) is the most common primitive malignant brain tumor. The GBM rapidly proliferates, invades and destroys surrounding brain tissues being nearly universally fatal in few months. Actual treatment options include surgery, radiotherapy, and chemotherapy using temozolomide (Stupp et al., 2005). As soon as the disease recurs, repeated surgery or administration of modified chemotherapy schemes give small chances of tumor growth control. Even with the most sophisticated treatments, the median overall survival for patients with GBM is actually estimated in approximately 15 months from diagnosis (Stupp et al., 2005).

Within the last few years, a more detailed knowledge of the genetic and molecular patterns of this cancer has led to laboratory's attempts in developing more targeted and effective therapies aiming to positively reverse its high mortality. While many important genetic features of GBM have been known for years or even decades through traditional methods, incremental technologies have allowed dramatic advances. New frontiers have been explored: the relatively recent discovery of microRNAs (miRNAs) has opened up a major new front in the war against GBM and other human tumors. A growing body of work is demonstrating key roles for them in GBM (Chan et al., 2005; Ciafre et al., 2005; Gillies & Lorimer, 2007; Godlewski et al., 2008; Kefas et al., 2008; Kefas et al., 2009; Li et al., 2009; Silber et al., 2008; Würdinger et al., 2008).

Noteworthy is the cancer genome atlas (TCGA), a joint comprehensive and coordinated effort of the National Cancer Institute (NCI) and the National Human Genome Research Institute (NHGRI), funded by the National Institutes of Health (NIH) in 2006 to thoroughly initially profile three cancer types systematically assessing the molecular basis and the entire spectrum of genomic changes involved in human tumors through the application of innovative genome analysis technologies, including large-scale genome sequencing (http://cancergenome.nih.gov). After the success of the pilot project, TCGA is now expanding its efforts to more than 20 different human tumors in order to yield accessible data set that will improve diagnosis, treatment, prognosis, and even prevention. TCGA has also included studies on miRNA expression with microarrays, copy number analysis with array comparative genomic hybridization (CGH), and sequencing of over 600 genes of banked high-quality tumor specimens.

We here reviewed current literature on the role of miRNAs in GBM emphasizing the potential implications of these molecules as biomarkers and targets for therapy.

2. Biogenesis and functions of microRNAs

The discovery of miRNAs dates back to 1993 when Lee et al. described a small RNA, lineage-deficient-4 (lin-4), with antisense complementarity to lin-14 involved in the regulation of developmental timing in Caenorhabditis elegans (Lee et al., 1993). At that time most investigators considered this small RNA as an oddity in worm genetics, but hundreds of these miRNAs were soon discovered in C. elegans and other animals by different laboratories (Lee & Ambros, 2001; Pasquinelli et al., 2000).

miRNAs consist of 18 to 25 nucleotides and represent a class of endogenous ribo-regulators that modulate gene expression via the RNA interference (RNAi) pathway. RNAi is a post-transcriptional silencing mechanism, present in most eukaryotic organisms, in which exposure to double-stranded RNA induces the sequence specific degradation of homologous messenger RNAs (mRNA). miRNAs act by base-pairing with their target mRNAs through perfect or nearly perfect complementarity particularly at the 3′ untranslated regions (UTRs) of the target mRNAs (Lai, 2002; Robins & Press, 2005) leading to their translational repression and/or direct cleavage (Meltzer, 2005).

To understand the mechanism of miRNA-mediated silencing, the basic steps of their biogenesis have to be summarized (Fig. 1). miRNAs originate from long primary miRNAs (pri-miRNAs) that are transcribed in the nucleus by the RNA polymerase II complex. miRNAs are then processed by a complex of the RNase III enzyme DROSHA and a double-stranded RNA binding domain possessing the protein DGCR8 (DiGeorge syndrome critical region gene 8), to 60-70 nucleotides precursor miRNA (pre-miRNA) intermediates. These hairpin-shaped pre-miRNAs are transported to the cytoplasm by Exportin-5 (Exp5) (a member of the Ran transport receptor family). Once in the cytoplasm, they are cleaved by DICER to generate 20 to 22 nucleotide duplexes bearing two nucleotide single-stranded 3′ extensions. Finally, the miRNA: miRNA* duplex is unwound into a mature miRNA and miRNA* by a helicase. Single strand miRNA is incorporated into a ribonucleoprotein effector complex, known as the RNA-induced silencing complex (RISC), whereas miRNA* is degraded. RISC identifies target messages based on complementarities between the "guide" miRNA and the mRNA and results in either endonucleolytic cleavage of targeted mRNA or translational repression.

There are estimates, in part based on computational methods, that mammalian genomes encode up to 1,000 unique miRNAs (http://www.microrna.org/microrna/home.do), which are predicted to regulate the expression of as much as 60% of gene (Friedmann et al., 2009). Though more than 600 miRNAs have been identified in humans, much remains to be understood about their precise cellular function and role in the development of diseases. miRNAs are implicated in the control of many fundamental cellular and biological processes such as the developmental timing, stem cell division, and apoptosis (Brennecke et al., 2003; Chen et al., 2004; Cuellar & McManus 2005; Harfe et al., 2005; Lim et al., 2005; Poy et al., 2004; Wilfred et al., 2007). Therefore changes in their expression may play a role in the development of diseases and cancer.

Calin and Croce first established a connection between microRNAs and cancer by showing that miR-15 and miR-16 are located on chromosome 13q14, a region deleted in more than half of B-cell chronic lymphocytic leukemia (CLL) (Calin & Croce, 2006). Cimmino et al. then demonstrated that expression of miR-15a and miR-16-1was inversely correlated with Bcl-2 expression in CLL and that both miRNAs negatively regulated Bcl-2 at a posttranscriptional level, so explaining the exact role of those miRNAs in CLL. Furthermore, Bcl-2 repression by these miRNAs induced apoptosis in a leukemic cell line model (Cimmino et al., 2005).

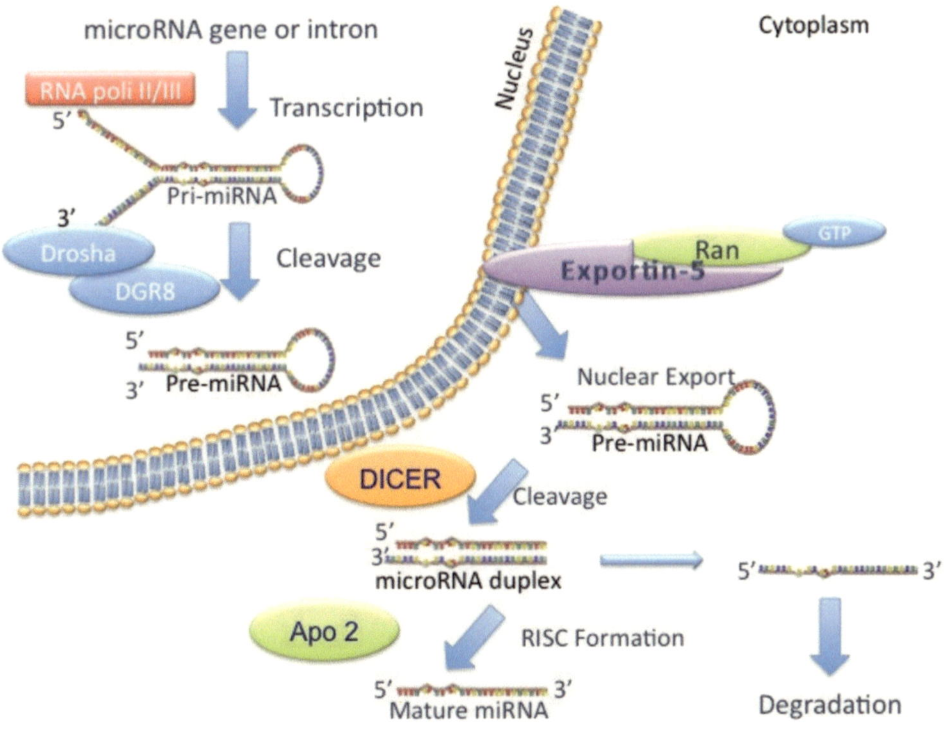

Fig. 1. Schematic representation of biogenesis of microRNA

3. MicroRNAs in brain cancer

Molecular-genetic, array-based gene profiling analysis of GBM, and gain- or loss-of-function study showed that specific deregulations in both mRNA and miRNAs are strongly associated with glioma development and progression (Juric et al., 2007; Kumar et al., 2007; Louis, 2006; Lukiw et al., 2009; Novakova et al., 2009; Pang et al., 2009; Tso et al., 2006; Zeng, 2009). It's possible to identify different subsets of miRNAs according to their main function into the development of GBM.

3.1 Oncogenes

The first oncomiR demonstrated as strongly overexpressed in GBM was miR-21 (Chan et al., 2005; Krichevsky et al., 2003) and it still remains the best characterized. miR-21 acts as oncogene in cultured GBM cells; moreover, it was found to be up-regulated yet in low-grade tumors (Conti et al., 2009). Its relevant targets appear to include tumor-suppressive genes (Frankel et al., 2008; Gabriely et al., 2008; Meng et al., 2007; Zhu et al., 2008). In fact, it has been demonstrated that inhibiting miR-21 by complementary antisense oligonucleotides in glioma cell lines decreases tumor cell viability inducing apoptosis both in vitro and in vivo settings (Chan et al., 2005, Corsten et al., 2007, Zhou et al., 2010). Recent researches showed how an overexpression of mir-21 could protect cultured human cells of GBM from temozolomide and taxol-induced apoptosis, suggesting a role in resistance to chemotherapeutic treatments (Ren et al., 2010; Shi et al., 2010). Even though an antiapoptotic role is likely for miR-21 in gliomas, other mechanisms are possible, because in Hela cells its down-regulation determines, instead, an increase in cell proliferation without affecting apoptosis. Meng et al. demonstrated that knock-down of miR-21 may render cholangiocarcinoma cells sensitive to gemcitabine whereas transfection of non-malignant cholangiocytes with the precursor of miR-21 renders them more resistant to this drug (Meng et al., 2007). This may be the result of downregulation of PTEN, the phosphatase that antagonizes the growth-promoting activity of the PI-3 kinase-Akt signaling pathway. It is noteworthy that PTEN was originally cloned as a oncosuppressor for brain tumors with point mutations occurring in 25% of cases. Further work by Frankel et al. on breast cancer cells (Frankel et al., 2008) and by Asangani et al. (Asangani et al., 2008) on colon cancer cells found that miR-21 overexpression leads to PDCD4 (programmed cell death 4) reduction, by direct interaction with its 3′ UTR, and that anti-miR-21 treatment is followed by an increase in endogenous PDCD4 protein levels. PDCD4 is a tumor suppressor known to be up-regulated during apoptosis and reduced in different tumors, and evidence demonstrates that miR-21 overexpression effects are at least in part due to PDCD4 down-regulation. Although this target has not been proven in brain tumors, it is possible that it may be relevant also in these tumor types, as a recent study demonstrated that most of the glioma samples analyzed lacked PDCD4 protein expression whereas adjacent normal glial tissues expressed high levels of it. An additional molecular mechanism, proving the oncogenic properties of miR-21 in an in-vivo xenograft breast cancer model, consists in targeting of the tumor suppressor protein tropomyosin 1 (TPM1) at the translational level. Tropomyosin is able per se to reduce tumor cell proliferation and anchorage independence, therefore explaining the effects on tumor growth exerted by miR-21 (Zhu et al., 2007).

miR-221 and miR-222 are two oncogenic miRNA overexpressed in GBM which enhance cell proliferation and survival (Ciafre et al., 2005; Felicetti et al., 2008; Galardi et al., 2007; Lee et al., 2007) targeting cell cycle inhibitors.

Gillies and Lorimer defined a specific function of miRNA 221 and 222 in GBM, showing that they repress expression of the cell cycle regulatory protein p27Kip1 (Gillies & Lorimer, 2007). The p27Kip1 gene is a member of the Cip/Kip family of cyclin-dependent kinase (CDK) inhibitors whose function is to negatively control cell cycle progression. The protein binds to CDK2 and cyclin E complexes to prevent cell cycle progression from G1 to S phase. p27Kip1 also acts as a tumor suppressor and its expression is often disrupted in human cancers. Analysis of the 3′ UTR of p27Kip1 suggests that repression of this protein is a consequence of direct binding of miRNA 221 and 222 to sites in the 3′ UTR. This mechanism was suggested contemporaneously and independently by le Sage et al. who demonstrated, using miRNA inhibitors, that some GBM cell lines require high activity of miR-221 and 222 to maintain low p27Kip1 levels and continuous proliferation, and that high levels of miR-221 and 222 seem to correlate with low levels of p27Kip1 protein in GBM (le Sage et al., 2007). Gonzalez et al. have previously shown that inhibition of cdk4 activity enhances translation of p27Kip1, providing a link between these two cell-cycle regulators (Gonzalez et al., 2003). This effect was shown to be mediated by the 3′ UTR of p27Kip1. The GBM cells used in that study were mutated at the INK4A/ARF locus and did not express the cdk4 inhibitor p16Ink4a (Ishii et al., 1999). This suggested the possibility that loss of cdk4 inhibition through INK4a/ARF mutations causes an increase in miR-221 levels, and a consequent decrease in p27Kip1. p27Kip1 is a well-known tumor suppressor down-regulated in many human tumors, and its expression in primary cancers is highly correlated with reduced patient survival.

Other oncomiR clusters affecting different targets that have been shown to be up-regulated in both GBM and other tumors are miR-10b (Ciafre et al., 2005; Ma et al., 2007; Silber et al., 2008) and the recently discovered miR-26a (Kim et al., 2010). miR-10b might play some role in the invasion of glioma cells by a positive regulation of RhoC (Sasayama et al., 2009) and urokinase-type plasminogen activator receptor (uPAR) and MMP-14 (Sun et al., 2011). miR-26a is a direct regulator of PTEN expression and is frequently amplified at the DNA level in human glioma, most often in association with monoallelic loss of PTEN (Huse et al., 2009).

3.2 Oncosuppressors

miR-34a is a well-characterized molecule playing a role as tumor suppressor. It has been found to be an important downstream mediator of p53 (He et al., 2007; Luan et al., 2010; Sun et al., 2008). Recent reports suggested a role for miR-34a in GBM (Li et al., 2009) and in vitro studies described that its overexpression results in inhibition of neoplastic cell growth and apoptosis (Luan et al., 2010).

Other studies identified miR-124 and miR-137 as potential oncosuppressors (Silber et al., 2008). miR-124 seems to be the most down-regulated miRNA in GBM as compared with low-grade gliomas and healthy brain tissue. Down-regulation of miR-124 allows cell cycle progression and increases tumorigenic power by preventing neuronal differentiation (Godlewski et al., 2008; Silber et al., 2008). In vitro, the expression of miR-137 was found to be increased up to 12-fold (Silber et al., 2008). Moreover, transfection of miRNA-124 or miRNA-137 induced morphological changes and enhanced marker expression consistent with neuronal differentiation in mouse and human GBM-derived neural stem cells, also inducing G1 cell cycle arrest in GBM cells (Silber et al., 2008). These results led to hypothesize that targeted delivery of miRNA-124 and/or miRNA-137 to GBM tumor cells may be therapeutically employed.

Also miRNA-128 is significantly down-regulated in vivo and in GBM cell lines resulting in proliferation of undifferentiated cells. Moreover, in human glioma cell cultures the overexpression of miR 128 specifically blocks glioma self-renewal factors. This implicates that miR-128 may be used against the "stem cell-like" characteristics of glioma cells (Godlewski et al., 2008). In addition, the down-regulation of miRNA-128 was found to inversely correlate with tumor grade (Cui et al., 2010).

miRNA-181 may also play a role in glioma development. Shi et al. reported the downregulation of miR-181 and 181b in both human gliomas and glioma cell lines (Shi et al., 2008), confirming the data of Ciafre et al. (Ciafre et al., 2005). Those authors showed that transfection of those miRNAs triggered growth inhibition and apoptosis, and inhibited invasion. Furthermore, miR-181a expression turned out to be inversely correlated with tumor grading whereas miR-181b was uniformly downregulated in gliomas with different grades of malignancy.

miR-184 is another putative suppressor of glioma progression. The expression of miR-184 is down-regulated during progression from low-grade to GBM. Furthermore, its over-expression significantly decreases cell viability and proliferation of neoplastic cells, suggesting an anti-proliferative tumor-suppressive role of this miRNA, through a possible regulation of c-Myc (Würdinger et al., 2008). Interestingly, miR-184 is able to increase and reduce apoptotic activity and invasive growth in different subset of cultured cells (Malzkorn et al., 2010).

3.3 Metabolism, angiogenesis, immunosuppression, treatment resistance

MicroRNAs have been linked specifically with a number of key features affecting the viability of GBM cells including metabolism, angiogenesis, immunosuppression, radio- and chemoresistance.

Aberrant metabolism is increasingly recognized as critical issue in GBM biology. A report recently showed how miRNAs are involved in its regulation. miR-451, a miRNA with a role in cell proliferation and migration, is influenced by glucose levels and metabolic stress typically presented in GBM (Godlewski et al., 2010). It has been demonstrated that an increased expression of mirR-451 inhibits cell growth, inducing G0/G1 phase transition arrest, and predisposes to apoptosis. Furthermore, it diminishes the invasive capacity of GBM cells (Nan et al., 2010).

Angiogenesis plays a pivotal role in the progression of most solid tumors, and miR-296 is up-regulated in GBM-associated endothelial cells promoting tumor angiogenesis (Würdinger et al., 2008).

Immunosuppression is another trait allowing tumors to grow, and miRNAs have been shown to play a role here as well: miR-222 and miR-339 were found to promote GBM immune evasion by down-regulating the immunologic molecule ICAM-1 (Ueda et al., 2009).

Treatment resistance is one of the principal challenges in GBM therapy, and early results of modern laboratory researches hint at a possible miRNAs involvement. In recent studies, a temozolomide-resistant GBM cell line was found to have several up-regulated miRNAs versus the parental line, including miR-21, miR-195, miR-455-3p, and miR-10a* (Shi et al., 2010; Ujifuku et al., 2010). Also during radiotherapy, miR-181a and miR-181b, usually down-regulated in GBM (Conti et al., 2009), may influence the sensitivity of this tumor to radiation (Slaby et al., 2010).

3.4 Prognosis and grading

A role for miRNAs as prognostic biomarkers as been suggested as well. Real-time PCR quantitative analysis revealed increased expression levels of miR-196 in GBM cells in comparison with both anaplastic astrocytomas and normal brain. Furthermore, this subset of neoplastic patients showed significantly poorer survival. The expression level of miR-196 was an independent predictor of overall survival (Guan et al., 2010).

miR-182 was markedly up-regulated both in glioma cell lines and in human tumor specimens. Quantitative PCR analysis showed that its expression was significantly upregulated in GBM compared with the adjacent healthy brain tissue. Furthermore, statistical analysis revealed a significant correlation between miR-182 expression and tumor grading placing miR-182 as independent prognostic indicator for disease progression and survival (Jiang et al., 2010).

Promising reliable biomarkers of GBM thoroughly studied so far are miR-21, miR-124 and miR-128.

As abovementioned, miR-21 acts as an oncogene whose inhibition in GBM cells induce apoptosis (Chan et al., 2005) and reduce tumor cells invasiveness (Gabriely et al., 2008).

Recent studies also identified as miR-21 targets some tumor suppressors (Papagiannakopoulos & Kosik, 2008) and inhibitors of matrix metalloproteinase (Gabriely et al., 2008). Moreover, its expression increases 5- to 100-fold during human glioma progression from lower grades to GBM (Chan et al., 2005), making miR-21 a consistent both diagnostic and prognostic marker.

miR-124 is downregulated in GBM. miR-124 has been identified as a suppressor of proteins that drive neural precursors toward non-neuronal fat (Makeyev et al., 2007). These data, together with the finding that one of the miR-124 targets is the oncogenic cyclin dependent kinase 6 (Pierson et al., 2008), support the role for miR-124 as a tumor suppressor and a potentially relevant biomarker in early diagnosis.

miR-128 is another neuron-specific miRNA involved in neural tissue differentiation. It acts as a tumor-suppressor gene and is downregulated in GBM (Ciafre et al., 2005; Godlewski et al., 2008). Recent studies have shown that it inhibits the cell cycle progression and GBM proliferation targeting a transcription factor (Zhang et al., 2009).

The study of epigenetics in GBM is another important frontier at a relatively early stage, and there are major discoveries yet to be made. Powerful input from this field has come during the last several years with the discovery of frequent methylation in GBM of the promoter of the MGMT gene (Gonzalez-Gomez et al., 2003). Found in about 30% of GBMs, MGMT promoter methylation appears to sensitize this subset to the effects of temozolomide and confers improved prognosis (Hegi et al., 2005). A recent survey addresses miR-181 as a predictive marker for the responsiveness to the combination of radiotherapy and temozolomide, founding it downregulated in this cohort of patients (Slaby et al., 2010).

Despite the abovementioned evidence, it is quite clear that the use of a single miRNA as biomarker presently lacks of sufficient sensitivity and specificity, whereas the study of multiple miRNAs expression will possibly be used as a cluster to increase accuracy (Kong, et al., 2009).

4. miRNAs: a future scenario

There is a desperate need for developing innovative therapies for GBM. The clinical potential of delivering tumor-suppressive miRNAs or inhibitors of oncogenic miRNAs has been recently advocated (Brown et al., 2007; Edge et al., 2008; Gomez-Manzano & Fueyo, 2010; Wu et al., 2009). The ability of individual miRNAs to target multiple genes/pathways and, at the same time, the capacity of multiple miRNAs in addressing the same 3' UTR of a single gene, could be a major advantage, especially given the therapeutic necessity of simultaneously targeting multiple pathways in a multifaceted disease such as GBM. Furthermore, small-molecule drugs can have advantages like oral bioavailability and ability to penetrate the blood-brain barrier.

miRNAs are all expressed endogenously and are supposed to be safe for normal cells; nonetheless, their off-target effects would likely be much higher than other gene therapies targeted on a single gene/protein. Despite promising in vitro results, the use of miRNAs for the treatment of brain tumors poses great difficulties. A lot of interrogatives still remain under debate, but the main question rounds on how many molecules can be delivered and what kind of vehicle should be used to achieve therapeutic effects. So far, there are no studies to answer those questions.

More interestingly, with recent advances in detecting and quantifying miRNAs in tissue, serum, and cerebrospinal fluid it appears increasingly likely that they would be clinically useful as specific and reliable biomarkers patterns for brain tumors and other cancer diseases (De Smaele et al., 2010). Actually, miRNAs possess tissue specific expression in different regions of CNS (Bak et al., 2008; Cao et al., 2006; Trivedi & Ramakrishna, 2009) and some of them have been found typically expressed in the human brain with low variability (Smirnova et al., 2005); moreover, they have also been demonstrated to be relevant for neural differentiation of embryonic stem cells (Smirnova et al., 2005) and in tumorigenesis. The feature conferring them this putative role in early diagnosis of malignant brain tumors is their scarce susceptibility to protease degradation. This aspect allows their detection not only from fresh specimens, but also from plasma and serum (Cortez & Calin, 2009) and even after formalin fixation (Hasemeier et al., 2008). As for blood samples, miRNAs have been found in a more stable form, compared to mRNA, that is protected from endogenous RNase denaturation, either free (Mitchell et al., 2008) or enveloped in exosomes (Simpson et al., 2009). Glioblastoma derived exosomes founded in blood samples contain specific miRNAs (Skog et al., 2008). Hence the possibility to detect non-invasively miRNA in patients affected by GBM by the use of real time PCR has made them ideal candidates as biomarkers. Therefore, there is a possibility that they may be used as early diagnostic tools or markers of treatment response.

In conclusion, the uncovering of miRNAs has added a new level of complexity to our understanding in genetics of tumors. At the same time, it revealed a new category of therapeutic targets. There are huge amounts of data from researches that are still to be systematized, and new findings on miRNAs involved in GBM are expected from further analysis.

5. References

Asangani, I.A., Rasheed S.A., Nikolova, D.A., Leupold, J.H., Colburn, N.H., Post, S., & Allgayer, H. (2008). MicroRNA-21 (miR-21) posttranscriptionally downregulates tumor suppressor Pdcd4 and stimulates invasion, intravasation and metastasis in colorectal cancer. *Oncogene* 27: 2128–2136.

Bak, M., Silahtaroglu, A., Moller, M., Christensen, M., Rath, M.F., Skryabin, B., Tommerup, N., & Kauppinen, S. (2008). MicroRNA expression in the adult mouse central nervous system. *RNA* 14: 432–444.

Brennecke, J., Hipfner, D.R., Stark, A., Russell, R.B., & Cohen, S.M. (2003). bantam encodes a developmentally regulated microRNA that controls cell proliferation and regulates the proapoptotic gene hid in Drosophila. *Cell* 113 (1): 25–36.

Brown, B.D., Gentner, B., Cantore, A., Colleoni, S., Amendola, M., Zingale, A., Baccarini, A., Lazzari, G., Galli, C., & Naldini, L. (2007). Endogenous microRNA can be broadly exploited to regulate transgene expression according to tissue, lineage and differentiation state. *Nat Biotechnol* 25: 1457–1467.

Calin, G.A., & Croce, C.M. (2006). MicroRNA signatures in human cancers. *Nat Rev Cancer* 6:857–866.

Cao, X., Yeo, G., Muotri, A.R., Kuwabara, T., & Gage, F.H. (2006). Noncoding RNAs in the mammalian central nervous system. *Annu Rev Neurosci* 29, 77–103.

Chan, J.A., Krichevsky, A.M., & Kosik, K.S. (2005). MicroRNA-21 is an antiapoptotic factor in human glioblastoma cells. *Cancer Res* 65(14): 6029-6033.

Chen, C.Z., Li, L., Lodish, H.F., & Bartel, D.P. (2004). MicroRNAs modulate hematopoietic lineage differentiation. *Science* 303(5654): 83–6.

Ciafre, S.A., Galardi, S., Mangiola, A., Ferracin, M., Liu, C.G., Sabatino, G., Negrini, M., Maira, G., Croce, C.M., & Farace, M.G. (2005). Extensive modulation of a set of microRNAs in primary glioblastoma. *Biochem Biophys Res Commun* 334(4): 1351-1358.

Cimmino, A., Calin, G.A., Fabbri, M., Iorio, M.V., Ferracin, M., Shimizu, M., Wojcik, S.E., Aqeilan, R.I., Zupo, S., Dono, M., Rassenti, L., Alder, H., Volinia, S., Liu, C.G., Kipps, T.J., Negrini, M., & Croce, C.M. (2005). miR-15 and miR-16 induce apoptosis by targeting BCL2. *Proc Natl Acad Sci USA* 102: 13944–13949.

Conti, A., Aguennouz, M., La Torre, D., Tomasello, C., Cardali, S., Angileri, F.F., Maio, F., Cama, A., Germanò, A., Vita, G., & Tomasello, F. (2009). miR-21 and 221 upregulation and miR-181b downregulation in human grade II–IV astrocytic tumors. *J Neurooncol* 93(3): 325-332.

Corsten, M.F., Miranda, R., Kasmieh, R., Krichevsky, A.M., Weissleder, R., & Shah, K. (2007). MicroRNA-21 knockdown disrupts glioma growth in vivo and displays synergistic cytotoxicity with neural precursor cell delivered S-TRAIL in human gliomas. *Cancer Res* 67: 8994–9000.

Cortez, M.A., & Calin, G.A. (2009). MicroRNA identification in plasma and serum: a new tool to diagnose and monitor diseases. *Expert Opin Biol Ther* 9: 703–711.

Cuellar, T.L., & McManus, M.T. (2005). MicroRNAs and endocrine biology. *J Endocrinol* 187(3): 327–332.

Cui, G.J. , Zhao, Y., Sethi, P., & Li, Y.Y. (2010). Micro-RNA-128 (miRNA-128) down-regulation in glioblastoma targets ARP5 (ANGPTL6), Bmi-1 and E2F-3a, key regulators of brain cell proliferation. *J Neurooncol* 98: 297–304.

De Smaele, E., Ferretti, E., & Gulino, A. (2010). MicroRNAs as biomarkers for CNS cancer and other disorders. *Brain Res* 18;1338: 100-111.

Edge, R.E., Falls, T.J., Brown, C.W., Lichty, B.D., Atkins, H., & Bell, J.C. (2008). A let-7 microRNA-sensitive vesicular stomatitis virus demonstrates tumor-specific replication. *Mol Ther* 16: 1437–1443.

Felicetti, F., Errico, M.C., Bottero, L., Segnalini, P., Stoppacciaro, A., Biffoni, M., Felli, N., Mattia, G., Petrini, M., Colombo, M.P., Peschle, C., & Carè, A. (2008). The promyelocytic leukemia zinc finger-microRNA-221/-222 pathway controls melanoma progression through multiple oncogenic mechanisms. *Cancer Res* 68: 2745–2754.

Frankel, L.B., Christoffersen, N.R., Jacobsen, A., Lindow, M., Krogh, A., & Lund, A.H. (2008). Programmed cell death 4 (PDCD4) is an important functional target of the microRNA miR-21 in breast cancer cells. *J Biol Chem* 283: 1026–1033.

Friedman, R.C., Farh, K.K., Burge, C.B., & Bartel, D.P. (2009). Most mammalian mRNAs are conserved targets of microRNAs. *Genome Res* 19 (1): 92–105.

Gabriely, G., Würdinger, T., Kesari, S., Esau, C.C., Burchard, J., Linsley, P.S., & Krichevsky, A.M. (2008). MiR-21 promotes glioma invasion by targeting MMP regulators. *Mol Cell Biol* 28: 5369–5380.

Galardi, S., Mercatelli, N., Giorda, E., Massalini, S., Frajese, G.V., Ciafrè, S.A., & Farace, M.G. (2007). miR-221 and miR-222 expression affects the proliferation potential of human prostate carcinoma cell lines by targeting p27Kip1. *J Biol Chem* 282: 23716–23724.

Gillies, J.K., & Lorimer, I.A. (2007). Regulation of p27Kip1 by miRNA 221/222 in glioblastoma. *Cell Cycle* 6(16): 2005-2009.

Godlewski, J., Nowicki, M.O., Bronisz, A., Williams, S., Otsuki, A., Nuovo ,G., Raychaudhury, A., Newton, H.B., Chiocca, E.A., & Lawler, S. (2008). Targeting of the Bmi-1 oncogene/stem cell renewal factor by microRNA-128 inhibits glioma proliferation and self-renewal. *Cancer Res* 68(22): 9125-9130.

Godlewski, J., Nowicki, M.O., Bronisz, A., Nuovo, G., Palatini, J., De Lay, M., Van Brocklyn, J., Ostrowski, M.C., Chiocca, E.A., & Lawler, S.E. (2010). MicroRNA-451 regulates LKB1/AMPK signaling and allows adaptation to metabolic stress in glioma cells. *Mol Cell* 37: 620–632.

Gomez-Manzano, C., & Fueyo, J. (2010). Oncolytic adenoviruses for the treatment of brain tumors. *Curr Opin Mol Ther* 12(5): 530-537.

Gonzalez, T., Seoane, M., Caamano, P., Vinuela, J., Dominguez, F., & Zalvide, J. (2003). Inhibition of Cdk4 activity enhances translation of p27kip1 in quiescent Rb-negative cells. *J Biol Chem* 278: 12688–12695.

Gonzalez-Gomez, P., Bello, M.J., Arjona, D., Lomas, J., Alonso, M.E., De Campos, J.M., Vaquero, J., Isla, A., Gutierrez, M., & Rey, J.A. (2003). Promoter hypermethylation of multiple genes in astrocytic gliomas. *Int J Oncol* 22(3): 601-608.

Guan, Y., Mizoguchi, M., Yoshimoto, K., Hata, N., Shono, T., Suzuki, S.O., Araki, Y., Kuga, D., Nakamizo, A., Amano, T., Ma, X., Hayashi, K., & Sasaki, T. (2010). MiRNA-196 is upregulated in glioblastoma but not in anaplastic astrocytoma and has prognostic significance. *Clin Cancer Res* 15;16(16): 4289-4297.

Harfe, B.D., McManus, M.T., Mansfield, J.H., Hornstein, E., & Tabin, C.J. (2005). The RNaseIII enzyme Dicer is required for morphogenesis but not patterning of the vertebrate limb. *Proc Natl Acad Sci USA* 102(31): 10898–10903.

Hasemeier, B., Christgen, M., Kreipe, H., & Lehmann, U. (2008). Reliable microRNA profiling in routinely processed formalin-fixed paraffin-embedded breast cancer specimens using fluorescence labelled bead technology. *BMC Biotechnol* 8: 90.

He, L., He, X., Lim, L.P., de Stanchina, E., Xuan, Z., Liang, Y., Xue, W., Zender, L., Magnus, J., Ridzon, D., Jackson, A.L., Linsley, P.S., Chen, C., Lowe, S.W., Cleary, M.A., & Hannon, G.J. (2007). A microRNA component of the p53 tumour suppressor network. *Nature* 447: 1130–1134.

Hegi, M.E., Diserens, A.C., Gorlia, T., Hamou, M.F., de Tribolet, N., Weller, M., Kros, J.M., Hainfellner, J.A., Mason, W., Mariani, L., Bromberg, J.E., Hau, P., Mirimanoff, R.O., Cairncross, J.G., Janzer, R.C., & Stupp, R. (2005). MGMT gene silencing and benefit from temozolomide in glioblastoma. *N Engl J Med* 352(10): 997-1003.

Huse, J.T., Brennan, C., Hambardzumyan, D., Wee, B., Pena, J., Rouhanifard, S.H., Sohn-Lee, C., le Sage, C., Agami, R., Tuschl, T., & Holland, E.C. (2009). The PTEN-regulating microRNA miR-26a is amplified in high-grade glioma and facilitates gliomagenesis in vivo. *Genes Dev* 1;23(11): 1327-1337.

Ishii, N., Maier, D., Merlo, A., Tada, M., Sawamura, Y., Diserens, A.C., & Van Meir, E.G. (1999). Frequent co-alterations of TP53, p16/ CDKN2A, p14ARF, PTEN tumor suppressor genes in human glioma cell lines. *Brain Pathol* 9: 469–479.

Jiang, L., Mao, P., Song, L., Wu, J., Huang, J., Lin, C., Yuan, J., Qu, L., Cheng, S.Y., & Li, J. (2010). miR-182 as a prognostic marker for glioma progression and patient survival. *Am J Pathol* 177(1): 29-38.

Juric, D., Bredel, C., Sikic, B.I., & Bredel, M. (2007). Integrated high resolution genome-wide analysis of gene dosage and gene expression in human brain tumors. *Methods Mol Biol* 377: 187–202.

Kefas, B., Godlewski, J., Comeau, L., Li, Y., Abounader, R., Hawkinson, M., Lee, J., Fine, H., Chiocca, E.A., Lawler, S., & Purow, B. (2008). microRNA-7 inhibits the epidermal growth factor receptor and the Akt pathway and is down-regulated in glioblastoma. *Cancer Res* 68(10): 3566-3572.

Kefas, B., Comeau, L., Floyd, D.H., Seleverstov, O., Godlewski, J., Schmittgen, T., Jiang, J., diPierro, C.G., Li, Y., Chiocca, E.A., Lee, J., Fine, H., Abounader, R., Lawler, S., & Purow, B. (2009). The neuronal microRNA miR-326 acts in a feedback loop with notch and has therapeutic potential against brain tumors. *J Neurosci* 29(48): 15161-15168.

Kim, H., Huang, W., Jiang, X., Pennicooke, B., Park , P.J., & Johnson M.D. (2010). Integrative genome analysis reveals an oncomir/oncogene cluster regulating glioblastoma survivorship. *Proc Natl Acad Sci USA* 107: 2183–2188.

Kong, W., Zhao, J.J., He, L., & Cheng, J.Q. (2009). Strategies for profiling microRNA expression. *J Cell Physiol* 218: 22–25.

Krichevsky, A.M., King, K.S., Donahue, C.P., Khrapko, K., & Kosik, K.S. (2003). A microRNA array reveals extensive regulation of microRNAs during brain development. *RNA* 9: 1274–1281.

Kumar, M.S., Lu, J., Mercer, K.L., Golub, T.R., & Jacks, T. (2007). Impaired microRNA processing enhances cellular transformation and tumorigenesis. *Nat Genet* 39: 673–677.

Lai, E.C. (2002). Micro RNAs are complementary to 30 UTR sequence motifs that mediate negative post-transcriptional regulation. *Nat Genet* 30: 363–364.

le Sage, C., Nagel, R., Egan, D.A., Schrier, M., Mesman, E., Mangiola, A., Anile, C., Maira, G., Mercatelli, N., Ciafre, S.A., Farace, M.G., & Agami, R. (2007). Regulation of the p27(Kip1) tumor suppressor by miR-221 and miR-222 promotes cancer cell proliferation. *EMBO J* 26: 3699–3708.

Lee, R.C., Feinbaum, R.L., & Ambros, V. (1993). The C. elegans heterochronic gene lin-4 encodes small RNAs with antisense complementarity to lin-14. *Cell* 75 (5): 843–854.

Lee, R.C., & Ambros, V. (2001). An extensive class of small RNAs in Caenorhabditis elegans. *Science* 294: 862–864.

Lee, E.J., Gusev, Y., Jiang, J., Nuovo, G.J., Lerner, M.R., Frankel, W.L., Morgan, D.L., Postier, R.G., Brackett, D.J., & Schmittgen T.D. (2007). Expression profiling identifies microRNA signature in pancreatic cancer. *Int J Cancer* 120: 1046–1054.

Li, Y., Guessous, F., Zhang, Y., Dipierro, C., Kefas, B., Johnson, E., Marcinkiewicz, L., Jiang, J., Yang, Y., Schmittgen, T.D., Lopes, B., Schiff, D., Purow, B., & Abounader, R. (2009). MicroRNA-34a inhibits glioblastoma growth by targeting multiple oncogenes. *Cancer Res* 69(19): 7569-7576.

Lim, L.P., Lau, N.C., Garrett-Engele, P., Grimson, A., Schelter, J.M., Castle, J., Bartel, D.P., Linsley, P.S., & Johnson, J.M. (2005). Microarray analysis shows that some microRNAs downregulate large numbers of target mRNAs. *Nature* 433(7027): 769–773.

Louis, D.N. (2006). Molecular pathology of malignant gliomas. *Annu Rev Pathol* 1: 97–117.

Luan, S., Sun, L., & Huang, F. (2010). MicroRNA-34a: a novel tumor suppressor in p53-mutant glioma cell line U251. *Arch Med Res* 41(2): 67-74.

Lukiw, W.J., Cui, J.G., Li, Y.Y., & Culicchia, F. (2009). Up-regulation of micro-RNA-221(miRNA-221; chr Xp11.3) and caspase-3 accompanies down-regulation of the survivin-1 homolog BIRC1 (NAIP) in glioblastoma multiforme (GBM). *J Neurooncol* 91: 27–32.

Ma, L., Teruya-Feldstein, J., & Weinberg, R.A. (2007). Tumour invasion and metastasis initiated by microRNA-10b in breast cancer. *Nature* 449: 682–688.

Makeyev, E.V., Zhang, J., Carrasco, M.A., & Maniatis, T. (2007). The MicroRNA miR-124 promotes neuronal differentiation by triggering brain-specific alternative pre-mRNA splicing. *Mol.Cell* 27: 435–448.

Malzkorn, B., Wolter, M., Liesenberg, F., Grzendowski, M., Stühler, K., Meyer, H.E., & Reifenberger, G. (2010). Identification and functional characterization of microRNAs involved in the malignant progression of gliomas. *Brain Pathology* 20: 539–550.

Meltzer, P.S. (2005). Cancer genomics: small RNAs with big impacts. *Nature* 435: 745–746.

Meng, F., Henson, R., Wehbe-Janek, H., Ghoshal, K., Jacob, S.T., & Patel, T. (2007). MicroRNA-21 regulates expression of the PTEN tumor suppressor gene in human hepatocellular cancer. *Gastroenterology* 133: 647–658.

microRNA.org-Targets and Expression. Date of access: November, 30, 2010, Available from http://www.microrna.org/microrna/home.do.

Mitchell, P.S., Parkin, R.K., Kroh, E.M., Fritz, B.R., Wyman, S.K., Pogosova-Agadjanyan, E.L., Peterson, A., Noteboom, J., O'Briant, K.C., Allen, A., Lin, D.W., Urban, N., Drescher, C.W., Knudsen, B.S., Stirewalt, D.L., Gentleman, R., Vessella, R.L., Nelson, P.S., Martin, D.B., & Tewari, M. (2008). Circulating microRNAs as stable blood-based markers for cancer detection. *Proc Natl Acad Sci USA* 105: 10513–10518.

Nan, Y., Han, L., Zhang, A., Wang, G., Jia, Z., Yang, Y., Yue, X., Pu, P., Zhong, Y., & Kang, C. (2010). MiRNA-451 plays a role as tumor suppressor in human glioma cells. *Brain Res* 4;1359: 14-21.

Novakova, J., Slaby, O., Vyzula, R., & Michalek, J. (2009). Micro RNA involvement in glioblastoma pathogenesis. *Biochem Biophys Res Commun* 386: 1–5.

Pang, J.C.S., Kwok, W.K., Chen, Z., & Ng, H.K. (2009). Oncogenic role of microRNAs in brain tumors. *Acta Neuropathol* 117: 599–611.

Papagiannakopoulos, T., & Kosik, K.S. (2008). MicroRNAs: regulators of oncogenesis and stemness. *BMC Med* 6, 15.

Pasquinelli, A.E., Reinhart, B.J., Slack, F., Martindale, M.Q., Kuroda, M.I., Maller, B., Hayward, D.C., Ball, E.E., Degnan, B., Müller, P., Spring, J., Srinivasan, A., Fishman, M., Finnerty, J., Corbo, J., Levine, M., Leahy, P., Davidson, E., & Ruvkun, G. (2000). Conservation of the sequence and temporal expression of let-7 heterochronic regulatory RNA. *Nature* 408(6808): 86–89.

Pierson, J., Hostager, B., Fan, R., & Vibhakar, R. (2008). Regulation of cyclin dependent kinase 6 by microRNA 124 in medulloblastoma. *J Neurooncol* 90, 1–7.

Poy, M.N., Eliasson, L., Krutzfeldt, J., Kuwajima, S., Ma, X., Macdonald, P.E., Pfeffer, S., Tuschl, T., Rajewsky, N., Rorsman, P., & Stoffel, M. (2004). A pancreatic islet-specific microRNA regulates insulin secretion. *Nature* 432(7014): 226–230.

Ren, Y., Zhou, X., Mei, M., Yuan, X.B., Han, L., Wang, G.X., Jia, Z.F., Xu, P., Pu, P.Y., & Kang, C.S. (2010). MicroRNA-21 inhibitor sensitizes human glioblastoma cells U251 (PTEN-mutant) and LN229 (PTEN-wild type) to taxol. *BMC Cancer* 31; 10:27.

Robins, H., & Press, W.H. (2005). Human microRNAs target a functionally distinct population of genes with AT-rich 30 UTRs. *Proc Natl Acad Sci USA* 102:15557–15562.

Sasayama, T., Nishihara, M., Kondoh, T., Hosoda, K., & Kohmura, E. (2009). MicroRNA-10b is overexpressed in malignant glioma and associated with tumor invasive factors, uPAR and RhoC. *Int J Cancer* 15;125(6): 1407-1413.

Shi, L., Cheng, Z., Zhang, J., Li, R., Zhao, P., Fu, Z., & You, Y. (2008). hsamir- 181a and hsa-mir-181b function as tumor suppressors in human glioma cells. *Brain Res* 1236: 185–193.

Shi, L., Chen, J., Yang, J., Pan, T., Zhang, S., & Wang, Z. (2010). MiR-21 protected human glioblastoma U87MG cells from chemotherapeutic drug temozolomide induced apoptosis by decreasing Bax/Bcl-2 ratio and caspase-3 activity. *Brain Res* 17;1352: 255-264.

Silber, J., Lim, D.A., Petritsch, C., Persson, A.I., Maunakea, A.K., Yu, M., Vandenberg, S.R., Ginzinger, D.G., James, C.D., Costello, J.F., Bergers, G., Weiss, W.A., Alvarez-Buylla, A., & Hodgson, J.G. (2008). miR-124 and miR-137 inhibit proliferation of glioblastoma multiforme cells and induce differentiation of brain tumor stem cells. *BMC Med* 6: 14.

Simpson, R.J., Lim, J.W., Moritz, R.L., & Mathivanan, S. (2009). Exosomes: proteomic insights and diagnostic potential. *Expert Rev Proteomics* 6: 267–283.

Skog, J., Würdinger, T., van Rijn, S., Meijer, D.H., Gainche, L., Sena-Esteves, M., Curry, W.T. Jr, Carter, B.S., Krichevsky, A.M., & Breakefield, X.O. (2008). Glioblastoma microvesicles transport RNA and proteins that promote tumour growth and provide diagnostic biomarkers. *Nat Cell Biol* 10: 1470-1476.

Slaby, O., Lakomy, R., Fadrus, P., Hrstka, R., Kren, L., Lzicarova, E., Smrcka, M., Svoboda, M., Dolezalova, H., Novakova, J., Valik, D., Vyzula, R., & Michalek, J. (2010). MicroRNA-181 family predicts response to concomitant chemoradiotherapy with temozolomide in glioblastoma patients. *Neoplasma* 57: 264–269.

Smirnova, L., Grafe, A., Seiler, A., Schumacher, S., Nitsch, R., & Wulczyn, F.G. (2005). Regulation of miRNA expression during neural cell specification. *Eur J NeuroSci* 21: 1469–1477.

Stupp, R., Mason, W.P., van den Bent, M.J., Weller, M., Fisher, B., Taphoorn, M.J., Belanger, K., Brandes, A.A., Marosi, C., Bogdahn, U., Curschmann, J., Janzer, R.C., Ludwin, S.K., Gorlia, T., Allgeier, A., Lacombe, D., Cairncross, J.G., Eisenhauer, E., & Mirimanoff, R.O. (2005). Radiotherapy plus concomitant and adjuvant temozolomide for glioblastoma. *N Engl J Med* 352(10): 987-996.

Sun, F., Fu, H., Liu, Q., Tie, Y., Zhu, J., Xing, R., Sun, Z., & Zheng, X. (2008). Downregulation of CCND1 and CDK6 by miR-34a induces cell cycle arrest. *FEBS Lett* 582: 1564–1568.

Sun, L., Yan, W., Wang, Y., Sun, G., Luo, H., Zhang, J., Wang, X., You, Y., Liu, N., Yang, Z. (2011). MicroRNA-10b induces glioma cell invasion by modulating MMP-14 and uPAR expression via HOXD10. *Brain Res* 15.

TCGA: The Cancer Genome Atlas. Date of access: November, 30, 2010, Available from: http://cancergenome.nih.gov.

Trivedi, S., & Ramakrishna, G. (2009). miRNA and neurons. *Int J Neurosci* 119: 1995–2016.

Tso, C.L., Freije, W.A., Day, A., Chen, Z., Merriman, B., & Perlina, A. (2006). Distinct transcription profiles of primary and secondary glioblastoma subgroups. *Cancer Res* 66: 159–167.

Ueda, R., Kohanbash, G., Sasaki, K., Fujitaa, M., Zhua, X., Kastenhuberb, E.R., McDonaldb, H.A., Potterb, D.M., Hamiltonb, R.L., Lotzef, M.T., Khane, S.A., Sobolb, R.W., & Okada, H. (2009). Dicer-regulated microRNAs 222 and 339 promote resistance of cancer cells to cytotoxic T-lymphocytes by down-regulation of ICAM-1. *Proc Natl Acad Sci USA* 106: 10746–10751.

Ujifuku, K., Mitsutake, N., Takakura, S., Matsuse, M., Saenko, V., Suzuki, K., Hayashi, K., Matsuo, T., Kamada, K., Nagata, I., & Yamashita, S. (2010). miR-195, miR-455-3p and miR-10a(*) are implicated in acquired temozolomide resistance in glioblastoma multiforme cells. *Cancer Lett* 296: 241–248.

Wilfred, B.R., Wang, W.X., & Nelson, P.T. (2007). Energizing miRNA research: a review of the role of miRNAs in lipid metabolism, with a prediction that miR-103/107 regulates human metabolic pathways. *Mol Genet Metab* 91(3): 209–217.

Wu, C., Lin, J., Hong, M., Choudhury, Y., Balani, P., Leung, D., Dang, L.H., Zhao, Y., Zeng, J., & Wang, S. (2009). Combinatorial control of suicide gene expression by tissue-specific promoter and microRNA regulation for cancer therapy. *Mol Ther* 17: 2058–2066.

Würdinger, T., Tannous, B.A., Saydam, O., Skog, J., Grau, S., Soutschek, J., Weissleder, R., Breakefield, X.O., & Krichevsky, A.M. (2008). miR-296 regulates growth factor receptor overexpression in angiogenic endothelial cells. *Cancer Cell* 14(5): 382-393.

Zeng, Y. (2009). Regulation of the mammalian nervous system by micro-RNAs. *Mol Pharmacol* 75: 259–264.

Zhang, Y., Chao, T., Li, R., Liu, W., Chen, Y., Yan, X., Gong, Y., Yin, B., Liu, W., Qiang, B., Zhao, J., Yuan, J., & Peng, X. (2009). MicroRNA-128 inhibits glioma cells proliferation by targeting transcription factor E2F3a. *J Mol Med* 87: 43–51.

Zhou, X., Zhang, J., Jia, Q., Ren, Y., Wang, Y., Shi, L., Liu, N., Wang, G., Pu, P., You, Y., & Kang, C. (2010). Reduction of miR-21 induces glioma cell apoptosis via activating caspase 9 and 3. *Oncol Rep* 24(1): 195-201.

Zhu, S., Si, M.L., Wu, H., & Mo, Y.Y. (2007). MicroRNA-21 targets the tumor suppressor gene tropomyosin 1 (TPM1). *J Biol Chem* 282: 14328–14336.

Zhu, S., Wu, H., Wu, F., Nie, D., Sheng, S., & Mo, Y.Y. (2008). MicroRNA-21 targets tumor suppressor genes in invasion and metastasis. *Cell Res* 18: 350–359.

Aknowledgement: the study was financed by COFIN 2008 prot. 2008979M8K-001 by Italian Ministry of University and Research

Part 6

WNT/β-Catenin / TCF Signaling Pathway - Gliomas

18

Gliomas: Role of Wnt/β-Catenin/ Tcf Signaling Pathway

Gangadhara Reddy Sareddy and Phanithi Prakash Babu
Department of Biotechnology, School of Life Sciences, University of Hyderabad, India

1. Introduction

1.1 Gliomas

Gliomas are the most common primary brain tumors and accounts for about 1.7% of all human neoplasms and 77% of all brain tumors. Gliomas have an annual incidence of 5-10 cases per 100,000 in western population and are a leading cause of death among children and adults diagnosed with a neoplasia of the brain. Gliomas are the heterogeneous group of tumors that are broadly classified into oligodendrogliomas, ependymomas, astrocytomas and mixed oligoastrocytomas based on the specific type of cell to which they closely resemble. According to World Health Organization (WHO) astrocytomas are divided into four clinical grades on the basis of analysis of the most malignant tumor region, number of mitoses, nuclear atypia, microvascular proliferation and presence of necrosis. These includes pilocytic astrocytoma (WHO grade I), diffuse astrocytoma (WHO grade II) anaplastic astrocytoma (WHO grade III) and glioblastoma multiforme (WHO grade IV). Glioblastoma multiforme (GBM) is most malignant, aggressive and devastating form with a worse prognosis. Patients with GBM have a mean survival of about 1 year, whereas patients with anaplastic astrocytomas survive for 2-3 years, and those with diffuse astrocytomas can survive for as long as 10-15 years (Ohgaki and Kleihues., 2009; Louis *et al.*, 2007).

Grade I tumors, also known as pilocytic astrocytomas are childhood brain tumors, benign in nature with circumscribed and well differentiated tumor margins. These tumors are curable by surgery and might represent a separate disease from the astrocytomas of other grades. Diffuse astrocytomas (grade II) are well differentiated and slow-growing tumors, predominantly manifested in young adults (~34 years). They exhibit consistent tendency to diffusely infiltrate surrounding brain structures and tends to progress to anaplastic astrocytoma and eventually to GBM. Characteristic molecular genetic features of diffuse astrocytomas are point mutations in the TP53 tumor suppressor gene (50-80%) and overexpression of PDGF-A and PDGFR-α is observed in astrocytic tumors of all stages (60%), but gene amplification was only detected in a small subset (<10%) of secondary GBM (Nupponen *et al.*, 2006). Anaplastic astrocytoma (grade III) arise *de novo* or from less malignant diffuse astrocytoma and shows tendency for malignant progression to GBM. Males are frequently affected and the mean age is 41 years. Anaplastic astrocytoma possesses higher frequency of TP53 mutations and other genetic changes include p16 and p19 deletion, RB alterations, and LOH on chromosome 19q (50%) (Nupponen *et al.*, 2006).

Glioblastomas are the heterogeneous intraparenchymal masses and the most common malignant primary brain tumors in adults. These tumors show the histological evidences of cellular polymorphism, nuclear atypia, mitotic activity, microvascular proliferation, vascular thrombosis and necrosis. Microscopically, they consists of several cell types: the glioma cell proper, hyper proliferative endothelial cells, macrophages and trapped cells of normal brain structures that are overrun by the invading glioma cells. Several histological characteristics are used to grade and define gliomas. These include regions of necrosis, in which necrotic areas are surrounded by densely packed tumor cell nuclei and are referred as "pseudopalisading" necrosis. In addition, the blood vessels both within and adjacent to the tumor are hypertrophied. Furthermore, the nuclei of tumor cells are extremely variable in size and shape, a characteristic called nuclear polymorphism. Tumor cells characteristically invade the adjacent normal brain parenchyma, migrating through the white matter tracts to collect around blood vessels, neurons and at the edge of the brain parenchyma in the subpial region (Kleihues and Ohgaki., 1999).

GBM may develop *de novo* (primary GBM) or from less malignant precursor lesion (secondary GBM). However, the majority of develop *de novo* with short clinical history usually less than 3 months. They may manifest at any age, but are more common in adults (~55 years) and males are more frequently affected. The secondary GBM occur in younger age group (~39 years), show a slightly more favorable outcome and develop far less often than primary GBM. The time interval for progression from diffuse low-grade astrocytoma to secondary GBM varies considerably (~4-5 years). However, with regard to histopathological and immunohistochemical features there are no differences between primary and secondary GBM (Kleihues and Ohgaki., 1999). Comparative gene expression analysis showed that primary and secondary GBM have distinct expression profiles, however, half of the clinically determined primary GBM has a similar pattern to the secondary GBM. These suggest that primary GBM may originate from a clinically undiagnosed lower grade lesion.

1.2 Genetic alterations associated with primary and secondary GBM

Primary and secondary GBM are distinct in their molecular features. Chromosomal aberrations of gliomas have been studied using karyotyping, comparative genomic hybridization (CGH), or chromosome painting. The chromosomal aberrations identified in primary GBM are distinct from those of secondary GBM. However, there are also chromosomal aberrations that are shared by both primary and secondary GBM. The most chromosomal aberrations associated with primary GBM are amplifications and gains of 7p, 12q13-21, and chromosome 19. The main chromosomal regions showing losses are 10q, 9p, 13q, and 22q. In addition primary GBM may harbors additional aberrations such as losses of 18q, 16p, and 19q, and gains of 20q, and 12q. Anaplastic astrocytomas associated with losses of 9p, 10q, 13q and gains of 1q, 7p, 11q, and Xq. Diffuse astrocytomas associated with gains of 3q, 4q, 7q, 12p, and 19p, and losses of Xp, 1p, and 19q.

The genetic hallmark of primary GBM that typically lack a TP53 mutation is MDM2 amplification/overexpression (50%). Additional genetic changes in primary GBM includes EGFR amplification (40% of cases) and/or overexpression (60%), CDKN2-A, CDKN2-B and PTEN mutations (30%), RB alteration, p16 deletion (30-40%) LOH on the entire chromosome 10 (50-80%). The sequence in which gene alterations are acquired is not known since these neoplasms develop very rapidly, without a clinically or histopathologically identifiable precursor lesion. The TP53 mutations are less common in primary GBM (<10%). Secondary

GBM frequently associate with mutations of gene TP53. These mutations in more than 90% cases are already present in the first biopsy of diffuse low grade or anaplastic astrocytoma. Most likely, the TP53 mutation is the initial gatekeeper lesion in astrocytic tumors, which then, through genetic instability undergoes malignant progression. The pathway to secondary glioblastoma is further characterized by LOH on chromosomes 19q and 10q (but not on the entire chromosome 10 as it is seen in primary GBM). Recently it was pointed out that genomic alterations of LOH 1p and 19q, which are observed in the majority of oligodendroglioma, may be observed in GBM. However, in contrast to oligodendroglioma, in GBM loss of 19q is more likely to be partial than complete and loss of 1p is uncommon (~10%). It was suggested that combined losses of chromosome arms 1p and 19q may indicate better prognosis and potential sensitivity to chemotherapy in GBM patients, while isolated loss of either 1p or 19q is of no prognostic significance. The IDH1 gene at 2q33 encodes isocitrate dehydrogenase 1 (IDH1) catalyzes the oxidative carboxylation of isocitrate to α-ketoglutarate, predominantly located in the cytosol. Recent studies demonstrated that IDH1 mutations are very early and frequent genetic alteration in low grade astrocytomas (80%), anaplastic astrocytomas and secondary glioblastomas. In contrast, IDH1 mutations are very rare (<5%) or absent in pilocytic astrocytomas and primary glioblastomas. Almost 60% of the low grade astrocytomas have both TP53 and IDH1 mutations (Ohgaki and Kleihues., 2009).

The progression of astrocytomas to more malignant forms results from the stepwise accumulation of genetic alterations and the consequent disruption of apoptotic pathway and augmentation of survival signaling. These genetic alterations in astrocytomas ultimately result in the abnormal activation of signal transduction pathways, downstream of receptor tyrosine kinases or disruption of cell cycle arrest pathways. For example, amplification or activating mutations of EGFR, over-expression of FGF, FGFR, PDGF and PDGFR due to either gene amplification or other epigenetic mechanisms, all lead to constitutive activation of corresponding receptor tyrosine kinase signaling. Subsequently, a number of downstream signal transduction pathways are activated, including the PI3K/AKT pathway, RAS/MAP kinase pathway, C-MYC pathway, protein kinase C pathway, and STAT pathways (Ohgaki and Kleihues., 2007).

1.3 Wnt signaling pathway

The Wnt proteins (the name derived from mouse Int-1 and Drosophila wingless) comprise a large family of protein ligands that affect diverse processes such as embryonic induction, generation of cell polarity, and the specification of cell fate (Logan *et al.*, 2004), tissue homeostasis and cancer. A number of Wnt genes, including Wnt2, Wnt7b and Wnt 5a, have been associated with abnormal proliferation of human breast tissue and other tumors. The Wnt receptor complex that activates the canonical pathway contains two components: a member of the Frizzled family and either one of two single-span transmembrane proteins, low density-lipoprotein receptor related proteins (LRP5 and LRP6). Once bound by their cognate ligands, the Fzd/LRP receptor complex activates the canonical signaling pathway. The central player of the canonical signaling pathway is β-catenin, a cytoplasmic protein whose stability is regulated by the "destruction complex". Within this complex the Axin and APC proteins form a scaffold that facilitates β-catenin phosphorylation by CK1α and GSK3β. Phosphorylated β-catenin is subsequently recognized and ubiquitinylated, and degrades in proteasomes. The resulting low levels of β-catenin allow the DNA binding Tcf/Lef proteins to interact with transcriptional co-repressors to block target genes expression. Interaction of Wnt ligand with its specific receptor complex containing a Frizzled family member and LRP5 or LRP6 triggers the formation of Dvl-Fzd complexes and the phosphorylation of LRP by CK1γ facilitating relocation of Axin to the membrane and inactivation of the destruction box. This allows β-catenin to accumulate and enter the nucleus, where it interacts with members of the Tcf/Lef family and converts them into potent transcriptional activators by displacing groucho/TLE proteins and recruiting an array of co-activator proteins including CBP, TBP, BRG1, BCL9/PYG, Legless, Mediator and Hyrax. This ensures efficient activation of Tcf target genes such as c-myc, n-myc, cyclinD1, c-jun, MMP7, VEGF, IL-8 etc (Moon *et al.*, 2004. The overview of Wnt signaling pathway is illustrated in figure 1.

1.4 Wnt signaling-neural stem cells-gliomas

During the development of nervous system neural precursor or progenitor cells (NPC) act as a source of various types of specialized cells in the brain. Several studies have suggested that these cells are able to self-renew, a hall mark of stem cells. Wnt signaling is a candidate pathway in controlling neural stem cells self-renewal and differentiation. Wnt signaling is required at several stages of central nervous system development. The neural stem cells and progenitor cells in the brain are at a risk of malignant transformation, presumably because of the fact that most of the oncogenic and developmental pathways that responsible for tumor formation are critical for the functions like cell survival, self renewal, proliferation and differentiation and neural stem cells exhibit least resistance in tumorigenesis, since they already have the ability to bypass apoptosis and senescence. The developmental pathways in particular Wnt signaling pathway critically regulate the self-renewal, proliferation and differentiation of neural stem cells and other progenitor cells in the brain. Deregulation of/or abnormal operation of this pathway potentially leads to the development of brain tumors.

2. Wnt/β-catenin/Tcf signaling pathway components in gliomas

The progression of low grade astrocytomas to higher grades results from the stepwise accumulation of genetic alterations and the consequent disruption of the apoptotic pathways and augmentation of survival signaling. Here investigations on the possible role of Wnt signaling pathway components were described in detail.

2.1 Extracellular Wnt signaling inhibitors

Wnt signaling pathway is inhibited by extracellular Wnt antagonists which are divided into two functional classes, the sFRP (secreted Frizzled Related Protein) class and the Dickkopf class. sFRP class includes sFRP family (sFRP1, sFRP2, sFRP3, sFRP4, and sFRP5), sizzled, sizzled2, crescent, WIF-1 (Wnt inhibitory factor-1) and cerebrus, which directly binds to Wnts, thereby altering their ability to bind to the receptor complex. Roth *et al.* (2000) investigated the role of sFRPs in glioma cell growth and motility. sFRP-1 and sFRP-2 are produced by the majority of malignant glioma cell lines and ectopic expression of sFRPs increased clonogenecity and enhanced resistance to serum starvation. In contrast, sFRPs do not modulate glioma cell susceptibility to apoptosis induced by the cytotoxic cytokines and cytotoxic drugs. sFRP-2 strongly promotes the growth of intracranial glioma xenografts in nude mice. In contrast, enhanced expression of sFRPs inhibits the motility of glioma cells *in vitro*. sFRP-mediated effects on glioma cells are accompanied by decreased expression and activity of matrix metalloproteinase-2 (MMP-2) and decreased tyrosine phosphorylation of β-catenin. This suggested that sFRPs promote survival under non-supportive conditions and inhibit the migration of glioma cells. Dickkopf family comprises four members (Dkk-1 to Dkk-4) and a unique Dkk-3-related protein named Soggy (sgy). The DKK family of glycoproteins curtails Wnt induced signals by binding to co-receptors LRP 5 and LRP 6. The human Dkk-1 (hDkk-1) gene, a transcriptional target of the p53 tumor suppressor, encodes a potent inhibitor of the Wnt signaling pathway and regulates the spatial patterning/morphogenesis of the mammalian central nervous system. Its induction was greatly enhanced following DNA damage and in response to other chemotherapeutic agents through p53 dependent mechanism. Shou *et al.* (2002) reported that over expression of DKK-1 significantly reduced the Wnt2 dependent β-catenin expression and sensitizes the glioblastoma cell lines to apoptosis in response to various chemotherapeutic agents that cause DNA alkylation and DNA damage. Muller *et al.* (2005) analyzed the DKK1 in series of 73 brain tumors for structural alterations in the entire coding sequence by single-strand conformation polymorphism and direct sequencing. They detected several sequence variants but no obvious mutations that affecting DKK1. REIC/Dkk-3 acts as a suppressor in various human cancers. Studies by Mizobuchi *et al.* (2007) showed that the expression levels of Dkk-3 were lower in human malignant glioma tissues compared to normal brain tissues and inversely correlated with the degree of malignancy. Dkk-3 expression levels were lower in glioma cell lines compared to normal human astrocytes. Knockdown of Dkk-3 using si-RNA resulted in increased survival cell index compared to control cells. Further, ectopic expression of Dkk-3 in glioblastoma cell lines showed the decreased survival index in a time dependent manner. In contrast forced expression of Dkk-3 does not alter the survival cell index in normal astrocytes. Overexpression of Dkk-3 induced the apoptosis in GBM cell lines through the activation of phosphor-JUN, caspase-9 and caspase-3 and also resulted in the reduction and degradation of β-catenin.

Wnt inhibitory factor-1 (WIF-1) is one of the secreted antagonists that can directly bind to Wnt proteins and inhibits the Wnt/β-catenin signaling. Down-regulation and promoter hypermethylation of WIF-1 have been reported in several human malignancies. Yang *et al.* (2010) reported that expression levels of WIF-1 mRNA and protein were significantly decreased in human astrocytomas compared to normal brain tissues and expression levels were negatively correlated with the histological malignancy astrocytomas. Further this reduced WIF-1 gene expression was associated with the hypermethylation of WIF-1 gene promoter. In contrast, no hypermethylation was observed in normal brain tissues. Hypermethylation was observed in 54.72% of astrocytoma samples, especially in 70% of high grade astrocytomas. Gotze *et al.*, (2009) investigated gliomas of different malignancy grades for promoter hypermethylation in members of the secreted frizzled-related protein (*SFRP1, SFRP2, SFRP4, SFRP5*), dickkopf (*DKK1, DKK3*) and naked (*NKD1, NKD2*) families of Wnt pathway inhibitors. They found that frequent promoter hypermethylation of Wnt pathway inhibitor genes in astrocytomas of varying grades. Hypermethylation of *SFRP1, SFRP2* and *NKD2* each occurred in more than 40% of the primary glioblastomas, while

DKK1 hypermethylation was found in 50% of secondary glioblastomas. Further, treatment of *SFRP1-*, *SFRP5-*, *DKK1-*, *DKK3-*, *NKD1-* and *NKD2*-hypermethylated U87-MG glioblastoma cells with demethylating agent 5-aza-2-deoxycytidine and with histone deacetylase inhibitor Trichostatin A resulted in increased expression of each gene. Furthermore, *SFRP1*-hypermethylated gliomas showed significantly lower expression of the respective transcripts when compared with unmethylated tumors. Similarly, Foltz *et al.*, (2010) studied epigenetic inactivation of Wnt pathway inhibitors in glioblastomas using a large-scale whole-genome approach. They found that three genes DKK1, SFRP1, and WIF1 were epigenetically silenced in glioblastomas and confirmed the decreased expression of these genes in GBM tumor tissue samples relative to normal brain tissue samples. Further, the expression of these genes is restored in T98G GBM cells by treatment Trichostatin A, but only DKK1 expression is restored by treatment with the 5-azacytidine. Ectopic expression of DKK1 significantly reduces colony formation and increases chemotherapy-induced apoptosis in T98G glioblastoma cells. While, ectopic expression of WIF1 and SFRP1 shows a relative lack of response. Chronic Wnt3a stimulation only partially reverses growth suppression after DKK1 reexpression, whereas a specific inhibitor of the JNK pathway significantly reversed the effect of DKK1 reexpression on colony formation and apoptosis in T98G cells. This support the potential growth-suppressive function for epigenetically silenced DKK1 in GBM and suggests that DKK1 restoration could modulate Wnt signaling through both canonical and noncanonical pathways. These investigations suggest an important role of epigenetic silencing of Wnt pathway inhibitor genes in gliomas, particularly in glioblastomas, with distinct patterns of hypermethylated genes distinguishing primary from secondary glioblastomas.

2.2 Wnt ligands and frizzled receptors

Wnt proteins are secreted glycoproteins which are modified through post-translational modifications such as palmitoylation, required for correct secretion and N-linked glycosylation which increases the stability of Wnts. These are categorized according to canonical and noncanonical based on the pathway activated by Wnts. It was reported that a number of Wnt genes, including Wnt1, Wnt2, Wnt3a, Wnt5a, Wnt7a, Wnt7b, Wnt 10b and Wnt13, have been associated with tumor development. There were several studies investigated the expression of Wnts in gliomas. Howng *et al.* (2002) studied the mRNA expression of Wnt1, Wnt5a, Wnt10b and Wnt13 in brain tumors. It was observed that Wnt 5a, Wnt10b, Wnt13 were expressed in most of the brain tumors, whereas Wnt1 was less expressed. Further no correlations were observed between Wnts expression and histopathological grading. Yu *et al.* (2007) showed that Wnt5a was upregulated in glioblastomas than that of lowgrade tumors and normal brain samples and overexpression of Wnt5a in glioblastoma cell lines increased the proliferation. Knockdown of Wnt5a using siRNA resulted in the reduction of proliferation of glioblastoma cell lines and also reduced the tumor growth *in vivo*. Pu *et al.* (2009) studied the mRNA expression of Wnt1, Wnt2, Wnt3, Wnt4, Wnt5a, Wnt10b and Wnt13 and frizzled receptors Fzd2 and Fzd5. The expression levels of Wnt2, Wnt5a and Fzd2 mRNA and protein were overexpressed in astrocytomas but not expressed in normal brain tissues and exhibited significant positive correlation with the degree of malignancy. Whereas, Wnt1 and Fzd5 were not expressed in gliomas and Wnt3, Wnt4, Wnt10b, Wnt13 expression were almost equally expressed in tumor and normal brain tissues. Knockdown of Wnt2 in glioma cell lines significantly downregulated the expression of Wnt2, β-catenin as well as expression of Fzd2, p-GSK3β, cyclin D1, PI3K, and p-Akt. Further, Wnt2 knockdown also resulted in the reduced cell viability, cell cycle arrest in Go/G1 phase with lowered S phase proportion, increase in apoptotic cell population and reduced invasive ability. In nude mice experiments of xenograft tumors, Wnt2 siRNA treatment slowdown the tumor growth and the tumor size was significantly lower than control treated. Also in this subcutaneous model the expression levels of Wnt2, fzd2, β-catenin and p-GSK3β were decreased following Wnt2 siRNA treatment and induce tumor cell apoptosis. Zhang *et al.* (2006) studied the role of Frizzled 9 in astrocytoma samples and reported that Frizzled 9 was upregulated in astrocytomas.

2.3 Dishevelled and FRAT-1

Dishevelled (Dvl) identified as positive regulator of Wnt signaling pathway positioning downstream of the frizzled receptor and upstream of β-catenin. Overexpression or constitutive activation of dishevelled promotes neoplastic transformation and its involvement has been reported in various human cancers. Dvl performs dual functions, on one hand it transduces Wnt signals to stabilize the β-catenin and on the other hand it relays the signals for the activation of Jun kinases. Three variants of Dvls were identified to date and their prominent role in tumor progression was reported in several human cancers. In canonical Wnt signaling Dvl interacts with Axin and dissociates the destruction complex by relocating the Axin to the cytoplasmic tail of LRP. Also by interaction with FRAT1/GBP it inhibits the GSK3β activity. These mechanisms lead to the stabilization of β-catenin levels in the cytoplasm. We studied (Sareddy *et al.*, 2009a) the expression status of Dvl variants in astrocytoma tissues and found that Dvl-3 was upregulated in tumor tissues while very low expression was observed in normal brain sample. The expression levels were progressively increased from low grade to high grade astrocytomas and showed significant positive correlation with the pathological grade of astrocytomas.

FRAT1 (frequently arranged in advanced T-cell lymphomas-1) is an inhibitor of GSK-3β and was identified as a positive regulator of Wnt/β-catenin pathway by inhibiting the GSK-3β activity there by stabilizing β-catenin. Its oncogenic role was established in several human cancers. In response to Wnt signaling activation Dishevelled protein recruits FRAT1 into the destruction complex which facilitates the dissociation of GSK3β from destruction complex, leading to the stabilization of β-catenin. Guo *et al.* (2010) found that FRAT1 was overexpressed in several human astrocytoma samples and showed the significant positive correlation with the pathological grading of astrocytomas. In normal brain samples FRAT1 expression was very low compared to tumor samples. FRAT1 immunoreactivity was also positively correlated with the β-catenin immunoreactivity.

2.4 AXIN-APC-GSK3β

Axin, a tumor suppressor was originally identified as an inhibitor of Wnt signaling and is central to the down regulation of β-catenin. Axin acts as a scaffolding protein which facilitates the phosphorylation of β-catenin by GSK3β and CK1α and subsequent proteasomal degradation. It is a core component of destruction complex and binds directly to β-catenin, APC, GSK3 β, CK1α and Dvl. It is often mutated in several human malignancies. Nikuseva Martic *et al.* (2010) examined the changes of Axin1 in 72 neuroepithelial brain tumors. LOH experiments showed the LOH of AXIN1 in 11.1% of brain tumors and majority proportion was distributed to glioblastomas (6.3%). Compared to healthy brain tissues Axin1 expression was down regulated in 65.5% of brain tumors, of which majority of them are astrocytomas. In most of the samples Axin was localized in the cytoplasm. It was also observed that β-catenin was localized mainly in nucleus or cytoplasm and nucleus. They also demonstrated that there was no difference in Axin protein levels in patients with AXIN1 LOH and patients without it. In contrast, relative β-catenin levels were significantly higher in patients with AXIN LOH in comparison to without it. Comparison of relative levels of β-catenin and AXIN1 revealed that they were significantly reversely proportional.

Adenomatous polyposis coli gene (APC) is a tumor suppressor and is often mutated in wide variety of human cancers. It was demonstrated that most of the colon and other human malignancies having highly constitutive β-catenin due to mutations in APC or β-catenin itself. Mutations in APC and β-catenin genes were noticed in the childhood brain tumor medulloblastoma but till to date no mutations were found in gliomas. However, recent reports provided the evidence that the APC mutations are in secondary brain metastasis rather than in primary tumors. Pecina-Slaus *et al.* (2010) analyzed exon 15 of the APC in a 49-year-old male patient with brain metastasis and its primary site was lung carcinoma. PCR method and direct DNA sequencing of the metastasis and autologous lymphocyte samples identified the presence of a somatic mutation at position 5883 G–A in the metastasis tissue. Interestingly, these authors observed that the lack of protein expression of APC, however, β-catenin localization was observed in the nucleus. The mutation is a silent mutation that might have consequences in the creation of a new splice site. To date no prominent mutations were observed in β-catenin but it was reported that β-catenin is mutated at S33 as sporadic event in a brain metastasis (Lee *et al.*, 2009). Further, this mutated β-catenin enhances the Tcf dependent promoter activity.

Glycogen synthase kinase 3 is a serine/threonine kinase regulates diverse signaling pathways involved in proliferation, apoptosis and cell cycle control. GSK3 has two isoforms include GSK3α, GSK3β which are functionally independent. It performs independent functions based on the cell type, and it described as a prosurvival factor in pancreatic cancer and as a pro-apoptotic factor in colon cancer and interconnects several pathways which plays major role in several human disorders. Korur *et al.* (2009) analyzed the role of GSK3β in malignant gliomas and reported that mRNA and protein levels of GSK-3β were overexpressed in human glioblastoma tissues compared to normal brain tissues. Direct inhibition of GSK3β activity by siRNA, the specific inhibitor SB216763, or lithium chloride (LiCl) induced tumor cell differentiation, tumor cell apoptosis and reduced the clonogenecity.

2.5 β-Catenin

β-Catenin was first identified as a member of Wnt signaling pathway. The β-catenin gene *CTNNb1* was localized at 3p2.1. β-catenin existed in two pools: one is located in the cytomembrane which involved in cell adhesion and other is in the cytoplasm or/and nucleus which is mainly involved in the regulation of Wnt pathway. It was identified that mutations in the β-catenin gene that affect specific serine and threonine residues abrogates the phosphorylation dependent degradation of β-catenin. These regulatory sequences are often mutated in wide variety of human cancers. It was noticed that colorectal tumors that contain APC mutations harbors low β-catenin mutations where as in tumors lacking APC, mutations in CTNNb1 was greatly increased. Dissociation of cytoplasmic inhibitory complex owing to the upstream activity of Wnt signals or mutations in APC and Axin leads to the cytosolic accumulation of β-catenin. The Oncogenic potential of β-catenin was extensively studied in wide variety of human cancers. We studied the expression levels of β-catenin mRNA and protein in 32 human astrocytoma samples and found that the mRNA and protein levels of β-catenin were elevated in astrocytoma samples while very low levels were observed in normal brain tissues. The expression levels of β-catenin were progressively increased form low grade astrocytomas to higher grades and positively correlated with the histological grading of astrocytomas. In most of the tumor sections β-catenin was accumulated in the nucleus and cytosol which is crucial in mediating Wnt pathway activity (Sareddy *et al.* 2009a). Moreover, we examined the β-catenin levels in the progression of ENU-induced gliomas in rat model. In this study, we identified that the levels of β-catenin were increased as tumor grows and correlated with malignant progression of gliomas (Sareddy *et al.* 2009b). Pu *et al.* (2009) also showed that knockdown of β-catenin using siRNA downregulated the expression of β-catenin, p-GSK3β, cyclin D1, PI3K, and pAKT and reduced the cell viability, arrest the cell cycle at G0/G1 phase with lowered S phase cells, increased the apoptotic cell population and inhibited the invasion of glioma cell lines. Further, treatment with β-catenin siRNA in subcutaneous xenograft model reduced and slowed down the tumor size and growth respectively. In these tumors β-catenin siRNA treatment caused the reduction in the levels of β-catenin, pGSK3β, PI3K, Wnt2 and Fzd2 and induced the apoptosis. Similar results were also observed by Liu *et al.* (2010), stating that expression levels of β-catenin mRNA and protein were elevated in astrocytomas in comparison with normal brain tissues and showed the positive correlation with the grade of the astrocytomas. β-catenin siRNA transfection into glioma cell lines inhibited the cell proliferation, induced the apoptosis, arrested the cell cycle in G0/G1 phase and downregulated the expression of β-catenin targets such as cyclin D1, c-jun and c-Myc. Zhang *et al.* (2009) studied the correlation between β-catenin distribution, tumor grade and patient 2 year survival. They found that there was no correlation between grade of the tumor and distribution of β-catenin. However, significant positive correlation was observed between levels of β-catenin and 2-year patient survival. The expression of β-catenin was not correlated with other clinicopathological characteristics such as tumor age, tumor size, and sex and tumor location. Further, survival analysis showed that patients with astrocytoma showing less expression of β-catenin tend to be associated with good prognosis, whereas, astrocytoma patients with high β-catenin expression associated with poor prognosis.

2.6 Lef-1 and Tcf-4

Lef/Tcf family transcription factors consist of four members: Lef-1, Tcf-1, Tcf-3 and Tcf-4. Lef/Tcf transcription factors belong to high mobility group (HMG) domain proteins that recognize the same DNA consensus motif through HMG box DNA-binding domain. Tcf-1 is predominantly expressed in cells of T cell lineage and Lef-1 is expressed in pre-B and T cells. Lack of Tcf-1 and Lef-1 augment the T cell development and arrest the development at earlier stages. Tcf-3 is expressed in somatic epithelium, keratinocytes of the skin. Tcf-4 is expressed in midbrain and in epithelium of intestine and mammary glands. Constitutive expression of Tcf-4 is essential for maintenance of gut epithelium, however, constitutive active β-catenin-Tcf-4 complexes were observed in colon carcinoma. In the absence of β-catenin, Tcf/Lef factors suppress the Wnt target gene expression by binding with members of the Groucho (Grg/TLE) family of transcriptional co-repressors. Translocation of β-catenin converts Tcf family proteins into potent transcriptional activators by displacing Groucho/TLE proteins and recruiting an array of co-activator proteins including CBP, TBP, BRG1, BCL9/PYG, Legless, Mediator and Hyrax (Barker and Clevers., 2006). β-catenin does not have a DNA binding domain, but it has a potent transcription activation domain. In general, Lef/Tcf transcription factors do not have a strong transcription activation domain, but they have a good DNA binding/bending domain. Thus, when β-catenin binds to Lef/Tcf proteins, a potent transcription regulatory complex is formed. We examined the expression levels of Lef1 and Tcf4 in human astrocytic samples and found that compared to normal brain tissues Lef1 and Tcf-4 expression levels were significantly elevated in astrocytomas and in most of the tumors these proteins were localized in the nucleus. The increased Tcf4 and Lef1 levels were significantly correlating with the pathological grade of astrocytomas. We also demonstrated the interaction of β-catenin with Tcf4 in the nuclear fractions of GBM tissues and in cell lines. In addition, we also found that the Lef-1 and tcf-4 levels were elevated in ENU-induced rat gliomas compared to control rats and protein levels were progressively increased form initial stage to advanced stages. Oncogenic activity of Wnt signaling is mediated through overexpression of their target genes cyclin D1, c-Myc, c-Jun, MMP2, N-Myc etc. These proteins play essential roles in the cell cycle progression, cell proliferation and survival. In our study we observed the elevated levels of cyclin D1, c-Myc, c-jun, N-Myc in astrocytomas of different clinical grade in comparison with normal brain samples. The protein levels were significantly correlating with the histological grading of astrocytomas and similar results were also observed in ENU-induced gliomas.

2.7 Pygopus 2

When β-catenin is accumulated and translocated to nucleus, β-catenin relieves the action of corepressors and recruits the array of coactivators to Tcf/Lef factors such as CBP, TBP, BRG1, Legless, Mediator, Hyrax, Bcl-9 (B-cell lymphoma-9), and pygopus. These coactivators are essential for β-catenin/Tcf dependent transcription. Wang *et al.* (2010) examined the pygopus 2 expression in human astrocytoma samples. Pygopus 2 levels were overexpressed in astrocytoma samples compared to controls and exhibited a positive correlation with tumor grade. Knockdown of pygopus with small hairpin RNA (shRNA) resulted in inhibition of cell proliferation, colony forming ability, BrdU incorporation and invasiveness of human and rat glioma cell lines. Knockdown of pygopus 2 also resulted in the arrest of cell cycle at G1 stage and this was associated with reduction of S phase cell population. Knockdown of pygopus 2 also leads to the decreased expression of Wnt target gene cyclin D1 without altering the β-catenin levels and its nuclear translocation. Further, Chen *et al.* (2010) examined the pygopus 2 role in rat glioma cell lines. Overexpression of pygopus significantly enhances the cell proliferation and cell cycle progression from G1 to S and this was associated with the elevation of cyclin D1 levels without altering the β-catenin levels. Moreover, pygo2 expression levels were significantly correlated with the expression of cyclin D1 in human glioma samples.

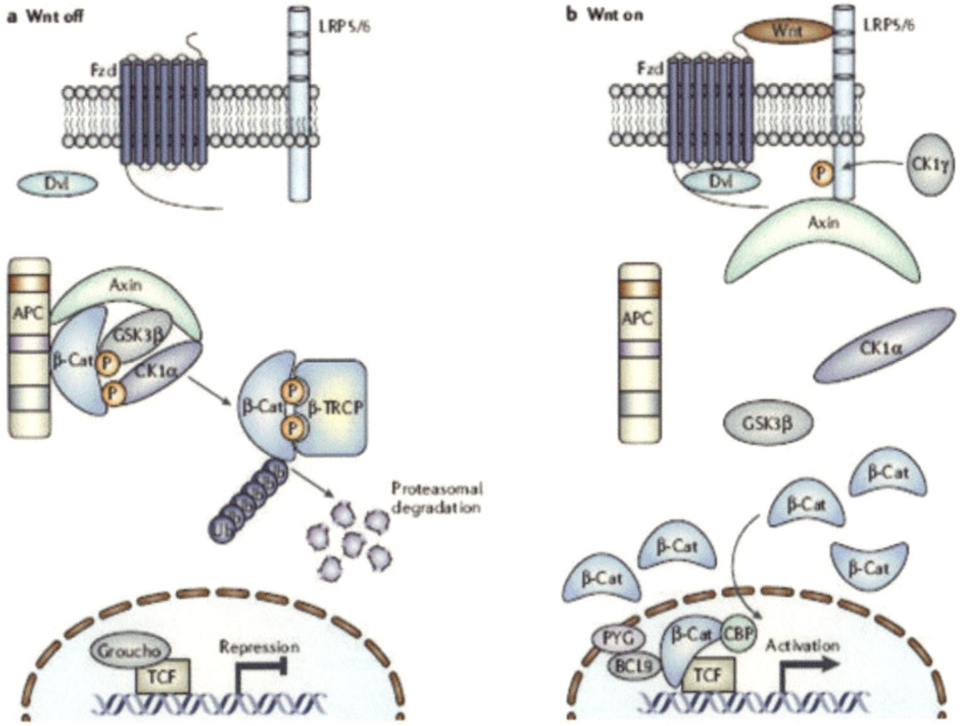

Fig. 1. **An overview of the Wnt signaling pathway**. **(a)** In the absence of a Wnt signal, β-catenin is captured by APC and axin within the destruction complex, facilitating its phosphorylation by the kinases CK1α and GSK3β. CK1α and GSK3β then sequentially phosphorylate a conserved set of serine and threonine residues at the amino terminus of β-catenin. This facilitates binding of the β-TRCP, which subsequently mediates the ubiquitinylation and efficient proteasomal degradation of β-catenin. The resulting β-catenin 'drought' ensures that nuclear DNA-binding proteins of the Tcf/Lef transcription factor family (TCF1, TCF3, TCF4 and LEF1) actively repress target genes by recruiting transcriptional co-repressors (Groucho/TLE) to their promoters and/or enhancers. **(b)** Interaction of a Wnt ligand with its specific receptor complex containing a Frizzled family member and LRP5 or LRP6 triggers the formation of Dvl–Fzd complexes and the phosphorylation of LRP by CK1γ, facilitating relocation of axin to the membrane and inactivation of the destruction box. This allows β-catenin to accumulate and enter the nucleus, where it interacts with members of the Tcf/Lef family. In the nucleus, β-catenin converts the Tcf proteins into potent transcriptional activators by displacing Groucho/TLE proteins and recruiting an array of coactivator proteins including CBP, TBP, BRG1, BCL9/PYG, Legless, Mediator and Hyrax. This ensures efficient activation of Tcf target genes such as c-MYC, which instruct the cell to actively proliferate and remain in an undifferentiated state. Following dissipation of the Wnt signal, β-catenin is evicted from the nucleus by the APC protein and Tcf proteins revert to actively repressing the target gene program. β-TRCP, β-transducin repeat-containing protein; APC, adenomatous polyposis coli; BCL9, B-cell lymphoma 9; CK1α, casein kinase 1α; CK1γ, casein kinase 1γ; CBP, CREB-binding protein; Fzd, Frizzled; Lef, lymphoid enhancer factor; LRP, low-density lipoprotein receptor-related protein; PYG, Pygopus; Tcf, T-cell factor. (This illustration is reproduced from Barker *et al.*, 2006).

3. Conclusion

In summary, recent activities that deal with the study of Wnt/β-catenin/Tcf signaling pathway in gliomas insist that this pathway is activated in human gliomas and involved in the malignant progression of gliomas. This pathway attracted as candidate therapeutic target and inhibition of this pathway may curtail the malignant progression of gliomas.

4. References

Barker, N., and Clevers, H. 2006. Mining the Wnt pathway for cancer therapeutics. Nat. Rev. Drug. Discov. 5: 997-1014.

Chen, Y. Y., Li, B. A., Wang, H. D., Liu, X. Y., Shen, S. H., Zhu, H. W., and Wang, H. D. 2011. The role of pygopus 2 in rat glioma cell growth. Med. Oncol.28:631–64.

Foltz, G., Yoon, J. G., Lee, H., Ma, L., Tian, Q., Hood, L., and Madan, A., 2010. Epigenetic regulation of Wnt pathway antagonists in human glioblastoma multiforme. Genes & Cancer 1: 81-90.

Gotze, S., Wolter, M., Reifenberger, G., Muller, O., and Sievers, S. 2010. Frequent promoter hypermethylation of Wnt pathway inhibitor genes in malignant astrocytic gliomas. Int. J. Cancer 126: 2584-2593.

Guo, G., Mao, X., Wang, P., Liu, B., Zhang, X., Jiang, X., Zhong, C., Huo, J., Jin, J., and Zhuo, Y. 2010. The expression profile of FRAT1 in human gliomas. Brain Res. 1320: 152-158.

Howng, S. L., Wu, C. H., Cheng, T. S., Sy, W. D., Lin, P. C., Wang, C., and Hong, Y. R. 2002. Differential expression of Wnt genes, beta-catenin and E-cadherin in human brain tumors. Cancer Lett. 183: 95-101.

Kleihues, P., and Ohgaki, H. 1999. Primary and secondary glioblastomas: From concept to clinical diagnosis. Neuro Oncol. 1: 44-51.

Korur, S., Huber, R. M., Sivasankaran, B., Petrich, M., Morin, P. Jr., Hemmings, B. A., Merlo, A., and Lino, M. M. 2009. GSK3beta regulates differentiation and growth arrest in glioblastoma. PLoS One 4: e7443.

Lee, C. I., Hsu, M. Y., Chou, C. H., Wang, C., Lo, Y. S., Loh, J. K., Howng, S. L., and Hong, Y. R. 2009. CTNNB1 (beta-catenin) mutation is rare in brain tumours but involved as a sporadic event in a brain metastasis. Acta Neurochir. 151: 1107-1111.

Liu, X., Wang, L., Zhao, S., Ji, X., Luo, Y., and Ling, F. 2010. beta-Catenin overexpression in malignant glioma and its role in proliferation and apoptosis in glioblastoma cells. Med. Oncol. 16: 75-79.

Logan, C. Y., and Nusse, R. 2004. The Wnt signaling pathway in development and disease. Annu. Rev. Cell. Dev. Biol. 20: 781-810.

Louis, D. N., Ohgaki, H., Wiestler, O. D., Cavenee, W. K., Burger, P. C., Jouvet, A., Scheithauer, B. W., and Kleihues, P. 2007. The 2007 WHO Classification of Tumours of the Central Nervous System. Acta Neuropathol. 114: 97–109.

Mizobuchi, Y., Matsuzaki, K., Kuwayama, K., Kitazato, K., Mure, H., Kageji, T., and Nagahiro, S. 2008. REIC/Dkk-3 induces cell death in human malignant glioma. Neuro Oncol. 10: 244-253.

Moon, R. T., Kohn, A. D., De Ferrari, G. V., and Kaykas, A. 2004. WNT and beta-catenin signalling: diseases and therapies. Nat. Rev. Genet. 5: 691-701.

Muller, W., Lass, U., Wellmann, S., Kunitz, F., and von Deimling, A. Mutation analysis of DKK1 and in vivo evidence of predominant p53-independent DKK1 function in gliomas. Acta Neuropathol. 109: 314-320.

Nikuseva Martic, T., Pecina-Slaus, N., Kusec, V., Kokotovic, T., Musinovic, H., Tomas, D., and Zeljko, M. 2010. Changes of AXIN-1 and beta-catenin in neuroepithelial brain tumors. Pathol. Oncol. Res. 16: 75-79.

Nupponen, N. N., and Joensuu, H. 2006. Molecular pathology of gliomas. Curr. Diagn. Pathol. 12: 394-402.

Ohgaki, H., and Kleihues, P. 2007. Genetic pathways to primary and secondary glioblastoma. Am. J. Pathol. 170: 1445-1453.

Ohgaki, H., and Kleihues, P. 2009. Genetic alterations and signaling pathways in the evolution of gliomas. Cancer Sci. 100: 2235-2241.

Pecina-Slaus, N., Majic, Z., Musani, V., Zeljko, M., and Cupic, H. 2010. Report on mutation in exon 15 of the APC gene in a case of brain metastasis. J. Neurooncol. 97: 143-148.

Pu, P., Zhang, Z., Kang, C., Jiang, R., Jia, Z., Wang, G., and Jiang, H. 2009. Downregulation of Wnt2 and beta-catenin by siRNA suppresses malignant glioma cell growth. Cancer Gene Ther. 16: 351-361.

Roth, W., Wild-Bose, C., Platten, M., Grimmel, C., Melkonyan, H.S., Dichgans, J., and Weller, M. 2000. Secreted Frizzled-related proteins inhibit motility and promote growth of human malignant glioma cells. Oncogene 19: 4210-4220.

Sareddy, G. R., Challa, S., Panigrahi, M., and Babu, P. P. 2009b. Wnt/beta-catenin/Tcf signaling pathway activation in malignant progression of rat gliomas induced by transplacental N-ethyl-N-nitrosourea exposure. Neurochem. Res. 34: 1278-1288.

Sareddy, G. R., Panigrahi, M., Challa, S., Mahadevan, A., and Babu, P. P. 2009a. Activation of Wnt/beta-catenin/Tcf signaling pathway in human astrocytomas. Neurochem. Int. 55: 307-317.

Shou, J., Ali-Osman, F., Muttani, A. S., Pathak, S., Fedi, P., and Srivenugopal, K. S. 2002. Human Dkk-1, a gene encoding a Wnt antagonist, responds to DNA damage and its overexpression sensitizes brain tumor cells to apoptosis following alkylation damage of DNA. Oncogene 21: 878-889.

Wang, Z. X., Chen, Y Y., Li, B. A., Tan, G. W., Liu, X. Y., Shen, S. H., Zhu, H. W., and Wang, H. D. 2010. Decreased pygopus 2 expression suppresses glioblastoma U251 cell growth. J. Neurooncol. 100: 31-41.

Yang, Z., Wang, Y., Fang, J., Chen, F., Liu, J., Wu, J., and Wang, Y. 2010. Expression and aberrant promoter mehtylation of Wnt inhibitory factor-1 in human astrocytomas. J. Exp. Clin. Cancer Res. 29: 26.

Yu, J. M., Jun, E. S., Jung, J. S., Suh, S. Y., Han, J. Y., Kim, J. Y., Kim, K. W., and Jung, J. S. 2007. Role of Wnt5a in the proliferation of human glioblastoma cell lines. Cancer Lett. 257: 172-181.

Zhang, L. Y., Jiang, L. N., Li, F. F., Li, H. Liu, F., Gu, Y., Song, Y., Zhang, F., Ye, J., and Li, Q. 2009. Reduced beta-catenin expression is associated with good prognosis in astrocytoma. Pathol. Oncol. Res. 16: 253-257.

Zhang, Z., Schittenhelm, J., Guo, K., Buhring, H. J., Trautmann, K., Meyermann, R., and Schluesener, H. J. 2006. Upregulation of frizzled 9 in astrocytomas. Neuropathol. Appl. Neurobiol. 32: 615-624.

Part 7

IGFBP2 - Gliomas

19

Insulin-Like Growth Factor Binding Protein-2: A Possible Regulator of Invasive Growth in Glioblastoma

Tsuyoshi Fukushima and Hiroaki Kataoka
Section of Oncopathology and Regenerative Biology, Department of Pathology, Faculty of Medicine, University of Miyazaki, Japan

1. Introduction

Glioblastoma is the most common malignant brain tumor and has an extremely lethal course (Clark *et al.*, 2010). Although genetic abnormalities in p53, Akt, phosphatase and tensin homolog deleted from chromosome 10 (PTEN), and epidermal growth factor receptor that are common to various cancers are also found in glioblastoma, the prime cause of glioblastoma's malignant features and conclusive treatment targets have yet to be determined. Better understanding of non-major signal pathways involved in glioblastoma could thus provide breakthroughs in treatment strategies. Insulin-like growth factor binding protein-2 (IGFBP2) was originally reported to be a modulator of the action of insulin-like growth factors (IGFs), but IGF-independent effects of IGFBP2 on cellular proliferation, apoptosis, metabolism, and mobility have since been reported in pathological conditions, including cancers. Recent studies of gene expression microarray revealed that elevated expression of IGFBP2 occurs in gliomas, and is associated with increasing grades of malignancy with significant overexpression in glioblastomas (Fuller *et al.*, 1999; Sallinen *et al.*, 2000). Subsequent studies have suggested that IGFBP2 may be one of the proteins that play an important role in malignant phenotypes of glioblastoma cells (Fukushima & Kataoka, 2007).

This chapter highlights key examples of recent biological and epidemiological research focusing on IGFBP2 in brain tumors and reviews more specialized studies on the fundamental role of IGFBP2 in glioma progression.

2. Structure and physiological functions of IGFBP2

2.1 Human insulin-like growth factor binding proteins (IGFBPs)

IGFBPs are a family of six proteins present in plasma and bodily fluids that bind insulin-like growth factor-I (IGF-I) and IGF-II with high affinity (Table 1) (Hwa *et al.*, 1999; Firth & Baxter, 2002; Fukushima & Kataoka, 2007). By interacting with IGFs, the IGFBPs modulate distribution and activity of IGFs in various tissues and bodily fluids, thereby controlling their biological function *in vivo* (Clemmons 1998; Kelley *et al.*, 2002). IGFBPs in IGFBP/IGF complexes can be cleaved at specific sites by various proteinases (Bunn *et al.*, 2003). This

IGFBP cleavage might be an important regulatory mechanism of pericellular IGF function, as IGFBP proteolysis releases IGF from the IGFBP/IGF complexes (Lee *et al.*, 1996; Bunn *et al.*, 2003; Fowlkes *et al.*, 2004; Mark *et al.*, 2005; Nakamura *et al.*, 2005). Therefore, IGFBPs both positively and negatively regulate IGF function.

	IGFBP1	IGFBP2	IGFBP3	IGFBP4	IGFBP5	IGFBP6
Gene location	7p13-p12	2q33-q34	7p13-p12	17q12-q21.1	2q33-q36	12q13
mRNA (kbp)	1.6	1.4	2.6	2.2	6.3	1
MW (kDa)	25	31	43-45	24	29	28-30
RGD motif	(+)	(+)				
Heparin binding	(+)	(+)	(+)	(+)	(+)	(+)
Phospho. site	(+)		(+)		(+)	
NLS			(+)		(+)	
N-Glycosylation			(+)	(+)		
O-Glycosylation					(+)	(+)

Table 1. Summary of IGFBP family. MW, molecular weight of mature protein. Phosopho. site, presumed phosphorylation site. NLS, nuclear localization signal.

2.2 Molecular properties and physiological functions of IGFBP2

2.2.1 Synthesis, structure and distribution of IGFBP2

The IGFBP2 precursor is 36-kDa (328 amino acid residues) in size and consists of a signal peptide and three distinct regions: the highly conserved N-terminal region (IGFBP homolog domain, amino acid residues 43-136); the highly conserved C-terminal region with a thyroglobulin type 1 repeat (amino acid residues 229-309); and an intervening region with four major cleavage sites (Bunn *et al.*, 2003; Mark *et al.*, 2005) (Figure 1). The N-terminal and C-terminal domains are cysteine-rich and globular, both of which have IGF-binding property. Mature IGFBP2 is a 31.4-kDa protein and is the second most abundant IGFBP found in serum.

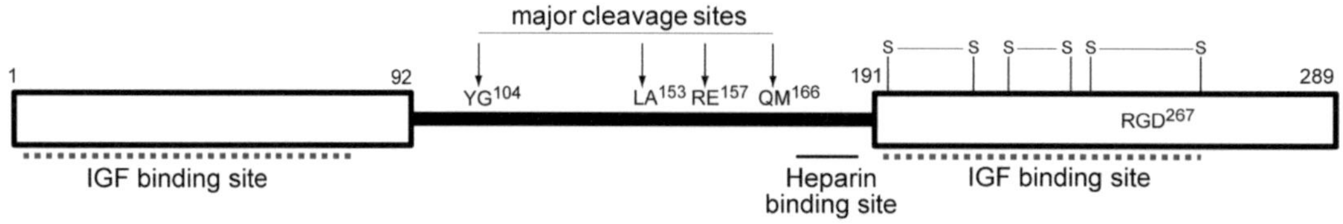

Fig. 1. Molecular structure of human IGFBP2. Amino acid positions of mature IGFBP2 protein are indicated. Integrin binding RGD motif is also shown.

Although IGFBP1, IGFBP3, and IGFBP5 each have phosphorylation sites, IGFBP2 does not. IGFBP2 does, however, have an arginine-glycine-aspartic acid (RGD) motif, which binds to cell surface integrins, and a heparin-binding domain, which facilitates association with extracellular matrices (Figure 1). Both regions are able to localize IGFBP2 and IGFBP2/IGF complexes on/around the cell surface (Schutt *et al.*, 2004; Russo *et al.*, 2005; Wang *et al.*, 2006). Among the six IGFBPs, only IGFBP1 and IGFBP2 possess a RGD motif (Table 1).

IGFBP2 is widely expressed in the fetus where its expression is reported to closely parallel that of IGF-II (Wood *et al*, 1992, 1993; Lee *et al.*, 1993). IGFBP2 is predominantly expressed in the early post-implantation epiblast, the apical ectodermal ridge, the progenitors of spleen and liver, and fetal astroglial cells (Wood *et al.*, 1992; Lee *et al.*, 1993). Fetal epithelial cells and epidermal progenitor cells abundantly express IGFBP2, which also participates in the regulation of hair follicle development (Harris *et al.*, 2010). The expression of IGFBP2 decreases significantly after birth, but gradually increases again, especially after the age of sixty, and found in plasma, seminal plasma, milk and cerebrospinal fluid (Blum *et al.*, 1993; Schwander & Mary, 1993; van den Beld *et al.*, 2003).

2.2.2 Regulation of IGFBP2 expression

The *IGFBP2* gene is located on chromosome 2q33-q34 near that of IGFBP5 (Garner *et al.*, 2008). The promoter region lacks TATA box and CAAT boxes, but contains GC-rich sequences and therefore putative Sp1 binding sites. Portions of the promoter responsible for dexamethasone-induced transcriptional activity and IGF-induced stimulation of transcription have also been reported (Mouhieddine *et al.*, 1996). Other possibly important promoter regions contain binding sites for AP-4 and nuclear factor κB (NF-κB) (Cazals *et al.*, 1999). The relationship between IGFBP2 expression and loss of tumor suppressor gene function has been recently elucidated (Perks *et al.*, 2007; Moore *et al.*, 2009) and hypoxic microenvironment may also upregulate *IGFBP2* gene expression (Feldser *et al.*, 1999). These lines of evidence indicate that upregulated *IGFBP2* gene expression should occur in injured tissue and particularly in tumors.

2.2.3 Proposed physiological functions of IGFBP2

By virtue of its IGF binding capacity, IGFBP2 was initially considered to be an inhibitory factor of IGFs, particularly of IGF-II with K_D values for IGF-I and IGF-II to be 1.14 and 0.37, espectively (Hwa *et al.*, 1999; Russo *et al.*, 2005). However, it was subsequently found to prolong the half-life of IGFs. The binding between IGFs and IGFBP2 is reversible, and IGFs are released when IGFBP2 is processed at its central region cleavage sites by serine proteinases including thrombin and prostate specific antigen (human tissue kallikrein 3) (Clemmons *et al.*, 1998; Cohen *et al.*, 1992, Zheng *et al.*, 1998) or matrix metalloproteinase (MMP) (Nakamura *et al.*, 2005). As IGFBP2 can associate with cell surface integrins via its RGD motif, IGFBP2 could in theory not only be an IGF inhibitor but also provide an IGF reservoir at the cell surface to maintain efficient IGF activity in the pericellular microenvironment. Therefore, interaction between integrins and IGFBP2, cleavage of IGFBPs by proteases, and other factors that could influence the affinity of IGFBP2 for IGFs may be important regulatory mechanisms of pericellular IGF function. On the other hand, IGFBP2 has also been reported in several studies to have a cytosolic or perinuclear localization, suggesting that IGFBP2 may also have IGF-independent functions (Hoeflich *et al.*, 2004; Fukushima & Kataoka, 2007; Migita et al., 2010).

IGFBP2 knockout mice are both viable and fertile, and do not show significant differences in prenatal or postnatal body growth (Wood *et al.*, 1993, 2000). However, detailed analyses of the knockout mice revealed decreased spleen weight and increased liver weight (Wood *et al.*, 2000). Interestingly, male IGFBP2 knockout mice have shorter femurs than their control mouse counterparts, and also have significantly enhanced levels of PTEN in their osteoblasts and osteoclasts (DeMambro *et al.*, 2008). Recent studies also revealed that IGFBP2 likely has a crucial regulatory role in glucose metabolism as might be expected since IGFBP2 is regulated by leptin, secreted by visceral white adipocytes, and contributes to the prevention of diet-induced obesity as well as having anti-diabetic effects (Hedbacker *et al.*, 2010; Li & Picard, 2010).

3. Roles of IGFBP2 in progression of gliomas

3.1 Expression of IGFBP2 in tumors

3.1.1 Enhanced expression of IGFBP2 in malignancies of various organs

To date, there is accumulating evidence to suggest that IGFBP2 is involved in tumor progression. Increased serum/plasma levels of IGFBP2 are associated with many malignant tumors of various organs, including prostate (Cohen *et al.*, 1993), ovary (Lancaster *et al.*, 2006), colon (Mishra *et al.*, 1998), breast (Busund *et al.*, 2005), lung (Lee *et al.*, 1999), skin (Harris *et al.*, 2010) and the central nervous system (Lin *et al.*, 2009). Upregulated IGFBP2 expression levels have been reported for various tumor tissues as well, and in many instances, these expression levels correlate with the grade of malignancy (Mishira *et al.*, 1998; Pekonen *et al.*, 1992; Fuller *et al.*, 1999; Rickman *et al.*, 2001; Sallinen *et al.*, 2000). Moreover, an inverse correlation between IGFBP2 and tumor suppressor genes, such as *PTEN* and *p16/INK4*, whose loss-of-function is frequently observed in malignant tumors, has also been reported (Perks *et al.*, 2007; Moore *et al.*, 2009). Indeed, induction of PTEN downregulates IGFBP2 expression in glioblastoma and prostate cancer cells (Levitt *et al.*, 2005; Mehrian-Shai *et al.*, 2007). On the other hand, the p53 tumor suppressor is suggested to be a transcription factor that stimulates IGFBP2 expression (Grimberg *et al.*, 2006). Hypoxia-induced expression of IGFBP2 mediated by hypoxia inducible factor 1α (HIF1α), has also been demonstrated (Feldser *et al.*, 1999). In sum, the expression of IGFBP2 can be significantly influenced by oncogenic genetic alteration and by a hypoxic tumor microenvironment, and many clinicopathological analyses strongly suggest that IGFBP2 participates in tumor progression.

3.1.2 Expression of IGFBP2 in gliomas and its correlation with histological grade

A consistent overexpression of IGFBP2 in glioblastoma was initially reported by Fuller *et al.* (1999) based on a gene expression profiling analysis. This finding has since been confirmed by many researchers and it is now well established that IGFBP2 expression in gliomas increases with tumor grade (Sallinen *et al.*, 2000; Rickman *et al.*, 2001; Elminger *et al.*, 2001; Fukushima & Kataoka, 2007). Indeed, IGFBP2 is one of the most powerful discriminators to distinguish glioblastomas from low-grade gliomas in proteomic analyses (Jiang *et al*, 2006). Regarding a possible mechanism for IGFBP2 overexpression in glioblastoma, Mehrian-Shai *et al.* (2007) have identified IGFBP2 as the most significant molecular signature for loss of PTEN and activation of the phosphatidylinositol 3-kinase (PI3K)/Akt pathway. Notably, glioblastoma is one of the cancers most commonly affected by PTEN abnormalities (Sulis & Parsons, 2003). Enhanced activation of NF-κB signaling pathway in glioblastoma cells (Wang *et al.*, 2004) may also be involved in the upregulation of *IGFBP-2* transcription (Cazals *et al.*, 1999).

The prognostic impact of IGFBPs expression in patients with newly diagnosed glioblastoma was recently reported (Santosh *et al.*, 2010), with protein expression of IGFBP2, IGFBP 3 and

IGFBP5 being significantly associated with shorter survival by univariate Cox regression analysis. However, multivariate Cox proportional hazards model showed that only IGFBP3 had independent prognostic impact. Plasma levels of IGFBP2 can also predict clinical outcomes of patients with glioblastoma (Lin *et al.*, 2009). In that study, preoperative plasma IGFBP2 levels were significantly higher in high-grade glioma patients compared to low-grade glioma patients, and are significantly correlated with recurrence and disease-free survival in glioblastoma patients.

3.1.3 Expression of IGFBP2 in other brain tumors

Analysis of tissue mRNA levels revealed that IGFBP2 expression is indicative of poor prognosis in patients with medulloblastoma (de Bont *et al.*, 2008). IGFBP2 is also expressed by meningiomas, and a high IGF-II/IGFBP2 mRNA ratio is a sign of biologically aggressive behavior in meningiomas (Nordqvist *et al.*, 1997). However, a subsequent study by the same group revealed that IGFBP6 mRNA is more informative than IGFBP2 for the evaluation of meningioma invasiveness (Nordqvist *et al.*, 2002).

3.2 Role of IGFBP2 in malignant progression of gliomas

3.2.1 Role for IGFBP2 in glioma development

As mentioned above, analyses of clinical samples revealed that IGFBP2 expression significantly correlates with disease progression of gliomas, suggesting a role for IGFBP2 in malignant progression. Furthermore, a recent study using a glial-specific transgenic (RCAS/Ntv-a) mouse system indicated that IGFBP2 in combination with platelet-derived growth factor-β (PDGFB) is also an oncogenic factor in glioma development (Dunlap *et al.*, 2007). In this model, the expression of oncogenic IGFBP2 is negatively regulated by *Ink4a-Arf*, and consequently, loss of *Ink4a-Arf* results in enhanced IGFBP2 expression (Moore *et al.*, 2009). Indeed, the *Ink4a-Arf* locus is frequently deleted in human gliomas and IGFBP2 expression is inversely correlated with $p16^{INK4a}$ status (Moore *et al.*, 2009).
Evidence regarding a role for IGFBP2 in glioma development also arose from a recent study of glioma stem cell (GSC) that was found to overexpress IGFBP2, which subsequently promoted GSC expansion and survival (Hsieh *et al.*, 2010). Notably Hedgehog-GLI1 signaling regulates human glioma growth, GSC self-renewal, and tumorigenicity (Clement *et al.*, 2007) and gene expression of IGFs and IGFBPs is upregulated by GLI transcription factors (Villani *et al.*, 2010). Therefore, an autocrine circuit of IGF/IGFBP2- or IGFBP2-induced signaling may be established in GSCs via activation of Hedgehog-GLI1 signaling, which may contribute to the stemness of GSCs.

3.2.2 Roles for IGFBP2 in malignant phenotypes of glioblastoma cells

Glioblastoma is a devastating brain tumor with extremely poor prognosis (Clarke *et al.*, 2010). Significant invasiveness into surrounding brain parenchyma, increased mitotic activity, sustained angiogenesis and necrosis surrounded by palisaded atypical tumor cells are histological hallmarks of this untreatable tumor. The major impediment to successful therapeutic intervention for glioblastomas is their diffuse invasive nature. An *in vitro* study using a human glioblastoma cell line engineered to overexpress IGFBP2 revealed that IGFBP2 enhances glioblastoma cell invasiveness (Wang *et al.*, 2003). Similarly, a study using human glioblastoma cell lines in which IGFBP2 expression was knocked down by consistent retroviral expression of IGFBP2 short hairpin RNA (shRNA) revealed that silencing of the IGFBP2 gene reduces *in vitro* invasiveness and *in vivo* aggressiveness of the cells (Fukushima *et al.*, 2007). Consistent with these studies, high levels of IGFBP2 expression were detected within the infiltrating tumor cells of human glioblastomas *in vivo* (de Groot *et al.*, 2010). Therefore, IGFBP2 has a crucial role in glioblastoma invasion.

IGFBP2 may also be implicated in glioblastoma angiogenesis. In a cDNA-array analysis of 53 patient biopsies, IGFBP2 was included in a prominent gene cluster that allowed discrimination between primary (*de novo*) and non-primary (secondary) glioblastomas (Godard *et al.*, 2003). This gene cluster is composed mostly of angiogenesis-related genes, including vascular endothelial growth factor (VEGF) and fms-related tyrosine kinase 1. Notably, *in situ* hybridization demonstrates coexpression of IGFBP2 and VEGF in pseudopalisading cells surrounding tumor necrosis, providing evidence for a possible involvement of IGFBP2 in angiogenesis (Godard *et al.*, 2003). It is reasonable to postulate that HIF1α is responsible for the concomitant expression of VEGF and IGFBP2 (Carmeliet *et al.*, 1998; Feldser *et al.*, 1999). In addition, an anti-apoptotic function of intracellular IGFBP2 was recently reported in lung cancer cells (Migita *et al.*, 2010), which may also have implications for the enhanced expression of IGFBP2 within glioblastoma cells around necrosis.

Taken together, these results strongly indicate that IGFBP2 has significant roles in the development of the malignant phenotypes of glioblastoma.

3.2.3 Potential mechanisms of IGFBP2 action in the invasive growth of glioblastoma cells

Interaction of IGFBP2 with components of the pericellular matrices results in local sequestration of IGFs and then in an enhancement of cellular IGF-induced signaling (Schutt *et al.*, 2004). Experiments using a cultured neuroblastoma cell line showed that the heparin binding domain of IGFBP2 is required for IGFBP2 association to pericellular matrices and for IGFBP2 to promote invasive growth via efficient pericellular localization of IGF-1 (Russo *et al.*, 2005).

However, IGF-independent actions of IGFBP2 may be equally or more important in glioblastoma biology, as has been amply demonstrated by recent research. Interaction of IGFBP2 RGD domain with integrin α5 induces outside-in signaling and may be essential for IGFBP2-induced glioma cell mobility (Wang *et al.*, 2006). Moreover, intracellular localization of IGFBP2 has been shown in glioblastoma cells and other tumor cells such as lung carcinoma, which appears to influence the cellular gene expression signature (Fukushima & Kataoka, 2007; Migita et al., 2010). Overexpression of IGFBP2 in the SNB19 human glioblastoma cell line revealed that IGFBP2 enhances the invasiveness of these cells by up-regulating expression of invasion-associated gene products, such as extracellular matrix-degrading protease, MMP-2 (Wang et al., 2003). We compared the expression profiles of two human glioblastoma cell lines, U251 and YKG-1, in the presence and absence of shRNA-induced silencing of IGFBP2 expression (Fukushima *et al.*, 2007). In both cell lines, expression levels of various genes were altered by IGFBP2 knockdown without apparent alteration of IGF signaling, suggesting that IGFBP2 influences transcriptional regulation of many genes in glioblastoma cells independent of IGF signaling. Among the genes influenced by *IGFBP2* silencing, the *CD24* gene was identified as a candidate downstream target of IGFBP2-induced signaling, and subsequent analysis revealed that

CD24 is critically involved in the invasiveness of U251 and YKG-1 cells (Fukushima *et al.*, 2007). CD24 is a heavily glycosylated, cell surface, glycosylphosphatidylinositol-anchored protein (Kristiansen *et al.*, 2004). While the precise mechanism by which CD24 induces cellular invasion is unclear, CD24 has been shown to recruit adhesion molecules to lipid rafts, thereby contributing to tumor cell migration, dissemination, and metastasis (Baumann *et al.*, 2005; Runz *et al.*, 2008). Of interest is a recent observation that a splice variant of *GLI1*, truncated *GLI1* (*tGLI1*), which is highly expressed in glioblastoma cells but not in normal cells, induces cellular migratory and invasive capabilities via upregulaton of CD24 in U87 glioblastoma cells (Lo *et al.*, 2009). As mentioned above, Hedgehog-GLI1 signaling is involved in glioma cell growth, expansion of GSC and induction of IGFBP2 expression (Clement *et al.*, 2007; Villani *et al.*, 2010). Therefore, Hedgehog-GLI1/IGFBP2/CD24 signaling may play a pivotal role in the invasive growth of glioblastoma cells.

The NF-κB pathway is another important candidate for the signaling involved in IGFBP2-induced phenotypes. In fact, NF-κB signaling is activated in glioblastomas and involved in invasion and angiogenesis of glioma cells (Wang *et al.*, 2004; Li *et al.*, 2007). While NF-κB is suggested to regulate *IGFBP2* gene expression in response to tissue injury (Cazals *et al.*, 1999), intracellular IGFBP2 itself is involved in the regulation of NF-κB signaling via binding to invasion inhibitory protein 45 (IIp45, also named migration and invasion inhibitor protein MIIP), which was identified by a yeast two-hybrid assay (Song *et al.*, 2003). The *IIp45* gene is located on chromosome 1p36 (Song *et al.*, 2003), a region that is frequently deleted in oligodendrogliomas and occasionally deleted in astrocytomas (Smith *et al.*, 1999). Decreased IIp45/MIIP levels were also observed in 15% of glioblastoma cases (Song *et al.*, 2003). IIp45/MIIP binds to the RGD motif of IGFBP2 and inhibits the interaction between IGFBP2 and integrin, which eventually may inhibit the expression of transcriptional NF-κB and its downstream genes involved in invasive glioma cell growth (Song *et al.*, 2003). It may be possible that upregulated NF-κB in the absence of IIp45/MIIP also stimulates IGFBP2 transcription and eventually establishes an autocrine stimulation circuit for invasive growth. Moreover, recent studies have indicated that IIp45/MIIP also interacts with intracellular proteins, such as Cdc20 and histon deacetylase 6 (HDAC6), and inhibits glioma cell proliferation and migration (Ji et al., 2010; Wu et al., 2010). Therefore, interaction between IIp45/MIIP and intracellular IGFBP2 may occur in glioblastoma cells, which may attenuate the function of IIp45/MIIP and thereby may enhance the cellular proliferation and migration.

We summarize hypothetical functions of IGFBP2 in the invasive growth of glioblastoma cells in Figure 2.

3.2.4 IGFBP2 as a therapeutic target for high-grade gliomas

We have shown above that IGFBP2 can provide crucial signaling during glioma development and can exhibit malignant phenotypes of glioblastoma. As such, IGFBP2 and its downstream targets may reasonably serve as novel therapeutic targets for glioblastoma. However, there have been limited attempts to target IGFBP2 for *in vivo* glioblastoma treatments. Moore *et al.* (2009) examined the effect of antisense IGFBP2 *in vivo* using PDGFB-induced glioma in *Ink4a-Arf*-null mice, and found that the inhibition of IGFBP2 expression confers a survival benefit. Therefore, IGFBP2 is a potential therapeutic target for *Ink4a-Arf*-dleted gliomas, such as anaplastic oligodendroglioma and glioblastoma (Moore *et al.*, 2009).

As a downstream molecule of IGFBP2 involved in invasiveness of glioblastoma cells, CD24 may also serve as a molecular target for glioblastoma treatment. Targeting CD24 by monoclonal antibodies, small interfering RNA or shRNA has been reported in xenograft models of human colorectal cancer, pancreatic cancer and ovarian cancer cell lines (Sagiv *et al.*, 2008; Su *et al.*, 2009). In those studies, retardation of tumorigenicity and significant reduction of tumor growth were observed *in vivo*, indicating that CD24 is a promising therapeutic target for treatment of cancer. As glioblastomas abundantly express CD24 as well as IGFBP2 (Fukushima *et al.*, 2007), we suggest that targeting CD24 may be a potential therapeutic approach against glioblastoma.

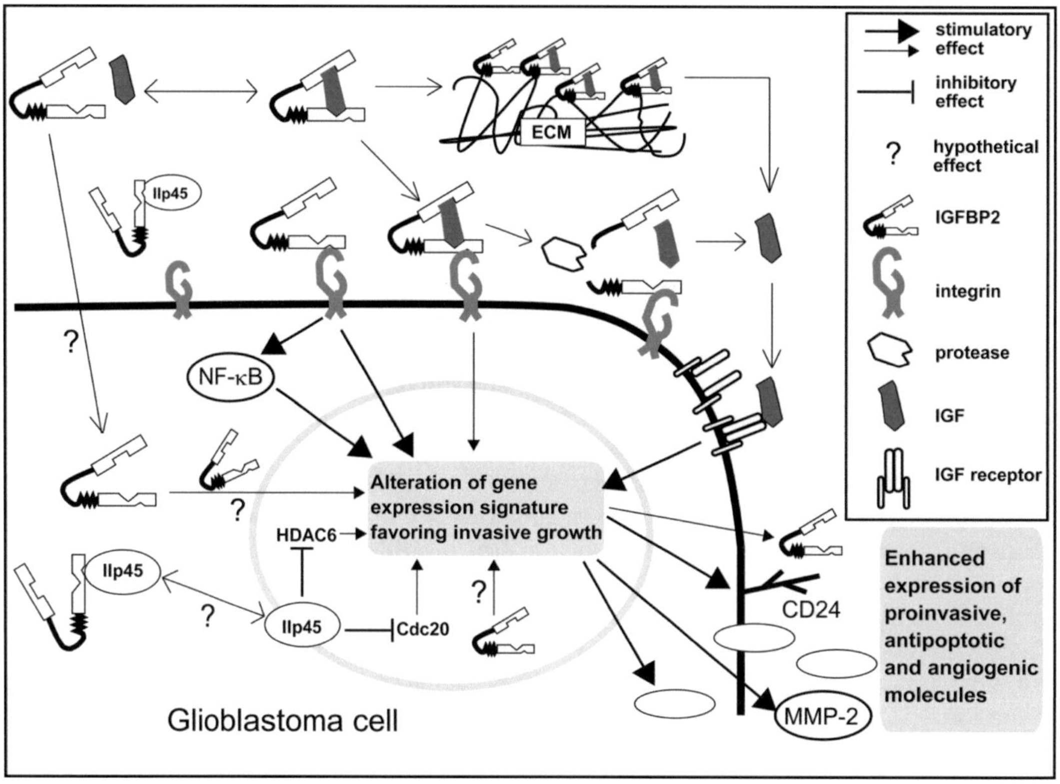

Fig. 2. Roles for IGFBP2 in the establishment of malignant phenotypes of glioblastoma cells. Both IGF-dependent and IGF-independent effects of IGFBP2 have been proposed. Integrin-mediated outside-in signaling and NF-κB signaling appear to be involved in the IGFBP2-induced effects, which eventually result in enhanced expression of proinvasive molecules, such as CD24 and MMP-2. While IIp45/MIIP may inhibit binding of IGFBP2 to integrin, it is possible to hypothesize that excess intracellular (intranuclear) IGFBP2 may suppress the inhibitory effects of IIp45/MIIP on Cdc20 and/or HDAC6-mediated cellular growth and migration. The upregulated NF-κB signaling enhances the expression of IGFBP2. Hypoxic microenvironment, loss of PTEN function and Hedgehog-GLI1 signaling might also be involved in the enhanced IGFBP2 expression in glioblastoma cells. Functions of intracellular and intranuclear IGFBP2 remain to be elucidated. ECM, extracellular matrix.

IGFBP2 may also be an attractive marker to influence glioblastoma treatment strategy decisions. Since high IGFBP2 levels serve as a marker for loss of PTEN function and PI3K/Akt activation, the clinical data linking IGFBP2 expression to poor prognosis may be due, at least in part, to the loss of PTEN function, which is well known to lead to aggressive behavior of gliomas (Levitt *et al.*, 2005; Mehrian-Shai, 2007). Therefore, measurements of IGFBP2 expression levels may be useful for estimating the functional PTEN status and PI3K/Akt activation levels in glioma, which in turn may be beneficial for organizing specific treatment strategies for each glioma case (Gonzalez & de Groot, 2008). Moreover, recent study suggests that IGFBP2 expression level may be a marker for DNA hypermethylation profiles in gliomas (Zheng *et al.*, 2011).

4. Conclusion

IGFBP2 is a pleiotropic protein that appears to be involved in many aspects of physiological and pathological processes and shows both positive and negative effects. Even in cancers, opposite effects of IGFBP2 are observed. For example, the growth of colorectal adenomas induced by chemical carcinogens in mice was inhibited upon crossing with IGFBP2 transgenic mice (Diehl *et al.*, 2008). In contrast, IGFBP2 exerts oncogenic effects in brain-specific transgenic mice (Dunlap *et al.*, 2007; Moore *et al.*, 2009). Thus, IGFBP2 shows both negative and positive effects on tumor growth, and these differences are probably dependent on cell type and pericellular environment. Despite the diverse effects of IGFBP2 on the biological behaviors of cancers, it has been clearly demonstrated that IGFBP2 is overexpressed in a wide variety of human malignancies, and evidence is rapidly accumulating to indicate that IGFBP2 is significantly involved in the progression of glioma and confers malignant phenotypes of glioblastoma cells. To clarify the molecular mechanisms underlying the effects of IGFBP2 on gliomas, not only the pericellular IGF-dependent and IGF-independent functions but also the functions of intracellular IGFBP2 should be defined (Figure 2). Additional information concerning the factors that directly regulate IGFBP2 overexpression in gliomas and those that are critically involved in the IGFBP2-mediated malignant features of glioblastoma cells is required and may lead to new therapeutic avenues for one of the most treatment-resistant human tumors.

5. Acknowledgment

We thank Drs. Makiko Kawaguchi, Yukihiro Haruyama and Hideo Takeshima for their valuable suggestions and Ms. Yasuko Tobayashi for her skillful technical assistance in our project. This work was supported in part by Grant-in-Aid for Scientific Research no. 20390114 (H. Kataoka) and for Young Scientists no. 22790384 (T. Fukushima) from the Ministry of Education, Science, Sports and Culture, Japan. The authors disclose no conflicts.

6. References

Baumann, P., Cremers, N., Kroese, F., Orend, G., Chiquet-Ehrismann, R., Uede, T., Yagita, H. & Sleeman, J.P. (2005). CD24 expression causes the acquisition of multiple cellular properties associated with tumor growth and metastasis. *Cancer Research*, Vol.65, No.23, pp. 10783-10793, ISSN 0008-5472

Bunn, R.C., John L. & Fowlkes, J.L. (2003). Insulin-like growth factor-binding protein proteolysis. *Trends in Endocrinology and Metabolism,* Vol.14, No.4, pp. 174-181, ISSN 1043-2760

Busund, L.T., Richardsen, E., Busund, R., Ukkonen, T., Bjornsen, T., Busch, C. & Stalsberg, H. (2005). Significant expression of IGFBP2 in breast cancer compared with benign lesions. *Journal of Clinical Pathology,* Vol.58, No.4, pp. 361-366, ISSN 0021-9746

Blum, W.F., Horn, N., Kratzsch, J., Jørgensen, J.O., Juul, A., Teale, D., Mohnike, K. & Ranke, M.B. (1993). Clinical studies of IGFBP-2 by radioimmunoassay. *Growth Regulation,* Vol.3, No.1, pp.100-104, ISSN 0956-523X

Carmeliet, P., Dor, Y., Herbert, J.M., Fukumura, D., Brusselmans, K., Dewerchin, M., Neeman, M., Bono, F., Abramovitch, R., Maxwell, P., Koch, C.J., Ratcliffe, P., Moons, L., Jain, R.K., Collen, D. & Keshert, E. (1998) Role of HIF-1α in hypoxia-mediated apoptosis, cell proliferation and tumour angiogenesis. *Nature,* Vol.394, No.6692, pp. 485-490, ISSN 0028-0836

Cazals, V., Nabeyrat, E., Corroyer, S., de Keyzer, Y. & Clement, A. (1999). Role for NF-kappa B in mediating the effects of hyperoxia on IGF-binding protein 2 promoter activity in lung alveolar epithelial cells. *Biochemical and Biophysical Research Communications,* Vol.1448, No.3, pp. 349-362, ISSN 0006-3002

Clarke, J., Butowski, N. & Chang S. (2010). Recent advances in therapy for glioblastoma. *Archives of Neurology,* Vol.67, No.3, pp. 279-283, ISSN 0003-9942

Clement, V., Sanchez, P., de Tribolet, N., Radovanovic, I., Ruiz, I. & Altaba, A. (2007). HEDGEHOG-GLI1 signaling regulates human glioma growth, cancer stem cell self-renewal, and tumorigenicity. *Current Biology,* Vol.17, No.2, pp. 165-172, ISSN 0960-9822

Clemmons, D.R. (1998). Role of insulin-like growth factor binding proteins in controlling IGF actions. *Molecular and Cellular Endocrinology,* Vol.140, No.1-2, pp. 19-24, ISSN 0303-7207

Cohen, P., Peehl, D. M., Graves, H.C., Rosenfeld, R.G. & Rosenfeld, R. G. (1994). Biological effects of prostate specific antigen as an insulin-like growth factor binding protein-3 protease. *Journal of Endocrinology,* Vol.142, No.3, pp. 407-415, ISSN 0022-0795

de Bont, J.M., van Doorn, J., Reddingius, R.E., Graat, G.H., Passier, M.M., den Boer, M.L. & Pieters, R. (2008). Various components of the insulin-like growth factor system in tumor tissue, cerebrospinal fluid and peripheral blood of pediatric medulloblastoma and ependymoma patients. *International Journal of Cancer,* Vol.123, No.3, pp. 594-600, ISSN 0020-7136

de Groot, J.F., Fuller, G., Kumar, A.J., Piao, Y., Eterovic, K., Ji ,Y. & Conrad, C.A. (2010). Tumor invasion after treatment of glioblastoma with bevacizumab: radiographic and pathologic correlation in humans and mice. *Neuro-Oncology,* Vol.12, No.3, pp.233-242, ISSN 1522-8517

DeMambro, V.E., Clemmons, D.R., Horton, L.G., Bouxsein, M.L., Wood, T.L., Beamer, W.G., Canalis, E. & Rosen, C.J. (2008). Gender-specific changes in bone turnover and skeletal architecture in igfbp-2-null mice. *Endocrinology,* Vol.149, No.5, pp. 2051-2561, ISSN 0013-7227

Diehl, D., Hessel, E., Oesterle, D., Renner-Müller, I., Elmlinger, M., Langhammer, M., Göttlicher, M., Wolf, E., Lahm, H. & Hoeflich, A. (2008). IGFBP-2 overexpression reduces the appearance of dysplastic aberrant crypt foci and inhibits growth of adenomas in chemically induced colorectal carcinogenesis. *International Journal of Cancer*, Vol.124, No.9, pp. 2220-2225, ISSN 0020-7136

Dunlap, S.M., Celestino, J., Wang, H., Jiang, R., Holland, E.C., Fuller, G.N. & Zhang, W. (2007). Insulin-like growth factor binding protein 2 promotes glioma development and progression. *Proceedings of the National Academy of Sciences of the United States of America* Vol.104, No.28, pp. 11736-11741, ISSN 0027-8424

Elmlinger, M.W., Deininger, M.H., Schuett, B.S., Meyermann, R., Duffner, F., Grote, E.H. & Ranke, M.B. (2001). *In Vivo* expression of insulin-like growth factor-binding protein-2 in human gliomas increases with the tumor grade. *Endocrinology*, Vol.142, No.4, pp.1652-1658, ISSN 0013-7227

Feldser, D., Agani F., Iyer, N.V., Pak, B., Ferreira, G. & Semenza, G.L. (1999). Reciprocal positive regulation of hypoxia-inducible factor 1alpha and insulin-like growth factor 2. *Cancer Research*, Vol.59, No.16, pp. 3915-3918, ISSN 0008-5472

Firth, S.M. & Baxter, R.C. (2002). Cellular Actions of the Insulin-Like Growth Factor Binding Proteins. *Endocrine Reviews*, Vol.23, No.6, pp. 824–854, ISSN 0163-769X

Fowlkes, J.L., Serra, D.M., Bunn, R.C., Thrailkill, K.M., Enghild, J.J. & Nagase, H. (2004). Regulation of insulin-like growth factor (IGF)-I action by matrix metalloproteinase-3 involves selective disruption of IGF-I/IGF-binding protein-3 complexes. *Endocrinology*, Vol.145, No.2, pp. 620-626, ISSN 0013-7227

Fukushima, T. & Kataoka, H. (2007). Roles of insulin-like growth factor binding protein-2 (IGFBP-2) in glioblastoma. *Anticancer Research*, Vol.27, No.6A, pp. 3685-3692, ISSN 0250-7005

Fukushima, T., Tezuka, T., Shimomura, T., Nakano, S. & Kataoka, H. (2007), Silencing of insulin-like growth factor-binding protein-2 in human glioblastoma cells reduces both invasiveness and expression of progression-associated gene CD24. *Journal of Biological Chemistry*, Vol. 282, No.25, pp. 18634-18644, ISSN 0021-9258

Fuller, G. N., Rhee, C. H., Hess, K. R., Caskey, L. S., Wang, R., Bruner, J. M., Yung, W. K., & Zhang, W. (1999). Reactivation of insulin-like growth factor binding protein 2 expression in glioblastoma multiforme: a revelation by parallel gene expression profiling. *Cancer Research*, Vol.59, No.17, pp. 4228-4232, ISSN 0008-5472

Garner, C.P., Ding, Y.C., John, E.M., Ingles, S.A., Olopade, O.I., Huo, D., Adebamowo, C., Ogundiran, T. & Neuhausen, S.L.(2008). Genetic variation in IGFBP2 and IGFBP5 is associated with breast cancer in populations of African descent. *Human Genetics*, Vol.123, No.3, pp. 247-255, ISSN 0340-6717

Godard, S., Getz, G., Delorenzi, M., Farmer, P., Kobayashi, H., Desbaillets, I., Nozaki, M., Diserens, A.C., Hamou, M.F., Dietrich, P.Y., Regli, L., Janzer, R.C., Bucher, P., Stupp, R., de Tribolet, N., Domany, E. & Hegi, M.E. (2003). Classification of human astrocytic gliomas on the basis of gene expression: a correlated group of genes with angiogenic activity emerges as a strong predictor of subtypes. *Cancer Research*, Vol.63, No.20, pp. 6613-6625, ISSN 0008-5472

Gonzalez, J. & de Groot, J. (2008) Combination therapy for malignant glioma based on PTEN status. *Expert Review of Anticancer Therapy*, Vol.8, No.11, pp. 1767-1779, ISSN 1473-7140

Grimberg, A., Coleman, C.M., Shi, Z., Burns, T.F., MacLachlan, T.K., Wang, W. & El-Deiry, W.S. (2006). Insulin-like growth factor factor binding protein-2 is a novel mediator of p53 inhibition of insulin-like growth factor signaling. *Cancer Biology & Therapy*, Vol.5, No.10, pp.1408-1414, ISSN 1538-4047

Harris, P.J., Takebe, N. & Ivy, S.P. (2010). Molecular conversations and the development of the hair follicle and basal cell carcinoma. *Cancer Prevention Research*, Vol.3, No.10, pp. 1217-1221, ISSN 1940-6207

Hedbacker, K., Birsoy, K., Wysocki, R.W., Asilmaz, E., Ahima, R.S., Farooqi, I.S. & Friedman, J.M.(2010). Antidiabetic effects of IGFBP2, a leptin-regulated gene. *Cell Metabolism*, Vol.11, No.1, pp. 11-22, ISSN 1550-4131

Hoeflich, A., Reisinger, R., Schuett, B.S., Elmlinger, M.W., Russo, V.C., Vargas, G.A., Jehle, P.M., Lahm, H., Renner-Muller, I. & Wolf, E. (2004). Peri/nuclear localization of intact insulin-like growth factor binding protein-2 and a distinct carboxyl-terminal IGFBP-2 fragment *in vivo*. *Biochemical and Biochemical and Biophysical Research Communications*, Vol.324, No.2, pp.705-710, ISSN 0006-291X

Hsieh, D., Hsieh, A., Stea, B. & Ellsworth, R. (2010). IGFBP2 promotes glioma tumor stem cell expansion and survival. *Biochemical and Biochemical and Biophysical Research Communications*, Vol.397, No.2, pp.367-372, ISSN 0006-291X

Hwa, V., Oh, Y. & Rosenfeld, R.G. (1999). The insulin-like growth factor-binding protein (IGFBP) superfamily. *Endocrinology Review*, Vol.20, No.6, pp. 761-787, ISSN 0163-769X

Ji, P., Smith, S.M., Wang, Y., Jiang, R., Song, S.W., Li, B., Sawaya, R., Bruner, J.M., Kuang, J., Yu, H., Fuller, G.N. & Zhang, W. (2010). Inhibition of gliomagenesis and attenuation of mitotic transition by MIIP. *Oncogene*, Vol.29, No.24, pp. 3501-3508, ISSN 0950-9232

Jiang, R., Mircean, C., Shmulevich, I., Cogdell, D., Jia, Y., Tabus, I., Aldape, K., Sawaya, R., Bruner, J.M., Fuller, G.N. & Zhang, W. (2006). Pathway alterations during glioma progression revealed by reverse phase protein lysate arrays. *Proteomics*, Vol.6, No.10, pp. 2964-2971, ISSN 1615-9853

Kelley, K.M., Schmidt, K.E., Berg, L., Sak, K., Galima, M.M., Gillespie ,C., Balogh, L., Hawayek, A., Reyes, J.A. & Jamison, M. (2002). Comparative endocrinology of the insulin-like growth factor-binding protein. *The Journal of Endocrinology*, Vol.175, No.1, pp. 3-18, ISSN 0022-0795

Kristiansen, G., Sammar, M. & Altevogt, P. (2004). Tumour biological aspects of CD24, a mucin-like adhesion molecule. *Journal of Molecular Histology*, Vo.35, No.3 , pp. 255-264, ISSN 1567-2379

Lancaster, J. M., Sayer, R. A., Blanchette, C., Calingaert, B., Konidari, I., Gray, J., Schildkraut, J., Schomberg, D. W., Marks, J. R., & Berchuck, A. (2006). High expression of insulin-like growth factor binding protein-2 messenger RNA in epithelial ovarian cancers produces elevated preoperative serum levels. *International Journal of Gynecological Cancer*, Vol.16, No.4, pp. 1529-1535, ISSN 1048-891X

Lee, C.Y. & Rechler, M.M. (1996). Proteolysis of insulin-like growth factor (IGF)-binding protein-3 (IGFBP-3) in 150-kilodalton IGFBP complexes by a cation-dependent protease activity in adult rat serum promotes the release of bound IGF-I. *Endocrinology*, Vol.137, No.5, pp. 2051-2058, ISSN 0013-7227

Lee, D.Y., Kim, S.J. & Lee, Y.C. (1999). Serum insulin-like growth factor (IGF)-I and IGF-binding proteins in lung cancer patients. *Journal of Korean Medical Science*, Vol.14, No.4, pp. 401-404, ISSN 1011-8934

Lee, W.H., Michels, K.M. & Bondy, C.A. (1993). Localization of insulin growth factor binding protein-2 messenger RNA during postnatal brain development: correlation with insulin-like growth factors I and II. *Neuroscience*, Vol.53, No.1, pp. 251-265, ISSN 251-265

Levitt, R.J., Georgescu, M.M. & Pollak, M. (2005). PTEN-induction in U251 glioma cells decreases the expression of insulin-like growth factor binding protein-2. *Biochemical and Biophysical Research Communications*, Vol.336, No.4, pp. 1056-1061, ISSN 0006-291X

Li, L., Gondi, C.S., Dinh, D.H., Olivero, W.C., Gujrati, M. & Rao, J.S. (2007). Transfection with anti-p65 intraantibody suppresses invasion and angiogenesis in glioma cells by blocking nuclear factor-κB transcriptional activity. *Clinical Cancer Research*, Vol.13, No.7, pp. 2178-2190, ISSN 1078-0432

Li, Z. & Picard, F. (2010). Modulation of IGFBP2 mRNA expression in white adipose tissue upon aging and obesity. *Hormone and Metabolic Research*, Vol.42, No.11, pp. 787-791, ISSN 0018-5043

Lin, Y., Jiang, T., Zhou, K., Xu, L,. Chen, B., Li, G., Qiu, X., Jiang, T., Zhang, W. & Song, S.W. (2009). Plasma IGFBP-2 levels predict clinical outcomes of patients with high-grade gliomas. *Neuro-Oncology*, Vol.11, No.5, pp. 468-476, ISSN 1522-8517

Lo, H.W., Zhu, H., Cao, X., Aldrich, A. & Ali-Osman, F. (2009) A novel splice variant of GLI1 that promotes glioblastoma cell migration and invasion. *Cancer Research*, Vol.69, No.17, pp. 6790-6798, ISSN 0008-5472

Mark, S., Kubler, B., Honing, S., Oesterreicher, S., John, H., Braulke ,T., Forssmann, W.G. & Standker, L. (2005). Diversity of human insulin-like growth factor (IGF) binding protein-2 fragments in plasma: primary structure, IGF-binding properties, and disulfide bonding pattern. *Biochemistry*, Vol.44, No.9, pp. 3644-3652, ISSN 0006-2960

Mehrian-Shai ,R., Chen, C.D., Shi, T., Horvath, S., Nelson, S.F., Reichardt, J.K. & Sawyers, C.L. (2007). Insulin growth factor-binding protein 2 is a candidate biomarker for PTEN status and PI3K/Akt pathway activation in glioblastoma and prostate cancer. *Proceedings of the National Academy of Sciences of the United States of America*, Vol.104, No.13, pp. 5563-5568, ISSN 0027-8424

Migita, T., Narita, T., Asaka, R., Miyagi, E., Nagano, H., Nomura, K., Matsuura, M., Satoh, Y., Okumura, S., Nakagawa, K., Seimiya, H. & Ishikawa, Y. (2010). Role of insulin-like growth factor binding protein 2 in lung adenocarcinoma: IGF-independent antiapoptotic effect via caspase-3. *American Journal of Pathology*, Vol.176, No.4, pp. 1756-1766, ISSN 0002-9440

Mishra, L., Bass, B., Ooi, B. S., Sidawy, A., & Korman, L. (1998), Role of insulin-like growth factor-I (IGF-I) receptor, IGF-I, and IGF binding protein-2 in human colorectal cancers. *Growth Hormone & IGF Research*, Vol.8, No.6, pp.473-479, ISSN 1096-6374

Moore, L.M., Holmes, K.M., Smith, S.M., Wu, Y., Tchougounova, E., Uhrbom, L., Sawaya, R., Bruner, J.M., Fuller, G.N. & Zhang, W. (2009). IGFBP2 is a candidate biomarker for Ink4a-Arf status and a therapeutic target for high-grade gliomas. *Proceedings of the National Academy of Sciences of the United States of America*, Vol.106, No.39, pp. 16675-16679, ISSN 0027-8424

Mouhieddine, O.B., Cazals, V., Kuto, E., Le, Bouc, Y. & Clement, A. (1996). Glucocorticoid-induced growth arrest of lung alveolar epithelial cells is associated with increased production of insulin-like growth factor binding protein-2. *Endocrinology*, Vol.137, No.1, pp.287-295, ISSN 0013-7227

Nakamura, M., Miyamoto, S., Maeda, H., Ishii, G., Hasebe, T., Chiba, T., Asaka, M. & Ochiai, A. (2005). Matrix metalloproteinase-7 degrades all insulin-like growth factor binding proteins and facilitates insulin-like growth factor bioavailability. *Biochem Biophys Research Communications*, Vol.333, No.3, pp. 1011-1016, ISSN 0006-291X

Nordqvist, A. C. & Mathiesen, T. (2002). Expression of IGF-II, IGFBP-2, -5, and -6 in meningiomas with different brain invasiveness. *Journal of Neurooncology*, Vol.57, No.1, pp. 19-26, ISSN 0167-594X

Nordqvist, A.C., Peyrard,M., Pettersson, H., Mathiesen, V.T., Collins, P., Dumanski, J.P. & Schaffing, M. (1997). A high ratio of insulin-like-growth factor II/insulin-like growth factor binding protein 2 messenger RNA as a marker for anaplasia in meningiomas. *Cancer Research*, Vol.57, No.13, pp.2611-2614, ISSN 0008-5472

Pekonen, F., Nyman, T., Ilvesmäki, V. & Partanen, S. (1992). Insulin-like growth factor binding proteins in human breast cancer tissue. *Cancer Research*, Vol.52. No.19, pp. 5204-5207, ISSN 0008-5472

Perks, C.M., Vernon, E.G., Rosendahl, A.H., Tonge, D. & Holly, J.M. (2007). IGF-II and IGFBP-2 differentially regulate PTEN in human breast cancer cells. *Oncogene* Vol.26, No.40, pp. 5966-5972, ISSN 0950-9232

Rickman, D. S., Bobek, M. P., Misek, D. E., Kuick, R., Blaivas, M., Kurnit, D. M., Taylor, J. & Hanash, S. M. (2001). Distinctive molecular profiles of high-grade and low-grade gliomas based on oligonucleotide microarray analysis. *Cancer Research*, Vol.61, No.18, pp.6885-6891, ISSN 0008-5472

Runz, S., Mierke, C.T., Joumaa, S., Behrens, J., Fabry, B. & Altevogt, P. (2008). CD24 induces localization of beta1 integrin to lipid raft domains. *Biochemical and Biophysical Research Communications*, Vol.365, No.1, pp.35-41, ISSN 0006-291X

Russo, V.C., Schütt, B.S., Andaloro, E., Ymer, S.I., Hoeflich, A., Ranke, M.B., Bach, L.A. & Werther, G.A. (2005). Insulin-like growth factor binding protein-2 binding to extracellular matrix plays a critical role in neuroblastoma cell proliferation, migration, and invasion. *Endocrinology*, Vol.146, No.10, pp. 4445-4455, ISSN 0013-7227

Sallinen, S. L., Sallinen, P. K., Haapasalo, H. K., Helin, H. J., Helen, P. T., Schraml, P., Kallioniemi, O. P. & Kononen, J. (2000). Identification of differentially expressed genes in human gliomas by DNA microarray and tissue chip techniques. *Cancer Research*, Vol.60, No.23, pp. 6617-6622, ISSN 0008-5472

Sagiv, E., Starr, A., Rozovski, R., Altevogt, P., Wang, T. & Arber, N. (2008). Targeting CD24 for treatment of colorectal and pancreatic cancer by monoclonal antibodies or small interfering RNA. *Cancer Research*, Vol.68, No.8, pp. 2803-2812, ISSN 0008-5472

Santosh, V., Arivazhagan, A., Sreekanthreddy, P., Srinivasan, H., Thota, B., Srividya, M.R., Vrinda, M., Sridevi, S., Shailaja, B.C., Samuel, C., Prasanna, K.V., Thennarasu, K., Balasubramaniam, A., Chandramouli, B.A., Hegde, A.S., Somasundaram, K., Kondaiah, P. & Rao, M.R. (2010). Grade-specific expression of insulin-like growth factor-binding proteins-2, -3, and -5 in astrocytomas: IGFBP-3 emerges as a strong predictor of survival in patients with newly diagnosed glioblastoma. *Cancer Epidemiology, Biomarkers & Prevention*, Vol.19, No.6, pp. 1399-1408, ISSN 1055-9965

Schutt, B.S., Langkamp, M., Rauschnabel, U., Ranke, M.B. & Elmlinger, M.W. (2004). Integrin-mediated action of insulin-like growth factor binding protein-2 in tumor cells. Journal of Molecular Endocrinology, Vol.32, No.3, pp. 859-868, ISSN 0952-5041

Schwander, J. & Mary, J.L. (1993). The RIA for IGFBP-2 in man--a meagre catch?, *Growth Regulation*, Vol.3, No.1, pp. 104-108, ISSN 0956-523X

Smith, J.S., Alderete, B., Minn, Y., Borell, T.J,. Perry, A., Mohapatra, G., Hosek, S.M., Kimmel, D., O'Fallon, J., Yates, A., Feuerstein, B.G., Burger, P.C., Scheithauer, B.W. & Jenkins, R.B. (1999). Localization of common deletion regions on 1p and 19q in human gliomas and their association with histological subtype. *Oncogene*, Vol.18, No.28, pp. 4144-4152, ISSN 0950-9232

Song, S.W., Fuller, G.N., Khan, A., Kong, S., Shen, W., Taylor, E., Ramdas, L., Lang, F. F. & Zhang, W. (2003) IIp45, an insulin-like growth factor binding protein 2 (IGFBP-2) binding protein, antagonizes IGFBP-2 stimulation of glioma cell invasion. *Proceedings of the National Academy of Sciences of the United States of America*, Vol.100, No.24, pp. 13970-13975, ISSN 0027-8424

Su, D., Deng, H., Zhao, X., Zhang, X., Chen, L., Chen, X., Li, Z., Bai, Y., Wang, Y., Zhong, Q., Yi, T., Qian, Z. & Wei, Y. (2009). Targeting CD24 for treatment of ovarian cancer by short hairpin RNA. *Cytotherapy*, Vo.11, No.5, pp. 642-652, ISSN 1465-3249

Sulis, M.L. & Parsons, R. (2003). PTEN: from pathology to biology. *Trends in Cell Biology*, Vol.13, No.9, pp. 478-483, ISSN 0962-8924

van den Beld, A.W., Blum, W.F., Pols, H.A., Grobbee, D.E. & Lamberts, S.W. (2003). Serum insulin-like growth factor binding protein-2 levels as an indicator of functional ability in elderly men. *European Journal of Endocrinology*, Vol.148, No.6, pp. 627–634, ISSN 0804-4643

Villani, R.M., Adolphe, C., Palmer, J., Waters, M.J. & Wainwright, B.J. (2010) Patched1 inhibits epidermal progenitor cell expansion and basal cell carcinoma formation by limiting Igfbp2 activity. *Cancer Prevention Research*, Vol.3, No.10, pp. 1222-1234, ISSN 1940-6207

Wang, G.K., Hu, L., Fuller, G.N. & Zhang, W. (2006). An interaction between insulin-like growth factor-binding protein 2 (IGFBP2) and integrin alpha5 is essential for

IGFBP2-induced cell mobility. *Journal of Biological Chemistry*, Vol.281, No.20, pp. 14085-14091, ISSN 0021-9258

Wang, H., Shen, W., Huang, H., Hu, L., Ramdas, L., Zhou, Y.H., Liao, W.S., Fuller, G.N. & Zhang, W. (2003). Insulin-like growth factor binding protein 2 enhances glioblastoma invasion by activating invasion-enhancing genes. *Cancer Research*, Vol.63, No.15, pp. 4315-4321, ISSN 0008-5472

Wang, H., Wang, H., Zhang, W., Huang, H.J., Liao, W.S.L. & Fuller, G.N. (2004). Analysis of the activation status of Akt, NFκB, and Stat3 in human diffuse gliomas. *Laboratory Investigation*, Vol.84, No. 8, pp.941-951, ISSN 0023-6837

Wood, T.L., Rogler, L.E., Czick, M.E., Schuller, A.G. & Pintar, J.E.. (2000). Selective alterations in organ sizes in mice with a targeted disruption of the insulin-like growth factor binding protein-2 gene. *Journal of Molecular Endocrinology*, Vol.14, No.9, pp. 1472-1482, ISSN 0952-5041

Wood, T.L., Rogler, L., Streck, R.D., Cerro, J., Green, B., Grewal, A. & Pintar, J.E. (1993). Targeted disruption of IGFBP-2 gene. *Growth Regulation*, Vol.3, No.1, pp. 5-8, ISSN 0956-523X

Wood, T. L., Streck, R. D. & Pintar, J. E. (1992). Expression of the IGFBP-2 gene in post-implantation rat embryos. *Development*, Vol.114, No.1, pp. 59-66, ISSN 0950-1991

Wu, Y., Song, S.W., Sun, J., Bruner, J.M., Fuller, G.N. & Zhang, W. (2010). IIp45 inhibits cell migration through inhibition of HDAC6. *Journal of Biological Chemistry*, Vol.285, No.6, pp. 3554-3560, ISSN 0021-9258

Zheng, B., Clark,e J.B., Busby, W.H., Duan, C., Clemmons, D.R. (1998). Insulin-like growth factor-binding protein-5 is cleaved by physiological concentrations of thrombin. *Endocrinology*, Vol.139, No.4, pp. 1708-1714. ISSN 0013-7227

Zheng, S., Houseman, E.A., Morrison, Z., Wrensch, M.R., Patoka, J.S., Ramos, C., Haas-Kogan, D.A., McBride, S., Marsit, C.J., Christensen, B.C., Nelson, H.H., Stokoe, D., Wiemels, J.L., Chang, S.M., Prados, M.D., Tihan, T., Vandenberg, S.R., Kelsey, K.T., Berger, M.S. & Wiencke, J.K. (2011). DNA hypermethylation profiles associated with glioma subtypes and EZH2 and IGFBP2 mRNA expression. *Neuro-Oncology*, Vol.13, No.3, pp. 280-289, ISSN 1522-8517

Part 8

IDHs Mutations- Gliomas

20

The Role of Isocitrate Dehydrogenase Mutations in Glioma Brain Tumors

Chi-Ming Chang, Kaiming Xu and Hui-Kuo G. Shu
Emory University
United States

1. Introduction

Isocitrate dehydrogenases (IDHs) are enzymes long known to biologists as a component of the tricarboxylic acid (TCA) cycle that converts isocitrate to α-ketoglutarate (α-KG) with production of NADH and/or NADPH. However, it was mainly viewed as a "housekeeping" gene by cancer biologists with no previously defined role in cancer. This changed in 2008 with the discovery that IDH1 was frequently mutated in glioblastoma multiformes (GBMs) (Parsons et al., 2008). IDH mutations have now also been found in lower grade gliomas as well as in acute myelocytic leukemias. The purpose of this chapter is to review the normal functions of the IDH isoforms and their role in glioma brain tumors from initial discovery of a specific mutation in IDH1 to what is currently known about the mechanisms of action of mutant IDHs.

2. Normal function of isocitrate dehydrogenases

2.1 Isocitrate dehydrogenase enzymatic activity and structure

IDH is an enzyme whose activity is to oxidatively decarboxylate isocitrate producing α-ketoglutarate (α-KG) and CO_2 (Haselbeck & McAlister-Henn, 1993). A schematic of this reaction with all the family members is shown (Fig. 1). During this process, NAD^+ or $NADP^+$ is reduced to NADH or NADPH, respectively, depending on the isoform that is catalyzing this reaction. The IDH1 and IDH2 isoforms are $NADP^+$ dependent and function as homodimers (Bailey & Colman, 1985; Kelly & Plaut, 1981). They are structurally related sharing approximately 70% sequence identity between the two isoforms (Xu et al., 2004). IDH1 is most highly expressed in liver while IDH2 show the greatest expression in muscle (Haselbeck et al., 1992; Jennings et al., 1994). However, both isoforms show moderate expression within a variety of other tissues including brain (Jennings et al., 1994). The IDH3 isoform is NAD^+ dependent, functions as a heterotetramer consisting of 2 α, 1 β and 1 γ subunits (Ramachandran & Colman, 1980), and is structurally unrelated to IDH1 and IDH2 (Nichols et al., 1993; Nichols et al., 1995). IDH3 is the classical TCA cycle enzyme and plays an integral role in cellular energy metabolism. Consequently, IDH3 is found predominantly in the mitochondria (Haselbeck & McAlister-Henn, 1993). IDH2 also localizes to the mitochondria and has a mitochondrial signal peptide at its N-terminus (Nekrutenko et al., 1998). By contrast, IDH1 is localized mainly in the cytoplasm but has a type 1 peroxisomal targeting sequence permitting localization in peroxisomes (Henke et al., 1998; Nekrutenko et al., 1998). The reactions catalyzed by IDH1/2 are reversible while the similar reaction catalyzed by IDH3 is irreversible. Because only IDH1 and IDH2 mutations have been shown to be important in malignancies, we will not be addressing IDH3 further.

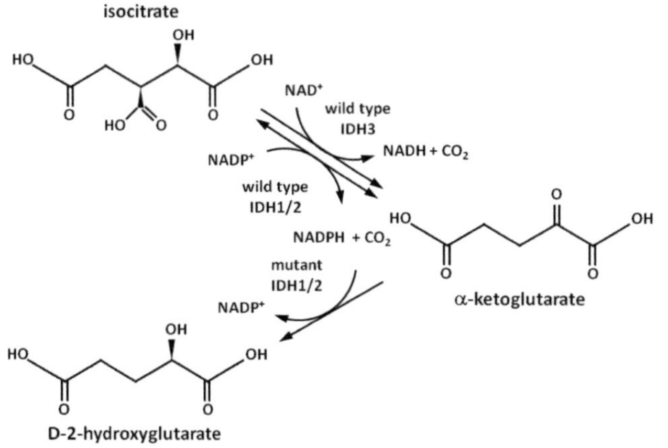

Fig. 1. Enzymatic activity of wild type and mutant IDH isoforms.

Structural characteristics of mammalian IDH1 and IDH2 are well-known with elucidation of their crystal structures (Ceccarelli et al., 2002; Xu et al., 2004). A cartoon representation of the IDH1 homodimer is shown (IDH2 structure is similar) (Fig. 2). These enzymes dimerize with two active site in an open, inactive conformation, which is maintained by an intramolecular interaction between a conserved serine at position 94 and aspartic acid at position 279 in IDH1 blocking access to the active site. The IDH homodimer shifts to the closed, active conformation when this serine:aspartic acid interaction is lost permitting entry of an isocitrate:metal ion complex into the active site. The reaction proceeds with formation of α-KG and NADPH which is released with either immediate reoccupation of the active site with another isocitrate:metal ion complex and $NADP^+$ or reassociation of the serine:aspartic acid interaction returning the enzyme back to an inactive state.

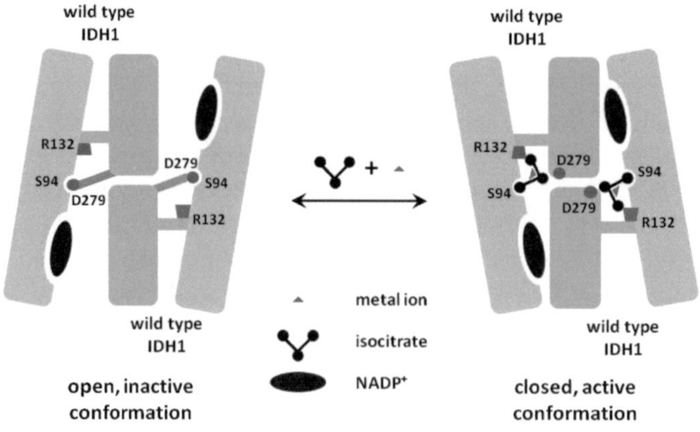

Fig. 2. Representation of wild type IDH1 homodimers shifting between the inactive and active conformations.

2.2 Normal function of isocitrate dehydrogenase in cellular metabolism

Both IDH1 and IDH2 play key roles in various cellular metabolic functions. They are involved in the oxidation of polyunsaturated fatty acids within peroxisomes (IDH1) and mitochondria (IDH2) by using the NADPH generated by their enzymatic activity (Minard & McAlister-Henn, 1999; van Roermund et al., 1998). In the liver, IDH1 is regulated by sterol regulatory element-binding proteins and also generates NADPH for peroxisomal lipogenesis (Shechter et al., 2003). In pancreatic islet cells, IDH1 has an important role in cellular glucose sensing as evidenced by impairment of glucose-stimulated insulin secretion after knockdown of IDH1 expression (Ronnebaum et al., 2006). Consistent with these functions, IDH1 transgenic mice display fatty livers, hyperlipidemia, obesity and higher glucose sensitivity on glucose tolerance testing consistent with enhanced insulin secretion (Koh et al., 2004). Finally, IDH2 has probable roles in the TCA cycle as evidenced by the lack of pathology in most normal tissues of certain retinitis pigmentosa patients with a homozygous IDH3 subunit defect (Hartong et al., 2008). The reverse reaction (producing isocitrate and $NADP^+$ from α-KG and NADPH) by IDH2 has been proposed as a way of limiting flux through the TCA cycle and dissipating the proton electrochemical gradient across the inner mitochondrial membrane with heat generation (Sazanov & Jackson, 1994). These various metabolic functions that have been defined to date show the central role that IDH1 and IDH2 play at the crossroads of lipid synthesis and carbohydrate utilization.

2.3 The role of isocitrate dehydrogenase in response to oxidative stress

IDH1/2 also likely plays a part in the oxidative stress response and helps limit damage from such insults. Consistent with this idea, Mailloux et al. found that oxidative stress enhances α-KG and NADPH production by IDH1/2 with a concomitant decrease in IDH3, α-KG dehydrogenase, and succinate dehydrogenase activities decreasing utilization of the TCA cycle (Mailloux et al., 2007). NADPH produced by IDH1/2 can also be used by glutathione reductase for converting the oxidized form of glutathione (GSSG) to the reduced form (GSH) that can neutralize free radicals and reactive oxygen species (Jo et al., 2001; Kehrer & Lund, 1994; Lee et al., 2002). While the pentose phosphate pathway is the major source of NADPH required for regeneration of GSH, IDH1/2 can also contribute to this NADPH pool (Winkler et al., 1986). In addition, Lee et al. were able to generate a series of NIH3T3 derviatives that expressed varying levels of IDH1 and found that the ratio of GSH:GSSG was directly correlated with IDH1 expression level consistent with a role of this enzyme in the regeneration of GSH (Lee et al., 2002). Reduced expression of both IDH1 and IDH2 results in higher levels of reactive oxygen species and greater oxidative damage in response to an oxidative insult (Jo et al., 2001; Lee et al., 2002). In fact, numerous reports have now demonstrated that overexpression of IDH1 and IDH2 can protect cells against a variety of insults that produce oxidative stress (Jo et al., 2002; Kim et al., 2007; Lee et al., 2004; Shin et al., 2004). Based on this wealth of evidence demonstrating a role in the response of IDH1/2 to oxidative damage, the $NADP^+$-dependent IDHs clearly have significant functions beyond energy metabolism and biosynthetic processes.

3. Isocitrate dehydrogenase mutations in glial and other neoplasms

3.1 Discovery of isocitrate dehydrogenase 1 mutations in glioblastomas

GBMs are highly aggressive brain tumors classified by the World Health Organization (WHO) grading system as grade IV astrocytomas (Louis et al., 2007). While outcomes for patients with this diagnosis have gradually improved with better surgical/radiation therapy techniques and temozolomide chemotherapy, median survival still remain only slightly longer than one year (Stupp et al., 2005). With recent genomic technology advances, projects were initiated to perform detailed genomic analysis of various malignancies including GBMs. This effort quickly bore fruit with the discovery by Parson et al. that IDH1 is frequently mutated in GBMs (Parsons et al., 2008). They performed an initial screen consisting of comprehensive analysis of 20,661 protein-coding genes in 22 GBM samples. This yielded 21 mutated genes that were further analyzed in a followup screen on 83 additional GBMs. In addition to finding expected mutations at several genes known to be important in GBMs, the IDH1 gene was surprisingly found to be altered in 11% of analyzed GBMs. Most striking, mutations were invariably at a highly conserved arginine at position 132 (R132) found in the isocitrate binding site and was mutated to either histidine (R132H) (10 of 12) or serine (R132S) (remaining 2). This unexpected finding implicated IDH1 in the development and/or maintenance of glial neoplasms.

Followup studies confirmed the presence of IDH mutations in GBMs (Balss et al., 2008; Hartmann et al., 2009; Sanson et al., 2009; Watanabe et al., 2009; Yan et al., 2009) (Table 1). GBMs are classified as primary (de novo) or secondary depending on whether they arise spontaneously or from malignant transformation of a low grade glioma. Interestingly, the frequency of IDH1 mutations was significantly higher in secondary (82%) than primary (6%) GBMs. Thus, the incidence of IDH mutations in an undifferentiated cohort of GBMs would depend on the distribution of primary and secondary tumors in that group. Of note, initial studies suggest that pediatric GBMs only rarely harbor IDH mutations (Antonelli et al., 2010; Balss et al., 2008; Paugh et al., 2010; Yan et al., 2009). However, a recent paper suggests that pediatric malignant glioma patients ≥ 14 years of age appear to harbor IDH mutations at a substantial rate (7 of 20) (Pollack et al., 2011). This result suggests that high-grade

WHO Grade	Tumor type	Balss/ Hartmann[1]	Yan[2]	Watanabe[3]	Sanson[4]	Total (percent)
IV	1° GBM	7/99	6/123	3/59	11/183	27/464 (5.8%)
	2° GBM	7/8	11/13	28/34	10/13	56/68 (82.4%)
III	AA	148/228	38/52	21/27	9/18	216/325 (66.5%)
	AOA	128/177	7/7	10/14	34/54	179/252 (71.0%)
	AO	130/174	34/36	6/8	24/49	194/267 (72.7%)
II	A	167/227	27/30	60/68	10/12	264/337 (78.3%)
	OA	63/76	3/3	16/17	26/34	108/130 (83.1%)
	O	111/128	43/51	31/39	41/54	226/272 (83.1%)
I	Pilocytic Astrocytoma	1/41	0/21	3/31	NT	4/93 (4.3%)
I-III	Ependymoma	0/31	0/30	0/24	NT	0/85 (0%)

[1] Combined results of Balss and Hartmann studies due to duplication of some cases (Balss et al., 2008; Hartmann et al., 2009), [2] (Yan et al., 2009), [3] (Watanabe et al., 2009), [4] (Sanson et al., 2009).
Abbreviations: WHO, World Health Organization; GBM, glioblastoma multiforme; AA, anaplastic astrocytoma; AOA, anaplastic oligoastrocytoma; AO, anaplastic oligodendroglioma; A, astrocytoma; OA, oligoastrocytoma; O, oligodendroglioma; NT, not tested.

Table 1. Frequency of IDH mutations in various glial brain tumors.

gliomas in younger pediatric patients may be a different entity that those presenting in late adolescence with the older pediatric patients likely having a tumor that may be more similar to such tumors that present in young adulthood (eg. 20-40 years of age).

3.2 Isocitrate dehydrogenase mutations in other gliomas

Since secondary GBMs have a high incidence of IDH mutations, these mutations were postulated to be present in low grade gliomas as well. As predicted, pooled results found IDH mutations in 65% to 80% of grade II/III astrocytomas (Table 1) (Balss et al., 2008; Hartmann et al., 2009; Sanson et al., 2009; Watanabe et al., 2009; Yan et al., 2009). Grade II/III oligodendrogliomas and oligoastrocytomas also had a high incidence of IDH1 mutations in the 70-85% range. Finally, pilocytic astrocytomas only rarely harbor IDH1 mutations (<5%) while no IDH1 mutations were found in ependymomas of any grade (Balss et al., 2008; Watanabe et al., 2009; Yan et al., 2009).

Although IDH1 and IDH2 reside largely in different subcellular compartments, they have the same enzymatic activity, utilize $NADP^+$, and are believed to provide some redundant function(s) in the cell. Therefore, Yan et al. also sequenced IDH2 in addition to IDH1 in their series of brain tumors and found that IDH2 was, in fact, mutated at a low frequency on arginine at position 172 (R172), the comparable residue to R132 of IDH1 (Yan et al., 2009). Based on pooled results from multiple studies examining glioma brain tumors, when IDH is mutated, IDH1 is affected 96% of the time and IDH2 is affected in only 4% of cases (Table 2) (Hartmann et al., 2009; Sonoda et al., 2009; Yan et al., 2009). In addition, mutation on one IDH isoform was always mutually exclusive for mutation on the other isoform.

Type	Balss[1]	Yan[2]	Hartman[3]	Sanson[4]	Sonoda[5]	Total (percent)
IDH1	221	161	716	155	39	1292
R132H	205	142	664	138	39	1188 (92.0%)
R132C	8	7	29	5	--	49 (3.8%)
R132L	1	7	2	2	--	12 (0.9%)
R132S	4	4	11	3	--	22 (1.7%)
R132G	2	1	10	7	--	20 (1.5%)
R132V	1	--	--	--	--	1 (0.1%)
IDH2	NT	9	31	NT	1	41
R172K	NT	4	20	NT	1	25 (61.0%)
R172M	NT	3	6	NT	--	9 (22.0%)
R172G	NT	2	--	NT	--	2 (4.9%)
R172W	NT	--	5	NT	--	5 (12.2%)

[1] (Balss et al., 2008), [2] (Yan et al., 2009), [3] (Hartmann et al., 2009), [4] (Sanson et al., 2009), [5] (Sonoda et al., 2009).

Abbreviations: IDH, isocitrate dehydrogenase; NT, not tested.

Table 2. Type and frequency of IDH1/IDH2 mutations in gliomas.

The frequency distribution of mutations in IDH1/2 is summarized on Table 2 (Balss et al., 2008; Hartmann et al., 2009; Sanson et al., 2009; Sonoda et al., 2009; Yan et al., 2009). The great majority of mutations at R132 in IDH1 and R172 in IDH2 result from single nucleotide changes within the codon. Possible changes at these codons are shown with the frequency they are observed (Fig. 3). It is interesting to note that nearly 92% of IDH1 mutations were to histidine. Thus, a very significant selective advantage must be at play for this particular point mutation. There may also be slight selection for alterations to cysteine with an increased incidence of between 2-4 fold higher than any of the other three observed amino acids although total number of cases are relatively small. Numbers for IDH2 mutations are also relatively small, but does suggest skewing towards mutation of R172 to lysine (R172K).

IDH1 type	Codon[132]	AA	Frequency of mutation	IDH2 type	Codon[172]	AA	Frequency of mutation
wild type IDH1	C•G•T	Arg	N/A	wild type IDH2	A•G•G	Arg	N/A
R132S	*A*•G•T	Ser	1.7%	conserved	*C*•G•G	Arg	N/A
R132G	*G*•G•T	Gly	1.5%	R172G	*G*•G•G	Gly	4.9%
R132C	*T*•G•T	Cys	3.8%	R172W	*T*•G•G	Trp	12.2%
R132H	C•*A*•T	His	92.0%	R172K	A•*A*•G	Lys	61.0%
not seen	C•*C*•T	Pro	0%	not seen	A•*C*•G	Thr	0%
R132L	C•*T*•T	Leu	0.9%	R172M	A•*T*•G	Met	22.0%
conserved	C•G•*A*	Arg	N/A	conserved	A•G•*A*	Arg	N/A
conserved	C•G•*C*	Arg	N/A	not seen	A•G•*C*	Ser	0%
conserved	C•G•*G*	Arg	N/A	not seen	A•G•*T*	Ser	0%
R132V	*G*•*T*•T	Val	0.1%				

Fig. 3. Possible mutations in codon 132 of IDH1 and codon 172 of IDH2 with observed frequency in glial neoplasms.

3.3 Isocitrate dehydrogenase mutations in other malignancies

After discovery of the specific IDH1 and IDH2 mutations in gliomas, there was significant interest to determine whether these mutations were also present in other malignancies. Despite screening of a large number of tumor specimens, very few non-glioma, solid malignancies were found to contain these mutations. One study found 2 of 75 (2.7%) prostate cancers with IDH1 mutations while a second study found a metastatic melanoma with an IDH1 mutant (Bleeker et al., 2009; Kang et al., 2009; Lopez et al., 2010). Kang et al. also found an IDH1 mutation in 1 of 60 cases of B-cell acute lymphoblastic leukemia (Kang et al., 2009). Mutations at both IDH1 and IDH2 have now been shown to be present in acute myelogenous leukemias (AMLs). Mardis et al. were the first to report that 16 of 188 (8.5%) primary, cytogenetically normal AMLs had mutation at R132 in IDH1 (Mardis et al., 2009). Likewise, Ward et al. found in their cohort that 6 of 60 (10%) karyotypically normal AMLs had the expected IDH1 mutation (Ward et al., 2010). They also found that these AMLs were actually more likely to harbor mutations in IDH2 with the previously defined R172K mutation seen in 5 cases and a new mutation altering arginine at position 140 to glutamine (R140Q). These specific mutations all resulted in elevated levels of 2-hydroxyglutarate (2-HG), a marker of mutant IDH activity (details of this enzymatic activity will be covered in section 4.3). Marcucci et al. reported similar results in a Cancer and Leukemia Group B study where out of 358 cases of cytogenetically normal AMLs, 47 had IDH1 mutations at R132, 13 had IDH2 mutations at R172 and 56 had IDH2 mutations at R140 (Marcucci et al., 2010). Based on these studies, it appears that ~30% of cytogenetically normal AMLs harbor mutations in IDH1/2. Also, whereas the great majority of IDH mutations found in gliomas involve IDH1, mutations of IDH in AML are more evenly distributed between IDH1 and IDH2 with a slight favoring of the latter. Unlike the case where IDH1 and IDH2 mutations were always mutually exclusive, rare instances of AMLs with both mutation present has been reported (Paschka et al., 2010).

3.4 Clinical outcomes in gliomas harboring isocitrate dehydrogenase mutations

With the identification of IDH1 mutations in GBMs, Parson et al. made an intriguing observation that patients with this mutation had a significantly better survival (Parsons et al., 2008). However, since their clinical series only included 11 patients with IDH1 mutations, this finding required validation. At this time, multiple reports have confirmed that IDH1/2 mutations predict for improved outcomes in patients with GBMs as well as lower grade glial neoplasms (Dubbink et al., 2009; Nobusawa et al., 2009; Sanson et al., 2009; Sonoda et al., 2009; Yan et al., 2009). A summary of these reports is shown on Table 3.

		Median OS[1] (n = # of pts)		
Publications	**Glioma type**	**wtIDH**	**mutIDH**	**P-value**
Parsons[2]	**GBM**	1.1 yrs (79)	3.8 yrs (11)	<0.001
Yan[3]	**GBM**	15 (115)	31 (14)	0.002
	AA	20 (14)	65 (38)	< 0.001
Sanson[4]	**GBM, 1°**	14 (172)	27.4 (11)	< 0.01
	Grade 3	19.4 (54)	81.1 (67)	< 0.001
	Grade 2	60.1 (23)	150.9 (77)	0.01
Nobusawa[5]	**GBM, all**	9.9 (186)	24.0 (17)	< 0.0001
	GBM, 1°	10.0 (185)	31.6 (9)	< 0.0001
Sonoda[6]	**GBM (1° and 2°)**	17 (57)	66 (5)	0.1
	AA	22 (8)	50 (13)	0.001
Dubbink[7]	**Grade 2**	48 (7)	98 (42)	0.003

[1] in months except when otherwise indicated, [2] (Parsons et al., 2008), [3] (Yan et al., 2009), [4] (Sanson et al., 2009), [5] (Nobusawa et al., 2009), [6] (Sonoda et al., 2009), [7] (Dubbink et al., 2009).
Abbreviations: OS, overall survival; wtIDH, wild type isocitrate dehydrogenase; mutIDH, mutant isocitrate dehydrogenase; GBM, glioblastoma multiforme; AA, anaplastic astrocytomas; yrs, years.

Table 3. Series reporting outcomes for glioma patients with IDH mutations.

3.5 Factors in gliomas correlating with isocitrate dehydrogenase mutations

Certain clinical characteristics and markers have been associated with the presence of IDH1 mutations in GBMs. Patients with tumors harboring this mutation tend to be younger with an average age in the 40-50 year range versus 60+ years in patients lacking this mutation (Nobusawa et al., 2009). Although IDH1 mutations were associated with a younger age, presence of this mutation was still independently prognostic. Patients with tumors containing IDH1 mutations were also more likely to have a longer duration of symptoms consistent with a slower growing, less aggressive tumor. In addition, the presence of IDH1 mutations appears to be associated with certain genetic abnormalities including *TP53* mutation, *PTEN* mutation, lack of *EGFR* amplification, loss of heterozygosity on 19q, and loss of *CDKN2A/B* (Nobusawa et al., 2009; Yan et al., 2009). These correlations are not surprising given the predominance of IDH1 mutation in secondary GBMs. However, even when only primary GBMs are considered, correlation between IDH mutations and *TP53* mutation/lack of *EGFR* amplification was maintained (Nobusawa et al., 2009).

3.6 Isocitrate dehydrogenase mutations associate with proneural glioblastomas

Expression profiling of a series of high-grade astrocytomas have permitted subclassification based on a molecular signature. Phillips et al. performed one such analysis whereby 115 grade 3 and 4 astrocytomas were evaluated (Phillips et al., 2006). Based on their analysis, 3 distinct subgroups termed proneural, proliferative and mesenchymal could be identified based on similarities in gene expression pattern. The proneural group had markedly better prognosis and expressed genes associated with normal brain and neurogenesis. The proliferative group had a poor prognosis and expressed genes in a pattern that resembled highly proliferative cell lines. The mesenchymal group likewise had a poor prognosis and expressed genes that resembled tissues of mesenchymal origin. Since this report, the National Institutes of Health (NIH) established The Cancer Genome Atlas (TCGA) program that was charged with generating comprehensive multi-dimensional maps of the key genomic changes in major types of cancers. GBM was chosen as the pilot disease for this program. The expression profiling of GBMs for TCGA also permitted classification into subtypes (proneural, neural, classical, mesenchymal) similar to that described by Phillips et al. (Fig. 4) (Phillips et al., 2006; Verhaak et al., 2010). Interestingly, IDH1 was mutated in 11 of 37 cases (30%) of proneural GBMs with only a single case of mutant IDH1 found outside of the proneural group with that case being classified in the neural group (Verhaak et al., 2010). This analysis also validated an association between mutations in *TP53* and the presence of IDH1 mutations that had previously been noted. A subsequent updated TCGA report continues to show a tight association between IDH1 mutation and this favorable GBM subtype (Noushmehr et al., 2010).

	Median Survival (mos)	*IDH1* mutation	*TP53* mutation
Proneural subtype PDGFR alterations IDH1 mutations	16.2 (n=57)	11/37 (30%)	20/37 (54%)
Neural subtype Neural markers	15.0 (n=33)	1/19 (5%)	4/19 (21%)
Mesenchymal subtype Mesenchymal markers NF1 deletion	15.0 (n=58)	0/38 (0%)	12/38 (32%)
Classical subtype Chromosome 10 loss Chromosome 7 amplification	12.2 (n=54)	0/22 (0%)	0/22 (0%)

Fig. 4. GBM subtypes with their characteristics as classified by TCGA analysis with survival outcomes and associations with IDH1 and TP53 mutations.

4. Functional consequence of isocitrate dehydrogenase mutations

4.1 Isocitrate dehydrogenase mutants lose normal enzymatic activity

Based on modeling studies, the side chain of R132 can form three hydrogen bonds with the α- and β-carboxyl groups of isocitrate while other residues within the binding site forms no more than two such bonds (Zhao et al., 2009). Thus, replacement of R132 is likely to impair interactions between isocitrate and this site. In fact, this residue in IDH1 has been previously mutated to glutamic acid (R132E) and resulted in almost complete abrogation of enzymatic activity (Jennings et al., 1997). Zhao et al. show that the activity of the R132H, R132C and R132S mutants dropped to less than 20% of the wild type IDH1 enzyme with a corresponding increase in the Km for isocitrate by 60 to 94-fold (Zhao et al., 2009). Porcine IDH2 have also been mutated at the site comparable to R172 in human IDH2 (R133Q) and found to have decreased activity and increased Km for isocitrate (Soundar et al., 2000). All of the mutations found in IDH1 at R132 and in IDH2 at R172 have now been tested and the normal enzymatic activity is impaired in each case (Ichimura et al., 2009; Zhao et al., 2009).

4.2 Possible dominant negative activity of mutant isocitrate dehydrogenase 1

Because R132 mutations were so specific and alterations in the second allele had not been seen, this had the profile of an activating mutation. This hypothesis appeared to be incorrect with the discovery that R132 mutations resulted in loss of enzymatic activity (see section 4.1) (Yan et al., 2009; Zhao et al., 2009). However, since homozygous deletions or other inactivating mutations of IDH1/2 had not been reported, the IDH1 R132 mutations (and the IDH2R172 mutations) were clearly acting in a more complex fashion. This was explained to some extent with the report that R132 IDH1 mutants can act as a dominant negative inhibitor (Zhao et al., 2009). To show this, His-tagged wild type IDH1 and FLAG-tagged R132H mutant were purified, mixed and subjected to affinity purification using nickel resin and anti-FLAG beads to obtain preparations of wild type homodimer, R132H homodimers and wild type:R132H heterodimers. The R132H homodimer was found to have no activity while the wild type:R132 heterodimer had 4% of the wild type homodimer activity. While this result partially explained how mutant IDH1 can act as a tumor suppressor in the absence of deletion of its second allele, this model was still not completely satisfying. In this model, mutant IDH1 needs to be in great excess (although amplification/overexpression has never been shown) or the wild type:mutant IDH1 interactions needs to be favored over wild type:wild type interactions (although such differential affinity has also never been demonstrated). In addition, the cellular metabolite profiles of cells engineered either to express the R132H mutant or to suppress expression of wild type IDH1 have been assessed and showed very little similarity again consistent with the putative dominant negative function of mutant IDH1 having little if any role *in vivo* (Reitman et al., 2011). Finally, Jin et al. found that the various IDH mutants did not associate with or inhibit the activity of the corresponding native IDH enzyme (Jin et al., 2011).

4.3 Isocitrate dehydrogenase mutations results in a neomorphic enzyme activity

Based on discussion in the previous section, if these mutations at R132 in IDH1 (or R172 in IDH2) were activating, it would better fit the available observations. Complicating this assertion, though, was the fact that the normal enzymatic activity of IDH1 was severely hampered when R132 was mutated. This hypothesis was finally proven with the report that 2-hydroxyglutarate (2-HG) accumulates in glioma cells that express the R132H mutant (Dang et al., 2010). In particular, the (R) enantiomer of 2-HG (D-2-hydroxyglutarate, D-2-HG) was detecetd with no (S) enantiomer (L-2-hydroxyglutarate, L-2-HG) found in mutant IDH1-expressing cells. Like previous investigators, Dang et al. found that the R132H mutant lost the ability to oxidative decarboxylate isocitrate to α–KG (Dang et al., 2010; Yan et al., 2009; Zhao et al., 2009). However, this mutant now gained a new activity, namely, the

NADPH-dependent reduction of α-KG to 2-HG (Fig. 1) (Dang et al., 2010). Importantly, coexpression of wild type IDH1 and the R132H mutant did not reduce this new enzymatic activity but actually appear to enhance it. This has led to the suggestion that heterodimers can more efficiently produce 2-HG due to higher local concentrations of α-KG and NADPH produced by the wild type partner (Fig. 5). The x-ray structures of wild type IDH1 and the R132H mutant have been compared (Dang et al., 2010; Xu et al., 2004). Overall, R132 acts as a gate-keeper residue orchestrating the hinge movement between an open and closed conformation with the histidine mutation favoring a shift to the closed conformation which may increase binding of a new substrate (α-KG) and cofactor (NADPH) (Fig. 5).

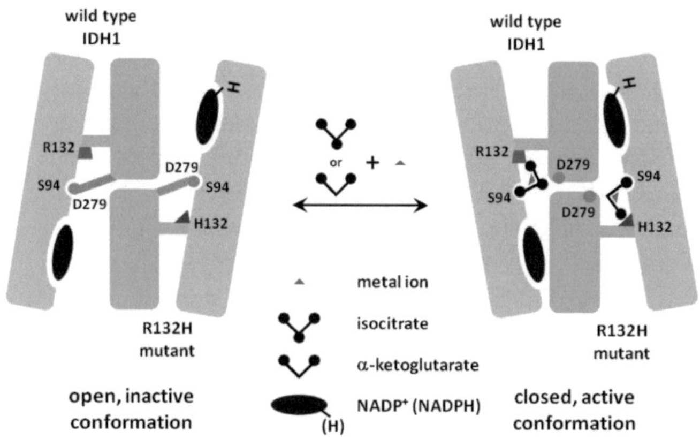

Fig. 5. Representation of wild type:R132H mutant IDH1 heterodimers shifting between the inactive and active conformations.

Ward et al. performed a comparable analysis of the R172K IDH2 mutant found in AMLs and gliomas (Ward et al., 2010). Similar to the finding of Dang et al., this IDH2 mutant also displayed α-KG-dependent NADPH consumption and accumulation of 2-HG within expressing cells and surrounding media (Dang et al., 2010; Ward et al., 2010). Interestingly, they also found that knockdown of both wild type IDH1 and IDH2 with siRNA dramatically decreased proliferative capacity of a cancer cell line (Ward et al., 2010). These findings provide another explanation for why the corresponding normal IDH allele is not deleted and actually appears to always be present with the mutant IDH allele. Finally, this study found a new mutant IDH2 (R140Q) that also resulted in accumulation of 2-HG in cytogenetically normal AMLs. R140 is also a highly conserved residue and structural modeling puts it immediately adjacent to R172 in the isocitrate binding site, which helps explain acquisition of this neomorphic enzymatic activity in R140 mutants. To date, R140 mutations in IDH2 have not been identified in gliomas. Based on previous discussions, IDH1 mutations at R132 and IDH2 mutations at R140 and R172 gain similar new enzymatic function. However, differences must still exist between these mutations due to the observed disparity in distribution of IDH1 and IDH2 mutations in gliomas (ratio of ~9:1) and AMLs (ratio of ~2:3). One factor for this difference may lie in their respective subcellular location. IDH1 is primarily cytosolic and peroxisomal where NADPH is more limiting while IDH2 is mitochondrial where NADPH is more readily available because it can be easily interchanged with NADH produced by IDH3 through the action of H^+-transhydrogenase (Sazanov & Jackson, 1994). Despite this, both mutant IDH1 and IDH2 can produce 2-HG, which can readily pass throughout the cell and even be secreted, and no definite functional differences between the two mutant enzymes have been demonstrated.

5. The effect of mutant isocitrate dehydrogenase on normal cellular functions

5.1 The effect of mutant isocitrate dehydrogenase on cellular metabolism

Mutant IDHs are clearly selected for in gliomas and AMLs. While wild type IDH1/2 have well-defined roles in metabolism, it remains unclear in what way expression of mutant IDHs will alter these various processes. One consequence of mutant IDH expression is decreased NADPH levels, which can potentially affect cellular biosynthetic processes such as lipogenesis. Similarly, depletion of cytosolic NADPH may be sensed in the cell as a low nutrient status leading to a response marked by increasing cellular nutrient consumption (eg. increase glucose transporters, increase throughput in the pentose phosphate pathway, etc.). These responses may provide malignant cells expressing mutant IDHs with a selective growth advantage. Reitman et al. have now profiled >200 metabolites in human oligodendroglioma cells engineered to express mutant IDH1 and IDH2 (Reitman et al., 2011). One striking finding from this study was that the profile of mutant IDH-expressing cells were very similar to those of corresponding cells treated with octyl-2-HG, a cell permeable precursor of 2-HG. This directly implicates this mutant IDH product as a key component of the cellular changes seen in mutant IDH-expressing cells. The main classes of changes found on this study include increases in free amino acids, increases in lipid precursors such as glycerol-phosphates and glycerophosphocholine, depletion of TCA cycle intermediaries and depletion of N-acetylated amino acids such as N-acetyl-aspartate and N-acetyl-aspartyl-glutamate, two of the most abundant compounds found in brain. Such widespread changes are likely a consequence of global changes in gene expression that will be discussed in sections 5.3-5.4 on epigenetic changes associated with mutant IDHs.

5.2 Mutant isocitrate dehydrogenase and hypoxia signaling

In addition to its effects on cellular metabolism, mutant IDHs may alter hypoxic response. Zhao et al. showed that expression of the R132H mutant in U87MG and 293T cells induced HIF-1α expression in a response that could be mitigated by treatment of cells with octyl-α-KG, a cell-permeable derivative of α-KG (Zhao et al., 2009). Prolyl hydroxylase utilizes α-KG to hydroxylate conserved prolines on HIF-1α leading to ubiquitination and subsequent rapid degradation (for review, see (Semenza, 2007)). Expression of the R132H mutant can theoretically deplete α-KG that is needed for HIF-1α proline hydroxylation or, alternatively, the 2-HG product of R132H may act as a competitive inhibitor of prolyl hydroxylase limiting HIF-1α proline hydroxylation. Since α-KG levels in mutant IDH1-expressing cells generally change very little while 2-HG levels rise tremendously (Dang et al., 2010), the latter hypothesis was more likely to be correct. Direct evidence for this have now been reported by Xu et al. whereby treatment of cells with octyl-2-HG induces HIF-1α in a process that is reversible with concomitant treatment with octyl-α-KG (Xu et al., 2011). The consequence of HIF-1α stabilization is induction of HIF-dependent genes such as vascular endothelial growth factor (VEGF), a pro-angiogenic factor, and glucose transporter 1 (glut1), which can alter metabolism and nutrient consumption (Zhao et al., 2009). While this HIF-1α response and its consequence is certainly intriguing, it still remains unclear how much of a role this induction actually plays in the tumorigenic process. HIF-1α and VEGF induction may contribute to the angiogenic phenotype seen in GBMs (for review, see (Van Meir et al., 2010)). However, since IDH mutation is a positive prognostic factor, that would suggest that HIF-1α induction is not a major function of IDH mutants (Nobusawa et al., 2009; Parsons et al., 2008; Yan et al., 2009). This is further supported by the lack of significant tumor angiogenesis in grade II and III gliomas of which >70% contain IDH mutations and the lack of HIF-1 target gene induction in AMLs with IDH mutation (Balss et al., 2008; Hartmann et al., 2009; Mardis et al., 2009; Yan et al., 2009).

5.3 Mutant isocitrate dehydrogenase is associated with a hypermethylation phenotype in gliomas

Association of IDH1 mutations with the proneural GBM subtype was a key finding from the assessment of GBMs in TCGA based mainly on expression profiling (Verhaak et al., 2010). Since that project acquired a host of genetic and epigenetic information about GBMs, investigators also looked for other factors that may associate with mutant IDH1. This culminated in work that found a glioma-CpG island methylator phenotype (G-CIMP) that defined a subgroup of GBMs that was tightly associated with IDH1 mutations (Noushmehr et al., 2010). Using the Illumina GoldenGate and/or Infinium methylation array platform, 272 TCGA GBM samples were assessed. Hypermethylation in a subset of loci was seen in 24 samples from this group that was reminiscent of the CpG island methylator phenotype (CIMP) previously described in colorectal cancer (Noushmehr et al., 2010; Toyota et al., 1999). 21 of 24 G-CIMP samples were classified as a proneural subtype and this represented approximately 30% of all proneural tumors. A subset of this cohort (207 samples) was then assessed for IDH mutations with the discovery of 18 IDH1 and no IDH2 mutations. Interestingly, all 18 tumors that had IDH1 mutations were labeled G-CIMP+ (18/23). Patients with proneural GBMs have been previously shown to have a better prognosis (Phillips et al., 2006; Verhaak et al., 2010). This study replicated that finding but found that G-CIMP positivity was an even stronger predictor of better outcomes (Noushmehr et al., 2010). Patients with G-CIMP+ proneural tumors (n=20) had a median survival of ~4 years while patients with G-CIMP- proneural tumors (n=49) did no better than patients with other subtypes (n=184) (median survivals of ~1 year). The association between mutant IDH1 and G-CIMP positivity also held in grade II and III gliomas and G-CIMP positivity still predicted for survival in the lower grade tumors. These results have now been replicated in an independent set of gliomas with the presence of IDH mutations correlating more strongly with hypermethylation than *TP53* mutation or lack of *EGFR* alterations (Christensen et al., 2011). Hypermethylation of the O-6-methylguanine-DNA-methyltransferase (MGMT) promoter is highly associated with better outcomes in patients with GBM (Hegi et al., 2005; Stupp et al., 2009). Given its prognostic value, MGMT methylation testing of has become relatively standard in the pathologic workup of GBMs. Although *MGMT* was not among the 50 most differentially hypermethylated genes on the TCGA study (Noushmehr et al., 2010), *MGMT* hypermethylation is correlated with IDH1 mutations in gliomas (Christensen et al., 2011; Laffaire et al., 2010; Sanson et al., 2009).

5.4 Mutant isocitrate dehydrogenase is associated with hypermethylation in AMLs

Previously, AMLs without known genetic or molecular features were found to be classifiable into five distinct clusters with particular epigenetic signatures (Figueroa et al., 2010b). Similar to the association of IDH1 mutation and G-CIMP, IDH1/2 mutations were also associated with certain DNA methylation patterns in AML (Figueroa et al., 2010a). In fact, AMLs with IDH mutations fell primarily in two epigenetically-defined clusters that tended toward increased DNA methylation, which was reminiscent of G-CIMP (Figueroa et al., 2010a; Noushmehr et al., 2010). Hypermethylation was associated with decreased expression of the relevant gene in the majority of cases. Unlike GBMs where >90% of IDH mutations were on IDH1, mutations in AMLs are more equally distributed permitting comparisons in the type of methylation phenotypes that arise. Despite the IDH isoforms localizing to different subregions of the cell, DNA methylation profile was not significantly different between the two IDH mutants (Figueroa et al., 2010a). Giving more support for IDH mutants having a causative role in increasing DNA methylation, engineered overexpression of mutant IDH1 or IDH2 both leads to increased 5-methylcytosine levels (Figueroa et al., 2010a). A mechanism for how the DNA hypermethylation phenotype arises in mutant IDH-expressing cells has been proposed and will be reviewed in section 6.2.

6. The role of 2-hydroxyglutarate in human malignancies

6.1 Genetic disorders that result in 2-hydroxyglutarate accumulation

With the identification of 2-HG as a novel tumor-associated metabolite, or oncometabolite, its effect on tumor cells has received increasing scrutiny. Two genetic defects have been described that involves accumulation of 2-HG and have been termed L-2- and D-2-hydroxyglutaric aciduria (L-2-HGA and D-2-HGA) based on which enantiomer of 2-HG accumulates (for reviews, see (Struys, 2006; Van Schaftingen et al., 2009)). They are rare neurometabolic disorders characterized by elevated 2-HG in bodily fluids including urine, plasma, and cerebrospinal fluid. L-2-HGA is the more common of the two. It is associated with L-2-HG dehydrogenase loss in virtually all cases resulting in the inability to oxidize L-2-HG to α-KG leading to L-2-HG accumulation. D-2-HGA is associated with either D-2-HG dehydrogenase loss or an R140 mutation in IDH2 both of which leads to D-2-HG accumulation (Kranendijk et al., 2010). L-2-HGA is the more severe of the two disorders and mainly affects the central nervous system with symptoms of hypotonia, tremors, and epilepsy that may progress to spongiform leukencephalopathy, muscular choreodystonia, mental retardation and psychomotor regression. Symptoms associated with D-2-HGA may be mild to nearly absent and include developmental delay, epilepsy, hypotonia, cardiomyopathy, and dysmorphic features. Interestingly, while IDH mutations result in D-2-HG accumulation, patients with L-2-HGA, and not D-2-HGA, have been reported to have a higher risk of developing malignant brain tumors (Aghili et al., 2009; Haliloglu et al., 2008). Thus mutant IDH likely has other effects beyond just production of the oncometabolite D-2-HG.

6.2 Inhibition of hydroxylases by 2-hydroxyglutarate

A major breakthrough in elucidating the function of 2-HG came with the discovery that this metabolite can inhibit the function of the TET dioxygenases (Xu et al., 2011). Members of the TET family have been shown to catalyze the conversion of 5-methylcytosine to 5-hydroxymethylcytosine (5-OH-MeC) in a reaction requiring α-KG, iron and oxygen (Ito et al., 2010; Tahiliani et al., 2009). While the physiologic significance of 5-OH-MeC has not been fully defined, it is believed to be an intermediate in the pathway that demethylates 5-methylcytosine. Thus, TET activity will result in decreased DNA methylation with potential widespread changes in gene expression. The first clue that 2-HG may be interacting with TET was the discovery that TET2 loss-of-function mutations seen in AML was mutually exclusive with IDH1/2 mutations (Of 375 cases, 57 were IDH mutants, 28 were TET2 mutants, 0 were both IDH and TET2 mutants) (Figueroa et al., 2010a). This result suggests that IDH1/2 mutations and TET2 mutations have overlapping roles in AML pathogenesis. Forced expression of TET2 also resulted in increased 5-OH-MeC levels and this could be blocked by cotransfection with mutant but not wild type IDH1. Xu et al. has now shown that 2-HG can act as a competitive inhibitor of multiple α-KG-dependent dioxygenases including the TET family of 5-methylcytosine hydroxylases, histone demethylases and even prolyl hydroxylases (see section 5.2) (Xu et al., 2011). Using an *in vitro* enzymatic assay, D-2-HG could inhibit the activity of TET1 and TET2 reducing 5-OH-MeC in a dose-dependent fashion. Interestingly, L-2-HG, which is not produced by mutant IDH, was actually even more effective at inhibiting the TET enzymes than the (D) enantiomer (Xu et al., 2011). This result may partially explain why malignant brain tumors were associated with the L-2-HGA but not the D-2-HGA genetic disorder.

6.3 Metabolic consequence of 2-hydroxyglutarate accumulation

As reviewed in section 5.1, direct treatment of cells with D-2-HG results in a metabolite profile, or metabolome that was similar to that found with mutant IDH1/2-expressing cells (Reitman et al., 2011). Of the 204 assessed biochemicals, from 107 to 130 were altered either up or down in the R132H-expressing or 2-HG-treated cells. Of these, 64 biochemical changes were shared between these cells. This number was much greater than the biochemical changes seen when comparing the R132H-expressing and the IDH1 knockdown cells where only 28 biochemicals were altered similarly. Likewise, mutant IDH2 (R172K) gave a profile similar to the R132H mutant. While these results suggest that D-2-HG is mediating some of the downstream effects of mutant IDH1/2, significant differences still exist thus highlighting 2-HG-independent effects of the mutant IDHs. One potential difference between these cells is that mutant IDH1 expression leads to glutamate depletion due to its conversion to α-KG and 2-HG while simply treating cells with 2-HG will not deplete glutamate. Some of the observed differences is consistent with this explanation as decreases in glutamate and several metabolites that are directly or indirectly derived from glutamate including glutathiones, N-acetylglutamate, N-acetyl-aspartyl-glutamate, α-KG, malate and fumarate are seen uniquely in mutant IDH1-expressing cells (Reitman et al., 2011). However, this explanation does not account for all the differences seen and mutant IDH expression is still likely to be causing some changes in the metabolite profile that is 2-HG-independent. These exact changes remain to be defined. The overall implication of these metabolite shifts on gliomagenesis is currently still largely unknown. However, there is an increasing recognition that changes in metabolism can have effects on tumorigenesis (for review, see (Vander Heiden et al., 2009)) and further research will likely begin to unravel the answers to these questions in the near future.

7. Diagnostic and therapeutic considerations with isocitrate dehydrogenase status in gliomas

7.1 Should routine testing for isocitrate dehydrogenase be performed?

Currently, determining the mutation status of IDH1/2 is not part of the standard molecular pathologic workup of gliomas. However, this is likely to change in the near future given the significant prognostic information the mutation status provides. With the high incidence of these IDH1/2 mutations in grade II and III gliomas (range from 66-83%) including astrocytomas, oligodendrogliomas and mixed oligoastrocytomas (Table 1), we would propose that all such tumors be assessed for these mutations. The incidence of these mutations is lower with GBMs so the decision to assess for such mutations remains an open question. Clearly, the incidence of IDH mutations in secondary GBMs is quite high, similar to that seen in lower grade gliomas. However, primary GBMs probably only contain IDH mutations in ~6% of cases (Table 1). Given this yield, we favor routine testing for IDH mutations in secondary but not primary GBMs. This view is based on the low potential yield of positive results in this GBM patient population and the fact that knowing the mutation status, while prognostic, will not alter the current therapeutic approach for these patients. However, if therapies that exploit the presence of these mutations are developed in the future, more comprehensive testing among all GBMs would be warranted.

7.2 Diagnostic tests used to detect mutant isocitrate dehydrogenase status

Determining the mutation status of IDH can be accomplished in a number of different ways. One standard approach is to detect for the mutant IDH protein. Currently, antibodies that recognize the mutant-specific epitope of the R132H IDH1 mutant have been reported (Capper et al., 2009; Kato et al., 2009). These antibodies have utility for western blotting of tumor cell lysates or immunohistochemical (IHC) staining of tumor tissue. While these methods utilize standard techniques familiar to pathology and molecular biology laboratories, they are limited by the fact that only the R132H mutant, which represents ~85% of IDH mutations in gliomas, can be identified (Table 2). Recently, an antibody specific for the altered epitope in the R132S IDH1 mutant was generated and found to be useful for western blotting and IHC staining (Kaneko et al., 2010). As more mutant-specific IDH1/2 antibodies become available, these antibodies and western blotting/IHC staining may be used to identify almost all potential cases with IDH1/2 mutations.

Alternatively, direct sequencing of the relevant regions in IDH1/2, or even the entire IDH1/2 genes, can be accomplished either from RNA or DNA harvested from the tumor. Improved genomic technologies have made these approaches very accessible both technically and costwise. Direct sequencing should theoretically provide 100% yield of mutations at the R132 residue of IDH1 and R140/R172 residues of IDH2. However, in practice, this may not be the case. Takano et al. reported their experience in comparing positive staining for IMab-1, an R132H-specific antibody, with results from routine direct sequencing of tumor DNA (Takano et al., 2010). In their study, only 9 of 12 cases detected as positive for expressing the R132H mutant on IHC staining turned out to be positive on initial screening with direct DNA sequencing. However, when the initial PCR product was subcloned, the IDH1-R132H could finally be detected in the three negative cases. This result indicates that tumor DNA was likely contaminated with a large amount of normal brain DNA making it difficult to detect the mutation on their initial screen. They conclude that IHC staining with the R132H antibody may be more sensitive than routine DNA sequencing for the detection of the IDH1-R132H mutant.

Finally, a mass spectrometry approach may be taken to detect for elevated D-2-HG in tumor lysate. This approach should permit detection of nearly all cases of mutant IDH1/2 since the neomorphic enzyme activity producing D-2-HG results with every mutation detected on R132 of IDH1 and R140/R172 of IDH2. Techniques for the detection both enantiomers of

2HG from urine or plasma using gas chromatography/mass spectrometry (GC/MS) or liquid chromatography/mass spectrometry (LC/MS) have been published and are routinely used by molecular genetics labs for the diagnosis of 2-hydroxyglutaric aciduria (Nyhan et al., 1995; Rashed et al., 2000). GC/MS and LC/MS have also been used by mutiple groups in the detection of 2-HG from media and lysates of cells grown in culture as well as of tumor tissue (Dang et al., 2010; Ward et al., 2010; Xu et al., 2011). These techniques should be rapidly adaptable for clinical use in the detection of the 2-HG metabolite in tumor lysates.

7.3 Future directions for mutant isocitrate dehydrogenase diagnostic testing

Because 2-HG is produced in the media of cells expressing mutant IDH1/2, this metabolite may be a good biomarker for detection of disease, response to therapy, and, potentially, long-term followup assessing for disease control. Although there are no current reports of this approach, mass spectrometry analysis of cerebrospinal fluid (CSF) may potentially be utilized for detecting 2-HG produced by gliomas of varying grades. Examining CSF for 2-HG have been proposed as a reliable screen for the detection of this tumor-specific metabolite and plans are in place to investigate this in more detail (Van Meir, 2011). Similarly, 2-HG elevations may be detected by mass spectrometry in other bodily fluids such as serum or urine as alternative means of detecting for tumors that express mutant IDH1/2. Finally, others have proposed using magnetic resonance spectroscopic imaging (MRSI) as a potential approach for noninvasive detection of 2-HG within tumors seen on MRI (Mao, 2011). Again, while interesting, significant research on the use of MRSI for detection of 2-HG will need to be accomplished before clinical use can be contemplated.

7.4 Therapeutic targeting of mutant isocitrate dehydrogenase status

The specific IDH mutations is a very attractive target for therapeutic manipulations. A variety of therapeutics approaches can be realistically taken to target this mutation. One obvious approach would be to directly target the mutant enzyme. This can potentially be accomplished by utilizing approaches that alter the expression of the mutant enzyme or developing therapeutic inhibitors of its neomorphic enzyme activity. Alternatively, approaches that target some of the downstream effects of this enzyme activity can be taken. This might include counteracting the pseudohypoxic state that results from 2-HG inhibition of prolyl hydroxylases that induces HIF-1α, reversing partially or fully the hypermethylation phenotype that results from 2-HG inhibition of the 5-methylcytosine hydroxylases, etc. However, caution must be taken with approaches that target these changes since such patients have been shown to have a better prognosis than their counterparts without IDH mutations (Nobusawa et al., 2009; Sanson et al., 2009; Yan et al., 2009). The main concern is that cellular changes that result from IDH mutations is actually driving increased sensitivity to current therapies and reversing some effects of these mutations may decrease response to such therapies potentially worsening patient outcomes. In addition, since mutant IDH1/2 is thought to mainly have a role in tumor initiation and not necessarily in tumor maintenance, blocking mutant IDH1/2 activity or its downstream consequences may not be a particularly effective therapy. Therefore, any potential therapeutic regimen that targets mutant IDH1/2 and/or its downstream effects needs to be carefully evaluated to assure that such therapies are not detrimentally affecting outcomes.

7.5 Therapeutic targeting of a metabolic dependency seen in tumors that express mutant isocitrate dehydrogenase

An alternative therapeutic approach might be to target a "weakness" that results from the adaptation of the cell to the presence of IDH mutations. Seltzer et al. recently proposed an interesting idea along this line whereby they sought to target a specific metabolic dependency found in mutant IDH1-expressing tumors (Seltzer et al., 2010). Previous work had demonstrated that the predominant source of cytoplasmic α-KG for mutant IDH1 is glutamine (Dang et al., 2010), which is converted to glutamate by glutaminase and then to α-KG by either glutamate oxaloacetate transaminase or glutamate dehydrogenase. They reasoned that inhibition of glutaminase (GLS) could severely limit the availability of α-KG for production of 2-HG by mutant IDH1, which could potentially have anti-tumor effects in mutant IDH1-expressing tumors. Exactly as predicted, inhibition of GLS either genetically with siRNA targeting GLS or chemically with bis-2-(5-phenylacetamido-1,2,4-thiadiazol-2-yl)ethyl sulfide (BPTES) resulted in growth inhibition of mutant but not wild type IDH1-expressing cells (Seltzer et al., 2010). However, this explanation does not fully resolve all their data since they also found that inhibition of glutamine uptake by glutamine deprivation did not have a similar selective effect on mutant IDH1-expressing cells. They speculate that the growth inhibitory effect mediated by glutaminase inhibition may be dictated by alteration in the balance of specific metabolites that are not altered when glutamine is simply limited. Overall, this novel approach provides an example of a therapy that can be developed to specifically target the growth of mutant IDH1-expressing tumors by exploiting a metabolic dependency found in these tumors.

8. Conclusion

Even though IDH mutations were discovered less than 3 years ago, researchers have already gained a wealth of knowledge about how they are functioning. It is clear that IDH mutants lose their normal enzymatic activity and gain a new one that results in production of 2-HG. As we reviewed in this chapter, 2-HG appears to inhibit a number of α-KG-dependent hydroxylases which can have broad-ranging effects on a host of cellular functions. These include epigenetic changes with implications for having global effects on gene expression and changes in the stability of factors such as HIF-1α which can also change gene expression for hypoxia-related genes producing a pseudohypoxic state that may detrimentally affect treatment response. Researchers are probably just scratching the surface about the potential cellular effects of 2-HG. It is also apparent that mutant IDHs probably have cellular effects beyond just producing 2-HG. Many of these 2-HG-independent effects still remain to be determined. Currently, assessing for IDH1/2 mutations can be readily done in a number of ways but still only provides prognostic information. As we gain a greater understanding of the many cellular effects of mutant IDHs and start to link them with mechanisms involved in the initiation and maintenance of glial neoplasms, then more novel therapeutic approaches that exploit the presence of these mutations may be developed for these tumors.

9. References

Aghili, M., Zahedi, F., & Rafiee, E. (2009). Hydroxyglutaric aciduria and malignant brain tumor: a case report and literature review. *J Neurooncol*, Vol. 91, pp. 233-236

Antonelli, M., Buttarelli, F.R., Arcella, A., Nobusawa, S., Donofrio, V., Oghaki, H., et al. (2010). Prognostic significance of histological grading, p53 status, YKL-40 expression, and IDH1 mutations in pediatric high-grade gliomas. *J Neurooncol*, Vol. 99, pp. 209-215

Bailey, J.M., & Colman, R.F. (1985). Affinity labeling of NADP+-specific isocitrate dehydrogenase by a new fluorescent nucleotide analogue, 2-[(4-bromo-2,3-dioxobutyl)thio]-1,N6-ethenoadenosine 2',5'-bisphosphate. *Biochemistry*, Vol. 24, pp. 5367-5377

Balss, J., Meyer, J., Mueller, W., Korshunov, A., Hartmann, C., & von Deimling, A. (2008). Analysis of the IDH1 codon 132 mutation in brain tumors. *Acta Neuropathol*, Vol. 116, pp. 597-602

Bleeker, F.E., Lamba, S., Leenstra, S., Troost, D., Hulsebos, T., Vandertop, W.P., et al. (2009). IDH1 mutations at residue p.R132 (IDH1(R132)) occur frequently in high-grade gliomas but not in other solid tumors. *Hum Mutat*, Vol. 30, pp. 7-11

Capper, D., Zentgraf, H., Balss, J., Hartmann, C., & von Deimling, A. (2009). Monoclonal antibody specific for IDH1 R132H mutation. *Acta Neuropathol*, Vol. 118, pp. 599-601

Ceccarelli, C., Grodsky, N.B., Ariyaratne, N., Colman, R.F., & Bahnson, B.J. (2002). Crystal structure of porcine mitochondrial NADP+-dependent isocitrate dehydrogenase complexed with Mn2+ and isocitrate. Insights into the enzyme mechanism. *J Biol Chem*, Vol. 277, pp. 43454-43462

Christensen, B.C., Smith, A.A., Zheng, S., Koestler, D.C., Houseman, E.A., Marsit, C.J., et al. (2011). DNA methylation, isocitrate dehydrogenase mutation, and survival in glioma. *J Natl Cancer Inst*, Vol. 103, pp. 143-153

Dang, L., White, D.W., Gross, S., Bennett, B.D., Bittinger, M.A., Driggers, E.M., et al. (2010). Cancer-associated IDH1 mutations produce 2-hydroxyglutarate. *Nature*, Vol. 465, pp. 966

Dubbink, H.J., Taal, W., van Marion, R., Kros, J.M., van Heuvel, I., Bromberg, J.E., et al. (2009). IDH1 mutations in low-grade astrocytomas predict survival but not response to temozolomide. *Neurology*, Vol. 73, pp. 1792-1795

Figueroa, M.E., Abdel-Wahab, O., Lu, C., Ward, P.S., Patel, J., Shih, A., et al. (2010a). Leukemic IDH1 and IDH2 mutations result in a hypermethylation phenotype, disrupt TET2 function, and impair hematopoietic differentiation. *Cancer Cell*, Vol. 18, pp. 553-567

Figueroa, M.E., Lugthart, S., Li, Y., Erpelinck-Verschueren, C., Deng, X., Christos, P.J., et al. (2010b). DNA methylation signatures identify biologically distinct subtypes in acute myeloid leukemia. *Cancer Cell*, Vol. 17, pp. 13-27

Haliloglu, G., Jobard, F., Oguz, K.K., Anlar, B., Akalan, N., Coskun, T., et al. (2008). L-2-hydroxyglutaric aciduria and brain tumors in children with mutations in the L2HGDH gene: neuroimaging findings. *Neuropediatrics*, Vol. 39, pp. 119-122

Hartmann, C., Meyer, J., Balss, J., Capper, D., Mueller, W., Christians, A., et al. (2009). Type and frequency of IDH1 and IDH2 mutations are related to astrocytic and oligodendroglial differentiation and age: a study of 1,010 diffuse gliomas. *Acta Neuropathol*, Vol. 118, pp. 469-474

Hartong, D.T., Dange, M., McGee, T.L., Berson, E.L., Dryja, T.P., & Colman, R.F. (2008). Insights from retinitis pigmentosa into the roles of isocitrate dehydrogenases in the Krebs cycle. *Nat Genet*, Vol. 40, pp. 1230-1234

Haselbeck, R.J., Colman, R.F., & McAlister-Henn, L. (1992). Isolation and sequence of a cDNA encoding porcine mitochondrial NADP-specific isocitrate dehydrogenase. *Biochemistry*, Vol. 31, pp. 6219-6223

Haselbeck, R.J., & McAlister-Henn, L. (1993). Function and expression of yeast mitochondrial NAD- and NADP-specific isocitrate dehydrogenases. *J Biol Chem*, Vol. 268, pp. 12116-12122

Hegi, M.E., Diserens, A.C., Gorlia, T., Hamou, M.F., de Tribolet, N., Weller, M., et al. (2005). MGMT gene silencing and benefit from temozolomide in glioblastoma. *N Engl J Med*, Vol. 352, pp. 997-1003

Henke, B., Girzalsky, W., Berteaux-Lecellier, V., & Erdmann, R. (1998). IDP3 encodes a peroxisomal NADP-dependent isocitrate dehydrogenase required for the beta-oxidation of unsaturated fatty acids. *J Biol Chem*, Vol. 273, pp. 3702-3711

Ichimura, K., Pearson, D.M., Kocialkowski, S., Backlund, L.M., Chan, R., Jones, D.T., et al. (2009). IDH1 mutations are present in the majority of common adult gliomas but rare in primary glioblastomas. *Neuro Oncol*, Vol. 11, pp. 341-347

Ito, S., D'Alessio, A.C., Taranova, O.V., Hong, K., Sowers, L.C., & Zhang, Y. (2010). Role of Tet proteins in 5mC to 5hmC conversion, ES-cell self-renewal and inner cell mass specification. *Nature*, Vol. 466, pp. 1129-1133

Jennings, G.T., Minard, K.I., & McAlister-Henn, L. (1997). Expression and mutagenesis of mammalian cytosolic NADP+-specific isocitrate dehydrogenase. *Biochemistry*, Vol. 36, pp. 13743-13747

Jennings, G.T., Sechi, S., Stevenson, P.M., Tuckey, R.C., Parmelee, D., & McAlister-Henn, L. (1994). Cytosolic NADP(+)-dependent isocitrate dehydrogenase. Isolation of rat cDNA and study of tissue-specific and developmental expression of mRNA. *J Biol Chem*, Vol. 269, pp. 23128-23134

Jin, G., Reitman, Z.J., Spasojevic, I., Batinic-Haberle, I., Yang, J., Schmidt-Kittler, O., et al. (2011). 2-hydroxyglutarate production, but not dominant negative function, is conferred by glioma-derived NADP-dependent isocitrate dehydrogenase mutations. *PLoS One*, Vol. 6, pp. e16812

Jo, S.H., Lee, S.H., Chun, H.S., Lee, S.M., Koh, H.J., Lee, S.E., et al. (2002). Cellular defense against UVB-induced phototoxicity by cytosolic NADP(+)-dependent isocitrate dehydrogenase. *Biochem Biophys Res Commun*, Vol. 292, pp. 542-549

Jo, S.H., Son, M.K., Koh, H.J., Lee, S.M., Song, I.H., Kim, Y.O., et al. (2001). Control of mitochondrial redox balance and cellular defense against oxidative damage by mitochondrial NADP+-dependent isocitrate dehydrogenase. *J Biol Chem*, Vol. 276, pp. 16168-16176

Kaneko, M.K., Tian, W., Takano, S., Suzuki, H., Sawa, Y., Hozumi, Y., et al. (2010). Establishment of a novel monoclonal antibody SMab-1 specific for IDH1-R132S mutation. *Biochem Biophys Res Commun*, Vol. 406, pp. 608-613

Kang, M.R., Kim, M.S., Oh, J.E., Kim, Y.R., Song, S.Y., Seo, S.I., et al. (2009). Mutational analysis of IDH1 codon 132 in glioblastomas and other common cancers. *Int J Cancer*, Vol. 125, pp. 353-355

Kato, Y., Jin, G., Kuan, C.T., McLendon, R.E., Yan, H., & Bigner, D.D. (2009). A monoclonal antibody IMab-1 specifically recognizes IDH1R132H, the most common glioma-derived mutation. *Biochem Biophys Res Commun*, Vol. 390, pp. 547-551

Kehrer, J.P., & Lund, L.G. (1994). Cellular reducing equivalents and oxidative stress. *Free Radic Biol Med*, Vol. 17, pp. 65-75

Kelly, J.H., & Plaut, G.W. (1981). Physical evidence for the dimerization of the triphosphopyridine-specific isocitrate dehydrogenase from pig heart. *J Biol Chem*, Vol. 256, pp. 330-334

Kim, S.Y., Lee, S.M., Tak, J.K., Choi, K.S., Kwon, T.K., & Park, J.W. (2007). Regulation of singlet oxygen-induced apoptosis by cytosolic NADP+-dependent isocitrate dehydrogenase. *Mol Cell Biochem*, Vol. 302, pp. 27-34

Koh, H.J., Lee, S.M., Son, B.G., Lee, S.H., Ryoo, Z.Y., Chang, K.T., et al. (2004). Cytosolic NADP+-dependent isocitrate dehydrogenase plays a key role in lipid metabolism. *J Biol Chem*, Vol. 279, pp. 39968-39974

Kranendijk, M., Struys, E.A., van Schaftingen, E., Gibson, K.M., Kanhai, W.A., van der Knaap, M.S., et al. (2010). IDH2 mutations in patients with D-2-hydroxyglutaric aciduria. *Science*, Vol. 330, pp. 336

Laffaire, J., Everhard, S., Idbaih, A., Criniere, E., Marie, Y., de Reynies, A., et al. (2010). Methylation profiling identifies 2 groups of gliomas according to their tumorigenesis. *Neuro Oncol*, Vol. 13, pp. 84-98

Lee, S.H., Jo, S.H., Lee, S.M., Koh, H.J., Song, H., Park, J.W., et al. (2004). Role of NADP+-dependent isocitrate dehydrogenase (NADP+-ICDH) on cellular defence against oxidative injury by gamma-rays. *Int J Radiat Biol*, Vol. 80, pp. 635-642

Lee, S.M., Koh, H.J., Park, D.C., Song, B.J., Huh, T.L., & Park, J.W. (2002). Cytosolic NADP(+)-dependent isocitrate dehydrogenase status modulates oxidative damage to cells. *Free Radic Biol Med*, Vol. 32, pp. 1185-1196

Lopez, G.Y., Reitman, Z.J., Solomon, D., Waldman, T., Bigner, D.D., McLendon, R.E., et al. (2010). IDH1(R132) mutation identified in one human melanoma metastasis, but not correlated with metastases to the brain. *Biochem Biophys Res Commun*, Vol. 398, pp. 585-587

Louis, D.N., Ohgaki, H., Wiestler, O.D., & Cavenee, W.K., (Eds.) (2007). *WHO classification of tumours of the central nervous system* (4th edn), IARC Press, Lyon, France

Mailloux, R.J., Beriault, R., Lemire, J., Singh, R., Chenier, D.R., Hamel, R.D., et al. (2007). The tricarboxylic acid cycle, an ancient metabolic network with a novel twist. *PLoS One*, Vol. 2, pp. e690

Mao, H. (2011). Personal communications

Marcucci, G., Maharry, K., Wu, Y.Z., Radmacher, M.D., Mrozek, K., Margeson, D., et al. (2010). IDH1 and IDH2 gene mutations identify novel molecular subsets within de novo cytogenetically normal acute myeloid leukemia: a Cancer and Leukemia Group B study. *J Clin Oncol*, Vol. 28, pp. 2348-2355

Mardis, E.R., Ding, L., Dooling, D.J., Larson, D.E., McLellan, M.D., Chen, K., et al. (2009). Recurring mutations found by sequencing an acute myeloid leukemia genome. *N Engl J Med*, Vol. 361, pp. 1058-1066

Minard, K.I., & McAlister-Henn, L. (1999). Dependence of peroxisomal beta-oxidation on cytosolic sources of NADPH. *J Biol Chem*, Vol. 274, pp. 3402-3406

Nekrutenko, A., Hillis, D.M., Patton, J.C., Bradley, R.D., & Baker, R.J. (1998). Cytosolic isocitrate dehydrogenase in humans, mice, and voles and phylogenetic analysis of the enzyme family. *Mol Biol Evol*, Vol. 15, pp. 1674-1684

Nichols, B.J., Hall, L., Perry, A.C., & Denton, R.M. (1993). Molecular cloning and deduced amino acid sequences of the gamma-subunits of rat and monkey NAD(+)-isocitrate dehydrogenases. *Biochem J*, Vol. 295 (Pt 2), pp. 347-350

Nichols, B.J., Perry, A.C., Hall, L., & Denton, R.M. (1995). Molecular cloning and deduced amino acid sequences of the alpha- and beta- subunits of mammalian NAD(+)-isocitrate dehydrogenase. *Biochem J*, Vol. 310 (Pt 3), pp. 917-922

Nobusawa, S., Watanabe, T., Kleihues, P., & Ohgaki, H. (2009). IDH1 mutations as molecular signature and predictive factor of secondary glioblastomas. *Clin Cancer Res*, Vol. 15, pp. 6002-6007

Noushmehr, H., Weisenberger, D.J., Diefes, K., Phillips, H.S., Pujara, K., Berman, B.P., et al. (2010). Identification of a CpG island methylator phenotype that defines a distinct subgroup of glioma. *Cancer Cell*, Vol. 17, pp. 510-522

Nyhan, W.L., Shelton, G.D., Jakobs, C., Holmes, B., Bowe, C., Curry, C.J., et al. (1995). D-2-hydroxyglutaric aciduria. *J Child Neurol*, Vol. 10, pp. 137-142

Parsons, D.W., Jones, S., Zhang, X., Lin, J.C., Leary, R.J., Angenendt, P., et al. (2008). An integrated genomic analysis of human glioblastoma multiforme. *Science*, Vol. 321, pp. 1807-1812

Paschka, P., Schlenk, R.F., Gaidzik, V.I., Habdank, M., Kronke, J., Bullinger, L., et al. (2010). IDH1 and IDH2 mutations are frequent genetic alterations in acute myeloid leukemia and confer adverse prognosis in cytogenetically normal acute myeloid leukemia with NPM1 mutation without FLT3 internal tandem duplication. *J Clin Oncol*, Vol. 28, pp. 3636-3643

Paugh, B.S., Qu, C., Jones, C., Liu, Z., Adamowicz-Brice, M., Zhang, J., et al. (2010). Integrated molecular genetic profiling of pediatric high grade gliomas reveals key differences with the adult disease. *J Clin Oncol*, Vol. 28, pp. 3061-3068

Phillips, H.S., Kharbanda, S., Chen, R., Forrest, W.F., Soriano, R.H., Wu, T.D., et al. (2006). Molecular subclasses of high-grade glioma predict prognosis, delineate a pattern of disease progression, and resemble stages in neurogenesis. *Cancer Cell*, Vol. 9, pp. 157-173

Pollack, I.F., Hamilton, R.L., Sobol, R.W., Nikiforova, M.N., Lyons-Weiler, M.A., Laframboise, W.A., et al. (2011). IDH1 mutations are common in malignant gliomas arising in adolescents: a report from the Children's Oncology Group. *Childs Nerv Syst*, Vol. 27, pp. 87-94

Ramachandran, N., & Colman, R.F. (1980). Chemical characterization of distinct subunits of pig heart DPN-specific isocitrate dehydrogenase. *J Biol Chem*, Vol. 255, pp. 8859-8864

Rashed, M.S., AlAmoudi, M., & Aboul-Enein, H.Y. (2000). Chiral liquid chromatography tandem mass spectrometry in the determination of the configuration of 2-hydroxyglutaric acid in urine. *Biomed Chromatogr*, Vol. 14, pp. 317-320

Reitman, Z.J., Jin, G., Karoly, E.D., Spasojevic, I., Yang, J., Kinzler, K.W., et al. (2011). Profiling the effects of isocitrate dehydrogenase 1 and 2 mutations on the cellular metabolome. *Proc Natl Acad Sci U S A*, Vol. 108, pp. 3270-3275

Ronnebaum, S.M., Ilkayeva, O., Burgess, S.C., Joseph, J.W., Lu, D., Stevens, R.D., et al. (2006). A pyruvate cycling pathway involving cytosolic NADP-dependent isocitrate dehydrogenase regulates glucose-stimulated insulin secretion. *J Biol Chem*, Vol. 281, pp. 30593-30602

Sanson, M., Marie, Y., Paris, S., Idbaih, A., Laffaire, J., Ducray, F., et al. (2009). Isocitrate dehydrogenase 1 codon 132 mutation is an important prognostic biomarker in gliomas. *J Clin Oncol*, Vol. 27, pp. 4150-4154

Sazanov, L.A., & Jackson, J.B. (1994). Proton-translocating transhydrogenase and NAD- and NADP-linked isocitrate dehydrogenases operate in a substrate cycle which contributes to fine regulation of the tricarboxylic acid cycle activity in mitochondria. *FEBS Lett*, Vol. 344, pp. 109-116

Seltzer, M.J., Bennett, B.D., Joshi, A.D., Gao, P., Thomas, A.G., Ferraris, D.V., et al. (2010). Inhibition of glutaminase preferentially slows growth of glioma cells with mutant IDH1. *Cancer Res*, Vol. 70, pp. 8981-8987

Semenza, G.L. (2007). Hypoxia-inducible factor 1 (HIF-1) pathway. *Sci STKE*, Vol. 2007, pp. cm8

Shechter, I., Dai, P., Huo, L., & Guan, G. (2003). IDH1 gene transcription is sterol regulated and activated by SREBP-1a and SREBP-2 in human hepatoma HepG2 cells: evidence that IDH1 may regulate lipogenesis in hepatic cells. *J Lipid Res*, Vol. 44, pp. 2169-2180

Shin, A.H., Kil, I.S., Yang, E.S., Huh, T.L., Yang, C.H., & Park, J.W. (2004). Regulation of high glucose-induced apoptosis by mitochondrial NADP+-dependent isocitrate dehydrogenase. *Biochem Biophys Res Commun*, Vol. 325, pp. 32-38

Sonoda, Y., Kumabe, T., Nakamura, T., Saito, R., Kanamori, M., Yamashita, Y., et al. (2009). Analysis of IDH1 and IDH2 mutations in Japanese glioma patients. *Cancer Sci*, Vol. 100, pp. 1996-1998

Soundar, S., Danek, B.L., & Colman, R.F. (2000). Identification by mutagenesis of arginines in the substrate binding site of the porcine NADP-dependent isocitrate dehydrogenase. *J Biol Chem*, Vol. 275, pp. 5606-5612

Struys, E.A. (2006). D-2-Hydroxyglutaric aciduria: unravelling the biochemical pathway and the genetic defect. *J Inherit Metab Dis*, Vol. 29, pp. 21-29

Stupp, R., Hegi, M.E., Mason, W.P., van den Bent, M.J., Taphoorn, M.J., Janzer, R.C., et al. (2009). Effects of radiotherapy with concomitant and adjuvant temozolomide versus radiotherapy alone on survival in glioblastoma in a randomised phase III study: 5-year analysis of the EORTC-NCIC trial. *Lancet Oncol*, Vol. 10, pp. 459-466

Stupp, R., Mason, W.P., van den Bent, M.J., Weller, M., Fisher, B., Taphoorn, M.J., et al. (2005). Radiotherapy plus concomitant and adjuvant temozolomide for glioblastoma. *N Engl J Med*, Vol. 352, pp. 987-996

Tahiliani, M., Koh, K.P., Shen, Y., Pastor, W.A., Bandukwala, H., Brudno, Y., et al. (2009). Conversion of 5-methylcytosine to 5-hydroxymethylcytosine in mammalian DNA by MLL partner TET1. *Science*, Vol. 324, pp. 930-935

Takano, S., Tian, W., Matsuda, M., Yamamoto, T., Ishikawa, E., Kaneko, M.K., et al. (2010). Detection of IDH1 mutation in human gliomas: comparison of immunohistochemistry and sequencing. *Brain Tumor Pathol*, Vol. 28, pp. 115-123

Toyota, M., Ahuja, N., Ohe-Toyota, M., Herman, J.G., Baylin, S.B., & Issa, J.P. (1999). CpG island methylator phenotype in colorectal cancer. *Proc Natl Acad Sci U S A*, Vol. 96, pp. 8681-8686

Van Meir, E.G. (2011). Personal communications

Van Meir, E.G., Hadjipanayis, C.G., Norden, A.D., Shu, H.K., Wen, P.Y., & Olson, J.J. (2010). Exciting new advances in neuro-oncology: the avenue to a cure for malignant glioma. *CA Cancer J Clin*, Vol. 60, pp. 166-193

van Roermund, C.W., Hettema, E.H., Kal, A.J., van den Berg, M., Tabak, H.F., & Wanders, R.J. (1998). Peroxisomal beta-oxidation of polyunsaturated fatty acids in Saccharomyces cerevisiae: isocitrate dehydrogenase provides NADPH for reduction of double bonds at even positions. *Embo J*, Vol. 17, pp. 677-687

Van Schaftingen, E., Rzem, R., & Veiga-da-Cunha, M. (2009). L: -2-Hydroxyglutaric aciduria, a disorder of metabolite repair. *J Inherit Metab Dis*, Vol. 32, pp. 135-142

Vander Heiden, M.G., Cantley, L.C., & Thompson, C.B. (2009). Understanding the Warburg effect: the metabolic requirements of cell proliferation. *Science*, Vol. 324, pp. 1029-1033

Verhaak, R.G., Hoadley, K.A., Purdom, E., Wang, V., Qi, Y., Wilkerson, M.D., et al. (2010). Integrated genomic analysis identifies clinically relevant subtypes of glioblastoma characterized by abnormalities in PDGFRA, IDH1, EGFR, and NF1. *Cancer Cell*, Vol. 17, pp. 98-110

Ward, P.S., Patel, J., Wise, D.R., Abdel-Wahab, O., Bennett, B.D., Coller, H.A., et al. (2010). The common feature of leukemia-associated IDH1 and IDH2 mutations is a neomorphic enzyme activity converting alpha-ketoglutarate to 2-hydroxyglutarate. *Cancer Cell*, Vol. 17, pp. 225-234

Watanabe, T., Nobusawa, S., Kleihues, P., & Ohgaki, H. (2009). IDH1 mutations are early events in the development of astrocytomas and oligodendrogliomas. *Am J Pathol*, Vol. 174, pp. 1149-1153

Winkler, B.S., DeSantis, N., & Solomon, F. (1986). Multiple NADPH-producing pathways control glutathione (GSH) content in retina. *Exp Eye Res*, Vol. 43, pp. 829-847

Xu, W., Yang, H., Liu, Y., Yang, Y., Wang, P., Kim, S.H., et al. (2011). Oncometabolite 2-hydroxyglutarate is a competitive inhibitor of alpha-ketoglutarate-dependent dioxygenases. *Cancer Cell*, Vol. 19, pp. 17-30

Xu, X., Zhao, J., Xu, Z., Peng, B., Huang, Q., Arnold, E., et al. (2004). Structures of human cytosolic NADP-dependent isocitrate dehydrogenase reveal a novel self-regulatory mechanism of activity. *J Biol Chem*, Vol. 279, pp. 33946-33957

Yan, H., Parsons, D.W., Jin, G., McLendon, R., Rasheed, B.A., Yuan, W., et al. (2009). IDH1 and IDH2 mutations in gliomas. *N Engl J Med*, Vol. 360, pp. 765-773

Zhao, S., Lin, Y., Xu, W., Jiang, W., Zha, Z., Wang, P., et al. (2009). Glioma-derived mutations in IDH1 dominantly inhibit IDH1 catalytic activity and induce HIF-1alpha. *Science*, Vol. 324, pp. 261-265

Part 9

BORIS as a Transcription Factor - Gliomas

21

The Expression of BORIS Protein in a Newly Established Primary Glioma Cell Culture Line

Siti Zawani Mohd Ramli[1], Shaharum Shamsuddin[1], Nik Norliza Hassan[1], Azmi Alias[3], Mohd Saffari Mohd Haspani[3] and Jafri Abdullah[2]

[1]*School of Health Sciences, Health Campus, Universiti Sains Malaysia, Kelantan,*
[2]*School of Medical Sciences, Health Campus, Universiti Sains Malaysia, Kelantan,*
[3]*Institut Kaji Saraf Tunku Abdul Rahman, Hospital Kuala Lumpur, Kuala Lumpur, Malaysia*

1. Introduction

1.1 Glioma

Malignant gliomas are the most common types of brain tumors in adults. These tumors are highly invasive and despite multi- modality treatment, the mean survival time of patients is still less than a year (Machado et al., 2005). Gliomas, a cancer of glial cells constitute more than 90% of all primary malignant central nervous system (CNS) tumors. Although gliomas are the most common major subgroup of primary nervous systems tumors, their etiology is less well understood than is the etiology of the other two major subgroups: meningiomas and neuromas. The development of glioma is a complex process with the involvement of both oncogenes and tumor suppressor genes in the accumulation of genetic lesions (Zhang et al., 2005). Brain tumors arise as a result of gradual accumulation of several genetic aberrations in precursor cells which can occur either at the chromosomal level or at the gene expression level (Furnari et al. 1995). Despite considerable efforts to unravel the etiologic basis for this cancer and attempts to find a cure, gliomas largely remain refractory to treatment. Except for a small percentage of cases, the tumors continue to show high morbidity and mortality (Wrensch et al. 2005). The identification and evaluation of the cellular sites in which such genes and their encoded proteins are expressed, could help us to determine how those cellular expression sites are linked to the convoluted circuits of neurons that control brain function. To date, there is major technological challenge in the capability to detect and map genes whose expression is altered either by the disease's process or by the cells adaptations to resist the disease's process (Bloom et al., 2004).

1.2 Primary culture

Primary culture is the initial culture established from an individual which represents the environment most closely related to the original cell. The availability of unlimited number of cells and the possibility of performing multiple, repetitive experiments over long period of time renders cultured tumor cells a valuable mean for preliminary assessments of new therapeutic agents (Bakir et al., 1998). Development of biotechnology methods including primary culture technique gives us the opportunity to study the malignant glioma in depth in order to understand the etiology of the brain tumor especially on gene regulations and cellular pathway mechanisms.

1.2.1 Primary culture: explant technique

Primary explant technique is one of the primary culture techniques. It was the original method developed by Harrison (1907) and Carrel (1912), and others for initiating a tissue culture. As originally performed, a fragment of tissue was embedded in blood plasma or lymph, mixed with heterologous serum and embryo extract, and placed on a coverslip that was inverted over a concative slide. The clotted plasma held the tissue in place, and the explant could be examined with a conventional microscope. The heterologous serum induced clotting of the plasma, the embryo extract and serum, together with the plasma, supplied nutrients and growth factors will stimulate cell migration from the explant. This technique is still being used but has been largely replaced by the simplified method. First of all, the tissue is chopped finely and rinsed, the pieces are seeded onto the surface of a culture flask or petri dish in a small volume of medium with a high concentration of serum, such that surface tension holds the pieces in place until they adhere spontaneously to the surface. Once this is archieved, outgrowth of cells usually follows.

1.3 Glioma primary culture

The established glioma primary culture gives us permanent material to examine the expression of proteins of interest and their functional characterization *in vivo* and *in vitro*. For that reason, we developed our very own primary culture of the cancerous glioma from local clinical tumor sample so as to understand better its genetic background and cellular development. Establishing primary glioma cell line in culture, the malignant cells will represent an excellent permanent representative material for molecular and cellular characterization of tumor supported with specific antigenic identification and biochemical characterization of cellular proliferation (Tomaso et al., 2000; Halfter et al., 1998; Pohl et al., 1999; Grippo et al., 2001; Machado et al., 2005). In this study, we used four well known antigens such as GFAP (Glial Fibrillary Acidic Protein), which has been shown to be a marker of glial cell origin (Zhang et al., 2005), S-100 protein which was originally identified as a brain specific marker (Machado et al., 2005), Vimentin which has been detected in a few primary cultured glioma (Bakir et al., 1998) and positive expression of BORIS protein in glioma (D'Arcy et al., 2006).

1.4 Transcription factor in cancer development

Cancer is known to be a pathophysiological condition with many different genes involved including transcription factor as a main. Transcription factor is a molecule that participates, alone or as part of a complex, in the binding to a gene's enhancer response element or promoter. Transcription factors also known as regulatory proteins which have an ability to bind to specific DNA sequences (Nebert, 2002). Transcription factor have two separate protein domains called a DNA binding domain and a regulatory domain. DNA binding domain binds to their specific DNA binding sites and the regulatory domain modulates transcription. The DNA binding domain interacts with the promoters and the regulatory domain allows interaction with other transcription factors. The binding of the transcription factors activates (or in some cases, to inhibits) transcription of the specific DNA with the ultimate outcome being the up- or down-regulation of expression of that gene (Nebert, 2002, Theresa Phillips, 2008) which leads to the production of the gene's end product; mainly in protein form or in certain circumstances without production of functional end product.

1.4.1 BORIS as a transcription factor and cancer testis antigen (CTA) family

BORIS is one of the transcription factors which believed to play role in cancer development. Human BORIS (Brother of the Regulator of Imprinted Sites) gene maps to chromosome 20q13.2 (Loukinov et al, 2002). This chromosome region is often amplified in many cancers and is believed to contain a dominant immortalising or transforming gene(s).

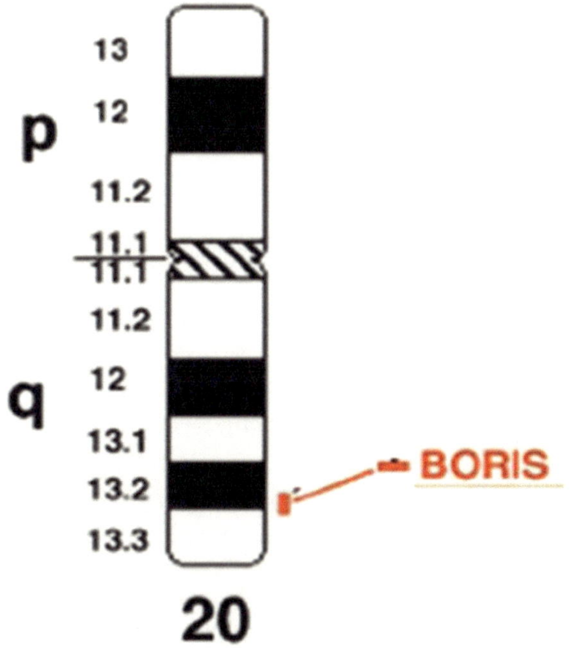

Fig. 1. BORIS map to cancer-associated 'hot spots' on HUMAN CHROMOSOME 20q13. (Modified from Klenova et al., 2002)

BORIS is a conserved, ubiquitous, and highly versatile 11-zinc-finger transcription factor involved in various aspects of gene regulation, forms methylation-sensitive insulators that regulate X chromosome inactivation and expression of imprinted genes. It is a multivalent Zinc Finger transcription factor which present only in the testis and expressed in a mutually exclusive manner with CTCF (CCCTC- binding factor) Zinc Finger transcription factor during spermatogenesis. BORIS is paralogous to CTCF and thus has the same DNA-binding potential, but with distinct amino and carboxy termini (Loukinov et al., 2002). Under normal physiologic conditions, BORIS is predominantly expressed during embryonic male germ cell development. However, BORIS is also expressed in tumors and cancer cell lines including glioma and it has been classified as a cancer-germ line or cancer-testis gene (Nguyen et al., 2008). Since BORIS bears the same DNA-binding domain that CTCF employs for recognition of methylation marks in the soma, it was identified as a candidate protein for the elusive epigenetic reprogramming factor acting in the male germ line (Loukinov et al., 2002). Other than glioma, recent studies reported that BORIS is aberrantly expressed in various cancer cell lines including uterine cancer and breast cancer (Klenova et al. 2002; Loukinov et al. 2002;Hoffmann et al., 2006; Risinger et al.; 2007, D'Arcy et al., 2008).

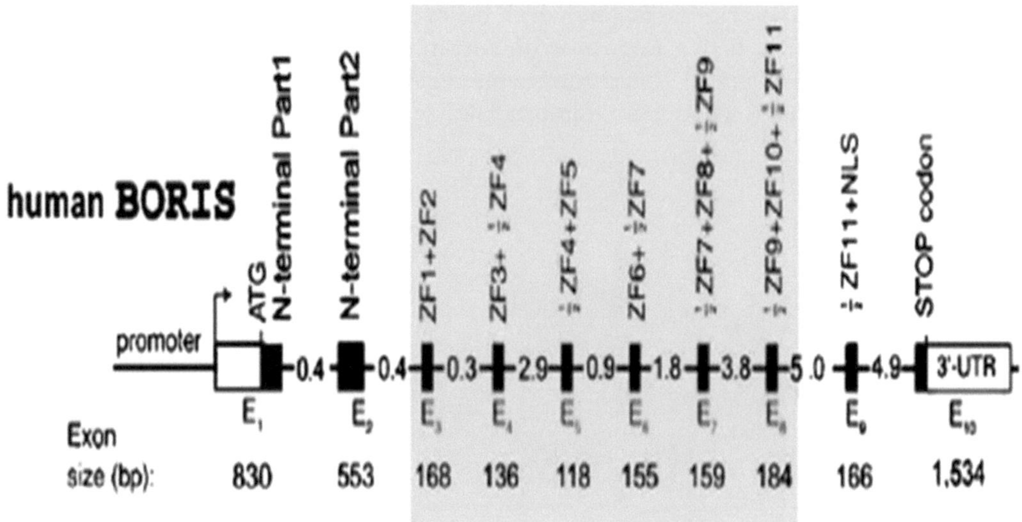

Fig. 2. Exon- Intron structure of BORIS is shown. The 11 Zn fingers are positioned in exons E3 through E8, with several individual fingers being separated between neighbouring exons. Exon 10 harbours the stop codon and a long 3'- UTR. (Klenova et al., 2002)

BORIS has been implicated in the initiation of a series of methylation events at the imprinting control regions, in the vicinity of the CTCF-/BORIS-binding sites which may be significant for cancer development (Jelinic and Shaw, 2007). However, recent study by Renaud et al. (2007) reveal that the regulation of BORIS activity is complex and being both promoter- and cell type-dependent. Varying promoter usage driving multiple BORIS transcripts influence many aspects of epigenetic reprogramming in normal development and also in tumorigenesis.

BORIS belongs to the cancer testis antigen (CTA) family which its genes products exhibit highly tissue-restricted expression and are immunogenic in cancer patients (Vatolin et al., 2005, Risinger et al., 2007). The function of the majority CTAs is still unknown; however, some CTAs may play role in a regulation of gene expression and others in gametogenesis (Old, 2001; Kalejs & Erenpreisa, 2005). The CTAs are attractive targets for developing cancer-specific therapy due to their highly restricted expression in normal tissues and broad expression in a wide range of tumors (Risinger et al., 2007). Studies by Hong et al., (2005) and Vatolin et al. (2005) reveal that the expression of BORIS correlated with and induced the expression of other cancer testis genes MAGE-A1 and NY-ESO-1.

The main focus of this study was to reveal the expression of BORIS protein as well as morphological characteristics of this newly established clinical derived glioma primary cell line. BORIS has been selected in this study due to its physical and functional related to CTCF, multifunctional transcription factor. BORIS which also known as CTCFL (CTCF-like), is the mammalian paralog of a highly conserved (Pugacheva et al., 2006), multi-functional chromatin factor encoded by a candidate tumor suppressor gene, CTCF; CCCTC- binding factor (Ohlsson et al., 2001). Loukinov et al., (2002) showed that, both BORIS and CTCF encode polypeptides of similar size that share a centrally positioned nearly identical DNA-binding domain (DBD). The DBD is composed of 11 Zn-fingers (11ZF), including ten of the classic DNA-binding C2H2-class and one (ZF 11) of the C2HC-class capable of binding both

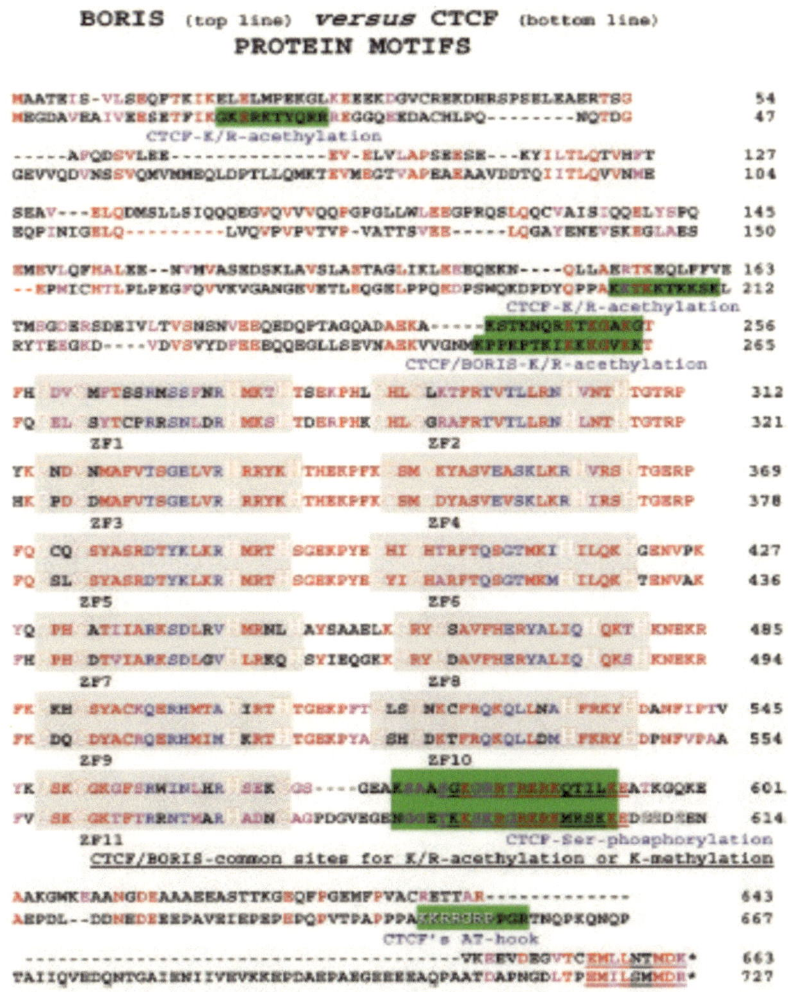

Fig. 3. Comparison of protein motifs in BORIS and CTCF. The best-fit alignment of the human CTCF and BORIS polypeptides produced by the GCG-package of programs with zero-penalty for the gap extension. Identical and similar amino acids are shown by red letters. The CxxC and HxxxH invariant residues involved in Zn-coordinated formation of the C2H2-ZF structures are shown by outlined letters in a bigger font. The near-identical ZFs, numbered 1-11, are highlighted by a gray background, and the critical base-recognizing residues at positions−1, 2, 3, and 6 inside of each ZF are shown by blue letters. Dashed lines show the gaps introduced to reveal minor similarities outside of the ZF-domains. The major Ser-phosphorylation sites and the putative additional DNA-binding 'AT-hook' motif, conserved in vertebrate CTCF proteins but absent in BORIS proteins, are shown by outlined letters. The most likely sites for K/R-acetylation and K-methylation, similar to those in the H3 and H4 histones, are highlighted in green. The experimentally determined acetylation site in the K/R-rich CTCF region downstream of the 11th ZF, and a homologous site in BORIS, are underlined in addition to green background that shows major H3-like putative K-methylation sites in both proteins. (Klenova et al., 2002)

single-strand DNA and RNA (Ladomery & Dellaire, 2002). It is remarkable that the 11 ZF DBD regions in BORIS and CTCF are encoded by genomic sequences, which present an accurate duplication of a region containing all ZF-coding exons of the CTCF gene from an early mammal. The accuracy of this duplication in the human genome was maintained to the extent that genomic nucleotide similarities between CTCF and BORIS at individual intron–exon junctions approach 100% identity at the single nucleotide level (Loukinov et al. 2002). Due to this shared DNA-recognition domain, BORIS can bind specifically to the same DNA target sequences that interact with CTCF. However, the consequences of BORIS or CTCF bound to the same site would be different because the amino- and carboxy-termini of BORIS and CTCF are totally unrelated (Klenova et al, 2002; Loukinov et al, 2002; Campbell et al., 2010). And the different functional outcomes depending on which one of the two paralogs occupies a CTCF/BORIS-11ZF binding site (Vatolin et al., 2005).

2. Materials and methods

2.1 Patient and tumor

Malignant glioma was obtained directly from the operation theater , Hospital Universiti Sains Malaysia Kubang Kerian, Malaysia with the permission from the Human Ethical Committee, Universiti Sains Malaysia (Reference number: USM/ PPSP/Ethics Com/ 2006 (179.5(2). The sample was derived from an adult male patient with recurrent glioblastoma multiforme. After surgery, the sample was immediately transferred into sterile falcon tube and transported in ice to the laboratory for subsequent culture. The cell line has been successfully cryopreserved and passaged up to 32 times.

2.2 Primary culture work

2.2.1 Preparation of sterile complete media RPMI 1640 (50mL)

10mL pre- warmed Fetal Bovine Serum (Sigma, USA) was poured into a sterile falcon tube (50mL). 1mL of penicillin-streptomycin and 100µL antibiotic cocktail (kanamycin, gentamycin, streptomycin, ampicillin, penicillin and chloramphenicol with total working concentration 50µg/ mL) (Sigma, USA) were added into the same falcon tube. Finally, RPMI 1640 with L-Glutamine and $NaHCO_3$ (HyClone, A Perbio Science Company) was added until the mixture volume became 50mL. Then, the completed media was dispensed into another sterile 50mL falcon tubes after filtering it through 0.22 micron (µm) membrane filter. The media was kept in 4^0C refrigerator until use.

2.2.2 Glioma culture

As for the primary culture technique, we chose the explant method developed by Harrison (1907) and Carrel (1912) for initiating the culture of clinically derived glioma tissue since it was a type of soft tissue and in most cases, we only managed to take out a very small amount. Based on local adaptation to our operation theatre (OT), we added a few extra steps to modify the standard explant method to reduce or to eliminate possible contamination at the early stage. For that purpose, the addition of antibiotic cocktail in the complete culture media and the pre-rinsing of the collected tissue with 70% ethanol before culturing in the flasks help us in achieving that goal. In addition, full cooperation from the neurosurgeons and OT staffs in avoiding cross contamination between surgical procedure, careful retrieval of the clinical sample from the patient's brain and careful transportation of collected sample from the OT to our culture laboratory also helped to reduce and eliminate contamination.

The tumor was given a quick rinse in 70% ethanol to disinfect all the possible microorganisms, followed by a brief rinse in sterile 1x PBS (Sigma, USA) to wash out the ethanol and also the blood. The tumor was then placed in a sterile petri dish filled with complete culture media and minced into fragments sized 1-2 mm by using a sterile blade in sterile complete medium RPMI 1640 with L-Glutamine and $NaHCO_3$ (refer to 2.2.1). The fragments were then layered on the bottom of plastic flasks (25 cm^2) and 3mL of the complete medium was poured gently into the flask to avoid detachment of the tissue fragments. The culture was incubated at 37°C in a humidified atmosphere of 5% CO_2 for about 5-7 days (Figure 1). Once the cells had migrated out and attached to the bottom of the flasks, medium was changed after intervals of 48- 72 hrs.

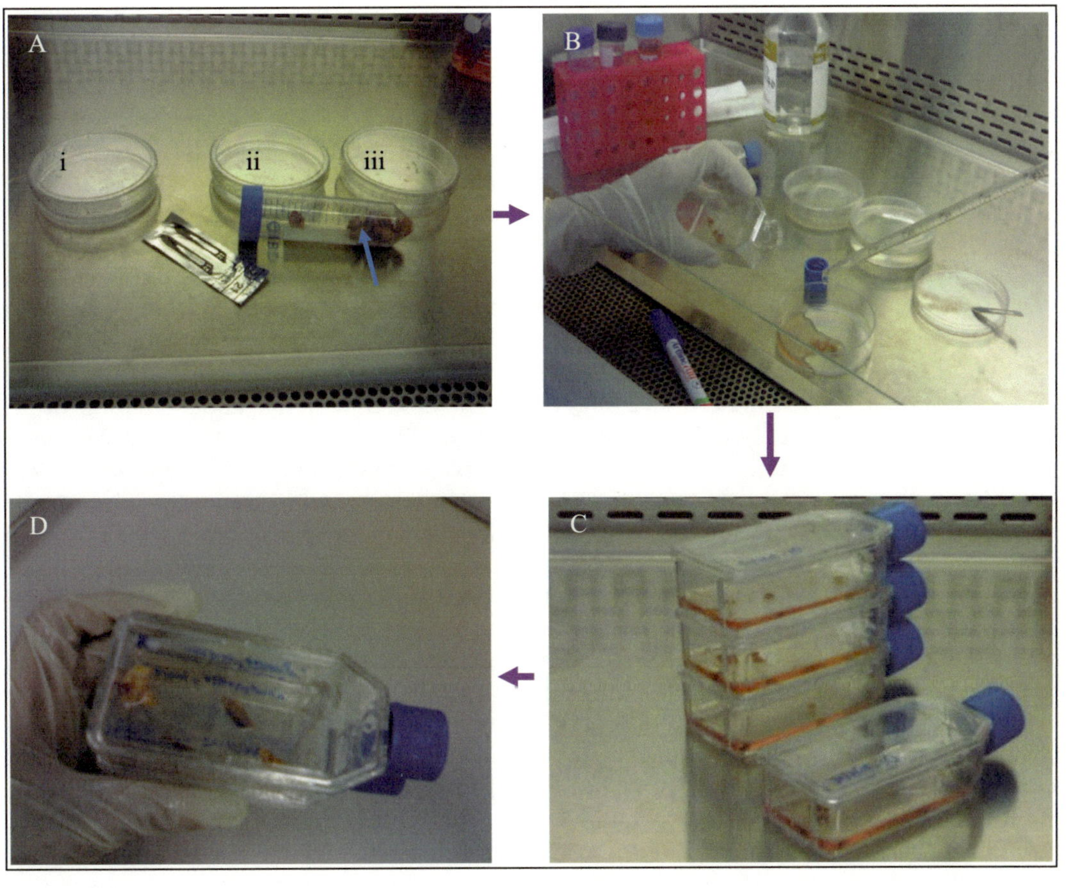

Fig. 4. Primary cell culture; steps in processing the clinical samples. (A) Materials used to culture clinical tissues (⟶); i- 70% ethanol to disinfect the tissues; ii- sterile PBS to rinse the tissues; iii- complete media RPMI 1640 wherein tissues been minced to small pieces. (B) Minced tissues transferred into cell culture flask with complete media RPMI 1640. (C) Volume of the complete media RPMI 1640 sufficient for the minced tissue contact to the bottom of the inner flask surface. (D) Labeled flask is ready to be placed in humid CO_2 incubator

When the primary culture reached confluence the cells were sub-cultured by treatment with 0.05% trypsin and 0.02% EDTA and maintained in the same medium. Subsequently the cultures were serially sub-cultured using the same procedure. Large quantities of this glioma cells were routinely frozen at various passage levels in 95% fetal bovine serum plus 5% DMSO (v/v) for future use.

2.3 Image analysis work: phase contrast microscopy

The cellular glioma cultured cells at various passages were grown in sterile cell culture flasks. The cultured cells were observed and photographed using an inverted microscope fitted with a camera (Axiovert 25 ZEISS with 0.5 X magnifier software evolution LC Kit and Image Pro- Express software).

2.4 Confirmation of cell line establishment based on marker antigen

2.4.1 ProteinExpression: SDS-PAGE & western blotting

The human malignant glioma cells were cultured in 75cm^2 flasks. Subconfluent tumor cells were collected after incubation with 0.25% trypsin and 0.02% EDTA, and washed once with pre- cooled PBS. The neutralization of the trypsin was done by the addition of pre-cooled complete medium. The detached cells suspension was spun down by centrifugation at 1500rpm for 5 minutes. The supernatant was discarded and the pellet was washed with pre-cooled sterile 1x PBS. Following centrifugation, the supernatant was discarded and the pellet was lyzed with pre- cooled radioimmunoprecipitation assay (RIPA) buffer (0.4 M NaCl, 50 mM Tris pH 7.5 (by HEPES), 1% NP- 40, 0.1% SDS, 0.1% Na deoxycholate, 1mM EDTA, 1mM PMSF) overnight at 4°C . The next day, the suspension was spun at 10, 000 rpm for 20 minutes at 4°C and the supernatant was then extracted. Protein samples with concentration of approximately 0.72 mg/mL were mixed with an equal volume of 2x loading dye/ treatment buffer and then heated at 95^{0}C for 5 minutes. Samples were electrophoresed in gradient (12.5% and 10%) SDS-PAGE. Once electrophoresis was completed, the proteins were visualized either by staining with commasie blue or by western blotting. SDS- PAGE used in this study was a modified of Laemmli system (Laemmli, 1970).

After electrophoresis, gels were electroblotted onto the PVDF membrane (MILLIPORE Immobilon P- Transfer membrane). The membrane was treated with 5% skim milk for 1 hour. After washing with the washing buffer, the membrane was then incubated with primary antibody; GFAP (abcam), Vimentin (abcam) or BORIS (Santa Cruz) for 1 hour at room temperature. Following three times (5 minutes each) washes in washing buffer, the membrane was treated with anti- mouse or anti- rabbit immunoglobulin antibody conjugated with Horse-Radish Peroxidase (HRP) for 1 hour at room temperature. A final wash was performed, and the membrane was equilibrated with detection buffer ECL solution (Immobilon Western Chemiluminescent HRP Substrate) for about 3 minutes and the membrane was placed in developing folder on the hypercassette (Amersham Life Science). In the dark room, the film (Kodak X- Omat LS Film Sigma- Aldrich) was exposed to the membrane for about 10 minutes before it was developed accordingly.

2.4.2 Immunocytochemistry

Immunocytochemical analysis of neuron- glial markers (Beta III- Tubulin, MAP2, Oligodendrocytes and GFAP) were performed using specific antibodies purchased ; neuron-glial cell marker sampler kit from Millipore, Chemicon whereas the other glial markers (S-

100 and vimentin) and BORIS were performed using specific antibodies purchased from Abcam and Santa Cruz respectively. IHC Select HRP/ DAB (Millipore, Chemicon) kit was used as the secondary antibody system in this analysis.

Briefly, cultured glioma cells were harvested at a specific passage, trypsinized and cultured in new chambered slides. When the cells in each chamber reached semi confluent, the medium was discarded, washed with sterile 1X PBS plus 0.05% tween 20. The slides were then fixed in cold methanol for 20 minutes at 4° C. After a thorough wash with 0.05% tween 20 in 1X PBS, the cells were treated with all of the above primary antibodies according to the manufacture's instructions. The bound primary antibody was detected using peroxidase labeled polymer conjugated to either mouse or rabbit secondary antibodies. Subsequently, the slides were incubated with a substrate mixture of 3, 3- diaminobenzidine (DAB) and 0.02% H_2O_2. Cells were then counterstained with haematoxylin. Negative control slide was also included by omission of the primary antibody.

2.5 Growth curve

Glioma cells were collected from the 16th passage for determination of growth curves. Briefly, semi confluent cultures were trypsinized and cells resuspended in complete medium for counting. Cells (1×10^4) were plated into each well of a 12-well plate and counts from triplicate wells were made daily for 8 days. Trypsinized cells were counted in haemocytometer chamber and numbers were averaged for each time interval. Cell population doubling time was calculated from the linear phase of the growth curve, and the saturation density was the plateau point on the growth curve after the linear growth phase.

2.6 Real-time PCR analysis

Total RNA from cell lines (~$1x10^7$ cells) were extracted using RNeasy Mini Kit (Qiagen, Germany) and checked for concentration, integrity and purity. Two microgram of total RNA was reverse transcribed into cDNA using Revert Aid H Minus First Strand cDNA Synthesis Kit (Fermentas, USA). The BORIS primers and probe were the same as previously published by D'Arcy et al., (2006); the sequences (64bp) were as follows, forward: 5'-CCCATTGTGCCACCATCA-3', reverse: AGCATGCAAGTTGCGCATAT--3', and probe: 6FAM-ACGGAAAAGCGACCTAC-MGB; they were purchased from Applied Biosystems, USA. Real-time PCR analysis with optimal condition was performed using Taqman probe Master Mix (ABI, USA) via Applied Biosystems 7500 Real-Time PCR System (USA). The Real-time PCR products were also subsequently subjected to 2% agarose gel electrophoresis for the confirmation of PCR amplicons.

3. Results and discussion

Working in a high humidity and tropical condition exposed our clinical sample to bacterial and fungal contamination. Indeed, it is one of the constraints in the establishments of any primary tumor culture taken from a clinical source. We established an antibiotic cocktail that we used in our initial complete media which consists of amphotericin B (fungizone), gentamycin, chloramphenicol, kanamycin and ampicilin. The concentration of the cocktail used in this study varies depending on the severity of contamination in the initial condition of our clinical samples. A referral to a comprehensive pharmacology guide for antibiotic-cellular incompatibilities information was very important when we were using two or more antibiotics in the same culture system because combined antibiotics frequently exert cytotoxic effects at lower concentrations than those indicated as appropriate for the individual antibiotics (Sigma-Aldrich.inc). In this case, we have started the cocktail addition at the lowest concentration possible.

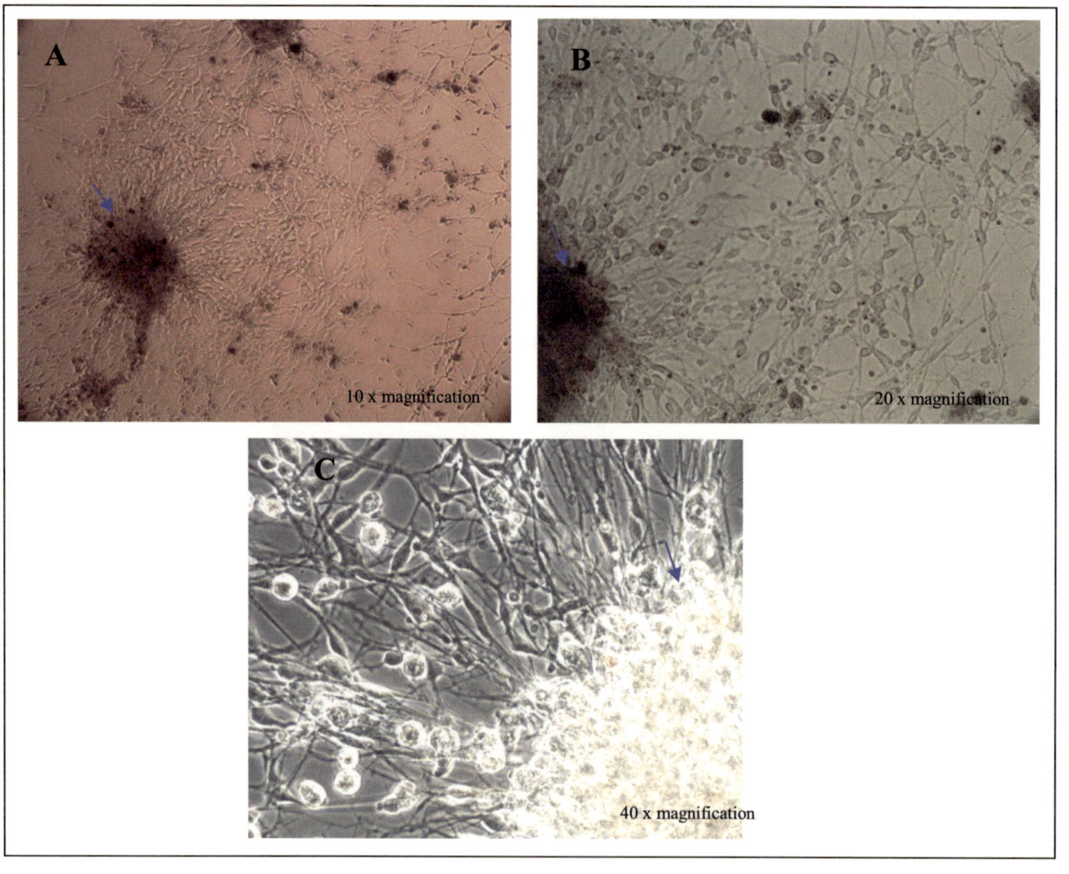

Fig. 5. Morphology of the clinical derived glioblastoma multiforme primary cell line at the initial stage; Attached tissue fragment (⟶). (A) 10 X magnification; (B) 20 X magnification; and (C) 40 X magnification.

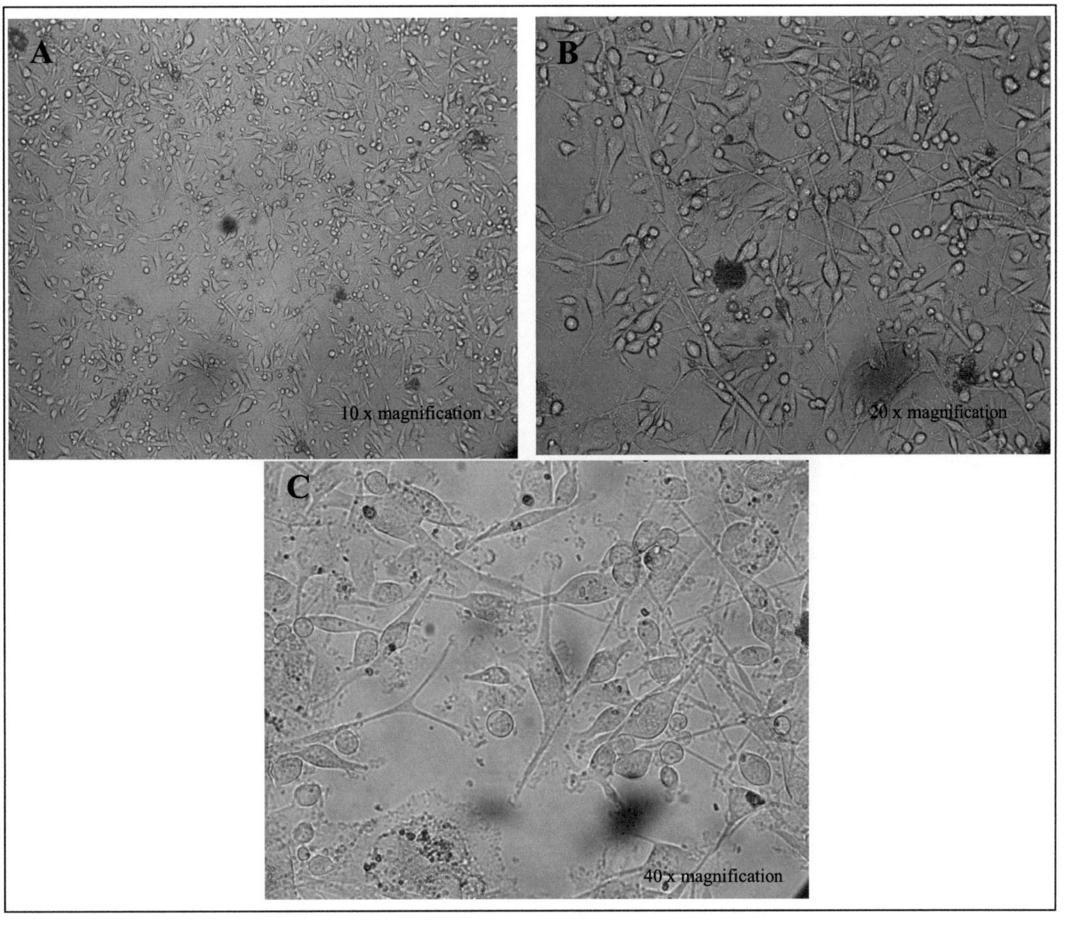

Fig. 6. Morphology of the clinical derived glioblastoma multiforme primary cell line at passage 1; rounded cells and dendritic-like cells with extensive cytoplasmatic prolongations (→).
(A) 10 X magnification; (B) 20 X magnification; and (C) 40 X magnification.

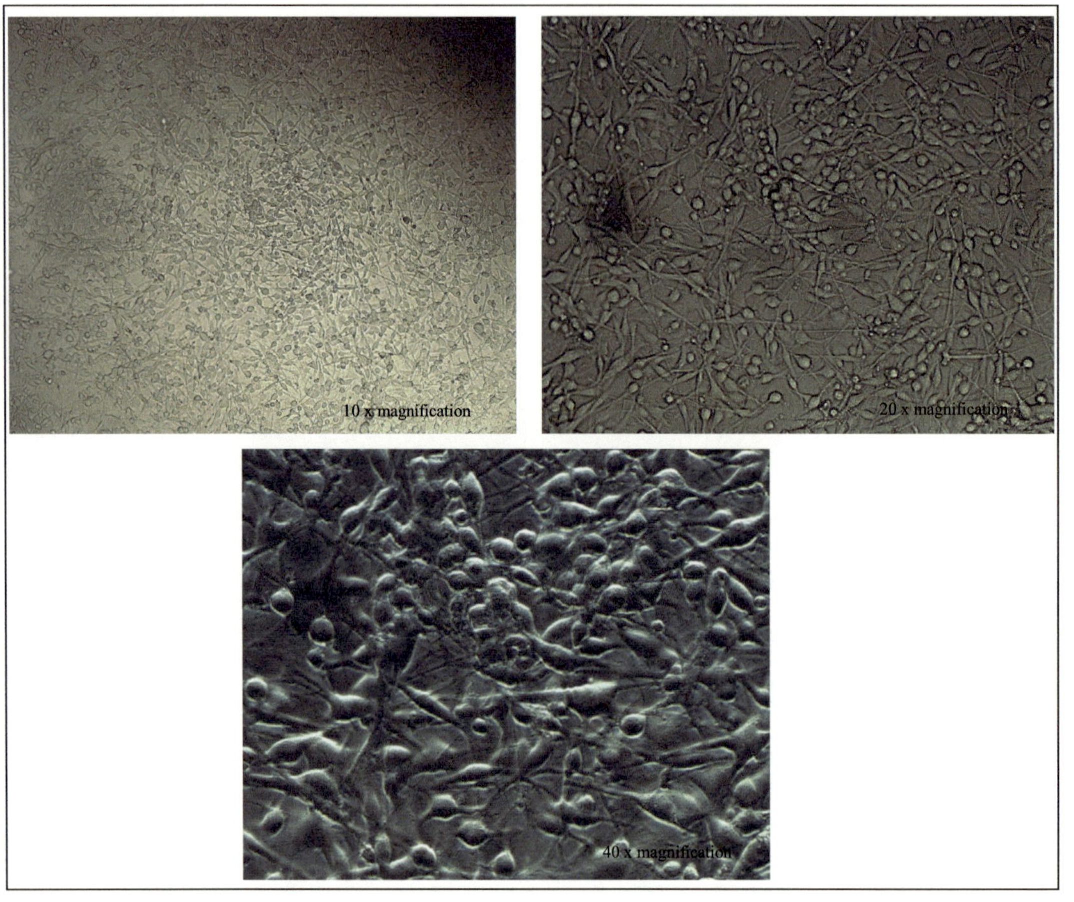

Fig. 7. Confluent monolayer of the clinical derived glioblastoma multiforme primary cell line with rounded and dendritic-like cells. (A) 10 X magnification; (B) 20 X magnification; and (C) 40 X magnification.

Variable morphological features could be found in the glioblastoma multiforme cells i.e small rounded cells and dendritic- like cells with extensive cytoplasmatic prolongations (figure 2, figure 3 and figure 4). Our finding was in agreement with other works in literature that showed evidences suggesting that some types of cancers, notably solid tumors,were not homogeneous in their cell composition but are composed of heterogeneous cell types (Bigner et al.,1979, 1981; Perzelova et al., 1998; Grippo et al., 2001; Machado et al., 2005). Similar morphological features were observed throughout serial passages, as described. This tumor cell line presented features of malignant glioma characterized by cell pleomorphism, necrosis and aggressive growth (Machado et al. 2005; Grippo MC et al. 2001). Low passage cultures grew slower than high passage cultures. This fact could indicated a perfect adaptation of cells to the culture conditions. This cell line would be useful for testing potential anticancer agents either *in vitro* or *in vivo*.

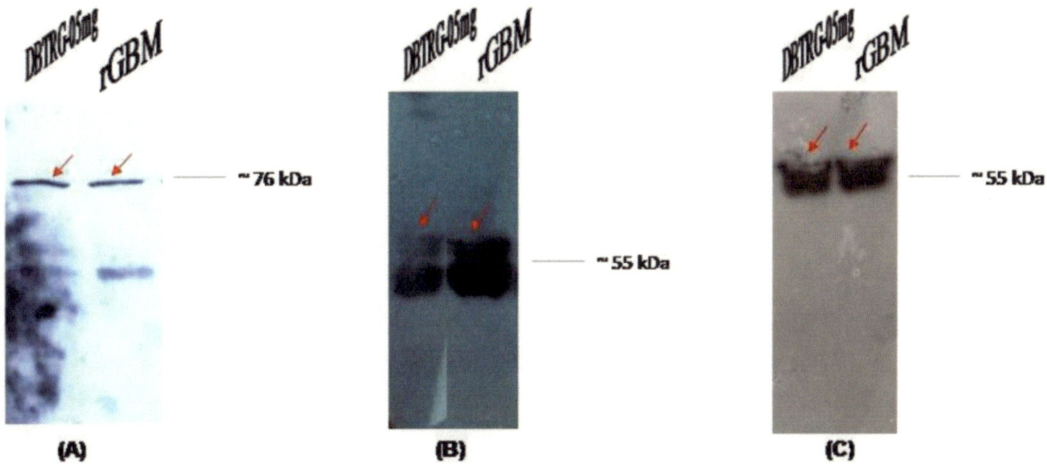

Fig. 8. Western Blotting of the clinical derived glioblastoma multiforme (rGBM) primary cell line.

Western blotting of total lysate of DBTRG-05MG (ATCC derived glioma) and primary culture cell glioblastoma multiforme (rGBM) separated in SDS-PAGE and probed with:

(A) α-BORIS polyclonal (dilution 1:500). The presence of BORIS is indicated by red arrow at ~76 kDa for both DBTRG-05MG and rGBM.

(B) α-GFAP monoclonal (dilution 1:500). The presence of GFAP is indicated by red arrow at ~50 kDa to ~57kDa for both DBTRG-05MG and rGBM.

(C) α-Vimentin monoclonal (dilution 1:500). The presence of vimentin is indicated by red arrow at ~50 to ~57 kDa for both DBTRG-05MG and rGBM.

Western blot analyses showed strong expression for BORIS protein (figure 8, A). BORIS is a CTCF paralog, which contains all eleven zinc fingers of CTCF, and has been shown to promote cell growth leading to transformation (Loukinov et al., 2002). One mechanism of action by which BORIS is thought to cause cancer through interference is the maintenance of an appropriate methylation pattern in the genome (Klenova et al., 2002). The detection of BORIS protein in glioblastoma multiforme suggested its potential as an early marker of this type of glioma since BORIS has been reported as an early tumor marker in breast cancer (D'Arcy et al., 2006). Western blot analysis also showed that the glioblastoma multiforme cell line retains the expression of GFAP (figure 5, B) which is a reliable marker of astrocytic cells (Moore 1965; Machado et al., 2005). However,literature has shown a negative correlation between the degree of malignancy and the expression of GFAP protein in the majority of human gliomas (Machado et al., 2005). We also showed that vimentin which has been identified in some human glioma cell lines (Roessmann et al., 1983; Rutka et al., 1998) was also detectable in this glioma cell line (figure 8, C). Machado et al., 2005 claimed that the effect of vimentin filaments on the invaginations or folding in the nucleus is not absolute and raised the possibility that this nuclear configuration could be an indirect effect of a metabolic difference between cells that contain or lack organized vimentin filaments. To all appearances, ours and previous study results indicated that the absence or presence of an organized vimentin filament network do not affect the shape of the cell. However, interestingly S100 protein that was originally identified as brain specific (Moore, 1965) and believed to be expressed in a few types of gliomas was not identified in this cell line. But still, literature has shown a negative correlation between the degree of malignancy and the expression of GFAP and S100 protein in the majority of human gliomas (Jacques et al., 1981; Duffy et al., 1982).

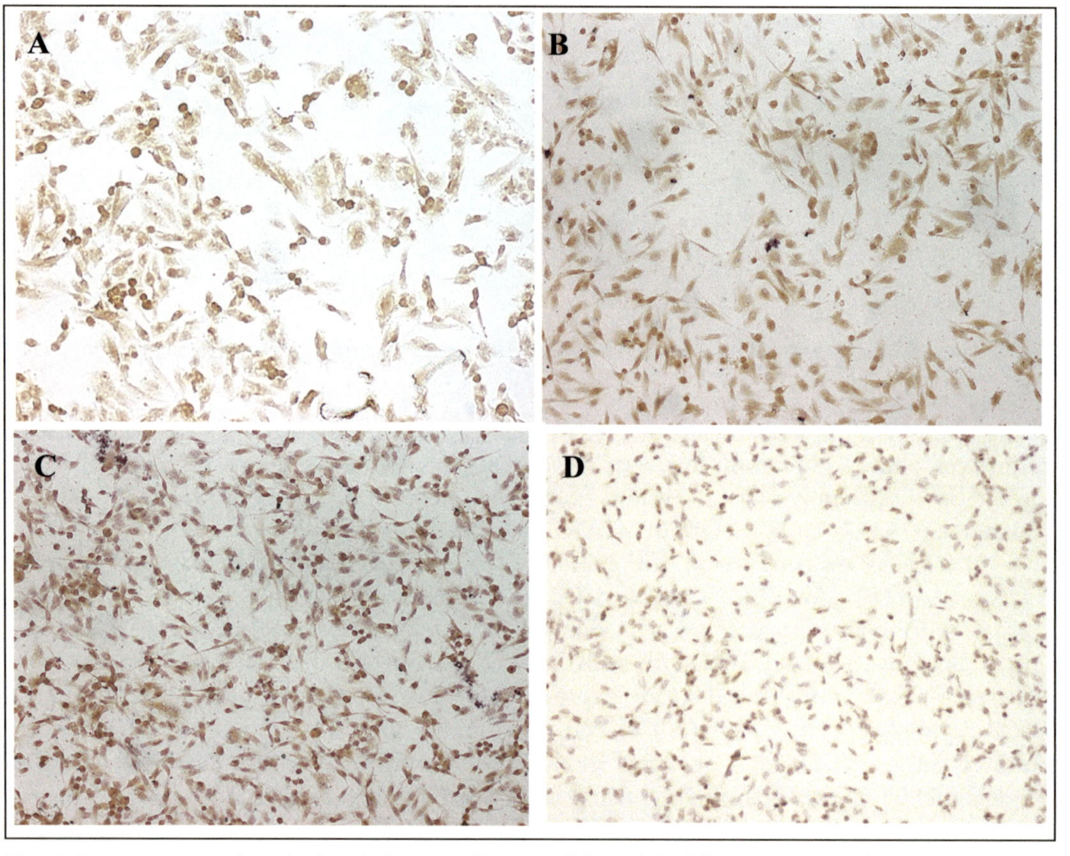

Fig. 9. Immunocytochemical staining in glioma cell line (glioblastoma multiforme) at passage 6 to passage 17 at 5 x magnification. Note the immunopositive staining for (A) BORIS, (B) GFAP and (C) B- tubulin. On the other hand, cells were S-100- negative stained (D). The negative control is the slide that stained with secondary antibody only.

Immunopositive (figure 9) and western blotting results for BORIS indicates that the tumor-antigenic polypeptide is expressed in the glioma cell lines. These results suggest that BORIS might play an important role in regulating the tumorigenesis pathway. And if that persists, BORIS can be manipulated as a biomarker in detecting the presence of tumoric condition in glial cells in an uninvasive way and at the very early stage. Deeper understanding of the place and the role of BORIS in that exact molecular pathway, gave us a good chance in preventing or disrupting the tumorigenesis pathway. This could lead to the application of genetic therapy in treating glioma patients. Understanding and moving towards that goal, require us to study deeper and not just stop at this preliminary study. This cell line showed negative expression of MAP-2, a neuron-marker which suggests that the tumor cell line is not originated from neuron cell and the negative expression of oligodendrocytes suggested that the cells absolutely not oligodendrocytes.

The newly established cells entered into an exponential growth phase at the 16th passage, when the cells grew aggressively in the culture. The high growth rate was observed for these successive passages when the population doubling time of the glioblastoma multiforme cell line was about 6 hrs at 37°C and the saturation cell density was reached at 3.3×10^5 cells/cm^2 (graph 1). The cells showed continuous progressive growth until day 7 without showing any sign of senescence. On the other hand, the growth kinetic of the DBTRG-05MG cells, used as a reference cells in this study, achieved population doubling time of approximately 34 to 41 hours. The saturation density of the cells reached 8.3×10^5 cells/ well (Kruise et al., 1992).

In comparison, DBTRG-05MG the well known established glioma cell line, introduced by Kruse et al. in 1992, showed rounded and spindle shape cells with fibroblast-like cells (figure 7).This is exactly different with our newly established clinically derived glioma but the heterogeneity of the morphology was in parallel with most studies done in glioma cells.

The study of characterization of the ATCC derived cell line also revealed positive expression of BORIS, GFAP, Vimentin (figure 8) and S100 proteins (Kruise et al., 1992). This profiling was in parallel with our newly established glioma cells with the exclusion of S100 protein. Figure 9 (D) showed our newly established cells immunonegative for S100 protein. The comparison of protein expression in both DBTRG-05MG the ATCC derived glioma cell line and our newly established glioma is shown and summarized in Figure 11 and Table 1.

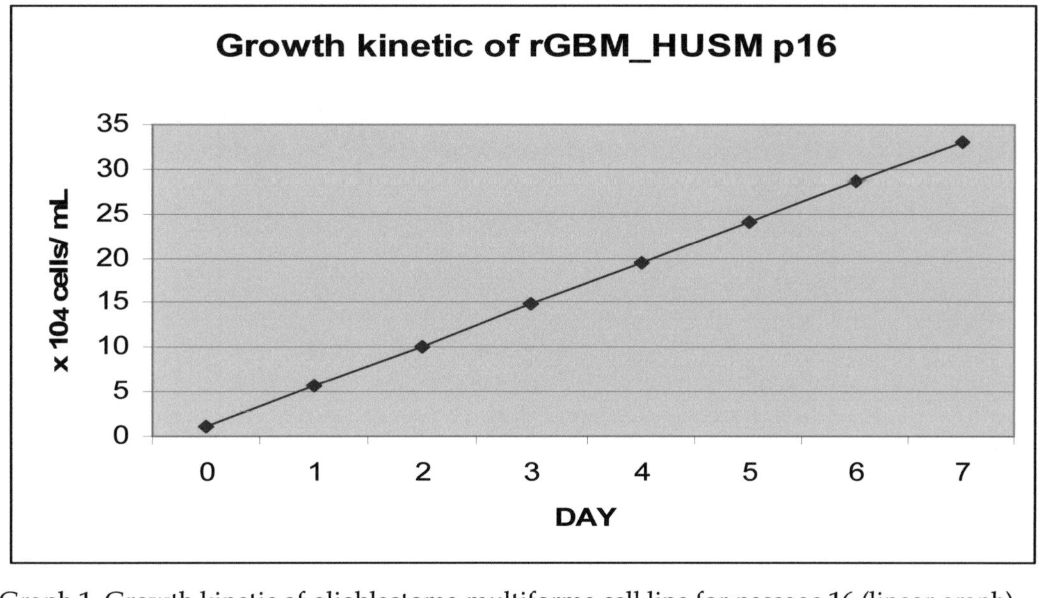

Graph 1. Growth kinetic of glioblastoma multiforme cell line for passage 16 (linear graph)

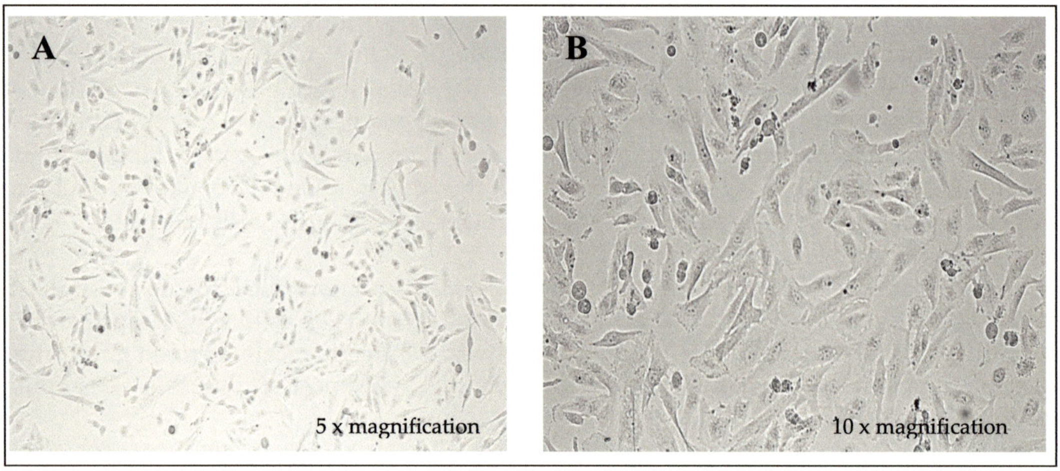

Fig. 10. Morphology of DBTRG-05MG (ATCC derived glioma cell line) under phase contrast microscopy. Rounded cell with fibroblastic-like cells.

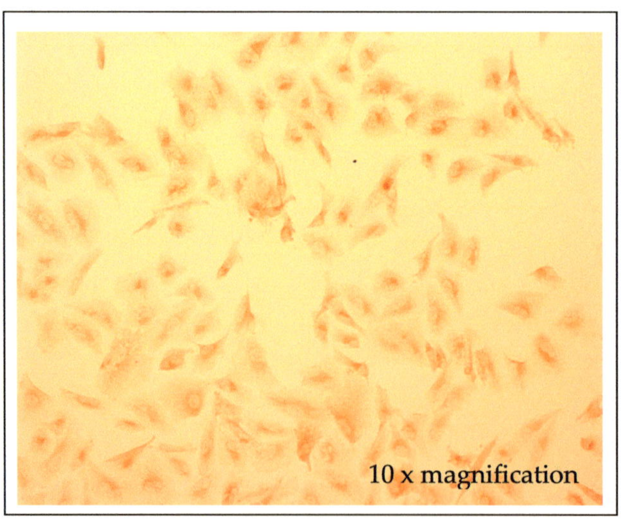

Fig. 11. Immunopositive of BORIS in DBTRG-05MG ATCC derived cell line. The negative control is the slide that stained with secondary antibody only (not shown).

Specificity	Cells	
	Clinically derived glioma (this study)	ATCC derived glioma (DBTRG-05MG)
BORIS	+	+ (Kruise et al., 1992)
GFAP	+	+ (this study)
Vimentin	+	+ (Kruise et al., 1992)
S100	-	+ (Kruise et al., 1992)

Table 1. The summary of protein studies based on immunocytochemistry and western blotting assay for established glioma cell line in comparison with the ATCC derived glioma cell line (adapted from Kruise et al., 1992).

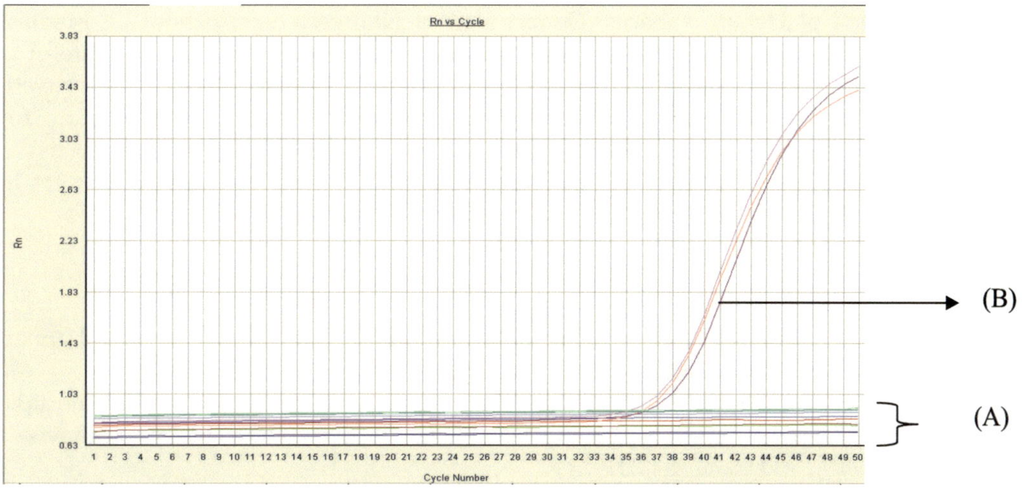

Fig. 12. Amplification plots of BORIS mRNA expression using Taqman probe master mix. The result showed that BORIS mRNA was unexpressed in DBTRG 05MG (ATCC derived glioma), ATCC derived normal osteoblast, ATCC derived normal glial cell lines and in no template controls (A). BORIS mRNA was expressed in positive control osteosarcoma U2OS cells (ATCC derived) detected at ~38 cycles (B).

The expression of BORIS mRNA was not found in DBTRG-05MG ATCC derived glioma cell line (Figure 12) although we observed the positive expression of BORIS protein in the same sample. Recently Hines et al., 2010 has reported that BORIS mRNA was not expressed in most human breast cancer cell lines and tumors. Furthermore expression of BORIS mRNA showed no significant difference between normal and prostate cancer tissues overall and no relationship was seen to clinical parameters (D'Arcy et al., 2006). This strengthened the study done by Renaud et al., in 2007 that BORIS involved in complex mechanism and it is promoter dependent gene. Therefore, at this stage we expected the undetected expression of BORIS mRNA in our newly established clinically derived glioma primary cell line with positive expression of BORIS protein in the same clinical derived sample.

4. Conclusion

We established our glioblastoma multiforme cell line with the basic characteristics including the morphology study, surface antigen profile, protein study and also the growth analysis. This cell line which was derived from our clinical sample would be useful for studies on the molecular basis of malignancy and progression of glioma as well as in studies of glioma treatment. BORIS has been shown to be expressed in our glioma primary cell line. This study has strengthened the suggestion of a previous study (D' Arcy et al., 2001) where BORIS could play an important role in the early diagnosis of glioma which requires further study with consideration of its complex behaviour in cancer development as well as the splice variants in promoter dependent gene.

5. Acknowledgement

This study was supported by Fundamental Research Grant Scheme (FRGS) and the Ministry of Science & Innovation, Malaysia for the National Science Fellowship (to support the postgraduate study of S.Z.M.R). We thank all the students and staffs of Molecular Biology Laboratory, School of Health Sciences, Department of Neurosciences, School Of Medical Sciences / Brain Mind Nexus., Universiti Sains Malaysia Health Campus. We are grateful to the technical staffs of the Craniofacial laboratory, School of Dental Science, USM Health Campus for their assistance with the inverted microscopy. We thank the Institute for Molecular Medicine (INFORMM), USM Health Campus for allowing us to use their tissue culture facilities. Special thanks to all the neurosurgeons, nurses and technical staffs in operation theater 15 (Neurosurgery), Hospital Universiti Sains Malaysia (HUSM).

6. References

Bakir A., Gezen F, Yildiz O., et al. 1998. Establishment and Characterization of a Human Glioblastoma Multiforme Cell Line. *Cancer Genet Cytogenet.*, 103, 46-51

Bigner DD, Bigner SH, Ponten J et al. 1981. Heterogeneity of genotypic and phenotypic characteristics of fifteen permanent cell lines derived from human gliomas. *J Neuropathol Exp Neurol*, 40, 201–229.

Bigner DD, Bullard D, Schold C, and Wikstrand C. 1979. Cellular heterogeneity and diversity as a basis for therapeutic resistance of human gliomas. In: *Paoletti P,Walker MD, and Butti G (Eds.).* Multidisciplinary Aspects of Brain Tumor Therapy, Elsevier, Amsterdam, 329–334

Campbell, A. E., Martinez, S. R. & Miranda, J. J. L. (2010). Molecular architecture of CTCFL. *Biochemical and Biophysical Research Communications,* In Press, Uncorrected Proof.

D'Arcy V, Abdullaev ZK, Pore N et al. 2006. The Potential of BORIS detected in the Leukocytes of Breast Cancer Patients as an Early Marker of Tumorigenesis. *Clinical Cancer Research*, 12, 5978-5986

D'Arcy, V., Pore, N., Docquier, F., Abdullaev, Z. K., Chernukhin, I., Kita, G. X., Rai, S., Smart, M., Farrar, D., Pack, S., Lobanenkov, V. & Klenova, E. (2008). BORIS, a paralogue of the transcription factor, CTCF, is aberrantly expressed in breast tumours (British Journal of Cancer (2008) 98 (571-579) doi: 10.1038/sj.bjc.6604181). *British Journal of Cancer,* 98(3), 676.

Di Tomaso E, Pang JCS, Ng HK et al. 2000. Establishment and characterization of a human cell line from paedriatic cerebellar glioblastoma multiform. *Neuropathol Appl Neurobiol*, 26, 22-30

Floyd E. Bloom, John H. Morrison, Jeff M. Redwine, John F. Reilly & G.Young, W. (2004). Neuroinformatics tools for visualizing gene expression in the brain. *DDT: BIOSILICO* 2(3).

Furnari FB, Huang HJ, Cavenee WK: Genetics and malignant progression of human brain tumours. *Cancer Surv* 1995, 25:233-275.

Grippo MC, Penteado PF, Carelli EF et al., 2001. Establishment and Partial Characterization of a Continuous Human Malignant Glioma Cell Line: NG97. *Cell Mol Neurobiol,* 21, 421-428.

Halfter H, Kremerskothen J, Weber J et al. 1998. Growth inhibition of newly established human glioma cell lines by leukemia inhibitory factor. *J Neuro-Oncol,* 39, 1-18.

Hines WC, Bazarov AV, Mukhopadhyay R, Yaswen P: BORIS (CTCFL) is not expressed in most human breast cell lines and high grade breast carcinomas. *PLoS One* 2010, 5:e9738.

Hoffmann, M. J., Müller, M., Engers, R. & Schulz, W. A. (2006). Epigenetic control of CTCFL/BORIS and OCT4 expression in urogenital malignancies. *Biochemical Pharmacology,* 72(11), 1577-1588.

Hong, J. A., Kang, Y., Abdullaev, Z., Flanagan, P. T., Pack, S. D., Fischette, M. R., Adnani, M. T., Loukinov, D. I., Vatolin, S., Risinger, J. I., Custer, M., Chen, G. A., Zhao, M., Nguyen, D. M., Barrett, J. C., Lobanenkov, V. V. & Schrump, D. S. (2005). Reciprocal binding of CTCF and BORIS to the NY-ESO-1 promoter coincides with derepression of this cancer-testis gene in lung cancer cells. *Cancer research,* 65(17), 7763-7774.

Jelinic, P. & Shaw, P. (2007). Loss of imprinting and cancer. *Journal of Pathology,* 211(3), 261-268.

Kalejs M, Erenpreisa J: Cancer/testis antigens and gametogenesis: a review and "brain-storming" session. *Cancer Cell Int* 2005, 5:4.

Klenova, E. M., Morse, H. C., Ohlsson, R. & Lobanenkov, V. V. (2002). The novel BORIS + CTCF gene family is uniquely involved in the epigenetics of normal biology and cancer. *Seminars in Cancer Biology,* 12(5), 399-414.

Kruise CA, Mitchell DH, Kleinschmidt-DeMasters et al. 1992. Characterization of a human glioma cell line DBTRG-05MG Groeth kinetics, karyotype, receptor expression, and tumor suppressor gene analysis.*In Vitro Cell. Dev. Biol.* 28A:609-614.

Laemmli, U.K., 1970 *Nature* 227:680-685.

Lei Zhang, Tetsu Yamane, Eiji Satoh, Kenichi Amagasaki, Tomoyuki Kawataki, Takayuki Asahara, Koro Furuya, Hideaki Nukui & Naganuma., H. (2005). Establishment and partial characterization of five malignant glioma cell lines. *Neuropathology,* 25136-143.

Loukinov DI, Pugacheva E, Vatolin S et al. 2002. BORIS, a novel male germ-line-specific protein associated with epigenetic reprogramming events, shares the same 11-zinc-finger domain with CTCF, the insulator protein involved in reading imprinting marks in the soma. Procedings of the National Academy of Sciences, 99, 6806- 6811.

Machado CML, Schenka A, Vassallo J et al. 2005. Morphological characterization of a human glioma cell line. *Cancer cell International,* 5:13.

Moore BW. 1965. A soluble protein characteristic of the nervous system. *Biochem. Biophys Res Commun*, 19, 739-744.

Nebert, D. W. (2002). Transcription factors and cancer: an overview. *Toxicology,* 181-182131-141.

Nguyen P, Bar-Sela G, Sun L et al. 2008. BAT3 and SET1A Form a Complex with CTCFL/BORIS To Modulate H3K4 Histone Dimethylation and Gene Expression, *Molecular and Cellular Biology,* nov 2008, p. 6720–6729

Ohlsson R, Renkawitz R, Lobanenkov V: CTCF is a uniquely versatile transcription regulator linked to epigenetics and disease. *Trends Genet* 2001, 17:520-527.

Old LJ: Cancer/testis (CT) antigens - a new link between gametogenesis and cancer. *Cancer Immun* 2001, 1:1.

Perzelova, A, Macikova I, Mraz P, Bizik I, and Steno J. 1998. Characterization of two new permanent glioma cell lines 8-MG-BA and 42-MGBA. *Neoplasma,* 45, 25–29.

Pohl U, Wick W, Weissenberger J et al. 1999. Characterization of Tu- a glioma cell line derived from a spontaneous tumor in GFAP-v-src-transgenic mice: comparison with established murine glioma cell lines. *Int J Oncol*, 15, 829-834.

Pugacheva, E. M., Kwon, Y.-W., Hukriede, N. A., Pack, S., Flanagan, P. T., Ahn, J.-C., Park, J. A., Choi, K.-S., Kim, K.-W., Loukinov, D., Dawid, I. B. & Lobanenkov, V. V. (2006). Cloning and characterization of zebrafish CTCF: Developmental expression patterns, regulation of the promoter region, and evolutionary aspects of gene organization. *Gene,* 375: 26-36.

Renaud, S., Pugacheva, E. M., Delgado, M. D., Braunschweig, R., Abdullaev, Z., Loukinov, D., Benhattar, J. & Lobanenkov, V. (2007). Expression of the CTCF-paralogous cancer-testis gene, brother of the regulator of imprinted sites (BORIS), is regulated by three alternative promoters modulated by CpG methylation and by CTCF and p53 transcription factors. *Nucleic Acids Research,* 35(21), 7372-7388.

Risinger, J. I., Chandramouli, G. V. R., Maxwell, G. L., Custer, M., Pack, S., Loukinov, D., Aprelikova, O., Litzi, T., Schrump, D. S., Murphy, S. K., Berchuck, A., Lobanenkov, V. & Barrett, J. C. (2007). Global expression analysis of cancer/testis genes in uterine cancers reveals a high incidence of BORIS expression. *Clinical Cancer Research,* 13(6), 1713-1719.

Roessmann U, Velasco ME, Gambetti P and Autilio-Gambetti L. 1983. Neuronal and astrocytic differentiation in human neuroepithelial neoplasms. An immunohistochemical study. *J Neuropathol Exp Neurol*, 42, 113-121.

Rutka JT, Ackerley C, Hubbard SL et al. 1998. Characterization of glial filament- cytoskeletal interactions in human astrocytomas: an immuno-ultrastructural analysis. *Eur J Cell Biol*, 76, 279-287.

Theresa Phillips, W. S. R. N. E. (2008), Vol. 1 *Nature Education*.

Vatolin, S., Abdullaev, Z., Pack, S. D., Flanagan, P. T., Custer, M., Loukinov, D. I., Pugacheva, E., Hong, J. A., Morse Iii, H., Schrump, D. S., Risinger, J. I., Barrett, J. C. & Lobanenkov, V. V. (2005). Conditional expression of the CTCF-paralogous transcriptional factor BORIS in normal cells results in demethylation and derepression of MAGE-A1 and reactivation of other cancer-testis genes. *Cancer research,* 65(17), 7751-7762.

Wrensch M, Fisher JL, Schwartzbaum JA, Bondy M, Berger M, Aldape KD: The molecular epidemiology of gliomas in adults. *Neurosurg Focus* 2005, 19:E5.

Part 10

miR-221/222 Cluster - Gliomas

22

MiR-221/222 Promote the Growth of Malignant Glioma Cells by Regulating Its Target Genes

Zhang Chunzhi[1,2], Jiang Tao[3], Wang Jinhuan[4], Cheng Jinquan[5], Pu Peiyu[2] and Kang Chunsheng[2]

[1]*Department of Radiation Oncology, Tianjin Huanhu hospital, Tianjin,*
[2]*Department of Neurosurgery, Laboratory of Neuro-Oncology, Tianjin Medical University General Hospital, Tianjin Key Laboratory of Nerve Injury, Variation and Regeneration, Tianjin,*
[3]*Department of Neurosurgery, Tiantan Hospital, Capital Medical University, Beijing,*
[4]*Department of Neurosurgery, Tianjin Huanhu hospital, Tianjin*
[5]*Department of Molecular Oncology, H.Lee Moffitt Cancer and Research Institute, Tampa,*
[1,2,3,4]*China*
[5]*USA*

1. Introduction

MicroRNAs (miRNAs or miRs) are a class of small noncoding RNAs of 19~22 nucleotides, and repress protein expression at the posttranscriptional level through imperfect or perfect base pairing with 3`untranslated region of the target mRNA in mammalian cells, leading to its reduced translation or mRNA degradation. Although miRs are thought to be involved in various biological processes, including development, differentiation, cell proliferation, cell death, and so on, accumulating evidence suggests that alterations of their expression may play a role in the development of human cancers(1-4). Specific miRNAs have been demonstrated to be deregulated in diverse cancer subtypes including lymphoma, colorectal cancer, lung cancer, breast cancer, papillary thyroid carcinoma, hepatocellular carcinoma, and glioblastoma(5-13). Ciafre et al. used microarray method to compare the global expression levels of 245 miRNAs in glioblastoma tissue with normal brain tissue and found that the expression of miR-221 was strongly upregulated in glioblastoma cells. They identified nine overexpression miRNAs including miR-221 and miR-222(miR-221/222) cluster (13). This chapter review how miR-221/222 cluster regulated glioma cell phenotype and it`s mechanism.

2. miR-221 and miR-222 cluster regulated glioma cell phenotype and it`s mechanism

In Ciafre study, they found that miR-221 and miR-222 overexpress in glioma tumor tissue and glioma cell line compare to normal brain tissue, as well as our microarray results. So, we question what biogenesis of miR-221 and miR-222 and this cluster miRs function.

2.1 Biogenesis of miR-221 and miR-222 and this tow miRs location

MiR-221, miR-222 genes are clustered chromosome Xp11.3 in tandem. When zhanglilei research retinitis pigmentosa, they discover miR-221 and miR-222 genes. Two miR genes are located near the telomeric end of deletion ~700bp apart(mir-221：45,361,839-45,361,948 and mir-222：45,362,675-45,362,784) (14). Like some other clustered miRNA genes, two miRNA genes is high similariry in sequence and they might be transcribed as polycistrons (Fig 1).

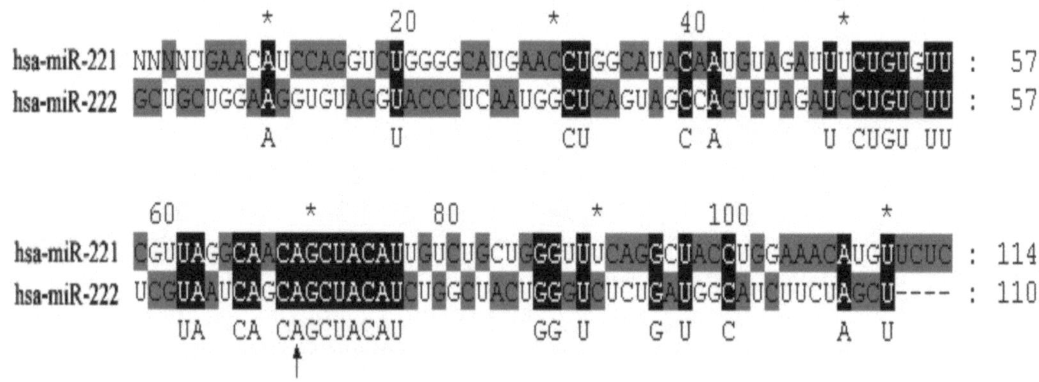

Fig. 1. A schematic representation defines the miR-221 and miR-222 sequences (arrow indicates identical seed sequences AGCUACAU as shown in GeneDoc, www.psc.edu/biomed /genedoc).

As well as the other miRs, biogenesis of miR-221 and miR-222 are a multi-step process beginning with transcription by RNA polymerase Ⅱ of a primary transcript, called pri-miRNA. This precursor is cleaved to form a 70nt long stem-loop precursor RNA(pre-miRNA) by an RNAse Ⅲ type endonuclease called Drosha inside the nucleus. RanGTP exportin 5 transports pre- miRNA to the cytoplasm, where another RNAse Ⅲ, Dicer, cleaves the stem-loop structure to produce 19~23 nucleotide miRNA duplexes. That one of the two RNA strands is then included into the RNA-induced silencing complex(RISC) form asymmetric RISC assembley. Asymmetric RISC assembley is also called miRNP. It inhibit translation or mRNA degradation by miRNA complete pairing or incomplete pairing with mRNA 3`UTRs.(15-17)

2.2 miR-221 and miR-222 cluster regulated glioma cell phenotype in vitro

We already proved that miR-221 and miR-222 upregulted in glioma compared to normal brain tissue, and knowed this two miRs biogenesis and location in chromosome. Furthermore, we ready to research how the cluster miRs affect glioma cell phenotype, including proliferation, cell cycle, apoptosis, invasion and radiosensitivity, *in vitro*.
Our previous work identified that a functional overlap between miR-221/222 in modulating glioma cell phenotype. So, we knocked down or ectopic express miR-221/222 to study their function. Firstly, by northern blot, it is identified that pMSCV-miR-221/222 increased miR-221 and miR-222 level and anti-miR-221/222(AS-miR-221/222 or As-miR-221/222) knocked down miR-221 and miR-222 level (not show).By MTT assay, the glioma U251 cell proliferation rate in different transfected cells was measured. It was shown that the cells transfected with anti-miR-221/222 were proliferated at a significantly lower rate than the other three groups (Figure 2).

Moreover, the cells transfected with pMSCV-miR-221/222 proliferated at a significantly higher rate than the control and the scramble groups (Figure 2). These data demonstrated that the growth rate of glioma cell could be co-modulated by miR-221 and miR-222. The result were also proved in the other tumors. Agami R et al found that miR-221 and miR-222 promote cancer cell proliferation(18). Frenquelli M et al also identified that miR-221 and miR-222 promote cancer cell proliferation in chronic lymphocytic leukemia(19). The same result were also proved in human prostate carcinoma cell lines, human thyroid papillary carcinomas, human colorectal carcinoma, and so on(20-22).

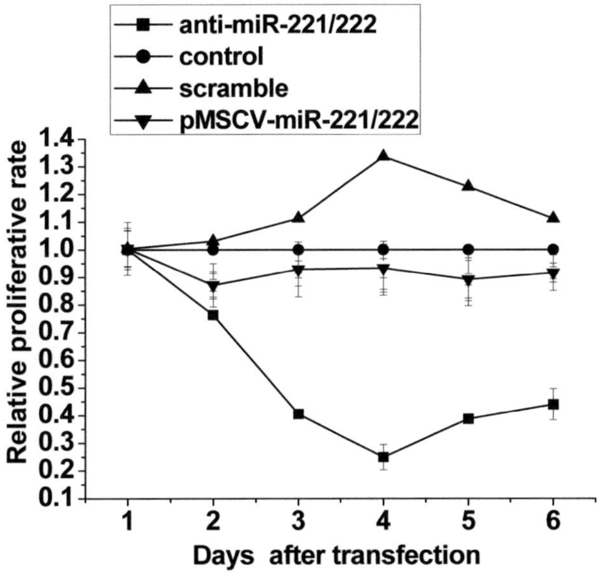

Fig. 2. As-miR-221/222 decrease cell proliferation. MTT assay show that the cells transfected with As-miR-221/222 were proliferated at a significantly lower rate than the other four groups. The latitudinal axis represented days after cell implantation in the 96-well plate. The cell proliferation rate in parental U251 glioma cells was presented as 100%.

The cell cycle distribution and cell apoptosis were analyzed by flow cytometry. The cell cycle distribution showed that the G0/G1 phase percentage of control, scramble treated cells was 28.6%, 26.0%, respectively; while the fraction of anti-miR-221/222 treated cells was 46.2% and the fraction of pMSCV-miR-221/222 treated cells was 22.3%. The S phase fraction in control, scramble treated cells, anti-miR-221/222 treated cells, pMSCV-miR-221/222 treated cells was 56.8%, 57.2%, 26.8%, 60%, respectively. No statistical significance of G2/M phase percentage was detected among the four groups (Fig. 3). Frenquelli M et al also identified that miR-221/222 promote cancer cell into S phase in chronic lymphocytic leukemia. They synchronized cells in the G1 phase and analyzed by flow cytometry the cell-cycle distribution at 4, 6, and 24 hours after cell-cycle block release. The result document that miR-221- and miR-222-transduced cells progressed more quickly through the cell-cycle phases (19). The same result was also proved in human prostate carcinoma cell lines, human thyroid papillary carcinomas, human colorectal carcinoma, and so on (20-22).

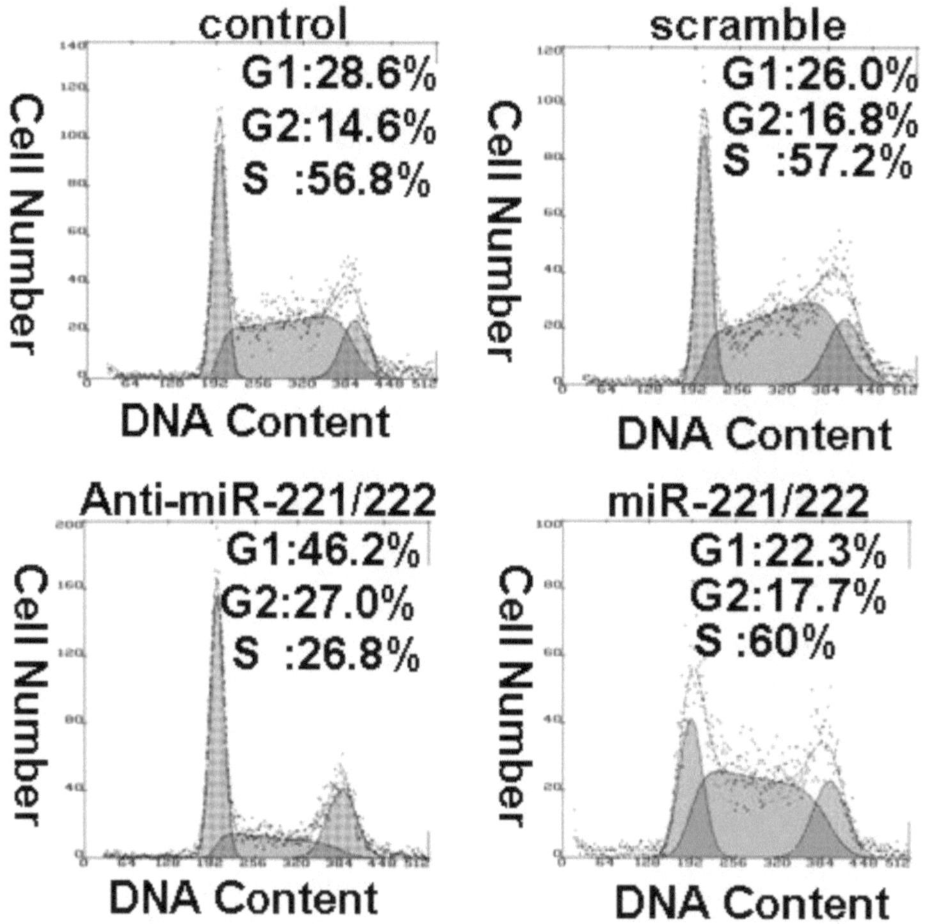

Fig. 3. Co-suppression of miR-221/222 expression by as-miR-221/222 induce G1 arrest in U251 cell. Transfected and control cells were harvested by trypsinization, washed and fixed overnight. Nuclei of cells were stained with propidium iodide, a total of 10,000 nuclei were examined. By flow cytometry analysis, the rate of cell in G1 in anti-miR-221/222 group was higher significantly than the other four groups.

Moreover, miR-221 and miR-222 inhibit glioma cell apoptosis. To examine biological significance of miR-221 and miR-222 in glioma, glioma U251 cells were treated with anti-miR-221 /222. Interestingly, annexin V-labeling revealed that knockdown of miR-221 and miR-222 significantly increased cell apoptosis compared to the cells treated with scramble oligonucleotide (Fig. 4). In addition, caspase 3/7 activity was also considerably elevated in miR-221 and miR-222 knocked down cells (Fig. 5). Since collapse of the mitochondrial membrane potential is one of the early events in apoptosis (23), we next examined whether miR-221 and miR-222 regulate mitochondrial membrane potential. The cells with depletion of miR-221 and miR-222 were stained with cationic dye JC-1. FACSCalibur analysis showed that the mitochondrial membrane potential was largely damaged when miR-221 and miR-222 were depleted (Fig. 6). These findings indicate that miR-221 and miR-222 play an important role in initiation of cell apoptosis(24).

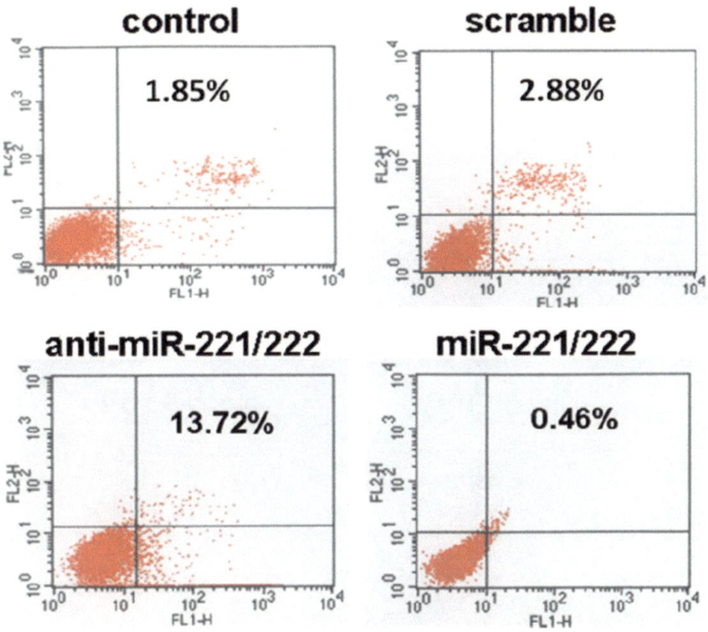

Fig. 4. Annexin V analysis showed that U251 cells transfected with As-miR-221/222 displayed significantly more apoptosis than the other three groups.

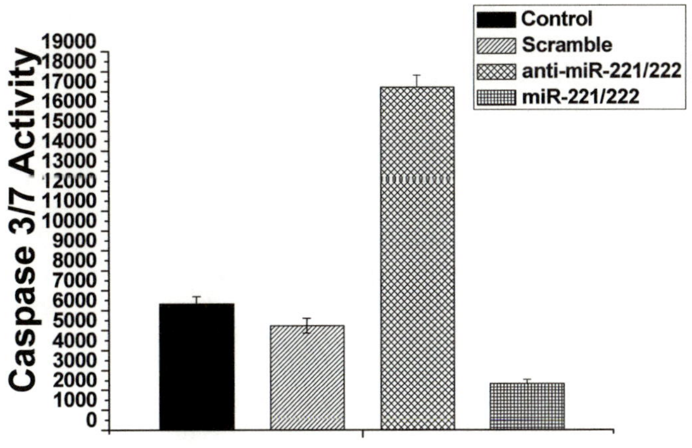

Fig. 5. Caspase 3/7 activity was considerably elevated in miR-221 and miR-222 knocked down cells compared to the other three group.

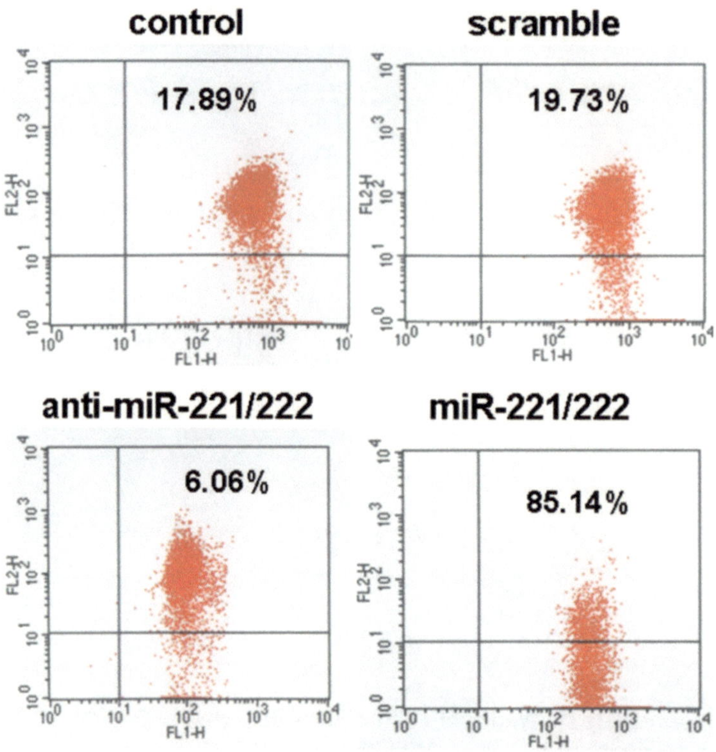

Fig. 6. U251 cells transfected with As-miR-221/222 showed a significantly greater collapse in mitochondrial membrane potential compared with the other four groups.

Furthermore, Garofalo M et al proved that miR-221/222 modulated TIMP3 expression by binding it`s 3`UTR (25). Whether miR-221/222 modulated TIMP3 expression to affect glioma cell invasion or not. To further explore the role of miR-221/222 in cell invasion, we performed gain-of-function and loss-of-function analyses by over-expressing or suppressing miR-221/222 with anti-miR-221/222 or pMSCV-miR-221/222, respectively. Interestingly, the transwell assay revealed that knockdown of miR-221/222 significantly decreased cell invasion potential compared with cells treated with scrambled oligonucleotide, whereas over-expression of miR-221/222 increased cell invasion (Fig. 7). Consistent with the results of the transwell assay, in the wound healing assay, repression of miR-221/222 significantly inhibited cell migration, while over-expression of miR-221/222 increased migration in U251 cells (Fig. 8). Therefore, miR-221 and miR-222 are required for glioma cell invasion.

In addition to modulating proliferation, cell cycle, apoptosis and invasion, whether miR-221 and miR-222 regulated glioma cell radiosensitivity or not. To test this hypothesis, we transfected AS-miR-221/-222 into U251 cells, then preformed the colony formation assay to elevated radiosensitivity. Figure 9 shows the survival curves for U251 cells transfected with control, anti-miR-221/-222, and scrambled oligonucleotides and then exposed to IR over a dose range of 0 to 6 Gy. We found that whereas scrambled oligonucleotides did not affect radiosensitivity, anti-miR-221/-222 transfection significantly decreased IR-induced survival. Radiation survival curves were characterized based on parameters such as the dose required to reduce survival to 37% of its value (D0), the surviving fraction at 2 Gy (SF2), and the sensitization enhancement ratio at 10% (SER10). The SER10 value for the U251 cells transfected with AS-miR-221/-222 was 1.97 (Table 1) ($p < 0.01$ compared to the controls), indicating a radiosensitization potential for targeting miR-221/-222. Collectively, these observations provide strong evidence for the role of miR-221/-222 in regulation of radiosensitivity.

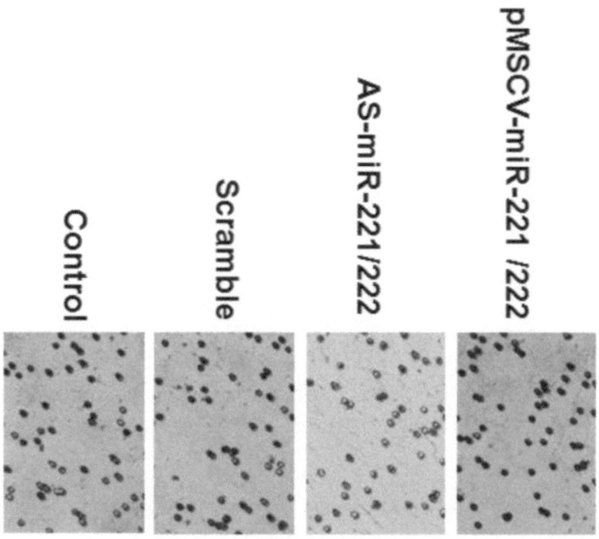

Fig. 7. The transwell assay revealed that knockdown of miR-221/222 significantly decreased cell invasion potential compared with cells treated with scrambled oligonucleotide, whereas over-expression of miR-221/222 increased cell invasion

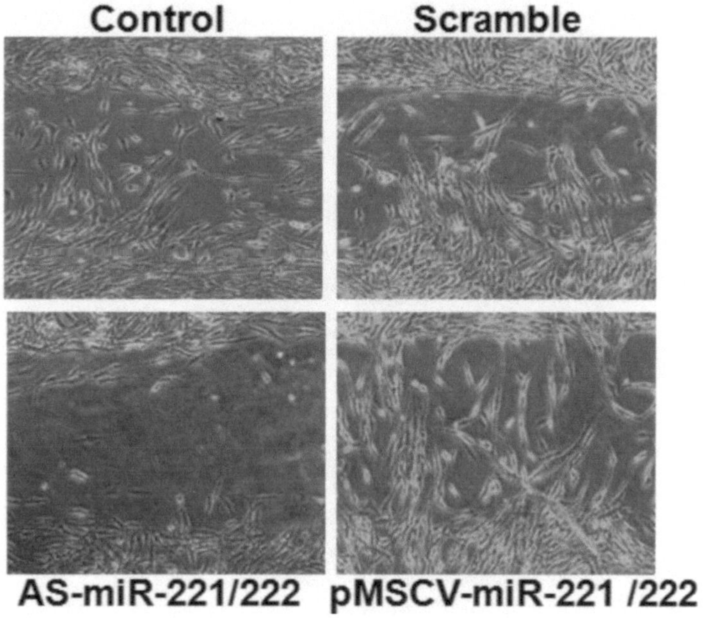

Fig. 8. The wound healing assay, repression of miR-221/222 significantly inhibited cell migration, while over-expression of miR-221/222 increased migration in U251 cells

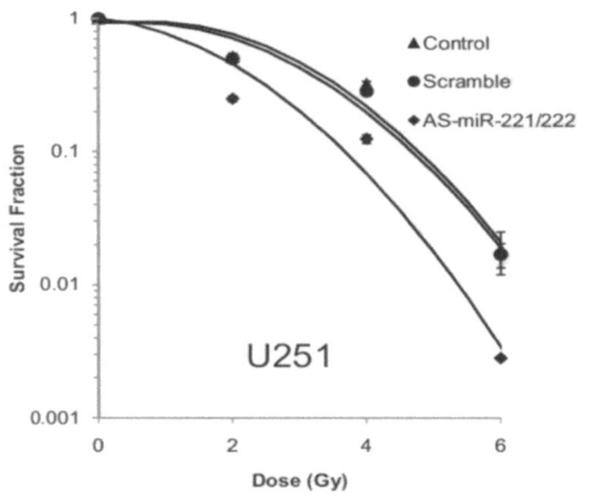

Fig. 9. miR-221/-222 knockdown leads to an increase of radiosensitivity. U251 cells stably transfected with control, AS-miR-221/-222, or scrambled ODN were exposed to 0 to 6 Gy IR and incubated for 2 weeks prior to fixation, staining, and assessment of colony formation. The clonogenic survival assays were performed in triplicate. Standard errors of the mean are shown by error bars.

Cell	Group	D_0	SF2	SER10
U251	Control	2.8827	0.51	1
	Scramble	2.649	0.49	1.0731
	AS-miR-221/-222	1.3656*	0.25*	1.9705*

Abbreviations: D0 = dose to reduce survival to 37% of its value; SF2 = surviving fraction at 2 Gy; SER10 = sensitizer enhancement ratio at 10% survival.* p<0.01.

Table 1. Radiosensitizing effects of respective cell lines

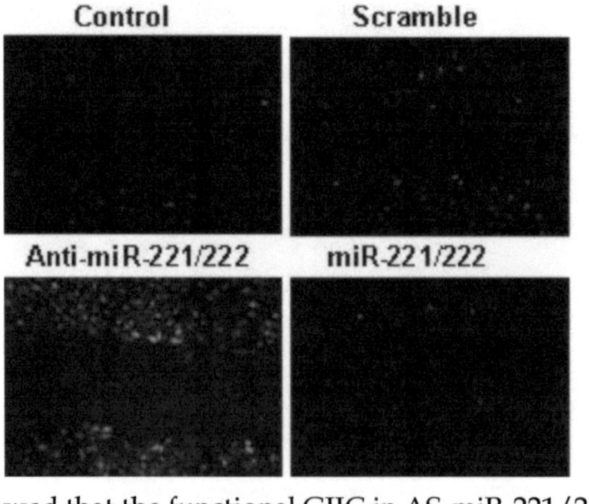

Fig. 10. SLDT assay showed that the functional GJIC in AS-miR-221/222 treated U251 cells were re-established, lucifer yellow was transferred to multiple rows of cells nearby the scrape border.

In addition, by Scrape loading and dye transfer (SLDT) assay, we found that miR-221 and miR-222 also regulated gap junction intercellular communication (GJIC) of glioma cell.

2.3 miR-221 and miR-222 cluster promote glioma growth in vivo

In vitro, miR-221/222 modulated glioma cell growth by regulating cell cycle, apoptosis, and invasion, and so on. Whether these results are right or not in vivo. Ciafre et al firstly proved that the anti-miR-221/222 antagomir treatment of established subcutaneous tumors derived from the highly aggressive PC3 cell line, naturally expressing high levels of miR-221/222, reduces tumor growth by increasing intratumoral p27 amount; this effect is long lasting, as it is detectable as long as 25 days after the treatment(26). We used 5-week-old female immune-deficient nude mice (BALB/C-nu) to perform related experiment. It were housed in microisolator individually ventilated cages with water and food. All experimental procedures were carried out according to the regulations and internal biosafety and bioethics guidelines of Tianjin Medical University and the Tianjin Municipal Science and Technology Commission. U251 glioma subcutaneous model was established as previously described (27). When the volumer of the subcutaneous tumor reached 50 mm^3, the mice were randomly divided into four groups (ten mice/group). A mixture of 5 µl oligonucleotides containing Scr, AS-miR-221, AS-miR-222 or equal mount of AS-miR-221/222 cluster and 10 µl Lipofectamine was injected into the xenograft tumor model using a multi-site injection manner. Mice in U251 control group received 10 µl of PBS only. Treatment was conducted one time every three days and five times in all (Please confirm if it is correct). The tumor volume was measured with a caliper every two days, using the formula volume = length × $width^2/2$.

Fluorescence in situ hybridization proved that As-miR-221 and As-miR-222 efficiently and specifically silenced endogenous miR-221 and miR-222, respectively, in xenograft tumor in vivo (Figure 11).Moveover, we have found that transfection of U251 cells with As-miR-221/222 mediated significant inhibition of tumor growth in a xenograft tumor mouse model (Figure 12). Tumor pathological examination of xenograft tumors demonstrated that, in control and scramble group, more neonatal micro-vessels, bigger tumor cell nucleus, deeper blue staining chromosome, more mitotic tumor cells and lesser necrosis focuses were

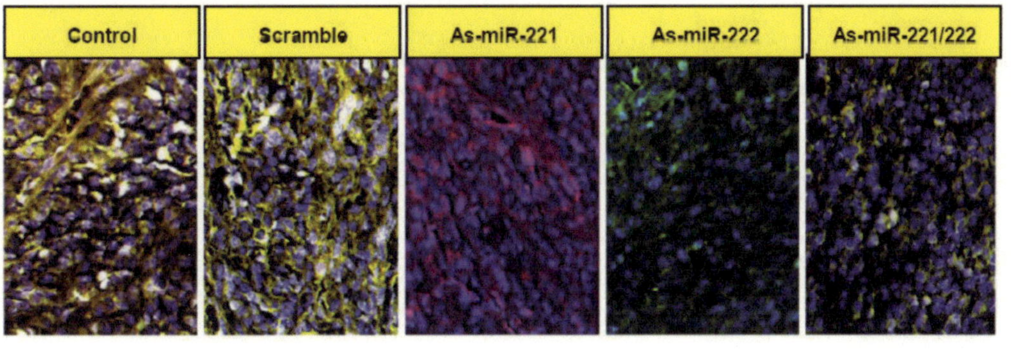

Fig. 11. Tumor pathological section of xenograft tumors show that miR-221 and miR-222 expression were knocked down by As-miR-221/222 in vivo by fluorescence in situ hybridization .

observed than in As-miR-221/222 treatment group (Figure13). All these morphological changes among the three different treated groups indicate that the xenograft tumor without effective As-miR-221/222 therapy can perform relative more malignant pathological manifestation. TUNEL assay analysis of xenograft tumor taken at 28 days after treatment revealed much more apoptosis in As-miR221/222 group when compared to tumors from scramble and control groups (Figure14). Also, the As-miR-221/222 treated tumors had a lower level of Ki-67 expression compared to the other four groups group. Tumor immunochemistry examination of xenograft tumors demonstrated that some protein expression level in As-miR-221/222 group was up-regulated significantly than the other four groups, such as p27, puma, PTEN, TIMP3, and so on. Some protein expression levels in As-miR-221/222 group was down-regulated significantly than the other four groups, such as CyclinD, MMP2, MMP9, pAkt, and so on (Figure 15).

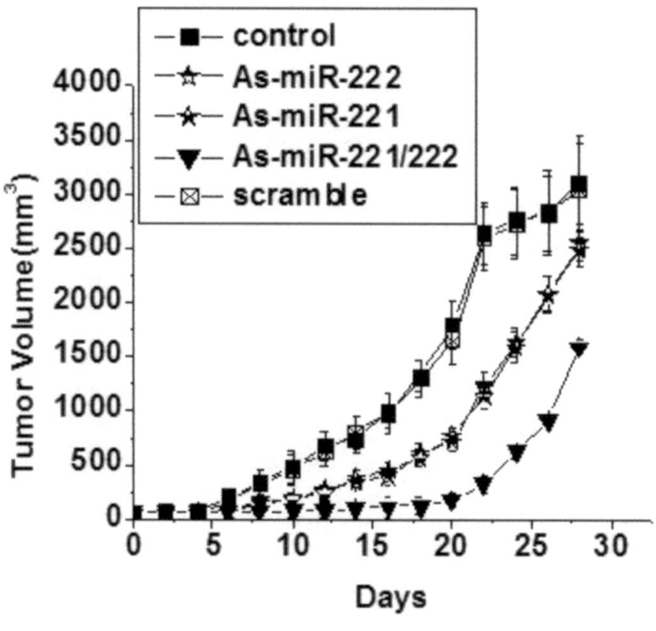

Fig. 12. Transfection of U251 cells with As-miR-221/222 mediated significant inhibition of tumor growth in a xenograft tumor mouse model.

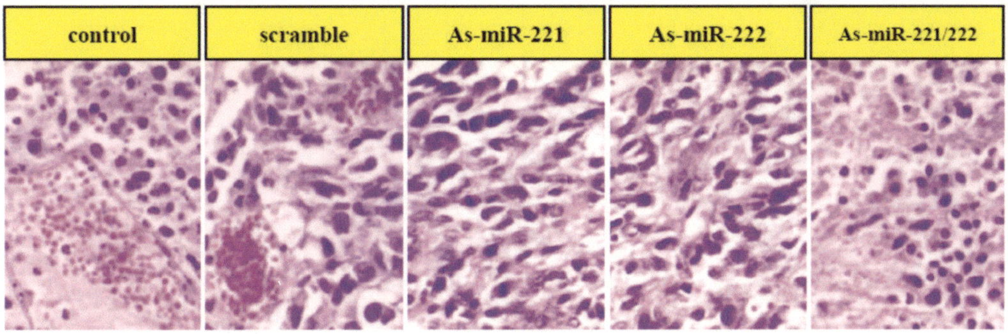

Fig. 13. Tumor pathological examination of xenograft tumors demonstrated that, in control and scramble group, more neonatal micro-vessels, bigger tumor cell nucleus, deeper blue staining chromosome, more mitotic tumor cells and lesser necrosis focuses were observed than in As-miR-221/222 treatment group.

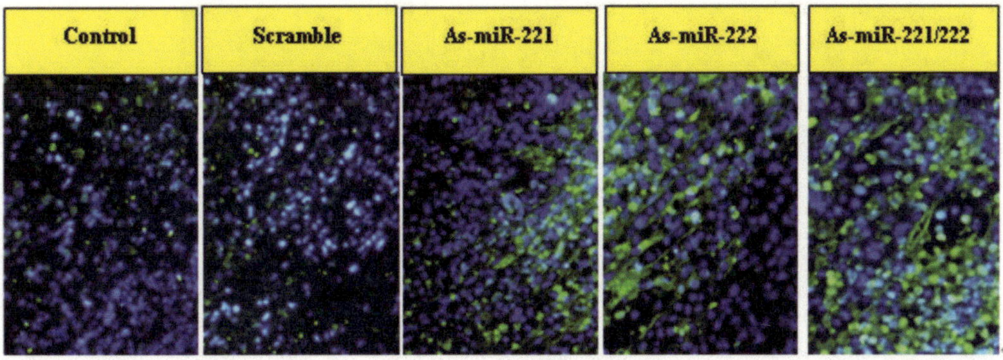

Fig. 14. TUNEL assay revealed much more apoptosis in As-miR221/222 group when compared to tumors from scramble and control groups.

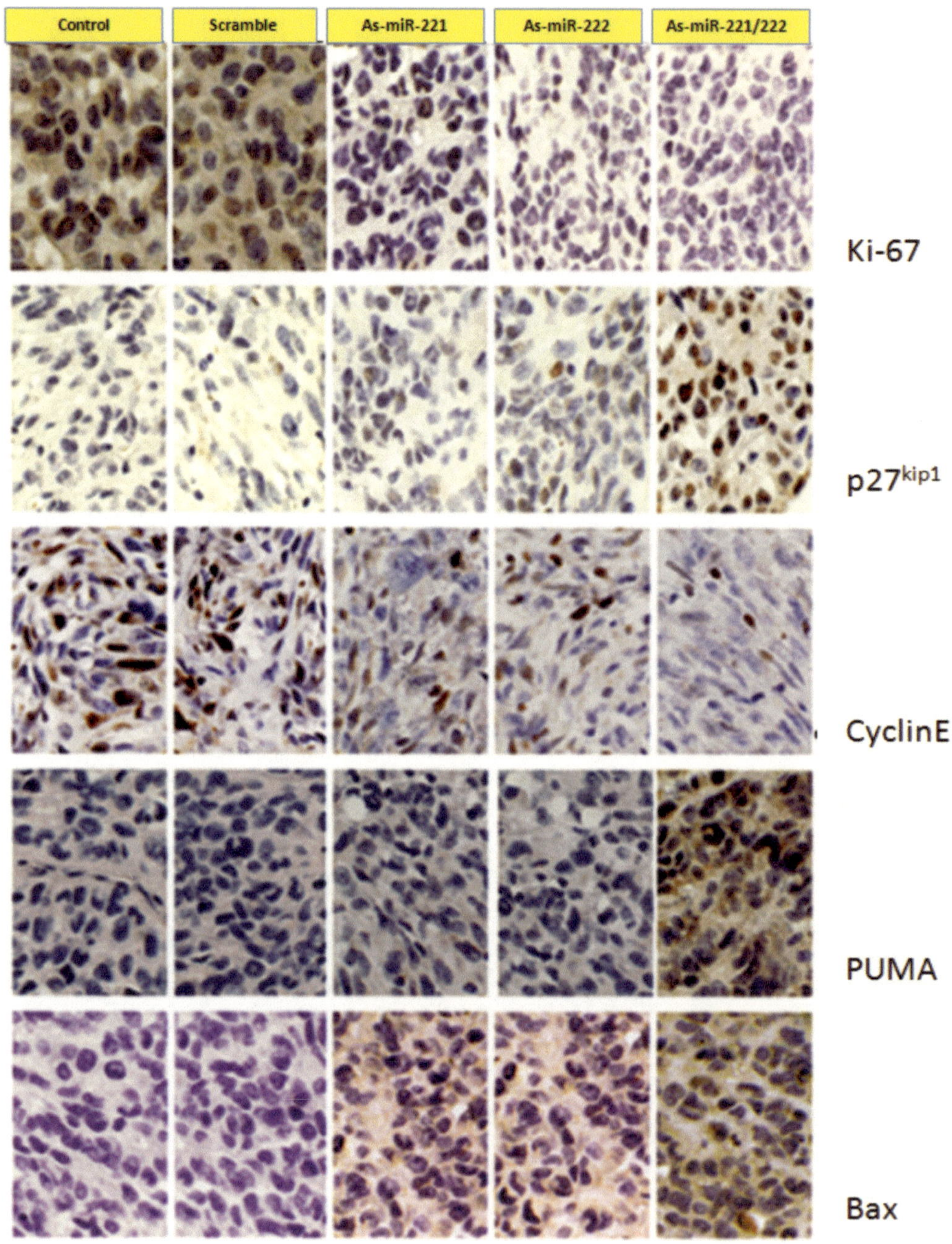
Control
Scramble
As-miR-221
As-miR-222
As-miR-221/222
Ki-67
p27kip1
CyclinE
PUMA
Bax

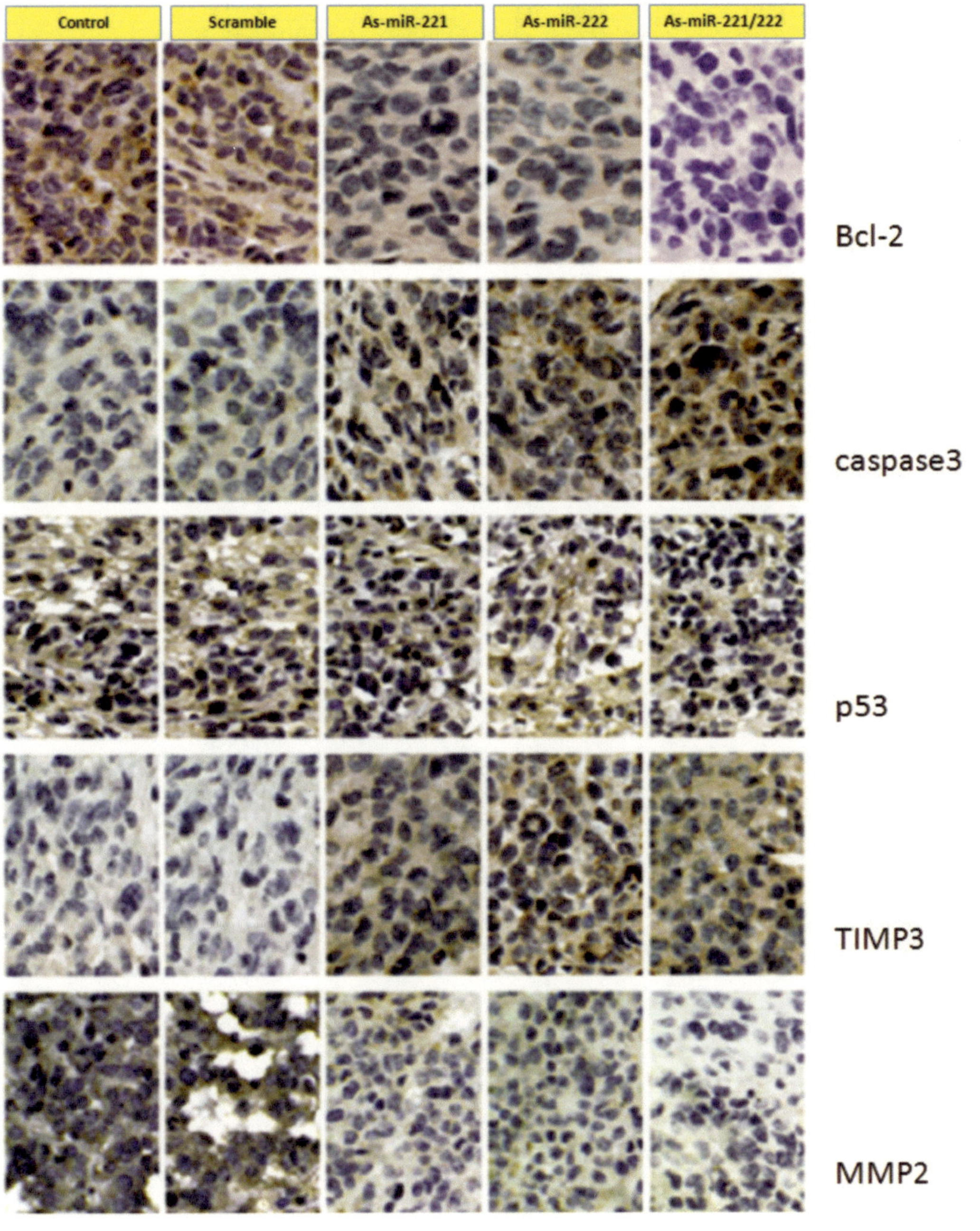
Control
Scramble
As-miR-221
As-miR-222
As-miR-221/222
Bcl-2
caspase3
p53
TIMP3
MMP2

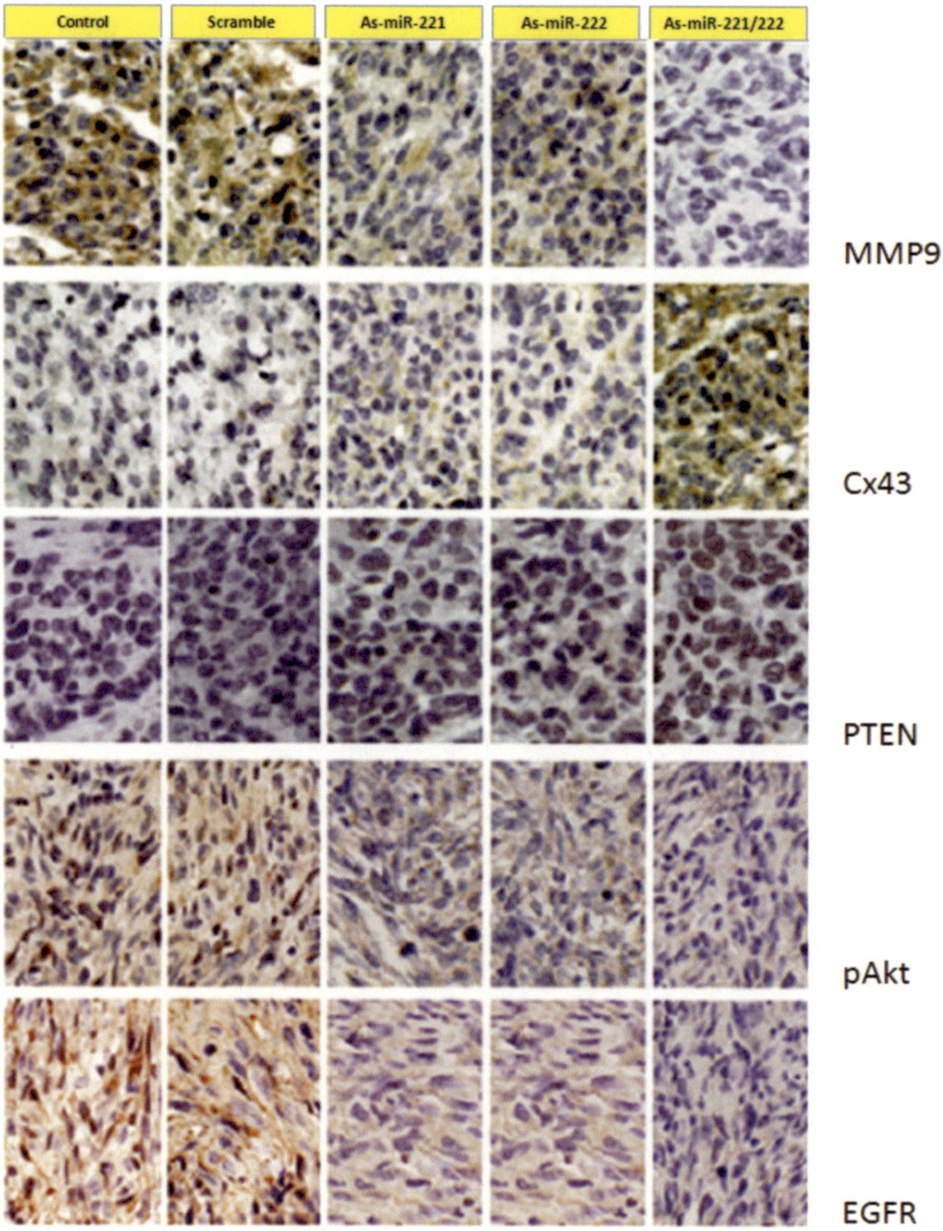

Fig. 15. Tumor immunochemistry examination of xenograft tumors demonstrated that some protein expression level in As-miR-221/222 group was up-regulated significantly than the other four groups and the other proteins expression level in As-miR-221/222 group was down-regulated.

2.4 The mechanism on miR-221 and miR-222 cluster modulate glioma cell malignant phenotype

MiRs repress protein expression at the posttranscriptional level through imperfect base pairing with 3`untranslated region of the target mRNA in mammalian cells, leading to its reduced translation in order to affect cell function. That is, function of miRs depend on function of it target. So, it is necessary to identify targets of miRs. Bioinformatic analysis is the most effective approach to study miRNAs. We search some target by miRs target database, such as PicTar, TargetScan, and so on. Then, by luciferase assay, these targets were identified. As for miR-221 and miR-222, we proved that p27, PUMA, PTEN, TIMP3 and Cx43 were some targets of miR-221 and miR-222 in glioma.

2.4.1 p27^{Kip1}

The p27^{Kip1} gene is a member of the cip/kip family of cyclin-dependent kinase (CDK) inhibitors that negatively control the cell cycle progression. The p27^{Kip1} binds to CDK2 and cyclin E complexes to prevent cell cycle progression from G1 to S phase (28,29). The p27^{Kip1} does not follow Knudson's classic ‘two-hit hypothesis’ of tumor suppression. The inactivation of p27^{Kip1} is not caused by direct mutations in the gene encoding p27Kip1. The homozygous loss or silencing of the locus in human tumors is extremely rare (30). A recent study demonstrated that the miR-221/222 cluster is an endogenous regulator of p27^{Kip1}, confirming the miRNA modulation may play a key role in the inactivation of p27^{Kip1} (31-34). However, that the miR-221/222 cluster affects tumor cell proliferation by regulating p27^{Kip1} in vivo has not been well documented.

2.4.2 PUMA

Puma was originally identified during large-scale analysis for novel p53-inducible genes and Bcl-2-interacting proteins. Puma is an extremely potent BH3-only protein, having the capacity to bind with high affinity to all known anti-apoptotic Bcl-2 proteins. In addition, Puma may also directly interact with and activate Bax/Bak, for example, through an interaction with the first α-helix of Bax. In keeping with its highly pro-apoptotic nature, Puma has been shown to have an essential role in the induction of apoptosis in numerous in vitro and in vivo systems and cell types including neurons, lymphocytes, thymocytes, fibroblasts and cardiomyocytes. Puma expression is regulated by transcription, and factors regulating Puma ranscription include p53, p73, E2F and FOXO3a (24,35).

2.4.3 PTEN

The PTEN (phosphatase and tensin homology) gene, located at 10q23.3, encodes a central domain with homology to the catalytic region of protein tyrosine phosphatases. It is important in the function of protein phosphatases and 3′ -phosphoinositol phosphatase acivities. It dephosphorylates phosphatidylinositol-3,4,5-triphosphate(PIP3), the second messenger produced by PI3K. In do so, PTEN negatively regulates the activity of the serine/threonine protein kinase, AKt(36-37). PTEN is inactivated in some malignant tumors, including glioblastoma 、 prostate cancer、 melanoma、 endometrial carcinoma and lung carcinoma. To restore PTEN expression become an approach which enhances cancer radiosensitivity instead of suppressing Akt activity in PTEN-deficient tumor cells(38).

2.4.4 TIMP3

Malignant glioma cells express certain known proteinases such as matrix metalloproteinases (MMPs), which have been implicated as important factors in regulating cell invasiveness in gliomas(39). MMPs are a family of at least 20 zinc-dependent endopeptidases collectively capable of degrading essentially all extracellular matrix(ECM) components, including collagents, fibronectin, laminin and basement membrance proteoglycans (40). Among the MMPs, attention has focused on gelatinases(MMP-2 and MMP-9) in human gliomas. A high level of MMP-2 expression was observed in the higher-grade gliomas, which correlated well with the malignant potential of human gliomas (41). A major mechanism for controlling MMPs activity in the pericellular space is mediated by the action of tissue inhibitors of metalloproteinases (TIMPs), which bind to active MMPs in a 1:1 molar stoichiometry (42). There are four family member, including TIMP-1, TIMP-2, TIMP-3, TIMP-4 (43). TIMP-3 is unique within the TIMP family as it remains closely associated to the extracellular matrix after being secreted by the cell (40, 44). In human gliomas, TIMP expression is reported to be down-regulated with increasing malignancy, including TIMP-3 (44).

2.4.5 Cx43

Cx genes have been demonstrated as tumor suppressor genes. Up to date, twenty members of Cx genes have been identified in mammalian tissues and they are expressed in tissue specific manner. Cx43 is the predominant form of Cxs expressed in astrocytes and also the constituent of connexons which compose the gap junction intercellular communication(GJIC) in brain (45, 46). Our previous study and other studies showed that Cx 43 expression was inversely correlated with the degree of malignancy of astrocytomas (47). In most malignant gliomas, Cx43 expression was reduced or deleted and GJIC was deficient (47).

In addition these target above, c-kit, p57, ERα,Bmf are also is some target of miR-221 and miR-222, but they are not proved in glioma until now (48-51).

2.5 Inter-relationship between miR-221 and miR-222 expression and global mRNA expression

Studies above have identified some targets of miR-221 and miR-222, such as p27, p57, and so on. Inter-relationship between miR-221 and miR-222 expression and global mRNA expression remains important as well. Here we knocked down miR-221 and miR-222 expression and found 158 differentially expressed genes with 2-fold changes in U251 glioma cells by microarray analysis. Using the KEGG pathway databases and BioCarta, we found that the IFN-α signaling pathway was the most significant pathway modulated by differentially expressed genes. STAT1 and STAT2 are core proteins in the IFN-α signaling pathway. By Western blotting and immunofluorescence, we found that STAT1 and STAT2 expression and phosphorylation were upregulated in U251 cells with knocked-down miR-221/222. Furthermore, tyrosine phosphorylation of STAT1 and STAT2 was present in the nucleus after repression of miR-221/222 expression in U251 cells. These data indicate for the first time a mechanism involving STAT1/2 upregulation under the transcriptional control of INF-αsignaling after knockdown of miR-221/222 cluster in U251 glioma cells.

2.6 Transcription factor modulate miR-221 and miR-222 expression

MiRNAs finely modulate virtually all physiological pathways in metazoans, and are deeply implicated in all main pathologies by regulating their taregets. But who regulate them expression. Ciafrè et al report that the ectopic modulation of NF-kB modifies miR-221/222 expression in prostate carcinoma and glioblastoma cell lines, where we had previously shown their oncogenic activity. We identify two separate distal regions upstream of miR-221/222 promoter which are bound by the NF-kB subunit p65 and drive efficient transcription in luciferase reporter assays; consistently, the site-directed mutagenesis disrupting p65 binding sites or the ectopical inhibition of NF-kB activity significantly reduce luciferase activity. In the most distal enhancer region, we also define a binding site for c-Jun, and we show that the binding of this factor cooperates with that of p65, fully accounting for the observed upregulation of miR-221/222. Thus, our work uncovers an additional mechanism through which NF-kB and c-Jun, two transcription factors deeply involved in cancer onset and progression, contribute to oncogenesis, by inducing miR-221/222 transcription (52).Moreover, Garofalo et al also identified that c-jun regulated miR-221 and miR-222 expression level.

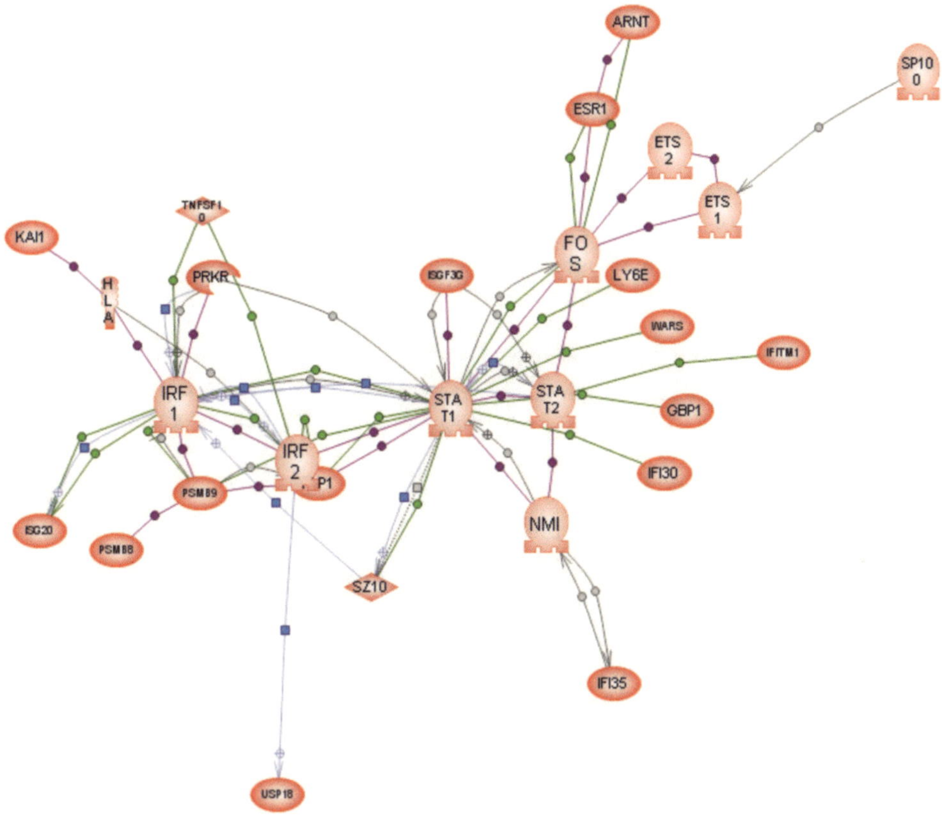

Fig. 16. Constructed network of miR-221/222-TFs-STAT1/2-gene expression. Genes involved in TF-gene expression in glioma U251 cells after repression of the miR-221/222 cluster, determining the cell death or survival through the INF- α pathway. Genes associated with eight TFs (FOS, ESR1,ETS2, IRF2, ARNT, ETS1, HOXC1, FOXN2) were manually identified via literature mining. IRF-1, STAT1 and STAT2 regulate the balance between miR-221/222-TFs and TF-gene expression, determining the cell death or survival through the INF-α pathway in glioma U251 cells. The INF- α pathway regulates cell survival negatively, via processes occurring in multiple intracellular compartments. Regulatory relationships are denoted by line colors, including the 28 genes and 64 verified modulation nodes.

3. Conclusion

In summary, We first identified that miR-221 and miR-222 play an role in malignant phenotype of glioma by increasing or knocking down miR-221 and miR-222. It was found that miR-221/222 increased cell proliferation, increased S phase proportionality, inhibited cell apoptosis, increased cell invasion and migration, enhanced radioresistance and reduced gap junction intercellular communication (GJIC) in glioma U251 cell. Furthermore, knockeddown miR-221/222 considerably decreases tumor growth in U251 cell xenograft model. Then, we identified that p27kip1, PUMA, PTEN, TIMP3 and Cx43 are some targets of miR-221 and miR-222. We also found that knocked down miR-221/222 changed some proteins expression. Taken together, our studies provide evidence that miR-221/222 regulate its target genes and its related transduction signal way to promote the growth of malignant glioma cells. So, we thought that miR-221 and miR-222 may serve as a novel therapeutic target for malignant gliomas.

4. Acknowledgment

Supported by China National Natural Scientific Found (30772231, 30901772), Tianjin Science and Technology Committee (07ZCGHHZ01000), and Program for New Century Excellent Talents in University (NCET-07-0615). The authors wish to thank Dr. R. Agami, Division of Tumor Biology, The Netherlands Cancer Institute, Amsterdam, Netherlands, for kindly providing the constructs of pGL3-p27-3'UTR and pGL3-p27-3'UTR-DM; and Dr. J.Q. Cheng, Molecular Oncology, H. Lee Moffitt Cancer Center, Tampa, USA, for kindly providing the protocol of miRNA Northern blotting. PH.D. Xu B, Department of Radiation Oncology, The Methodist Hospital Research Institute, Houston, TX, USA, for help in studying glioma cell radiosensitivity.

5. References

[1] Osada H, Takahashi T. MicroRNAs in biological processes and carcinogenesis. Carcinogenesis 2007,28:2-12.
[2] Zhang BH, Pan XP, Cobb GP, Anderson TA. MicroRNA as oncogenes and tumor suppressors. Developmental Biology. 2007,302:1-12.
[3] Dalmay T, Edwards DR. MicroRNAs and the hallmarks of cancer. Oncogene. 2006,25:6170-6175.
[4] Chen CZ. MicroRNAs as Oncogenes and Tumor Suppressors. New England Med, 2005, 353:1768-1771.
[5] George A .Calin, Carlo M.Croce, MicroRNA signatures in human cancers, Nature Reviews Cancer 6(2006)857-866.
[6] Metzler M, Wilda M, Busch K, Viehmann S, Borkhardt A, High expression of precursor microRNA-155/BIC RNA in children with Burkitt lymphoma, Genes Chromosomes Cancer 39(2004)167-169
[7] Michael MZ, O' Connor SM, van Holst Pellekaan NG, Young GP, James RJ, Reduced accumulation of specific microRNAs in colorectal neoplasia, Mol Cancer Res 1(2003) 882- 891.

[8] Takamizawa J, Konishi H, Yanagisawa K, Tomida S, Osada H, Endoh H, Harano T,Yatabe Y, Nagino M, Nimura Y, Mitsudomi T, Takahashi T, Reduced expression of the let-7 microRNAs in human lung cancers in association with shortened postoperative survival, Cancer Res 64(2004) 3753-3756.

[9] Iorio MV, Ferracin M, Liu CG, Veronese A, Spizzo R, Sabbioni S, Magri E,Pedriali M, Fabbri M, Campiglio M, Ménard S, Palazzo JP, Rosenberg A, Musiani P, Volinia S, Nenci I, Calin GA, Querzoli P, Negrini M, Croce CM, MicroRNA gene expression deregulation in human breast cancer, Cancer Res 65(2005)7065-7070.

[10] He H, Jazdzewski K, Li W, Liyanarachchi S, Nagy R, Volinia S, Calin GA, Liu CG, Franssila K, Suster S, Kloos RT, Croce CM, de la Chapelle A, The role of microRNA genes in papillary thyroid carcinoma, Proc Natl Acad Sci U S A 102(2005)19075-19080

[11] Murakami Y, Yasuda T, Saigo K, Urashima T, Toyoda H, Okanoue T, Shimotohno K, Comprehensive analysis of microRNA expression patterns in hepatocellular carcinoma and non-tumorous tissues, Oncogene 25(2006)2537-2545.

[12] Chan JA, Krichevsky AM, Kosik KS, MicroRNA-21 is an antiapoptotic factor in human glioblastoma cells, Cancer Res 65(2005)6029-6033.

[13] Ciafrè SA, Galardi S, Mangiola A, Ferracin M, Liu CG, Sabatino G, Negrini M,Maira G, Croce CM, Farace MG, Extensive modulation of a set of microRNAs in primary glioblastoma, Biochem Biophys Res Commun 334(2005)1351-1358.

[14] Zhang lilei, Wang tao, Wright AF, et al. A microdeletion in Xp11.3 accounts for co-segregation of retinitis pigmentosa and mental retardation in a large kindred. American Journal of Medical Genetics.2006,140A:349-357.

[15] Branislav Kusenda, Marek Mraz, Jiri Mayer, et al. MicroRNA biogenesis, functionality and cancer relevance. Biomed Pap Med Fac Univ Palacky Olomouc Czech Repub. 2006, 150:205-215.

[16] Mishima T, Mizuguchi Y, Kawahigashi Y, et al. RT-PCR-based analysis of microRNA (miR-1 and -124) expression in mouse CNS. Brain Res, 2007,1131:37-43.

[17] Berezikov E, Thuemmler F, Van Laake LW, et al. Diversity of microRNAs in human and chimpanzee brain. Nat Genet,2006 ,38:1375-1377.

[18] le Sage C, Nagel R, Egan DA, Schrier M, Mesman E, Mangiola A, Anile C, Maira G, Mercatelli N, Ciafrè SA, Farace MG, Agami R, Regulation of the p27(Kip1) tumor suppressor by miR 221 and miR 222 promotes cancer cell proliferation, EMBO J 26(2007)3699-3708.

[19] Frenquelli M, Muzio M, Scielzo C, Fazi C, Scarfo` L, Rossi L, Ferrari G, Ghia P, Caligaris-Cappio F. MicroRNA and proliferation control in chronic lymphocytic leukemia: functional relationship between miR-221/222 cluster and p27. Blood.2010, 115: 3949-3959.

[20] Galardi S, Mercatelli N, Giorda E, Massalini S, Frajese GV, Ciafrè SA, Farace MG, miR-221 and miR-222 expression affects the proliferation potential of human prostate carcinoma cell lines by targeting p27Kip1, J Biol Chem 282(2007)23716-23724.

[21] Visone R, Russo L, Pallante P, Martino ID, Ferraro A, Leone V, Borbone E, Petrocca F,Alder H, Croce2 CM, Fusco A. MicroRNAs (miR)-221 and miR-222, both overexpressed in human thyroid papillarycarcinomas, regulate p27Kip1 protein levels and cell cycle. Endocrine-Related Cancer.2007,14:791–798.

[22] Sun K, Wang W, Zeng J, Wu C, Lei S, Li G. MicroRNA-221 inhibits CDKN1C/p57 expression in human colorectal carcinoma. Acta Pharmacologica Sinica (2011) 32: 375–384.

[23] Yee KS, Wilkinson S, James J, Ryan KM, Vousden KH: PUMA- and Baxinduced autophagy contributes to apoptosis. Cell Death Differ. 2009,16:1135-1145.

[24] Zhang C, Zhang J, Zhang A, Han L, Jia Z, Yang W, Wang G, You Y, Pu P, Cheng J, Kang C. MiR-221 and miR-222 target PUMA to induce Cell suvivalI in glioblastoma. Molecular Cancer. 2010,9:229.

[25] Garofalo M, Leva GD, Romano G, Nuovo G, Suh SS, Ngankeu A, Taccioli C, Pichiorri F, Alder H, Secchiero P, Gasparini P, Gonelli A, Costinean S, Acunzo M, Condorelli G, Croce CM. MiR-221&222 regulate TRAIL-resistance and enhance tumorigenicity through PTEN and TIMP3 down-regulation. Cancer Cell. 2009 , 16: 498–509.

[26] Mercatelli N, Coppola V, Bonci D, Miele F, Costantini A, Guadagnoli M, Bonanno E, Muto G, Frajese GV, Maria RD, Spagnoli LG, Farace MG, Ciafre SA. The Inhibition of the Highly Expressed Mir-221 and Mir-222 Impairs the Growth of Prostate Carcinoma Xenografts in Mice. PLoS one. 2008,3: e4029.

[27] Kang CS, Zhang ZY, Jia ZF, Wang GX, Qiu MZ, Zhou HX, Yu SZ, Chang J, Jiang H, Pu PY. Suppression of EGFR expression by antisense or small interference RNA inhibits U251 glioma cell growth in vitro and in vivo, Cancer Gene Ther.2006, 13:530-538.

[28] Blain SW, Scher HI, Cordon-Cardo C and Koff A. p27 as a target for cancer therapeutics. Cancer Cell.2003,3: 111-115.

[29] Chu IM, Hengst L and Slingerland JM. The Cdk inhibitor p27 in human cancer: prognostic potential andrelevance to anticancer therapy. Nat Rev. 2008, 8: 253-267.

[30] Philipp-Staheli J, Payne SR and Kemp CJ. p27Kip1: regulation and function of a haploin-sufficient tumor suppressor and its misregulation in cancer. Exp Cell Res.2001,264: 148-168.

[31] Le Sage C, Nagel R, Egan DA, Schrier M, Mesman E, Mangiola A, Anile C, Maira G, Mercatelli N, Ciafre SA, Farace MG and Agami R. Regulation of the p27 (Kip1) tumor suppressor by miR-221 and miR-222 promotes cancer cell proliferation. EMBO J.2007,26: 3699-3708.

[32] Galardi S, Mercatelli N, Giorda E, Massalini S, Frajese GV, Ciafre SA and Farace MG. miR-221 and miR-222 expression affects the proliferation potential of human prostate carcinoma cell lines by targeting p27Kip1. J Biol Chem.2007,282: 23716-23724.

[33] Garofalo M, Quintavalle C, Di Leva G, Zanca C, Romano G, Taccioli C, Liu CG, Croce CM and Condorelli G. MicroRNA signatures of TRAIL resistance in human non-small cell lung cancer. Oncogene . 2008 , 27:3845-3855.

[34] Chunzhi Zhang, Chunsheng Kang, Yongping You , Peiyu Pu, Weidong Yang, Peng Zhao, Guangxiu Wang, Anling Zhang, Zhifan Jia, Lei Han, Hao Jiang. Co-suppression of miR-221/222 cluster suppresses human glioma cells growth by targeting p27kip1 in vitro and in vivo. International Journal of Oncology. 2009, 34:1653-1660.

[35] Fricker M, O'Prey J, Tolkovsky AM and Ryan KM. Phosphorylation of Puma modulates its apoptotic function by regulating protein stability. Cell Death and Disease.2010, 1: e59

[36] Sun YL, LK.St.Clair D, Fang F, Warren GW, Rangnekar VM, Crooks PA, St.Clair WH. The radiosensitization effect of parthenolide in prostate cancer cells is mediated by nuclear factor-κB inhibition and enhanced by the presence of PTEN. Mol Cancer Ther. 2007,6:2477-2486.

[37] Jiang ZB, Pore N, Cerniglia GJ, Mick R, Georgescu MM, Bernhard EJ, Hahn SM, Gupta AK, Maity A. Phosphatase and tensin homologye deficiency in glioblastoma confers resistance to radiation and temozolomide that is reversed by the protease inhibitor nelfinavir. Cancer Res.2007,67:4467-4473.

[38] Pappas G, Zumstrin LA, Munshi A, Hobbs M, Meyn RE. Adenoviral-mediated PTEN expression radiosensitizes non-small cell lung cancer cells by suppressing DNA repair capacity. Cancer Gene Therapy.2007,14:543-549.

[39] Hsun-Jin Jan, Chin-Cheng Lee, Yung-Luen Shih, Dueng-Yuan Hueng, Hsin-I Ma, Jing-Huei Lai, Hen-Wei Wei and Horng-Mo Lee. Osteopontin regulates human glioma cell invasiveness and tumor growth in mice. Neuro-Oncology.2010,12:58-70.

[40] Paula Lam, Kar Sian Lim, Suk Mei Wang, Kam M.Hui. A mictoarry study to charaterize the molecular mechanism to TIMP-3-mediated tumor rejection. Molecular Therapy. 2005,12:144-152.

[41] Levicar N, Nuttall RK, Lah TT. Proteases in brain tumor progression. Acta Neurochir(Wien). 2003,145:825-838.

[42] Jiang Y, Goldberg I.D, Shi Y.E. Complex role of tissue inhibitor of metalloproteinases in cancer. Oncogene.2002,21:2245-2252.

[43] Brew.K, Dinakarpandian.D, Nagase.H. Tissue inhibitors of metalloproteinase: evolution, structure and function. Biochim. Biophys. Acta.2000,1477:267-283.

[44] Martine LM, Gianni D, Tung CH, Idema S, Schagen HE, Carette JE, Quax HA, Beusechem WV, Vandertop WP, Dirven MF, Chiocca EA, Gerritsen WR. Tissue inhibitor of metalloproteinase-3 expression from an oncolytic adenovirus inhibits matrix metalloproteinase activity in vivo without affecting antitumoral efficacy in malignant glioma. Cancer Res.2005,65:9398-9405.

[45] Yamasaki, H, Naus, CC. Role of connexin genes in growth control. Carcinogenesis 1996, 17: 1199–1213.

[46] Medina R, Zaidi SK, Liu CG, Stein JL, van Wijnen AJ, Croce CM, Stein GS. MicroRNAs 221 and 222 bypass quiescence and compromise cell survival. Cancer Res. 2008, 68: 2773-2780.

[47] Pu PY, Xia ZB, Yu SZ, Huang Q. Altered expression of Cx43 in astrocytic tumors. Clin Neurol Neurosurg 2004, 107: 49-54.

[48] Mayoral RJ, Monticelli S. Stable overexpression of miRNAs in bone marrow-derived murine mast cells using lentiviral expression vectors. Methods Mol Biol. 2010;667:205-14.

[49] Fornari F, Gramantieri L, Ferracin M, Veronese A, Sabbioni S, Calin GA, Grazi GL, Giovannini C, Croce CM, Bolondi L, Negrini M. MiR-221 controls CDKN1C/p57 and CDKN1B/p27 expression in human hepatocellular carcinoma. Oncogene. 2008 , 27:5651-5661.

[50] Zhao JJ, Lin J, Yang H, Kong W, He L, Ma X, Coppola D, Cheng JQ. MicroRNA-221/222 negatively regulates estrogen receptor alpha and is associated with tamoxifen resistance in breast cancer.J Biol Chem. 2008 ,283:31079-1086.

[51] Gramantieri L, Fornari F, Ferracin M, Veronese A, Sabbioni S, Calin GA, Grazi GL, Croce CM, Bolondi L, Negrini M.MicroRNA-221 targets Bmf in hepatocellular carcinoma and correlates with tumor multifocality. Clin Cancer Res. 2009 Aug 15;15(16):5073-81.

[52] Galardi S, Mercatelli N, Farace MG, Ciafrè SA. NF-kB and c-Jun induce the expression of the oncogenic miR-221 and miR-222 in prostate carcinoma and glioblastoma cells. Nucleic Acids Research, 2011, doi:10.1093/nar/gkr006

Part 11

EGFR /EGFRvIII Amplification - Glioblastoma

23

Primary Glioblastoma with Different Patterns of *EGFR* Amplification and the Relationship with Gene Expression Profile

Concha Lopez-Gines, Rosario Gil-Benso, Daniel Monleon, Jose Gonzalez-Darder and Miguel Cerda-Nicolas
Department of Pathology, University of Valencia. Fundación HCU, Labim, Department of Neurosurgery. Hospital Clínico Universitario, Spain

1. Introduction

Glioblastoma multiforme (GBM) is the most common intracranial tumor and the most aggressive of all gliomas. These tumors are very heterogeneous both histopathological and genetic. There is no consistent theory today that can explain the etiology of glioblastoma. A number of factors, both environmental and genetic, have been suggested as potential causes of the tumor. It is possibly a combination of both which initiates and triggers the pathogenesis of tumor and the sequence of genetic alterations that lead to the genesis of neoplasia. They represent 60% of all astrocytic tumors and between 12-15% of all intracranial tumors. Three new patients per 100,000 people are diagnosed every year.

Among its clinical features, age is particularly important for their development and survival. Although the tumor may arise at any age, most cases occur in adults (45-75 years). The average onset is between 53 and 62 years depending on the series (Kleihues et al., 2002, Ohgaki et al., 2004). The presence of tumor is much less frequent at earlier ages. Only 22% of cases involved patients younger than 45 years. It has been reported that cases between 0 and 20 years old only represent 3-8% of the total (Dohrmann et al., 1976). This frequency of cases in the late adulthood may indicate the need for a relatively important period of time before the accumulation of genetic damage leading to tumor formation. As for the sex of the patients there is a preference for males, about 1.5 men for every woman (Kleihues et al., 2002).

Glioblastoma is an almost exclusively supratentorial tumor, affecting both cerebral hemispheres, with a similar spatial distribution to low-grade astrocytoma and anaplastic astrocytoma, being the most affected regions the frontal, temporal and parietal lobes (Dohrmann and et al., 1976; Russell & Rubinstein, 1989). The symptoms usually develop through a short history and in most cases do not exceed 3 months. The literature reflects that 50% of cases are under the threshold of 3 months (Russell & Rubinstein, 1989). The speed of onset of symptoms can be explained by the rapid growth and by the high invasiveness and infiltration of the tumor.

The three types of treatment (surgery, radiotherapy and chemotherapy) commonly used in the treatment of other malignancies, are also used as therapeutic strategies for glioblastoma.

Metastases are rarely found, probably due to the short survival time of these patients. The removal of a tumor produces large symptomatic relief and a slight increase in survival, but practically no cure. The high infiltration capacity of the tumor and the proximity of functionally important brain regions make surgical resection unable to eliminate all tumor cells, which produce relapses in short periods of time. Radiation therapy has also shown some efficacy in improving survival time. Likewise, chemotherapy strategies active in other tumors, have shown a relative efficacy in glioblastoma (Walker et al.., 1978, Walker et al., 1980, Yung et al., 2000; Balañá et al., 2004).

The biological aggressiveness of glioblastoma multiforme makes the survival of patients short, about a year, this being significantly lower than that observed for grade II and grade III astrocytomas (5 and 3 years respectively) (Jelsma & Bucy, 1969, Sant et al., 1988, Kallio et al., 1991, Ohgaki et al., 2004).

From a histopathological point of view, glioblastoma is considered in the group of astrocytic gliomas and is the most malignant tumor in this group. According to the latest ranking of the World Health Organization (Louis et al., 2007), the tumor is classified as grade IV. It may show up as a lesion with high heterogeneity both intratumoral and intertumoral. This heterogeneity is represented by the variability of cell populations and their degree of differentiation.

Glioblastoma may be the final stage of a progression that can result from less malignant lesions (Scherer, 1940). Low-grade astrocytoma, classified as grade II, is the first step on the scale of malignancy of astrocytomas, which already makes clear the invasive nature of the tumor. This tumor shows a slight increase in cellularity and diffuse compared to normal surrounding tissue. Vascularization in these cases becomes slightly hyperplasic in any of the three variants: fibrillary, protoplasmic and gemistocytic. Microscopically, despite the invasive nature, has low destructive power and distorts little the adjacent brain structures (Russell & Rubinstein, 2006).

Although sharing some common ground with low-grade astrocytoma, anaplastic astrocytoma represents a further step in the progressive increase in cellularity, reflected in the degree of anaplasia, the cellular and nuclear pleomorphism and increased proliferative rates, and already considered as malignant astrocytoma, grade III in the WHO classification (Louis et al., 2007).

Finally, a last step in the malignant progression of the lesion, which reflects the changes with respect anaplastic astrocytoma, is morphologically expressed in a predominance of anaplastic cells and vascular proliferation with vascular hyperplasia and glomerular formations, besides the presence of necrosis

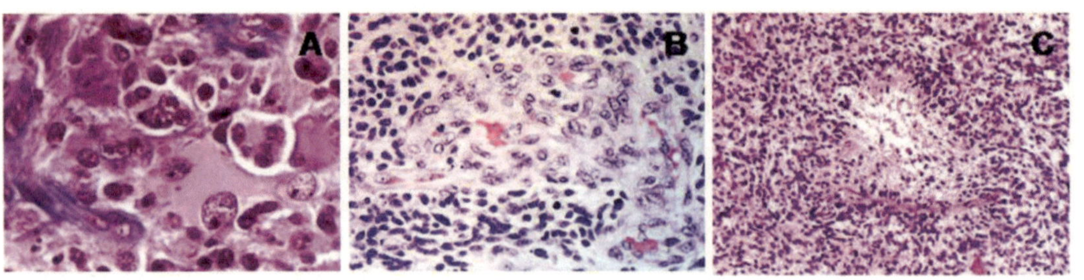

Fig. 1. Histopathological features of glioblastoma with HE techniques. A) Anaplastic histological pattern. B) Pseudoglomerular vascular hyperplasia. C) Pseudoempalizada necrosis

The glioblastoma tumor cells differentially express glial fibrillary acidic protein (GFAP). GFAP is an antigen protein that is present in astroglial cells and is part of the structure of gliofilaments. The intensity and extent of GFAP expression is highly variable (Kleihues and Cavanee, 2000). Tumor cells usually retain some astrocytic differentiation and are strongly positive, especially gemistocytic. Undifferentiated small cells stain more weakly or are clearly negative. Multinucleated giant cells are the most variable in their expression of GFAP. Within a tumor, there may also coexist regions with no GFAP expression. As the tumor progresses, there is a tendency towards the lack of GFAP expression, but this fact is not considered to have prognostic value (Schmitt, 1983).

In these tumors, Ki-67 rates are high ranging between 15-20% (Burger et al., 1986, Karamitopoulou et al., 1994). Both the number of mitosis and the proliferative rates vary depending on the tumor region studied. The spindle-like cells and the undifferentiated small cells seem to show a marked proliferative activity and may therefore have a more aggressive behavior. However, gemistocytic tumors show a lesser degree of proliferation. The determination of proliferative activity may be indicative of tumor behavior and provide additional information on the morphological diagnosis (Watanabe et al., 1997).

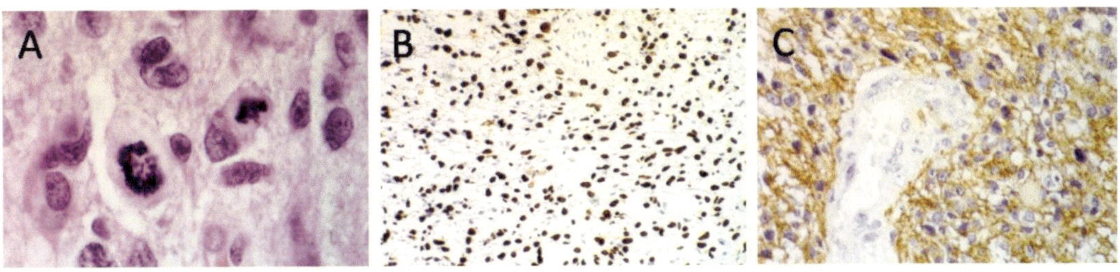

Fig. 2. Morphological and immunohistochemical features of glioblastomas. A) Mitosis in tumor cells. B) Positive expression Ki-67/MIB-1. C) GFAP positive expression.

According to the clinical concepts of Scherer (1940) with respect primary and secondary glioblastoma, most cases develop rapidly without clinical, radiological or morphological evidence of a less malignant precursor. This type of glioblastoma is considered primary or de novo glioblastoma, if also the diagnosis of glioblastoma was obtained in the first biopsy. In these cases, the tumor rapidly develops after a short history of less than 3 months in most cases. The diagnosis of secondary glioblastoma is performed only in cases with histopathological evidence of an earlier low-grade astrocytoma or anaplastic astrocytoma. In these cases, the tumor develops slowly and is considered to have arisen from the glioblastoma tumor progression of lower primary malignancy. Using these criteria, secondary glioblastomas are much less common than primary, reaching only 5% of the total (Dropcho & Soong, 1996, Ohgaki & Kleihues, 2005).

Besides the difference in the diagnosis and progression of primary and secondary glioblastoma, there are also differences in the distribution of age and sex in the two types of tumors. Primary glioblastoma affects older patients with a mean age of 62, while secondary glioblastoma affects middle-aged patients with a mean of 45 years. The distribution between the sexes is also different, dominated by men in cases of primary glioblastoma (M:F 1.5), and women in secondary (F:M 0.65) (Ohgaki & Kleihues, 2005).

A difference between the two subtypes is also observed in terms of survival. Primary glioblastoma has a median survival time shorter (4.7 months) than secondary glioblastoma

(7.8 months). This difference in survival may be due to the difference in the age at which they occur. In fact, there is no significant difference after an adjustment for age (Ohgaki & Kleihues, 2005).

Primary and secondary glioblastomas are two tumor subtypes indistinguishable from a histopathological point of view.

Taking these differences and clinical presentation, the group of Kleihues et al (1997), studied the distribution of molecular features known for glioblastomas, in each of these two subtypes. These authors performed a separation of primary and secondary glioblastomas based on two different histogenetic pathways. Amplification / overexpression of EGFR and *TP53* mutation are considered the pillars of the two proposed genetic pathways for the formation of the two subtypes of glioblastomas. In principle, they were also considered mutually exclusive.

Further studies were to define more precisely the presence of these molecular alterations. Amplification in primary glioblastomas and / or overexpression of EGFR occurred in about 40% of cases. Mutations in *TP53*, however, are features of secondary glioblastomas and appeared in 65% of cases, being much less frequent in primary glioblastomas (28% of cases) (Ohgaki et al., 2004, Ohgaki & Kleihues, 2005).

This chapter is organized as follow: In the 2nd section, we have realised a description on cytogenetic and molecular characteristics of glioblastoma. We analyzed the presence of numerical chromosomal aberrations by applying cytogenetic methods in cultured cells and centromeric DNA probes specific for chromosomes 7 and 10 in material proceeding from smear preparations; and we have studied the association between these parameters. Then, in the 3rd section, characteristics of epidermal growth factor receptor gene (EGFR) and its implication in the pathways of signalization are illustrated. We have investigated the expression of activated ERK1/2 in glioblastomas using western blot analysis and immunohistochemistry, and assessed the relationship between activated ERK1/2 and genetic factors such as *EGFR* amplification, *TP53* mutation and alteration of 9p21 locus genes, as well as clinicopathological parameters. In section 4, we presented the histopathological and genetic findings of primary glioblastomas. The association between cases with *EGFR* gene amplification and cases without *EGFR* amplification with cytogenetic parameters, *TP53* mutations, *MDM2* and *CDK4* amplification, and cell cycle regulatory genes located at 9p21, was evaluated. A second aim of this study was to investigate the relationship between such genetic variations and clinical and pathological data. For last, in section 5, we investigated differences in the pattern of *EGFR* amplification in the glioblastoma. We performed FISH analysis with an *EGFR* probe in metaphases of primary cultured cells and in paraffin sections from 60 cases of primary glioblastomas. We also aimed to compare the *EGFR* copy number alterations, mRNA level and protein expression status and to correlate the FISH data with the clinical and histopathological parameters in the glioblastoma multiforme.

2. Genetic hallmarks in glioblastomas

The glioblastoma is characterized by intratumoral heterogeneity with regard to both histomorphology and genetic changes. Cytogenetically, the GBM displays highly complex karyotypes, with numerous structural and numerical aberrations, the presence of double minutes, as well as differences in ploidy level. The most common numerical chromosome aberrations are +7, +8, -9, -10, -13, -14, -22 and loss of a sex chromosome. Structural changes involve predominantly the following chromosome arms: 1q, 2q, 6q, 7p, 7q, 9p, 14q, 17p and 18p (Jenkins et al., 1989, Bigner et al., 1990, Mitelman et al., 2004, Lopez-Gines et al., 2006). However, in vitro tissue culturing for karyotype analysis may result in the selective growth of cells with the highest proliferative activity, and these cells may not be representative of the primary tissue (Heim et al., 1989, Moertel et al., 1993).

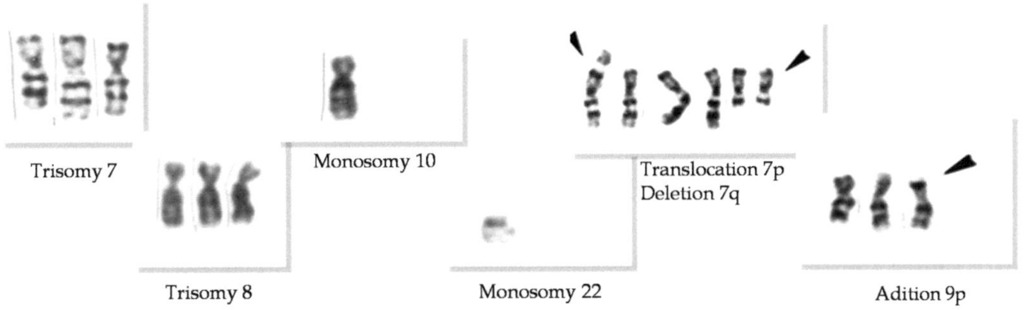

Fig. 3. Cytogenetic alterations in glioblastomas

By minimizing any in vitro culture artefact, fluorescence in situ hybridization (FISH) may more accurately depict the chromosome aberrations in tissues, like the brain, in which cellular turnover is low. These studies showed different aneuploidy for chromosomes 1, 7, 10, 17, X, and Y in astrocytomas, and in all of them the over-representation of chromosome 7 and the under-representation of chromosome 10 are the most common in GBM (Arnoldus et al., 1992, Wernicke et al., 1997, Amalfitano et al., 2000, Koschny et al., 2002, Lopez-Gines et al., 2005). FISH on interphase cells is a powerful tool for detecting different chromosome aberrations, because it can detect chromosomal changes on a cell-by-cell basis. The FISH studies of GBM have also found, that trisomy for chromosome 7 and/or monosomy for chromosome 10 are the principal anomalies, but very few of them have been carried out on about smear preparations; this is a good material and a rapid method for to detection aneuploidy, with control by hematoxilyin-eosin for the presence of tumoral cells in the preparation. According to a few publications, the association between trisomy/polisomy 7 and monosomy 10 is very different, 35-80% depending on the methods used (Steilen-Gimbel et al., 1996, Nishizaki et al., 2002, Lopez-Gines et al., 2005). The studies using karyotype analysis consider trisomy/polisomy 7 to be an early change and monosomy 10 as a progression-associated aberration (Rey et al., 1987, Bigner et al., 1990). On the contrary, other studies with FISH have suggested that in tumorigenesis, monosomy 10 may be an earlier change than the abnormalities in chromosome 7, because cases with monosomy 10 but without trisomy 7 were observed (Steilen-Gimbel et al., 1996, Amalfitano et al., 2000). It is possible that the association of both is necessary in tumorigenesis of GBM.
At the molecular level the glioblastoma multiforme has been studied extensively and the most commonly affected genes are the following:

- Loss of heterozygosity (LOH): LOH on chromosome arm 10q is the most frequent gene alteration for both primary and secondary glioblastomas; it occurs in 60-90% of cases. This mutation appears to be specific for glioblastoma multiforme and is found rarely in other tumor grades. This mutation is associated with poor survival (Fujisawa et al., 1999, Tada et al., 2001).

- Epidermal growth factor receptor (*EGFR*) gene: This oncogene is frequently amplified/overexpressed and mutated in glioblastoma. This alteration is observed in 40-50% of these tumors (Wong et al., 1992, Ekstrand et al., 1994, Wang et al., 1994).
- *TP53* tumor suppressor gene: Appears to be deleted or altered in approximately 25-40% of all glioblastoma multiformes, more commonly in secondary glioblastoma (Yoon et al., 2001, Houiller et al.., 2006).
- *PTEN: A*lso known as *MMAC* and *TEP1,* encodes a tyrosine phosphatase located at band 10q23.3. *PTEN* mutations have been found in as many as 30% of glioblastomas, more commonly in primary glioblastoma (Karlbom et al., 1993, Lin et al., 1998).
- *MDM2:* Amplification or overexpression of *MDM2* is the second most common gene amplification in glioblastoma and is observed in 10-15% of patients. Some studies show that this mutation has been associated with a poor prognosis (Reifenberger et al., 1994).
- Platelet-derived growth factor–alpha (*PDGF-alpha*) gene: The *PDGF* gene acts as a major mitogen for glial cells by binding to the *PDGF* receptor (PDGFR). Amplification or overexpression of PDGFR is typical (60%) in the pathway leading to secondary glioblastomas (Hermanson et al., 1992; Varela et al., 2004).
- Additional genetic alterations in primary glioblastomas include *INK4A* deletions (30-40%), and retinoblastoma (*RB*) gene protein alterations (Quelle et al., 1995, Stott et al., 1998, Ichimura et al., 1996).

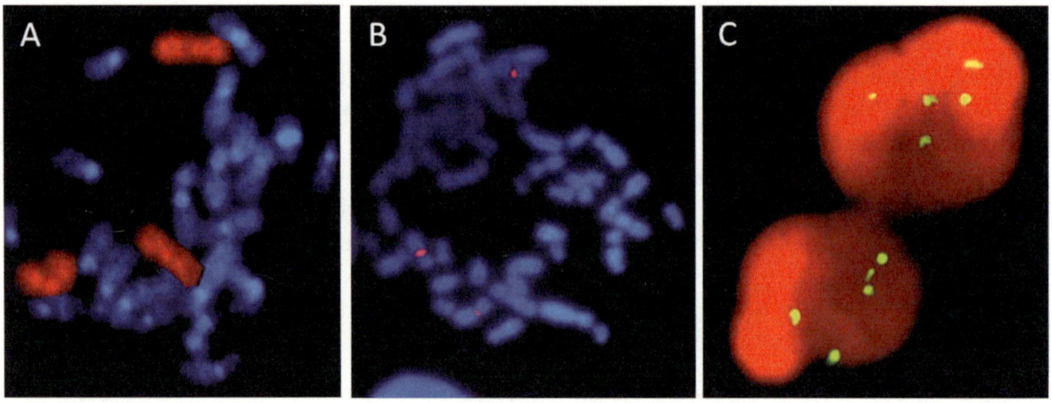

Fig. 4. FISH analysis. A) Metaphase with trisomy 7 (painting probe). B) Metaphase with trisomy 7 (probe centromere of chromosome 7). C) Interphase nuclei with polysomy of chromosome 7.

3. Epidermal growth factor receptor gene and pathways of signalization in glioblastoma multiforme

The EGFR receptor is encoded by the gene c-erbB-1 or Her-1, located on chromosome 7 in the 7p12 region (Kondo et al., 1983). EGFR was the first receptor in which the ability to phosphorylate tyrosine residues in a portion of the molecule was detected. Their activation by the ligand leads to an increase in DNA synthesis, and consequently to an increase in cell proliferation and a decrease in apoptotic activity. This stimulation of cell division begins in the actions of its tyrosine kinase activity (Carpenter & Cohen, 1990).

The oncogenic properties of EGFR receptor are associated with a constitutive and uncontrolled increase in its phosphorylation catalytic activity. The reversible phosphorylation of proteins is one of the major mechanisms for protein regulation and for control of cell physiology. The phosphorylation of certain residues of a protein can regulate its activity, its interaction with other proteins, its structure and its location. Hence, protein kinases and phosphatases are an important part in its control.

The kinases that phosphorylate tyrosine are involved in the initial steps of transmitting signals within the cell, resulting from ligand binding to the receptor (Ullrich & Schlessinger, 1990).

Phosphorylated tyrosine residues serve to the receptor as recruitment and association site for cytosolic proteins, which are activated in turn by new phosphorylations. The association of a protein to the receptor also produces the approximation of soluble proteins from the cytoplasm and thus facilitates this interaction. This will initiate the signaling pathways mediated by these molecules.

Transduction pathways that are activated in this way include the route PI3 kinase/AKT, the Ras/MAP kinase, route c-myc, protein kinase C route and route STAT. All these paths induce the cell to activate transcription of specific genes that produce cell proliferation, apoptosis resistance, invasion, metastasis and angiogenesis, ultimately leading to malignant transformation (Dai et al., 2001; Arteaga, 2002, Rao & James, 2004). Therefore, the intracellular domain of the receptor has an extracellular signal transmitted to the cell nucleus via phosphorylation cascades.

The signaling pathway RAS/RAF is altered in many tumor types, including glioblastomas. This signaling pathway through MAP kinases is involved in cell proliferation. ERK1 and ERK2 are the best studied kinases in solid tumors. ERK1/2 are activated by phosphorylation of tyrosine and threonine residues. Dual phosphorylation is necessary for full activation of ERK1/2. When ERK1/2 is activated migrates into the nucleus and phosphorylates transcription factors which affect the expression of certain genes and ultimately cell growth (Canagarajah et al., 1997, Jelinek et al., 1996). In our work we have observed that in many cases the amplification of *EGFR* is related to the dual activation of ERK1/2. Additionally, if the amplification of *EGFR* is linked to deletions or p16 gene methylation, the relationship with activation of ERK1/2 is more significant (Lopez-Gines et al., 2008).

Major intracellular signaling pathways related to aging and apoptosis involve the enzyme phosphatidylinositol 3-kinase PI3-K. This kinase phosphorylates inositol phospholipids instead of proteins, and also acts on Akt by phosphorylation. Akt itself phosphorylates MDM2, which enters the nucleus where it accumulates, causing inhibition of *TP53* (Honda et al., 1997; Roth et al., 1998).

Nuclear factor NFkB is an important mediator in the regulation of *TP53* and in the Akt signaling pathway. This regulation is achieved through an essential component of NFkB activation cascade, the protein RIP1 (death domain-containing receptor kinase interacting protein 1). RIP1 activates NFkB which causes an increase in MDM2 gene expression by inhibiting the action of *TP53* (Park et al., 2009).

Conversely, in the *P13-K/PTEN/AKT* pathway, *PTEN* tumor suppressor plays also an important role. This tumor gene encodes a phosphatase that dephosphorylates PI3-K, thus preventing the phosphorylation of Akt, and thus favoring *TP53* action. PTEN produces a negative control on Akt kinase pathway, by its action opposite to PI3-K. Therefore, alterations in this gene have a negative effect on TP53 and therefore influence the aging processes and apoptosis, and the cell migration and tumor invasion (Li et al., 1997; Knobbe et al., 2002).

The genetic pathway *TP53/MDM2* is also regulated by p14/ARF. p14 is a repressor of *MDM2*. If p14 does not exert its proper function, it will trigger an excess of free *MDM2* and consequently inactivation of TP53. The alterations of these genes are diverse. p14, which acts as a suppressor gene, typically exhibits some deletions. MDM2, on the other hand, with oncogenic activity is often amplified whereas *TP53* can show different types of mutations (Stott et al., 1998, Ichimura et al., 2000).

Finally, another pathway affected in glioblastomas is p16/Rb/*CDK4*, which controls the G1-S transition in the cell cycle and hence proliferation. In glioblastomas this pathway is impaired because p16, which normally acts as a tumor suppressor gene, has deletions. Additionally, *CDK4* amplifications are also present, giving the cells oncogenic activity. The disturbance causes Rb to be continuously phosphorylated, and as a result there is an uncontrolled cell division (Reifenberger et al., 1994, Rollbrocker et al., 1996).

All these molecules could be therapeutic targets in a tumor as aggressive as this that we are studying.

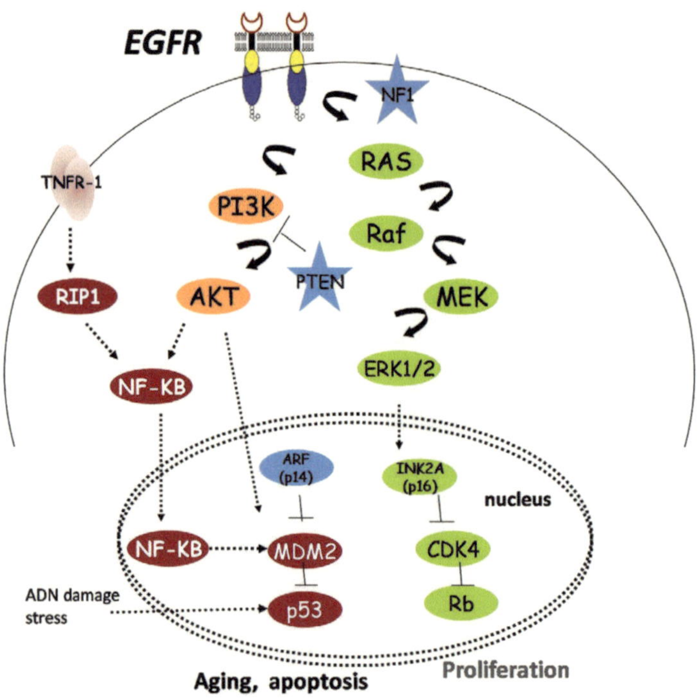

Fig. 5. Pathways of signalization in glioblastoma multiforme

Most gene amplification events in astrocytoma in general and in glioblastoma specifically, involve the EGFR gene. These gene amplification phenomena involve the duplication of certain regions of DNA that leads to the existence of multiple copies of a gene. *EGFR* amplification was an early genetic alteration involved in tumorigenesis of glioblastoma (Márquez et al., 2004).

The vast majority of authors place the percentage of glioblastomas with EGFR amplification around 40-50% (Ekstrand et al., 1992, Diedrich et al., 1995, Shinojima et al., 2003). However, some studies extend this range up to 73% (Márquez et al., 2004). These differences have been attributed to the different methodologies used (PCR, FISH, Southern blot). *EGFR* amplification has been observed in association with the increase in the number of copies of chromosome 7, both total or partial, which is the most common karyotypic abnormality found in glioblastoma (Hurtt et al., 1992, Rao & James, 2004).

An increase in EGF receptor expression and its natural ligands has been observed using immunohistochemical techniques. This expression is not limited to the membrane, but also observed in the nucleus of tumor cells (Libermann et al., 1985, Ekstrand et al., 1991; Shinojima et al., 2003, Márquez et al., 2004).

This increase coincides with the amplification of the gene encoding the receptor (Shinojima et al., 2003, Varela et al., 2004, Márquez et al., 2004, Lopez-Gines et al., 2005). On the contrary, no expression of this marker is present in normal tissue (Márquez et al., 2004).

The combined increase in the expression of ligands and receptors has led to the assumption that there is a loop autocrine/paracrine growth which stimulates neoplasic growth. Thus, by the autocrine stimulation the cell induces autoproliferation in response to their own growth factors and by the paracrine stimulation there is induction of proliferation in response to factors secreted by neighboring cells and adjacent. In any case, there is an activation of the machinery of the cell cycle and uncontrolled cell proliferation. In fact there are several studies that support the importance of the system EGF/EGFR in the tumorigenesis of glioblastoma, due to the strong coexpression of EGF receptor and its respective ligands EGF and TGF-α (Ekstrand et al , 1991; Shinojima et al., 2003).

Half of the glioblastoma cases with EGFR amplification also exhibit rearrangements of the gene, which results in a considerable variety of qualitative and structural alterations of the receptor, prompted by different mutations that can undergo the gene (Ekstrand et al., 1992, Shinojima et al., 2003, Rao & James, 2004).

The gene sequences which are amplified in glioblastoma are frequently mutated and code protein variants shorter than the native protein (Frederick et al., 2000; Shinojima et al., 2003). These mutations can affect both the 5 'region and the 3' region of the gene. Thus, the mutant protein can be affected at both the extracellular and the intracellular domain. On the other hand, the reading frame is not usually affected by these mutations (Eley et al., 1998, Frederick et al., 2000).

The most common rearrangement is a variant called EGFRvIII, a receptor with a molecular weight of 140-155 kDa that is expressed together with the normal 170 kDa protein (Sugawa et al., 1990, Sugawa et al., 1998; Wikstrand et al., 1998). This rearrangement has also been seen in other tumors where EGFR is also overexpressed (Eley et al., 1998; Arteaga, 2002). This mutation lacks a portion of the ligand binding extracellular domain as a result of genomic deletions that eliminate exons 2-7 in the EGFR mRNA (Frederick et al., 2000; Collins, 2002; Shinojima et al., 2003). This gives this form of the receptor a number of features distinct to those of the normal EGFR (Collins, 2002; Shinojima et al., 2003).

4. Primary glioblastomas with and without *EGFR* amplification

The pathogenic mechanisms leading to the development and progression of glioblastoma are still unclear. *EGFR* amplification has been identified as a genetic hallmark of primary glioblastoma and occurs in approximately 40-60% of primary glioblastomas, but rarely in secondary glioblastomas (Houiller et al., 2006, TCGA, 2008). Generally, primary glioblastomas with *EGFR* amplification show EGFR overexpression, and 70% to 90% of those with EGFR overexpression have *EGFR* amplification (Liu et al., 2004). This oncogenetic pathway, is heavily involved in this variant of glioblastoma. However, there exist primary glioblastomas with no amplification/overexpression of the *EGFR*.

In our previous works, *EGFR* amplification was observed in 53% of the tumors, and 80% of them presented EGFR overexpression. On the other hand, 47% of our primary glioblastomas showed no *EGFR* amplification and 67% of them showed no overexpression. We studied the association between cases with *EGFR* gene amplification and cases without *EGFR* amplification with cytogenetic parameters, *TP53* mutations, *MDM2* and *CDK4* amplification, and cell cycle regulatory genes located at 9p21. Furthermore, we investigated the relationship between such genetic variations and clinical and pathological data (Benito et al., 2009).

At clinipathological level, the age distribution of cases with *EGFR* amplification closely follows that of patients with primary glioblastomas (60 years), and patients of less than 35 years of age are more infrequent. In our results, the mean age of the group with *EGFR* amplification was 57.2 years and only one patient was under 35 years of age. However, the mean age for the group of cases without *EGFR* amplification was 49.8 years and four patients were under 35 years of age. The rest of the clinicopathological findings on primary glioblastomas with and without *EGFR* amplification did not show any significant differences, although, interestingly, patients with *EGFR* amplification survived for the shortest time.

Cytogenetically, glioblastomas have shown many numerical and structural anomalies (Bigner et al., 1990, Lopez-Gines et al., 2006). In our study, the number of karyotypes with anomalies was greater in the group without *EGFR* amplification. Trisomy 7, monosomy 10 and monosomy 22 were observed in both groups, and the structural alterations of chromosomes 1, 7 and 9 were more frequent in the first group. Every case with dmin had *EGFR* amplification.

FISH on interphase cells is a powerful tool for detecting different chromosome aberrations, because it can detect chromosome changes on cell-by-cell bases. The FISH studies into primary glioblastomas have also found that trisomy for chromosome 7 and/or monosomy for chromosome 10 are the principal anomalies. In our cases, we found a high percentage (85%) of trisomy/polisomy and 70% of monosomy 10, higher in fact than those found by conventional cytogenetic analysis. Likewise, the association of both trisomy/polisomy 7 and monosomy 10 were present in 59% of the cases. In our study, both amplified and non-amplified tumors showed trisomy/polysomy of chromosome 7 and monosomy of chromosome 10. This fact suggests that these alterations could be an initial event in the tumorigenesis of glioblastoma.

At a molecular level, a close association between *EGFR* amplification and *CDKN2A* (*INK4a/ARF*) deletions is a frequent alteration in glioblastomas. Homozygous *INK4a/ARF* deletions were more frequent in primary than in secondary glioblastomas, but there was no significant difference in the overall frequency of these alterations (homozygous deletion and promoter methylation) between primary and secondary glioblastomas (Ohgaki & Kleihues, 2007). In our results on primary glioblastomas, both cases with and without *EGFR* amplification showed similar percentages of *INK4a/ARF* deletions, but the promoter methylation of *INK4a* was more frequent in the group of cases with *EGFR* amplification. As a consequence of *CDKN2A* deletions, there is a disruption of both *RB1/CDK4/P16* and *P53/MDM2/p14* pathways. *MDM2* facilitates the ubiquitin-mediated degradation of p53, which is inhibited by *p14/ARF*. This fact probably explains why both *MDM2* amplification and *INK4a/ARF* are mutually exclusive. The amplification of *MDM2* is present in less than 10% of glioblastomas, exclusively in primary glioblastomas that lack a *TP53* mutation (Houiller et al., 2006, Ohgaki & Kleihues, 2007). In our series, *MDM2* amplification was present in 11% of the cases, all of them with *EGFR* amplification and without deletions of *INK4a/ARF*. *CDK4* promotes the phosphorylation of the Rb protein and is inhibited by p16 protein, a product of the INK4a tumor suppressor gene. Again, both alterations result in a redundant effect. In our cases, *CDK4* amplification and *INK4a/ARF* deletions were mutually exclusive, and all cases except one were present with *EGFR* amplification. We also found tightly associated *MDM2* and *CDK4* amplifications, suggesting that both genes, which map close together to the same region on 12q13, are frequently included in the same amplicon.

	mut *TP53*	del 9p21	met 9p21	- chro 10	+ chro 7	amp *CDK4*	amp *MDM2*
amp *EGFR*	4	10	18	31	42	6	9
mut *TP53*		2	8	17	18	2	0
del 9p21			4	17	16	0	0
met 9p21				24	25	2	2
- chro 10					57	3	0
+ chro 7						10	11
amp *CDK4*							7

Table 1. Co-presence of genetic alterations in glioblastomas (expressed in %).

Finally, the *TP53* pathway plays a crucial role in the development of secondary glioblastomas, *TP53* mutations being the first detectable genetic alteration. However, although this event also occurs in primary glioblastomas, it does so at a lower frequency (<30% of the cases). In our study, 18% of primary glioblastomas showed *TP53* mutations. Furthermore, we have been found two glioblastomas showing both concurrent *EGFR* amplification and *TP53* mutation.

The first case, arising *de novo* in a 51-years old woman, expressed GFAP, S100, vimentin, and had p53_LI of 27%. EGFR was overexpressed. The cytogenetic analysis showed a hypertriploid complex karyotype with rearrangements of chromosomes 1, 7, 8, and 11, and dmin. FISH studies using centromeric DNA probes for chromosomes 7 and 10 showed trisomy 7 and monosomy 10 in the majority of the cells. Molecular biology showed *EGFR* amplification, and a C176R TP53 mutation; furthermore, aberrant hypermehylation in the promoter region of p14 gene was demonstrated.

The second case arising three years later than a previous anaplastic astrocytoma in a 38-year old man, expressed GFAP, S-100, vimentin, and had p53_LI of 26%. EGFR was overexpressed. The karyotype was hypodiploid, with a t(9;18) and rearrangements of chromosomes 2, 13, and 14. Disomy 7/monosomy 10 was confirmed by FISH. At molecular level the tumor showed *EGFR* amplification and a R282W TP53 mutation.

Hypermethylation of promoter region of p16 gene was also observed. These cases showed, in common, monosomy of chromosome 10, hypermethylation in the INK4A locus, *EGFR* amplification and *TP53* mutation (Gil-Benso et al., 2007).
Our results suggest that, in primary glioblastomas, there exists a subgroup of cases closely linked with *EGFR* amplification. However, there is another subgroup of cases without *EGFR* amplification with some different clinical and genetic characteristics. This second group might include the increased activation or expression of other growth factor receptors observed in these tumors such as PDGFR or IGFR, although they are only amplified in a low percentage of cases.

Group	Clinical characteristics	Histophatological characteristics	Genetic alterations
1 Amplification *EGFR*	**Primary glioblastoma Mean age: 57 years Mean survival: 10.5** months	**Mean Ki-67 : 31 Sobreexpresión EGFR p53 index: low**	**Citogenetics:+7,-10,-22 Structural: # 1, 9, dmin Amplification: *MDM2,CDK4* del 9p21; met 9p21**
2 No amplification *EGFR*	**Primary/secondary glioblastoma Mean age: 49 years Mean survival: 11** months	**Mean Ki-67 : 24 No EGFR sobreexpresión p53 index: high**	**Citogenetics: +7, -10, -14, -15, -17, -22, Structural: # 1, 6, 11, 12 del 9p21**

Table 2. Characteristics of glioblastomas with and without *EGFR* amplification

5. Patterns of *EGFR* amplification and gene expression profile

Amplifications are mutations that result in multiple copies of genes in chromosomal regions (amplicons) and induce overexpression in cancer cells. The amount of overexpressed genes in amplified regions varies between different types of cancers, and gene expression in general was significantly regulated by DNA copy number alterations (Schwab, 1998, Myllykangas & Knuutila, 2006). Chromosomal abnormalities associated with DNA amplification can be organized as extrachromosomal copies, called double minutes (dmin); in tandem arrays as head-to-tail or inverted repeats within a chromosome, often forming a cytologically visible, homogeneously staining region (HSR); or distributed at various locations in the genome (distributed insertions) (Schwab,1998, Kuwahara et al., 2004, Albertson, 2006). *MYCN, ERBB2* and *EGFR* are the most frequently amplified genes in cancers.
According to the breakage-fusion-bridge (BFB) model of amplification, the initiating event in HSR formation is double chromatid breakage at a fragile site or telomere erosion (Coquelle et al., 1997, Murnane & Sabatier, 2004), fused sister chromatids and breaking of the anaphase bridges (Shimizu et al., 2005). BFB cycles could then result in inverted amplified structures (Toledo et al., 1992), and the mutated sister chromatids are distributed

to the daughter cells giving rise to intra-tumor heterogeneity (Gisselsson et al., 2000). Gene amplifications are also acquired by selection and unequal segregation of circular extrachromosomal chromatin (dmin and episomes). These elements are formed by looping out from the chromosomes. Dmin and episomes may also relocate in the genome after DNA double-stranded breaks to form HSR or distributed insertions (Schwab, 1999, Kuwahara et al., 2004). Instead of these above-mentioned mechanisms, N-myc duplication located at 2p24 has been described in neuroblastoma cell lines, as studied by FISH (Corvi et al., 1995). Large direct duplications may arise by unequal sister-chromatid exchange and appear to play a role during the initial stages in amplification. It is unclear whether duplication represents a prelude to amplification or an alternative pathway for activating the oncogenic potential of *MYC*. (Corvi et al., 1995, Schwab, 2004).

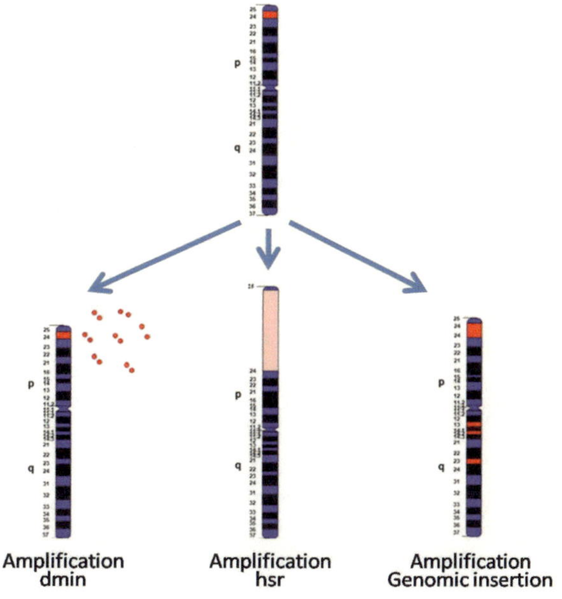

Fig. 6. Patterns of gene amplification: dmin, hsr and genomic insertion.

The first evidence of gene amplification in glioblastoma was provided by cytogenetic analyses which exhibited the presence of dmin, found in up to 50% of tumors (Bigner & Volgelstein, 1990; Thiel et al., 1992).

Molecular studies demonstrated the amplification of several genes in these tumors, especially of the EGFR gene; the amplified sequences were found located on dmin in a small number of cases, by in situ hybridization of tumor metaphases (Muleris et al., 1994, Vogt et al., 2004). However, studies by FISH in interphase nuclei are more frequent, displaying a considerable heterogeneity of *EGFR* copy number (Sauter et al., 1996, Vogt et al., 2004, Layfield et al., 2006, Mizoguchi et al., 2006). The large fraction of cases presenting a diffuse rather than a clustered pattern of amplification within single cells supports the notion that the most common pattern of *EGFR* amplification in glioblastoma biopsies is as double minutes, which ranged in size from 0.7 to 2.1 Mb and in level of amplification from 8-to-63-fold (Vogt et al., 2004). The FISH signals differed from case to case, intense and multiple, double, faint and single. This suggests the complexity of dmin formation since both their size and the number of *EGFR* copies they contain, vary. Cell to cell variations are also likely to exist for a given tumor (Sauter et al., 1996).

Molecular screening for gene amplification revealed the frequent amplification of the *EGFR*, observed in about 35%-70% of glioblastomas (Sauter et al., 1996, Okada et al., 2003, Ohgaki and Kleihues, 2007). Differences in the frequency of *EGFR* amplification are most likely due to the different methods used, such as Southern blot, polymerase chain reaction (PCR), and fluorescent in situ hybridization.

EGFR protein overexpresssion is usually associated with gene amplification in glioblastomas and these two parameters have been studied as a potential prognostic indicator (Shinojima et al., 2003, Layfield et al., 2006). The majority of GBMs with EGFR amplification also contain the mutant EGFR gene, EGFRvIII, which is characterized by the deletion of exons 2-7, resulting in an in frame deletion variant that has a truncated extracellular domain with ligand-independent constitutive activity.

Overexpression of wild-type EGFR was not found to be an independent prognostic indicator of survival in several studies, and one study was inconclusive (Simmons et al., 2001, Shinojima et al., 2003). Four studies identified EGFR as a negative prognostic indicator of survival, one of which showed the effect only in patients younger than 45. In some of these studies, analysis was limited by small sample size, uncharacterized extent of surgical resection, and variable postoperative treatment. The prognostic impact of EGFRvIII has not been as extensively studied, but in the study that addressed this variable, the presence of EGFRvIII was found to be an independent and significant unfavorable prognosticator of survival (Ekstrand et al., 1991, Simmons et al., Smith et al., 2001, Arteaga et al., 2002, Marquez et al., 2004). *EGFR* amplification and EGFRvIII have been shown to increase glioma proliferation and invasion *in vitro*; therefore logically EGFR and/or EGFRvIII expression could exhibit a proclivity towards the development of multifocal disease, gliomatosis cerebri or ependymal seeding.

In our study we performed FISH analysis with an *EGFR* specific probe in metaphases of primary cultured cells and in paraffin sections from 60 cases of primary glioblastomas, in order to investigate differences in the pattern of *EGFR* amplification in this tumor. We compared the *EGFR* copy number alterations and gene expression with the clinical and histopathological parameters in this subset of tumors.

5.1 Methodology

5.1.1 Histopathological study

Tissue removed from the patient during the surgical resection was divided into three fragments, one for histopathological and immunohistochemical study, one for culture, and the other was frozen and stored at -80ºC until molecular analysis and DNA extraction were performed.

The tumoral tissue was fixed in neutral-buffered formalin during the first 48h, embedded in paraffin, sectioned and stained with HE. The samples were categorized according to the WHO classification and diagnosed as glioblastoma multiforme (Louis et al., 2007). Mitotic index values were obtained by counting the total number of mitotic figures in the tumor cells in 20 high-power fields (HPF) and in two different sections. The values are the mean number of mitoses per 10 HPF.

The immunohistochemical study was performed on paraffin-embedded sections using the avidin-biotin peroxidase method. The study was carried out with antibodies against glial

fibrillary acidic protein (GFAP) (Dako, Glostrup, Denmark), Ki-67 (MIB-1, Dako, Glostrup, Denmark), p53 (Dako, Glostrup, Denmark), and monoclonal mouse antihuman EGFR (clone H11, Dako, Glostrup, Denmark) that recognizes the wild-type EGFR and the deletion mutant form of the receptor (EGFRvIII).
Proliferation index was evaluated using MIB-1 antibody staining, and was calculated by determining the percentage of immunopositive nuclei. EGFR expression was scored according to the intensity of staining and number of staining cells, as: 0 (no staining), 1 (light or focal), 2 (moderate) and 3 (strong). Scores of 0 or 1 were defined as no overexpression; scores of 2 and 3 as overexpression (Shinojima et al., 2003).

5.1.2 Cytogenetic analysis and fluorescence in situ hybridization

Cytogenetic analyses were performed by short-term culture of the tumors. Fresh tumor samples were disaggregated with 2mg/mL of collagenase II. The cells were seeded in flasks using RPMI-1640 medium supplemented with 20% foetal bovine serum, L- glutamine, and antibiotics. The cells were processed after 72 h of culture by a standard technique. Air dried slides were banded by trypsin-Giemsa. Karyotypic analyses were performed according to ISCN (1995).

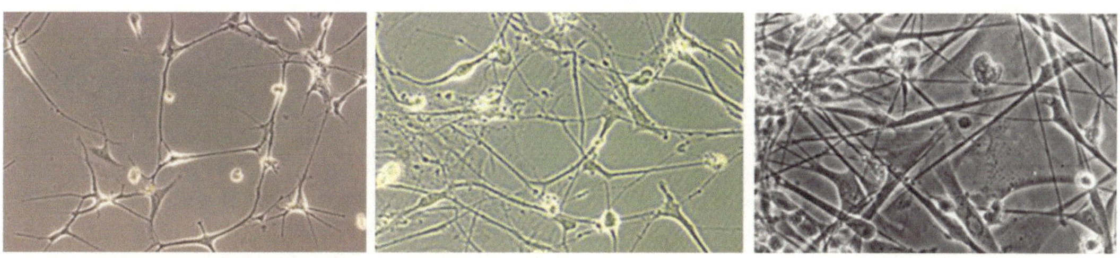

Fig. 7. Cultured cells of glioblastoma

To evaluate EGFR gene status, dual-color FISH was performed on cultured cells and on paraffin sections. FISH was carried out using the LSR EGFR Spectrum Orange/CEP 7 Spectrum Green Probe from Vysis (Abbott Laboratories, Downers Grove, IL, USA. Cat. No. 32-191053).

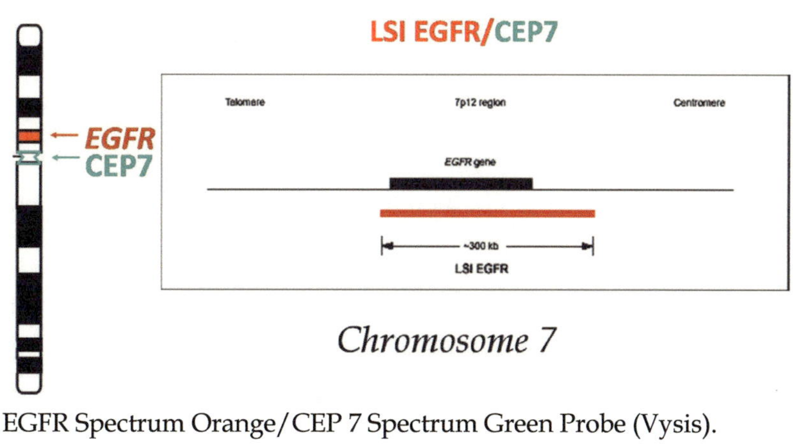

Fig. 8. LSR EGFR Spectrum Orange/CEP 7 Spectrum Green Probe (Vysis).

Cultured cells were treated with Colcemid (0.02 μg/mL) (Gibco BRL, Grand Island, NY, USA) for 80 minutes, and chromosomes were prepared by conventional fixation. The paraffin embedded tissues were cut at 5-μm and mounted on Superfrost/Plus microscope slides. Hybridizations were performed according to the instructions that accompany the probe. Counterstaining of nuclei was carried out using DAPI. The fluorescent signal was detected using a photomicroscope Axioplan 2 and Axiophot 2 (Zeiss) equipped with a set of the appropriate filters. Signals were counted in 100-200 cultured cell nuclei, in all the possible metaphases and in 100 non-overlapping tumor cell nuclei in the paraffin sections. The mean signal number for the EGFR gene and CEP 7 was calculated for each case, as well as the EGFR gene/CEP 7 ratio. The EGFR gene was scored as amplified in individual cells when the EGFR/control signal ratio was greater than 2 (Layfield et al., 2006).

5.1.3 Real-time quantitative PCR

Tumor DNA was extracted from 10-15 mg using DNeasy kit extraction (Qiagen, Valencia, CA). Quantitative PCR was performed using an ABI Prism 7900 HT Fast Real-Time PCR System (Applied Biosystem, Foster City, CA) to analyze *EGFR* copy number. Primer sequences for *EGFR* were: forward GTGCAGATCGCAAAGGTAATČAG; reverse GCAGACCGCATGT GAGGAT; and probe FAM-CCCCTCCCCGTATCTC-MGB. Primer sequences for *RNase P* and *GAPDH* used as references genes were purchased to TaqMan RNase P and GAPDH Detection Reagents (P/N: 4316831).
Target and reference genes were amplified in separate wells. Each 20 μl assay contained 20 ng of genomic DNA, 900 nM each of forward and reverse primers for the gene (*RNasa P*, and *GAPDH* as reference gene, and *EGFR* as target gene), and 250 nM of labelled gene specific probe in 1x TaqMan Universal PCR Master Mix. The TaqMan universal PCR Master Mix (Applied Biosystems) contained AmpliTaq Gold DNA polymerase, AmpErase uracyl-N-Glycosylase, deoxynucleotide triphospates with dUTP that replace dTTP, and optimized buffers.
Individual samples were run in triplicate. PCR conditions were: 2 min at 50°C (initial incubation for activate AmpErase), 10 min at 95°C (Activation of AmpliTaq Gold DNA Polymerase) followed by 40 cycles of 15 sec at 95°C (melt) and 1 min at 60°C (anneal/extend). Real Time data was collected by the SDS 2.1 software. Each replicate was normalized to reference gene (*RNasa P* and *GAPDH*) to obtain ΔCt, and average ΔCt for each sample (from the 3 replicates) was calculated. All samples were normalized to a calibrator sample to determine ΔΔCt. Relative quantity is $2^{-\Delta\Delta Ct}$, and copy number is 2x (Relative quantity) (Livak & Schmittgen, 2001).
Theoretically, a normal sample has two copies for each gene. Such an assumption is right in cell lines, but taking into consideration that human tumor tissue samples may be contaminated by normal cells, we use a copy number range approach and consider: Homozigous Deletion (HD) 0 - 0.4; Borderline HD-Loss of Heterozigosity (LOH) > 0.4 - 0.6; LOH > 0.6 – 1.4; Borderline LOH-Normal > 1.4 – 1.6; Normal > 1.6 - 2.4; Borderline Amplification > 2.4 – 2.6; and Amplification > 2.6.

5.1.4 Single nucleotide polymorphism (SNPs) array analysis for assessment of EGFR copy number status

Nucleic Acid Isolation and microarray experiment: Fresh frozen tumor tissues (10-20 mg) from patients with glioblastoma were used to extract high molecular weight, genomic DNA using DNeasy kit extraction (Qiagen, Valencia, CA). DNA quality was assessed by

electrophoresis in 1% of agarose gel. Two hundred and fifty DNA nanograms were used for hybridization on Genechip Human Mapping 100K as recommended by the manufacturer (Affymetrix, Santa Clara, CA). The mapping 100K set provides a broad coverage of the human genome (92%), with an average distance between SNPs of 23.6 Kb. This set includes two arrays, each with more than 50,000 SNPs. The processing was performed following the manufacturer's guidelines. Arrays were scanned by means of a GeneChip Scanner 3000, and GeneChip Operating software was used to define Absent or Present Call and generate CEL files.
Data Analysis: CEL files were imported into dChipSNP arrays analysis software (Lin et al., 2004). Arrays were normalized against the array with median overall intensity (Baseline array) employing the *Invariant set* normalization method (Li & Wong 2001a). Probe set signal intensity was obtained by using a model based on expression index (PM/MM) method (Li & Wong, 2001b). Average array call rate was > 95 %. We employ a Hidden-Markov model to identify LOH regions from unpaired tumor samples, taking into account SNP intermarker distance, SNP heterozigosity rates, and the haplotype structure of the genome (Beroukhim et al., 2006). We used 60 CEPH parents as normal reference genotype and we removed inferred LOH regions consistent with 95% of homozygous markers in normal reference samples. Copy number alterations at each SNP locus were determined using the probe level signal intensity data. Reference signal distribution was obtained using a trimmed analysis with 80 % of the samples.

5.1.5 EGFR mRNA expression

Nucleic acid isolation: RNA was extracted from 19 glioblastoma samples. Five pilocytic astrocytomas without *EGFR* amplification were used as reference. For total RNA extraction, 10-20 mg of frozen tumor samples were homogenized with Ultra Turrax and total RNA was isolated using mirVANA kit (Ambion Inc, Austin, TX) following the manufacturer's instructions. Purified RNA was quantified by UV absorbance at 260 and 280 nm and RNA quality was assessed using a spectrophotometer and Agilent 2100 Bioanalyzer (Agilent Technologies, Palo Alto, CA). Samples with 28S/18S ratio of ≥ 1.1 and no evidence of ribosomal peak degradation were included.
Microarray experiments: Total RNA (1-15µg) was used to generate double-stranded cDNA. cDNA synthesis and cRNA labelling were performed using the protocol for one-cycle cDNA synthesis. Biotin-labeled cRNA (20 µg) was fragmented and hybridized overnight to Affymetrix HU133plus2.0 genechip. Protocols were performed as recommended by Affymetrix. Arrays were washed, stained with streptavidin phycoerythrin and scanned to generate an image file. Scan quality was assessed by the inspection of visible microarray artifacts, grid placement, background intensity, and housekeeping gene expression. GeneChip operating software (GCOS) was used to define Absent or Present Call and generate CEL files. Arrays with < 30% "Present" call for the 47,000 probe sets and signal 3′/5′ratio of GDAPH control 0.5 ≤ ratio ≤ 4.5 were omitted.
Data analysis: CEL files were imported into dCHIP program. Arrays were normalized against the array with median overall intensity (Baseline array) employing the *Invariant set* normalization method (Li & Wong 2001a). Probeset signal intensity was obtained by using a model based on expression index (PM/MM) method (Li & Wong, 2001b). EGFR probesets with Present Call and expression level ≥10 in ≥ 45 % samples were selected. Probesets that pass established criteria were: 1565484_x_at; 201983_s_at; 201984_s_at; 211551_at; 211607_x_at.

5.1.6 Statistical analysis

In this study we used no parametric test for Ki67 levels, *EGFR* copy number, EGFR transcript expression, and percentage of cells found to be *EGFR* amplification by FISH. First, the Kruskal-Wallis test was used to assess significant differences among established groups, and then the comparisons among the pairs of groups were assessed by means of the Mann-Whitney U test. We used the Bonferroni method to correct the p-values in order to avoid type I error.

Pearson´s coefficient was used to assess the significant correlation between: *EGFR* copy number measured by qPCR, EGFR transcript expression and percentage of *EGFR* positive cells measured by FISH. The significance of the differential protein expression was contrasted by comparing the *EGFR* amplification type using Fischer´s exact test (one-tailed). Survival curves for amplification types, KPS groups (≤80, >80), and age (<55, ≥55 years) were evaluated by the Kaplan-Meier method and were compared with the log-rank test. The statistical tests significance was determined at p-value ≤ 0.05. The analysis was performed with SPSS 15.0 software (SPSS Inc., Chicago, IL).

5.2 Levels of *EGFR* amplification in glioblastoma

Sixty glioblastomas were analyzed successfully by FISH in cultured cells and paraffin sections. We have analyzed the type of *EGFR* amplification, the fraction of amplified cells, and the number of signals of *EGFR* in each tumor.

On basis of the *EGFR* status, the gene copy number and the type of amplification, the cases were categorized into three groups: GBM-h: high level EGFR gene amplification and dmin, **GBM-l:** low level EGFR gene amplification and insertions, and GBM-n: no EGFR gene amplification (Lopez-Gines et al., 2010).

GBM-h: The 47% of the cases was included in this group. The 50% of patients were male and 50% female. Patient age ranged from 38 to 72, with a mean age of 56 years. Survival ranged from 1 to 24 months, with a mean of 9 months.

Histologically, all tumors demonstrated features of glioblastoma with pleomorphic, astrocytic tumor cells, prominent microvascular proliferation, and necrosis. In every case, the expression of GFAP was confirmed in the neoplastic cells. The number of mitoses ranged between 1 and 20, with a mean of 7. The mean Ki-67 of the tumors was 38%; range: 10-80%.

The type of amplification was dmin with a variable number of copies affecting over 25% of the cells in most cases. Only two cases contained less than 10% of amplified cells in paraffin sections.

By using SNP arrays, we inferred the presence of frequent copy number gains in the region of the *EGFR* locus. In tumor samples, an excess of EGFR gene copies was identified by copy number variation from the reference set and from the copy number of the control samples. Gene copy numbers at 7p12.1 were validated by quantitative PCR. Every case showed a strong correlation of these values with the copies demonstrated by FISH (Pearson's correlation coefficient= 0.77; p-value≤ 0.01).

Gene expression have a significant, positive correlation between the *EGFR* copy number and the transcript gene expression (Pearson's correlation coefficient = 0.75; p-value≤ 0.01). The higher percentage of cases of amplified *EGFR* detected by FISH was correlated with a higher gene expression (Pearson's correlation coefficient = 0.85; p-value≤ 0.01).

The EGFR protein expression was evaluated by immunohistochemistry. Cases with a high level of amplification, manifested EGFR overexpression (except in two cases).

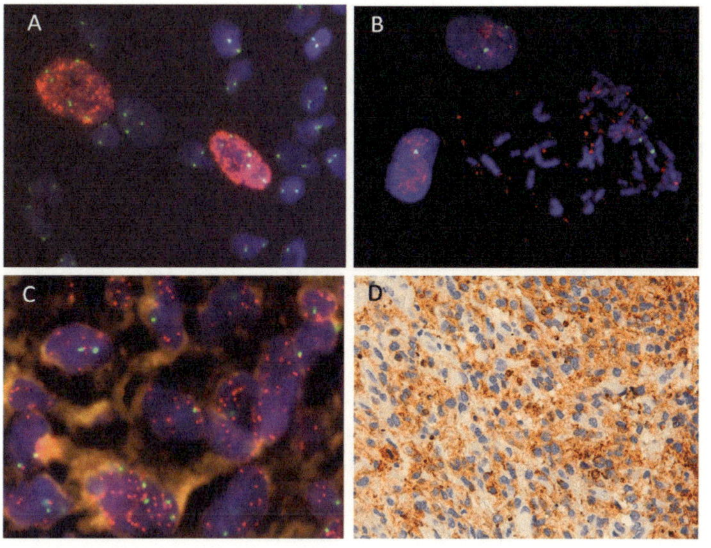

Fig. 9. High-level of amplification of the *EGFR* present in GBM-h group. Probe for EGFR and centromere 7 were labelled with red and green respectively. A) Interphase nuclei of cultured cells. B) Metaphase showing trisomy 7 and *EGFR* amplification as dmin C) Nuclei in paraffin sections showing high level of amplification. Probe for EGFR and centromere 7 were labelled with red and green respectively. D) Immunoreactivity for EGFR: Strong staining.

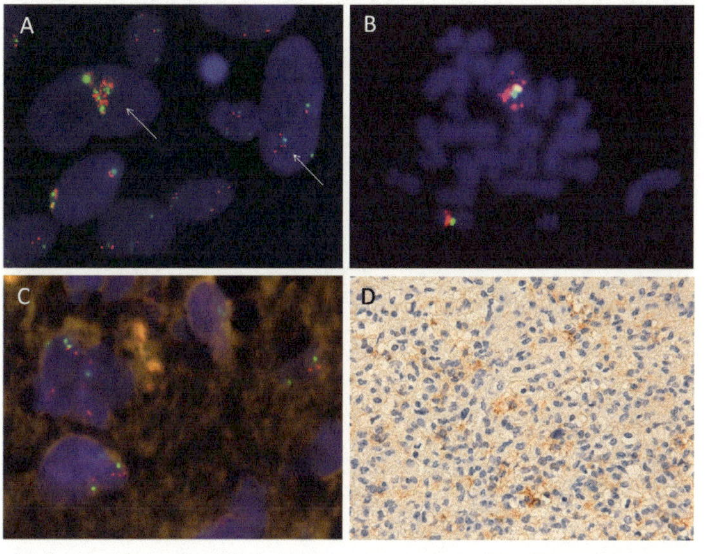

Fig. 10. Low-level of amplification of the *EGFR* present in GBM-l group. A) Different interphase nuclei of cultured cells showing low-level (arrow) of amplification. B) Metaphase spread with extra copies of *EGFR* inserted in p and q arms of chromosomes 7. C) Tumoral cells in paraffin section with low-level amplification/copy number gains with other cells exhibiting a normal copy number of the EGFR gene. D) Immunoreactivity for EGFR with focal staining.

GBM-l: The 21% of the cases was included in this group. The 69% of patients were male and 31% female. Patient age ranged from 24 to 73, with a mean age of 48 years. Survival ranged from 3 to 23 months, with a mean of 12 months.

Histologically, all tumors demonstrated features of glioblastoma with pleomorphic, astrocytic tumor cells, prominent microvascular proliferation, and necrosis. In every case, the expression of GFAP was confirmed in the neoplastic cells. The number of mitoses ranged between 0 and 20, with a mean of 4. The mean Ki-67 of the tumors was 24%; range: 5-50%. The type of amplification showed extra copies of *EGFR* inserted in different locus of chromosome 7, both in p and q arms. In this form of amplification, the number of copies was small, and the percentage of cells with *EGFR* amplification, rarely affects more than 15% of the cells. These cases presented low values validated by quantitative PCR. The increase in mRNA caused by amplification is not always proportional to the number of gene copies. Non increase of RNA expression was found in this group. The EGFR protein expression was variable, only one third of the cases scored EGFR overexpression.

GBM-n: The 32% of the cases was included in this group. The 63% of patients were male and 37% female. Patient age ranged from 22 to 76, with a mean age of 49 years. Survival ranged from 3 to 24 months, with a mean of 11 months.

Histologically, all tumors demonstrated features of glioblastoma with pleomorphic, astrocytic tumor cells, prominent microvascular proliferation, and necrosis. In every case, the expression of GFAP was confirmed in the neoplastic cells. The number of mitoses ranged between 0 and 10, with a mean of 3.The mean Ki-67 of the tumors was 23%; range: 5-50%.

These cases without *EGFR* amplification presented the values of quantitave PCR nearly 2, and non increase of RNA expression was found. The immunohistochemistry analysis showed no overexpression in 79% of cases and overexpression in 21% of cases.

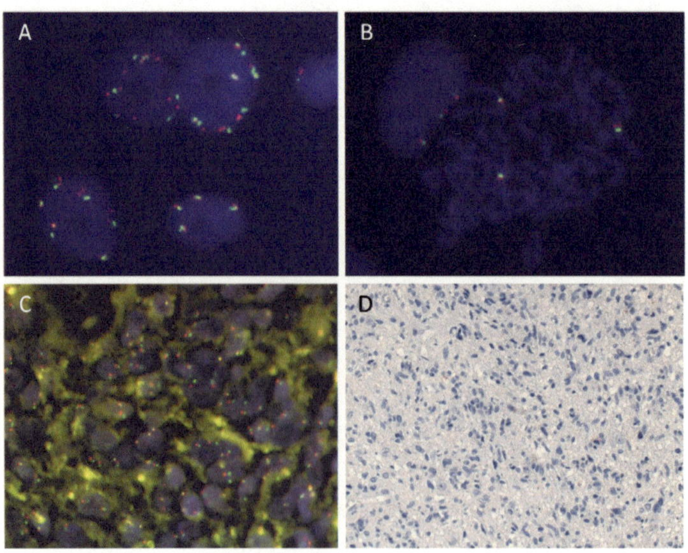

Fig. 11. No amplification of the *EGFR* present in GBM-n group. A) Different interphase nuclei of cultured cells showing no amplification. B) Metaphases spread with three centromeres of chromosome 7 and three copies of *EGFR*. C) Non-amplified tumoral cells of paraffin sections. D) No immunoexpression for EGFR

On the basis of these results, the model of amplification of group GBM-l could correspond to a variant of the distributed insertion mechanism, or a consequence of a process of duplication like the one demonstrated in neuroblastoma cell lines (Corvi et al., 1995), and we suggest that this mechanism could be considered as an early stage of amplification in glioblastoma. This hypothesis is corroborated by the findings of both status of amplification, dmin, and extra copies located in chromosome 7, in two cases. In glioblastomas, the cut-points that define amplification are controversial (Smith et al., 2001, Layfield et al., 2006), although the most commonly accepted criteria is that *EGFR* amplification exists when the EGFR gene/chromosome per cell ratio was ≥2, or ≥15 copies of *EGFR* per cell in ≥10% of analyzed cells (Capuzzo et al., 2005, Nagasaka et al., 2007).

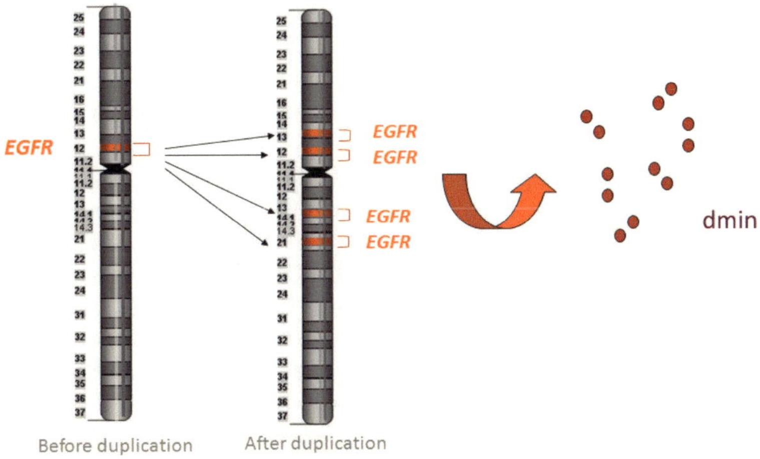

Fig. 12. Model of amplification of *EGFR* correspond to a variant of the distributed insertion mechanism.

In addition, there was considerable heterogeneity in the centromere 7 (CEP7) copy number in these tumors. The relationship between trisomy/polysomy of chromosome 7 and EGFR gene amplification has been analyzed. In our study, both amplified and non-amplified tumors showed trisomy/polysomy of chromosome 7. This fact suggests that this alteration could be an initial event in the tumorigenesis of glioblastoma.

Cases	Status *EGFR*	Copies *EGFR* (% cases)			CEP 7 (% cases)				% of cells		q-PCR	EGFR expression	
		2-10	6-25	25->100	dis	dis/tri	tri	tri/pol	1-20	25-95		0-1	2-3 (%cases)
46%	Amplification dmin	0	0	100	6	6	50	38	12	88	19-227.8	3	97
22%	Amplification insertion	0	100	0	10	30	30	30	80	20	3.3 - 7.2	69	31
32%	No amplification	100	0	0	8	0	46	46	-	-	2.1 -3.1	79	21

Table 3. Characterization of the three types of *EGFR* amplification found in glioblastoma

5.3 Statistical correlation of *EGFR* copy alterations with clinicopathological parameters

The Kruskal Wallis test was used to assess the differences among the three amplification groups and it showed significant differences in the percentage of cells with positive *EGFR* amplification detected by FISH, the *EGFR* copy number quantified by PCR, and the EGFR transcript expression assessed by microarrays (p-value ≤ 0.01). In the percentage of *EGFR* positive cells and *EGFR* copy number, all bilateral comparisons of the three amplification groups showed statistically significant differences, after the Bonferroni correction (GBM-h vs GBM-l, GBM-h vs GBM-n, GBM-l vs GBM-n) (p-value ≤ 0.01). The EGFR expression values of amplification types GBM-h and GBM-l were statistically significant after the Bonferroni correction (p-value ≤ 0.01). No significant differences were found between types GBM-l and GBM-n. The mean Ki-67 value of group GBM-h exhibited statistically significant differences with respect the rest (p-value < 0.05). Ki-67 mean values for the different groups were 38% for the GBM-h group, 24% for the GBM-l group and 23% for the GBM-n group.

None of the survival curves showed any significant differences in established groups according to *EGFR* amplification type, and age (<55, ≥55 years). As we expected, younger patients (<55 years) showed a slightly higher survival rate. Interestingly, patients with *EGFR* amplification type GBM-h survived for the shortest time, a mean of 9 months.

Amplification in general and amplicons in particular are important for both prognosis and targeted therapies. Specific amplicons, such as *MYCN* in neuroblastomas, and *MYC* and *ERBB2* in breast cancer, also have prognostic significance (Albertson, 2006). *EGFR* amplification status has been studied as a potential prognostic indicator. The majority of the early reports showed that amplification of the *EGFR* was associated with a poorer prognosis than that associated with non-amplified glioblastomas (Simmons et al., 2001, Shinojima et al., 2003). Other studies failed to confirm this relationship. Our study did not show that the type of *EGFR* amplification led to significant differences in survival rates; although, interestingly, patients of group GBM-h, with *EGFR* amplification type dmin survived for the shortest time.

6. Conclusion

Glioblastoma multiforme is characterized by intratumoral heterogeneity in both histomorphological and genetic changes, displaying a wide variety of numerical chromosome aberrations, the most common of which are trisomy 7 and monosomy 10. The amplification of the epidermal growth factor receptor (EGFR) gene is the most frequently reported genetic abnormality.

Our studies about histopathological and genetical characterization of glioblastoma multiforme suggest that, in primary glioblastomas, there exists a subgroup of cases closely linked with *EGFR* amplification. However, there is another subgroup of cases without *EGFR* amplification with some different clinical and genetic characteristics. This second group might include the increased activation or expression of other growth factor receptors observed in these tumors such as PDGFR or IGFR, although they are only amplified in a low percentage of cases.

Furthermore, we proposed that *EGFR* amplification is an important and frequent pathway in glioblastomas. This amplification is expressed as dmin in a subset of glioblastoma, but we have observed another type of amplification of the EGFR gene. This is seen at chromosome level as distributed insertions of this gene in chromosome 7 itself. Detection of this pattern of amplification of *EGFR* may further improve the prognostic value of genomic diagnosis of this disease.

Since amplification is often associated with poor prognosis and is a mechanism of resistance to therapies, it will be important to identify the genes or pathways (or both) that promote amplification in tumors, so that they might be targeted as part of a combination therapy to prevent the evolution of resistance to drugs designed to arrest or eradicate the tumor.

7. Acknowledgment

This work was supported by a grant from FIS PI020228, FEDER-FSE (2000-2006), FIS, PI061134 (2006-2009), SAF2008-00270, GV-AP119/10, ACOMP2011-237, and PROMETEO11/2011/083.

We thank Ana Clari, Mercedes Salinas, Eva Serna, and Jose Benavent for their technical assistance.

8. References

Albertson, DG. (2006). *Gene amplification in cancer.* Trends in Genetics, 22:447-455.

Amalfitano, G.; Chatel, M.; Paquis, P.; & Michiels, JF. (2000). *Fluorescence in situ hybridization study of aneuploidy of chromosomes 7, 10, X, and Y in primary and secondary glioblastomas.* Cancer Genet Cytogenet, 116:6-9.

Arnoldus, EP.; Wolters, LB.; Voormolen, JH.; van Duinen, SG.; Raap, AK.; van der Ploeg, M.; & Peters, AC. (1992). *Interphase cytogenetics: a new tool for the study of genetic changes in brain tumors.* J Neurosurg, 76:997-1003.

Arteaga, CL. (2002). *Epidermal growth factor receptor dependence in human tumors: more than just expression?* Oncologist, 7 Suppl 4:31-39.

Balana, C.; López-Pousa, A.; Berrocal, A.; Yaya-Tur, R.; Herrero, A.; Garcia, JL.; Martin-Broto, J.; Benavides, M.; Cerdá-Nicolás, M.; Ballester, R.; Balart, J.;& Capellades, J. (2004). *Phase II study of temozolomide and cisplatin as primary treatment prior to radiotherapy in newly diagnosed glioblastoma multiforme patients with measurable disease. A study of the Spanish Medical Neuro-Oncology Group (GENOM).* J Neurooncol, 70:359-369.

Benito, R.; Gil-Benso, R.; Quilis, V.; Pérez, V.; Gregori-Romero, M.; Roldan, P.; González-Darder, J.; Cerdá-Nicolás, M.; & López-Ginés, C. (2010). *Primary glioblastomas with and without EGFR amplification: relationship to genetic alterations and clinicopathological features.* Neuropathology. 30:392-400.

Beroukhim, R.; Ling, M.; Park, Y.; Hao, K.; Zhao, X.; Garraway, LA.; Fox, E.; Hochberg, EP.; Mellinghoff, IK.; Hofer, MD.; Descazeaud, A.; Rubin, MA.; Meyerson, M.; Sellers, WR.; & Li, C. (2006). *Inferreing LOH from Unpaired tumours using High Density Oligonucleotide SNP arrays.* PLoS Computational Biology, 2; 5.

Bigner, SH.; & Vogelstein, B. (1990). *Cytogenetics and molecular genetics of human brain tumors.* Brain Pathol, 1:12-18.

Bigner, SH.; Mark, J.; & Bigner DD. (1990). *Cytogenetics of human brain tumors.* Cancer Genet Cytogenet, 47:141-154.

Burger, PC.; Shibata, T.; & Kleihues, P. (1986). *The use of the monoclonal antibody Ki-67 in the identification of proliferating cells: application to surgical neuropathology.* Am J Surg Pathol, 10:611-617.

Canagarajah, BJ.; Khokhlatchev, A.; Cobb, MH.; & Goldsmith, EJ. (1997). *Activation mechanism of the MAP kinase ERK2 by dual phosphorylation.* Cell, 90:859-869.

Carpenter, G.; & Cohen, S. (1990). Epidermal growth factor. J Biol Chem, 265:7709-7712.

Collins, VP. (2002). *Cellular mechanisms targeted during astrocytoma progression.* Cancer Lett, 188:1-7.

Coquelle, A.; Pipiras, E.; Toledo, F.; Buttin, G.; & Debatisse, M. (1997). *Expression of fragile sites triggers intrachromosomal mammalian gene amplification and sets boundaries to early amplicons.* Cell, 89:215-225.

Corvi, R.; Savelyeva, L.; & Schwab, M. (1995). *Duplication of N-MYC at its resident site 2p24 may be a mechanism of activation alternative to amplification in human neuroblastoma cells.* Cancer Res, 55:3471-3474.

Dai, C.; & Holland, EC. (2001). *Glioma models.* Biochim Biophys Acta, 1551: M19-27.

Diedrich, U.; Lucius, J.; Baron, E.; Behnke, J.; Pabst, B.; & Zoll, B. (1995). *Distribution of epidermal growth factor receptor gene amplification in brain tumours and correlation to prognosis.* J Neurol, 242:683-688.

Dohrmann, GJ.; Farwell, JR.; & Flannery, JT. (1976). *Glioblastoma multiforme in children.* J Neurosurg, 44:442-448.

Dropcho, EJ.; & Soong, SJ. (1996). *The prognostic impact of prior low grade histology in patients with anaplastic gliomas: a case-control study.* Neurology, 47:684-690.

Ekstrand, AJ.; Longo, N.; Hamid, ML.; Olson, JJ.; Liu, L.; Collins, VP.; & James, CD. (1994). *Functional characterization of an EGF receptor with a truncated extracellular domain expressed in glioblastomas with EGFR gene amplification.* Oncogene, 9:2313-2320.

Ekstrand, A.J.; Sugawa, N.; James, CD.; & Collins, VP. (1992). *Amplified and rearranged epidermal growth factor receptor genes in human glioblastomas reveal deletions of sequences encoding portions of the N- and/or C-terminal tails.* Proc Natl Acad Sci U S A, 89:4309-4313.

Eley, G.; Frederick, L.; Wang, XY.; Smith, DI.; & James, CD. (1998). *3' end structure and rearrangements of EGFR in glioblastomas.* Genes Chromosomes Cancer, 23:248-254.

Frederick, L.; Eley, G.; Wang, XY.; & James, CD. (2000). Analysis of genomic rearrangements associated with EGRFvIII expression suggests involvement of Alu repeat elements. Neuro-oncol, 2:159-163.

Fujisawa, H.; Kurrer, M.; Reis, RM.; Yonekawa, Y.; Kleihues, P.; & Ohgaki H. (1999). *Acquisition of the glioblastoma phenotype during astrocytoma progression is associated with loss of heterozygosity on 10q25-qter.* Am J Pathol, 155:387-394.

Gil-Benso, R.; López-Ginés, C.; Benito, R.; López-Guerrero.; JA, Callaghan, RC.; Pellin, A.; Roldan, P.; & Cerdá-Nicolás, M. (2007). *Concurrent EGFR amplification and TP-53 mutation in glioblastomas.* Clin Neuropathol, 26(5):224-231.

Gisselsson, D.; Pettersson, L.; Hoglund, M.; Heidenblad, M.; Gorunova, L.; & Wiegant, J. (2000). *Chromosomal breakage-fusion-bridge events cause genetic intratumor heterogeneity.* Proc Natl Acad Sci USA, 97:5357-5362.

Heim, S.; Mandahl, N.; Jin, Y.; Stromblad, S.; Lindstrom, E.; Salford, LG.; & Mitelman, F. (1989). *Trisomy 7 and sex chromosome loss in human brain tissue.* Cytogenet Cell Genet, 52:136-138.

Hermanson, M.; Funa, K.; Hartman, M.; Claesson-Welsh, L.; Heldin, C. H.; Westermark, B.; & Nister, M. (1992). *Platelet-derived growth factor and its receptors in human glioma tissue: expression of messenger RNA and protein suggests the presence of autocrine and paracrine loops.* Cancer Res, 52:3213-3219.

Honda, R.; Tanaka, H.; & Yasuda, H. (1997). *Oncoprotein MDM2 is a ubiquitin ligase E3 for tumor suppressor p53.* FEBS Lett, 420:25-27.

Houillier, C. ; Lejeune, J. ; & Benouaich-Amiel, A. (2006). *Prognostic impact of molecular markers in a series of 220 primary glioblastomas.* Cancer, 106:2218-2223.

Hurtt, MR.; Moossy, J.; Donovan-Peluso, M.; & Locker, J. (1992). *Amplification of epidermal growth factor receptor gene in gliomas: histopathology and prognosis.* J Neuropathol Exp Neurol, 51:84-90.

Ichimura, K.; Schmidt, EE.; Goike, HM.; & Collins, VP. (1996). *Human glioblastomas with no alterations of the CDKN2A (p16INK4A, MTS1) and CDK4 genes have frequent mutations of the retinoblastoma gene.* Oncogene, 13:1065-1072.

ISCN 1995. *An International System for Human Cytogenetic Nomenclature.* ISBN: 978-3-8055-6226-3 Basel, Switzerland: Karger.

Jelinek, T.; Dent, P.; Sturgill, TW.; & Weber, MJ. (1996). *Ras-induced activation of Raf-1 is dependent on tyrosine phosphorylation.* Mol Cell Biol, 16:1027-1034.

Jelsma, R.; & Bucy, PC. (1969). *Glioblastoma multiforme: its treatment and some factors effecting survival.* Arch Neurol, 20:161-171.

Jenkins, RB.; Kimmel, DW.; Moertel, CA.; Schultz, CG.; Scheithauer, BW.; Kelly, PJ.; & Dewald, GW. (1989). *A cytogenetic study of 53 human gliomas.* Cancer Genet Cytogenet, 39:253-279.

Kallio, M.; Sankila, R.; Jaaskelainen, J.; Karjalainen, S.; & Hakulinen, TA. (1991). *Population-based study on the incidence and survival rates of 3857 glioma patients diagnosed from 1953 to 1984.* Cancer, 68:1394-1400.

Karamitopoulou, E.; Perentes, E.; Diamantis, I.; & Maraziotis, T. (1994). *Ki-67 immunoreactivity in human central nervous system tumors: a study with MIB 1 monoclonal antibody on archival material.* Acta Neuropathol (Berl), 87:47-54.

Karlbom, AE.; James, CD.; Boethius, J.; Cavenee, WK.; Collins, VP.; Nordenskjold, M.; Larsson, C. (1993). *Loss of heterozygosity in malignant gliomas involves at least three distinct regions on chromosome 10.* Hum Genet, 92:169-74

Kleihues, P.; & Ohgaki, H. (1997). *Genetics of glioma progression and the definition of primary and secondary glioblastoma.* Brain Pathol, 7:1131-1136.

Kleihues, P.; Louis, DN.; Scheithauer, BW.; Rorke, LB.; Reifenberger, G.; Burger, PC.; & Cavenee, WK. (2002). *The WHO classification of tumors of the nervous system.* J Neuropathol Exp Neurol, 61:215-225.

Kleihues, P.; Louis, DN.; Scheithauer, BW.; Rorke, LB.; Reifenberger, G.; Burger, PC.; & Cavenee, WK. (2002). *The WHO classification of tumors of the nervous system.* J Neuropathol Exp Neurol, 61: 215-225.

Knobbe, CB.; Merlo, A.; & Reifenberger, G. (2002). *Pten signaling in gliomas.* Neuro-oncol, 4: 196-211.

Kondo, I,; & Shimizu, N. (1983). *Mapping of the human gene for epidermal growth factor receptor (EGFR) on the p13 leads to q22 region of chromosome 7.* Cytogenet Cell Genet, 35:9-14.

Koschny, R.; Koschny, T.; Froster, UG.; Krupp, W.; & Zuber MA. (2002). *Comparative genomic hybridization in glioma: a meta-analysis of 509 cases.* Cancer Genet Cytogenet, 135:147-159.

Kuwahara, Y.; Tanabe, C.; Ikeuchi, T.; Aoyagi, K.; Nishigaki, M.; Sakamoto, H.; Hoshinaga. K.; Yoshida, T.; Sasaki, H.; & Terada, M. (2004). *Alternative mechanisms of gene amplification in human cancers.* Genes, Chromosomes & Cancer, 41:125-132.

Layfield, LJ.; Willmore, C.; Tripp, S.; Jones, C.; Jensen, RL. (2006). *Epidermal growth factor receptor gene amplification and protein expression in glioblastoma multiforme*. Appl Immunohistochem Mol Morphol, 14:91-96.

Li, C.; & Wong, WH. (2001a). *Model based analysis of oligonucleotide arrays: Expression index computation and outlier detection*. Proc. Natl Acad Sci, 98;31-36.

Li, C.; & Wong, WH. (2001b). *Model based analysis of oligonucleotide arrays: model validation, design issues and standard error application*. Li C. and Wong WH. Genome Biology, 2: 8-14.

Li, J.; Yen, C.; Liaw, D.; Podsypanina, K.; Bose, S.; Wang, SI.; Puc, J.; Miliaresis, C.; Rodgers, L.; McCombie, R.; Bigner, SH.; Giovanella, BC.; Ittmann, M.; Tycko, B.; Hibshoosh, H.; Wigler, MH.; & Parsons, R. (1997). *PTEN, a putative protein tyrosine phosphatase gene mutated in human brain, breast, and prostate cancer*. Science, 275:1943-1947.

Libermann, T.A.; Nusbaum, HR.; Razon, N.; Kris, R.; Lax, I.; Soreq, H.; Whittle, N.; Waterfield, MD.; Ullrich, A.; & Schlessinger, J. (1985). *Amplification and overexpression of the EGF receptor gene in primary human glioblastomas*. J Cell Sci Suppl, 3:161-172.

Lin, H.; Bondy, ML.; Langford, LA.; Hess, KR.; Delclos, GL.; Wu, X.; Chan, W.; Pershouse, MA.; Yung, WK.; & Steck, PA. (1998). *Allelic deletion analyses of MMAC/PTEN and DMBT1 loci in gliomas: relationship to prognostic significance.* Clin Cancer Res, 4:2447-2454.

Lin, M.; Wei, LJ.; Sellers, WR.; Lieberfarb, M.; Wong, WH.; & Li, C. (2004). *dChipPSNP: Significance curve and clustering of SNP-array-based loss-of-heterozigosity data*. Bioinformatics, 20:1233-1240.

Livak, KJ.; & Schmittgen, TD. (2001). *Analysis of Relative Gene Expression data using Real-Time Quantitative PCR and the* $2^{-\Delta\Delta Ct}$ *Method*. Methods, 25:402-408.

López-Ginés, C.; Cerdá-Nicolás, M.; Gil-Benso, R.; Pellin, A.; López-Guerrero, JA.; Callaghan, R.; Benito, R.; Roldan, P.; Piquer, J.; Llacer, J.; & Barberá, J. (2005). *Association of chromosome 7, chromosome 10 and EGFR gene amplification in glioblastoma multiforme*. Clin Neuropathol, 24:209-218.

López-Ginés, C.; Cerdá-Nicolás, M.; Gil-Benso, R.; Pellin, A.; López-Guerrero, JA.; Benito, R.; del Rey, J.; Miro, R.; Roldan, R.; & Barberá, J. (2006). *Primary glioblastoma with EGFR amplification and a ring chromosome 7 in a young patient.* Clin Neuropathol, 25 (4):193-199.

López-Ginés, C.; Gil-Benso, R.; Benito, R.; Mata, M.; Pereda, J.; Sastre, J.; Roldan, P.; Gonzalez-Darder, J.; & Cerdá-Nicolás, M. (2008). *The activation of ERK1/2 MAP kinases in glioblastoma pathobiology and its relationship with EGFR amplification*. Neuropathology, 28:507-515.

López-Ginés, C.; Gil-Benso, R.; Ferrer-Luna, R.; Benito, R.; Serna, E.; González-Darder, J.; Quilis, V.; Monleón, D.; Celda, B.; & Cerdá-Nicolás, M. (2010). *Novel pattern of EGFR amplification in glioblastoma and the relationship of gene copy number with gene expression profile*. Modern Pathology, 23:856-865.

Louis, D.; Ohgaki, H.; Wiestler, O.; & Cavenee, W. (2007). *WHO classification of tumors of the nervous system*. IARC, 4th edition.

Marquez, A.; Wu, R.; Zhao, J.; Tao, J.; & Shi, Z. (2004). *Evaluation of epidermal growth factor receptor (EGFR) by chromogenic in situ hybridization (CISH) and immunohistochemistry (IHC) in archival gliomas using bright-field microscopy*. Diagn Mol Pathol, 13:1-8.

Mitelman, F.; Johansson, B.; & Mertens, F. (2004) editors Mitelman *database of chromosome aberration in cancer*. http://cgap.ncbi.nih.gov/chromosomes/mitelman.

Mizoguchi, M.; Betensky, RA.; Batchelor, TT.; Bernay, DC.; Louis, DN.; & Nutt, CL. (2006). *Activation of STAT3, MAPK, and AKT in malignant astrocytic gliomas: correlation with EGFR status, tumor grade, and survival*. J Neuropathol Exp Neurol, 65:1181-1188.

Moertel, CA.; Dahl, RJ.; Stalboerger, PG.; Kimmel, DW.; Scheithauer, BW.; & Jenkins, RB. (1993). *Gliosis specimens contain clonal cytogenetic abnormalities*. Cancer Genet Cytogenet, 67:21-27.

Muleris, M.; Almeida, A.; Dutrillaux, AM.; Pruchon, E.; Vega, F.; Delattre, JY.; Poisson, M.; Malfoy, B.; & Dutrillaux, B. (1994). *Oncogene amplification in human gliomas: a molecular cytogenetic analysis*. Oncogene, 9:2717-2722.

Murnane, JP.; & Sabatier, L. (2004). *Chromosome rearrangements resulting from telomere dysfunction and their role in cancer*. Bioessays, 26:1164-1174.

Myllykangas, S.; & Knuutila, S. (2006). *Manifestation, mechanism and mysteries of gene amplifications*. Cancer Letters, 232:79-89.

Nagasaka, T., Gunji, M., & Hosokai, N. (2007). *FISH 1p/19q deletion/imbalance for molecular subclassification of glioblastoma*. Brain Tumor Pathol, 24:1-5.

Nakamura, M.; Watanabe, T.; Klangby, U.; Asker, C.; Wiman, K.; Yonekawa, Y.; Kleiues, P.; & Ohgaki, H. (2001). *p14ARF deletion and methylation in genetic pathways to glioblastomas*. Brain Pathol, 11:159-168.

Nishizaki, T.; Harada, K.; Kubota, H.; Furuya, T.; Suzuki, M.; & Sasaki, K. (2002). *Chromosome instability in malignant astrocytic tumors detected by fluorescence in situ hybridization*. J Neurooncol, 56:159-165.

Ohgaki, H.; & Kleihues, P. (2007). *Genetic pathways to primary and secondary glioblastoma*. The Am J Pathol, 170:1445-1453.

Ohgaki, H.; & Kleihues, P. (2005). *Population-based studies on incidence, survival rates, and genetic alterations in astrocytic and oligodendroglial gliomas*. J Neuropathol Exp Neurol, 64:479-489.

Ohgaki, H.; Dessen, P.; Jourde, B.; Horstmann, S.; Nishikawa, T.; Di Patre, PL.; Burkhard, C.; Schuler, D.; Probst-Hensch, NM.; Maiorka, PC.; Baeza, N.; Pisani, P.; Yonekawa, Y.; Yasargil, MG.; Lutolf, UM.; & Kleihues, P. (2004). *Genetic pathways to glioblastoma: a population-based study*. Cancer Res, 64:6892-6899.

Okada, Y.; Hurwitz, EE.; Esposito, JM.; Brower, MA.; Nutt, CL.; & Louis, DN. (2003). *Selection pressures of TP53 mutation and microenvironmental location influence epidermal growth factor receptor gene amplification in human glioblastomas*. Cancer Res, 63:413-416.

Park, S.; Hatanpaa, KJ.; Xie, Y.; Mickey, BE.; Madden, CJ.; Raisanen, JM.; Ramnarain, DB.; Xiao, G.; Saha, D.; Boothman, DA.; Zhao, D.; Bachoo, RM.; Pieper, RO.; & Habib, AA. (2009). *The receptor interacting protein 1 inhibits p53 induction through NF-kappaB activation and confers a worse prognosis in glioblastoma*. Cancer Res, 69(7):2809-2816.

Quelle, DE. ; Zindy, F. ; Ashmun, RA. ; & Sherr, CJ. (1995). *Alternative reading frames of the INK4a tumor suppressor gene encode two unrelated proteins capable of inducing cell cycle arrest*. Cell, 83:993-1000.

Rao, RD.; & James, CD. (2004). *Altered molecular pathways in gliomas: an overview of clinically relevant issues*. Semin Oncol, 31:595-604.

Reifenberger, G.; Reifenberger, J.; Ichimura, K.; Meltzer, PS.; & Collins, VP. (1994). *Amplification of multiple genes from chromosomal region 12q13-14 in human malignant gliomas: preliminary mapping of the amplicons shows preferential involvement of CDK4, SAS, and MDM2.* Cancer Res, 54:4299-4303.

Rey, JA.; Bello, MJ.; de Campos, JM.; Kusak, ME.; Ramos, C.; & Benitez, J. (1987). *Chromosomal patterns in human malignant astrocytomas.* Cancer Genet Cytogenet, 29:201-221.

Rollbrocker, B.; Waha, A.; Louis, DN.; Wiestler, OD.; & von Deimling, A. (1996). *Amplification of the cyclin-dependent kinase 4 (CDK4) gene is associated with high cdk4 protein levels in glioblastoma multiforme.* Acta Neuropathol (Berl), 92:70-74.

Roth, J.; Dobbelstein, M.; Freedman, DA.; Shenk, T.; & Levine, AJ. (1998). *Nucleo-cytoplasmic shuttling of the hdm2 oncoprotein regulates the levels of the p53 protein via a pathway used by the human immunodeficiency virus rev protein.* Embo J, 17:554-564.

Russell, DS.; & Rubinstein, LS. (1989). *Pathology of tumors of the nervous system.* ISBN 9780340581131, 5th ed. Baltimore: Williams & Williams.

Russell, DS.; & Rubinstein, LS. (2006). *Pathology of tumors of the nervous system.* ISBN 0340810076, 7th ed. London: Hodder Arnold.

Sant, M.; Crosignani, P.; Bordo, BM.; Nicola, G.; Bianchi, M.; & Berrino, F. (1988). *Incidence and survival of brain tumors: a population-based study.* Tumori, 74:243-252.

Sauter, G.; Maeda, T.; & Waldman, FM. (1996). *Short communication: Patterns of epidermal growth factor receptor amplification in malignant gliomas.* American Journal of Pathology, 148:1047-1053.

Scherer, HJ. (1940). *Cerebral astrocitomas and their derivatives.* Am J Cancer, 40: 159-198.

Schmitt, HP. (1983). *Rapid anaplastic transformation in gliomas of adulthood. "Selection" in neuro-oncogenesis.* Pathol Res Pract, 176: 313-323.

Schwab, M. (1998). *Amplification of oncogenes in human cancer cells.* Bioessays, 20:99-102.

Schwab, M. (1999). *Oncogene amplification in solid tumors.* Cancer Biology, 9:319-325.

Schwab, M. (2004). MYCN in neuronal tumours. Cancer Letters 204:179-187.

Shinojima, N.; Tada, K.; Shiraishi, S.; Kamiryo, T.; Kochi, M.; Nakamura, H.; Makino, K.; Saya, H.; Hirano, H.; Kuratsu, J.; Oka, K.; Ishimaru, Y.; & Ushio, Y. (2003). *Prognostic value of epidermal growth factor receptor in patients with glioblastoma multiforme.* Cancer Res, 63:6962-6970.

Simmons, ML.; Lamborn, KR.; Takahashi, M.; Chen, P.; Israel, MA.; Berger, MS.; Godfrey, T.; Nigro, J.; Prados, M.; Chang, S.; Baeker, FG.; & Aldape, K. (2001). *Analysis of complex relationships between age, p53, epidermal growth factor receptor, and survival in glioblastoma patients.* Cancer Res, 61:1122-1128.

Smith, JS.; Tachibana, I.; Pohl, U.; Lee, HK.; Thanarajasingam, U.; Portier, BP.; Ueki, K.; Ramaswamy, S.; Billings, SJ.; Mohrenweiser, HW.; Louis, DN.; & Jenkins, RB. (2001). *PTEN mutation, EGFR amplification, and outcome in patients with anaplastic astrocytoma and glioblastoma multiforme.* J Natl Cancer Inst, 93:1246-1256.

Steilen-Gimbel, H.; Henn, W.; Kolles, H.; Moringlane, JR.; Feiden, W.; Steudel, WI.; & Zang, KD. (1996). *Early proliferation enhancement by monosomy 10 and intratumor heterogeneity in malignant human gliomas as revealed by smear preparations from biopsies.* Genes Chromosomes Cancer, 16:180-184.

Stott, FJ.; Bates, S.; James, MC.; McConnell, BB.; Starborg, M.; Brookes, S.; Palmero, I.; Ryan, K.; Hara, E.; Vousden, KH.; & Peters, G. (1998). *The alternative product from the human CDKN2A locus, p14(ARF), participates in a regulatory feedback loop with p53 and MDM2.* Embo J, 17:5001-5014.

Sugawa, N.; Ekstrand, AJ.; James, CD.; & Collins, VP. (1990). *Identical splicing of aberrant epidermal growth factor receptor transcripts from amplified rearranged genes in human glioblastomas.* Proc Natl Acad Sci U S A, 87: 8602-8606.

Sugawa, N.; Yamamoto, K.; Ueda, S.; Morita, N.; Kita, M.; Nishino, H.; Fushiki, S.; & Okabe, T. (1998). *Function of aberrant EGFR in malignant gliomas.* Brain Tumor Pathol, 15:53-57.

Tada, K.; Shiraishi, S.; Kamiryo, T.; Nakamura, H.; Hirano, H.; Kuratsu, J.; Kochi, M.; Saya, H.; & Ushio, Y. (2001). *Analysis of loss of heterozygosity on chromosome 10 in patients with malignant astrocytic tumors: correlation with patient age and survival.* J Neurosurg, 95:651-659.

TCGA (The Cancer Genome Atlas Research Network). *Comprehensive genomic characterization defines human glioblastoma genes and core pathways.* (2008). Nature, 455:1061-1068.

Thiel, G.; Losanowa, T.; Kintzel, D.; Nisch, G.; Martin, H.; Vorpahl, K.; & Witkowski, R. (1992). Karyotypes in 90 human gliomas. Cancer Genet Cytogenet, 58:109-120.

Toledo, F.; Le Roscouet, D. ; Buttin, G. ; & Debatisse, M. (1992). *Co-amplified markers alternate in megabase long chromosomal inverted repeats and cluster independently in interphase nuclei at early steps of mammalian gene amplification.* Eur Mol Biol Org J, 11:2665-2673.

Ullrich, A.; & Schlessinger, J. (1990). *Signal transduction by receptors with tyrosine kinase activity.* Cell, 61:203-212.

Varela, M.; Ranuncolo, S. M.; Morand, A.; Lastiri, J.; De Kier Joffe, EB.; Puricelli, LI.; & Pallotta, MG. (2004). *EGF-R and PDGF-R, but not bcl-2, overexpression predict overall survival in patients with low-grade astrocytomas.* J Surg Oncol, 86:34-40.

Vogt, N.; Lefèvre, SH.; Apiou, F.; Dutrillaux, AM.; Cör, A.; Leuraud, P.; Poupon, MF.; Dutrillaux, B.; Debatisse, M.; & Malfoy, B. (2004). *Molecular structure of double-minute chromosomes bearing amplified copies of the epidermal growth factor receptor gene in gliomas.* PNAS, 101:11368-11373.

Walker, MD.; Alexander, E.Jr.; Hunt, WE.; MacCarty, CS.; Mahaley, MS.Jr.; Mealey, J.Jr.; Norrell, HA.; Owens, G.; Ransohoff, J.; Wilson, CB.; Gehan, EA.; & Strike, TA. (1978). *Evaluation of BCNU and/or radiotherapy in the treatment of anaplastic gliomas. A cooperative clinical trial.* J Neurosurg, 49:333-343.

Walker, MD.; Green, SB.; Byar, DP.; Alexander, E.Jr.; Batzdorf, U.; Brooks, WH.; Hunt, WE.; MacCarty, CS.; Mahaley, MS.Jr.; Mealey, J.Jr.; Owens, G.; Ransohoff, J. 2nd; Robertson, JT.; Shapiro, WR.; Smith, KR.Jr.; Wilson, CB.; & Strike, TA. (1980). *Randomized comparisons of radiotherapy and nitrosoureas for the treatment of malignant glioma after surgery.* N Engl J Med, 303:1323-1329.

Wang, XY.; Smith, DI.; Frederick, L.; & James, CD. (1998). *Analysis of EGF receptor amplicons reveals amplification of multiple expressed sequences.* Oncogene, 16:191-195.

Watanabe, K.; Tachibana, O.; Yonekawa, Y.; Kleihues, P.; & Ohgaki, H. (1997a). *Role of gemistocytes in astrocytoma progression.* Lab Invest, 76:277-284.

Wernicke, C.; Thiel, G.; Lozanova, T.; Vogel, S.; & Witkowski, R. (1997). *Numerical aberrations of chromosomes 1, 2, and 7 in astrocytomas studied by interphase cytogenetics.* Genes Chromosomes Cancer, 19:6-13

Wikstrand, CJ.; Reist, CJ.; Archer, GE.; Zalutsky, MR.; & Bigner, DD. (1998). *The class III variant of the epidermal growth factor receptor (EGFRvIII): characterization and utilization as an immunotherapeutic target.* J Neurovirol, 4:148-158.

Wong, AJ.; Ruppert, JM.; Bigner, SH.; Grzeschik, CH.; Humphrey, PA.; Bigner, DS.; & Vogelstein, B. (1992). *Structural alterations of the epidermal growth factor receptor gene in human gliomas.* Proc Natl Acad Sci USA, 89:2965-2969.

Yoon, KS.; Lee, MC.; Kang, SS.; Kim, JH.; Jung, S.; Kim,YJ.; Lee JH.; Ahn, KY.; Lee, JS.; & Cheon, JY. (2001) *p53 mutation and epidermal growth factor receptor overexpression in glioblastoma.* J Korean Med Sci, 16:481-488.

Yung, W.K.; Albright, RE.; Olson, J.; Fredericks, R.; Fink, K.; Prados, MD.; Brada, M.; Spence, A.; Hohl, RJ.; Shapiro, W.; Glantz, M.; Greenberg, H.; Selker, RG.; Vick, NA.; Rampling, R.; Friedman, H.; Phillips, P.; Bruner, J.; Yue, N.; Osoba, D.; Zaknoen, S.; & Levin, VA. (2000). *A phase II study of temozolomide vs. procarbazine in patients with glioblastoma multiforme at first relapse.* Br J Cancer, 83: 588-593.

24

Nuclear Signaling of EGFR and EGFRvIII in Glioblastoma

Anupama E. Gururaj, Oliver Bögler and Khatri Latha
Department of Neurosurgery, University of Texas M. D. Anderson Cancer Center, Houston, Texas, USA

1. Introduction

The pivotal role of kinases in signal transduction and cellular regulation has lent them considerable appeal as therapeutic targets across a broad spectrum of cancers. The epidermal growth factor receptor (EGFR) was the first receptor tyrosine kinase to be discovered and remains the most investigated. Most of the mechanistic principles of receptor tyrosine kinases were first established with the EGFR family as a model. EGFR is a single pass transmembrane receptor with two extracellular, cysteine-rich regions involved in ligand binding, and intervening region important for receptor dimerization, an intracellular tyrosine kinase domain, and a number of intracellular sites for autophosphorylation, phosphorylation by other kinases, and docking of signaling components. Three additional EGFR family members have been identified, human epidermal growth factor receptor (erbB or HER) 2, 3 and 4. In many cell types, including those of epithelial and mesenchymal lineages, receptors of the HER family transduce signals from the cell surface to the intracellular domain, regulating normal cell growth, lineage determination, repair and functional differentiation. A range of growth factors serves as ligands for these receptors, although none have been identified for the HER2 receptor. Ligands for HER1/EGFR include epidermal growth factor (EGF) and transforming growth factor-α (TGF-α), and heregulins serve as ligands for both HER3 and HER4. Binding of a ligand to a HER family member leads to receptor homodimerization, or heterodimerization with another HER receptor, bringing about receptor phosphorylation. Ligand binding to HER1, HER3 or HER4 induces rapid receptor dimerization, with a marked preference for HER2 as a partner(Graus-Porta et al., 1997). Moreover, HER2-containing heterodimers generate intracellular signals that are significantly more potent than signals emanating from other HER combinations. Of the receptor dimers, HER3 homodimers cannot initiate signal transduction.The differing signaling characteristics of the HER family members are thought to be due to their different ligand-binding affinities and the type of phosphorylated homo- or heterodimer formed, and the resulting intracellular signaling events. Two of the key pathways involved in this cascade are the ras-raf-mitogen-activated protein kinase (MAPK) pathway, which affects DNA synthesis and cell proliferation, and the phosphatidylinositol 3-kinase (PI3-K)/Akt pathway, which plays a role in cell metabolism and survival (Yarden and Sliwkowski, 2001; Bange et al., 2001).

Functional dysregulation of the EGFR family is frequently observed in human cancers, suggesting that its signal modulates processes that play a pivotal role in tumorigenesis and disease progression. Activating mutations, gene amplification and overexpression of HER family kinases have been implicated as integral contributors to a variety of epithelial cancers, including breast, colon, pancreas, lung, and squamous cancers and also glioblastomas(Yarden, 2001; Foley et al., 2010; Yarom and Jonker, 2011; Wheeler et al., 2010; Dobashi et al., 2011; Machiels and Schmitz, 2011; Hwang, 2008). This is highlighted by HER1/EGFR overexpression or activation by autocrine or paracrine growth factor loops in at least 50% of epithelial malignancies, HER2 amplification and overexpression in approximately 20-25% of breast cancers and variable HER3 and HER4 expression in breast and other cancers. Overexpression and/or activation of HER1/EGFR, HER2/neu and HER3 have been correlated with poor prognosis. In contrast, it is unclear whether HER4 induces cell division or differentiation, and there is controversy regarding its role in breast cancer, with conflicting reports associating overexpression with shorter or prolonged survival (Normanno et al., 2006). Therefore, attenuation of HER family signaling is a developing strategy for the management of human malignancies and is the subject of a number of ongoing clinical trials.

Signaling from the plasma membrane by receptor tyrosine kinases (RTKs) to initiate downstream events that bring about their biological effects is well established. In the past decade, it has become increasingly apparent that several RTKs also move to several intracellular compartments, with nuclear localization in many cases being necessary for full function of the receptors. Access to the inside of the cell by the RTKs has in fact been shown to contribute to genesis and progression of a variety of human tumors (Carpenter, 2003). Accruing evidence points to a scenario where nuclear localization of EGFR in different tumor types has impact on not only the tumor grade but also on the resistance of tumors to therapies (Lo et al., 2006b; Wang and Hung, 2009). Here we critically evaluate the existing literature regarding intracellular localization of EGFR and its importance to cancer, and discuss future directions for the field. Further, the opportunity for targeting nuclear translocation of EGFR to develop therapeutics for intervention during critical stages of development and progression of neoplasms should be evaluated. There are numerous excellent recent reviews of HER family biology, signaling and therapeutic targeting (Yarden, 2001; Yarden and Sliwkowski, 2001; Foley et al., 2010; Yarom and Jonker, 2011; Wheeler et al., 2010; Hwang, 2008). This chapter will provide an overview of aberrant EGFR signaling in the biology of gliomas highlighting several key developments in the rapidly evolving area of HER family biology with specific reference to new localization of EGFR and the integral role of these receptors in malignant transformation and as targets of cancer therapy specifically in glioblastomas.

2. EGFR in glioma

Although a large number of other genetic alterations also occur in GBM, EGFR represents the most frequently amplified gene (2008; Hatanpaa et al., 2010). In fact, in primary GBM, it has been noted for about two decades and confirmed recently with two large-scale cancer genomics studies that EGFR amplification and mutation is a recurrent occurrence, being detected in about 40% of the samples (2008; Parsons et al., 2008). However, this is a rare event in low-grade gliomas (Ohgaki and Kleihues, 2007), suggesting a causal role for aberrant EGFR signaling in the pathogenesis of primary GBM. The resulting dysregulation of the signal transduction process affects gene transcription and protein translation, stimulating tumor cell proliferation, tumorigenesis, migration, adhesion and angiogenesis, and inhibiting apoptosis (Huang et al., 2009). Recent research has shown an unfavorable prognostic relationship between EGFR amplification and overall survival in patients with GBM (Aldape et al., 2004; Heimberger et al., 2005; Pelloski et al., 2007). EGFR expression is also associated with enhanced resistance to radiation in malignant GBM cells *in vitro* and is correlated with poor radiographic response to radiation therapy in some patients with GBM (Nakamura, 2007; Hatanpaa et al., 2010). EGFR dysregulation in GBM result from a number of different mechanisms. Primarily, gene amplification causes EGFR overexpression, which correlates with disease progression, poor prognosis and reduced sensitivity to chemotherapy. In addition, overproduction of EGFR ligands, such as TGF-α and EGF can cause autocrine receptor activation, enhancing transformation and leading to independent tumor cell growth. Further, activating mutations in EGFR generates EGFR mutants that demonstrate constitutive activity resulting in activation of the downstream intracellular cascade without ligand binding and insensitivity to regulation by normal cellular controls (Hwang, 2008).

While there are various mutant forms of EGFR in GBM, the most prevalent and well studied EGFR mutation is EGFRvIII (Hwang, 2008). EGFRvIII is detected in about half of all tumors with EGFR amplification (Aldape et al., 2004; Heimberger et al., 2005). Immunohistochemical and quantitative PCR studies of human GBM biopsies suggest that in most tumors the overexpression or amplification of EGFRvIII occurs concurrently with that of EGFR. Only in about 10% of glioblastomas does overexpression or amplification of EGFRvIII exceed that of the wild-type receptor (Sugawa et al., 1990; Furnari et al., 2007). In addition to GBM, EGFRvIII has been detected in several human cancers including NSCLC and breast carcinomas (Moscatello et al., 1995; Ge et al., 2002; Ji et al., 2006; Sasaki et al., 2007). Structurally, EGFRvIII exhibits a large inframe deletion of the extracellular ligand binding domain which results from the elimination of a 801 base pair (nucleotide positions 275–1075) DNA fragment containing exons 2–7 of the gene (Sugawa et al., 1990; Ekstrand et al., 1991; Wong et al., 1992; Frederick et al., 2000). This partial deletion of the ligand-binding domain renders EGFRvIII ligand insensitive and also constitutively activated. The ability of this variant to 'switch on' cell signaling without ligand stimulation, albeit at low levels, results in increased oncogenic signaling and aggressive behavior in tumors that express it (Huang et al., 1997; Nishikawa et al., 1994; Chu et al., 1997). Further, it has a low rate of receptor endocytosis, so is not readily attenuated and/or down-regulated (Chu et al., 1997; Huang et al., 1997). EGFRvIII correlates with advanced disease and resistance to therapy (Hwang, 2008). Several studies have found that it enhances tumorigenicity in human glioma xenografts in mice. The introduction of EGFRvIII into glioma cells enhances tumorigenicity, proliferation, migration, and inhibits apoptosis (Huang et al., 1997; Nagane et al., 1996; Nagane et al., 2001). In a transgenic mouse model, EGFRvIII was found to contribute to glioma progression in the presence of other predisposing genetic changes, such as mutated RAS, but failed to initiate tumors on its own (Holland et al., 1998; Bachoo et al., 2002; Ding et al., 2003). Furthermore, there is growing evidence from *in vitro* studies in human glioblastoma cells, human tumor xenografts in animal models, and in patients with GBM, to suggest that EGFRvIII promotes tumor growth and progression in part via constitutive activation of the phosphatidylinositol 3-kinase (PI3K)/Akt pathway (Choe et al., 2003; Aldape et al., 2004; Mizoguchi et al., 2006; Pedersen et al., 2005; Huang et al., 2007). The role of the mitogen-activated protein kinase (MAPK)/ERK 1/2 signal transduction pathway downstream of EGFRvIII is still unclear. Constitutive activity as well as impaired attenuation has been implicated as mechanisms for the enhancement of human glioblastoma cell tumorigenicity by EGFRvIII as compared to wild-type EGFR. Further, it has been recently demonstrated that EGFRvIII overexpression results in secretion of IL-6 and other cytokines to potentiate tumorigenesis in a paracrine manner (Inda et al., 2010). These data may explain the observation that patients with EGFRvIII-expressing tumors have a shorter interval to clinical relapse and poorer survival than patients with EGFRvIII-negative tumors. For GBM patients who survive 1 year or longer after diagnosis, the expression of EGFRvIII is also an independent negative prognostic indicator of survival (Aldape et al., 2004; Heimberger et al., 2005; Pelloski et al., 2007), which makes EGFRvIII an ideal target for antitumor therapy.

Signaling pathways are complex, multidimensional events that frequently converge, diverge, and cross talk with one another. The traditional cellular functions of EGFR and EGFRvIII has been reviewed elsewhere; this review focuses specifically on the role played by EGFR and EGFRvIII in the nuclear compartment as well as its nuclear downstream effectors in a number of human malignancies, and the possible novel therapeutic opportunities provided for development of anti-tumor agents.

3. EGFR/EGFRvIII in mitochondria

In the past decade, it has become increasingly apparent that several RTKs, including EGFR act also from intracellular organelles wherein they elicit biological effects that are uniquely distinct from their cell-surface functions. In addition to translocation to the nucleus (which is described in detail in the next sections), EGFR also localizes to the mitochondria, where it interacts with COXII and regulates cell survival in an EGFR Tyr845-dependent manner (Boerner et al., 2004). Src can activate EGFR by phosphorylating it on the Tyr845 and interestingly, the kinetics of mitochrondrial localization of both EGFR and Src (which also undergoes mitochondrial import) seem to be similar suggesting that they might translocate in the same complex (Demory et al., 2009). While the complete mechanism by which EGFR translocates to the mitochondria has not yet been defined, a recent investigation revealed that both EGFR and Src kinase activity was essential for mitochondrial translocation. Further, the same group identified that a mitochondrial localization signal in the juxtamembrane region of EGFR (residues 645 to 666) as well as the endocytic pathway are important for the movement of EGFR to the mitochondrion (Demory et al., 2009). Since the fusion of endosomes with mitochondria has not been demonstrated, the actual process by which endosomal EGFR moves to the mitochondria is still open to investigation. However, it was also shown that EGFR interacted with Tom40 (Demory et al., 2009), the pore component of the TOM complex and an outer mitochondrial membrane transport protein that is necessary for transport of newly synthesized mitochondrial proteins encoded by nuclear DNA. This suggests that EGFR could utilize the TOM complex to enter the mitochondria. Further, a report also demonstrated that EGFR translocates to the mitochondrion during autophagy where it again promoted cell survival (Yue et al., 2008), implying that mitochondrial localization of EGFR could potentially be an important survival strategy for cells. The same study showed that EGFR mitochondrial translocation can be increased by the mTOR inhibitor, rapamycin, and decreased by the topoisomerase inhibitor, etoposide, and by 3'-methyladenine, an inhibitor of autophagy. The reported link between autophagy and mitochondrial EGFR is particularly interesting due to the recent observation that apoptotic stress induces EGFR mitochondrial transport. Given the pivotal role that mitochondria plays in intrinsic apoptosis, a study by Cao et al (Cao et al., 2011) show that not only EGFR but EGFRvIII can also translocate to the mitochondria when induced by apoptosis-inducing agents and EGFR kinase inhibitors(Iressa) and that tumor cells with accumulated mitochondrial EGFRvIII are resistant to apoptosis induced by these agents. These results implicate mitochondrial EGFR/EGFRvIII in the modulation of mitochondria-mediated apoptosis. Taken together these studies suggest that tumor cells re-program their intracellular trafficking of EGFR/EGFRvIII by increasing its mitochondrial accumulation, as a mechanism for escape from therapy- and stress-induced apoptosis and growth suppression.

4. EGFR in the nuclear compartment

In addition to ligand recognition, binding, and initiation of intracellular signaling cascades, receptor tyrosine kinases such as the EGFR family have newly emerging roles in the regulation of nuclear functions through their direct translocation to the cell nucleus. Broadly speaking two kinds of nuclear translocation have been identified: EGFR, HER2 and HER3 have been found as full-length proteins in the nuclear compartment and this will be our focus here; in contrast HER4 nuclear translocation and transactivation functions occur through a separate mechanism involving cleavage by matrix metalloprotease of the extracellular domain upon receptor activation, and cleavage of the intracellular domain by gamma secretase, releasing a protein fragment that translocates to the nucleus (Carpenter, 2003). This carboxyl-terminal HER4 fragment then associates with the WW-domain-containing transcriptional regulatory protein YAP (Yes-associated protein) and acts as a co-transcriptional activator (Ni et al., 2001). The physiological and clinical importance of nuclear EGFR has been underscored by the observation that presence of EGFR in the nuclear compartment in tumor biopsies correlates strongly with poor prognosis and resistance to standard treatment modalities (Wang and Hung, 2009).

4.1 Nuclear localization and function

Almost two decades of research have documented the presence of EGFR and its ligand EGF in the nucleus. Early studies focused on EGF localization and demonstrated that nuclear presence of intact EGF was dependent on the expression of EGFR (Rakowicz-Szulczynska et al., 1986; Rakowicz-Szulczynska et al., 1989). The use of labeled EGF enabled definitive documentation that nuclear EGF was derived from extracellularly added ligand (Rakowicz-Szulczynska et al., 1989). The same studies demonstrated that the nuclear membranes and isolated chromatin contained EGFR which was indistinguishable from plasma membrane localized EGFR both biochemically and immunologically (Rakowicz-Szulczynska et al., 1989; Oksvold et al., 2002; Cao et al., 1995; Marti et al., 1991; Marti and Wells, 2000). Further, EGF could stimulate phosphorylation of nuclear EGFR and other nuclear proteins in isolated nuclei and nuclear membranes, and could be specifically inhibited by monoclonal antibodies directed against the extracellular domain of cell surface EGFR (Holt et al., 1994).
In normal tissues, nuclear expression of EGFR has been shown to be associated with the acquisition of proliferative capabilities of the cell. In hepatocytes which start proliferating after hepatectomy, nuclear EGFR was detected. In contrast, quiescent hepatocytes did not show nuclear EGFR (Marti et al., 1991). EGFR was also identified in the nucleus of mouse

lung epithelial cells where it was shown to respond to neuregulin stimulation(Zscheppang et al., 2006). Additionally, functional nuclear EGFR was demonstrated in human placenta where its role as a transcription factor was put forth (Cao et al., 1995). Further, nuclear localization of EGFR was demonstrated in primary human umbilical venous endothelial cells (HUVEC) and arterial endothelial cells (HUAEC) derived from early fetal gestation (Bueter et al., 2006).

Three basic functions of nuclear EGFR have been defined thus far (Figure 1). They are

1. gene regulation/transactivation,
2. tyrosine phosphorylation of target proteins and
3. protein-protein interactions leading to DNA repair

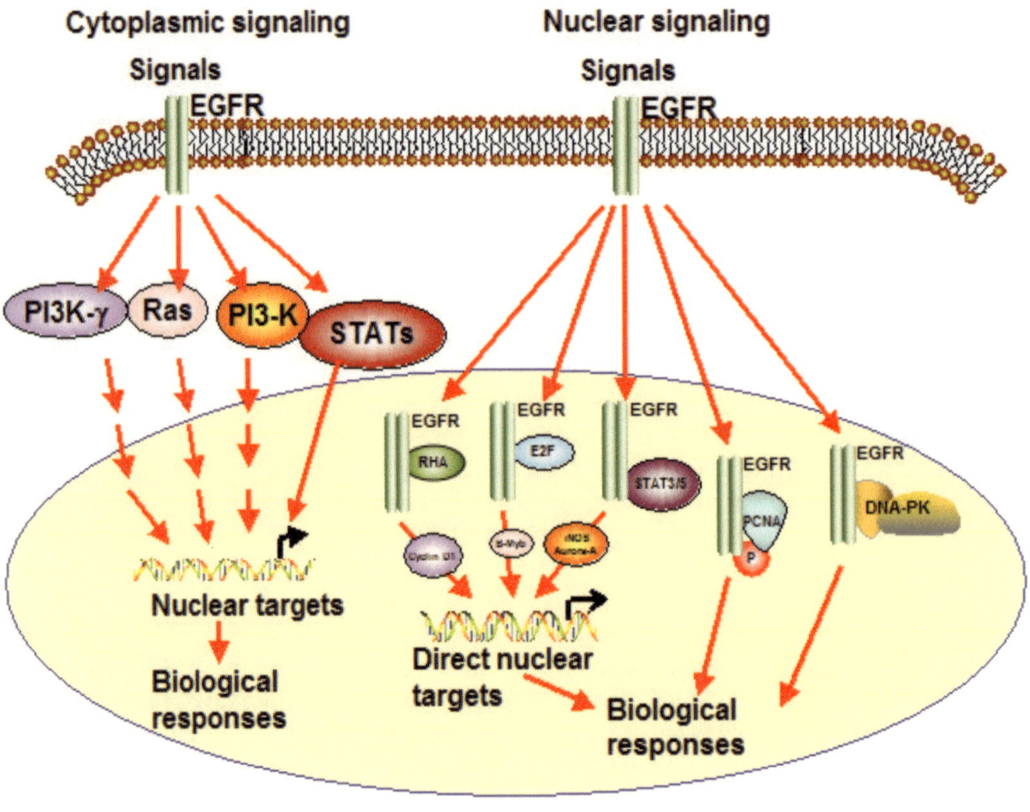

Fig. 1. Schematic representation of nuclear functions of EGFR. The cartoon shows both traditional cytoplasmic signaling eliciting nuclear effects as well as the more recently identified nuclear translocation and direct nuclear effects. Adapted from (Lo et al., 2006c)

4.1.1 Regulation of transcription

Although nuclear localization and potential transcriptional activity of EGFR had been noted in previous publications, Lin et al. demonstrated for the first time the presence of a strong transactivation domain in the C-terminal Pro-rich domain of EGFR, which mediated nuclear transactivation functions in a sequence-specific fashion (Lin et al., 2001). Although an EGFR mutant which lacked the transmembrane domain could also translocate to the nucleus, this movement required both wild type EGFR and active ligand signaling (Marti and Wells, 2000). Upon ligand stimulation, EGFR translocated to the nucleus and associated with an A/T-rich sequence (ATRS) in the cyclin D1 promoter, resulting in transcriptional activation of cyclin D1. This study thus defined a direct link between nuclear EGFR function and cell proliferation specifically in tumors (Lin et al., 2001). Interestingly, it had been shown about a decade earlier that for induction of a mitogenic response, amphiregulin, one of the ligands of EGFR, had to undergo nuclear translocation where it bound to AT-rich DNA sequences (Kimura, 1993). Since EGFR lacks a putative DNA-binding domain, the wide-held idea in the field is that EGFR first associates with DNA-binding transcription factors and then enhances target gene transcription via their intrinsic transactivational activity. Another mechanism underlying nuclear EGFR-mediated gene regulation could be attributed to its interaction with mucin 1 (MUC1) wherein there is increased accumulation of chromatin-bound EGFR on cyclin D1 promoter and significant co-localization with phosphorylated RNA polymerase II, a marker of active transcription (Bitler et al., 2010). A recent study showed that EGFR was also able to associate with ATRS sites on DNA by association with RNA helicase A (RHA), a DNA and RNA binding protein (Huo et al., 2010). This association was found to be absolutely necessary for EGFR recruitment to the ATRS site of cyclin D1 promoter and partially necessary for recruitment onto another ATRS-containing promoter of inducible nitric oxide synthase (iNOS) gene (Huo et al., 2010). The partial role of RHA in EGFR regulation of iNOS could be because nuclear EGFR has been shown to get recruited to iNOS promoter via physical protein-protein interaction with the well characterized transcription factor, signal transducer and activator of transcription 3 (STAT3) (Lo et al., 2005a). Physical interaction and functional cooperation of EGFR with STAT3 at the cytoplasmic level is very well characterized. According to this classical model, active EGFR at the plasma membrane binds to the SH2 domain of STAT3, via the two docking autophosphorylated tyrosines (Tyr1068 and Tyr1086)(Shao et al., 2003). This interaction leads to the phosphorylation of STAT3 at Tyr705 and its activation. The dimeric STAT complex translocates to the nucleus, where it binds to specific DNA promoter sequences, recruits other transcriptional regulators, and activates the transcription of multiple genes important for cell survival (Shao et al., 2003). However, data now show that EGFR can interact with STAT3 in the nucleus where they form a complex that functions as a transcriptional activator for the iNOS gene (Lo et al., 2005a) and the Cox-2 gene (Lo et al., 2010), allowing for the possibility that STAT activation is not an exclusively plasma membrane/cytosolic event. Further, iNOS gene expression was also induced by nuclear EGFR in reactive astrocytes of human glaucomatous optic nerve head, implying an important role for nuclear EGFR in other diseases besides cancers (Liu and Neufeld, 2003). Furthermore, cooperation of nuclear EGFR with the transcription factor E2F1 activates expression of B-Myb, a positive regulator of G1/S cell-cycle progression (Hanada et al., 2006). Thus, B-Myb joins cyclin D1 as another transcriptional target of nuclear EGFR that promotes cell proliferation.

Another member of the STAT family that associates with EGFR in both the cytoplasmic and nuclear compartment is STAT5. There are two STAT5 proteins, STAT5A and STAT5B, which are encoded by two distinct but closely related genes. STAT5A has a higher DNA-binding affinity than STAT5B, and it is mostly involved in prolactin-directed mammary gland maturation (Grimley et al., 1999), whereas STAT5B is believed to be involved in the response to the growth hormone. Similar to STAT3, unphosphorylated STAT5 is present in the nucleus and cytoplasm, and it constitutively shuttles in and out of the nucleus (Zheng et al., 2002). The N terminus is required for the constitutive nuclear import of STAT5, although the precise nature of its nuclear import domain remains to be determined. Following tyrosine phosphorylation, STAT5 accumulates in the nucleus where it induces its biological effects by transcriptional control of target genes (Debierre-Grockiego, 2004). As observed with STAT3, EGFR interacts with STAT5 on the ATRS motif to transactivate the Aurora-A promoter . Increased expression of the Aurora-A gene induced centrosome amplification and microtubule disorder (Hung et al., 2008). Further, studies from our laboratory have shown that EGFR can also associate with STAT5b to regulate Bcl-XL expression (Latha et. al., manuscript in preparation). Our study also showed a significant correlation between phosphoSTAT5b and EGFR expression in human GBMs. Furthermore, semi-quantitative scoring showed that patients whose tumors had detectable phosphoSTAT5 had a worse clinical outcome when compared to patients whose tumors had no detectable phosphoSTAT5 (Latha et. al., manuscript in preparation).

4.1.2 Nuclear substrates of EGFR

That the nucleus is an important site of direct action on the part of EGFR is supported by studies showing that exogenously added EGF can stimulate autophosphorylation of the EGFR, along with stimulation of phosphorylation of other non-EGF-binding proteins in isolated nuclei and nuclear membranes (Holt et al., 1994). Further, use of monoclonal antibody directed against the extracellular domain of EGFR inhibited the phosphorylation induced by EGF in isolated nuclei (Holt et al., 1994; Cao et al., 1995). Thus, apart from functioning as a transcriptional coregulator to modulate gene expression, the regulated kinase activity of EGFR in the nucleus can control the activation state of nuclear factors and thereby gene expression as well as other functions of such nuclear factors. The only direct nuclear substrate identified thus far is proliferating cell nuclear antigen (PCNA) (Wang et al., 2006). Wang et al. showed that nuclear EGFR phoshorylates chromatin-bound PCNA on Tyr211, and this phosphorylation is required for maintaining PCNA function on chromatin. Inhibition of the phosphorylation led to degradation of the chromatin-bound, but not the unbound, form of PCNA in a proteasome-dependent manner and consequently suppressed its function in DNA synthesis and DNA damage repair (Wang et al., 2006). This important finding raised the possibility that additional nuclear proteins may be phosphorylated by nuclear EGFR and their functions, stability, and/or subcellular localization altered as a consequence of tyrosine phosphorylation. Future efforts are needed to explore this possibility.

4.1.3 Regulation of DNA repair by nuclear EGFR

In addition to ligand-induced accumulation of EGFR in the nucleus, EGFR has been demonstrated to escape receptor degradation after internalization and translocate to the nucleus in response to stress signals such as ionizing radiation, heat shock, H_2O_2, and cisplatin (Rodemann et al., 2007). Specifically, ionizing radiation causes nuclear transport of EGFR via caveolin and protein kinase C dependent mechanisms (Khan et al., 2006). Further, radiation has also been shown to drive EGFR translocation from the perinuclear region to the nucleoplasm via a process involving generation of free radicals (Dittmann et al., 2005a). Also, ultraviolet irradiation has been shown to induce EGFR nuclear translocation in human keratinocytes (Xu et al., 2009). In addition, Bandyopadhyay et al. reported that nuclear EGFR can influence DNA repair directly via physical interaction with DNA-dependent kinase (DNA-PK). They showed that cetuximab, an EGFR neutralizing antibody could decrease nuclear DNA-PK protein and kinase activity (Bandyopadhyay et al., 1998). Cetuximab treatment was also shown to block nuclear shuttling of EGFR and increased sensitivity to radiation-induced cell death in these cells (Dittmann et al., 2005b). It was also shown that the presence of EGFR in the nucleus resulted in activation of DNA-PK as shown by its phosphorylation on Thr2609. In the same study, it was again demonstrated that nuclear EGFR binds to the catalytic subunit DNA-PKs, and the regulatory subunit Ku70 of DNA-PK (Dittmann et al., 2005b). Nuclear EGFR has been shown to associate with p53 and MDC1 protein, an essential protein for the recruitment of DNA repair foci, following irradiation and treatment with the radioprotector Bowman-Birk proteinase inhibitor (Gueven et al., 1998; Dittmann et al., 2008a). Another radioprotector O-phospho-l-tyrosine (P-Tyr) has been shown to activate PKCepsilon, which triggers nuclear EGFR accumulation and concurrent phosphorylation of DNA-PK at amino acid residue Thr2609, and leads to repair of DNA double-strand breaks (Dittmann et al., 2007). Together these observations suggest an important role of nuclear EGFR for regulation of DNA repair following treatment with genotoxic substances.

4.2 Mechanism of nuclear transport

The intact EGFR protein containing both intracellular and extracellular domains moves to the nucleus in a ligand-bound form and the mechanism of this translocation is still incompletely understood. A seminal study very clearly demonstrated that intact EGFR bound by monoclonal antibodies directed against extracellular residues can accumulate specifically in the nucleus only in EGFR-expressing cells (Holt et al., 1994). This provided the first clue that endocytic events associated with the plasma membrane receptor could lead to intracellular trafficking and the delivery of EGFR to the nucleus. Further studies have convincingly demonstrated that a novel pathway exists by which internalized EGFR in the early endosomes is transferred into the nucleus instead of lysosomes or being recycled to the cell surface. Inhibition of receptor endocytosis using a dominant-negative dynamin mutant, which abrogates the formation of clathrin-coated pits from the cell surface, blocks the nuclear transport of EGFR (Lo et al., 2006a). Further, EGFR has been shown to colocalize with EEA1, an early endosomal marker in the nuclear compartment (Giri et al., 2005; Lo et al., 2006a). Thus, it seems clear that EGFR utilizes the endocytic pathway for its translocation into the nucleus, though additional routes cannot be excluded.

Nuclear localization requires recognition by the cellular nuclear import machinery and, in particular, by members of the nuclear localization sequence (NLS)-recognizing IMP superfamily. The best-understood NLS dependent nuclear import pathway is that mediated by the IMPα/β heterodimer. After irradiation, it was demonstrated that EGFR is found in complex with Importin α and RAN-GTP. It was also shown that EGFR-dependent activation of the PI3K/AKT signaling pathway was important for this association (Dittmann et al., 2005a). A prerequisite for Importin binding is the presence of an NLS within the cargo protein. EGFR has been shown to contain a tripartite NLS in its juxtamembrane region that mediates the nuclear translocation. EGFR has also been demonstrated to interact with importins $\alpha 1/\beta 1$ for which the NLS appears to be indispensable (Lo et al., 2006a; Lin et al., 2001; Hsu and Hung, 2007). Interestingly, another group studying nuclear transport of

EGFR following irradiation observed phosphorylation of EGFR at residue T654, which is located within the EGFR NLS. Furthermore, the same group identified PKCepsilon as the kinase responsible for this modification (Wanner et al., 2008). Nuclear EGFR accumulation results from a balance of import and export processes. Recent evidence also showed that the CRM1 is involved in nuclear-cytoplasmic shuttling of EGFR (Lo et al., 2006a). Existence of nuclear export sequences within EGFR sequence, however, has not yet been demonstrated.

While the above delineated mechanisms shed light on the mechanics of nuclear translocation of EGFR, it still is unclear how a transmembrane receptor is processed into a nuclear non-membrane-bound receptor. A protein translocon mediates the trafficking of protein complexes into and out of lipid bilayers. It was first suggested by Liao & Carpenter that the Sec61 translocon could mediate nuclear transport of EGFR (Liao and Carpenter, 2007). The Sec61 translocon is located in the endoplasmic reticulum and mediates the trafficking of secretory and transmembrane proteins into the ER during protein sythesis. This translocon is bidirectional and functions also, as part of the ERAD pathway, to retrotranslocate malfolded transmembrane proteins from the ER to the cytoplasm. Studies showed that radiation and EGF induced trafficking of EGFR to the ER membrane presumably via membrane fusion of the late edosomes to the golgi apparatus where it interacted with the Sec61 translocon. The data showed that knock-down of a Sec61 subunit abrogates both EGFR nuclear localization and EGF induction of cyclin D1 (Liao and Carpenter, 2007). While it has been proposed that Sec61 associated EGFR is retrotranslocated to the cytoplasm and subsequently imported into the nucleus via Importinβ and the nuclear pore complex (NPC), a recent study showed that Sec61β present in the inner nuclear membrane (INM) mediates retrotranslocation of EGFR from the INM into the nucleus (Wang et al., 2010b). Since the ER membrane system is contiguous with the outer nuclear membrane (ONM) and it is known that the ONM connects to the INM at the NPCs, it presents a model where EGFR is traficked first to ER via the endocytic machinery, then to the INM and then released into the nucleus by retrograde translocation at the NPC (Figure 2).

4.3 Nuclear EGFR in the clinical setting

Over the last 20 years, multiple reports have demonstrated beyond doubt that EGFR can translocate into the nuclear compartment where it has specific functions as outlined above. Concurrent studies have also identified that nuclear localization of EGFR is a common component of numerous cancer types. In addition to rapidly proliferating cells, nuclear EGFR has been detected in glioma as well as cancers of the breast, epidermoid, bladder, ovary, and oral cavity (Wang and Hung, 2009).

Increased nuclear EGFR expression is a prognostic feature in multiple tumor types correlating with parameters of known prognostic significance, such as tumor grade, stage and metastasis and is also associated with resistance to standard therapy such as radiation and cisplatin (Wang and Hung, 2009; Hwang, 2008). Analysis of nuclear localization of EGFR in human breast carcinoma biopsy samples demonstrated that nuclear EGFR levels inversely correlated with survival and correlation existed between nuclear localization of EGFR and markers of proliferation such as Cyclin D1 (that was shown to be a transcriptional target of EGFR in the same study) and Ki-67 (Lin et al., 2001). A follow up study also showed positive correlation between nuclear EGFR, Cyclin D1 and RHA expression in breast tumors (Huo et al., 2010). Early investigations revealed that cases with high nuclear EGFR demonstrated a trend towards poor survival in oral carcinomas (Lo et al., 2005b). This was later corroborated by studies that showed that nuclear EGFR was associated with increased local recurrence rate and inversely correlated with disease free survival (Psyrri et al., 2005). A study in esophageal squamous cell carcinoma using antibodies specific for phosphorylated EGFR showed that pEGFR not only localized to the nucleus but also correlated with higher TNM stage, nodal metastasis, and poor patient outcome (Hoshino et al., 2007). A follow up analysis by the same group showed that there was a strong correlation between nuclear EGFR and PCNA as well as nuclear ERK2 and non-nuclear EGFR (Psyrri et al., 2008). The above study was in line with earlier findings that PCNA is a substrate for EGFR in the nucleus and PCNA Tyr211 phosphorylation was associated with pronounced increase in cell proliferation and worse survival of breast cancer patients (Wang et al., 2006). A recent study also demonstrated that an inverse correlation exists between increased nuclear localization of EGFR and overall survival in ovarian tumor samples (Xia et al., 2009).

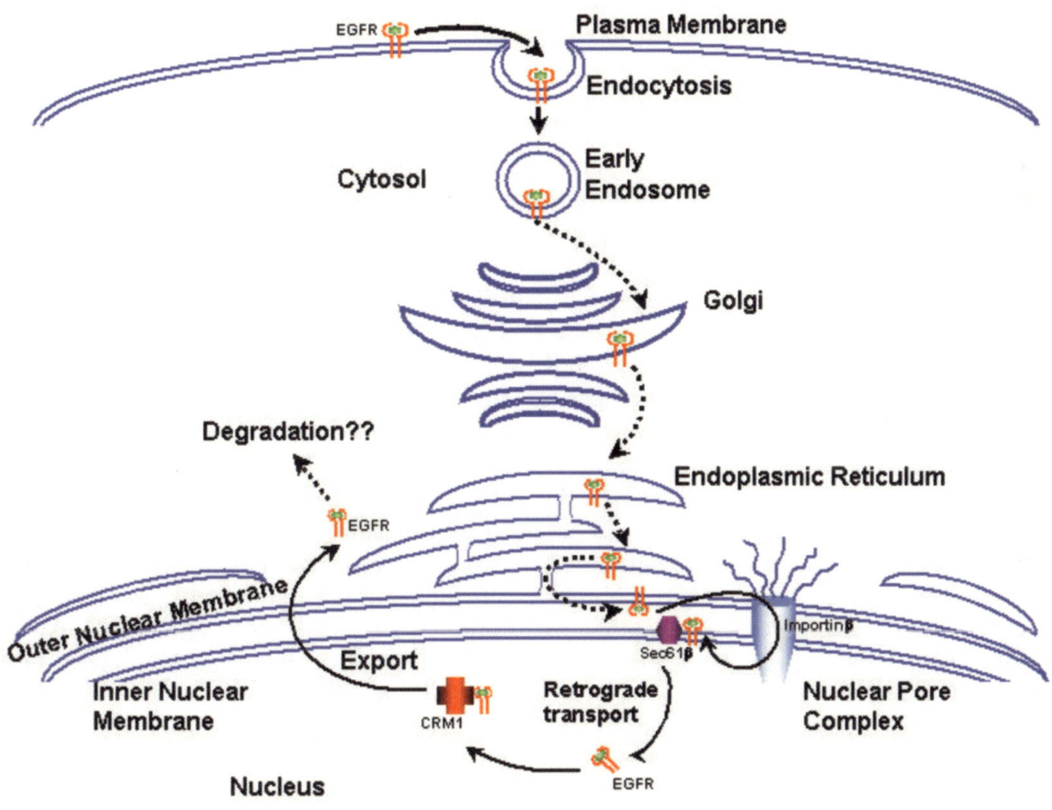

Fig. 2. A cartoon depicting the transport of EGFR from the plasma membrane to the nucleus. The current model shows the role of endocytosis for movement of EGFR to the early endosome, Golgi and thereafter, to the ER. From the ER, it is assumed that EGFR moves to the ONM and then via the NPC and Importinβ to the INM. On INM, it associates with Sec61β and through retrograde transport is released into the nucleoplasm. Nuclear export occurs via CRM1. The dotted lines represent potential pathways while solid lines depict pathways that have been experimentally proved. After (Wang et al., 2010a)

These clinical correlations of nuclear EGFR expression underscore the importance of examining the role of nuclear EGFR in other cancers especially those of epithelial origin as well as other human diseases. In this context, interestingly in addition to cancers, localization of EGFR in the nuclear compartment has also been implicated in glaucoma and neuropathy of the optic nerve (Liu and Neufeld, 2003). While the above studies indicate that nuclear EGFR is a prognostic indicator for poor clinical outcome and nuclear expression of EGFR is associated with cancer development, all the studies have been correlative studies. Mechanistic investigations delineating oncogenic capacity of nuclear EGFR are still limited and need to be further addressed. Further, a systematic approach has, yet to be conducted to identify nuclear EGFR target genes. Knowledge of the target genes will advance our understanding of the nature and effect of nuclear EGFR on cell physiology, provide novel insights into the role of nuclear EGFR in human cancers, and help clarify some of the molecular mechanisms underlying the observed association between nuclear EGFR and poor clinical outcome.

5. Role of EGFRvIII in the nucleus

A substantial body of evidence suggests that the EGFRvIII contributes a strong oncogenic signal in GBM while simultaneously protecting them from conventional therapy (Hwang, 2008; Gan et al., 2009). Two recent reports briefly described the nuclear localization of EGFRvIII in glial cells as well as glioblastoma (de, I et al., 2008; Lo et al., 2010). In glioblastoma, nuclear EGFRvIII was found to form a complex with STAT3 as was observed for EGFR. The EGFRvIII-STAT3 oncogenic complex was found to be essential for EGFRvIII induced transformation of astrocytes (de, I et al., 2008). Further, the second report of EGFRvIII nuclear localization showed that the EGFRvIII-STAT3 transcriptional complex could get recruited onto the promoter of Cox2 gene in glioma cells and increase transcription of Cox2 (Lo et al., 2010). Likewise, our finding that EGFRvIII binds STAT5b and positively regulates the transcription of Aurora A and Bcl-XL is the first demonstration of a role for EGFR/STAT5 pathway in the nucleus. Importantly, we show that nuclear EGFRvIII cooperates with STAT5b to regulate the Bcl-XL promoter and its expression in gliomas (Latha et. al., manuscript in preparation). This suggests that nuclear EGFR and EGFRvIII may be acting in concert with several members of the STAT family to generate a specific facet of its oncogenic signal in the nucleus and they also provide a potential role for combination therapy targeting EGFR/EGFRvIII and STAT5.The above studies suggest that the EGFRvIII-STAT family axis is important in gliomas. Although the above studies have shown nuclear translocation of EGFRvIII, the mechanism of translocation as well as the oncogenic role of EGFR in the nucleus remains unkown. Our recent investigation has shown that in gliomas, nuclear EGFRvIII as well as EGFR is membrane-derived and cycling of EGFRvIII and EGFR between the cytoplasm and nucleus is dependent on Importinβ and CRM1. Moreover, by manipulating EGFRvIII such that it is restricted to either the nucleus or the cytoplasm followed by functional studies, we show that nuclear EGFRvIII drives tumor formation. There is dramatic attenuation in the tumorigenic capacity of EGFRvIII upon blockade of its nuclear translocation in glioma cells (Gururaj et. al., manuscript in preparation). This suggests that while only a fraction of EGFRvIII or EGFR is in the nucleus, signaling here may be particularly important as it offers direct access to transcriptional regulators such as members of the STAT family. Taken together, these data provide an important insight into a new signaling node that may make a unique and key contribution to the oncogenic signal from overactive and mutant EGFR.

Nuclear expression EGFRvIII has also been described in prostate cancer (Edwards et al., 2006) and invasive breast cancer. In hormone-refractory prostate cancer, nuclear expression of EGFRvIII was associated with decreased time to death from relapse and decreased overall survival (Edwards et al., 2006). EGFRvIII is associated with radioresistance as well as chemoresistance (Huang et al., 2009; Schmidt and Lichtner, 2002; Chakravarti et al., 2004), which may be related to nuclear localization, in light of the finding that EGFR's association with nuclear targets is key to its ability to protect cells from DNA damaging agents, discussed above. *In vitro* studies using established glioma cell lines have shown that EGFRvIII confers resistance to cisplatin (Nagane et al., 1998; Nagane et al., 2000; Lammering et al., 2001; Lammering et al., 2003; Stea et al., 2003) and IR . Further, xenograft studies have shown that EGFR-specific inhibitors (small-molecule as well as α-EGFR antibodies) significantly enhance the efficacy of radiotherapy (Chakravarti et al., 2004; Harari and Huang, 2000). Also, EGFRvIII expression has been shown to enhance radioresistance by promoting the rapid repair of radiation-induced DNA double-strand breaks (Mukherjee et al., 2009). In line with this, a recent study showed that as with EGFR, EGFRvIII associates with DNA-PKcs after radiation and cisplatin treatment. They also showed that EGFRvIII not only conferred resistance to the two treatment modules but also significantly increased the activity of DNA-PKcs in cells (Liccardi et al., 2011). Recently, two independent studies showed that nuclear EGFR contributes to resistance to cisplatin treatment and cetuximab treatment (Hsu et al., 2009; Li et al., 2009). One of the studies also demonstrated that nuclear EGFR is required for DNA repair (Hsu et al., 2009). However, the role of nuclear EGFRvIII in either chemo- or radiation resistance in GBM is yet to be explored.

6. Nuclear EGFR/EGFRvIII and therapeutics

Since EGFR function is aberrantly regulated in a majority of the different epithelial cancers, attenuation of EGFR signaling is one of the key strategies for the management of human malignancies. Various therapeutic strategies have been developed to block EGFR signaling, with the most frequent strategies involving humanized monoclonal antibodies directed against EGFR, and small molecule tyrosine kinase inhibitors that target the enzymatic activity of the tyrosine kinase domain.

Anti-receptor antibodies including cetuximab bind to the receptor extracellular domain and induce internalization and degradation, thus effectively blocking receptor activation of subsequent cellular signaling cascades. Cetuximab is currently used in combination with chemotherapy for treatment of metastatic colorectal cancers with EGFR expression and wt-KRAS genotype as well as recurrent or metastatic head and neck squamous cell carcinoma (HNSCC). It is also indicated in treatment along with radiation for locally advanced HNSCC. As monotherapy, it is used in treatment of patients who have failed platinum based therapy of metastatic colorectal cancers. With respect to nuclear translocation of EGFR and cetuximab, there are conflicting data. In the context of radiation induced nuclear translocation, it was shown that cetuximab treatments results in accumulation of cytoplasmic EGFR and blockade of EGFR transport into the nucleus following radiation (Dittmann et al., 2005b). In contrast, a more recent study showed that cetuximab, like EGF, can induce nuclear localization of EGFR (Liao and Carpenter, 2009). However, it is to be noted that in this study, it was also shown that while EGF induced translocation required kinase activity, cetuximab induced translocation was kinase independent (Liao and Carpenter, 2009). This could be due to a fundamental difference either in the trafficking or conformation of EGF- and cetuximab- bound EGFR and warrants further investigation. Of interest is another study demonstrating that cells which acquire resistance to cetuximab show increased localization of EGFR in the nuclear compartment (Li et al., 2009). Further, expression of EGFR tagged with NLS that show increased nuclear localization render cells resistant to cetuximab treatment both *in vitro* and in xenograft studies (Li et al., 2009). Collectively, these data suggest that the mechanisms of the effect of cetuximab on EGFR nuclear transport are likely to be complex and dependent on cellular context. Further research is necessary to clarify the role and effect of cetuximab in nuclear translocation of EGFR. Interestingly, a recent study also showed that a monoclonal antibody which recognizes EGFRvIII and activated EGFR, Mab 806, and which has been demonstrated to inhibit the growth of tumors expressing EGFRvIII or overexpressing EGFR, can sensitize radioresistant glioma cells expressing EGFRvIII (Johns et al., 2010). These findings provide a strong rationale for the study of nuclear EGFRvIII in resistance to therapy which has not been addressed thus far.

Small molecule inhibitors such as erlotinib act against the cytoplasmic tyrosine kinase domain and inhibit the enzymatic activity of EGFR and so cytoplasmic signaling. Erlotinib is used as monotherapy for locally advanced or metastatic non-small cell lung cancer patients who have failed chemotherapy regimen and also for pancreatic cancer patients who have advanced local disease, metastasis or non-resectable tumors. However, there is insufficient evidence for using combinations of erlotinib with either chemotherapy or radiotherapy in patients and needs to be further investigated. Lapatinib, a dual EGFR and HER2 tyrosine kinase inhibitor, can sensitize cells to fluoropyrimidines possibly by inhibiting nuclear translocation of both EGFR and HER2 (Kim et al., 2009). Also, a recent study showed that nuclear EGFR is required for tumor resistance to DNA damage induced by the DNA alkylator, cisplatin (Hsu et al., 2009). Interestingly, a COX2 inhibitor, celecoxib has been shown to radiosensitize tumor cells by inhibiting radiation-induced nuclear EGFR translocation and DNA repair. Since this action of celecoxib did not correlate with COX2 expression, it is suggested that it could be a COX2 independent mechanism (Dittmann et al., 2008b). Another investigation demonstrated that the Src family kinase inhibitor, dasatinib could resensitize cells that were cetuximab resistant by inhibiting nuclear transport of EGFR (Li et al., 2009). While the above studies encourage the use of combination therapy to address treatment resistance by keeping EGFR out of the nucleus, we must proceed with caution since we are yet to understand the nuclear functions of EGFR in a comprehensive manner. Furthermore, such knowledge holds out the hope of leading to new targets that could be exploited in new combinations in the future.

7. Conclusion

Recent research has further strengthened the case for an important role of the EGFR family in a variety of cancers. It has also broadened our understanding of where these proteins may be active, by showing that in addition to propagating cytoplasmic signaling events, EGFR can also control other functions directly by translocating into the nuclear or mitochondrial compartment. Direct action within the nucleus could be a means by which the receptor achieves selectivity, specificity, and efficiency of gene activation not possible through shared transcription factors and second messenger/phosphorylation cascade systems. It may also represent an ancient signaling connection between the limiting membrane and the genetic material and other vital cellular complexes that predate the evolution of intracellular, membrane bound organelles. Understanding the nuclear functions of EGFR as well as the mechanisms of its nuclear trafficking provides the hope of novel avenues for therapeutic interventions in various tumor types. Further, nuclear EGFR itself could be a new clinically relevant target with the potential to find application specifically in chemo- and radio-resistant tumors. However, to evaluate the fitness of nuclear EGFR as a target, a selective inhibitor of EGFR transport needs to be identified. Thus, the current challenge in the field is to gain substantial knowledge about the functions as well as translocation of EGFR and define its role in cancer prognosis, targeting, and therapeutic sensitization.

8. Acknowledgment

We are indebted to Dr. Mien-Chie Hung for helpful discussions and to the National Cancer Institute of the National Institutes of Health for support of our research via RO1CA108500 (O.B.), P50CA127001 (O.B. and A.G.) and through The University of Texas M.D. Anderson's Cancer Centre Support Grant CA016672.

9. References

(2008). *Nature* Comprehensive genomic characterization defines human glioblastoma genes and core pathways. 455 1061-1068.

Aldape KD, Ballman K, Furth A, Buckner JC, Giannini C, Burger PC, Scheithauer BW, Jenkins RB, and James CD. (2004). *J. Neuropathol. Exp. Neurol.* Immunohistochemical detection of EGFRvIII in high malignancy grade astrocytomas and evaluation of prognostic significance. 63 700-707.

Bachoo RM and others. (2002). *Cancer Cell* Epidermal growth factor receptor and Ink4a/Arf: convergent mechanisms governing terminal differentiation and transformation along the neural stem cell to astrocyte axis. 1 269-277.

Bandyopadhyay D, Mandal M, Adam L, Mendelsohn J, and Kumar R. (1998). *J Biol Chem* Physical interaction between epidermal growth factor receptor and DNA-dependent protein kinase in mammalian cells. 273 1568-1573.

Bange J, Zwick E, and Ullrich A. (2001). *Nat Med* Molecular targets for breast cancer therapy and prevention. 7 548-552.

Bitler BG, Goverdhan A, and Schroeder JA. (2010). *J Cell Sci* MUC1 regulates nuclear localization and function of the epidermal growth factor receptor. 123 1716-1723.

Boerner JL, Demory ML, Silva C, and Parsons SJ. (2004). *Mol Cell Biol* Phosphorylation of Y845 on the epidermal growth factor receptor mediates binding to the mitochondrial protein cytochrome c oxidase subunit II. 24 7059-7071.

Bueter W, Dammann O, Zscheppang K, Korenbaum E, and Dammann CE. (2006). *Cytokine* ErbB receptors in fetal endothelium--a potential linkage point for inflammation-associated neonatal disorders. 36 267-275.

Cao H, Lei ZM, Bian L, and Rao CV. (1995). *Endocrinology* Functional nuclear epidermal growth factor receptors in human choriocarcinoma JEG-3 cells and normal human placenta. 136 3163-3172.

Cao X, Zhu H, Ali-Osman F, and Lo HW. (2011). *Mol Cancer* EGFR and EGFRvIII undergo stress- and EGFR kinase inhibitor-induced mitochondrial translocalization: A potential mechanism of EGFR-driven antagonism of apoptosis. 10 26.

Carpenter G. (2003). *Curr Opin Cell Biol* Nuclear localization and possible functions of receptor tyrosine kinases. 15 143-148.

Chakravarti A, Dicker A, and Mehta M. (2004). *Int J Radiat Oncol Biol Phys* The contribution of epidermal growth factor receptor (EGFR) signaling pathway to radioresistance in human gliomas: a review of preclinical and correlative clinical data. 58 927-931.

Choe G and others. (2003). *Cancer Res* Analysis of the phosphatidylinositol 3'-kinase signaling pathway in glioblastoma patients in vivo. 63 2742-2746.

Chu CT, Everiss KD, Wikstrand CJ, Batra SK, Kung HJ, and Bigner DD. (1997). *Biochem J* Receptor dimerization is not a factor in the signalling activity of a transforming variant epidermal growth factor receptor (EGFRvIII). 324 (Pt 3) 855-861.

de l, I, Konopka G, Puram SV, Chan JA, Bachoo RM, You MJ, Levy DE, Depinho RA, and Bonni A. (2008). *Genes Dev.* Identification of a PTEN-regulated STAT3 brain tumor suppressor pathway. 22 449-462.

Debierre-Grockiego F. (2004). *Apoptosis.* Anti-apoptotic role of STAT5 in haematopoietic cells and in the pathogenesis of malignancies. 9 717-728.

Demory ML and others. (2009). *J Biol Chem* Epidermal growth factor receptor translocation to the mitochondria: regulation and effect. 284 36592-36604.

Ding H and others. (2003). *Cancer Res* Oligodendrogliomas result from the expression of an activated mutant epidermal growth factor receptor in a RAS transgenic mouse astrocytoma model. 63 1106-1113.

Dittmann K, Mayer C, Fehrenbacher B, Schaller M, Raju U, Milas L, Chen DJ, Kehlbach R, and Rodemann HP. (2005a). *J Biol Chem* Radiation-induced epidermal growth factor receptor nuclear import is linked to activation of DNA-dependent protein kinase. 280 31182-31189.

Dittmann K, Mayer C, Kehlbach R, and Rodemann HP. (2008a). *Radiother Oncol* The radioprotector Bowman-Birk proteinase inhibitor stimulates DNA repair via epidermal growth factor receptor phosphorylation and nuclear transport. 86 375-382.

Dittmann K, Mayer C, and Rodemann HP. (2005b). *Radiother Oncol* Inhibition of radiation-induced EGFR nuclear import by C225 (Cetuximab) suppresses DNA-PK activity. 76 157-161.

Dittmann K, Mayer C, Wanner G, Kehlbach R, and Rodemann HP. (2007). *Radiother Oncol* The radioprotector O-phospho-tyrosine stimulates DNA-repair via epidermal growth factor receptor- and DNA-dependent kinase phosphorylation. 84 328-334.

Dittmann KH, Mayer C, Ohneseit PA, Raju U, Andratschke NH, Milas L, and Rodemann HP. (2008b). *Int J Radiat Oncol Biol Phys* Celecoxib induced tumor cell radiosensitization by inhibiting radiation induced nuclear EGFR transport and DNA-repair: a COX-2 independent mechanism. 70 203-212.

Dobashi Y, Koyama S, Kanai Y, and Tetsuka K. (2011). *Front Biosci.* Kinase-driven pathways of EGFR in lung carcinomas: perspectives on targeting therapy. 16 1714-1732.

Edwards J, Traynor P, Munro AF, Pirret CF, Dunne B, and Bartlett JM. (2006). *Clin Cancer Res* The role of HER1-HER4 and EGFRvIII in hormone-refractory prostate cancer. 12 123-130.

Ekstrand AJ, James CD, Cavenee WK, Seliger B, Pettersson RF, and Collins VP. (1991). *Cancer Res.* Genes for epidermal growth factor receptor, transforming growth factor alpha, and epidermal growth factor and their expression in human gliomas in vivo. 51 2164-2172.

Foley J, Nickerson NK, Nam S, Allen KT, Gilmore JL, Nephew KP, and Riese DJ. (2010). *Semin. Cell Dev Biol* EGFR signaling in breast cancer: bad to the bone. 21 951-960.

Frederick L, Eley G, Wang XY, and James CD. (2000). *Neuro. Oncol.* Analysis of genomic rearrangements associated with EGRFvIII expression suggests involvement of Alu repeat elements. 2 159-163.

Furnari FB and others. (2007). *Genes Dev.* Malignant astrocytic glioma: genetics, biology, and paths to treatment. 21 2683-2710.

Gan HK, Kaye AH, and Luwor RB. (2009). *J Clin Neurosci.* The EGFRvIII variant in glioblastoma multiforme. 16 748-754.

Ge H, Gong X, and Tang CK. (2002). *Int J Cancer* Evidence of high incidence of EGFRvIII expression and coexpression with EGFR in human invasive breast cancer by laser capture microdissection and immunohistochemical analysis. 98 357-361.

Giri DK, Ali-Seyed M, Li LY, Lee DF, Ling P, Bartholomeusz G, Wang SC, and Hung MC. (2005). *Mol Cell Biol* Endosomal transport of ErbB-2: mechanism for nuclear entry of the cell surface receptor. 25 11005-11018.

Graus-Porta D, Beerli RR, Daly JM, and Hynes NE. (1997). *EMBO J* ErbB-2, the preferred heterodimerization partner of all ErbB receptors, is a mediator of lateral signaling. 16 1647-1655.

Grimley PM, Dong F, and Rui H. (1999). *Cytokine Growth Factor Rev* Stat5a and Stat5b: fraternal twins of signal transduction and transcriptional activation. 10 131-157.

Gueven N, Dittmann K, Mayer C, and Rodemann HP. (1998). *Int J Radiat Biol* Bowman-Birk protease inhibitor reduces the radiation-induced activation of the EGF receptor and induces tyrosine phosphatase activity. 73 157-162.

Hanada N, Lo HW, Day CP, Pan Y, Nakajima Y, and Hung MC. (2006). *Mol. Carcinog.* Co-regulation of B-Myb expression by E2F1 and EGF receptor. 45 10-17.

Harari PM and Huang SM. (2000). *Clin Cancer Res* Modulation of molecular targets to enhance radiation. 6 323-325.

Hatanpaa KJ, Burma S, Zhao D, and Habib AA. (2010). *Neoplasia* Epidermal growth factor receptor in glioma: signal transduction, neuropathology, imaging, and radioresistance. 12 675-684.

Heimberger AB, Hlatky R, Suki D, Yang D, Weinberg J, Gilbert M, Sawaya R, and Aldape K. (2005). *Clin. Cancer Res.* Prognostic effect of epidermal growth factor receptor and EGFRvIII in glioblastoma multiforme patients. 11 1462-1466.

Holland EC, Hively WP, Depinho RA, and Varmus HE. (1998). *Genes Dev* A constitutively active epidermal growth factor receptor cooperates with disruption of G1 cell-cycle arrest pathways to induce glioma-like lesions in mice. 12 3675-3685.

Holt SJ, Alexander P, Inman CB, and Davies DE. (1994). *Biochem Pharmacol* Epidermal growth factor induced tyrosine phosphorylation of nuclear proteins associated with translocation of epidermal growth factor receptor into the nucleus. 47 117-126.

Hoshino M and others. (2007). *Pathobiology* Nuclear expression of phosphorylated EGFR is associated with poor prognosis of patients with esophageal squamous cell carcinoma. 74 15-21.

Hsu SC and Hung MC. (2007). *J. Biol. Chem.* Characterization of a novel tripartite nuclear localization sequence in the EGFR family. 282 10432-10440.

Hsu SC, Miller SA, Wang Y, and Hung MC. (2009). *Am. J Transl Res* Nuclear EGFR is required for cisplatin resistance and DNA repair. 1 249-258.

Huang HS and others. (1997). *J. Biol. Chem.* The enhanced tumorigenic activity of a mutant epidermal growth factor receptor common in human cancers is mediated by threshold levels of constitutive tyrosine phosphorylation and unattenuated signaling. 272 2927-2935.

Huang PH, Mukasa A, Bonavia R, Flynn RA, Brewer ZE, Cavenee WK, Furnari FB, and White FM. (2007). *Proc Natl Acad Sci U S A* Quantitative analysis of EGFRvIII cellular signaling networks reveals a combinatorial therapeutic strategy for glioblastoma. 104 12867-12872.

Huang PH, Xu AM, and White FM. (2009). *Sci Signal.* Oncogenic EGFR signaling networks in glioma. 2 re6.

Hung LY, Tseng JT, Lee YC, Xia W, Wang YN, Wu ML, Chuang YH, Lai CH, and Chang WC. (2008). *Nucleic Acids Res.* Nuclear epidermal growth factor receptor (EGFR) interacts with signal transducer and activator of transcription 5 (STAT5) in activating Aurora-A gene expression. 36 4337-4351.

Huo L and others. (2010). *Proc Natl Acad Sci U S A* RNA helicase A is a DNA-binding partner for EGFR-mediated transcriptional activation in the nucleus. 107 16125-16130.

Hwang,Y. L. K. G. A. R. M. a. B. O. 2008. Aberrant EGFR Signaling in Glioma: biology and clinical implications. in *CNS cancer, Models, Markers, Prognostic Factors, Targets and Therapeutic Approaches.* (ed. E Van Meir), Springer Science + Business Media.

Inda MM and others. (2010). *Genes Dev* Tumor heterogeneity is an active process maintained by a mutant EGFR-induced cytokine circuit in glioblastoma. 24 1731-1745.

Ji H and others. (2006). *Proc Natl Acad Sci U S A* Epidermal growth factor receptor variant III mutations in lung tumorigenesis and sensitivity to tyrosine kinase inhibitors. 103 7817-7822.

Johns TG, McKay MJ, Cvrljevic AN, Gan HK, Taylor C, Xu H, Smyth FE, and Scott AM. (2010). *Int J Radiat Oncol Biol Phys* MAb 806 enhances the efficacy of ionizing radiation in glioma xenografts expressing the de2-7 epidermal growth factor receptor. 78 572-578.

Khan EM, Heidinger JM, Levy M, Lisanti MP, Ravid T, and Goldkorn T. (2006). *J Biol Chem* Epidermal growth factor receptor exposed to oxidative stress undergoes Src- and caveolin-1-dependent perinuclear trafficking. 281 14486-14493.

Kim HP and others. (2009). *PLoS. One.* Lapatinib, a dual EGFR and HER2 tyrosine kinase inhibitor, downregulates thymidylate synthase by inhibiting the nuclear translocation of EGFR and HER2. 4 e5933.

Kimura H. (1993). *Proc Natl Acad Sci U S A* Schwannoma-derived growth factor must be transported into the nucleus to exert its mitogenic activity. 90 2165-2169.

Lammering G, Hewit TH, Valerie K, Contessa JN, Amorino GP, Dent P, and Schmidt-Ullrich RK. (2003). *Oncogene* EGFRvIII-mediated radioresistance through a strong cytoprotective response. 22 5545-5553.

Lammering G, Valerie K, Lin PS, Mikkelsen RB, Contessa JN, Feden JP, Farnsworth J, Dent P, and Schmidt-Ullrich RK. (2001). *Clin Cancer Res* Radiosensitization of malignant glioma cells through overexpression of dominant-negative epidermal growth factor receptor. 7 682-690.

Li C, Iida M, Dunn EF, Ghia AJ, and Wheeler DL. (2009). *Oncogene* Nuclear EGFR contributes to acquired resistance to cetuximab. 28 3801-3813.

Liao HJ and Carpenter G. (2007). *Mol Biol Cell* Role of the Sec61 translocon in EGF receptor trafficking to the nucleus and gene expression. 18 1064-1072.

Liao HJ and Carpenter G. (2009). *Cancer Res* Cetuximab/C225-induced intracellular trafficking of epidermal growth factor receptor. 69 6179-6183.

Liccardi G, Hartley JA, and Hochhauser D. (2011). *Cancer Res* EGFR nuclear translocation modulates DNA repair following cisplatin and ionizing radiation treatment. 71 1103-1114.

Lin SY, Makino K, Xia W, Matin A, Wen Y, Kwong KY, Bourguignon L, and Hung MC. (2001). *Nat. Cell Biol.* Nuclear localization of EGF receptor and its potential new role as a transcription factor. 3 802-808.

Liu B and Neufeld AH. (2003). *Neurobiol. Dis.* Activation of epidermal growth factor receptor signals induction of nitric oxide synthase-2 in human optic nerve head astrocytes in glaucomatous optic neuropathy. 13 109-123.

Lo IIW, Ali-Seyed M, Wu Y, Bartholomeusz G, Hsu SC, and Hung MC. (2006a). *J. Cell Biochem.* Nuclear-cytoplasmic transport of EGFR involves receptor endocytosis, importin beta1 and CRM1. 98 1570-1583.

Lo HW, Cao X, Zhu H, and Ali-Osman F. (2010). *Mol. Cancer Res.* Cyclooxygenase-2 Is a Novel Transcriptional Target of the Nuclear EGFR-STAT3 and EGFRvIII-STAT3 Signaling Axes. 8 232-245.

Lo HW, Hsu SC, and Hung MC. (2006b). *Breast Cancer Res. Treat.* EGFR signaling pathway in breast cancers: from traditional signal transduction to direct nuclear translocalization. 95 211-218.

Lo HW, Hsu SC, and Hung MC. (2006c). *Breast Cancer Res. Treat.* EGFR signaling pathway in breast cancers: from traditional signal transduction to direct nuclear translocalization. 95 211-218.

Lo HW, Hsu SC, li-Seyed M, Gunduz M, Xia W, Wei Y, Bartholomeusz G, Shih JY, and Hung MC. (2005a). *Cancer Cell* Nuclear interaction of EGFR and STAT3 in the activation of the iNOS/NO pathway. 7 575-589.

Lo HW, Xia W, Wei Y, Ali-Seyed M, Huang SF, and Hung MC. (2005b). *Cancer Res.* Novel prognostic value of nuclear epidermal growth factor receptor in breast cancer. 65 338-348.

Machiels JP and Schmitz S. (2011). *Curr Opin Oncol* Molecular-targeted therapy of head and neck squamous cell carcinoma: beyond cetuximab-based therapy.

Marti U, Burwen SJ, Wells A, Barker ME, Huling S, Feren AM, and Jones AL. (1991). *Hepatology* Localization of epidermal growth factor receptor in hepatocyte nuclei. 13 15-20.

Marti U and Wells A. (2000). *Mol Cell Biol Res Commun* The nuclear accumulation of a variant epidermal growth factor receptor (EGFR) lacking the transmembrane domain requires coexpression of a full-length EGFR. 3 8-14.

Mizoguchi M, Betensky RA, Batchelor TT, Bernay DC, Louis DN, and Nutt CL. (2006). *J Neuropathol. Exp Neurol.* Activation of STAT3, MAPK, and AKT in malignant astrocytic gliomas: correlation with EGFR status, tumor grade, and survival. 65 1181-1188.

Moscatello DK, Holgado-Madruga M, Godwin AK, Ramirez G, Gunn G, Zoltick PW, Biegel JA, Hayes RL, and Wong AJ. (1995). *Cancer Res* Frequent expression of a mutant epidermal growth factor receptor in multiple human tumors. 55 5536-5539.

Mukherjee B and others. (2009). *Cancer Res* EGFRvIII and DNA double-strand break repair: a molecular mechanism for radioresistance in glioblastoma. 69 4252-4259.

Nagane M, Coufal F, Lin H, Bogler O, Cavenee WK, and Huang HJ. (1996). *Cancer Res* A common mutant epidermal growth factor receptor confers enhanced tumorigenicity on human glioblastoma cells by increasing proliferation and reducing apoptosis. 56 5079-5086.

Nagane M, Levitzki A, Gazit A, Cavenee WK, and Huang HJ. (1998). *Proc Natl Acad Sci U S A* Drug resistance of human glioblastoma cells conferred by a tumor-specific mutant epidermal growth factor receptor through modulation of Bcl-XL and caspase-3-like proteases. 95 5724-5729.

Nagane M, Lin H, Cavenee WK, and Huang HJ. (2001). *Cancer Lett* Aberrant receptor signaling in human malignant gliomas: mechanisms and therapeutic implications. 162 Suppl S17-S21.

Nagane M, Pan G, Weddle JJ, Dixit VM, Cavenee WK, and Huang HJ. (2000). *Cancer Res* Increased death receptor 5 expression by chemotherapeutic agents in human gliomas causes synergistic cytotoxicity with tumor necrosis factor-related apoptosis-inducing ligand in vitro and in vivo. 60 847-853.

Nakamura JL. (2007). *Expert Opin Ther Targets.* The epidermal growth factor receptor in malignant gliomas: pathogenesis and therapeutic implications. 11 463-472.

Ni CY, Murphy MP, Golde TE, and Carpenter G. (2001). *Science* gamma -Secretase cleavage and nuclear localization of ErbB-4 receptor tyrosine kinase. 294 2179-2181.

Nishikawa R, Ji XD, Harmon RC, Lazar CS, Gill GN, Cavenee WK, and Huang HJ. (1994). *Proc Natl Acad Sci U S A* A mutant epidermal growth factor receptor common in human glioma confers enhanced tumorigenicity. 91 7727-7731.

Normanno N and others. (2006). *Gene* Epidermal growth factor receptor (EGFR) signaling in cancer. 366 2-16.

Ohgaki H and Kleihues P. (2007). *Am. J Pathol* Genetic pathways to primary and secondary glioblastoma. 170 1445-1453.

Oksvold M, Huitfeldt H, Stang E, and Madshus I. (2002). *Nat Cell Biol* Localizing the EGF receptor. 4 E22-E23.

Parsons DW and others. (2008). *Science* An integrated genomic analysis of human glioblastoma multiforme. 321 1807-1812.

Pedersen MW, Pedersen N, Damstrup L, Villingshoj M, Sonder SU, Rieneck K, Bovin LF, Spang-Thomsen M, and Poulsen HS. (2005). *J Cell Biochem* Analysis of the epidermal growth factor receptor specific transcriptome: effect of receptor expression level and an activating mutation. 96 412-427.

Pelloski CE and others. (2007). *J. Clin. Oncol.* Epidermal growth factor receptor variant III status defines clinically distinct subtypes of glioblastoma. 25 2288-2294.

Psyrri A, Egleston B, Weinberger P, Yu Z, Kowalski D, Sasaki C, Haffty B, Rimm D, and Burtness B. (2008). *Cancer Epidemiol Biomarkers Prev* Correlates and determinants of nuclear epidermal growth factor receptor content in an oropharyngeal cancer tissue microarray. 17 1486-1492.

Psyrri A, Yu Z, Weinberger PM, Sasaki C, Haffty B, Camp R, Rimm D, and Burtness BA. (2005). *Clin Cancer Res* Quantitative determination of nuclear and cytoplasmic epidermal growth factor receptor expression in oropharyngeal squamous cell cancer by using automated quantitative analysis. 11 5856-5862.

Rakowicz-Szulczynska EM, Otwiaska D, Rodeck U, and Koprowski H. (1989). *Arch. Biochem Biophys* Epidermal growth factor (EGF) and monoclonal antibody to cell surface EGF receptor bind to the same chromatin receptor. 268 456-464.

Rakowicz-Szulczynska EM, Rodeck U, Herlyn M, and Koprowski H. (1986). *Proc Natl Acad Sci U S A* Chromatin binding of epidermal growth factor, nerve growth factor, and platelet-derived growth factor in cells bearing the appropriate surface receptors. 83 3728-3732.

Rodemann HP, Dittmann K, and Toulany M. (2007). *Int J Radiat Biol* Radiation-induced EGFR-signaling and control of DNA-damage repair. 83 781-791.

Sasaki H, Kawano O, Endo K, Yukiue H, Yano M, and Fujii Y. (2007). *Oncol Rep* EGFRvIII mutation in lung cancer correlates with increased EGFR copy number. 17 319-323.

Schmidt M and Lichtner RB. (2002). *Drug Resist. Updat.* EGF receptor targeting in therapy-resistant human tumors. 5 11-18.

Shao H, Cheng HY, Cook RG, and Tweardy DJ. (2003). *Cancer Res* Identification and characterization of signal transducer and activator of transcription 3 recruitment sites within the epidermal growth factor receptor. 63 3923-3930.

Stea B, Falsey R, Kislin K, Patel J, Glanzberg H, Carey S, Ambrad AA, Meuillet EJ, and Martinez JD. (2003). *Cancer Lett* Time and dose-dependent radiosensitization of the glioblastoma multiforme U251 cells by the EGF receptor tyrosine kinase inhibitor ZD1839 ('Iressa'). 202 43-51.

Sugawa N, Ekstrand AJ, James CD, and Collins VP. (1990). *Proc. Natl. Acad. Sci. U. S. A* Identical splicing of aberrant epidermal growth factor receptor transcripts from amplified rearranged genes in human glioblastomas. 87 8602-8606.

Wang SC and Hung MC. (2009). *Clin Cancer Res* Nuclear translocation of the epidermal growth factor receptor family membrane tyrosine kinase receptors. 15 6484-6489.

Wang SC and others. (2006). *Nat. Cell Biol.* Tyrosine phosphorylation controls PCNA function through protein stability. 8 1359-1368.

Wang YN, Yamaguchi H, Hsu JM, and Hung MC. (2010a). *Oncogene* Nuclear trafficking of the epidermal growth factor receptor family membrane proteins. 29 3997-4006.

Wang YN, Yamaguchi H, Huo L, Du Y, Lee HJ, Lee HH, Wang H, Hsu JM, and Hung MC. (2010b). *J Biol Chem* The translocon Sec61beta localized in the inner nuclear membrane transports membrane-embedded EGF receptor to the nucleus. 285 38720-38729.

Wanner G, Mayer C, Kehlbach R, Rodemann HP, and Dittmann K. (2008). *Radiother Oncol* Activation of protein kinase Cepsilon stimulates DNA-repair via epidermal growth factor receptor nuclear accumulation. 86 383-390.

Wheeler DL, Dunn EF, and Harari PM. (2010). *Nat Rev Clin Oncol* Understanding resistance to EGFR inhibitors-impact on future treatment strategies. 7 493-507.

Wong AJ, Ruppert JM, Bigner SH, Grzeschik CH, Humphrey PA, Bigner DS, and Vogelstein B. (1992). *Proc. Natl. Acad. Sci. U. S. A* Structural alterations of the epidermal growth factor receptor gene in human gliomas. 89 2965-2969.

Xia W, Wei Y, Du Y, Liu J, Chang B, Yu YL, Huo LF, Miller S, and Hung MC. (2009). *Mol. Carcinog.* Nuclear expression of epidermal growth factor receptor is a novel prognostic value in patients with ovarian cancer. 48 610-617.

Xu Y, Shao Y, Zhou J, Voorhees JJ, and Fisher GJ. (2009). *J Cell Biochem* Ultraviolet irradiation-induces epidermal growth factor receptor (EGFR) nuclear translocation in human keratinocytes. 107 873-880.

Yarden Y. (2001). *Eur J Cancer* The EGFR family and its ligands in human cancer. signalling mechanisms and therapeutic opportunities. 37 Suppl 4 S3-S8.

Yarden Y and Sliwkowski MX. (2001). *Nat Rev Mol Cell Biol* Untangling the ErbB signalling network. 2 127-137.

Yarom N and Jonker DJ. (2011). *Discov. Med* The role of the epidermal growth factor receptor in the mechanism and treatment of colorectal cancer. 11 95-105.

Yue X, Song W, Zhang W, Chen L, Xi Z, Xin Z, and Jiang X. (2008). *Autophagy* Mitochondrially localized EGFR is subjected to autophagic regulation and implicated in cell survival. 4 641-649.

Zscheppang K, Korenbaum E, Bueter W, Ramadurai SM, Nielsen HC, and Dammann CE. (2006). *Pediatr. Pulmonol.* ErbB receptor dimerization, localization, and co-localization in mouse lung type II epithelial cells. 41 1205-1212.

Part 12

AP-1 Transcription Factor - Glioblastoma

25

Ap 1 in Glioblastomas

Densie Smith[1,2] and Bruce Bejcek[2]
[1]*W. M. Keck Center for Transgene Research University of Notre Dame South Bend, IN*
[2]*Department of Biological Sciences Western Michigan University, Kalamazoo, MI, USA*

1. Introduction

Although the origins of cancer can be exceptionally complex due to the range of genes that may be involved it is also apparent that there are "consensus" genes, ones that are frequently mutated. The AP-1 family of transcription factors represent a set of proteins that are commonly involved in cancers as well as other developmental and pathological conditions including heart development, apoptosis, and hepatogenesis (reviewed in (1). Although defined as a protein that can bind to a consensus sequence in a variety of promoters, AP-1 is in fact a series of heterodimmers that are created between at least 7 distinct proteins including c-jun, junB, Fos, FosB, Fra1,Fra2 and the Maf family of proteins (2). Each of these proteins is the product of distinct genes and although they are different at the amino acid level they share homology and structural similarities including a leucine zipper, transactivation domain and a basic region. Expression of these different proteins is tightly controlled and they may be expressed at different times of development and in different tissues. Control of AP-1 activity revolves around the control of these protein's transcription, translation and post-translation modification

There have been several reports that have detailed the role that some of the family members may play in several tumors. Through the use of dominant negative mutants for c-jun it has been demonstrated that this protein is necessary for tumor survival while inhibition of jun-B may enhance tumor survival (3-5). In all of these experiments it is not clear if any of the other family members that comprise AP-1 are actually present in the cell and if they might play roles as well. Instead of developing dominant negative mutants that could mask the role that the other family members play in tumorigenesis we have taken the approach of creating a series of either siRNAs or shRNAs to investigate the role that each of these family members play in a glioblastoma cell line. Our results demonstrate that in the U87-MG cell line all family members are expressed. However the necessity of each these members varies greatly for cell proliferation and survival.

2. Materials and methods

Cells and transfections: Cell lines U87-MG, U118-MG and U373-MG were obtained from the American Type Culture Collection and maintained according to their instructions. Cells transfections, selections in geneticin sulfate and secreted alkaline phosphatase assays were performed as essentially as described (6)

shRNA: siRNAs were developed by Elbashir using the methods described by (7, 8). At 63-190 nucletoides downstream of the start codon a 19 nucleotide sequence was chosen. This sequence began with an adenine dimer and had a 47-80% GC content. Controls were created from these sequences by randomizing the order of the bases. Both the selected shRNA sequence and its cognate control were compared to the nucleotide databases at the National Institute for Biotechnoilogy using the BLAST program (9). Only those sequences that were unique were used for oligonucleotides synthesis. These sequences were then used to direct the synthesis of oligonucleotides. In addition to the shRNA sequences these oligonucleoitides contained a short region that resulted in a hairpin region. Oligonucleotides were ligated into pBluescript that contained an H1 promoter (10) and pSuperiorneo (Oligoengines). Clones were verified by sequence analysis.
Cell growth assays. Cells were seeded into 96 well plates. On day 0 cells were dosed with media that contained the control solvent or media that contained 2μg/ml doxycycline . Medium was replenished every 2 days thereafter with the appropriate additions. Cell division was determined using the 10 μl per well of CCK8 (Dojindo) a formazan dye based assay. After 1 hour of incubation with the dye the amount of dye converted was measured by spectrophotometry at a wavelength of 459 nm.
Western blots. Western blots were performed essentially as described (6). Protein amounts in each sample were determined using the BCA assay (Pierce) with bovine serum albumin as a standard. Antibodies to c-jun, c-fos (Upstate Biotechnologies) JunB, JunD, FosB, Fra-1 and Fra-2 (Santa Cruz), and cleaved PARP (Cell Signalling Technologies) were purchased.
Caspase assays. Assays for activated caspase 3 and 7 were performed using the Apo-ONE kit (Promega). Lysates from induced cells were compared to cells that were not induced with 2μg/ml of doxycyclin. Assays were read on a Perkin Elmer LS-50B fluorometer with an excitation wavelength of 485nm and an emission wavelength of 530nm according to manufacturer's recommendations.

3. Results

To determine if the transcription factor AP-1 was present at elevated levels in glioblastomas we transfected a reporter plasmid, pAP-1SEAP, or a control plasmid pTal into the glioblastoma cell lines U87-MG, U118-MG and U373-MG. After 24 hour cells were harvested, the amounts of protein and β-galactosidase measured. Identical amounts of protein were then used for a secreted alkaline phosphatase assay and the assay results normalized to the specific activity of β-galactosidase. The results are presented in Fig.1 and demonstrate that the levels of AP-1 were significantly elevated in both U87-Mg and U118-MG cells. U373-MG cells did not have elevated levels of SEAP indicating that they did not have activated Ap-1 (data not shown). The AP-1 activity was sensitive to genistein indicating the possible involvement of a tyrosine kinase in activating the AP-1 pathway. We have obtained similar results with NF-κB activation (6). When compared to a control cell line, MCF-10A, which is a cell line derived from normal breast epithelium, U87-MG and U118-MG Ap-1 levels also appeared elevated (data not shown).
Although it was clear that AP-1 levels were elevated at least in the two glioblastomas cell lines it was not clear which of the family members of AP-1 might be present and the contribution that each family member was making. To determine what roles each individual

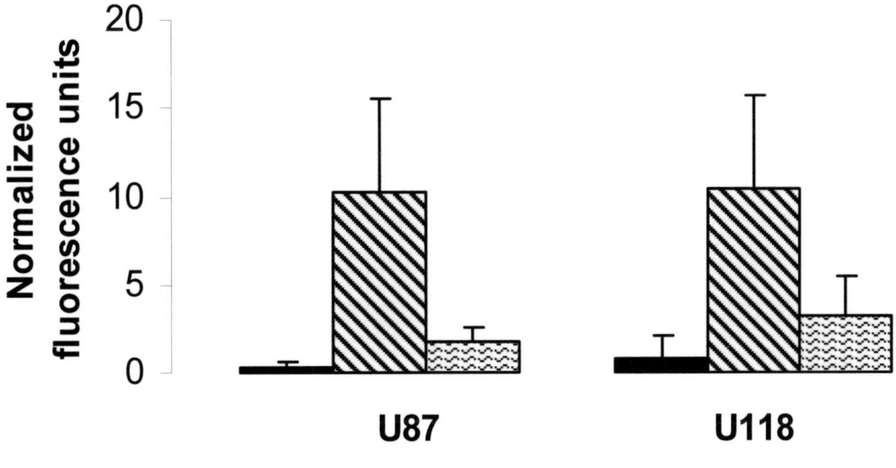

Fig. 1. AP-1 is elevated in the glioblastoma cell lines U87-MG and U118-MG. Cells were co-transfected with either the pTAL (black bars), or pAP1SEAP (diagonal striped bars), or pAP1SEAP in the presence of genistein (horizontal striped bars) and a plasmid that constitutively expressed the β-galactosidase protein. Media was assayed for the presence of secreted alkaline phosphatase and the values were normalized to the specific activity of β–galactosidase levels from cell lysates. Levels of SEAP in pAP1SEAP transfected cells were statistically significantly different from either the pTAL control or the cells treated with genistein (p0.05).

Protein	siRNA Sequence
c-jun-1	GATCCCAACCTGGCCGACCCACTGGTTCAAGAGACCAGTGGGTCGGCCAGGTTTTTTGGAAA GGGTTGGACCGGCTGGGTGACCAAGTTCTCTGGTCACCCAGCCGGTCCAAAAAACCTTTTCGA
c-junC-1	GATCCCCAAGACTACGCGCTCCGCGCTTCAAGAGAGCGCGGAGCGCGTAGTCTTTTTTGGAAA GGGTTCTGATGCGCGAGGCGCGAAGTTCTCTCGCGCCTCGCGCATCAGAAAAAACCTTTTCGA
JunD-1	GATCCCCAAGCCTGCGGCCGCGCCGCTTCAAGAGAGCGGCGCGGCCGCAGGCTTTTTTGGAAA GGGTTCGGACGCCGGCGCGGCGAAGTTCTCTCGCCGCGCCGGCGTCCGAAAAAACCTTTTCGA
JunDC-1	GATCCCCGCCGCGCCGGCGTCCGAATTCAAGAGATTCGGACGCCGGCGCGGCGTTTTTGGAAA GGGGCGGCGCGGCCGCAGGCTTAAGTTCTCTAAGCCTGCGGCCGCGCCGCAAAAACCTTTTCGA
JunB-1	GATCCCCAAGCGCCTGGGGCTCGCGGTTCAAGAGACCGCGAGCCCCAGGCGCTTTTTTGGAAA GGGTTCGCGGACCCCGAGCGCCAAGTTCTCTGGCGCTCGGGGTCCGCGAAAAAACCTTTTCGA
JunBC-1	GATCCCCGCGGCGGAGGCATCCGTCGTTCAAGAGACGACGGATGCCTCCGCCGCTTTTTGGAAA GGGCGCCGCCTCCGTAGGCAGCAAGTTCTCTGCTGCCTACGGAGGCGGCGAAAAACCTTTTCGA
Fra2-1	GATCCCCAACGCCATCACGACCAGCCTTCAAGAGAGGCTGGTCGTGATGGCGTTTTTTGGAAA GGGTTGCGGTAGTGCTGGTCGGAAGTTCTCTCCGACCAGCACTACCGCAAAAAACCTTTTCGA
Fra2C-1	GATCCCCCCGACCAGCACTACCGCAATTCAAGAGATTGCGGTAGTGCTGGTCGGTTTTTGGAAA GGGGGCTGGTCGTGATGGCGTTAAGTTCTCTAACGCCATCACGACCAGCCAAAAACCTTTTCGA
Fra1-1	GATCCCCAAGTTCCACCTGGTGCCAATTCAAGAGATTGGCACCAGGTGGAACTTTTTTGGAAA GGGTTCAAGGTGGACCACGGTTAAGTTCTCTAACCGTGGTCCACCTTGAAAAAACCTTTTCGA
Fra1C-1	GATCCCCTCATCAGTCATCAGGCCCATTCAAGAGATGGGCCTGATGACTGATGATTTTTGGAAA GGGAGTAGTCAGTAGTCCGGGTAAGTTCTCTACCCGGACTACTGACTACTAAAAACCTTTTCGA
c-fos-1	GATCCCCAAGGCTGGCTTCCCGTCGCTTCAAGAGAGCGACGGGAAGCCAGCCTTTTTTGGAAA GGGTTCCGACCGAAGGGCAGCGAAGTTCTCTCGCTGCCCTTCGGTCGGAAAAAACCTTTTCGA
c-fosC-1	GATCCCCGATCAGGTCGCCTCTGCCGTTCAAGAGACGGCAGAGGCGACCTGATCTTTTTGGAAA GGGCTAGTCCAGCGGAGACGGCAAGTTCTCTGCCGTCTCCGCTGGACTAGAAAAACCTTTTCGA
FosB-1	GATCCCCAAGCTGATTCTGTACAGCGTTCAAGAGACGCTGTACAGAATCAGCTTTTTTGGAAA GGGTTCGACTAAGACATGTCGCAAGTTCTCTGCGACATGTCTTAGTCGAAAAAACCTTTTCGA
FosBC-1	GATCCCCTTTAGCACCTAGGAGCATGTTCAAGAGACATGCTCCTAGGTGCTAAATTTTTGGAAA GGGAAATCGTGGATCCTCGTACAAGTTCTCTGTACGAGGATCCACGATTTAAAAACCTTTTCGA

shRNA sequences. Sequences for the shRNAs are given in table 1.

Table 1. Sequences of the siRNAs that were synthesized. The designation of c indicates control oligonucleotides that are scrambled. Note that the overhanging ends are compatible with HindII and BglII sites in the vectors that were used.

family member might be playing in the increased levels of AP-1 we designed a series of shRNAs that were directed specifically to each individual family member (Table 1). We then tested these constructs in both transient expression and in stable expression assays. Western blotting demonstrated that all of the family members were present in the U87-MG cells that there were no family members that were expressed. Furthermore, levels of these proteins could be reduced with either transient or stable expression studies as compared to cognate controls (Fig. 2).

To determine what effect, if any, this reduction in protein might have on AP-1 activity we transfected into cells the pAP1-SEAP reporter plasmid or its control pTAL. From this assay it became apparent that the contributions that the different AP-1 family members had on AP-1 levels were quite variable and ranged from a low of 7% for JunB to 84% for c-Fos.

We were interested what the affect was of inhibiting these proteins would have on the cells in stable assays. Transient transfections could only allow us to assay the affects of the shRNA constructs on a potentially minor proportion of the population of cells. By creating stable transfectants we could investigate the role of some of these proteins consistently within a population. The shRNAs for c-Jun and c-Fos were cloned into a modified pSuperior neo vector that we created so that it expressed the hygromycin resistance gene in place of

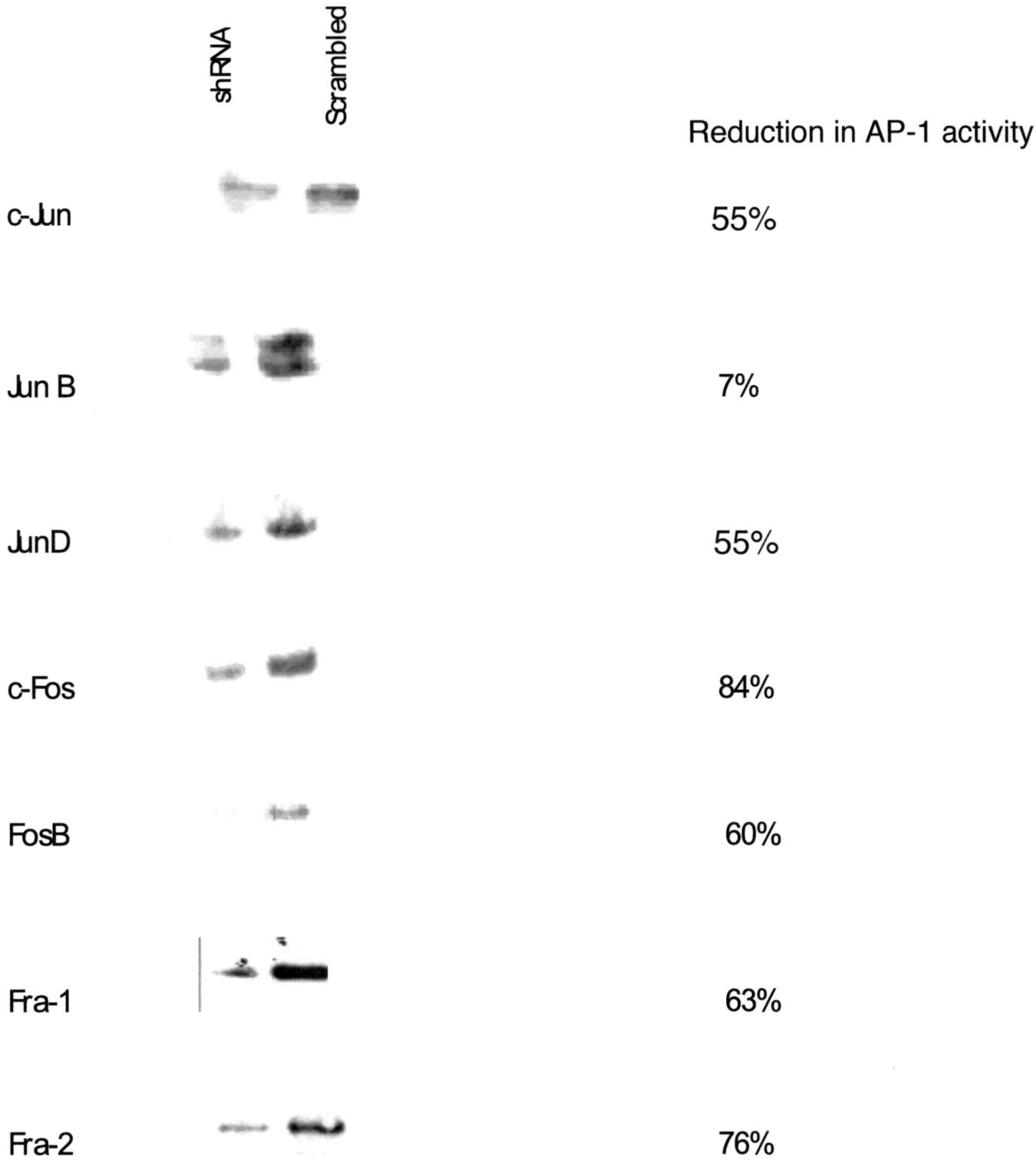

Fig. 2. Expression of AP-1 family members transiently transfected with plasmids that either expressed shRNA or the scrambled control shRNA. Cels were transfected with indicated plasmids and lysates were tested for expression of the various family members by western blot analysis of whole cell lysates. Cells were also transfected with the pAP1SEAP reporter plasmid and the media assayed for SEAP.

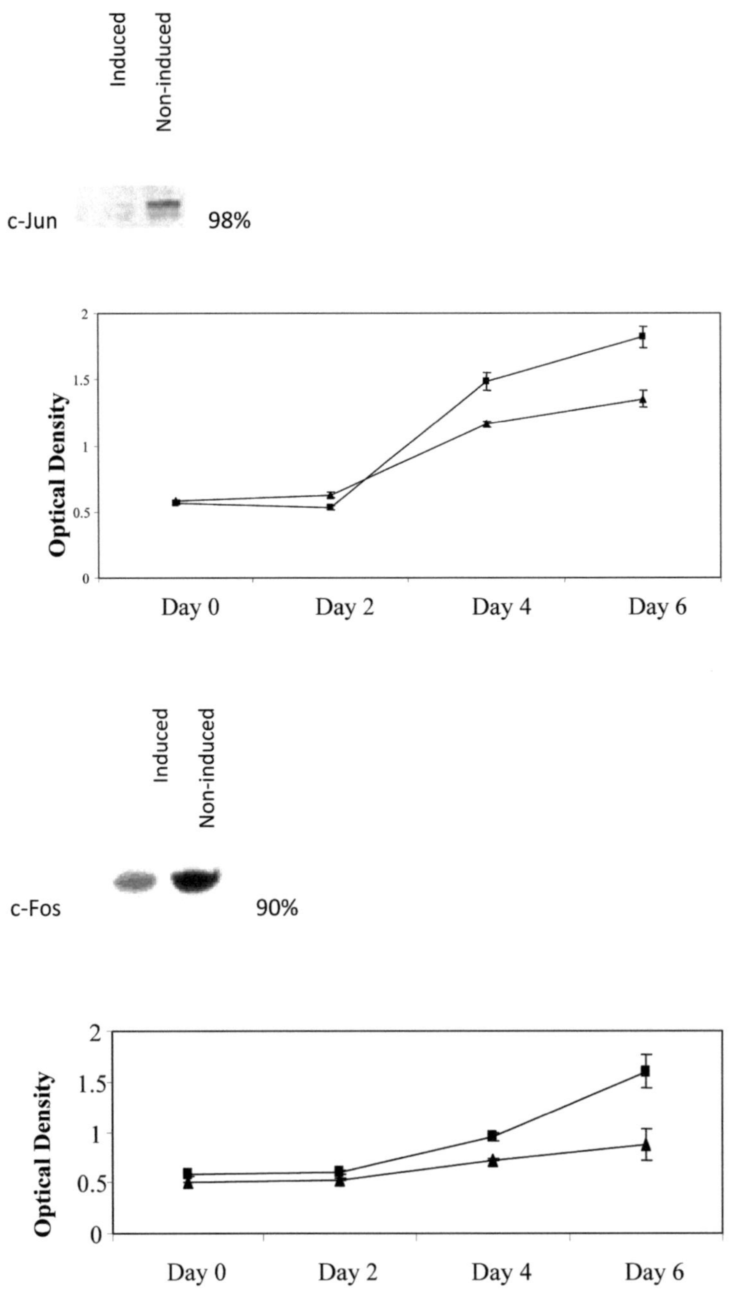

Fig. 3. Stable transfection and inhibition of cell doubling with c-Jun and c-Fos shRNAs. U87-MG cells that expressed the pTET-ON plasmid were transfected with the pSuperior constructs of the shRNAs for c-Jun and c-fos shRNAs or their cognate controls. Cells selected in hygromycin were then tested for their ability to replicate in the presence or absence of the inducer for shRNA, doxtcyclin. In both cases day 6 values are statistically significantly different between the control and shRNA expressing cells ($p<0.05$).

the neo resistance gene. The promoter in this vector that drives the expression of the shRNAs is an H1 promoter that has additional sequences that make is responsive to the Tet repressor. Cell lines of U87-MG were created that expressed the Tet repressor and these were transfected and selected so that they also carried either the c-Fos or c-Jun shRNAs that were used in the transient assays described above. As expected induction of the shRNA expression with doxycycline resulted in depression of c-Jun (90%) and c-Fos (98%) protein levels as compared to their uninduced controls (Fig. 3a). To determine what effect this type of reduction would have on the ability of the cells to divide cells were treated with doxycycline and their division measured over a period of several days using a formazan dye derivative. The results (Fig. 3b) demonstrate that a reduction in c-Fos and c-Jun did have a modest but statistically significant suppressive affect on cell division which was not seen in the cells that were transfected with the scrambled control oligonucleotides. If doxycycline was removed part way through the assay this effect was not seen indicating that the effect could be cytostatic as opposed to resulting in apoptosis or cell death. However, western blots of the cell lines demonstrated that they had increased levels of cleaved PARP and caspase 3,7 activity indicating that at least some of the cells were undergoing apoptosis in response to expression of the shRNAs.

4. Discussion

AP-1 is a transcription factor that is frequently up regulated in a variety of tumors. In this study we determined that AP-1 is up regulated in some glioblastoma cell lines. Transcription factors are typically defined by the sequences that they are capable of binding even though the transcription factor itself may be composed of several different but related polypeptides. The purpose of this study was to determine if the cell lines that expressed higher levels of activated AP-1 only expressed certain family members. Similar to what we previously found with the NF-κB family of transcription factors (6), most if not all of the family members of AP-1 were present in these cells and they appeared to play a role in the level of AP-1 that was found within the cell. Although inhibition of c-Jun, JunD, c-Fos, FosB, Fra-1 and 2 all had similar effects on the levels of AP-1, inhibition of JunB did not have a substantial impact on AP-1 levels indicating that certain family members were not as important for the AP-1 effect on the cells. This is in contrast to previous findings that JunB had an antagonistic effect to c-Jun on cells (4). Whether our results differ due to the fact that we used established cell lines as opposed to fresh tumor tissue is unclear.

5. References

[1] Shaulian, E. & Karin, M. (2002) *Nat. Cell Biol.* 4, E131-E136.
[2] Eychène, A., Rocques, N. & Pouponnot, C. (2008) *Nat. Rev. Cancer* 8, 683-693.
[3] Olive, M., Krylov, D., Echlin, D. R., Gardner, K., Taparowsky, E. & Vinson, C. (1997) *J. Biol. Chem.* 272, 18586-18594.
[4] Jin, J. Y., Ke, H., Hall, R. P. & Zhang, J. Y. (2011) *J. Invest. Dermatol.* 131, 1149-1158.
[5] Shaulian, E. (2010) *Cell Signal.* 22, 894-899.
[6] Smith, D. I., Shimamura, T., Barbera, S. & Bejcek, B. E. (2008) *Mol. Cell Biochem.* 307, 141-147.

[7] Elbashir, S. M., Lendeckel, W. & Tuschl, T. (2001) *Genes Devel.* 15, 188-200.
[8] Elbashir, S. M., Harborth, J., Lendeckel, W., Yalcin, A., Weber, K. & Tuschl, T. (2001) *Nature* 411, 494-498.
[9] Altschul, S. F., Madden, T. L., Schaffer, A. A., Zhang, J., Zhang, Z., Miller, W. & DJ, L. (1997) *Nucleic Acids Res* 25, 3389-3402.
[10] Brummelkamp, T. R., Bernards, R. & Agami, R. (2002) Science 296, 550-553.

Part 13

Musashi1 RNA-Binding Protein - Glioblastoma

26

The Musashi1 RNA-Binding Protein: A Critical Regulator in Glioblastoma

Dat T. Vo[1,2], Devraj Sandhu[1],
Jonathan A. Gelfond[3] and Luiz O. Penalva[1,2]
[1]*Greehey Children's Cancer Research Institute*
[2]*Department of Cellular and Structural Biology*
[3]*Department of Epidemiology and Biostatistics*
University of Texas Health Science Center at San Antonio
United States of America

1. Introduction

Musashi1 (Msi1) is an evolutionary conserved RNA-binding protein that plays important roles in neural stem cell maintenance, nervous system development, and tumorigenesis. In glioblastoma, Msi1 is found to be highly expressed and to control a network of cancer-related genes. In this chapter, we will review the participation of RNA-binding proteins in tumorigenesis and the role of Msi1 in stem cells and in glioblastoma. Furthermore, we will discuss the results of a study done with The Cancer Genome Atlas (TCGA) dataset to map genes highly correlated in expression with Msi1 as an avenue to understand its function in gliomagenesis.

2. Musashi1 and RNA-binding proteins

2.1 RNA-binding proteins

RNA-binding proteins (RBPs) are instrumental in RNA metabolism, from biogenesis to degradation affecting molecular processes associated with mRNA capping, 3′ end formation, splicing, transport, localization, stability, and translation (**Figure 1**). RNA-binding proteins associate with target RNA ligands forming the so-called ribonucleoprotein complexes (RNPs). Changes that affect RBP expression and/or function, either temporally or spatially, can have a profound impact on the fate of their target RNAs.

Recent genomic analyses suggest that RNA-binding proteins target mRNAs that code for proteins of similar function, forming the so-called RNA operon (Keene, 2007). In this scenario, RNA-binding proteins coordinate the expression of newly synthesized transcripts in order to ensure the needs of the cells are met. This relationship is not linear and any particularly mRNA may be bound by many different RNA-binding proteins thus forming a higher order of regulation termed the RNA regulon. Since RNA-binding proteins regulate large subsets of mRNA, it is conceivable that changes in expression or function can have a profound impact on human disease.

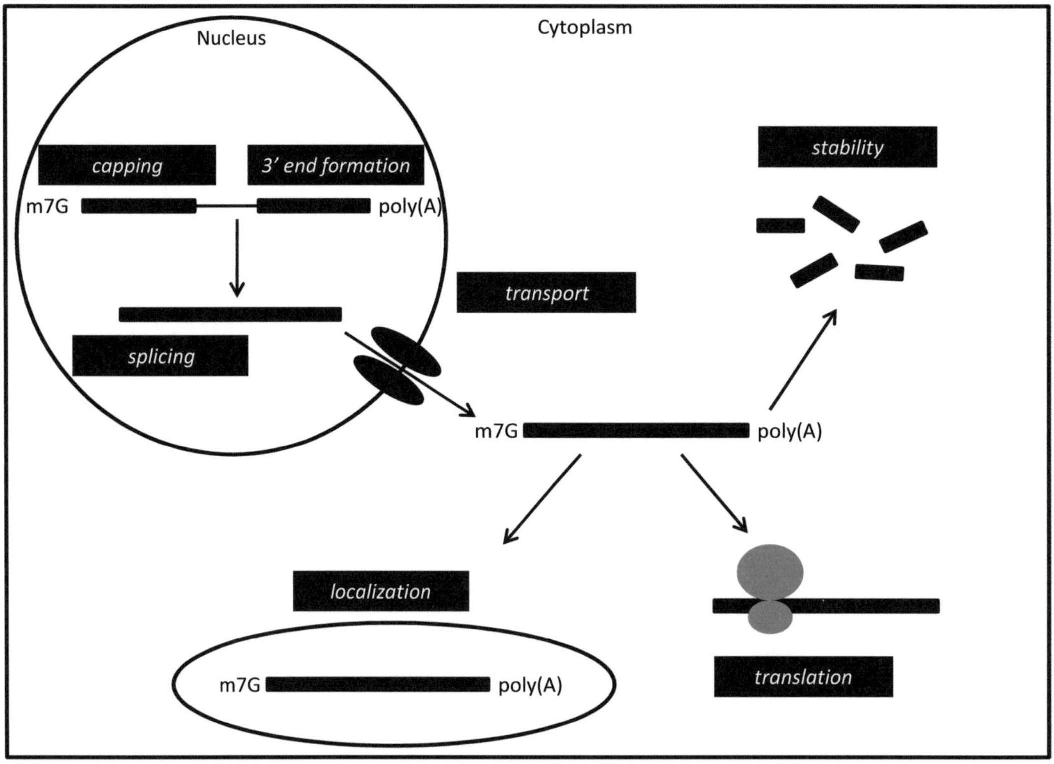

Fig. 1. RNA-binding proteins have diverse functions in RNA metabolism. A schematic of the life cycle of an mRNA and various functions, in black boxes, where RNA-binding proteins participate is shown. m7G denotes the 7-methylguanosine cap and poly(A) denotes the poly(A) tail of mRNAs.

2.2 RNA-binding proteins and cancer

RNA-binding proteins can regulate operons formed by mRNAs involved in cell proliferation, apoptosis, growth, angiogenesis, and invasion/metastasis, processes which, if dysregulated can lead to or potentiate cancer (Lukong et al., 2008). In recent times, the recognition of the impact RNA-binding proteins have on tumorigenesis has been emerging. For example, eIF4E is an important RNA-binding protein that acts downstream of the mTOR pathway (Wendel et al., 2007). This protein functions normally as a component of the translation initiation complex. When elevated, eIF4e contributes to tumor formation by increasing the translation of oncogenes and genes involved in cell proliferation.

It is estimated that the human genome encodes ~1000 different RNA-binding proteins. A recent study from our lab utilized a comprehensive *in silico* approach to analyze the expression pattern of RNA-binding proteins in normal and tumor tissues (Galante et al., 2009). In this study, we analyzed 383 RNA-binding proteins in 12 different tissue/tumor types. 53 proteins have been shown to be aberrantly expressed in at least two tumor types, with the majority of them being upregulated, suggesting that RNA-binding proteins may be oncogenic or potentiate certain characteristics in cancer. One example is Musashi1, whose increased expression pattern has been shown in malignancies such as glioblastoma, medulloblastoma, breast, and colon cancer (Kanemura et al., 2001; Toda et al., 2001; Sureban et al., 2008; Wang et al., 2010).

2.3 The Musashi1 RNA-binding protein

Musashi (Msi) is an evolutionarily conserved RNA-binding protein (RBP) that controls translation through its interaction with specific motifs located in the 3′ untranslated region of target messenger mRNAs (Okano et al., 2005). Msi1 represses the translation of Numb (Imai et al., 2001), a negative regulator of Notch, $p21^{Cip1}$, an inhibitor of cyclin-dependent kinases (Battelli et al., 2006), and doublecortin (Dcx), a microtubule-binding protein involved in neural stem cell migration (Horisawa et al., 2009), but promotes the translation of Robo3, a receptor involved in axonal guidance (Kuwako et al., 2010). Additional targets for Msi1, many of which pertain to the cell cycle, apoptosis, proliferation and differentiation were identified by RIP-chip analysis (de Sousa Abreu et al., 2009). The ability of Msi1 to either positively or negatively control protein expression suggests the duality of its function in translation. Musashi1 inhibits translation through its interaction with poly (A)-binding protein (PABP), thus disrupting the formation of an active translation complex (Kawahara et al., 2008). The mechanism by which Msi1 activates translation is not yet known.

Msi1 was identified in *Drosophila* as a protein involved in sensory organ development and asymmetric cell division (Nakamura et al., 1994). In *Drosophila,* mutations in Musashi results in a double sensory shaft. The name Musashi is a tribute to the famous 17th century samurai, Miyamoto Musashi, who developed the two sword technique. In metazoans, Musashi has two paralogs, Msi1 and Msi2, which have similar RNA-binding properties (Sakakibara et al., 1996; Sakakibara et al., 2001; Sakakibara et al., 2002). Although Msi1 and Msi2 have differing patterns of expression and roles within the cell (Aubert et al., 2003; Chan et al., 2006; Siddall et al., 2006; Sugiyama-Nakagiri et al., 2006; Sgubin et al., 2007; Kharas et al., 2010), both Msi1 and Msi2 are required for brain stem cell self-renewal (Sakakibara et al., 2002). In mammalian cells, Msi1 denotes multipotent stem cells in the brain (Sakakibara et al., 1996; Keyoung et al., 2001; McGuckin et al., 2004; Uchida et al., 2004), intestine (Kayahara et al., 2003; Nishimura et al., 2003; Sakatani et al., 2005) , breast (Clarke, 2005; Wang et al., 2008), and hair follicles (Sugiyama-Nakagiri et al., 2006).

2.4 Function of Musashi1 in normal and cancer stem cells

In breast cancer cells, Musashi1 maintains the expression of the embryonic stem cell (ESC) markers c-Myc, Nanog, Sox2, Bmi1 and Oct4 (Wang et al., 2010). These markers when collectively expressed in differentiated cells were able to reprogram cells, conferring them stem-like characteristics (Yu et al., 2007; Gonzalez et al., 2009; Yu et al., 2009; Stadtfeld et al., 2010). An embryonic stem cell signature in breast cancer is associated with a lower five-year survival rate (Wang et al., 2010). The expression of embryonic stem cell markers are usually found in other malignant tumors such as cervical cancer, retinoblastoma, poorly differentiated lung cancer, medulloblastoma, glioblastoma, bladder cancer, and basal-type breast cancer, and predicts lower overall survival (Ben-Porath et al., 2008; Hassan et al., 2009; Hemmati et al., 2003; Seigel et al., 2007; Stevenson et al., 2009; Ye et al., 2008).

Msi1 expression is particularly important for the proper development of the brain as suggested by a genetically engineered *msi1*$^{-/-}$ in a C57BL6 background which results in a mouse with obstructive hydrocephalus and ependymal abnormalities (Sakakibara et al., 2002). Additionally, Msi1 is known as a neural stem cell marker useful for studying the

migration and biology of neural stem/progenitor cells during development (Kaneko et al., 2000; Chan et al., 2006). In a recent study, Msi1 was shown to be required for neuronal migration of precerebellar neurons via its target gene, Robo3 (Kuwako et al., 2010). Robo3 is a receptor found on astrocytes and is required to receive signals from migrating neurons through the secretion of the Slit1 diffusable protein. Slit1 signals the change of astrocyte morphology to create astrocytic tunnels, allowing migrating neurons to navigate through the dense meshwork of the adult brain (Kaneko et al., 2010).
Consistent with its role in self-renewal, Msi1 expression is positively correlated with a label-retaining and side population human breast epithelial cells enriched in ERα, $p21^{Cip1}$, CK19 and double-positive CK14/CK18 progenitor cells (Smalley and Clarke, 2005; Clarke et al., 2005). When Msi1 is overexpressed in murine mammary epithelial cells, $CD24^{hi}/Sca\text{-}1^{+}$, $CD24^{hi}/CD29^{+}$, $CK14^{+}/CK18^{+}$ and $CK6^{+}$ and $CK19^{+}$ expression is enhanced in mammary stem and progenitor cells (Glazer et al., 2008; Wang et al., 2008). Msi1 acts in a unique autocrine pathway which consists of increased secretion of the growth factor Proliferin, loss of the Wnt inhibitor DKK3, activation of Wnt and Notch signaling (Glazer et al., 2008; Wang et al., 2008). This results in a gene expression profile indicative of the cell cycle, growth factor signaling, invasion, adhesion, survival and embryonic stem cells. In addition, $CD24^{+}/CD29^{hi}$ mouse mammary cells contain multipotent self-renewing mammary stem cells which can reconstitute a complete mammary gland from a single mammary stem cell and represent a cancer stem cell population in tumors from MMTV-Wnt1 and p53-null in murine breast cancer models (Shackleton et al., 2006; Zhang et al., 2008). CD24 expression is controlled through the IGF2 receptor which binds to Proliferin and coexpressed in Msi1-positive cells (Glazer et al., 2008; Wang et al., 2008). In colon cancer, high expression of Msi1 is observed as a result of increased IGF2 expression in intestinal crypt cells due to loss of imprinting, thus predisposing the crypt cells to become malignant (Sakatani et al., 2005; Cui et al., 2006). Loss of imprinting of *IGF2* is observed in other cancers such as medulloblastoma (Corcoran et al., 2008). In studies done in our lab using the cross-linked and immunoprecipitation, or CLIP analysis in U251 glioblastoma cells, IGF2 was identified as a potential target of Musashi1 (Penalva lab, unpublished results), suggesting a potential mechanism by which Msi1 may control tumor progression.

3. Musashi1 as a critical regulator in brain tumors

Musashi1 expression has been seen to be elevated in brain tumors such as glioma and medulloblastoma. In gliomas, high Msi1 expression was identified as a poor prognostic factor (Kanemura et al., 2001). In *in vivo* xenograft models, silencing of Musashi1 by small interfering RNAs caused a reduction in tumor growth of both glioblastoma and medulloblastoma cells (Penalva lab, unpublished results). We summarized below the connections between Msi1 and brain tumor-related pathways.

3.1 Notch pathway

Musashi1 and Notch 1 expression correlate in areas of tumor proliferation and infiltration (Kanemura et al., 2001). Furthermore, suppression subtractive hybridization experiments established an association between Msi1 and Notch pathway activation in medulloblastoma cells (Yokota et al., 2004). Notch is a well-conserved signaling pathway that regulates cell fate, cell proliferation, and cell death during development (Artavanis-Tsakonas et al., 1999). Upon binding, cleavage of the Notch receptor occurs in two separate events. The first event is catalyzed by the ADAM-family of metalloproteinases. The second event is catalyzed by the γ-secretase protein complex; this complex consists of four proteins, presenilin, nicastrin, PEN2, and APH2 (Fortini, 2002). Cleavage by the γ-secretase protein complex releases the Notch intracellular domain, or NICD, which then localizes in the nucleus and transactivates transcription (Schweisguth, 2004). Musashi1 interacts with the Notch pathway via post-transcriptional regulation of the negative Notch regulator, Numb. Upon binding to the 3′ untranslated region of Numb, Musashi1 causes translational repression, thus effectively releasing Notch inhibition (Imai et al., 2001).

3.2 Wnt pathway

Wnt is an essential signaling pathway required for developmental processes such as body axis specification and morphogenic signaling (Cadigan and Nusse, 1997). Wnt is a family of secreted cysteine-rich glycoproteins that act in a paracrine-like fashion over short distances to activate signaling pathways. Msi1 influences Wnt pathway activation by repressing the translation of p21, a cyclin-dependent kinase inhibitor, required for the transition between the G_1 and S phase of the cell cycle (Battelli et al., 2006). Additionally, p21 negatively regulates Wnt4 transcription, thus connecting cell cycle regulation with the Wnt signaling pathway (Devgan et al., 2005).

3.3 Hedgehog pathway

The Hedgehog pathway initiates with the secretion of Hedgehog ligand from different tissues during development (Ingham and McMahon, 2001). Upon binding, the Hedgehog ligand inactivates the Patched-1 Hedgehog receptor, leading to the release of the catalytic inhibition on the Smoothened G-protein-coupled receptor signal transduction molecule (Villavicencio et al., 2000; Chen et al., 2002). This event activates the Hedgehog signal transduction cascade with the subsequent activation of transcription by the glioma-associated oncogene zinc finger transcription factor GLI2 and GLI3 of Hedgehog target genes (Dahmane et al., 2001). Msi1 interacts with the Hedgehog pathway by interfering with the expression of several key Hedgehog components such as SMO and GLI1. Morover, inhibition of Msi1 causes increased sensitivity to cyclopamine, a Hedgehog pathway inhibitor, resulting in a decrease in cell proliferation (Sanchez-Diaz et al., 2008).

3.4 Mining through the cancer genome atlas

To better understand the participation of Msi1 in glioblastoma, we conducted an expression correlation study to identify genes closely associated with Msi1. Glioblastoma (GBM) data from The Cancer Genome Atlas (TCGA) consortium was collected representing microarrays performed on GBM in nearly 500 patients (The Cancer Genome Atlas Research Network, 2008). The microarray results were downloaded from 7 distinct batches of experiments and then filtered for only those tumors assayed by the Agilent 244K platform and then combined to form a single dataset comprising expression results for 17815 genes across all patients. Due to data access restrictions patients could not be stratified by age, gender, or race. The data were re-normalized using quantile normalization, and the correlation with Msi1 and all other genes was computed for each batch stratum. The mean correlation across batches was computed for each gene, and the absolute value of the correlation was used to sort the genes from most correlated to least correlated with MSI1.

The genes with significant expression correlation with Musahi1 (~250 genes) were then analyzed for ontological information pertaining to disease states (**Figure 2 and 3**), biological processes (**Figure 4**), and functional association using Ariadne Genomics Pathway Studio (**Figure 5**). Identified genes were not found to have significant change in correlation levels across the four known subtypes of glioblastoma tumors (Classical, Mesenchymal, Proneural, and Neural) as defined by the TCGA (Parsons et al., 2008). Approximately 10% of the genes were shown to have interactions with other genes within the group (**Figure 5**). Major nodes in this network include CSF3 (Granulocyte colony stimulating factor), GnRH (Gonadotropin-releasing hormone), RARA (Retinoic acid receptor alpha), and RELB. All of these genes have a strong positive correlation with MSI1 expression in the TCGA expression data.

Disease State	Gene Symbol (Positive Correlation with MSI1)	Gene Symbol (Negative Correlation with MSI1)
Neoplasms	ALOX12, CSF3, CX3CL1, CYP2S1, ERCC2, FCGR1A, FPR1, GATA5, GNRH2, HOXB9, IL1F7, INHBC, MOS, MSMB, NOTCH3, PPY, RARA, RASSF3, RELB, SFTPA1, SOCS1, TFF2, TSPO, TYROBP, WNT3A	AKT3, CNTN1, CTGF, LIG4, MAPK9, MBD1, PIK3CB, SNIP1, SPIN1, TRIM37
Death	ALOX12, CSF3, CX3CL1, ERCC2, FCGR1A, NOTCH3, RARA, RELB, SFTPA1, SLC4A1, SOCS1, TYROBP	ATE1, CTCF, GRM1, MAPK9, PIK3CB
Inflammation	ALOX15, CCL24, CSF3, CX3CL1, DEFB4A, FCGR1A, FPR1, GNRH1, IL12RB1, RELB, RETNLB, SFTPA1, SOCS1, TFF2, TYROBP, VSIG4	MAPK9
Breast Neoplasms	CSF3, DPF3, ERCC2, GNRH1, GNRH2, HOXB9, NOTCH3, NOTCH4, OPRL1, RARA, RELB, TFF2, TSPO, WNT3A	AKT3, MAPK9, SLC39A6
Infection	CSF3, CST5, CX3CL1, DEFB4A, FCGR1A, FPR1, GNRH1, IL12RB1, PGLYRP4, PRSS22, RETNLB, SFTPA1, SOCS1, TYROBP, VSIG4	MAPK9
Wounds and Injuries	ALOX12, ALOX15, CCL24, CSF3, CX3CL1, DEFB4A, FCGR1A, FPR1, NOTCH3, RELB, RETNLB, SFTPA1, SOCS1, TFF2, TSPO	GRM1, MAPK9
Diabetes Mellitus	ALOX12, ALOX15, CSF3, CX3CL1, GNRH1, NEUROG3, NOTCH3, PPY, RETNLB, SOCS1	LIG4, MAPK9
Adenocarcinoma	ALOX12, CSF3, CX3CL1, GNRH1, HOXB9, MSMB, NOTCH3, SFTPA1, SLC4A1	
Prostatic Neoplasms	ALOX12, ALOX15, CSF3, GNRH1, MRGPRE, MSMB, RELB, WNT3A	AKT3, PIK3CB
Pancreatic Neoplasms	ALOX15, CX3CL1, GNRH1, LRG1, NOTCH3, PPY, TFF2	MBD1
Neutrophil Infiltration	ALOX15, CCL24, CSF3, DEFB4A, FCGR1A, FPR1	
Bone Resorption	CSF3, CX3CL1, NOTCH3, RELB, SOCS1, WNT3A	
Myeloid Leukemia	CSF3, RARA, SLC4A1, SOCS1	
B-Cell Lymphoma	FCGR1A, SLC4A1, SPIB	CTCF

Fig. 2. Msi1-correlated genes are involved in disease processes. The table above shows the incidence of genes from the TCGA data set shown to be correlated with MSI1 in various diseases. Genes in red were positively correlated with MSI1 expression while genes in green were negatively correlated with MSI1 expression.

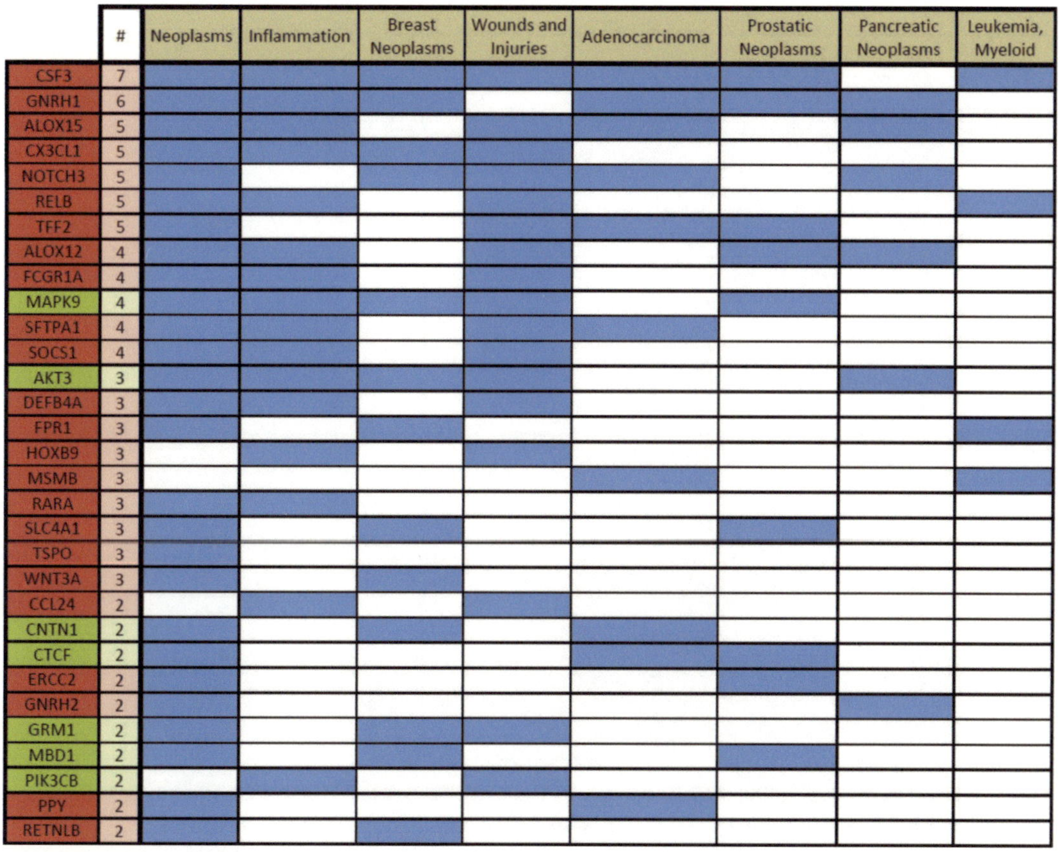

Fig. 3. Msi1-correlated genes have implication in important disease states. Genes and Disease were sorted by incidence count which is also given adjacent to or bellow each group respectively. Genes in red were positively correlated with MSI1 expression while genes in green were negatively correlated with MSI1 expression.

3.5 Genes that correlate with Msi1 expression are important players in glioblastoma

Among the genes identified in the TCGA analysis, a few should be highlighted based on its importance and role in gliomagenesis. We will summarize the functions of granulocyte colony stimulating factor 3 (CSF3), gonadotropin-releasing hormone (GnRH), retinoic acid receptor alpha (RARA), Notch3/4, DNA ligase IV (LIG4), excision repair cross-complementing rodent repair deficiency, complementation group 2 (ERCC2), and (C-X3-C motif) ligand 1 (CX3CL1).

3.5.1 Granulocyte colony stimulating factor 3

Granulocyte colony stimulating factor (CSF3) is a cytokine that controls the production, differentiation, and function of granulocytes. In the central nervous system, CSF3 plays an important role by inducing neurogenesis, maintain neuroplasticity, halting tissue degradation through inhibition of apoptosis and promoting cell survival through the MAPK, PI3K, and Akt pathways (Schneider et al., 2005).

Pathway	Gene Symbol (Positive Correlation with MSI1)	Gene Symbol (Negative Correlation with MSI1)
Cell Cycle Regulation	ADRA1D, ALOX12, ALOX15, BEST4, CCL24, CHRNE, CLCN1, CSF3, CX3CL1, DEFB4A, ERCC2, FCGR1A, FPR1, GALK1, GNRH1, GNRH2, HOXB9, IL12RB1, IL17RE, IL1F7, INHBC, KCNK7, KRT6B, MOS, MRGPRX3, MSI1, MSMB, NEUROG3, NFKBID, NOTCH3, NOTCH4, OPRL1, OR10J5, PPY, RARA, RASSF3, RASSF5, RELB, RETNLB, SCN4A, SFTPA1, SLC4A1, SOCS1, SPIB, TFF2, TSHB, TSPO, TYROBP, VSIG4, WNT3A	AKT3, ATE1, CDC40, CHRM5, CNTN1, CP110, CTCF, DPEP1, GRM1, KCNAB1, KPNA6, LIG4, MAPK9, PIK3CB, RSBN1, SLC39A6, SNIP1, SNX19, SPNS1, STXBP5, TRIM23, TRIM37, UBR5
Cell Proliferation	ADRA1D, ALOX12, ALOX15, BAALC, CCL24, CD320, CSF3, CX3CL1, DEFB4A, DHH, FCGR1A, FPR1, GALK1, GATA5, GNRH1, GNRH2, HOXB9, IL12RB1, KRT6B, MOS, MSMB, NEUROG3, NOTCH3, NOTCH4, OPRL1, RARA, RASSF3, RELB, RETNLB, SFTPA1, SLC4A1, SOCS1, SPATA12, TFF2, TSPO, TYROBP, VSIG4, WNT3A	AKT3, CHRM5, CNTN1, CTCF, GRM1, LIG4, MAPK9, PIK3CB, PSMD6, PUM2, SNIP1, UBR5
Apoptosis	ADRA1D, ALOX12, ALOX15, CSF3, CST5, CX3CL1, DEFB4A, ERCC2, FCGR1A, FPR1, GJB3, GNRH1, GNRH2, MAP3K9, MOS, MSMB, NEUROG3, NOTCH3, NOTCH4, OPA3, PROKR2, RARA, RASSF3, RASSF5, RELB, RETNLB, RPL13A, SFTPA1, SOCS1, TFF2, TSPO, TYROBP, WNT3A	AKT3, CTCF, GRM1, LIG4, MAPK9, MBD1, NEK1, PIK3CB, SLC39A6, SPIN1, SPNS1
Cell Differentiation	ADRA1D, ALOX15, BAALC, CD320, CSF3, CST5, CX3CL1, DHH, FCGR1A, FOXE3, FPR1, GATA5, GNRH1, HOXB9, IL12RB1, LCE3B, LRG1, MOS, MRPL12, MSMB, NEUROG3, NOTCH3, NOTCH4, RARA, RELB, RETNLB, SFTPA1, SOCS1, SPIB, TFF2, TSPO, TYROBP, VSIG4, WNT3A	AKT3, CNTN1, CTCF, MAPK9, MBD1, PUM2, UBR5
Sonic Hedgehog Pathway	ALOX15, CLCN1, CSF3, CX3CL1, DEFB4A, DHH, FCGR1A, FOXE3, FPR1, GALK1, GNRH1, GNRH2, HOXB9, MOS, NFKBID, NOTCH3, RARA, RELB, SFTPA1, TSHB, TSPO, WNT3A	AKT3, GRM1, MAPK9, RSBN1, SNIP1, STXBP5, UBR5
Notch Pathway	ALOX12, CHRNE, CSF3, CX3CL1, DEFB4A, FCGR1A, FPR1, GNRH1, GNRH2, MOS, NOTCH3, NOTCH4, RARA, RASSF3, RASSF5, RELB, SFTPA1, SLC4A1, SOCS1, TFF2, TSHB, TSPO, TYROBP, WNT3A	AP1AR, CDC40, CNTN1, MAPK9, PIK3CB
Cell Survival	ADRA1D, ALOX12, CSF3, CX3CL1, FCGR1A, GNRH1, MSMB, NOTCH3, RARA, RELB, SOCS1, SPIB, TSPO, WNT3A	AKT3, CTCF, GRM1, LIG4, MAPK9, PIK3CB
Neurogenesis	CSF3, NEUROG3, NOTCH3, RARA, WNT3A	GRM1, LIG4, MBD1

Fig. 4. Msi1-correlated genes are involved in many cancer-related processes. The table above shows the incidence of genes correlated with MSI1 in various pathways. Genes in red were positively correlated with MSI1 expression while genes in green were negatively correlated with MSI1 expression.

3.5.2 Gonadotropin-releasing hormone

Gonadotropin-releasing hormone (GnRH) is a tropic peptide hormone that facilitates the release of follicle-stimulating hormone and luteinizing hormone from the anterior pituitary. GnRH-mediated signaling may be important for the growth and maintenance of gliomas. The use of the GnRH agonist Zoladex results in inhibition of cell proliferation in two glioblastoma cell lines (U87MG and U373) thus presenting GnRH signaling as a potential therapeutic target (Marelli et al., 2009).

3.5.3 Retinoic acid receptor alpha

Retinoic acid receptor alpha (RARA) is a ligand-dependent nuclear receptor that upon binding to retinoic acid, can affect processes such as development, differentiation, apoptosis, and transcription of clock genes. Glioblastoma is extremely sensitive to retinoic acid, which flattens cell morphology, forming intercellular cross-bridges, and reduces anchorage-independent growth (Mukherjee and Das, 1995). Treatment of glioblastoma cells *in vitro* results in growth arrest and induces differentiation through the Notch pathway (Ying et al., 2011).

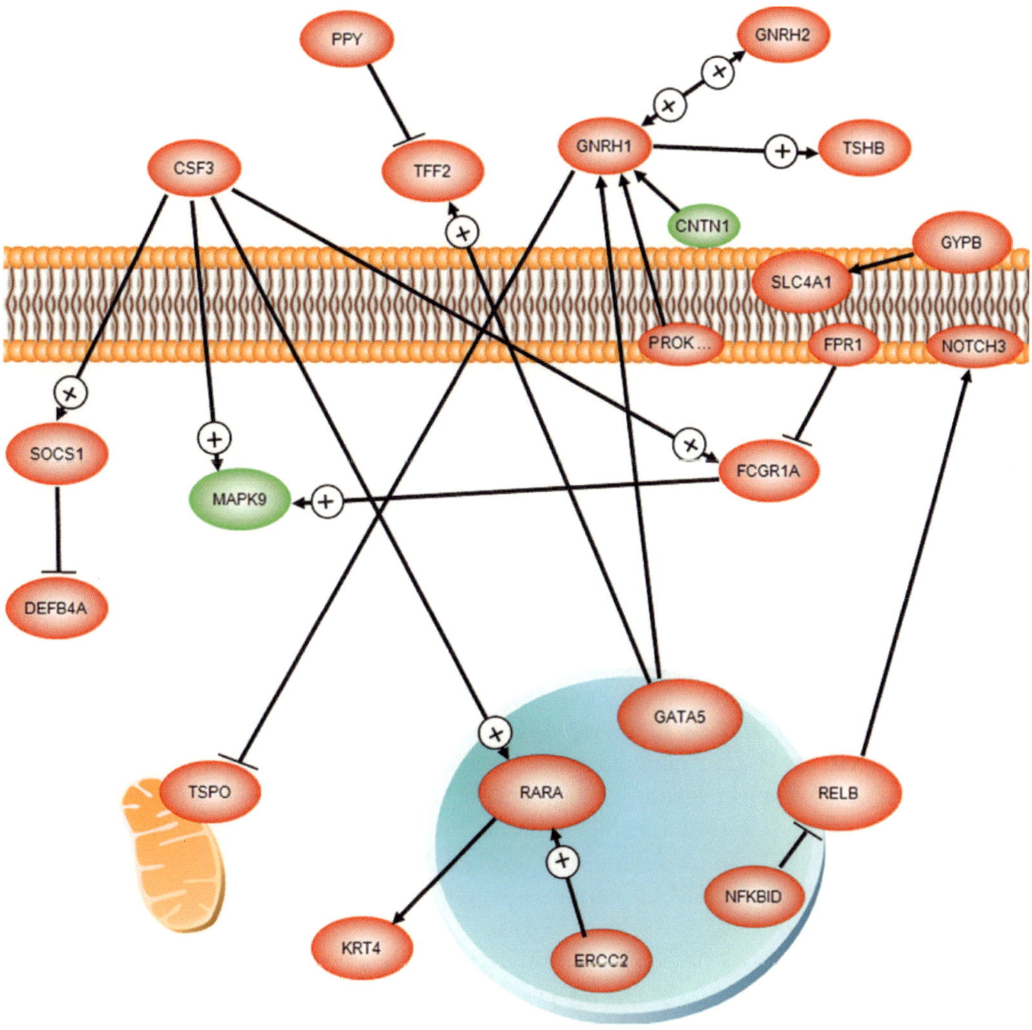

Fig. 5. Msi1-correlated genes interact in a wide network in glioblastoma. The image above shows the interactions amongst genes from the TCGA data set shown to be correlated with Msi1. Genes in red were positively correlated with Msi1 expression while genes in green were negatively correlated with Msi1 expression. The mitochondria, nucleus, and cell membrane are shown and genes are placed accordingly. Connections that involved positive changes in expression / up regulation are drawn with a "plus" symbol while those involving negative changes in expression / down regulation are shown with a bar. If no information was present or the effect was unclear only the direction of the connection was shown with an arrow.

3.5.4 Notch receptors

Notch3 and Notch4 receptors have been previously implicated in association with Msi1. Msi1 has been previously demonstrated to negatively affect Numb expression, a negative effector of the Notch pathway. Notch3 and Notch4 have previously been demonstrated to play important roles in the tumorigenesis and glioblastoma biology. Enhanced Notch3/4 expression is observed in astrocytomas and medulloblastomas in part due to the loss of the FBXW7, a Skp1-Cul1-F-box E2 ubiquitin ligase (Hagedorn et al., 2007; Xu et al., 2009). Notch3 activation has been implicated in gliomagenesis (Pierfelice et al., 2011).

3.5.5 DNA repair enzymes

A hurdle in treatment of glioblastoma with adjuvant chemotherapy or radiation therapy is the enhanced ability for the cell to repair DNA resultant of damage induced by the chemotherapeutic or radiation. Two genes, LIG4 and ERCC2, are found to be correlated with Msi1. LIG4, or DNA ligase IV, expression causes cells to be resistant to treatment by the nitrosourea chloroethylating agent, nimustine (ACNU) through the role of DNA ligase IV in nonhomologous end joining and siRNA silencing of LIG4 results in increased cell death when induced with ACNU (Kondo et al., 2010). In human genetic studies, polymorphisms of LIG4, particularly SNP2 rs3093739:T>C, was associated with increased risk for developing gliomas, probably due to increased DNA damage and the inability for the cell to repair the damage effectively, thus leading to tumor formation (Liu et al., 2008). ERCC2, or excision repair cross-complementing rodent repair deficiency, complementation group 2, is another DNA repair gene whose expression is associated with Msi1. ERCC2 is involved in transcription-coupled nucleotide excision repair through its binding to the basal transcription factor BTF2/TFIIH complex. Allelic loss of ERCC2 is associated with a younger age of diagnosis of glioma; however, the loss of the ERCC2 gene is not associated with a difference in response to therapy or survival (Liang et al., 1995). More recently, polymorphisms in the ERCC2 gene have been revealed. Particularly, homozygosity at codon 156 for the silent AA allele results in high incidences of glioma (odds ratio 2.3), probably through an alteration in relationship with a currently unidentified gene and ERCC2 (Caggana et al., 2001). In a follow up study, it was seen that a single nucleotide polymorphism, rs13181, for ERCC2 confers a significant, protective effect (McKean-Cowdin et al., 2009).

3.5.6 Chemokine (C-X3-C motif) ligand 1

Glioblastoma also have an enhanced ability to invade adjacent normal brain tissue; one gene that has been implicated in invasion is the chemokine ligand, CX3CL1 chemokine (C-X3-C motif) ligand 1 gene mediating the cross-talk between neurons and microglia. The chemokine receptor CX3CR1 and the ligand, CX3CL1, expression is increased in human glioblastoma samples and neural cancer stem cells at the mRNA and protein level (Erreni et al., 2010; Locatelli et al., 2010). The high expression levels are inversely correlated with patient overall survival (Erreni et al., 2010). CX3CL1 is localized in the outer layer of cells of glioblastoma tumorspheres, suggesting the involvement of the chemokine system in intracellular adhesion (Erreni et al., 2010). The high levels of CX3CL1/CX3CR1 results in the recruitment of glioma-infiltrating microglia, which displays high levels of adhesion and migration *in vitro*; this suggests an important role for the chemokine system in tumor promotion (Held-Feindt et al., 2010).

4. Conclusion

Musashi1 plays a role in glioblastoma and other tumor types by affecting a complex network of genes implicated in numerous cancer-related processes and biological pathways. This is evident from the TCGA study we discussed in this chapter. Further wet-lab experimentation is required to understand the different branches of Musashi1 regulation and hopefully to provide insight for the development of novel glioblastoma therapeutics.

5. Acknowledgement

The work here is supported by grants from the Children's Brain Tumor Foundation and Association for Research of Childhood Cancer.

6. References

Artavanis-Tsakonas S, Rand MD, Lake RJ (1999) Notch signaling: cell fate control and signal integration in development. Science 284:770-776.

Aubert J, Stavridis MP, Tweedie S, O'Reilly M, Vierlinger K, Li M, Ghazal P, Pratt T, Mason JO, Roy D, Smith A (2003) Screening for mammalian neural genes via fluorescence-activated cell sorter purification of neural precursors from Sox1-gfp knock-in mice. Proc Natl Acad Sci U S A 100 Suppl 1:11836-11841.

Battelli C, Nikopoulos GN, Mitchell JG, Verdi JM (2006) The RNA-binding protein Musashi-1 regulates neural development through the translational repression of p21WAF-1. Mol Cell Neurosci 31:85-96.

Ben-Porath I, Thomson MW, Carey VJ, Ge R, Bell GW, Regev A, Weinberg RA (2008) An embryonic stem cell-like gene expression signature in poorly differentiated aggressive human tumors. Nat Genet 40:499-507.

Cadigan KM, Nusse R (1997) Wnt signaling: a common theme in animal development. Genes Dev 11:3286-3305.

Caggana M, Kilgallen J, Conroy JM, Wiencke JK, Kelsey KT, Miike R, Chen P, Wrensch MR (2001) Associations between ERCC2 polymorphisms and gliomas. Cancer Epidemiol Biomarkers Prev 10:355-360.

Chan C, Moore BE, Cotman CW, Okano H, Tavares R, Hovanesian V, Pinar H, Johanson CE, Svendsen CN, Stopa EG (2006) Musashi1 antigen expression in human fetal germinal matrix development. Exp Neurol 201:515-518.

Chen JK, Taipale J, Cooper MK, Beachy PA (2002) Inhibition of Hedgehog signaling by direct binding of cyclopamine to Smoothened. Genes Dev 16:2743-2748.

Clarke RB (2005) Isolation and characterization of human mammary stem cells. Cell Prolif 38:375-386.

Clarke RB, Spence K, Anderson E, Howell A, Okano H, Potten CS (2005) A putative human breast stem cell population is enriched for steroid receptor-positive cells. Dev Biol 277:443-456.

Corcoran RB, Bachar Raveh T, Barakat MT, Lee EY, Scott MP (2008) Insulin-like growth factor 2 is required for progression to advanced medulloblastoma in patched1 heterozygous mice. Cancer Res 68:8788-8795.

Cui J, Han SY, Wang C, Su W, Harshyne L, Holgado-Madruga M, Wong AJ (2006) c-Jun NH(2)-terminal kinase 2alpha2 promotes the tumorigenicity of human glioblastoma cells. Cancer Res 66:10024-10031.

Dahmane N, Sanchez P, Gitton Y, Palma V, Sun T, Beyna M, Weiner H, Ruiz i Altaba A (2001) The Sonic Hedgehog-Gli pathway regulates dorsal brain growth and tumorigenesis. Development 128:5201-5212.

de Sousa Abreu R, Sanchez-Diaz PC, Vogel C, Burns SC, Ko D, Burton TL, Vo DT, Chennasamudaram S, Le SY, Shapiro BA, Penalva LO (2009) Genomic analyses of musashi1 downstream targets show a strong association with cancer-related processes. J Biol Chem 284:12125-12135.

Devgan V, Mammucari C, Millar SE, Brisken C, Dotto GP (2005) p21WAF1/Cip1 is a negative transcriptional regulator of Wnt4 expression downstream of Notch1 activation. Genes Dev 19:1485-1495.

Erreni M, Solinas G, Brescia P, Osti D, Zunino F, Colombo P, Destro A, Roncalli M, Mantovani A, Draghi R, Levi D, Rodriguez YBR, Gaetani P, Pelicci G, Allavena P (2010) Human glioblastoma tumours and neural cancer stem cells express the chemokine CX3CL1 and its receptor CX3CR1. Eur J Cancer 46:3383-3392.

Fortini ME (2002) Gamma-secretase-mediated proteolysis in cell-surface-receptor signalling. Nat Rev Mol Cell Biol 3:673-684.

Galante PA, Sandhu D, de Sousa Abreu R, Gradassi M, Slager N, Vogel C, de Souza SJ, Penalva LO (2009) A comprehensive in silico expression analysis of RNA binding proteins in normal and tumor tissue: Identification of potential players in tumor formation. RNA Biol 6:426-433.

Glazer RI, Wang XY, Yuan H, Yin Y (2008) Musashi1: a stem cell marker no longer in search of a function. Cell Cycle 7:2635-2639.

Gonzalez F, Barragan Monasterio M, Tiscornia G, Montserrat Pulido N, Vassena R, Batlle Morera L, Rodriguez Piza I, Izpisua Belmonte JC (2009) Generation of mouse-induced pluripotent stem cells by transient expression of a single nonviral polycistronic vector. Proc Natl Acad Sci U S A 106:8918-8922.

Hagedorn M, Delugin M, Abraldes I, Allain N, Belaud-Rotureau MA, Turmo M, Prigent C, Loiseau H, Bikfalvi A, Javerzat S (2007) FBXW7/hCDC4 controls glioma cell proliferation in vitro and is a prognostic marker for survival in glioblastoma patients. Cell Div 2:9.

Hassan KA, Chen G, Kalemkerian GP, Wicha MS, Beer DG (2009) An embryonic stem cell-like signature identifies poorly differentiated lung adenocarcinoma but not squamous cell carcinoma. Clin Cancer Res 15:6386-6390.

Held-Feindt J, Hattermann K, Muerkoster SS, Wedderkopp H, Knerlich-Lukoschus F, Ungefroren H, Mehdorn HM, Mentlein R (2010) CX3CR1 promotes recruitment of human glioma-infiltrating microglia/macrophages (GIMs). Exp Cell Res 316:1553-1566.

Hemmati HD, Nakano I, Lazareff JA, Masterman-Smith M, Geschwind DH, Bronner-Fraser M, Kornblum HI (2003) Cancerous stem cells can arise from pediatric brain tumors. Proc Natl Acad Sci U S A 100:15178-15183.

Horisawa K, Imai T, Okano H, Yanagawa H (2009) 3'-Untranslated region of doublecortin mRNA is a binding target of the Musashi1 RNA-binding protein. FEBS Lett 583:2429-2434.

Imai T, Tokunaga A, Yoshida T, Hashimoto M, Mikoshiba K, Weinmaster G, Nakafuku M, Okano H (2001) The neural RNA-binding protein Musashi1 translationally regulates mammalian numb gene expression by interacting with its mRNA. Mol Cell Biol 21:3888-3900.

Ingham PW, McMahon AP (2001) Hedgehog signaling in animal development: paradigms and principles. Genes Dev 15:3059-3087.

Kaneko N, Marin O, Koike M, Hirota Y, Uchiyama Y, Wu JY, Lu Q, Tessier-Lavigne M, Alvarez-Buylla A, Okano H, Rubenstein JL, Sawamoto K (2010) New neurons clear the path of astrocytic processes for their rapid migration in the adult brain. Neuron 67:213-223.

Kaneko Y, Sakakibara S, Imai T, Suzuki A, Nakamura Y, Sawamoto K, Ogawa Y, Toyama Y, Miyata T, Okano H (2000) Musashi1: an evolutionally conserved marker for CNS progenitor cells including neural stem cells. Dev Neurosci 22:139-153.

Kanemura Y, Mori K, Sakakibara S, Fujikawa H, Hayashi H, Nakano A, Matsumoto T, Tamura K, Imai T, Ohnishi T, Fushiki S, Nakamura Y, Yamasaki M, Okano H, Arita N (2001) Musashi1, an evolutionarily conserved neural RNA-binding protein, is a versatile marker of human glioma cells in determining their cellular origin, malignancy, and proliferative activity. Differentiation 68:141-152.

Kawahara H, Imai T, Imataka H, Tsujimoto M, Matsumoto K, Okano H (2008) Neural RNA-binding protein Musashi1 inhibits translation initiation by competing with eIF4G for PABP. J Cell Biol 181:639-653.

Kayahara T, Sawada M, Takaishi S, Fukui H, Seno H, Fukuzawa H, Suzuki K, Hiai H, Kageyama R, Okano H, Chiba T (2003) Candidate markers for stem and early progenitor cells, Musashi-1 and Hes1, are expressed in crypt base columnar cells of mouse small intestine. FEBS Lett 535:131-135.

Keene JD (2007) RNA regulons: coordination of post-transcriptional events. Nat Rev Genet 8:533-543.

Keyoung HM, Roy NS, Benraiss A, Louissaint A, Jr., Suzuki A, Hashimoto M, Rashbaum WK, Okano H, Goldman SA (2001) High-yield selection and extraction of two promoter-defined phenotypes of neural stem cells from the fetal human brain. Nat Biotechnol 19:843-850.

Kharas MG, Lengner CJ, Al-Shahrour F, Bullinger L, Ball B, Zaidi S, Morgan K, Tam W, Paktinat M, Okabe R, Gozo M, Einhorn W, Lane SW, Scholl C, Frohling S, Fleming M, Ebert BL, Gilliland DG, Jaenisch R, Daley GQ (2010) Musashi-2 regulates normal hematopoiesis and promotes aggressive myeloid leukemia. Nat Med 16:903-908.

Kondo N, Takahashi A, Mori E, Noda T, Su X, Ohnishi K, McKinnon PJ, Sakaki T, Nakase H, Ono K, Ohnishi T (2010) DNA ligase IV is a potential molecular target in ACNU sensitivity. Cancer Sci 101:1881-1885.

Kuwako K, Kakumoto K, Imai T, Igarashi M, Hamakubo T, Sakakibara S, Tessier-Lavigne M, Okano HJ, Okano H (2010) Neural RNA-binding protein Musashi1 controls midline crossing of precerebellar neurons through posttranscriptional regulation of Robo3/Rig-1 expression. Neuron 67:407-421.

Liang BC, Ross DA, Reed E (1995) Genomic copy number changes of DNA repair genes ERCC1 and ERCC2 in human gliomas. J Neurooncol 26:17-23.

Liu Y, Zhou K, Zhang H, Shugart YY, Chen L, Xu Z, Zhong Y, Liu H, Jin L, Wei Q, Huang F, Lu D, Zhou L (2008) Polymorphisms of LIG4 and XRCC4 involved in the NHEJ pathway interact to modify risk of glioma. Hum Mutat 29:381-389.

Locatelli M, Boiocchi L, Ferrero S, Martinelli Boneschi F, Zavanone M, Pesce S, Allavena P, Maria Gaini S, Bello L, Mantovani A (2010) Human glioma tumors express high levels of the chemokine receptor CX3CR1. Eur Cytokine Netw 21:27-33.

Lukong KE, Chang KW, Khandjian EW, Richard S (2008) RNA-binding proteins in human genetic disease. Trends Genet 24:416-425.

Marelli MM, Moretti RM, Mai S, Muller O, Van Groeninghen JC, Limonta P (2009) Novel insights into GnRH receptor activity: role in the control of human glioblastoma cell proliferation. Oncol Rep 21:1277-1282.

McGuckin CP, Forraz N, Allouard Q, Pettengell R (2004) Umbilical cord blood stem cells can expand hematopoietic and neuroglial progenitors in vitro. Exp Cell Res 295:350-359.

McKean-Cowdin R, Barnholtz-Sloan J, Inskip PD, Ruder AM, Butler M, Rajaraman P, Razavi P, Patoka J, Wiencke JK, Bondy ML, Wrensch M (2009) Associations between polymorphisms in DNA repair genes and glioblastoma. Cancer Epidemiol Biomarkers Prev 18:1118-1126.

Mukherjee P, Das SK (1995) Action of retinoic acid on human glioblastoma-astrocytoma--14 cells in culture. Neoplasma 42:123-128.

Nakamura M, Okano H, Blendy JA, Montell C (1994) Musashi, a neural RNA-binding protein required for Drosophila adult external sensory organ development. Neuron 13:67-81.

Nishimura S, Wakabayashi N, Toyoda K, Kashima K, Mitsufuji S (2003) Expression of Musashi-1 in human normal colon crypt cells: a possible stem cell marker of human colon epithelium. Dig Dis Sci 48:1523-1529.

Okano H, Kawahara H, Toriya M, Nakao K, Shibata S, Imai T (2005) Function of RNA-binding protein Musashi-1 in stem cells. Exp Cell Res 306:349-356.

Parsons DW et al. (2008) An integrated genomic analysis of human glioblastoma multiforme. Science 321:1807-1812.

Pierfelice TJ, Schreck KC, Dang L, Asnaghi L, Gaiano N, Eberhart CG (2011) Notch3 activation promotes invasive glioma formation in a tissue site-specific manner. Cancer Res 71:1115-1125.

Sakakibara S, Nakamura Y, Satoh H, Okano H (2001) RNA-binding protein Musashi2: developmentally regulated expression in neural precursor cells and subpopulations of neurons in mammalian CNS. J Neurosci 21:8091-8107.

Sakakibara S, Nakamura Y, Yoshida T, Shibata S, Koike M, Takano H, Ueda S, Uchiyama Y, Noda T, Okano H (2002) RNA-binding protein Musashi family: roles for CNS stem cells and a subpopulation of ependymal cells revealed by targeted disruption and antisense ablation. Proc Natl Acad Sci U S A 99:15194-15199.

Sakakibara S, Imai T, Hamaguchi K, Okabe M, Aruga J, Nakajima K, Yasutomi D, Nagata T, Kurihara Y, Uesugi S, Miyata T, Ogawa M, Mikoshiba K, Okano H (1996) Mouse-Musashi-1, a neural RNA-binding protein highly enriched in the mammalian CNS stem cell. Dev Biol 176:230-242.

Sakatani T, Kaneda A, Iacobuzio-Donahue CA, Carter MG, de Boom Witzel S, Okano H, Ko MS, Ohlsson R, Longo DL, Feinberg AP (2005) Loss of imprinting of Igf2 alters intestinal maturation and tumorigenesis in mice. Science 307:1976-1978.

Sanchez-Diaz PC, Burton TL, Burns SC, Hung JY, Penalva LO (2008) Musashi1 modulates cell proliferation genes in the medulloblastoma cell line Daoy. BMC Cancer 8:280.

Schneider A, Kruger C, Steigleder T, Weber D, Pitzer C, Laage R, Aronowski J, Maurer MH, Gassler N, Mier W, Hasselblatt M, Kollmar R, Schwab S, Sommer C, Bach A, Kuhn HG, Schabitz WR (2005) The hematopoietic factor G-CSF is a neuronal ligand that counteracts programmed cell death and drives neurogenesis. J Clin Invest 115:2083-2098.

Schweisguth F (2004) Regulation of notch signaling activity. Curr Biol 14:R129-138.

Seigel GM, Hackam AS, Ganguly A, Mandell LM, Gonzalez-Fernandez F (2007) Human embryonic and neuronal stem cell markers in retinoblastoma. Mol Vis 13:823-832.

Sgubin D, Aztiria E, Perin A, Longatti P, Leanza G (2007) Activation of endogenous neural stem cells in the adult human brain following subarachnoid hemorrhage. J Neurosci Res 85:1647-1655.

Shackleton M, Vaillant F, Simpson KJ, Stingl J, Smyth GK, Asselin-Labat ML, Wu L, Lindeman GJ, Visvader JE (2006) Generation of a functional mammary gland from a single stem cell. Nature 439:84-88.

Siddall NA, McLaughlin EA, Marriner NL, Hime GR (2006) The RNA-binding protein Musashi is required intrinsically to maintain stem cell identity. Proc Natl Acad Sci U S A 103:8402-8407.

Smalley MJ, Clarke RB (2005) The mammary gland "side population": a putative stem/progenitor cell marker? J Mammary Gland Biol Neoplasia 10:37-47.

Stadtfeld M, Maherali N, Borkent M, Hochedlinger K (2010) A reprogrammable mouse strain from gene-targeted embryonic stem cells. Nat Methods 7:53-55.

Stevenson M, Mostertz W, Acharya C, Kim W, Walters K, Barry W, Higgins K, Tuchman SA, Crawford J, Vlahovic G, Ready N, Onaitis M, Potti A (2009) Characterizing the Clinical Relevance of an Embryonic Stem Cell Phenotype in Lung Adenocarcinoma. Clin Cancer Res 15:7553-7561.

Sugiyama-Nakagiri Y, Akiyama M, Shibata S, Okano H, Shimizu H (2006) Expression of RNA-binding protein Musashi in hair follicle development and hair cycle progression. Am J Pathol 168:80-92.

Sureban SM, May R, George RJ, Dieckgraefe BK, McLeod HL, Ramalingam S, Bishnupuri KS, Natarajan G, Anant S, Houchen CW (2008) Knockdown of RNA binding protein musashi-1 leads to tumor regression in vivo. Gastroenterology 134:1448-1458.

The Cancer Genome Atlas Research Network (2008) Comprehensive genomic characterization defines human glioblastoma genes and core pathways. Nature 455:1061-1068.

Toda M, Iizuka Y, Yu W, Imai T, Ikeda E, Yoshida K, Kawase T, Kawakami Y, Okano H, Uyemura K (2001) Expression of the neural RNA-binding protein Musashi1 in human gliomas. Glia 34:1-7.

Uchida K, Mukai M, Okano H, Kawase T (2004) Possible oncogenicity of subventricular zone neural stem cells: case report. Neurosurgery 55:977-978.

Villavicencio EH, Walterhouse DO, Iannaccone PM (2000) The sonic hedgehog-patched-gli pathway in human development and disease. Am J Hum Genet 67:1047-1054.

Wang XY, Yin Y, Yuan H, Sakamaki T, Okano H, Glazer RI (2008) Musashi1 modulates mammary progenitor cell expansion through proliferin-mediated activation of the Wnt and Notch pathways. Mol Cell Biol 28:3589-3599.

Wang XY, Penalva LO, Yuan H, Linnoila RI, Lu J, Okano H, Glazer RI (2010) Musashi1 regulates breast tumor cell proliferation and is a prognostic indicator of poor survival. Mol Cancer 9:221-232.

Wendel HG, Silva RL, Malina A, Mills JR, Zhu H, Ueda T, Watanabe-Fukunaga R, Fukunaga R, Teruya-Feldstein J, Pelletier J, Lowe SW (2007) Dissecting eIF4E action in tumorigenesis. Genes Dev 21:3232-3237.

Xu P, Yu S, Jiang R, Kang C, Wang G, Jiang H, Pu P (2009) Differential expression of Notch family members in astrocytomas and medulloblastomas. Pathol Oncol Res 15:703-710.

Ye F, Zhou C, Cheng Q, Shen J, Chen H (2008) Stem-cell-abundant proteins Nanog, Nucleostemin and Musashi1 are highly expressed in malignant cervical epithelial cells. BMC Cancer 8:108.

Ying M, Wang S, Sang Y, Sun P, Lal B, Goodwin CR, Guerrero-Cazares H, Quinones-Hinojosa A, Laterra J, Xia S (2011) Regulation of glioblastoma stem cells by retinoic acid: role for Notch pathway inhibition. Oncogene.

Yokota N, Mainprize TG, Taylor MD, Kohata T, Loreto M, Ueda S, Dura W, Grajkowska W, Kuo JS, Rutka JT (2004) Identification of differentially expressed and developmentally regulated genes in medulloblastoma using suppression subtraction hybridization. Oncogene 23:3444-3453.

Yu J, Hu K, Smuga-Otto K, Tian S, Stewart R, Slukvin, II, Thomson JA (2009) Human induced pluripotent stem cells free of vector and transgene sequences. Science 324:797-801.

Yu J, Vodyanik MA, Smuga-Otto K, Antosiewicz-Bourget J, Frane JL, Tian S, Nie J, Jonsdottir GA, Ruotti V, Stewart R, Slukvin, II, Thomson JA (2007) Induced pluripotent stem cell lines derived from human somatic cells. Science 318:1917-1920.

Zhang M, Behbod F, Atkinson RL, Landis MD, Kittrell F, Edwards D, Medina D, Tsimelzon A, Hilsenbeck S, Green JE, Michalowska AM, Rosen JM (2008) Identification of tumor-initiating cells in a p53-null mouse model of breast cancer. Cancer Res 68:4674-4682.

Part 14

GSK3b Acts Like Tumor Promoter - GBM

The Pivotal Roles of GSK3β in Glioma Biology

Mitsutoshi Nakada[1], Toshinari Minamoto[2], Ilya V. Pyko[1],
Yutaka Hayashi[1] and Jun-ichiro Hamada[1]
[1]*Department of Neurosurgery, Graduate School of Medical Science and*
[2]*Divisions of Translational and Clinical Oncology and Surgical Oncology,*
Cancer Research Institute, Kanazawa University, Kanazawa,
Japan

1. Introduction

Glioblastoma (GBM) is the most common malignant primary brain tumor in adults and one of the most lethal of all human cancers. Despite substantial advances in surgical intervention and combining radiotherapy regimens with new generation chemotherapies, the median survival for these patients is still about 15 months (Nagane, 2011). In recent years, cancer treatments using molecularly targeted drugs that act against the respective molecules have been successful, although successful molecular targeted therapies for glioma have yet to be established. Because the mechanisms underlying glioma formation and progression are complex, many candidate target molecules are identified as potential therapeutic targets (Nakada M et al., 2011). To date, the benefit of molecularly targeted therapies is limited, although there are many completed and on-going clinical trials (Quant & Wen, 2010). Thus, promising molecular targets should be identified to establish innovative molecularly targeted therapies against GBM.

Glycogen synthase kinase 3β (GSK3β) is a serine-threonine protein kinase originally identified for its inhibitory role in the conversion of glucose to glycogen via phosphorylation and inactivation of glycogen synthase. Recent studies suggest a conflicting role of GSK3β in various human cancers, either as a tumor suppressor or tumor promoter. Emerging evidence suggests that GSK3β is a tumor promoter in glioma, acting to regulate and link key players that control proliferation, resistance to radiochemotherapy, activation of invasion, and anti-apoptosis (Kotliarova et al., 2008; Miyashita et al., 2009a; Nowicki et al., 2008). The combined anti-proliferative and anti-invasive properties of small molecule GSK3β inhibitors make them an attractive treatment modality for controlling GBM.

The aim of this chapter is to highlight important aspects of the biology of GSK3β, focusing on the pathological role, signal transduction, and possibility of being a molecular target for GBM.

2. General knowledge of GSK3β

GSK3 was discovered in 1980 as a kinase that phosphorylates glycogen synthase, a key enzyme involved in glycogen synthesis (Embi et al., 1980). GSK3 is evolutionarily conserved and consists of 2 distinct isoforms encoded by 2 different genes, GSK3α and GSK3β, in mammals (Woodgett, 1991). GSK3 is ubiquitously expressed, and is highly enriched in the brain. Compared with GSK3α, the GSK3β protein lacks 60 amino acid residues at the N terminus, resulting in a lower molecular weight for GSK3β (46.7 kDa). The 2 isoforms share extensive homology, most notably in the kinase domain (ATP binding site), which shares 97% homology. Initially, the primary function attributed to GSK3 was negative regulation of glycogen synthesis through phosphorylation and inactivation of glycogen synthase. However, further studies have uncovered additional functions of GSK3, such as cell cycle regulation, proliferation, differentiation, apoptosis, and migration. Despite high homology, the 2 isoforms are not functionally redundant, as demonstrated by gene knockout studies (Hoeflich et al., 2000).

2.1 Biological characteristics of GSK3β

Although the differences in functional roles of the 2 isoforms are not fully elucidated, research thus far has primarily focused on GSK3β. GSK3β is subject to multiple levels of regulation mediated by its phosphorylation, subcellular localization, and protein–protein interactions. GSK3β protein itself undergoes multiple phosphorylation events, which impact its activity depending on the amino acid being modified (Doble & Woodgett, 2003). Tyrosine phosphorylation of the GSK3β kinase domain at Tyr216 leads to its activation (Dajani et al., 2001), whereas phosphorylation of the N-terminal Ser9 results in inhibition of its activity and plays an important role in the regulation of GSK3β function (Stambolic & Woodgett, 1994) (Figure 1).

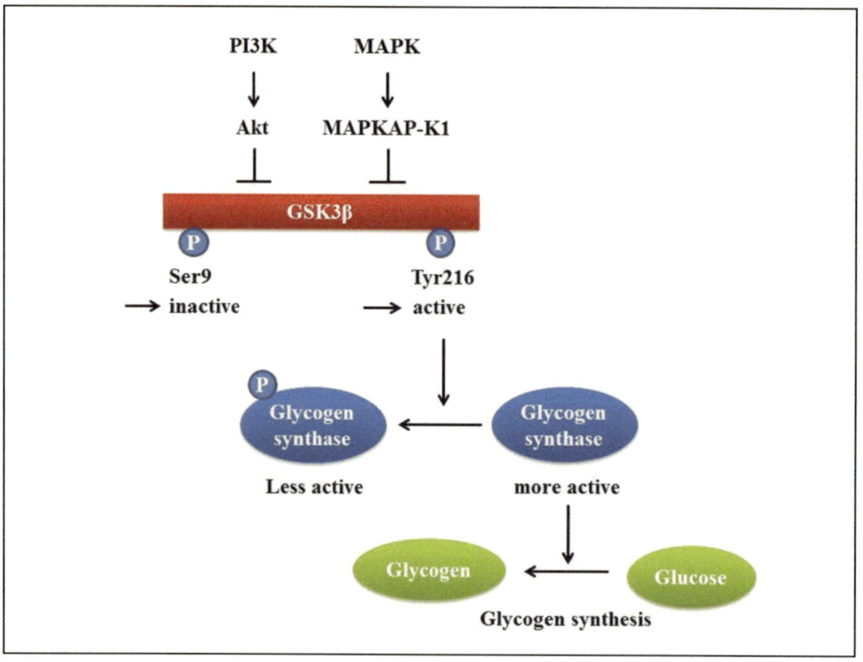

Fig. 1. Phosphorylation and activation of GSK3β. Akt and MAPKAP-K1 phosphorylate Ser9 of GSK3β, resulting in inhibition of activity. The inhibition of GSK3β decreases the phosphorylation of glycogen synthase, leading to an increase in the active form, since phosphorylated glycogen synthase is less active. As a result, glycogen synthesis is promoted. MAPK: mitogen-activated protein kinase, MAPKAP-K1: MAPK-activated protein kinase-1 (also called RSK), Circled P: phosphorylation.

One of the main regulators of GSK3β activity is the phosphoinositide 3-kinase (PI3-kinase)/Akt pathway. PI3-kinase–induced activation of Akt mediates Ser9 phosphorylation of GSK3β (Cross et al., 1995; Pap & Cooper, 1998), resulting in the inhibition of GSK3β activity. GSK3β can also be phosphorylated at Ser9 by the most downstream kinase of the classical mitogen-activated protein kinase (MAPK) cascade, called MAPK-activated protein kinase-1 (MAPKAP-K1, also called RSK) (Frame & Cohen, 2001). Apart from this, GSK3β functions as a suppressor protein in the Wnt signaling pathway, which is the protein network associated with embryo development and cancer progression (Cook et al., 1996; Manoukian & Woodgett, 2002; Fuchs et al., 2005). The Wnt pathway was found to have essential roles in promoting the survival, proliferation, differentiation, and migration of cells in many different tissues, including nervous tissue, as well as in synapse formation in the nervous system. Briefly, the Wnt pathway involves the inhibition of an inhibitor, leading to activation of a transcription factor. When Wnt signal is absent, GSK3β associates with other proteins (e.g., axin, adenomatous polyposis coli [APC]) and functions as a critical mediator of the pathway. In this situation, the proto-oncoprotein β-catenin is constitutively phosphorylated, rapidly removed by degradation, and thus, will not build up in the cell to a significant level (Hagen & Vidal-Puig, 2002). In contrast, when Wnt binds to frizzled (Frz), its receptor, dishevelled (Dsh) is recruited to the cell membrane. GSK3β is inhibited by the activation of Dsh. Consequently, β-catenin, having escaped ubiquitination-dependent proteasomal degradation mediated by GSK3β phosphorylation, accumulates in the cytoplasm. It is subsequently shifted to the nucleus, where it assembles with other proteins (e.g., T-cell factor [Tcf]/lymphoid enhancer factor [Lef]) to switch on transcription of specific target genes, leading to its function as an oncoprotein. In this mechanism, GSK3β is thought of as a tumor suppressor protein (Figure 2).

GSK3β acts as a downstream regulatory switch that determines the output of numerous signaling pathways initiated by diverse stimuli (Frame & Cohen, 2001). Phosphorylation of GSK3β (Ser9) leads to the dephosphorylation of substrates, including glycogen synthase and translation factor eukaryotic protein synthesis initiation factor-2B (eIF-2B) (Welsh et al., 1998), resulting in their functional activation and consequent increase in glycogen synthesis, release of a number of transcription factors from tonic inhibition, and protein synthesis (Cohen & Frame, 2001). Thus, GSK3β affects both key components of the response to stimuli, reprogramming of gene expression, and activation of protein synthesis. Additionally, GSK3β phosphorylates a broad range of substrates: c-myc (Gregory et al., 2003), c Jun (Boyle et al., 1991), c-Myb (Kitagawa et al., 2010), cyclin D1 (Diehl et al., 1998), Cdc25A (Kang et al., 2008), nuclear factor of activated T-cells (Beals et al., 1997), heat shock factor-1 (He et al., 1998; Xavier et al., 2000), Mcl-1 (Ding et al., 2007), cAMP response element-binding protein (Bullock & Habener, 1998), and so on. GSK3β can target these substrates for degradation or inactivation, resulting in inhibition of cell proliferation and self-renewal. GSK3β also regulates nuclear factor (NF)-κB stability and activity (Demarchi et al., 2003; Hoeflich et al., 2000). These findings identified GSK3β as a key determinant in both physiological and pathological conditions, such as glycogen metabolism, insulin signaling, cell fate, neuronal function, and oncogenesis.

2.2 Physiological function

GSK3β participates in a number of different cellular pathways in a context-dependent manner and is implicated in the regulation of a wide range of cellular processes, including apoptosis, cell proliferation, and migration. Multiple lines of evidence indicate that the function of GSK3β is opposing in different cell types. This functional dichotomy suggests that the function of GSK3β seems to be dependent on cell-types and/or cell conditions, which are physiological and pathological.

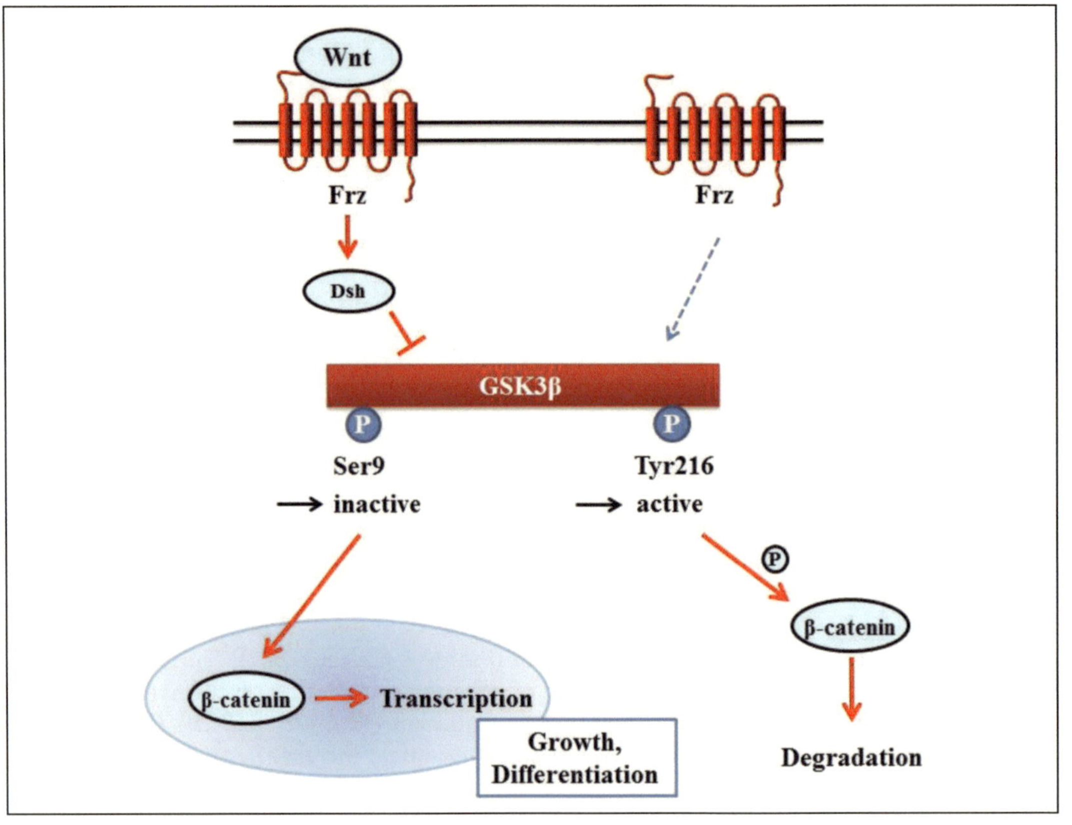

Fig. 2. Role of GSK3β in the Wnt pathway. When Wnt signal is absent, GSK3β promotes the proteasomal degradation of β-catenin. In contrast, when Wnt binds to frizzled (Frz), its receptor, dishevelled (Dsh) is recruited to the cell membrane. GSK3β is inhibited by the activation of Dsh. Consequently, β-catenin accumulates in the cytoplasm and is subsequently translocated into the nucleus to switch on Tcf/Lef-dependent transcription of specific target genes, leading it to act as an oncoprotein. Note that there are other regulatory components of each pathway; this schema was simplified for clarity.

2.2.1 Apoptosis

GSK3β is a component of signaling cascades involved in the process of apoptosis (Iqbal & Grundke-Iqbal, 2008) and is a critical downstream element of the PI3-kinase/Akt cell survival pathway (Pap & Cooper, 1998). Transient overexpression of GSK3β was found to induce spontaneous apoptosis in PC12 cells, used as a model system for neuronal differentiation, in a caspase-3-dependent manner (Pap & Cooper, 1998). Inhibition of GSK3β activity prevented cell death by blocking mitochondrial membrane potential changes and subsequent caspase-9 and caspase-3 activation in murine TSM1 neuronal cells (Petit-Paitel et al., 2009).

2.2.2 Proliferation

GSK3β is involved in cell proliferation through the canonical Wnt/β-catenin signaling pathway. GSK3β inhibition promotes translocation of dephosphorylated and stabilized β-catenin to the nucleus and its interaction with transcription factors, resulting in the induction of genes responsible for cell proliferation. Lithium chloride (LiCl), a chemical GSK3β inhibitor, significantly increased the proliferative potency of thyrocytes that appeared to be mediated by β-catenin (Rao et al., 2005). Similarly, the small molecule 6-bromoindirubin-3′-oxime (BIO), a specific inhibitor for GSK3, promotes proliferation in mammalian cardiomyocytes by elevated β-catenin activity (Tseng et al., 2006). In addition, it is known that inhibition of GSK3β promotes vascular cell proliferation, suggesting that active GSK3β inhibits angiogenesis (Hou et al., 2010). GSK3β signaling also plays an essential role in regulating the differentiation and proliferation of adult neural stem cells. Inhibition of GSK3β results in transcriptional activation of distinct target genes via β-catenin, leading to an increase in the number of neurons that differentiated from neurospheres (Maurer et al., 2007).

2.2.3 Migration

It has also been shown that, during cell migration, GSK3β plays a positive role in activating Rac, a Rho family member, and ADP-ribosylation factor 6 (Arf6), a related small GTPase, in adherent cells. Rac is responsible for forming lamellipodia during cell migration. Arf6 is also involved in vesicle trafficking, membrane ruffling, as well as lamellipodia formation (Turner & Brown, 2001). It has been shown that GSK3β activity is required for keratinocytes to form lamellipodia and migrate directionally in response to wound signaling (Koivisto et al., 2003). Similarly, GSK3β activates Rac in response to wound signaling in intestinal epithelial cells. When GSK3β is inhibited, and thus Rac activation prevented, these cells stop moving (Vaidya et al., 2006). Although the mechanisms by which guanine nucleotide exchange factor (GEF) and GTPase-activating protein (GAP) regulate Rac or Arf6 have been extensively studied, no direct evidence has demonstrated that GSK3β modifies these GEFs and GAPs.

Focal adhesion kinase (FAK) is another candidate that contributes to the regulation of cell migration by GSK3β. FAK tyrosine phosphorylation and Rac activation were suppressed in GSK3β knocked-down HeLa S3 (human cervical carcinoma cell line) cells, suggesting that GSK3β mediates the disassembly of focal adhesions to promote cell migration (Kobayashi et al., 2006). In contrast, Bianchi et al. showed that GSK3β reduces FAK kinase activity and cell motility in rat fibroblasts and HEK-293 (human embryonic kidney 293) cells. The influence of GSK3β on migration of various types of cells (e.g., neoplastic and non-neoplastic) appears to be complex. Further identification of additional GSK3β targets and more detailed studies of the pathways affecting cell migration will be necessary to clarify the function of GSK3β in cell migration (Sun et al., 2009).

2.3 Pathological function

GSK3β is ubiquitously expressed at high levels in the brain. Numerous studies have indicated that GSK3β is involved in key functions of the brain and is associated with a variety of neurological disorders like Alzheimer, Parkinson, and Huntington diseases, as well as affective disorders and other neurodegenerative disorders (Grimes & Jope, 2001; Jope & Roh, 2006). Additionally, it is not surprising that GSK3β has been implicated in glucose intolerance, considering its primary role is as a negative regulator of insulin-mediated glycogen synthesis and glucose homeostasis. Indeed, the activity of GSK3β has been reported in type II diabetes mellitus and obese animal models (Eldar-Finkelman et al., 1999; Nikoulina et al., 2000). GSK3β is also involved in inflammation that accompanies various kinds of diseases (reviewed in Jope et al., 2007). GSK3β inhibition attenuates activation of the pro-inflammatory transcription factor NF-κB and activates the immunomodulatory transcription factor β-catenin (Gong et al., 2008). GSK3β inhibition also induces secretion of the anti-inflammatory cytokine IL-10 (Hu et al., 2006).

More recent studies indicate a role for GSK3β in the control of neoplastic transformation and tumor development (reviewd in Miyashita et al., 2009b). Overexpression and activation of GSK3β was confirmed in various kinds of cancers such as colorectal, stomach, pancreatic, and liver cancers, as well as leukemia and GBM (Shakoori et al., 2005; Shakoori et al., 2007; Wang et al., 2008; Miyashita et al., 2009a; Mai et al., 2009). Previous studies have shown that inhibition of GSK3β suppresses cancer cell proliferation and induces apoptosis (Ougolkov et al., 2005; Ougolkov et al., 2007). In these cancers, the function of GSK3β is critical for malignant phenotype with respect to proliferation and invasion. Accumulated evidence supports the role of GSK3β in the regulation of apoptosis and proliferation appears to be diverse between physiological and pathological conditions.

However, the exact role of GSK3β in malignancies remains highly controversial due to the conflicting results from different tumor models. It has been shown that GSK3β is a tumor suppressor protein that controls cellular fate determination and stem cell maintenance through inhibition of the Wnt, Hedgehog, and Notch pathways. These pathways are aberrantly activated in several cancers (Saldanha, 2001; Waaler et al., 2011). This suggests that GSK3β inhibitors could exert a therapeutically negative, pro-survival effect on tumor cells. In addition, some studies found that GSK3β is part of a tumor suppressor complex consisting of axin and APC that phosphorylates the oncoprotein β-catenin and that, when GSK3β is inactivated, could possibly lead to tumor promotion (Hinoi et al., 2000; Rask et al., 2003). Available evidence indicates that GSK3β may function as a "tumor suppressor" for certain types of tumors such as skin and mammary tumors (Farago et al., 2005; Ma et al., 2007). These findings suggest that the mechanisms underlying the function of GSK3β as a tumor promoter or suppressor might depend on cell type and tissue context.

3. GSK3β biology in glioma

Recently, 3 independent research groups, including our group, simultaneously reported that GSK3β is a key promoter of malignant GBM phenotypes and is thus a promising candidate for molecular-targeted therapy (Kotliarova et al., 2008; Nowicki et al., 2008; Miyashita et al., 2009a).

3.1 Expression and activation

GSK3β is consistently expressed in primary GBM (Korur et al., 2009; Li et al., 2010). High expression levels of GSK3β and phosphorylated GSK3β (Tyr216) were detected in GBM compared with non-neoplastic brain tissues (Miyashita et al., 2009a). This finding identified GSK3β as an important regulator of malignant phenotype in GBM cells. GSK3β is constitutively active in GBM cells, despite the fact that PI3K/Akt, which can inhibit GSK3β activity, is a major signaling pathway in GBM. It is possible that an undetermined pathway other than that mediated by Akt prevents GSK3β Ser9 phosphorylation (Shakoori et al., 2005), allowing GSK3β to be constitutively active in GBM cells.

3.2 Localization in tumor cells

Overexpression of GSK3β was observed in the cytoplasm of neoplastic cells in GBM, whereas only weak expression was observed in the cytoplasm of neurons from non-neoplastic tissue (Miyashita et al., 2009a).

3.3 Function

GSK3β function in glioma has been investigated by inhibiting GSK3β using small interfering RNA (siRNA), the small-molecule inhibitors LiCl or thiazolidinediones (TZD), and a small heterocyclic compound first described as a non-ATP competitive inhibitor of GSK3β. Inhibition of GSK3β activity attenuated proliferation, inhibited cell survival, enhanced tumor cell apoptosis, induced tumor cell differentiation, impaired formation of neurospheres, and reduced clonogenicity of GBM cells in a dose-dependent manner (Aguilar-Morante et al., 2010; Korur et al., 2009; Kotliarova et al., 2008; Miyashita et al., 2009a) (Table 1). The cytotoxic effects are directly correlated with decreased enzyme-activating phosphorylation of GSK3β (Tyr216) (Kotliarova et al., 2008). Furthermore, specific pharmacologic GSK3β inhibitors and siRNA knockdown of GSK3β reduced glioma cell motility (Nowicki et al., 2008). Importantly, administration of a highly specific GSK3β inhibitor, AR-A014418 (Bhat et al., 2003), at a low dose sensitized GBM cells to chemotherapeutic agents such as temozolomide and ionizing radiation, resulting in reduced cell viability (Miyashita et al., 2009a).

	Inhibitory effect of GSK3β	Target molecules
Apoptosis	promotion	c-myc activation induction of Bax, Bim, DR4/DR5 and TRAIL increase of p53 and p21 expression decrease of Rb phosphorylated fractions stabilization of PTEN
Proliferation	inhibition	reduction of intracellular NF-κB activity
Invasion	inhibition	Rac1 inactivation?
Stemness	reduction of the number and volume of neurospheres induction of differentiation suppression of differentiation	 increase of differentiation markers interruption of cyclin D1 proteolysis
Metabolism	increase of intracellular glycogen	inhibition of glycogen synthase phosphorylation dissociation of HKII from outer mitochondrial membrane
Chemosensitivity	enhancement	methylation of MGMT promoter?
Radiosensitivity	enhancement	unknown
Neuroprotection	protection of hippocampal neurons from apoptosis	acceleration of double strand-break repair efficiency

Bax: BCL2-associated X protein, Bim: BCL2 interacting protein, DR4/DR5: death receptor4/ death receptor5, HKII: hexokinase-II, MGMT: O6-methylguanine-DNA methyltransferase, NF-κB: nuclear factor-kappa B, PTEN: Phosphatase and tensin homolog, Rb: Retinoblastoma protein, TRAIL: TNF-related apoptosis-inducing ligand

Table 1. Disadvantageous effects of GSK3β inhibition for glioma

4. GSK3β-mediated signaling in glioma

4.1 Apoptosis

The molecules associated with GSK3β were also assessed by GSK3β inhibition. Several signaling pathways are associated with the decreased cell survival related to GSK3β inhibition. Inhibition of GSK3β activates the oncogenic transcription factor c-myc, leading to the induction of apoptosis promoting factors such as Bax, Bim, DR4/DR5, and tumor necrosis factor (TNF)-related apoptosis-inducing ligand (TRAIL), as well as subsequent cytotoxicity (Kotliarova et al., 2008). In addition, inhibition of GSK3β was associated with increased expression of p53 and p21 in GBM cells with wild-type p53. Simultaneously, the phosphorylated fraction of retinoblastoma protein (Rb) (inactive form) decreased, which associated with down-regulation of cyclin-dependent kinase 6 (CDK6) (Miyashita et al., 2009a). It has been reported that decreased phosphorylation of Rb (activation of Rb) could be attributed to the down-regulation of CDK6 (Classon & Harlow, 2002). These signaling pathways probably induce apoptosis by inhibition of GSK3β in GBM cells. In contrast to the GSK3β phosphorylates the Thr366 residue of PTEN that negatively regulates PI3K and then reduces Akt activity. Blocking phosphorylation of PTEN by either mutating or inhibiting GSK3β in GBM cell lines leads to stabilization of the PTEN protein (Maccario et al., 2007). In this situation, PTEN can work stably as a suppressor for PI3K/Akt, leading to apoptosis (Figure 3).

4.2 Proliferation

One of the major targets of GSK3β is NF-κB, which is an intracellular protein complex that controls DNA transcription and is a pro-survival factor in glioma (Kasuga et al., 2004; Robe et al., 2004). Inhibition of GSK3β activity by GSK3β-specific inhibitors such as LiCl and by GSK3β siRNA caused a dramatic decrease in intracellular NF-κB activity in U251, T98, and U87 GBM cell lines (Kotliarova et al., 2008). NF-κB inhibition then resulted in decreased glioma cell survival *in vitro* and inhibition of tumor growth *in vivo* (Kotliarova et al., 2008) (Figure 3). TZD-8 can inhibit GSK3β activity not only by directly interacting with this enzyme, but also by phosphorylating the Ser9 residue of GSK3β via MAPK pathway activation. TZD-8 suppresses the growth of glioma cells *in vivo* and exerts anti-proliferative and pro-apoptotic activities in glioma cells *in vitro* (Aguilar-Morante et al., 2010). These effects were accompanied by an activation of the MAPK signaling pathway, concomitant phosphorylation of Ser9, inactivation of GSK3β, and an inhibition of NF-κB activity. These results are consistent with previously published data, showing that an activation of MAPK is associated with a reduction in cell survival in different tumor cell lines, including GBM cell lines (Tewari et al., 2008). In contrast, GSK3β inhibition promotes entrance of β-catenin to the nucleus and the interaction of β-catenin with transcription factors. While this could promote cell proliferation, it does not take place, presumably, because of the simultaneous action of other pathways, which inhibit glioma cell proliferation (Kotliarova, 2008).

4.3 Migration/invasion

Specific inhibitors and siRNA knockdown of GSK3β both reduced glioma cell motility. The effects are dose dependent and reversible (Nowicki et al., 2008). However, the mechanisms underlying the effect of GSK3β on glioma cell migration and invasion required further study. Migration of GBM cells requires the formation of lamellipodia at the cell front and stress fibers consisting of actomyosin at the rear; contraction of these stress fibers causes the cell to reacquire front-rear symmetry. The migrating morphology of GBM cells is dependent

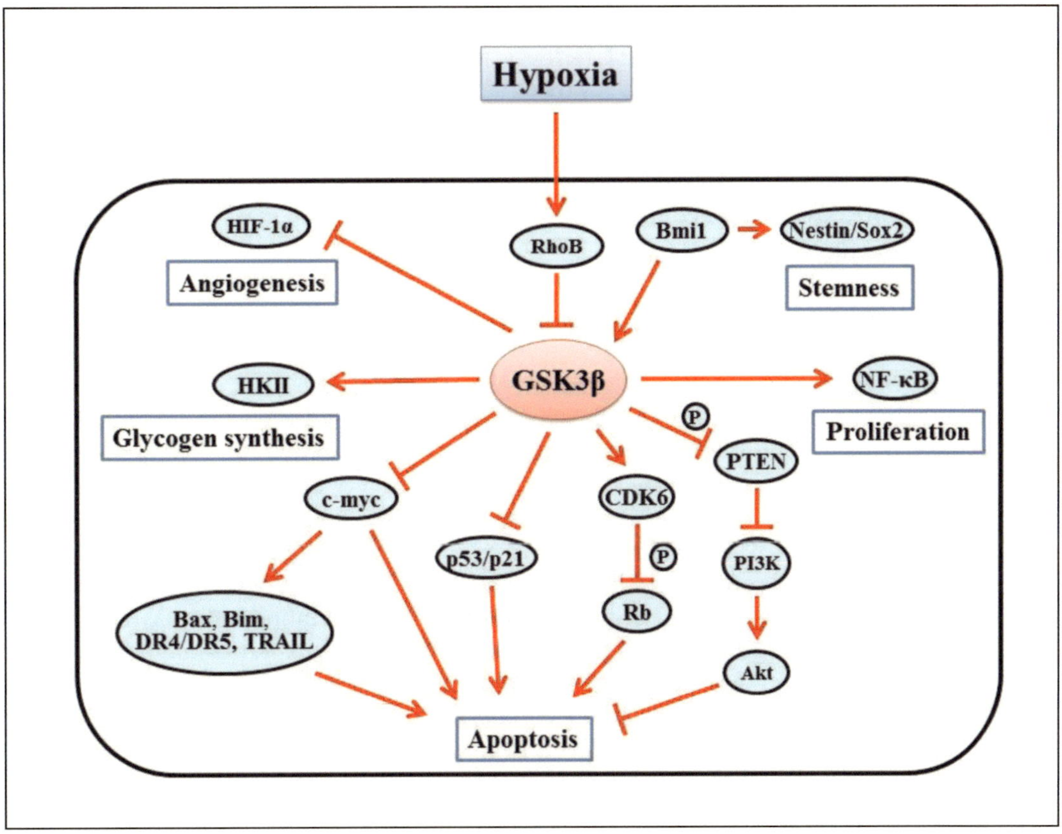

Fig. 3. GSK3β-mediated signaling in glioma. The signaling pathways associated with apoptosis, proliferation, angiogenesis, cell stemness, and glycogen synthesis are depicted. **Apoptosis**: GSK3β activity results in c-myc inhibition that consequently decreases expression of Bax, Bim, DR4/DR5, and TRAIL, preventing subsequent cytotoxicity. GSK3β increases the levels of Rb phosphorylation, resulting in Rb inactivation. Decreased Rb phosphorylation is associated with down-regulation of CDK6. GSK3β destabilizes PTEN, which negatively regulates PI3K and reduces Akt activity. **Proliferation**: siRNA targeting GSK3β causes a dramatic decrease in intracellular NF-κB activity. NF-κB inhibition results in decreased glioma cell survival. **Angiogenesis**: Hypoxia activates RhoB. HIF-1α may be regulated by RhoB through the Akt/GSK3β pathway under hypoxic conditions, although there is no data proving direct inhibition of HIF-1α by GSK3β. **Stemness**: Expression of GSK3β is reduced by down-regulation of polycomb group protein Bmi1. Inhibition of Bmi1 induces a differentiation phenotype and reduces expression of Nestin and Sox2 in glioma cells. **Glycogen synthesis**: GSK3β stabilizes HKII on the outer mitochondrial membrane, thereby supporting glycolysis. Bax: BCL2-associated X protein, Bim: BCL2 interacting protein, DR4/DR5: death receptor 4/death receptor 5, HIF-1α: hypoxia-inducible factor 1α, HKII: hexokinase-II, NF-κB: nuclear factor-kappa B, PI3K: phosphatidylinositol 3-kinases, PTEN: phosphatase and tensin homolog, Rb: retinoblastoma protein, RhoB: Ras homolog gene family member B, Sox2: SRY (sex determining region Y)-box 2, TRAIL: tumor necrosis factor (TNF)-related apoptosis-inducing ligand, Circled P, phosphorylation.

on the balance between Rac1, whose activity is largely responsible for lamellipodia formation, and RhoA, which is related to stress fiber formation. Interference with lamellipodia by the inhibition of Rac1 reduces migration. This also causes GBM cells to acquire a relatively round shape without extending cell processes (Chuang et al., 2004). In contrast, collapse of actin stress fiber formation by the inhibition of RhoA promotes migration (Salhia et al., 2005). As LiCl treatment is associated with a marked change in GBM cell morphology, with cells retracting their long extensions at their leading edge and losing lamellipodia formation (Nowicki et al., 2008), GSK3β signaling may involve small GTPases such as Rac1 and RhoA.

4.4 Angiogenesis (signal induced by hypoxia)

A hypoxic microenvironment is a striking characteristic of GBM that is the collective consequence of morphologically and functionally immature neovascularization, irregular blood flow, anemia, and high oxygen consumption due to rapidly proliferating malignant cells (Jensen, 2009). The hypoxic microenvironment is a powerful stimulus for the expression of genes involved in tumor cell proliferation and angiogenesis (Carmeliet et al., 1998). Hypoxia markedly increases the inactive GSK3β fraction and decreases the active GSK3β fraction in U87 GBM cells. In U87 cells under hypoxia, depletion of Ras homolog gene family member B (RhoB) by siRNA decreases the inactive form of GSK3β and increases active GSK3β. At the same time, RhoB inhibition induces degradation of hypoxia-inducible factor 1α (HIF-1α) in the proteasome (Skuli et al., 2006). These experimental data suggest that GSK3β controls RhoB-dependent HIF-1α stabilization under hypoxic conditions (Figure 3). The transcription factor, HIF-1, is an essential regulator of oxygen homeostasis by controlling a battery of target genes involved in angiogenesis, glycolysis, proliferation, and pH regulation (Semenza, 2009). According to this mechanism, it was shown that inhibition of RhoB in GBM xenografts leads to a decrease in vessel density (Ader et al., 2003). Considering the role of RhoB in the stimulation of angiogenesis, as well as the presumed connection between RhoB expression and GSK3β activity, it is reasonable to speculate that GSK3β activity in hypoxic conditions can regulate angiogenesis in GBM. However, the precise effect of GSK3β inhibition on angiogenesis has yet to be identified.

4.5 Cell stemness

GSK3β activity appears to regulate glioma stem cell populations. GSK3β protein, as well as stem cell markers Nestin and Notch2, are highly expressed in CD133+ populations, which was identified as a surface marker of cancer stem cells in brain tumors (Singh et al., 2004). Down-regulating GSK3β specifically decreased the subpopulation of cancer cells, with a 50–60% depletion of CD133+ cells that possessed a cancer stem cell-like signature. This depletion was attributed to the differentiation of the cell subtype. Additionally, reduction of Nestin in GBM stem cell cultures treated with GSK3β inhibitor at the molecular level indicated loss of cell stemness (Aguilar-Morante, 2010). Indeed, inhibition of GSK3β reduces the GBM stem cell pool and induces phenotypic switch towards differentiation in GBM cell cultures. This increases the expression of differentiation markers such as neuronal marker β-tubulin III, oligodendrocyte-specific marker CNPase, and astrocytic marker GFAP (Korur et al., 2009). One explanation for this mechanism is as follows. shRNA-mediated depletion of Bmi1, a polycomb group protein that is required for neural stem cell self-renewal, reduced expression of GSK3β in glioma. This decreased expression of Sox2 and Nestin in glioma cells and induced cell differentiation, suggesting a putative functional link between GSK3β and Bmi1 in glioma cell stemness (Figure 3).

Neurosphere formation is a representative feature of glioma stem cells. GSK3β inhibition significantly reduced the number and volume of neurospheres in glioma cells (Korur et al., 2009). Primary neurosphere cultures treated with TZD-8 failed to give rise to secondary neurospheres, indicating that self-renewing stem cells are lost under TZD-8 treatment (Aguilar-Morante et al., 2010). TZD-8 inhibits the proliferation and expansion of these neurospheres and hampered their capacity for self-renewal, suggesting that TZD-8 could reduce the tumor-initiating cells (Aguilar-Morante et al., 2010). Furthermore, reduction in the levels of Nestin protein in GBM stem cell cultures treated with TZD-8 indicated a loss of cell stemness induced by GSK3β inhibition (Aguilar-Morante et al., 2010). Taken together, GSK3β activation is identified as a key element in maintaining stem cell-like characteristics in a subset of glioma cells, providing these cells with a higher self-renewal capacity.

In contrast, there is a recent contradictory report showing that forced expression of GSK3β induces cellular differentiation of malignant glioma cells to normal astrocytes. Conversely, GSK3β suppression inhibits differentiation and is accompanied by the interruption of cyclin D1 proteolysis, which is necessary for the astrocytic differentiation of malignant glioma cells (Li et al., 2010). The exact mechanisms underlying the effect of GSK3β on glioma cell differentiation require more detailed study.

4.6 Metabolism

Increased glycolysis is characteristic of malignancy. Glioma cell growth is closely associated with glucose metabolism. Down-regulation of GSK3β activity results in changes of intracellular glucose metabolism (Kotliarova et al., 2008). The activity of mitochondrial hexokinase, an enzyme that localizes at the outer mitochondrial membrane and metabolizes glucose in rapidly-growing glioma cells, is about 3 times higher than that in slow-growing cells. Consistently, the intracellular glucose concentration is undetectable in rapidly-growing glioma cells, suggesting that glucose catabolism is activated in these cells (Nagamatsu et al., 1996). The dissociation of hexokinase from the outer mitochondrial membrane by GSK3β inhibition is partially responsible for the reduction in intracellular glucose concentration (Kotliarova et al., 2008). However, the reduction of intracellular glucose after GSK3β inhibition is mainly due to decreased GSK3β-dependent glycogen synthase phosphorylation. This leads to glycogen synthase activation and consequently to the increased intracellular glycogen (Figure 1). Further studies are necessary to examine whether the forced glucose consumption and subsequent accumulation of glycogen by GSK3β inhibition affects the glioma phenotype. However, it may be possible that GBM cells cannot use glucose effectively for cell proliferation and survival due to the lack of glucose under the condition induced by GSK3β inhibition.

4.7 Chemosensitivity

One of the potential molecules involved in the chemosensitization associated with GSK3β inhibition in GBM cells is O6-methylguanine-DNA methyltransferase (MGMT), a DNA repair enzyme and major determinant of temozolomide cytotoxicity. Recently, clinical research has revealed that the methylation status of the MGMT promoter is associated with the prognostic outcome of GBM patients treated with temozolomide (Hegi et al., 2005). Reduction of MGMT expression induced by p53 in GBM cells renders them sensitive to temozolomide (Natsume et al., 2005). It is reasonable to speculate that increased expression of p53 by GSK3β inhibition enhances temozolomide chemosensitivity through the reduction of MGMT (Miyashita et al, 2009a).

4.8 Neuroprotection

Radiation is a standard post-operative therapy for patients with GBM. Intellectual impairment, reduction in performance IQ, memory loss, and dementia have been reported after exposure of the brain to radiation. However, the exact mechanisms of radiation-induced brain injury remain unknown and prevention of cranial radiation-induced morbidity remains challenging. Recent studies indicate that inhibition of GSK3β protects hippocampal neurons from radiation–induced apoptosis and attenuation of neurocognitive dysfunction resulting from cranial radiation (Thotala et al., 2008; Yang et al., 2011). Inhibition of GSK3β accelerated double strand-break repair efficiency in irradiated mouse hippocampal neurons, whereas, none of these effects were observed in GBM cells, suggesting potential clinical application of neuroprotection with GSK3β inhibitors during cranial radiation.

5. GSK3β as a therapeutic target

In the field of medicinal chemistry, GSK3β has recently emerged as one of the most attractive therapeutic targets for the development of selective inhibitors as promising new drugs for diabetes. Several potent GSK3 inhibitors have been developed by pharmaceutical companies in preclinical models for diabetes treatment. Apart from this, inhibitors of GSK3β have enormous potential as therapeutics for a number of serious pathologies, including Alzheimer's disease, bipolar disorders, chronic inflammatory processes, and cancer. GSK3β inhibitors are being actively developed as drugs for the treatment of these various disorders. The therapeutic effect of GSK3β inhibition has been confirmed to inhibit inflammation in several studies (Jope et al., 2007). Concerns for the therapeutic use of GSK3β inhibitors remain because they may activate oncogenic (e.g., Wnt) signaling, thus promoting cell proliferation. Certainly, however, this concern has not deterred preclinical studies of GSK3β inhibitors in the treatment of many types of cancers, as discussed above, or Phase II clinical trials for the treatment of neurological diseases (Chico et al., 2009).

5.1 GSK3β-targeted therapy for cancers in clinic

The need for accurate determination of GSK3β status is illustrated by the excellent results of therapies targeting GSK3β in clinic. These strategies have been shown to benefit only tumors overexpressing the GSK3β protein. In other words, tumors that do not express GSK3β do not benefit from GSK3β-targeted therapies. To date, there are no clinical trial reports describing the use of specific GSK3β inhibitors for cancers, although many basic research results identified GSK3β as a tumor promoter and suitable candidate for targeted treatment. Chemical drugs already prescribed for other diseases were shown to have an inhibitory effect on GSK3β.

5.1.1 Lithium chloride (LiCl)

LiCl is highly effective in the treatment of bipolar disorder (Bowden et al., 2005). Results from an epidemiological study indicated that cancer prevalence in psychiatric patients on long-term LiCl medication was lower than in the general population (Cohen et al., 1998), suggesting that administration of LiCl induces cell differentiation and inhibits proliferation and, therefore, might effectively inhibit tumor formation and progression. GSK3β has emerged as a key target that is central to the effects of LiCl treatment. There are 2 mechanisms by which LiCl inhibits GSK3β (Figure 4). Firstly, LiCl promotes Ser9 phosphorylation in GSK3β, resulting in a less active form of GSK3β (Jope, 2003). Secondly, LiCl blocks the function of activated GSK3β by competing with magnesium ions (Mg^{2+}) (Jope, 2003). Mg^{2+} is required for activated GSK3β to phosphorylate its substrates, which are involved in the propagation of chemical signals required for cell survival, proliferation, and differentiation. As a consequence of these inhibitory effects, GSK3β can no longer regulate many important biological processes. It is notable that LiCl protects hippocampal neurons from radiation-induced apoptosis by promoting the DNA repair pathway, probably a result of the effect of GSK3β inhibition (Yang et al., 2009; Yang et al., 2011).

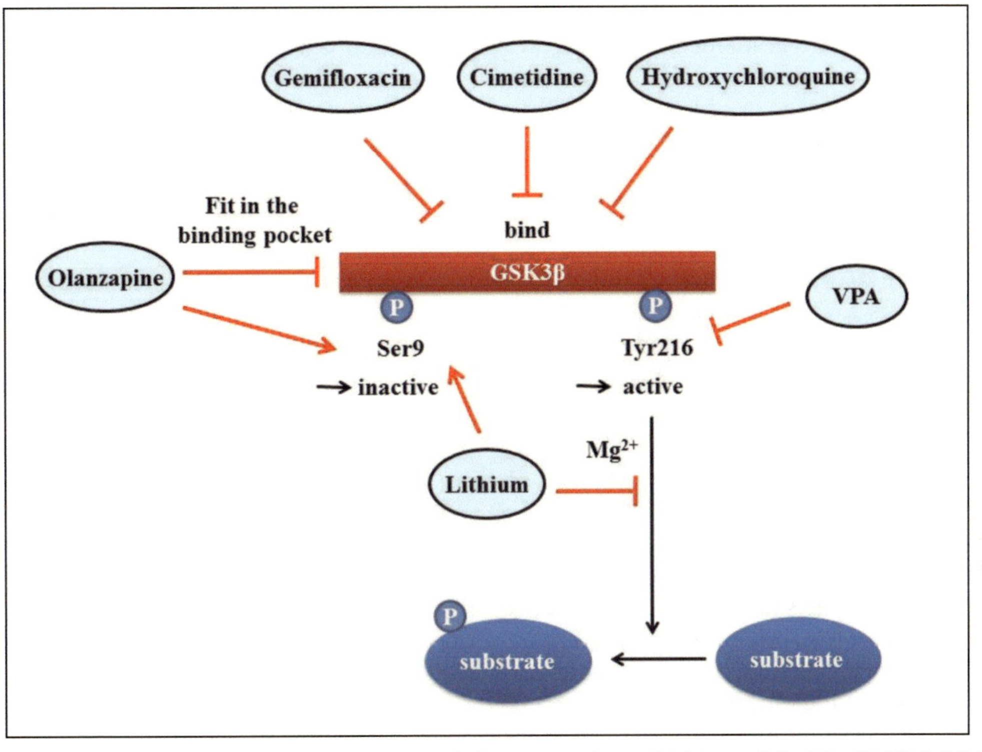

Fig. 4. Therapeutic mechanism of GSK3β inhibition in clinic. Lithium chloride (LiCl) inhibits phosphorylation of GSK3β substrates by competing with Mg^{2+}, which is required for GSK3β-dependent substrate phosphorylation. Simultaneously, LiCl and olanzapine increase the phosphorylation of the Ser9 residue. Valproic acid (VPA) inhibits GSK3β by direct interaction. LiCl and VPA show additive effects on GSK3β inhibition. Like a pharmacological GSK3β inhibitor AR-A014418, olanzapine can be successfully docked within the adenosine triphosphate (ATP)-binding pocket of GSK3β. Cimetidine, gemifloxacin, and hydroxychloroquine are potent GSK3β inhibitors with at least 2 distinct binding modes accessible to ligands within the GSK3β binding pocket. Circled P, phosphorylation.

5.1.2 Valproic acid (VPA)

VPA is now an established drug for the treatment of epileptic seizures (absence, tonic-clonic, and complex partial seizures) and mania in bipolar disorder (Kostrouchova & Kostrouch, 2007). VPA affects multiple cell regulatory pathways. The best substantiated molecular mechanism of VPA action is its inhibitory effect on histone deacetylase (HDAC) activity, a key regulator in the dynamics of chromatin structure and function. It was proposed that VPA activates Wnt-dependent gene expression through inhibition of HDAC, which generated interest for its use in cancer therapy (Phiel et al., 2001). Apart from this, VPA, like LiCl, exerts significant inhibitory effects on the activity of GSK3β both directly *in vitro* and also on endogenous GSK3β in intact human neuroblastoma SY5Y cells (Chen et al., 1999) (Figure 4). The dual inhibition of HDAC and GSK3β by VPA may provide a basis for its anticancer activity. As expected, clinical trials using VPA for cancer showed some effects (Chateauvieux et al., 2010).

Significant inhibitory effects for GSK3β are clearly observed at VPA concentrations approximating those attained clinically during treatment. Furthermore, addition of LiCl at therapeutic concentrations results in additive inhibitory effects to that of VPA. These additive effects of LiCl and VPA on GSK3β suggest that the 2 drugs may exert their effects at different sites, but additional studies will be necessary to establish this definitively (Chen et al., 1999).

5.1.3 Olanzapine

Olanzapine is broadly used for patients with schizophrenia. Recently, olanzapine was identified as a GSK3β inhibitor by a docking simulation experiment, which validates the interaction between the drug and its target molecule. Olanzapine, as well as the well-known GSK3β inhibitor AR-A014418, were found to readily fit within the adenosine triphosphate (ATP)-binding pocket of GSK3β and to inhibit its activity (Mohammad et al., 2008). Additionally, the administration of olanzapine, similar to LiCl, increased phospho-Ser9-GSK3β in brain (Li et al., 2007) (Figure 4). The inhibition of GSK3β by olanzapine was accompanied by a decrease in the blood glucose level and accumulation of glycogen in the liver in a dose-dependent manner. This is consistent with the effect of GSK3β inhibition (Mohammad et al., 2008). Olanzapine-induced low blood glucose level is also consistent with clinical reports (Budman & Gayer, 2001). This result contrasts that of a previous report, where olanzapine induced hyperglycemia as a major side effect (Fertig et al., 1998). The molecular mechanism of these contradictory findings is currently unknown.

On the basis of the reported reduced cancer risk in schizophrenic patients (Catts et al., 2008), a recent study demonstrated the anti-tumor effect of a number of antipsychotic drugs, including olanzapine, except for risperidone (Wiklund et al., 2010). The effect of these drugs against cancer cells was associated with changes in the expression of genes acting on cholesterol homeostasis and the biophysical properties of the cellular membrane. Inhibition of GSK3β activity might be an alternate mechanism by which olanzapine acts against cancer.

5.1.4 Cimetidine

Cimetidine was the first registered histamine H2 receptor antagonist, and its frequent prescription was based on its clinical effectiveness in healing gastrointestinal ulcers by inhibiting gastric acid secretion (Somogyi & Gugler, 1983). Cimetidine has been demonstrated to possess anti-tumor activity against colon, gastric, and kidney cancers and melanomas. This activity involves a number of different mechanisms of action, including blocking the cell growth-promoting activity of histamine (Lefranc et al., 2006). With respect to GBM, cimetidine combined with temozolomide was superior to temozolomide alone in extending the survival of nude mice with human GBM cells orthotopically xenografted into their brain (Lefranc et al., 2005).

In silico screening is a powerful method to analyze large chemical databases in order to identify possible new drug candidates. Recently, *in silico* screening revealed that cimetidine, as well as hydroxychlorquine (an antimalarial and anti-lupus erythematosus agent) and gemifloxacin (a new quinolone antibiotic), have an inhibitory effect on GSK3β (Taha et al., 2008) (Figure 4).

5.1.5 Enzastaurin

Enzastaurin, a selective serine/threonine protein kinase inhibitor already under clinical evaluation to treat recurrent GBM, potently inhibits GSK3β in addition to its primary target, protein kinase C (PKC) β. In phase I/II clinical trials, enzastaurin showed potentially encouraging efficacy in a subset of patients with recurrent malignant glioma, but does not appear to have enough single-agent activity to be useful as a monotherapy (Kreisl et al., 2009; Kreisl et al., 2010). In this trial, phosphorylation of GSK3β in peripheral blood mononuclear cells was identified as a potential biomarker of drug activity.

6. Perspective

GSK3β has been recognized as a key component in a wide range of cellular functions and is involved in the vast number of signaling pathways that converge on this enzyme, and subsequently, an even greater number of biological targets. GSK3β is undoubtedly a promising target not only for diabetes, bipolar disorder, Alzheimer's, and several other neurological disorders, but also for human cancers, including GBM, on the basis of the accumulated evidence. Inhibitors of GSK3β have enormous therapeutic potential. Of great importance is understanding the precise molecular mechanisms of GSK3β-mediated signal transduction, including signaling elements involved in proliferation, apoptosis, invasion, differentiation, chemosensitivity, radiosensitivity, and neuroprotection, as well as the precise functions of GSK3β proteins in cellular responses induced in human normal and malignant cell types. The emerging understanding of GSK3β function would also give rise to new insights in tumor biology. In the future, it is hoped that increasing knowledge of GSK3β will be translated into molecularly targeted therapies against intractable cancers represented by glioblastoma multiforme.

7. References

Ader, I., Delmas, C., Bonnet, J., Rochaix, P., Favre, G., Toulas, C. & Cohen-Jonathan-Moyal, E. (2003). Inhibition of Rho pathways induces radiosensitization and oxygenation in human glioblastoma xenografts. *Oncogene*. Vol. 22, No. 55, pp. 8861-8869, ISSN: 0950-9232

Aguilar-Morante, D., Morales-Garcia, J.A., Sanz-SanCristobal, M., Garcia-Cabezas, M.A., Santos, A. & Perez-Castillo, A. (2010). Inhibition of glioblastoma growth by the thiadiazolidinone compound TZD-8. *PLoS One*. Vol. 5, No. 11, pp. e13879, ISSN: 1932-6203

Beals, C.R., Sheridan, C.M., Turck, C.W., Gardner, P. & Crabtree, G.R. (1997). Nuclear export of NF-ATc enhanced by glycogen synthase kinase-3. *Science*. Vol. 275, No. 5308, pp. 1930-1934, ISSN: 0036-8075

Bhat, R., Xue, Y., Berg, S., Hellberg. S., Ormö, M., Nilsson, Y., Radesäter, A.C., Jerning, E., Markgren, P.O., Borgegård, T., Nylöf, M., Giménez-Cassina, A., Hernández, F., Lucas, J.J., Díaz-Nido, J. & Avila, J. (2003). Structural insights and biological effects of glycogen synthase kinase 3-specific inhibitor AR-A014418. *J Biol Chem*. Vol. 278, No. 46, pp. 45937–45945, ISSN: 0021-9258

Bowden, C.L., Grunze, H., Mullen, J., Brecher, M., Paulsson, B., Jones, M., Vagero, M. & Svensson, K. (2005). A randomized, double-blind, placebo-controlled efficacy and safety study of quetiapine or lithium as monotherapy for mania in bipolar disorder. *J Clin Psychiatry*. Vol. 66, No. 1, pp. 111-121, ISSN: 0160-6689

Boyle, W.J., Smeal, T., Defize, L.H., Angel, P., Woodgett, J.R., Karin, M. & Hunter, T. (1991). Activation of protein kinase C decreases phosphorylation of c-Jun at sites that negatively regulate its DNA-binding activity. *Cell*. Vol. 64, No. 3, pp. 573-584, ISSN: 0092-8674

Budman, C.L. & Gayer, A.I. (2001). Low blood glucose and olanzapine. *Am J Psychiatry*. Vol. 158, No. 3, pp. 500-501, ISSN: 0002-953X

Bullock, B.P. & Habener, J.F. (1998). Phosphorylation of the cAMP response element binding protein CREB by cAMP-dependent protein kinase A and glycogen synthase kinase-3 alters DNA-binding affinity, conformation, and increases net charge. *Biochemistry*. Vol. 37, No. 11, pp. 3795-3809, ISSN: 0006-2960

Catts, V.S., Catts, S.V., O'Toole, B.I. & Frost, A.D. (2008). Cancer incidence in patients with schizophrenia and their first-degree relatives—a meta-analysis. *Acta Psychiatry Scand*. Vol. 117, No. 5, pp. 323-336, ISSN: 1600-0447

Carmeliet, P., Dor, Y., Herbert, J.M., Fukumura, D., Brusselmans, K., Dewerchin, M., Neeman, M., Bono, F., Abramovitch, R., Maxwell, P., Koch, C.J., Ratcliffe, P., Moons, L., Jain, R.K., Collen, D. & Keshert, E. (1998). Role of HIF-1alpha in hypoxia-mediated apoptosis, cell proliferation and tumour angiogenesis. *Nature*. Vol. 394, No. 6692, pp. 485-490, ISSN: 0028-0836

Chateauvieux, S., Morceau, F., Dicato, M. & Diederich, M. (2010). Molecular and therapeutic potential and toxicity of valproic acid. *J Biomed Biotechnol*. Vol. 2010, No. pp., ISSN: 1110-7251

Chen, G., Huang, L.D., Jiang, Y.M. & Manji, H.K. (1999). The mood-stabilizing agent valproate inhibits the activity of glycogen synthase kinase-3. *J Neurochem*. Vol. 72, No. 3, pp. 1327-1330, ISSN: 0022-3042

Chico, L.K., Van Eldik, L.J. & Watterson, D.M. (2009). Targeting protein kinases in central nervous system disorders. *Nat Rev Drug Discov*. Vol. 8, No. 11, pp. 892-909, ISSN: 1474-1784

Chuang, Y.Y., Tran, N.L., Rusk, N., Nakada, M., Berens, M.E. & Symons, M. (2004). Role of synaptojanin 2 in glioma cell migration and invasion. *Cancer Res*. Vol. 64, No. 22, pp. 8271-8275, ISSN: 0008-5472

Classon, M. & Harlow, E. (2002). The retinoblastoma tumour suppressor in development and cancer. *Nat Rev Cancer*. Vol. 2, No. 12, pp. 910-917, ISSN: 1474-175X

Cohen, P. & Frame, S. (2001). The renaissance of GSK3. *Nat Rev Mol Cell Biol*. Vol. 2, No. 10, pp. 769-776, ISSN: 1471-0072

Cohen, Y., Chetrit, A., Sirota, P. & Modan, B. (1998). Cancer morbidity in psychiatric patients: influence of lithium carbonate treatment. *Med Oncol*. Vol. 15, No. 1, pp. 32-36, ISSN: 1357-0560

Cook, D., Fry, M.J., Hughes, K., Sumathipala, R., Woodgett, J.R. & Dale, T.C. (1996). Wingless inactivates glycogen synthase kinase-3 via an intracellular signalling pathway which involves a protein kinase C. *EMBO J*. Vol. 15, No. 17, pp. 4526-4536, ISSN: 0261-4189

Cross, D.A., Alessi, D.R., Cohen, P., Andjelkovich, M. & Hemmings, B.A. (1995). Inhibition of glycogen synthase kinase-3 by insulin mediated by protein kinase B. *Nature*. Vol. 378, No. 6559, pp. 785-789, ISSN: 0028-0836

Dajani, R., Fraser, E., Roe, S.M., Young, N., Good, V., Dale, T.C. & Pearl, L.H. (2001). Crystal structure of glycogen synthase kinase 3 beta: structural basis for phosphate-primed substrate specificity and autoinhibition. *Cell*. Vol. 105, No. 6, pp. 721-732, ISSN: 0092-8674

Demarchi, F., Bertoli, C., Sandy, P. & Schneider, C. (2003). Glycogen synthase kinase-3 beta regulates NF-kappa B1/p105 stability. *J Biol Chem*. Vol. 278, No. 41, pp. 39583-39590, ISSN: 0021-9258

Diehl, J.A., Cheng, M., Roussel, M.F. & Sherr, C.J. (1998). Glycogen synthase kinase-3beta regulates cyclin D1 proteolysis and subcellular localization. *Genes Dev*. Vol. 12, No. 22, pp. 3499-3511, ISSN: 0890-9369

Ding, Q., He, X., Hsu, J.M., Xia, W., Chen, C.T., Li, L.Y., Lee, D.F., Liu, J.C., Zhong, Q., Wang, X. & Hung, M.C. (2007). Degradation of Mcl-1 by beta-TrCP mediates glycogen synthase kinase 3-induced tumor suppression and chemosensitization. *Mol Cell Biol*. Vol. 27, No. 11, pp. 4006-4017, ISSN: 0270-7306

Doble, B.W. & Woodgett, J.R. (2003). GSK-3: tricks of the trade for a multi-tasking kinase. *J Cell Sci*. Vol. 116, No. Pt 7, pp. 1175-1186, ISSN: 0021-9533

Eldar-Finkelman, H., Schreyer, S.A., Shinohara, M.M., LeBoeuf, R.C. & Krebs, E.G. (1999). Increased glycogen synthase kinase-3 activity in diabetes- and obesity-prone C57BL/6J mice. *Diabetes*. Vol. 48, No. 8, pp. 1662-1666, ISSN: 0012-1797

Embi, N., Rylatt, D.B. & Cohen, P. (1980). Glycogen synthase kinase-3 from rabbit skeletal muscle. Separation from cyclic-AMP-dependent protein kinase and phosphorylase kinase. *Eur J Biochem*. Vol. 107, No. 2, pp. 519-527, ISSN: 0014-2956

Farago, M., Dominguez, I., Landesman-Bollag, E., Xu, X., Rosner, A., Cardiff, R.D. & Seldin, D.C. (2005). Kinase-inactive glycogen synthase kinase 3beta promotes Wnt signaling and mammary tumorigenesis. *Cancer Res*. Vol. 65, No. 13, pp. 5792-5801, ISSN: 0008-5472

Fertig, M.K., Brooks, V.G., Shelton, P.S. & English, C.W. (1998). Hyperglycemia associated with olanzapine. *J Clin Psychiatry*. Vol. 59, No. 12, pp. 687-689, ISSN: 0160-6689

Frame, S. & Cohen, P. (2001). GSK3 takes centre stage more than 20 years after its discovery. *Biochem J*. Vol. 359, No. Pt 1, pp. 1-16, ISSN: 0264-6021

Fuchs, S.Y., Ougolkov, A.V., Spiegelman, V.S. & Minamoto, T. (2005). Oncogenic β-catenin signaling networks in colorectal cancer. *Cell Cycle*. Vol. 4, No. 11, pp. 1522-1539, ISSN: 1551-4005

Gong, R., Rifai, A., Ge, Y., Chen, S. & Dworkin, L.D. (2008). Hepatocyte growth factor suppresses proinflammatory NFkappaB activation through GSK3beta inactivation in renal tubular epithelial cells. *J Biol Chem*. Vol. 283, No. 12, pp. 7401-7410, ISSN: 0021-9258

Gregory, M.A., Qi, Y. & Hann, S.R. (2003). Phosphorylation by glycogen synthase kinase-3 controls c-myc proteolysis and subnuclear localization. *J Biol Chem*. Vol. 278, No. 51, pp. 51606-51612, ISSN: 0021-9258

Grimes, C.A. & Jope, R.S. (2001). The multifaceted roles of glycogen synthase kinase 3beta in cellular signaling. *Prog Neurobiol*. Vol. 65, No. 4, pp. 391-426, ISSN: 0301-0082

Hagen, T. & Vidal-Puig, A. (2002). Characterisation of the phosphorylation of beta-catenin at the GSK-3 priming site Ser45. *Biochem Biophys Res Commun*. Vol. 294, No. 2, pp. 324-328, ISSN: 0006-291X

He, B., Meng, Y.H. & Mivechi, N.F. (1998). Glycogen synthase kinase 3beta and extracellular signal-regulated kinase inactivate heat shock transcription factor 1 by facilitating the disappearance of transcriptionally active granules after heat shock. *Mol Cell Biol*. Vol. 18, No. 11, pp. 6624-6633, ISSN: 0270-7306

Hegi, M.E., Diserens, A.C., Gorlia, T., Hamou, M.F., de Tribolet, N., Weller, M., Kros, J.M., Hainfellner, J.A., Mason, W., Mariani, L., Bromberg, J.E., Hau, P., Mirimanoff, R.O., Cairncross, J.G., Janzer, R.C. & Stupp, R. (2005). MGMT gene silencing and benefit from temozolomide in glioblastoma. *N Engl J Med*. Vol. 352, No. 10, pp. 997-1003, ISSN: 1533-4406

Hinoi, T., Yamamoto, H., Kishida, M., Takada, S., Kishida, S. & Kikuchi, A. (2000). Complex formation of adenomatous polyposis coli gene product and axin facilitates glycogen synthase kinase-3 beta-dependent phosphorylation of beta-catenin and down-regulates beta-catenin. *J Biol Chem*. Vol. 275, No. 44, pp. 34399-34406, ISSN: 0021-9258

Hoeflich, K.P., Luo, J., Rubie, E.A., Tsao, M.S., Jin, O. & Woodgett, J.R. (2000). Requirement for glycogen synthase kinase-3beta in cell survival and NF-kappaB activation. *Nature*. Vol. 406, No. 6791, pp. 86-90, ISSN: 0028-0836

Hou, X., Kumar, A., Lee, C., Wang, B., Arjunan, P., Dong, L., Maminishkis, A., Tang, Z., Li, Y., Zhang, F., Zhang, S.Z., Wardega, P., Chakrabarty, S., Liu, B., Wu, Z., Colosi, P., Fariss, R.N., Lennartsson, J., Nussenblatt, R., Gutkind, J.S., Cao, Y. & Li, X. (2010). PDGF-CC blockade inhibits pathological angiogenesis by acting on multiple cellular and molecular targets. *Proceedings of the National Academy of Sciences of the United States of America*. Vol. 107, No. 27, pp. 12216-12221, ISSN: 1091-6490

Hu, X., Paik, P.K., Chen, J., Yarilina, A., Kockeritz, L., Lu, T.T., Woodgett, J.R. & Ivashkiv, L.B. (2006). IFN-gamma suppresses IL-10 production and synergizes with TLR2 by regulating GSK3 and CREB/AP-1 proteins. *Immunity*. Vol. 24, No. 5, pp. 563-574, ISSN: 1074-7613

Iqbal, K. & Grundke-Iqbal, I. (2008). Alzheimer neurofibrillary degeneration: significance, etiopathogenesis, therapeutics and prevention. *J Cell Mol Med*. Vol. 12, No. 1, pp. 38-55, ISSN: 1582-1838

Jensen, R.L. (2009). Brain tumor hypoxia: tumorigenesis, angiogenesis, imaging, pseudoprogression, and as a therapeutic target. *J Neurooncol*. Vol. 92, No. 3, pp. 317-335, ISSN: 1573-7373

Jope, R.S. (2003). Lithium and GSK-3: one inhibitor, two inhibitory actions, multiple outcomes. *Trends Pharmacol Sci*. Vol. 24, No. 9, pp. 441-443, ISSN: 0165-6147

Jope, R.S. & Roh, M.S. (2006). Glycogen synthase kinase-3 (GSK3) in psychiatric diseases and therapeutic interventions. *Curr Drug Targets*. Vol. 7, No. 11, pp. 1421-1434, ISSN: 1873-5592

Jope, R.S., Yuskaitis, C.J. & Beurel, E. (2007). Glycogen synthase kinase-3 (GSK3): inflammation, diseases, and therapeutics. *Neurochem Res*. Vol. 32, No. 4-5, pp. 577-595, ISSN: 0364-3190

Kang, T., Wei, Y., Honaker, Y., Yamaguchi, H., Appella, E., Hung, M.C. & Piwnica-Worms, H. (2008). GSK-3 beta targets Cdc25A for ubiquitin-mediated proteolysis, and GSK-3 beta inactivation correlates with Cdc25A overproduction in human cancers. *Cancer Cell*. Vol. 13, No. 1, pp. 36-47, ISSN: 1535-6108

Kasuga, C., Ebata, T., Kayagaki, N., Yagita, H., Hishii, M., Arai, H., Sato, K. & Okumura, K. (2004). Sensitization of human glioblastomas to tumor necrosis factor-related apoptosis-inducing ligand (TRAIL) by NF-kappaB inhibitors. *Cancer Sci*. Vol. 95, No. 10, pp. 840-844, ISSN: 1347-9032

Kitagawa, K., Kotake, Y., Hiramatsu, Y., Liu, N., Suzuki, S., Nakamura, S., Kikuchi, A. & Kitagawa, M. (2010). GSK3 regulates the expressions of human and mouse c-Myb via different mechanisms. *Cell Div*. Vol. 5, No. pp. 27, ISSN: 1747-1028

Kobayashi, T., Hino, S., Oue, N., Asahara, T., Zollo, M., Yasui, W. & Kikuchi, A. (2006). Glycogen synthase kinase 3 and h-prune regulate cell migration by modulating focal adhesions. *Mol Cell Biol*. Vol. 26, No. 3, pp. 898-911, ISSN: 0270-7306

Koivisto, L., Alavian, K., Hakkinen, L., Pelech, S., McCulloch, C.A. & Larjava, H. (2003). Glycogen synthase kinase-3 regulates formation of long lamellipodia in human keratinocytes. *J Cell Sci*. Vol. 116, No. Pt 18, pp. 3749-3760, ISSN: 0021-9533

Korur, S., Huber, R.M., Sivasankaran, B., Petrich, M., Morin, P., Jr., Hemmings, B.A., Merlo, A. & Lino, M.M. (2009). GSK3beta regulates differentiation and growth arrest in glioblastoma. *PLoS One*. Vol. 4, No. 10, pp. e7443, ISSN: 1932-6203

Kostrouchova, M. & Kostrouch, Z. (2007). Valproic acid, a molecular lead to multiple regulatory pathways. *Folia Biol (Praha)*. Vol. 53, No. 2, pp. 37-49, ISSN: 0015-5500

Kotliarova, S., Pastorino, S., Kovell, L.C., Kotliarov, Y., Song, H., Zhang, W., Bailey, R., Maric, D., Zenklusen, J.C., Lee, J. & Fine, H.A. (2008). Glycogen synthase kinase-3 inhibition induces glioma cell death through c-MYC, nuclear factor-kappaB, and glucose regulation. *Cancer Res*. Vol. 68, No. 16, pp. 6643-6651, ISSN: 1538-7445

Kreisl, T.N., Kim, L., Moore, K., Duic, P., Kotliarova, S., Walling, J., Musib, L., Thornton, D., Albert, P.S. & Fine, H.A. (2009). A phase I trial of enzastaurin in patients with recurrent gliomas. *Clin Cancer Res*. Vol. 15, No. 10, pp. 3617-3623, ISSN: 1078-0432

Kreisl, T.N., Kotliarova, S., Butman, J.A., Albert, P.S., Kim, L., Musib, L., Thornton, D. & Fine, H.A. (2010). A phase I/II trial of enzastaurin in patients with recurrent high-grade gliomas. *Neuro Oncol*. Vol. 12, No. 2, pp. 181-189, ISSN: 1523-5866

Lefranc, F., James, S., Camby, I., Gaussin, J.F., Darro, F., Brotchi, J., Gabius, J. & Kiss, R. (2005). Combined cimetidine and temozolomide, compared with temozolomide alone: significant increases in survival in nude mice bearing U373 human glioblastoma multiforme orthotopic xenografts. *J Neurosurg*. Vol. 102, No. 4, pp. 706-714, ISSN: 0022-3085

Lefranc, F., Yeaton, P., Brotchi, J. & Kiss, R. (2006). Cimetidine, an unexpected anti-tumor agent, and its potential for the treatment of glioblastoma (review). *Int J Oncol*. Vol. 28, No. 5, pp. 1021-1030, ISSN: 1019-6439

Li, X., Rosborough, K.M., Friedman, A.B., Zhu, W. & Roth, K.A. (2007). Regulation of mouse brain glycogen synthase kinase-3 by atypical antipsychotics. *Int J Neuropsychopharmacol*. Vol. 10, No. 1, pp. 7-19, ISSN: 1461-1457

Li, Y., Lu, H., Huang, Y., Xiao, R., Cai, X., He, S. & Yan, G. (2010). Glycogen synthase kinases-3beta controls differentiation of malignant glioma cells. *Int J Cancer*. Vol. 127, No. 6, pp. 1271-1282, ISSN: 1097-0215

Ma, C., Wang, J., Gao, Y., Gao, T.W., Chen, G., Bower, K.A., Odetallah, M., Ding, M., Ke, Z. & Luo, J. (2007). The role of glycogen synthase kinase 3beta in the transformation of epidermal cells. *Cancer Res*. Vol. 67, No. 16, pp. 7756-7764, ISSN: 0008-5472

Maccario, H., Perera, N.M., Davidson, L., Downes, C.P. & Leslie, N.R. (2007). PTEN is destabilized by phosphorylation on Thr366. *Biochem J*. Vol. 405, No. 3, pp. 439-444, ISSN: 1470-8728

Mai, W., Kawakami, K., Shakoori, A., Kyo, S., Miyashita, K., Yokoi, K., Jin, M., Shimasaki, T., Motoo, Y. & Minamoto, T. (2009). Deregulated GSK3 beta sustains gastrointestinal cancer cells survival by modulating human telomerase reverse transcriptase and telomerase. *Clin Can Res*. Vol. 15, No. 22, pp. 6810-6819, ISSN: 1078-0432

Manoukian, A.S. & Woodgett, J.R. (2002). Role of glycogen synthase kinase-3 in cancer: regulation by Wnts and other signaling pathways. *Adv Cancer Res*. Vol. 84, No. pp. 203-229, ISSN: 0065-230X

Maurer, M.H., Bromme, J.O., Feldmann, R.E., Jr., Jarve, A., Sabouri, F., Burgers, H.F., Schelshorn, D.W., Kruger, C., Schneider, A. & Kuschinsky, W. (2007). Glycogen synthase kinase 3beta (GSK3beta) regulates differentiation and proliferation in neural stem cells from the rat subventricular zone. *J Proteome Res*. Vol. 6, No. 3, pp. 1198-1208, ISSN: 1535-3893

Miyashita, K., Kawakami, K., Nakada, M., Mai, W., Shakoori, A., Fujisawa, H., Hayashi, Y., Hamada, J. & Minamoto, T. (2009a). Potential therapeutic effect of glycogen synthase kinase 3beta inhibition against human glioblastoma. *Clin Cancer Res*. Vol. 15, No. 3, pp. 887-897, ISSN: 1078-0432

Miyashita, K., Nakada, M., Shakoori, A., Ishigaki, Y., Shimasaki, T., Motoo, Y., Kawakami, K. & Minamoto, T. (2009b). An emerging strategy for cancer treatment targeting aberrant glycogen synthase kinase 3 beta. *Anticancer Agents Med Chem*. Vol. 9, No. 10, pp. 1114-1122, ISSN: 1875-5992

Mohammad, M.K., Al-Masri, I.M., Taha, M.O., Al-Ghussein, M.A., Alkhatib, H.S., Najjar, S. & Bustanji, Y. (2008). Olanzapine inhibits glycogen synthase kinase-3beta: an investigation by docking simulation and experimental validation. *Eur J Pharmacol*. Vol. 584, No. 1, pp. 185-191, ISSN: 0014-2999

Nagamatsu, S., Nakamichi, Y., Inoue, N., Inoue, M., Nishino, H. & Sawa, H. (1996). Rat C6 glioma cell growth is related to glucose transport and metabolism. *Biochem J*. Vol. 319 (Pt 2), No. pp. 477-482, ISSN: 0264-6021

Nagane, M. (2011). Neuro-oncology: continuing multidisciplinary progress. *Lancet Neurol*. Vol. 10, No. 1, pp. 18-20, ISSN: 1474-4465

Nakada M, Kita D, Watanabe T, Hayashi Y, Teng L, Pyko IV, Hamada JI. (2011). Target signaling pathways in glioma. *Cancers*. in press.

Natsume, A., Ishii, D., Wakabayashi, T., Tsuno, T., Hatano, H., Mizuno, M. & Yoshida, J. (2005). IFN-beta down-regulates the expression of DNA repair gene MGMT and sensitizes resistant glioma cells to temozolomide. *Cancer Res*. Vol. 65, No. 17, pp. 7573-7579, ISSN: 0008-5472

Nikoulina, S.E., Ciaraldi, T.P., Mudaliar, S., Mohideen, P., Carter, L. & Henry, R.R. (2000). Potential role of glycogen synthase kinase-3 in skeletal muscle insulin resistance of type 2 diabetes. *Diabetes*. Vol. 49, No. 2, pp. 263-271, ISSN: 0012-1797

Nowicki, M.O., Dmitrieva, N., Stein, A.M., Cutter, J.L., Godlewski, J., Saeki, Y., Nita, M., Berens, M.E., Sander, L.M., Newton, H.B., Chiocca, E.A. & Lawler, S. (2008). Lithium inhibits invasion of glioma cells; possible involvement of glycogen synthase kinase-3. *Neuro Oncol*. Vol. 10, No. 5, pp. 690-699, ISSN: 1522-8517

Ougolkov, A.V., Fernandez-Zapico, M.E., Savoy, D.N., Urrutia, R.A. & Billadeau, D.D. (2005). Glycogen synthase kinase-3beta participates in nuclear factor kappaB-mediated gene transcription and cell survival in pancreatic cancer cells. *Cancer Res*. Vol. 65, No. 6, pp. 2076-2081, ISSN: 0008-5472

Ougolkov, A.V., Bone, N.D., Fernandez-Zapico, M.E., Kay, N.E. & Billadeau, D.D. (2007). Inhibition of glycogen synthase kinase-3 activity leads to epigenetic silencing of nuclear factor kappaB target genes and induction of apoptosis in chronic lymphocytic leukemia B cells. *Blood*. Vol. 110, No. 2, pp. 735-742, ISSN: 0006-4971

Pap, M. & Cooper, G.M. (1998). Role of glycogen synthase kinase-3 in the phosphatidylinositol 3-Kinase/Akt cell survival pathway. *J Biol Chem*. Vol. 273, No. 32, pp. 19929-19932, ISSN: 0021-9258

Petit-Paitel, A., Brau, F., Cazareth, J. & Chabry, J. (2009). Involvment of cytosolic and mitochondrial GSK-3beta in mitochondrial dysfunction and neuronal cell death of MPTP/MPP-treated neurons. *PLoS One*. Vol. 4, No. 5, pp. e5491, ISSN: 1932-6203

Phiel, C.J., Zhang, F., Huang, E.Y., Guenther, M.G., Lazar, M.A. & Klein, P.S. (2001). Histone deacetylase is a direct target of valproic acid, a potent anticonvulsant, mood stabilizer, and teratogen. *J Biol Chem*. Vol. 276, No. 39, pp. 36734-36741, ISSN: 0021-9258

Quant, E.C. & Wen, P.Y. (2010). Novel medical therapeutics in glioblastomas, including targeted molecular therapies, current and future clinical trials. *Neuroimaging Clin N Am*. Vol. 20, No. 3, pp. 425-448, ISSN: 1557-9867

Rao, A.S., Kremenevskaja, N., Resch, J. & Brabant, G. (2005). Lithium stimulates proliferation in cultured thyrocytes by activating Wnt/beta-catenin signalling. *Eur J Endocrinol*. Vol. 153, No. 6, pp. 929-938, ISSN: 0804-4643

Rask, K., Nilsson, A., Brannstrom, M., Carlsson, P., Hellberg, P., Janson, P.O., Hedin, L. & Sundfeldt, K. (2003). Wnt-signalling pathway in ovarian epithelial tumours: increased expression of beta-catenin and GSK3beta. *Br J Cancer*. Vol. 89, No. 7, pp. 1298-1304, ISSN: 0007-0920

Robe, P.A., Bentires-Alj, M., Bonif, M., Rogister, B., Deprez, M., Haddada, H., Khac, M.T., Jolois, O., Erkmen, K., Merville, M.P., Black, P.M. & Bours, V. (2004). In vitro and in vivo activity of the nuclear factor-kappaB inhibitor sulfasalazine in human glioblastomas. *Clin Cancer Res*. Vol. 10, No. 16, pp. 5595-5603, ISSN: 1078-0432

Saldanha, G. (2001). The Hedgehog signalling pathway and cancer. *J Pathol*. Vol. 193, No. 4, pp. 427-432, ISSN: 0022-3417

Salhia, B., Rutten, F., Nakada, M., Beaudry, C., Berens, M., Kwan, A. & Rutka, J.T. (2005). Inhibition of Rho-kinase affects astrocytoma morphology, motility, and invasion through activation of Rac1. *Cancer Res*. Vol. 65, No. 19, pp. 8792-8800, ISSN: 0008-5472

Semenza, G.L. (2009). Regulation of oxygen homeostasis by hypoxia-inducible factor 1. *Physiology (Bethesda)*. Vol. 24, No. pp. 97-106, ISSN: 1548-9213

Shakoori, A., Ougolkov, A., Yu, Z.W., Zhang, B., Modarressi, M.H., Billadeau, D.D., Mai, M., Takahashi, Y. & Minamoto, T. (2005). Deregulated GSK3beta activity in colorectal cancer: its association with tumor cell survival and proliferation. *Biochem Biophys Res Commun*. Vol. 334, No. 4, pp. 1365-1373, ISSN: 0006-291X

Shakoori, A., Mai, W., Miyashita, K., Yasumoto, K., Takahashi, Y., Ooi, A., Kawakami, K. & Minamoto, T. (2007). Inhibition of GSK-3 beta activity attenuates proliferation of human colon cancer cells in rodents. *Cancer Sci*. Vol. 98, No. 9, pp. 1388-1393, ISSN: 1347-9032

Singh, S.K., Hawkins, C., Clarke, I.D., Squire, J.A., Bayani, J., Hide, T., Henkelman, R.M., Cusimano, M.D. & Dirks, P.B. (2004). Identification of human brain tumour initiating cells. *Nature*. Vol. 432, No. 7015, pp. 396-401, ISSN: 1476-4687

Skuli, N., Monferran, S., Delmas, C., Lajoie-Mazenc, I., Favre, G., Toulas, C. & Cohen-Jonathan-Moyal, E. (2006). Activation of RhoB by hypoxia controls hypoxia-inducible factor-1alpha stabilization through glycogen synthase kinase-3 in U87 glioblastoma cells. *Cancer Res*. Vol. 66, No. 1, pp. 482-489, ISSN: 0008-5472

Somogyi, A. & Gugler, R. (1983). Clinical pharmacokinetics of cimetidine. *Clin Pharmacokinet*. Vol. 8, No. 6, pp. 463-495, ISSN: 0312-5963

Stambolic, V. & Woodgett, J.R. (1994). Mitogen inactivation of glycogen synthase kinase-3 beta in intact cells via serine 9 phosphorylation. *Biochem J*. Vol. 303 (Pt 3), pp. 701-704, ISSN: 0264-6021

Sun, T., Rodriguez, M. & Kim, L. (2009). Glycogen synthase kinase 3 in the world of cell migration. *Dev Growth Differ*. Vol. 51, No. 9, pp. 735-742, ISSN: 1440-169X

Taha, M.O., Bustanji, Y., Al-Ghussein, M.A., Mohammad, M., Zalloum, H., Al-Masri, I.M. & Atallah, N. (2008). Pharmacophore modeling, quantitative structure-activity relationship analysis, and in silico screening reveal potent glycogen synthase kinase-3beta inhibitory activities for cimetidine, hydroxychloroquine, and gemifloxacin. *J Med Chem*. Vol. 51, No. 7, pp. 2062-2077, ISSN: 0022-2623

Tewari, R., Sharma, V., Koul, N. & Sen, E. (2008). Involvement of miltefosine-mediated ERK activation in glioma cell apoptosis through Fas regulation. *J Neurochem*. Vol. 107, No. 3, pp. 616-627, ISSN: 1471-4159

Thotala, D.K., Hallahan, D.E. & Yazlovitskaya, E.M. (2008). Inhibition of glycogen synthase kinase 3β attenuates neurocognitive dysfunction resulting from cranial irradiation. *Cancer Res*. Vol. 68, No. 14, pp. 5859-5868, ISSN: 1538-7445

Tseng, A.S., Engel, F.B. & Keating, M.T. (2006). The GSK-3 inhibitor BIO promotes proliferation in mammalian cardiomyocytes. *Chem Biol*. Vol. 13, No. 9, pp. 957-963, ISSN: 1074-5521

Turner, C.E. & Brown, M.C. (2001). Cell motility: ARNO and ARF6 at the cutting edge. *Curr Biol*. Vol. 11, No. 21, pp. R875-877, ISSN: 0960-9822

Vaidya, R.J., Ray, R.M. & Johnson, L.R. (2006). Akt-mediated GSK-3beta inhibition prevents migration of polyamine-depleted intestinal epithelial cells via Rac1. *Cell Mol Life Sci*. Vol. 63, No. 23, pp. 2871-2879, ISSN: 1420-682X

Waaler, J., Machon, O., von Kries, J.P., Wilson, S.R., Lundenes, E., Wedlich, D., Gradl, D., Paulsen, J.E., Machonova, O., Dembinski, J.L., Dinh, H. & Krauss, S. (2011). Novel synthetic antagonists of canonical Wnt signaling inhibit colorectal cancer cell growth. *Cancer Res*. Vol. 71, No. 1, pp. 197-205, ISSN: 1538-7445

Wang, Z., Smith, K.S., Murphy, M., Piloto, O., Somervaille, T.C. & Cleary, M.L. (2008). Glycogen synthase kinase 3 in MLL leukaemia maintenance and targeted therapy. *Nature*. Vol. 455, No. 7217, pp. 1205-1209, ISSN: 1476-4687

Welsh, G.I., Miller, C.M., Loughlin, A.J., Price, N.T. & Proud, C.G. (1998). Regulation of eukaryotic initiation factor eIF2B: glycogen synthase kinase-3 phosphorylates a conserved serine which undergoes dephosphorylation in response to insulin. *FEBS Lett*. Vol. 421, No. 2, pp. 125-130, ISSN: 0014-5793

Wiklund, E.D., Catts, V.S., Catts, S.V., Ng, T.F., Whitaker, N.J., Brown, A.J. & Lutze-Mann, L.H. (2010). Cytotoxic effects of antipsychotic drugs implicate cholesterol homeostasis as a novel chemotherapeutic target. *Int J Cancer*. Vol. 126, No. 1, pp. 28-40, ISSN: 1097-0215

Woodgett, J.R. (1991). cDNA cloning and properties of glycogen synthase kinase-3. *Methods Enzymol*. Vol. 200, No. pp. 564-577, ISSN: 0076-6879

Xavier, I.J., Mercier, P.A., McLoughlin, C.M., Ali, A., Woodgett, J.R. & Ovsenek, N. (2000). Glycogen synthase kinase 3beta negatively regulates both DNA-binding and transcriptional activities of heat shock factor 1. *J Biol Chem*. Vol. 275, No. 37, pp. 29147-29152, ISSN: 0021-9258

Yang, E.S., Wang, H., Jiang, G., Nowsheen, S., Fu, A., Hallahan, D.E. & Xia, F. (2009). Lithium-mediated protection of hippocampal cells involves enhancement of DNA-PK-dependent repair in mice. *J Clin Invest*. Vol. 119, No. 5, pp. 1124-1135, ISSN: 1558-8238

Yang, E.S., Nowsheen, S., Wang, T., Thotala, D.K. & Xia, F. (2011). Glycogen synthase kinase 3{beta} inhibition enhances repair of DNA double-strand breaks in irradiated hippocampal neurons. *Neuro Oncol.* in press, ISSN: 1523-5866

Part 15

Astrocytomas - Regulatory Components and Effector Pathways

The Role of Matrix Metalloproteinases and Tissue Inhibitors of Metalloproteinases in the Progression of Astrocytomas

Fábio Motta et al.*
Federal University of Piauí, Parnaíba
Brazil

1. Introduction

Neoplasms of the central nervous system (CNS) constitute a group of tumors that are heterogeneous in epidemiology, biological behavior, genetic alterations, histological type, tumor location, pattern of spread, clinical presentation, natural history, age of occurrence, and prognosis (Behin et al., 2003; Louis, 2006; Stroher et al., 2000). According to the 2010 Surveillance Epidemiology and End Results [SEER] data, there were approximately 22,020 deaths from cancers of the brain and nervous system in the U.S. As reported by Binder et al., (2003) and Wrensch et al., (2002), some 7 to 16 cases of primary CNS tumors per 100,000 person-years are diagnosed in adults; approximately 50% of these cases are metastatic tumors, according to Hill et al. 1999.

CNS tumors are the third leading cause of cancer deaths in middle-aged adults, the second most common cause of death in children, and the most common solid tumor in children (Giles, 1995; Heuer et al., 2007). The incidence of CNS tumors in children and adolescents is approximately 2.7 cases per 100,000 patients per year. This figure accounts for 16% of the neoplasms within this group, making CNS tumors the second most frequent type of cancer (after leukemia) in young patients (20 years old and younger). The mortality rate observed with CNS tumors is one of the highest among childhood cancers. Diagnosis and treatment improvements, however, has contributed to the survival of these patients (Potter et al., 1998).

Epidemiological studies have shown a slight increase in the incidence of CNS tumors during the 1980s and 1990s in children and the elderly (Fisher et al. 2007; Swensen & Bushouse 1998). The apparent increase in the number of cases of CNS cancers is directly linked to the implementation of high-resolution neuroimaging tools, such as Magnetic Resonance Imaging (MRI) and Computed Tomography (CT), which have impacted the clinical diagnosis of neurological diseases (Cristensen et al., 2003; Fisher et al., 2007). Another

* Renata Canalle[1], France Yoshioka[1], Giovanny Pinto[1], Lúcia Harada[2], Carlotti Jurnior[3], Elvis Valera[3], Carlos Scrideli[3] and Luiz Tone[3]
[1]*Federal University of Piauí, Parnaíba, Brazil*
[2]*Federal University of Pará, Belém, Brazil*
[3]*University of São Paulo, Ribeirão Preto, Brazil*

important cause for the apparent increase in the incidence of brain tumors is the recent inclusion of low-grade neoplasms, which were not previously counted in the population-based registries (Linet et al., 1999).

Brain tumors have different incidence rates in different populations, with the highest rates in developed countries. Some factors have influenced the increased incidence in these countries, such as the increased accessibility of medical care and the implementation of cutting-edge technologies in health.However, cultural influences and ethnic or geographical differences cannot be disregarded as risk factors (Davis, 2007; Ohgaki & Kleihues, 2005). The incidence of brain tumors in Japan, for example, is less than half that of the northern European countries. In the U.S., neuroepithelial tumors are found more frequently in Caucasians than in blacks, Hispanics and Asians (SEER, 2010; Wrensch et al., 2002).

The etiologic factors of CNS tumors are not well established, and several studies have sought to elucidate the risk factors for these cancers. Some of the possible factors are shown in Table 1. Among the numerous associations that have been studied, the ones that definitely cause primary CNS tumors are the hereditary syndromes (tuberous sclerosis and neurofibromatosis Types 1 and 2) and ionizing radiation used for therapeutic purposes (Davis, 2007; Guney et al. 2001; Skalr, 2002)

Hereditary syndromes**
Family history of brain tumors
Constitutive polymorphisms
Lymphocyte mutagen sensitivity
Prior cancers
Infectious agents or immunological response
Allergies
Head trauma
Epilepsy, seizures, or convulsions
Drugs and medications
Diet and vitamins
Tobacco smoke exposure
Alcohol
Hair dyes and sprays
Traffic-related air pollution
Occupational and industrial exposures
Ionizing radiation**
Cellular telephones
Other radio frequency exposures
Power frequency electromagnetic fields

Table 1. Factors that have been studied in relation to the risk of primary tumors of the neuroepithelial tissue or meninges (adapted from Wrensh et al., 2002). **These factors have been shown to cause primary brain tumors.

The anatomical and pathological classifications of clinical brain tumors are complex and controversial, especially with regard to mixed tumors. As a result, the histological classification of brain tumors has been subject to constant review from the first attempt at histological classification proposed by Bailey & Cushing until today (Louis et al. 2007; Wrensh et al., 2002).

The histological classification of brain tumors currently adopted by the World Health Organization (WHO) divides these entities according to the predominant cell type in the lesions. This classification extends the concept of the degree of malignancy by incorporating data from phenotypic and molecular changes observed in these tumors. The WHO classification organizes brain tumors into neuroepithelial tumors of peripheral nerves, tumors of the meninges, lymphomas and hematological malignancies, germ cell tumors and metastatic tumors of the sellar region, with a total of over 100 distinct histological entities (Louis et al. 2007; Kleihues et al., 2002).

CNS tumors that originate from neuroepithelial tissue, generically called gliomas, are the CNS neoplasms that are most frequently encountered in children and adults. The subtypes have different biological behaviors and are distinguished by their histological characteristics, such as nuclear atypia, mitotic index, blood microvessel formation and necrosis. Such peculiarities are also used to assess the degree of malignancy according to the standards adopted by the WHO (Louis, 2006; Kleihues et al., 2002). Table 2 shows the WHO classification for neuroepithelial tumors in simplified form.

Neuroepithelial tumors	
Astrocytic tumors	
Pilocytic astrocytoma	9421/1*
Diffuse astrocytoma	9420/3
Anaplastic astrocytoma	9401/3
Glioblastoma	9440/3
Gliomatosis cerebri	9381/3
Oligodendroglial tumors	
Oligodendroglioma	9450/3
Anaplastic oligodendroglioma	9382/3
Ependymal tumors	
Ependymoma	9391/3
Anaplastic ependymoma	9392/3
Myxopapillary ependymoma	9394/1

Neuroepithelial tumors	
Subependymoma	9383/1
Choroid plexus tumors	
Choroid plexus papilloma	9390/0
Atypical choroid plexus papilloma	9390/1
Choroid plexus carcinoma	9390/3
Mixed gliomas of uncertain origin	
Astroblastoma	9430/3
Angiocentric glioma	9431/1
Chordoid gliomas of the third ventricle	9444/1
Neuronal and mixed neuronal-glial tumors	
Ganglioglioma	9505/1
Anaplastic ganglioglioma	9505/3
Central neurocytoma	9506/1
Embryonal tumors	
Medulloblastoma	9470/3
Medulloepithelioma	9501/3
Atypical teratoid/rhabdoid tumor	9508/3

Table 2. WHO classification for neuroepithelial tumors. * International Classification of Diseases - Oncology (ICD-O) (adapted from Louis et al., 2007).

1.1 Astrocytic tumors

The astrocytic tumors are derived from astrocytes, the principal glial support cells. These tumors are the most common primary brain tumors. They present extensive heterogeneity, differing in the location, age, extent, invasive potential, clinical course and tendency to progress (Khatua et al., 2003; Wang et al., 2003). Classically, astrocytomas are divided according to the degree of malignancy: pilocytic astrocytoma (Grade I), fibrillar diffuse astrocytoma (Grade II), anaplastic astrocytoma (Grade III) and glioblastoma multiforme (Grade IV).

The pilocytic astrocytomas are rare neoplasms, with an estimated incidence of less than 1 case per 100.000 person-years. They are predominantly pediatric tumors and are usually located in the cerebral hemispheres, with no infiltrative and circumscribed lesions. They are slow-growing and rarely lead to malignant transformation. Thus, these diffuse astrocytoma tumors are considered to be low-grade malignant neoplasms (Evren-Keles, et al., 2004). Although these neoplasms display benign behavior when located in the cerebral hemispheres, the same cannot be said when the lesions occur in the visual pathways or hypothalamus.

Histologically, pilocytic astrocytomas are presented as tumors of low to moderate cellularity. They consist of astrocytes with regular, uniform nuclei and little atypia. They are characterized by the presence of numerous Rosenthal fibers, which are protein inclusions within their astrocytic prolongations (Strother et al., 2000). Surgery is the recommended treatment for these lesions and is curative in most cases.

Chemotherapy has been used in specific cases, especially in children, with tumors of the optic tracts who experience progression after an initial period of observation and potential deterioration of vision (Packer et al., 1997).

Diffuse or fibrillary astrocytomas (Grade II) are less frequent in children, and commonly affecting young adults. Histologically, these tumors have increased cellularity, often do not exhibit microcysts or Rosenthal fibers, tend to undergo anaplastic transformation more frequently and they are more infiltrative (Behin et al., 2003).

Anaplastic astrocytomas (Grade III) are infiltrative, have a high proliferative potential and affect mainly adults. This type of tumor is associated with a shorter survival time than the two previously mentioned; presenting the three- or four-year survival in 70% of the cases. Surgery remains the best treatment option and this should target as wide an area as possible (Behin et al., 2003).

Grade IV astrocytoma, more commonly called glioblastoma multiforme, is most frequent in adults and is the most aggressive tumor of this lineage; it corresponds to approximately 50% of the malignant tumors of the CNS. It is clinically aggressive, highly invasive and capable of invading extra-axially. This neoplasm often appears in adulthood, after 40 years of age, which does not mean it is exclusive to this age group (Binder et al., 2003).

The histological features of glioblastoma multiforme are hypercellularity, cellular atypia and anaplasia, frequent nuclear mitotic figures, necrosis and endothelial proliferation. (Behin et al., 2003; Strother et al., 2000).

The optimal treatment is surgery, but many patients with neurological problems, the very elderly (over 80 years), and those at high risk of complications from anesthesia should be carefully evaluated; in many cases, biopsy is most suitable. Local radiotherapy is also indicated, even in cases where there is no indication for surgery.

Glioblastomas may arise from the transformation of low-grade or anaplastic tumors (in which case they are called secondary glioblastomas), or they can be primary (in which case they are called primary glioblastomas) (Kleihues et al., 2000). Although this classification is widely accepted in clinical practice, the designation of primary or secondary glioblastomas is more conceptual than diagnostic and has no pratical impact on treatment. The molecular analysis of these tumors has led to a classification based on the genetic alterations commonly found in them, which can distinguish primary from secondary glioblastomas (Figure 1) (Kleihues & Ohgaki, 2007).

2. The Extracellular Matrix (ECM)

The ECM consists of a complex network of proteins and proteoglycans, secreted by the connective tissue, whose purpose is to support the tissues that make up an organism. This network of proteins has a decisive influence on various biological activities (Giancotti et al. 1999; Matrisian, 1990).

The degradation of the ECM is a physiological process that is strictly controlled by the dynamic equilibrium between the activity of matrix metalloproteinases (MMPs) and tissue inhibitors of metalloproteinases (TIMPs). The cell-ECM interactions send signals promoting cell differentiation, migration and mobility that are necessary for cell homeostasis (Chang & Werb, 2001). MMPs degrade the ECM proteins and pericellular microenvironment, activating growth factors and adhesion molecules. These events are essential for a variety of physiological processes, such as embryonic development, remodeling, tissue repair and angiogenesis (Chakraborti et al. 2003; Löffek et al. 2010; Matrisian, 1990).

The disordered destruction of the ECM plays a crucial role in the development of various pathologies, such as liver fibrosis, aneurysms, periodontosis, rheumatoid arthritis, multiple sclerosis, cystic fibrosis and tumor formation. The development of tumors is highly dependent on the microenvironment because the production and/or uncontrolled activation of proteolytic enzymes involved in the degradation and remodeling of the ECM are the determining factors in tumor development (Overall et al., 2002; Pollet et al. 2004).

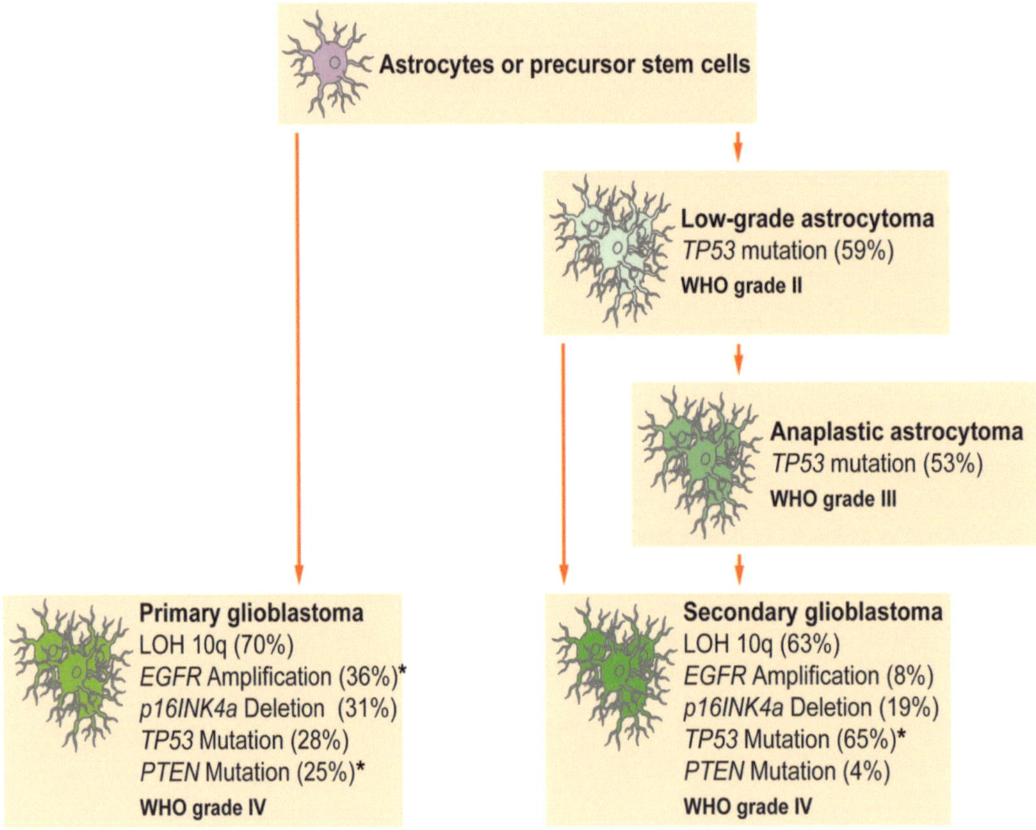

Fig. 1. The genetic pathways involved in the development of primary and secondary glioblastomas (adapted from Ohgaki & Kleihues, 2007).

2.1 Matrix metalloproteinases

The metalloproteinases are divided according to their biochemical characteristics as follows: MMPs; a disintegrin and metalloproteinases (ADAMs); and ADAMs with thrombospondin domains (ADAMS-TS) (Malemud, 2006; Werb, 1997).

MMPs are zinc-dependent (Zn^{+2}) peptidases with highly conserved substrate specificity that are capable of degrading proteoglycans, laminin, fibronectin, gelatin and fibrillar collagen (Types I, II, III, V and XI) on the basal membrane and in the ECM (Curran & Murray, 2000, Yong et al., 1998). There are more than 20 known members of this family of proteases. Mammalian MMPs are classified into soluble (secreted) and membrane (MT-MMPs) (Amalinei et al. 2007; Pei et al. 2000; Seiki, 1999).

Soluble MMPs are synthesized as pro-enzymes, while the MT-MMPs are activated in the intracellular space and expressed on the cell surface as active enzymes. These MMPs are divided into four subclasses according to their structural and functional characteristics: collagenases, gelatinases, stromelysins, and matrilysins (Nabeshima et al., 2002; Nagase & Woessner, 1999; Visse & Nagase, 2003).

The degradation of ECM is a physiological process that is strictly controlled by the dynamic equilibrium between the activity of matrix metalloproteinases (MMPs) and tissue inhibitors of metalloproteinases (TIMPs). The cell–ECM interactions send signals that promote cell differentiation, migration and mobility, which are necessary for cell homeostasis (Chang & Werb, 2001). MMPs degrade ECM proteins and the pericellular microenvironment, activating growth factors and adhesion molecules. These events are essential for a variety of physiological processes, such as embryonic development, remodeling, tissue repair and angiogenesis (Chakraborti et al. 2003; Löffek et al. 2010; Matrisian, 1990).

The general structure of MMPs consists of three domains that are highly conserved among this family but still distinct: a pro-N-terminal domain, a catalytic domain, and a C-terminal domain that contains the conserved hemopexin (HEXGHXXGXXH) motif (the matrilysins subfamilies do not have this motif). The histidine residues (H) contained in the hemopexin domain are involved in binding to Zn^{+2}, which is required for its proteolytic activity. The pro-domain of MMPs also contains a highly conserved PRCGVDP motif that bonds covalently to Zn^{+2}, keeping the protein in its non-activated zymogen form. Gelatinases have a binding site for fibronectin in the catalytic domain that confers specificity to the substrate (Figure 2) (Nakada et al. 1999; Pollet et al. 2004; Vihinen & Kalahari, 2002).

The collagenase subfamily includes MMP-1, MMP-8, MMP-13 and MMP-18, which exhibit biochemical characteristics that allow them to cleave interstitial collagen I, II and III in a site-specific N-terminal domain. Interstitial collagen I is one of the most abundant substances in the human body, so collagenases play an important role in the process of remodeling and degrading the ECM (Curran & Murray, 2000; Visse & Nagase, 2003).

The gelatinases include gelatinase A (MMP-2) and gelatinase B (MMP-9). These enzymes are specialized in degrading Type IV collagen, the main constituent of the basement membrane of cerebral blood vessels. As previously mentioned, these enzymes have three repeats of a fibronectin domain in their catalytic domains, which allows the gelatinases to bind to laminins and gelatin (Yong et al., 1998).

MMP-2, is a 72-kDa gelatinase, encoded on human chromosome 16q13 and constitutively expressed in variety of cell types. This enzyme has the ability to degrade collagen V, VII, XI and fibronectin. MMP-2 also mediates proliferation, adhesion and cell migration. This enzyme is secreted in its inactive form and gains catalytic activity by interacting with the complex formed by membrane metalloproteinase 1 (MT1-MMP, or MMP-14) and TIMP-2 (Chintala et al., 1999).

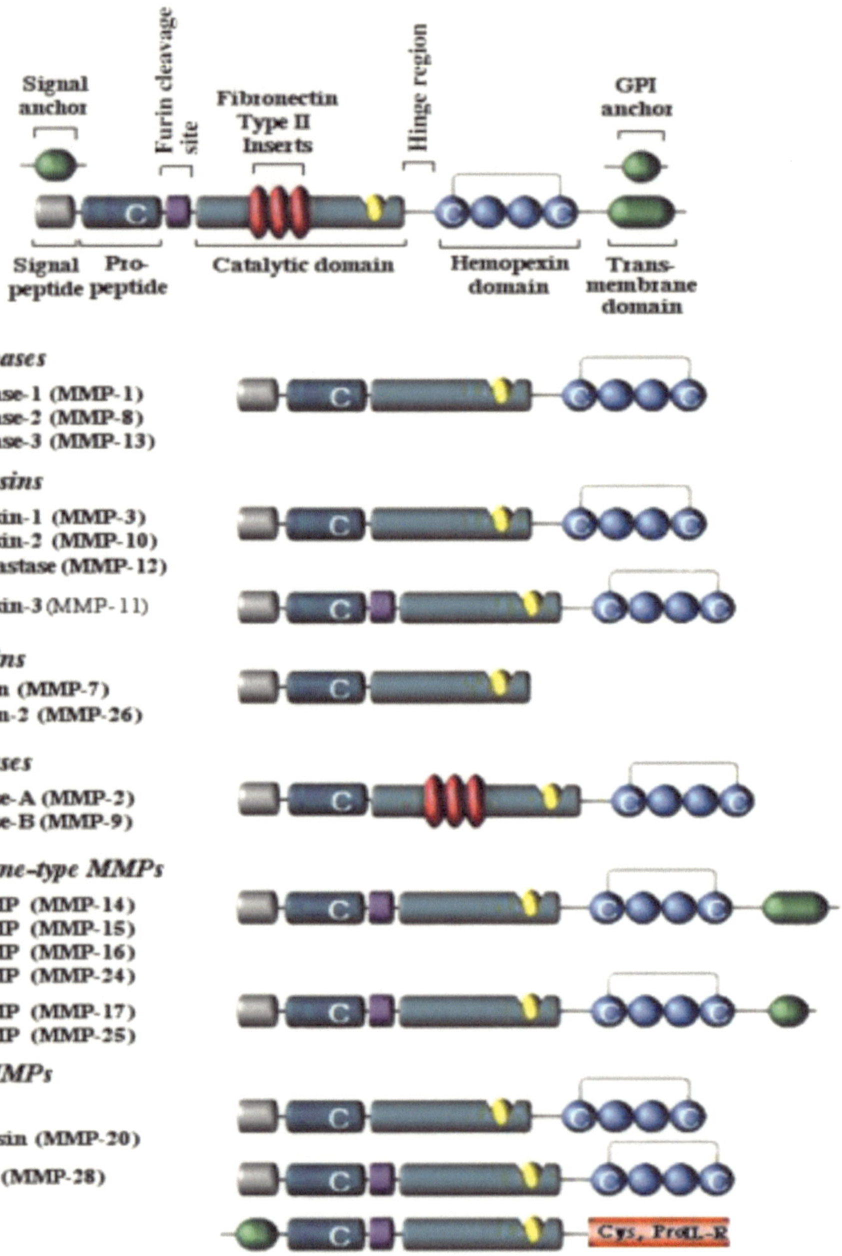

Fig. 2. The general structure of MMPs and their subfamilies (Vihinen & Kalahari, 2002).

MMP-9 is a 90–110-kDa protein encoded in the region 20q11.2-13.1. This enzyme is also secreted as a zymogen that can be stored in an active or latent form in the cytosol. The expression of MMP-9 is not constitutive and may be influenced by many factors, such as cell growth, cytokine signaling, cell–cell adhesion and cell–ECM interactions. The mechanism of protease activation thus involves a complex web of interactions with other MMPs and TIMPs (Amalinei et al. 2007; Chintala et al. 1999).

The stromelysins group is composed of the following proteases: MMP-3 (stromelysin-1), MMP-10 (stromelysin-2); and MMP-11 (stromelysis-3). These proteases have similar substrates, but MMP-3 has higher proteolytic activity than the other stromelysins. MMP-3 is expressed in several cell types and acts on the following ECM components: collagen, gelatin, elastin, fibronectin, and vitronectin. In addition to digesting the ECM components, MMP-3 participates in the activation of pro-MMP-1 and pro-MMP-9 (Egeblad & Werb, 2002).

The membrane-MMP subfamily consists of six MT-MMPs (MT1-MMP through MT6-MMP) and two glycosylphosphatidylinositol (GPI)-anchored MMPs (MMP-17 and MMP-25). One of the most prominent members of this subfamily is MT1-MMP (MMP-14), whose substrates are collagen Types I, II and III, gelatin, fibronectin and laminin (Koshikawa et al., 2000).

MT1-MMP is considered a multifunctional molecule. It is directly involved in cell growth, inflammation, the formation of new vessels, and the processes of cell adhesion and migration. Consequently, it plays a role in the formation of metastases (Shiomi & Okada, 2003; Yana & Seiki, 2002).

Its interactions with MT1-MMP cause TIMP-2 to play a crucial role in the activation of pro-MMP-2. The catalytic domain of MT1-MMP binds to the N-terminal domain of TIMP-2, causing the C-terminal region of TIMP-2 to become capable of connecting to the hemopexin domain of pro-MMP-2. The location of this protease in the membrane plays a role in pericellular proteolysis because this molecule activates pro-MMP-2, enabling it to use exogenous substrates to mediate the processes of invasion and metastasis. (Sternlicht & Werb, 2001; Sounni et al., 2003).

The expressions of MMPs are under the control of a sophisticated genetic mechanism. Under basal circumstances, levels of MMPs are relatively low; however, the expression of MMPs is increased by the processes of ECM remodeling that result from physiological or pathological conditions. The expression of some subfamilies of MMPs is tissue-specific. The regulation of the expressions of MMPs occurs by three main routes: transcriptional regulation of MMPs; activation of pro-enzymes, and inhibition by the action of TIMPs (Nagase et al., 2006; Yong et al. 1998).

2.1.1 Transcriptional regulation of MMP genes

The transcription factors that regulate MMP gene expression include activating protein-1 (AP-1), polyoma enhancer activator 3 (PEA3), SP1, β-catenin/Tcf-4 and NF-κB, these factors seem to have synergistic effects on MMP gene regulation. Based on the composition of their regulatory elements, the promoters of these genes can be divided into Classes I, II and III (Yan & Bold, 2007).

The Class I promoters contain a TATA box at position -30 (relative to the transcription start site) and an AP1-binding site at position -70. Many of these promoters also contain a binding site for PEA3 that is adjacent to the AP1 site. The Class II promoters also have a TATA box but without the proximal AP1 site. The regulation of these promoters is relatively simple and it is distinct from the regulation of the Class I promoters (Benbow & Brinckerhoff, 1997; Chakraborti et al., 2003).

The third and final group of promoters does not have a TATA box, meaning that transcription begins at multiple sites. However, the SP1 family of transcription factors, which bind close to the GC box, . controls the regulation of this group. The FOS and JUN proteins actively participate in the transcription regulatory mechanism by forming a heterodimer that binds to the AP1 sites and stimulates the transcription of MMPs in response to inflammatory cytokines (Matrisian, 1990). The structural differences between the MMP promoters are shown in Figure 3.

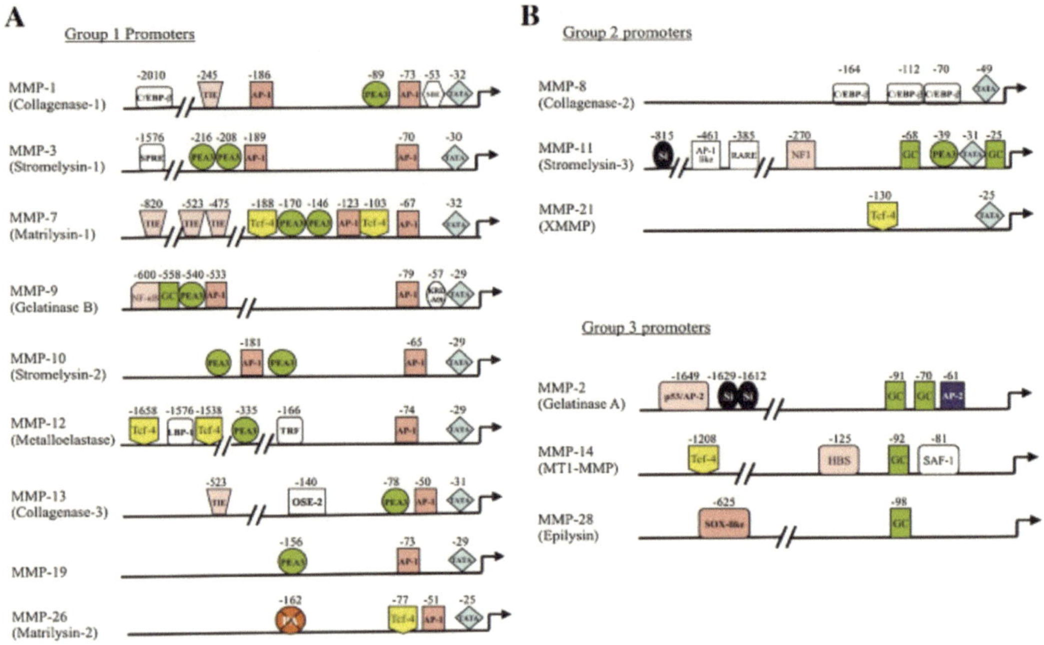

Fig. 3. The types and structures of the MMP-gene promoters (adapted from Yan & Bold, 2007).

2.1.2 Activation of proenzymes

MMPs are synthesized as zymogens. These enzymes can be activated by proteases in vivo or in vitro after exposure to chemical agents, such as thiol compounds ($HgCl_2$ and N-ethylmaleimide), SDS, reactive oxygen species, and exposure to heat or acidic pH. Activation in vivo occurs in the extracellular space and requires breaking the zinc–cysteine complex to expose its catalytic site. The cysteine residue (C) of the PRCGVPD sequence in the pro-domain interacts with the catalytic portion of the Zn^{2+} while maintaining the pro-MMPs in latent form. The disruption of this C–Zn^{2+} interaction results in a partial activation of the intermediate form of the enzyme, leading to the autocatalysis of the pro-peptide region that provides full activity to the enzyme. This mechanism allows the pro-MMPs to be activated by multiple agents, as mentioned above (Ra & Parks, 2007; Van Wart & Birkedal-Hansen, 1990).

The plasminogen/urokinase system is also an important physiological activator of pro-MMPs. The plasminogen activator of urokinase is associated with the membrane, thus creating an activation site for pro-MMPs and the subsequent renewal of the ECM. Plasmin can activate pro-MMP-1, pro-MMP-3, pro-MMP-7, pro-MMP-9, pro-MMP-10 and pro-MMP-13 (Nagase et al., 2006).

Most pro-MMPs that are secreted into the extracellular space are activated. Some pro-MMPs have a furin domain (KCKR) that allows them to be activated by furin in the intracellular space. These pro-enzymes include pro-MMP-11, MT-MMPs, pro-MMP-23 and pro-MMP-28 (Amalinei et al., 2007; Satmenkovic, 2003).

The activation of pro-MMP-2 is mediated by the MT-MMPs, with the exception of MT4-MMP, and it depends on the participation of TIMP-2. Pro-MMP-2 forms a complex with

TIMP-2 through its C-terminal domain, allowing the N-terminal domain of TIMP-2 to bind to MT1-MMP on the cell surface. The complex containing MT1-MMP, TIMP-2, and pro-MMP-2 is then presented to an adjacent free MT1-MMP, which activates the pro-MMP-2. The hemopexin domain seems to facilitate this activation process (Jo et al., 2000).

2.2 Tissue inhibitors of metalloproteinases

The TIMPs constitute the third regulatory level of MMP expression. These proteins are major physiological inhibitors of MMPs. The TIMPs are low-molecular-weight, 21-30 kDa, molecules that have approximately 12 cysteine residues that are involved in disulfide bridges, six of which are responsible for the formation of two domains that are essential for the interaction of these molecules with MMPs. The C-terminal domain is responsible for the interaction with and activation of pro-MMPs and for the subcellular localization of these proteins. The N-terminal domain acts as an independent unit that inhibits the activity of MMPs (Baker et al., 2002; Brew et al. 2000).

Blocking the proteolytic activity of both soluble and membrane-bound MMPs is accomplished by TIMPs through the formation of monocovalent complexes at a 1:1 ratio between the catalytic site of MMPs and the N-terminus of TIMPs. The amino groups and carbonyl groups of the cysteine residues in the N-terminus of TIMPs act together to chelate the Zn^{2+} in the catalytic domain of MMPs, making Zn^{2+} unavailable to activate the MMPs (Nagase et al., 2006; Visse & Nagase, 2003).

Four TIMPs, designated as TIMP-1 through TIMP-4, have been characterized in humans. They are resistant to heat denaturation and proteolytic degradation. These proteins are expressed in a variety of cell types and fluids (Gómez et al., 1997). Although all TIMPs are capable of inhibiting all the MMPs that have been studied, they differ in many aspects, such as solubility, the complementary nature of the pro-enzymes and the regulation of expression. TIMP-1, TIMP-2 and TIMP-4 are present in the soluble form, while TIMP-3 is connected to the ECM (Lamfers et al., 2005). The expression of TIMP-1 is inducible. This molecule has weak inhibitory action against MMP-19 and MT-MMPs (MT-MMP1, MT-MMP-2, MT-MMP-3 and MT-MMP-5) and even inhibits ADAM -10. The expression of TIMP-2 is constitutive, and it has strong inhibitory action against the MT-MMPs. TIMP-3 may also inhibit other members of the ADAM family, such as ADAM-17, ADAMTS-4 and ADAMTS-5, and the inhibitory effects of this molecule on MMP-9 are greater than those observed for TIMP-1 and TIMP-2. TIMP-4 expression is inducible, and it appears to inhibit the activities of MMPs constitutively. Table 3 presents some of the molecular characteristics and biological properties of TIMPs.

The TIMPs have also the ability to form complexes with pro-MMPs, thus regulating their activation. TIMP-1 preferentially forms complexes with pro-MMP-9, and TIMP-2 binds preferentially to pro-MMP-2 to facilitate its activation (Baker et al., 2002). TIMP-3 binds to both pro-MMP-2 and pro-MMP-9 (Bigg et al., 1997), and TIMP-4 can bind to the C-terminal domain of pro-MMP-2 (Butler et al., 1999).

The inhibition of MMPs is not unique to TIMPs. Molecules such as α-macroglobulin, general protease inhibitors, β-amyloid precursors linked to the cell membrane, and the membrane protein RECK play the same. RECK is a GPI-type, membrane-anchored protein that decreases the catalytic activity of MMP-2, MMP-9 and MT1-MMP and can overcome the angiogenic activity in neoplastic processes, leading to the death of tumor cells (Oh et al., 2001). A scheme for the interaction between the activation and inhibition of MMPs by TIMPs is presented in Figure 4.

	TIMP-1	TIMP-2	TIMP-3	TIMP-4
Chromosomal location	Xp11.23-11.4	17q23-17q25	22q12.1-22q13.2	3p25
mRNA (kb)	0,9	3,5	5,0	1,4
Molecular weight (kDa)	28,5	21	22/27	22
Protein localization	Soluble	Soluble	ECM	Soluble
Associated pro-MMPs	pro-MMP9	pro-MMP2	pro-MMP2/9	pro-MMP2
Gene Expression	Induced	Constitutive	Induced	Induced
Tumorigenic effects	Inhibition	Inhibition	Inhibition	Inhibition
Metastases	Stimulates	____	____	Stimulates

Table 3. The molecular and biological characteristics of TIMPs (adapted from Baker et al., 2002).

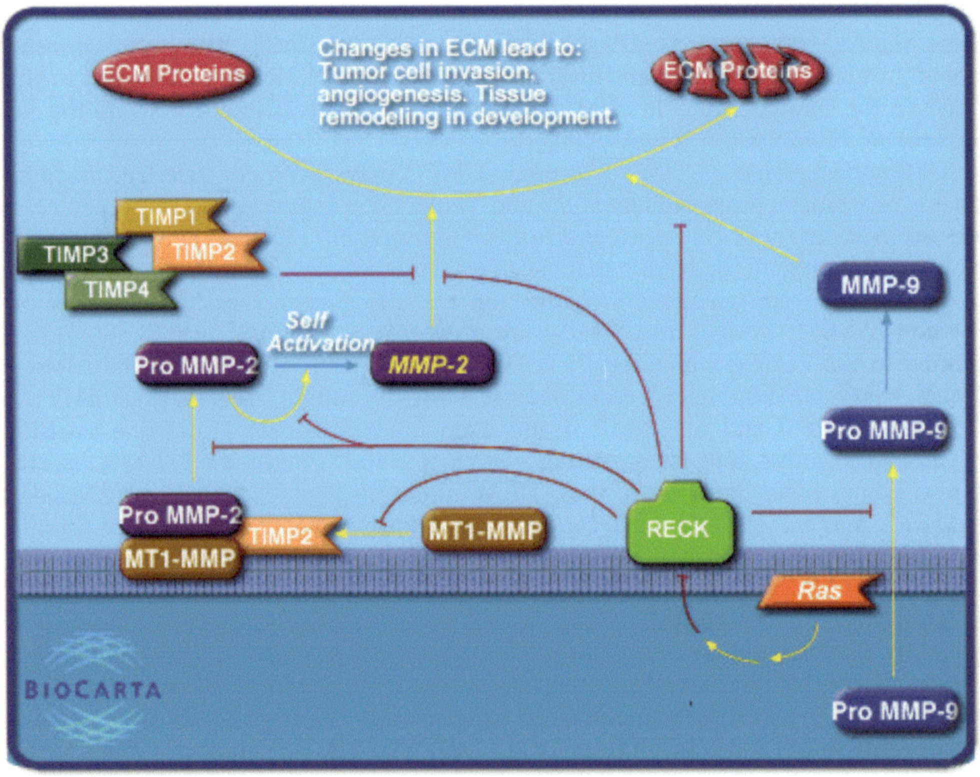

Fig. 4. MMPs are a class of proteases secreted by tumor cells. RECK is a membrane-anchored inhibitor of MMPs. It inhibits MMP-2, MMP-9 and MT1-MMP. Soluble, secreted MMP inhibitors, TIMPs, have also been identified. They appear to be less active at inhibiting MMPs and are perhaps even essential for MMP maturation. The inhibition of MMPs by RECK inhibits invasion of tissues, metastasis and tumor angiogenesis and is essential for normal development. (www.biocarta.com).

The main function of TIMPs is to act as natural receptor inhibitors of metalloproteinases. However, some studies have attributed other functions to TIMPs. Some of these functions are related to inhibiting MMPs and others are independent of it, such as promoting cell proliferation, anti-apoptosis activity and anti-angiogenesis (Chang & Werb, 2001; Chirco et al., 2006).

The induction of cell proliferation by TIMPs was first described for TIMP-1 and TIMP-2; they enhance the effect of erythropoietin in the proliferation and differentiation of erythroid progenitors. This property was observed not only in this cell type but also in keratinocytes, chondrocytes, epithelial cells and cancer cells (Hayakawa et al. 1992; Murat et al., 1993). In addition to promoting cell proliferation, the TIMPs may also modulate apoptosis in various ways, including opposing effects. TIMP-1 and TIMP-2 are involved in resistance to apoptosis in normal and cancer cells. The effect of TIMP-3 is different because it promotes apoptosis in smooth muscle cells, inducing the shedding of the ECM from transformed cells (Baker et al., 1998).

The effects of TIMP-4 in modulating apoptosis are contradictory; fibroblast-transformed heart tissue appear to be induced to apoptosis by TIMP-4, and the protein seems to have an inhibiting effect on apoptosis when hyperexpressed in breast-tumor cell lines (Baker et al., 2002).

Angiogenesis is described as the biological process of new capillary formation from existing vessels, which occurs in normal and pathological events. The TIMPs have anti-angiogenic activity, as was first demonstrated for TIMP-1 and TIMP-2. When hyperexpressed, they reduce angiogenic activity in pancreatic adenocarcinomas (Bloomston et al., 2002). TIMP-3 also has anti-angiogenesis and anti-invasion activities. For example, it reduces the invasiveness of the HT1080 cell line derived from fibrosarcoma and the expression of MMP-9, a molecule with known angiogenic activity (Lamfers et al., 2005). These observations corroborate the notion that the imbalance between the expressions of MMPs and TIMPs has a decisive role in the initiation and development of neoplastic processes.

2.3 The role of MMPs in progression of astrocytic tumors

Since the discovery of MMPs in 1962 by Gross and LaPierre, these enzymes have attracted great interest among researchers for their involvement in various physiological and pathological events. However, only in the 1980s, MMPs were discovered to be involved in the development and progression of tumors, a function that is widely studied to this day (Bourboulia & Stetler-Stevenson, 2010; Matrisian et al., 1986).

The invasive properties of CNS tumors are of great clinical importance because they contribute to the aggressive behavior of these tumors (Rao, 2003). For reasons still not well clarified yet , most primary neuroepithelial tumors do not evolve into metastatic disease. However, these tumors invade surrounding tissues, infiltrate their cells into normal tissue and (more rarely) spread along the neuro-axis into the cerebrospinal fluid.

The mechanism of astrocytic-tumor invasion is a complex process in which tumor cells separate from the parental tumor and rejoin the ECM. This process is associated with an increase in cell motility and with the ability of tumor cells to hydrolyze proteins, carbohydrates and proteoglycans in the ECM. These cells perform this task through the excessive production of proteases that modify the ECM, thus creating access to the surrounding tissues and promoting migration to other parts of the brain (Levicar et al., 2003).

MMPs are among the proteases that can degrade the ECM in brain tissue. The integrity of the ECM depends on a dynamic balance between MMP and TIMP activities. The loss of this balance can lead to the creation of a permissive environment for the initiation and development of a neoplastic process in brain tissue. MMPs, TIMPs and cell adhesion molecules are involved in the development of CNS malignancies (Forsyth et al. 1999; Mohana et al. 1995; Nakada et al. 2001; Rooprai et al., 1998). Changes in the expression of these proteins appear to be directly linked to the invasiveness of tumor cells. Classically, MMPs are considered to be responsible for promoting tumor growth, while TIMPs are thought to block the invasive ability of tumors (Amalinei et al. 2010; Deryugina & Quinley, 2006).

High-grade astrocytomas and medulloblastomas are neuroepithelial tumors of different cellular origins and are highly invasive. The degradation of the ECM is a prerequisite for invasion by these tumors. Among the MMPs that are commonly associated with the progression of astrocytic tumors are the gelatinases and the membrane MMPs, especially MT1-MMP1. Gelatinases A (MMP-2) and B (MMP-9) are undoubtedly the most well-studied MMPs in CNS tumors, and they have been identified as important factors in the development of high-grade gliomas (Munaut et al. 2003; Pagenstecher et al. 2001; Zhao, et al., 2007). This observation is directly linked to the invasive nature of these tumors because the expression levels of these gelatinases are generally low in normal brain tissue (Van Meter et al., 2001).

A study by Jäälinojä et al. (2000) demonstrated that the high expression of MMP-2 is a characteristic of highly malignant tumors and is associated with poor patient survival, similar data were also observed by Kunishio et al. (2003), who used immunohistochemistry analysis to show that MMP-2 and MMP-9 are not associated with increased aggressiveness in astrocytic tumors.

Komatsu et al. (2004) studied the expression of MMP-2 and MMP-9 in human gliomas by using two different techniques, RQ-PCR and immunohistochemistry, the results revealed no correlation between the expression of MMP-2 protein and the degree of malignancy. However, quantitative analysis of the mRNA showed that tumors of the highest grade, such as glioblastomas, express much higher levels of the MMP-2 and MMP-9 genes than do low-grade tumors. This study clearly demonstrated that methodological differences may explain some of the conflicting results found in the literature.

Increased levels of MMP-2 and MMP-9 and their relationships with astrocytic tumors of greater aggressiveness and invasiveness have also been reported by a number of authors, such as Forsyth et al. (1999), Lampert et al. (1998), Munaut et al. (2003), Pagenstecher et al. (2001) and Wang et al. (2003). Wild-Bode et al. (2001) reported that the overexpression of MMP-2 and MMP-9 is the best predictor of cell invasion by high-grade gliomas.

Another important result that highlights the prognostic significance of elevated MMP-9 expression was discovered by Hormigo et al. (2006), who found elevated MMP-9 protein in the serum of patients suffering from high-grade astrocytomas, which was not observed in low-grade tumors or in non-neoplastic tissue. These authors also suggested that MMP-9 can be used as a biomarker in the management of glioblastoma patients.

The analysis of *MMP-9* expression conducted by our group revealed that this gene is expressed more highly in astrocytic tumors than in non-tumor tissue. The expression is much greater in tumors with the highest degree of malignancy, especially glioblastomas, than in low-grade astrocytomas. Our study also revealed that pilocytic astrocytomas arising in the optic tracts, hypothalamus and pituitary gland, which appear to exhibit more aggressive behavior, show higher expressions of *MMP-9* than do the tumors that originate in the cerebral hemispheres (unpublished data). These observations suggest that overexpression of *MMP-9* is one of the main mechanisms necessary to increase the invasiveness and aggressiveness of CNS tumors. Our data also show that overexpression of MMP-9 in patients suffering from glioblastomas is significantly associated with decreased overall survival, as shown in Figure 5 (unpublished data). A multivariate analysis suggested that overexpression of MMP-9 is an independent prognostic factor of paramount importance in the management of glioblastoma patients. These observations support the hypothesis that abnormal expression of MMP-9 is a determinant of aggressiveness in astrocytic tumors.

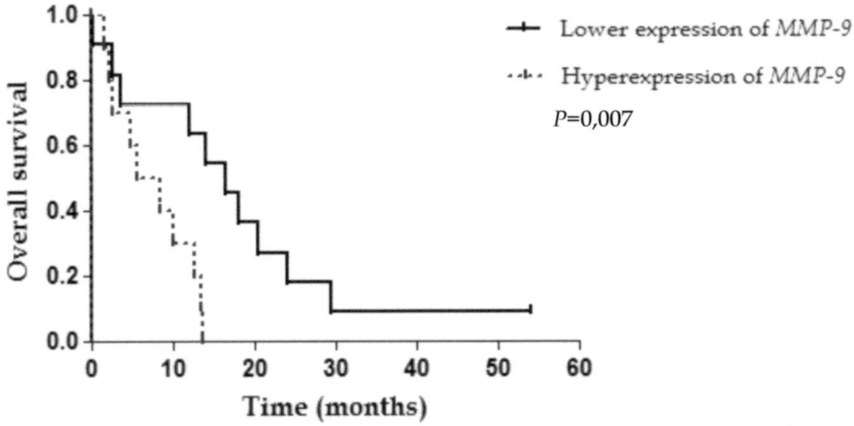

Fig. 5. The Overall survival of glioblastoma patients. The patients who overexpress the MMP-9 gene have significantly lower survival than patients with no marked upregulation of this gene (unpublished data).

Our observations suggest that overexpression of *MMP-9* increases the invasiveness of astrocytic tumors, making it a potential target for combating these neoplasms. Other authors, such as Vince et al. (2001), have found higher levels of expression of this gelatinase in medulloblastomas than in glioblastomas. They also observed that MMP-2 is more commonly found in areas of intense proliferative activity, while MMP-9 is associated with sites of angiogenesis, a typical feature of the invasive capacity of these tumors. Angiogenesis is highly dependent on the migration and invasion of endothelial cells into tissues. The ECM sequesters and stores angiogenesis-promoting factors, such as VEGF, bFGF and TGF1, which are released during the proteolytic degradation of the ECM. Accordingly, MMPs play a critical role in the process of angiogenesis. MMPs both promote and inhibit angiogenesis (Jain et al. 2007; Rundhaug, 2005; Zhao et al., 2008).

Gelatinases are the main promoters of the invasion of endothelial cells in the CNS (Lakka et al., 2005). MMP-2 is constitutively expressed by endothelial cells and interacts with thrombin, which is present at high levels in angiogenic sites. This interaction leads to activation of protein C on the surface of the endothelium. Activated protein C interacts with latent MMP-2 to increase its protease activity, thus allowing the endothelial cells to degrade the basement membrane. MMP-9 is then activated by intracellular vesicles secreted from endothelial cells to enhance the degradation of basement membrane. When the basement membrane reaches the interstice, the abundant collagen Type I contributes to the prolonged activation of MMP-2, thus consolidating the process of angiogenesis (Nguyen et al., 2001).

Glioblastomas are astrocytic tumors with increased invasive behavior, this property is closely related to their high vascularization. In vivo and in vitro, MMP-2 and MMP-9 are hyperexpressed in endothelial cells of glioblastomas (Vince et al., 2001; Zhao et al., 2010). The direct involvement of these proteins in angiogenesis may explain our observation of increased expression of MMP-2 and MMP-9 mRNA in highly malignant tumors (unpublished data). Similar results were found by Munaut et al. (2003), who also observed that overexpression of *MMP-2* and *MMP-9* is correlated with overexpression of VEGF in glioblastomas, a key mediator of angiogenesis.

Elevated expression of MMP-2 and MMP-9 and its clinical and biological implications for other cancers have been reported in several studies. Cho et al. (2007) reported that overexpression of MMP-9 is associated with poor prognosis in colorectal tumors. Similar observations were obtained by Kawata et al. (2007) for renal tumors and Iniesta et al. (2007) for non–small cell lung cancer.

Like the gelatinases, MT1-MMP is considered to be a promoter of tumor cell invasion and a facilitator of metastasis. MT1-MMP promotes the acquisition of invasive capacity in both normal and neoplastic cells through its ability to degrade pericellular collagen. It also facilitates angiogenesis by activating endothelial cells. This activity has been documented both in vivo and in vitro (Martin & Matrisian, 2007). The pro-invasive activity of MT1-MMP has been associated by some authors with invasion and progression in other tumors, such as neck tumors by Zhai et al. (2005) and astrocytic tumors by Forsyth et al. (1999); Nakada et al. (1999, 2001) and Kong et al. (2007).

Among the studies that have found a direct relationship between the increased expression of *MT1-MMP* and the evolution of gliomas, that of Nuttall et al. (2003) stands out because it found a greater than 21-fold increase in the level of MT1-MMP mRNA in glioblastomas relative to non-tumor brain tissue. The overexpression of *MT1-MMP* was also reported in a glioblastoma cell line (U251), the most invasive of the strains tested by the authors. This increase in the level of *MT1-MMP* was accompanied by the overexpression of *MMP-2* and *MMP-9* and of genes related to angiogenesis, such as VEGF. Munaut et al. (2003) also reported that strong expression of VEGF is accompanied by overexpression of MMP-2, MMP-9 and MT1-MMP and that these proteins act synergistically to create a permissive environment for glioblastoma cell invasion. Pagenstecher et al. (1999) also observed that the levels of MMP expression in pilocytic astrocytomas are comparable to those observed in anaplastic astrocytomas and glioblastomas, suggesting that this molecule is a major player in the progression of astrocytic tumors.

Arroyo et al. (2007) and Basile et al. (2007) demonstrated that MT1-MMP plays a crucial role in angiogenesis and that this protein is usually hyperexpressed at sites of neoangiogenesis. We believe that our observations are related to the level of vascularization of these tumors, and high-grade pilocytic astrocytomas have a significant level of vascularization. The overexpression of MT1-MMP and its relationship with the aggressive behavior of tumors have also been described in soft tissue cancers Roebuck et al. (2005) and more recently by Sroka et al. (2008) in prostate tumors.

2.4 The role of TIMPs in the progression of astrocytic tumors.

A high level of TIMP expression may occur in two distinct contexts: (1) as part of the defense mechanisms of the host tissue against the invasion; and (2) as promoter, either directly or indirectly, of cell growth in the tumor mass that helps the tumor progress and invade adjacent structures (Brand, 2002). The latter property directly promotes the evolution of these lesions to higher-malignancy tumors.

TIMP-1 is involved in a series of biological and pathological processes, including growth-promoting activity, inhibition of angiogenesis and changes in cell morphology. In the CNS, this molecule seems to possess the neuroprotective effect of maintaining the blood–brain barrier by its inherent inhibitory action on MMPs. TIMP-1 also has the distinguishing characteristic of not being able to inhibit MT1-MMP, in contrast to other TIMPs (Duffy et al., 2008). TIMP-1 is also involved in the development of neuroepithelial tumors (Gardner & Ghorpade, 2003; Lampert et al. 1998; Kakagawa et al. 1994; Pagentecher et al. 1999). Groft et al. (2001) showed that overexpression of TIMP-1 is associated with malignancy in gliomas and that TIMP-1 is detected mainly near the sites of blood vessel formation. These observations could be a result of interactions with pro-MMP-9 and the angiogenesis-promoting ability of this MMP. Huang et al (2005) and Pagentecher et al. (1999) found higher levels of TIMP-1 expression in pilocytic astrocytomas and glioblastomas. This result seems contradictory, but it may act to offset the simultaneous increases in the expression of MMP-9 and TIMP-1 because TIMP-1 preferentially inhibits MMP-9. The results of Pagentecher et al. (1999) also showed that this overexpression is linked to sites of neoangiogenesis.

Overexpression of *TIMP-1* appears to be an important prognostic factor for patients with breast cancer, since those patients with greater expression of this gene have higher survival rates (Nakopoulou et al., 2003). However, we found no similar reports for astrocytic tumors.

TIMP-2 preferentially inhibits MMP-2 and activates pro-MMP-2 by forming complexes with MT1-MMP. Béliveau et al. (1999), Huang et al. (2005) and Nakada et al. (2001) suggests that there is an inverse correlation between the expression of TIMP-2 and the degree of malignancy in CNS tumors. This result may be related to the antagonistic effects of these genes in the classical biological behavior of astrocytic tumors, in which MMPs act as promoters of invasion and TIMPs as blockers of tumor growth. Nuttal et al. (2003) has also detected high levels of TIMP-2 mRNA and protein expression in non-neoplastic brain-tissue samples. The in vitro protective effects of TIMP-2 were also described by Papi et al. (2007) in experiments using cells derived from gliomas. Moreover, Saxena et al. (1999) found a positive correlation between the expressions of TIMP-2 and MMP-2 and the degree of malignancy of CNS tumors, in which the highest levels of expression of these genes are primarily found in recurrent tumors. The increased expression of *TIMP-2* in these tumors may be related to defense against invasion or, more precisely, to the attempt to block the proteolytic activity of MMP-2, which facilitates tumor invasion. Other associations between the expression of TIMP-2 and survival in patients affected by CNS tumors have not been found. Curran et al. (2004) observed that the loss of TIMP-2 expression contributes significantly to the low survival rate of patients suffering from colorectal tumors.

The loss of TIMP-3 expression is related to cancer development, and normal brain tissue has high levels of TIMP-3. This physiological inhibitor of MMPs antagonizes the activity of most metalloproteinases, thereby leading to the inhibition of tumor growth, angiogenesis, invasion and metastasis formation. The overexpression of this gene in tumor cells seems to promote apoptosis and suppress early tumor growth (Hoe et al., 2007).

A study using microarray analysis that was conducted by Bozinov et al. (2008) showed that *TIMP-3* is one of the genes preferentially expressed in less-malignant CNS tumors. Huang et al. (2003) also observed that non-neoplastic tissue has low expression of TIMP-3. Furthermore, Lampert et al. (1998) and Pangestecher et al. (1999) found no variation in the gene expression levels between gliomas and suggested that this observation is consistent with constitutive expression. The protective effect of TIMPs against invasion by glioma cells was demonstrated by Lamfers et al. (2005), who used an adenovirus to transfer the gene for TIMP-3 into cultured cells, which resulted in increased expression of the gene and a reduction in the invasive capacity of the cells. The main cause of the decreased expression of *TIMP-3* is the hypermethylation of its promoter region. Gonzalez-Gomez et al. (2003a, 2003b) have shown that the promoter region of this gene is hypermethylated in glioblastomas, especially in secondary glioblastomas, and in medulloblastomas. Nakamura et al. (2005) have also found that the loss of heterozygosity in region 22q12.3, the region containing the TIMP- gene, is a frequent event in glioblastomas. These authors also suggested that these molecular alterations may be the primary cause of decreased expression of TIMP-3 in high-grade astrocytic tumors. Nakamura et al. (2005) have shown that hypermethylation of TIMP-3, and the consequent reduced expression of the gene, is an important factor in the poor survival of patients affected by highly malignant tumors. Correlations between decreased expression of this gene and low survival rates have also been observed in colorectal cancer (Hilska et al., 2007), non–small cell lung cancer (Mino et al., 2007) and bladder carcinomas (Hoque et al., 2008).

TIMP-4 has been studied less than the other TIMPs. It was discovered by Greene et al. (1996), who identified an expressed sequence tag (EST) with that was closely related to that of other TIMPs. This EST was identified and cloned in cDNA libraries from the human heart. They identified low levels of this transcript in a variety of tissues and organs, such as kidney and placenta, and did not observe expression of the gene in tissues derived from brain, lung, thymus or liver. These authors suggested that the contribution of TIMP-4 to maintaining the homeostasis of the ECM is tissue-specific. Bigg et al. (1997) also showed that TIMP-4 has a strong affinity for pro-MMP-2 and that, together with TIMP-2, it participates in the activation of pro-gelatinase A. The literature addressing the involvement of TIMP-4 in the development and progression of CNS tumors is sparse. Groft et al. (2001) have identified an inverse relationship between the expression of TIMP-4 and malignant CNS tumors. Microarray data obtained by Rorive et al. (2006) also show that TIMP-4 is preferentially expressed in pilocytic astrocytomas relative to normal brain tissue, Grade II astrocytomas and high-grade astrocytomas (Grades III and IV).The elevated expression of TIMP-4 in samples with low invasive potential compared to more aggressive tumors is not unique to CNS tumors. Similar findings have also been observed in studies of cells derived from breast tumors (Wang et al., 1997), prostate tumors (Lee et al., 2006) and rectal tumors (Hilska et al., 2007), in which the authors also observed that patients with higher expressions of TIMP-4 showed increased survival. However, our data revealed no relationship between the expression of *TIMP-4* and patient survival. These findings suggest that the supposed protection afforded by the overexpression of TIMP-4 is directly related to the ability of this molecule to promote the apoptosis of tumor cells (Guo et al., 2004).

The inherent properties of TIMPs can be exploited to achieve therapeutic benefits in various diseases. The role of the MMP/TIMP balance in blocking or even reversing tumor progression has led to the development of synthetic inhibitors of MMPs (ISMPs). Clinical trials evaluating the ISMPs, like batimastat and marimastat for cancer treatment have shown encouraging results, although they are less effective in advanced cancers and do have some side effects (Baker et al., 2002).

However, the results observed in animal models have shown that the use of Chantix prevented tumor growth and vascularization of pre-malignant tumors (Bergers et al. 1999; Mucha et al., 2007). TIMP gene therapy has also emerged as an important therapy for certain cancers, such as prostate (Deng et al., 2008) and hepatocellular carcinoma (Xia et al., 2006).

3. Conclusion

Recent advances in genetics and molecular biology have provided a great leap in understanding the molecular events responsible for the development and progression of brain tumors. The assessment of the level of expression of genes involved in the creation and maintenance of tumors of the nervous system can provide accurate information as which genes are involved in the development of a specific type of CNS tumor and to determine the molecular pathways that may become targets for therapy. Thereby, improving the prognosis of patients affected by this neoplasia, and their chances of cure. In this scenario the imbalance in the expression of MMPs and TIMPs seems to be an important clue to the progression, and therefore the aggressiveness, of astrocytic tumors. The invasive nature of these tumors is a major constraint on the efficacy of available therapies, especially for highly malignant astrocytomas. Therefore, a complete understanding of the interaction between the molecules that promote and block the migration routes of tumor cells will contribute significantly to developing new therapies to combat the progression of CNS tumors.

4. References

Amalinei, C., Caruntu, I.D. & Balan, R.A. (2007). Biology of metalloproteinases. *Rom J Morphol Embryol*, Vol.48, No.4, pp. 323-334

Amalinei, C., Caruntu, I.D., Giusca, S.E. & Balan, R.A. (2010). Matrix metalloproteinases involvement in pathologic conditions. *Rom J Morphol Embryol*, Vol.51, No.2, pp. 215-228

Arroyo, A.G., Genis, L., Gonzalo, P., Matias-Roman, S., Pollan, A. & Galvez, B.G. (2007). Matrix metalloproteinases: new routes to the use of MT1-MMP as a therapeutic target in angiogenesis-related disease. *Curr Pharm Des*, Vol.13, No.17, pp. 1787-1802

Baker, A.H., Zaltsman, A.B., George, S.J. & Newby, A.C. (1998). Divergent effects of tissue inhibitor of metalloproteinase-1, -2, or -3 overexpression on rat vascular smooth muscle cell invasion, proliferation, and death in vitro. TIMP-3 promotes apoptosis. *J Clin Invest*, Vol.101, No.6, pp. 1478-1487

Baker, A.H., Edwards, D.R. & Murphy, G. (2002). Metalloproteinase inhibitors: biological actions and therapeutic opportunities. *J Cell Sci*, Vol.115, No.Pt 19, pp. 3719-3727

Basile, J.R., Holmbeck, K., Bugge, T.H. & Gutkind, J.S. (2007). MT1-MMP controls tumor-induced angiogenesis through the release of semaphorin 4D. *J Biol Chem*, Vol.282, No.9, pp. 6899-6905

Behin, A., Hoang-Xuan, K., Carpentier, A.F. & Delattre, J.Y. (2003). Primary brain tumours in adults. *Lancet*, Vol.361, No.9354, pp. 323-331

Beliveau, R., Delbecchi, L., Beaulieu, E., Mousseau, N., Kachra, Z., Berthelet, F., Moumdjian, R. & Del Maestro, R. (1999). Expression of matrix metalloproteinases and their inhibitors in human brain tumors. *Ann N Y Acad Sci*, Vol.886, pp. 236-239

Benbow, U. & Brinckerhoff, C.E. (1997). The AP-1 site and MMP gene regulation: what is all the fuss about? *Matrix Biol*, Vol.15, No.8-9, pp. 519-526

Bergers, G., Javaherian, K., Lo, K.M., Folkman, J. & Hanahan, D. (1999). Effects of angiogenesis inhibitors on multistage carcinogenesis in mice. *Science*, Vol.284, No.5415, pp. 808-812

Bigg, H.F., Shi, Y.E., Liu, Y.E., Steffensen, B. & Overall, C.M. (1997). Specific, high affinity binding of tissue inhibitor of metalloproteinases-4 (TIMP-4) to the COOH-terminal hemopexin-like domain of human gelatinase A. TIMP-4 binds progelatinase A and the COOH-terminal domain in a similar manner to TIMP-2. *J Biol Chem*, Vol.272, No.24, pp. 15496-15500

Binder Dk.(2003). Aggressive glial Neoplasm. In: *Textbook of neurological surgery – principles and practice.* Batjer AZ\HH, Loftus CM. pp. (1270-1280), Lippincott Williams and Wilkins, ISBN 0781712718, Philadelphia

Bloomston, M., Shafii, A., Zervos, E.E. & Rosemurgy, A.S. (2002). TIMP-1 overexpression in pancreatic cancer attenuates tumor growth, decreases implantation and metastasis, and inhibits angiogenesis. *J Surg Res*, Vol.102, No.1, pp. 39-44

Bourboulia, D. & Stetler-Stevenson, W.G. Matrix metalloproteinases (MMPs) and tissue inhibitors of metalloproteinases (TIMPs): Positive and negative regulators in tumor cell adhesion. *Semin Cancer Biol*, Vol.20, No.3, pp. 161-168

Bozinov, O., Kohler, S., Samans, B., Benes, L., Miller, D., Ritter, M., Sure, U. & Bertalanffy, H. (2008). Candidate genes for the progression of malignant gliomas identified by microarray analysis. *Neurosurg Rev*, Vol.31, No.1, pp. 83-89; discussion 89-90

Brand, K. (2002). Cancer gene therapy with tissue inhibitors of metalloproteinases (TIMPs). *Curr Gene Ther*, Vol.2, No.2, pp. 255-271

Brew, K., Dinakarpandian, D. & Nagase, H. (2000). Tissue inhibitors of metalloproteinases: evolution, structure and function. *Biochim Biophys Acta*, Vol.1477, No.1-2, pp. 267-283

Butler, G.S., Apte, S.S., Willenbrock, F. & Murphy, G. (1999). Human tissue inhibitor of metalloproteinases 3 interacts with both the N- and C-terminal domains of gelatinases A and B. Regulation by polyanions. *J Biol Chem*, Vol.274, No.16, pp. 10846-10851

Chakraborti, S., Mandal, M., Das, S., Mandal, A. & Chakraborti, T. (2003). Regulation of matrix metalloproteinases: an overview. *Mol Cell Biochem*, Vol.253, No.1-2, pp. 269-285

Chang, C. & Werb, Z. (2001). The many faces of metalloproteases: cell growth, invasion, angiogenesis and metastasis. *Trends Cell Biol*, Vol.11, No.11, pp. S37-43

Chintala, S.K., Tonn, J.C. & Rao, J.S. (1999). Matrix metalloproteinases and their biological function in human gliomas. *Int J Dev Neurosci*, Vol.17, No.5-6, pp. 495-502

Chirco, R., Liu, X.W., Jung, K.K. & Kim, H.R. (2006). Novel functions of TIMPs in cell signaling. *Cancer Metastasis Rev*, Vol.25, No.1, pp. 99-113

Cho, Y.B., Lee, W.Y., Song, S.Y., Shin, H.J., Yun, S.H. & Chun, H.K. (2007). Matrix metalloproteinase-9 activity is associated with poor prognosis in T3-T4 node-negative colorectal cancer. *Hum Pathol*, Vol.38, No.11, pp. 1603-1610

Christensen, H.C., Kosteljanetz, M. & Johansen, C. (2003). Incidences of gliomas and meningiomas in Denmark, 1943 to 1997. *Neurosurgery*, Vol.52, No.6, pp. 1327-1333; discussion 1333-1324

Curran, S. & Murray, G.I. (2000). Matrix metalloproteinases: molecular aspects of their roles in tumour invasion and metastasis. *Eur J Cancer*, Vol.36, No.13 Spec No, pp. 1621-1630

Curran, S., Dundas, S.R., Buxton, J., Leeman, M.F., Ramsay, R. & Murray, G.I. (2004). Matrix metalloproteinase/tissue inhibitors of matrix metalloproteinase phenotype identifies poor prognosis colorectal cancers. *Clin Cancer Res*, Vol.10, No.24, pp. 8229-8234

Davis, F.S. (2007). Epidemiology of brain tumors. *Expert Rev Anticancer Ther*, Vol.7, No.12 Suppl, pp. S3-6

Deng, X., He, G., Levine, A., Cao, Y. & Mullins, C. (2008). Adenovirus-mediated expression of TIMP-1 and TIMP-2 in bone inhibits osteolytic degradation by human prostate cancer. *Int J Cancer*, Vol.122, No.1, pp. 209-218

Deryugina, E.I. & Quigley, J.P. (2006). Matrix metalloproteinases and tumor metastasis. *Cancer Metastasis Rev*, Vol.25, No.1, pp. 9-34

Duffy, M.J., McGowan, P.M. & Gallagher, W.M. (2008). Cancer invasion and metastasis: changing views. *J Pathol*, Vol.214, No.3, pp. 283-293

Egeblad, M. & Werb, Z. (2002). New functions for the matrix metalloproteinases in cancer progression. *Nat Rev Cancer*, Vol.2, No.3, pp. 161-174

Evren-Keles G.(2004). Supratentorial gliomas. In: *Pediatric CNS tumors*. Gupta N, Banerjee AB, Haas-Kogan D, pp. 7-26. Springer-Verlag, ISBN 978354087973,Berlin

Fisher, J.L., Schwartzbaum, J.A., Wrensch, M. & Wiemels, J.L. (2007). Epidemiology of brain tumors. *Neurol Clin*, Vol.25, No.4, pp. 867-890, vii

Forsyth, P.A., Wong, H., Laing, T.D., Rewcastle, N.B., Morris, D.G., Muzik, H., Leco, K.J., Johnston, R.N., Brasher, P.M., Sutherland, G. & Edwards, D.R. (1999). Gelatinase-A (MMP-2), gelatinase-B (MMP-9) and membrane type matrix metalloproteinase-1 (MT1-MMP) are involved in different aspects of the pathophysiology of malignant gliomas. *Br J Cancer*, Vol.79, No.11-12, pp. 1828-1835

Gardner, J. & Ghorpade, A. (2003). Tissue inhibitor of metalloproteinase (TIMP)-1: the TIMPed balance of matrix metalloproteinases in the central nervous system. *J Neurosci Res*, Vol.74, No.6, pp. 801-806

Giancotti, F.G. & Ruoslahti, E. (1999). Integrin signaling. *Science*, Vol.285, No.5430, pp. 1028-1032

Giles, G.G. (1995). The epidemiology of central nervous system tumours;trends and risk factors. *J Clin Neurosci*, Vol.2, No.3, pp. 191-205

Gomez, D.E., Alonso, D.F., Yoshiji, H. & Thorgeirsson, U.P. (1997). Tissue inhibitors of metalloproteinases: structure, regulation and biological functions. *Eur J Cell Biol*, Vol.74, No.2, pp. 111-122

Gonzalez-Gomez, P., Bello, M.J., Arjona, D., Lomas, J., Alonso, M.E., De Campos, J.M., Vaquero, J., Isla, A., Gutierrez, M. & Rey, J.A. (2003). Promoter hypermethylation of multiple genes in astrocytic gliomas. *Int J Oncol*, Vol.22, No.3, pp. 601-608

Gonzalez-Gomez, P., Bello, M.J., Lomas, J., Arjona, D., Alonso, M.E., Aminoso, C., De Campos, J.M., Vaquero, J., Sarasa, J.L., Casartelli, C. & Rey, J.A. (2003). Epigenetic changes in pilocytic astrocytomas and medulloblastomas. *Int J Mol Med*, Vol.11, No.5, pp. 655-660

Greene, J., Wang, M., Liu, Y.E., Raymond, L.A., Rosen, C. & Shi, Y.E. (1996). Molecular cloning and characterization of human tissue inhibitor of metalloproteinase 4. *J Biol Chem*, Vol.271, No.48, pp. 30375-30380

Groft, L.L., Muzik, H., Rewcastle, N.B., Johnston, R.N., Knauper, V., Lafleur, M.A., Forsyth, P.A. & Edwards, D.R. (2001). Differential expression and localization of TIMP-1 and TIMP-4 in human gliomas. *Br J Cancer*, Vol.85, No.1, pp. 55-63

Guo, P., Imanishi, Y., Cackowski, F.C., Jarzynka, M.J., Tao, H.Q., Nishikawa, R., Hirose, T., Hu, B. & Cheng, S.Y. (2005). Up-regulation of angiopoietin-2, matrix metalloprotease-2, membrane type 1 metalloprotease, and laminin 5 gamma 2 correlates with the invasiveness of human glioma. *Am J Pathol*, Vol.166, No.3, pp. 877-890

Hayakawa, T., Yamashita, K., Tanzawa, K., Uchijima, E. & Iwata, K. (1992). Growth-promoting activity of tissue inhibitor of metalloproteinases-1 (TIMP-1) for a wide range of cells. A possible new growth factor in serum. *FEBS Lett*, Vol.298, No.1, pp. 29-32

Heuer, G.G., Jackson, E.M., Magge, S.N. & Storm, P.B. (2007). Surgical management of pediatric brain tumors. *Expert Rev Anticancer Ther*, Vol.7, No.12 Suppl, pp. S61-68

Hill, J.R., Kuriyama, N., Kuriyama, H. & Israel, M.A. (1999). Molecular genetics of brain tumors. *Arch Neurol*, Vol.56, No.4, pp. 439-441

Hilska, M., Roberts, P.J., Collan, Y.U., Laine, V.J., Kossi, J., Hirsimaki, P., Rahkonen, O. & Laato, M. (2007). Prognostic significance of matrix metalloproteinases-1, -2, -7 and -13 and tissue inhibitors of metalloproteinases-1, -2, -3 and -4 in colorectal cancer. *Int J Cancer*, Vol.121, No.4, pp. 714-723

Hoe, H.S., Cooper, M.J., Burns, M.P., Lewis, P.A., van der Brug, M., Chakraborty, G., Cartagena, C.M., Pak, D.T., Cookson, M.R. & Rebeck, G.W. (2007). The metalloprotease inhibitor TIMP-3 regulates amyloid precursor protein and apolipoprotein E receptor proteolysis. *J Neurosci*, Vol.27, No.40, pp. 10895-10905

Hoque, M.O., Begum, S., Brait, M., Jeronimo, C., Zahurak, M., Ostrow, K.L., Rosenbaum, E., Trock, B., Westra, W.H., Schoenberg, M., Goodman, S.N. & Sidransky, D. (2008). Tissue inhibitor of metalloproteinases-3 promoter methylation is an independent prognostic factor for bladder cancer. *J Urol*, Vol.179, No.2, pp. 743-747

Hormigo, A., Gu, B., Karimi, S., Riedel, E., Panageas, K.S., Edgar, M.A., Tanwar, M.K., Rao, J.S., Fleisher, M., DeAngelis, L.M. & Holland, E.C. (2006). YKL-40 and matrix metalloproteinase-9 as potential serum biomarkers for patients with high-grade gliomas. *Clin Cancer Res*, Vol.12, No.19, pp. 5698-5704

Huang, H., Hara, A., Homma, T., Yonekawa, Y. & Ohgaki, H. (2005). Altered expression of immune defense genes in pilocytic astrocytomas. *J Neuropathol Exp Neurol*, Vol.64, No.10, pp. 891-901

Iniesta, P., Moran, A., De Juan, C., Gomez, A., Hernando, F., Garcia-Aranda, C., Frias, C., Diaz-Lopez, A., Rodriguez-Jimenez, F.J., Balibrea, J.L. & Benito, M. (2007). Biological and clinical significance of MMP-2, MMP-9, TIMP-1 and TIMP-2 in non-small cell lung cancer. *Oncol Rep*, Vol.17, No.1, pp. 217-223

Jaalinoja, J., Herva, R., Korpela, M., Hoyhtya, M. & Turpeenniemi-Hujanen, T. (2000). Matrix metalloproteinase 2 (MMP-2) immunoreactive protein is associated with poor grade and survival in brain neoplasms. *J Neurooncol*, Vol.46, No.1, pp. 81-90

Jain, R.K., di Tomaso, E., Duda, D.G., Loeffler, J.S., Sorensen, A.G. & Batchelor, T.T. (2007). Angiogenesis in brain tumours. *Nat Rev Neurosci*, Vol.8, No.8, pp. 610-622

Jo, Y., Yeon, J., Kim, H.J. & Lee, S.T. (2000). Analysis of tissue inhibitor of metalloproteinases-2 effect on pro-matrix metalloproteinase-2 activation by membrane-type 1 matrix metalloproteinase using baculovirus/insect-cell expression system. *Biochem J*, Vol.345 Pt 3, pp. 511-519

Kawata, N., Nagane, Y., Hirakata, H., Ichinose, T., Okada, Y., Yamaguchi, K. & Takahashi, S. (2007). Significant relationship of matrix metalloproteinase 9 with nuclear grade and prognostic impact of tissue inhibitor of metalloproteinase 2 for incidental clear cell renal cell carcinoma. *Urology*, Vol.69, No.6, pp. 1049-1053

Khatua, S., Peterson, K.M., Brown, K.M., Lawlor, C., Santi, M.R., LaFleur, B., Dressman, D., Stephan, D.A. & MacDonald, T.J. (2003). Overexpression of the EGFR/FKBP12/HIF-2alpha pathway identified in childhood astrocytomas by angiogenesis gene profiling. *Cancer Res*, Vol.63, No.8, pp. 1865-1870

Kleihues, P., Louis, D.N., Scheithauer, B.W., Rorke, L.B., Reifenberger, G., Burger, P.C. & Cavenee, W.K. (2002). The WHO classification of tumors of the nervous system. *J Neuropathol Exp Neurol*, Vol.61, No.3, pp. 215-225; discussion 226-219

Komatsu, K., Nakanishi, Y., Nemoto, N., Hori, T., Sawada, T. & Kobayashi, M. (2004). Expression and quantitative analysis of matrix metalloproteinase-2 and -9 in human gliomas. *Brain Tumor Pathol*, Vol.21, No.3, pp. 105-112

Kong, L., Li, Q., Wang, L., Liu, Z. & Sun, T. (2007). The value and correlation between PRL-3 expression and matrix metalloproteinase activity and expression in human gliomas. *Neuropathology*, Vol.27, No.6, pp. 516-521

Koshikawa, N., Giannelli, G., Cirulli, V., Miyazaki, K. & Quaranta, V. (2000). Role of cell surface metalloprotease MT1-MMP in epithelial cell migration over laminin-5. *J Cell Biol*, Vol.148, No.3, pp. 615-624

Kunishio, K., Okada, M., Matsumoto, Y. & Nagao, S. (2003). Matrix metalloproteinase-2 and -9 expression in astrocytic tumors. *Brain Tumor Pathol*, Vol.20, No.2, pp. 39-45

Lakka, S.S., Gondi, C.S. & Rao, J.S. (2005). Proteases and glioma angiogenesis. *Brain Pathol*, Vol.15, No.4, pp. 327-341

Lamfers, M.L., Gianni, D., Tung, C.H., Idema, S., Schagen, F.H., Carette, J.E., Quax, P.H., Van Beusechem, V.W., Vandertop, W.P., Dirven, C.M., Chiocca, E.A. & Gerritsen, W.R. (2005). Tissue inhibitor of metalloproteinase-3 expression from an oncolytic adenovirus inhibits matrix metalloproteinase activity in vivo without affecting antitumor efficacy in malignant glioma. *Cancer Res*, Vol.65, No.20, pp. 9398-9405

Lampert, K., Machein, U., Machein, M.R., Conca, W., Peter, H.H. & Volk, B. (1998). Expression of matrix metalloproteinases and their tissue inhibitors in human brain tumors. *Am J Pathol*, Vol.153, No.2, pp. 429-437

Lee, S., Desai, K.K., Iczkowski, K.A., Newcomer, R.G., Wu, K.J., Zhao, Y.G., Tan, W.W., Roycik, M.D. & Sang, Q.X. (2006). Coordinated peak expression of MMP-26 and TIMP-4 in preinvasive human prostate tumor. *Cell Res*, Vol.16, No.9, pp. 750-758

Levicar, N., Nuttall, R.K. & Lah, T.T. (2003). Proteases in brain tumour progression. *Acta Neurochir (Wien)*, Vol.145, No.9, pp. 825-838

Linet, M.S., Ries, L.A., Smith, M.A., Tarone, R.E. & Devesa, S.S. (1999). Cancer surveillance series: recent trends in childhood cancer incidence and mortality in the United States. *J Natl Cancer Inst*, Vol.91, No.12, pp. 1051-1058

Loffek, S., Schilling, O. & Franzke, C.W. Biological role of matrix metalloproteinases: a critical balance. *Eur Respir J*, pp.

Louis, D.N. (2006). Molecular pathology of malignant gliomas. *Annu Rev Pathol*, Vol.1, pp. 97-117

Louis, D.N., Ohgaki, H., Wiestler, O.D., Cavenee, W.K., Burger, P.C., Jouvet, A., Scheithauer, B.W. & Kleihues, P. (2007). The 2007 WHO classification of tumours of the central nervous system. *Acta Neuropathol*, Vol.114, No.2, pp. 97-109

Malemud, C.J. (2006). Matrix metalloproteinases (MMPs) in health and disease: an overview. *Front Biosci*, Vol.11, pp. 1696-1701

Martin, M.D. & Matrisian, L.M. (2007). The other side of MMPs: protective roles in tumor progression. *Cancer Metastasis Rev*, Vol.26, No.3-4, pp. 717-724

Matrisian, L.M., Bowden, G.T., Krieg, P., Furstenberger, G., Briand, J.P., Leroy, P. & Breathnach, R. (1986). The mRNA coding for the secreted protease transin is expressed more abundantly in malignant than in benign tumors. *Proc Natl Acad Sci U S A*, Vol.83, No.24, pp. 9413-9417

Matrisian, L.M. (1990). Metalloproteinases and their inhibitors in matrix remodeling. *Trends Genet*, Vol.6, No.4, pp. 121-125

Mino, N., Takenaka, K., Sonobe, M., Miyahara, R., Yanagihara, K., Otake, Y., Wada, H. & Tanaka, F. (2007). Expression of tissue inhibitor of metalloproteinase-3 (TIMP-3) and its prognostic significance in resected non-small cell lung cancer. *J Surg Oncol*, Vol.95, No.3, pp. 250-257

Mohanam, S., Wang, S.W., Rayford, A., Yamamoto, M., Sawaya, R., Nakajima, M., Liotta, L.A., Nicolson, G.L., Stetler-Stevenson, W.G. & Rao, J.S. (1995). Expression of tissue inhibitors of metalloproteinases: negative regulators of human glioblastoma invasion in vivo. *Clin Exp Metastasis*, Vol.13, No.1, pp. 57-62

Mucha, S.A., Melen-Mucha, G., Godlewski, A. & Stepien, H. (2007). Inhibition of estrogen-induced pituitary tumor growth and angiogenesis in Fischer 344 rats by the matrix metalloproteinase inhibitor batimastat. *Virchows Arch*, Vol.450, No.3, pp. 335-341

Munaut, C., Noel, A., Hougrand, O., Foidart, J.M., Boniver, J. & Deprez, M. (2003). Vascular endothelial growth factor expression correlates with matrix metalloproteinases MT1-MMP, MMP-2 and MMP-9 in human glioblastomas. *Int J Cancer*, Vol.106, No.6, pp. 848-855

Murate, T., Yamashita, K., Ohashi, H., Kagami, Y., Tsushita, K., Kinoshita, T., Hotta, T., Saito, H., Yoshida, S., Mori, K.J. & et al. (1993). Erythroid potentiating activity of tissue inhibitor of metalloproteinases on the differentiation of erythropoietin-responsive mouse erythroleukemia cell line, ELM-I-1-3, is closely related to its cell growth potentiating activity. *Exp Hematol*, Vol.21, No.1, pp. 169-176

Nabeshima, K., Inoue, T., Shimao, Y. & Sameshima, T. (2002). Matrix metalloproteinases in tumor invasion: role for cell migration. *Pathol Int*, Vol.52, No.4, pp. 255-264

Nagase, H. & Woessner, J.F., Jr. (1999). Matrix metalloproteinases. *J Biol Chem*, Vol.274, No.31, pp. 21491-21494

Nagase, H., Visse, R. & Murphy, G. (2006). Structure and function of matrix metalloproteinases and TIMPs. *Cardiovasc Res*, Vol.69, No.3, pp. 562-573

Nakada, M., Nakamura, H., Ikeda, E., Fujimoto, N., Yamashita, J., Sato, H., Seiki, M. & Okada, Y. (1999). Expression and tissue localization of membrane-type 1, 2, and 3 matrix metalloproteinases in human astrocytic tumors. *Am J Pathol*, Vol.154, No.2, pp. 417-428

Nakada, M., Kita, D., Futami, K., Yamashita, J., Fujimoto, N., Sato, H. & Okada, Y. (2001). Roles of membrane type 1 matrix metalloproteinase and tissue inhibitor of metalloproteinases 2 in invasion and dissemination of human malignant glioma. *J Neurosurg*, Vol.94, No.3, pp. 464-473

Nakagawa, T., Kubota, T., Kabuto, M., Sato, K., Kawano, H., Hayakawa, T. & Okada, Y. (1994). Production of matrix metalloproteinases and tissue inhibitor of metalloproteinases-1 by human brain tumors. *J Neurosurg*, Vol.81, No.1, pp. 69-77

Nakamura, M., Ishida, E., Shimada, K., Kishi, M., Nakase, H., Sakaki, T. & Konishi, N. (2005). Frequent LOH on 22q12.3 and TIMP-3 inactivation occur in the progression to secondary glioblastomas. *Lab Invest*, Vol.85, No.2, pp. 165-175

Nakopoulou, L., Giannopoulou, I., Lazaris, A., Alexandrou, P., Tsirmpa, I., Markaki, S., Panayotopoulou, E. & Keramopoulos, A. (2003). The favorable prognostic impact of tissue inhibitor of matrix metalloproteinases-1 protein overexpression in breast cancer cells. *Apmis*, Vol.111, No.11, pp. 1027-1036

Nguyen, M., Arkell, J. & Jackson, C.J. (2001). Human endothelial gelatinases and angiogenesis. *Int J Biochem Cell Biol*, Vol.33, No.10, pp. 960-970

Nuttall, R.K., Pennington, C.J., Taplin, J., Wheal, A., Yong, V.W., Forsyth, P.A. & Edwards, D.R. (2003). Elevated membrane-type matrix metalloproteinases in gliomas revealed by profiling proteases and inhibitors in human cancer cells. *Mol Cancer Res*, Vol.1, No.5, pp. 333-345

Oh, J., Takahashi, R., Kondo, S., Mizoguchi, A., Adachi, E., Sasahara, R.M., Nishimura, S., Imamura, Y., Kitayama, H., Alexander, D.B., Ide, C., Horan, T.P., Arakawa, T., Yoshida, H., Nishikawa, S., Itoh, Y., Seiki, M., Itohara, S., Takahashi, C. & Noda, M. (2001). The membrane-anchored MMP inhibitor RECK is a key regulator of extracellular matrix integrity and angiogenesis. *Cell*, Vol.107, No.6, pp. 789-800

Ohgaki, H. & Kleihues, P. (2005). Epidemiology and etiology of gliomas. *Acta Neuropathol*, Vol.109, No.1, pp. 93-108

Ohgaki, H. & Kleihues, P. (2007). Genetic pathways to primary and secondary glioblastoma. *Am J Pathol*, Vol.170, No.5, pp. 1445-1453

Overall, C.M. & Lopez-Otin, C. (2002). Strategies for MMP inhibition in cancer: innovations for the post-trial era. *Nat Rev Cancer*, Vol.2, No.9, pp. 657-672

Packer, R.J., Ater, J., Allen, J., Phillips, P., Geyer, R., Nicholson, H.S., Jakacki, R., Kurczynski, E., Needle, M., Finlay, J., Reaman, G. & Boyett, J.M. (1997). Carboplatin and vincristine chemotherapy for children with newly diagnosed progressive low-grade gliomas. *J Neurosurg*, Vol.86, No.5, pp. 747-754

Pagenstecher, A., Wussler, E.M., Opdenakker, G., Volk, B. & Campbell, I.L. (2001). Distinct expression patterns and levels of enzymatic activity of matrix metalloproteinases and their inhibitors in primary brain tumors. *J Neuropathol Exp Neurol*, Vol.60, No.6, pp. 598-612

Papi, A., Bartolini, G., Ammar, K., Guerra, F., Ferreri, A.M., Rocchi, P. & Orlandi, M. (2007). Inhibitory effects of retinoic acid and IIF on growth, migration and invasiveness in the U87MG human glioblastoma cell line. *Oncol Rep*, Vol.18, No.4, pp. 1015-1021

Pei, D., Kang, T. & Qi, H. (2000). Cysteine array matrix metalloproteinase (CA-MMP)/MMP-23 is a type II transmembrane matrix metalloproteinase regulated by a single cleavage for both secretion and activation. *J Biol Chem*, Vol.275, No.43, pp. 33988-33997

Polette, M., Nawrocki-Raby, B., Gilles, C., Clavel, C. & Birembaut, P. (2004). Tumour invasion and matrix metalloproteinases. *Crit Rev Oncol Hematol*, Vol.49, No.3, pp. 179-186

Potter, R. (1998). Tumours of central nervous system, in: *A Cancer in children – clinical management*, Voûte PA, Kalifa C, Barret, pp. (172-192), Oxford University Press, ISBN 0198529325,USA

Ra, H.J. & Parks, W.C. (2007). Control of matrix metalloproteinase catalytic activity. *Matrix Biol*, Vol.26, No.8, pp. 587-596

Rao, J.S. (2003). Molecular mechanisms of glioma invasiveness: the role of proteases. *Nat Rev Cancer*, Vol.3, No.7, pp. 489-501

Roebuck, M.M., Helliwell, T.R., Chaudhry, I.H., Kalogrianitis, S., Carter, S., Kemp, G.J., Ritchie, D.A., Jane, M.J. & Frostick, S.P. (2005). Matrix metalloproteinase expression is related to angiogenesis and histologic grade in spindle cell soft tissue neoplasms of the extremities. *Am J Clin Pathol*, Vol.123, No.3, pp. 405-414

Rorive, S., Maris, C., Debeir, O., Sandras, F., Vidaud, M., Bieche, I., Salmon, I. & Decaestecker, C. (2006). Exploring the distinctive biological characteristics of pilocytic and low-grade diffuse astrocytomas using microarray gene expression profiles. *J Neuropathol Exp Neurol*, Vol.65, No.8, pp. 794-807

Rundhaug, J.E. (2005). Matrix metalloproteinases and angiogenesis. *J Cell Mol Med*, Vol.9, No.2, pp. 267-285

Saxena A, Robertson , J., Kufta, C. (1995). Increased expression of gelatinase A and TIMP-2 in primary human glioblastomas. *Int J Oncol* Vol.7, pp. 469–473

Seiki, M. (1999). Membrane-type matrix metalloproteinases. *Apmis*, Vol.107, No.1, pp. 137-143

Shiomi, T. & Okada, Y. (2003). MT1-MMP and MMP-7 in invasion and metastasis of human cancers. *Cancer Metastasis Rev*, Vol.22, No.2-3, pp. 145-152

Sklar, C.A. (2002). Childhood brain tumors. *J Pediatr Endocrinol Metab*, Vol.15 Suppl 2, pp. 669-673

Sounni, N.E., Janssen, M., Foidart, J.M. & Noel, A. (2003). Membrane type-1 matrix metalloproteinase and TIMP-2 in tumor angiogenesis. *Matrix Biol*, Vol.22, No.1, pp. 55-61

Sroka, I.C., McDaniel, K., Nagle, R.B. & Bowden, G.T. (2008). Differential localization of MT1-MMP in human prostate cancer tissue: role of IGF-1R in MT1-MMP expression. *Prostate*, Vol.68, No.5, pp. 463-476

Stamenkovic, I. (2003). Extracellular matrix remodelling: the role of matrix metalloproteinases. *J Pathol*, Vol.200, No.4, pp. 448-464

Sternlicht, M.D. & Werb, Z. (2001). How matrix metalloproteinases regulate cell behavior. *Annu Rev Cell Dev Biol*, Vol.17, pp. 463-516

Swensen, A.R. & Bushhouse, S.A. (1998). Childhood cancer incidence and trends in Minnesota, 1988-1994. *Minn Med*, Vol.81, No.12, pp. 27-32

Van Wart, H.E. & Birkedal-Hansen, H. (1990). The cysteine switch: a principle of regulation of metalloproteinase activity with potential applicability to the entire matrix metalloproteinase gene family. *Proc Natl Acad Sci U S A*, Vol.87, No.14, pp. 5578-5582

VanMeter, T.E., Rooprai, H.K., Kibble, M.M., Fillmore, H.L., Broaddus, W.C. & Pilkington, G.J. (2001). The role of matrix metalloproteinase genes in glioma invasion: co-dependent and interactive proteolysis. *J Neurooncol*, Vol.53, No.2, pp. 213-235

Vihinen, P. & Kahari, V.M. (2002). Matrix metalloproteinases in cancer: prognostic markers and therapeutic targets. *Int J Cancer*, Vol.99, No.2, pp. 157-166

Vince, G.H., Herbold, C., Klein, R., Kuhl, J., Pietsch, T., Franz, S., Roosen, K. & Tonn, J.C. (2001). Medulloblastoma displays distinct regional matrix metalloprotease expression. *J Neurooncol*, Vol.53, No.2, pp. 99-106

Visse, R. & Nagase, H. (2003). Matrix metalloproteinases and tissue inhibitors of metalloproteinases: structure, function, and biochemistry. *Circ Res*, Vol.92, No.8, pp. 827-839

Wang, M., Liu, Y.E., Greene, J., Sheng, S., Fuchs, A., Rosen, E.M. & Shi, Y.E. (1997). Inhibition of tumor growth and metastasis of human breast cancer cells transfected with tissue inhibitor of metalloproteinase 4. *Oncogene*, Vol.14, No.23, pp. 2767-2774

Wang, M., Wang, T., Liu, S., Yoshida, D. & Teramoto, A. (2003). The expression of matrix metalloproteinase-2 and -9 in human gliomas of different pathological grades. *Brain Tumor Pathol*, Vol.20, No.2, pp. 65-72

Werb, Z. (1997). ECM and cell surface proteolysis: regulating cellular ecology. *Cell*, Vol.91, No.4, pp. 439-442

Wild-Bode, C., Weller, M. & Wick, W. (2001). Molecular determinants of glioma cell migration and invasion. *J Neurosurg*, Vol.94, No.6, pp. 978-984

Wrensch, M., Minn, Y., Chew, T., Bondy, M. & Berger, M.S. (2002). Epidemiology of primary brain tumors: current concepts and review of the literature. *Neuro Oncol*, Vol.4, No.4, pp. 278-299

Xia, D., Yan, L.N., Xie, J.G., Tong, Y., Yan, M.L., Wang, X.P., Zhang, M.M. & Zhao, L.Y. (2006). Overexpression of TIMP-1 mediated by recombinant adenovirus in hepatocellular carcinoma cells inhibits proliferation and invasion in vitro. *Hepatobiliary Pancreat Dis Int*, Vol.5, No.3, pp. 409-415

Yan, C. & Boyd, D.D. (2007). Regulation of matrix metalloproteinase gene expression. *J Cell Physiol*, Vol.211, No.1, pp. 19-26

Yana, I. & Seiki, M. (2002). MT-MMPs play pivotal roles in cancer dissemination. *Clin Exp Metastasis*, Vol.19, No.3, pp. 209-215

Yong, V.W., Krekoski, C.A., Forsyth, P.A., Bell, R. & Edwards, D.R. (1998). Matrix metalloproteinases and diseases of the CNS. *Trends Neurosci*, Vol.21, No.2, pp. 75-80

Zhai, Y., Hotary, K.B., Nan, B., Bosch, F.X., Munoz, N., Weiss, S.J. & Cho, K.R. (2005). Expression of membrane type 1 matrix metalloproteinase is associated with cervical carcinoma progression and invasion. *Cancer Res*, Vol.65, No.15, pp. 6543-6550

Zhao, J.X., Yang, L.P., Wang, Y.F., Qin, L.P., Liu, D.Q., Bai, C.X., Nan, X., Shi, S.S. & Pei, X.J. (2007). Gelatinolytic activity of matrix metalloproteinase-2 and matrix metalloproteinase-9 in rat brain after implantation of 9L rat glioma cells. *Eur J Neurol*, Vol.14, No.5, pp. 510-516

Zhao, Y., Xiao, A., diPierro, C.G., Carpenter, J.E., Abdel-Fattah, R., Redpath, G.T., Lopes, M.B. & Hussaini, I.M. (2010). An extensive invasive intracranial human glioblastoma xenograft model: role of high level matrix metalloproteinase 9. *Am J Pathol*, Vol.176, No.6, pp. 3032-3049

Part 16

Medulloblastoma - Regulatory Components and Effector Pathways

29

Medulloblastoma – Genetic Alterations

Esther Manor[1] and Lipa Bodner[2]
[1]*Genetic Laboratories, Institute of Human Genetics, Soroka University Medical Center*
Ben Gurion University of the Negev
[2]*Department of Oral and Maxillofacial Surgery, Soroka University Medical Center*
Ben Gurion University of the Negev
Israel

1. Introduction

Medulloblastoma (MB) is an embryonal brain tumor of the cerebellum. MB accounts for 4-6% of all primary intracranial tumors. It is the most common malignant brain tumor in children it represents 15-30% of all pediatric brain tumors, with 85% of MBs being diagnosed in patients younger then 18 years of age. The peak incidence occurs between the ages 3-9 years, with about 35% metastasis disease(Crawford *et al.*, 2007; Polkinghorn and Tarbell 2007; Rossi et al., 2008).

In contrast, medulloblastoma is rare in adults and accounts for less than1% of primary intracranial malignancies in this age group (Brandes et al 2009; Louis 2007; Padovani et al 2007).

Based on histopathological features, the 2007 WHO classification of CNS tumors (Louis et al.,2007; Gilbertson and Ellison 2008), has separated MB into five recognizable subtypes: the classic tumor which is the most common subtype of MB in general and in children in particular. The other four variants are: 1. desmoplastic/nodular which is the second most common (10-20% of the cases) in very young patients and adults, 2. MB with extensive nodularity is predominantly observed in infants (less then 3 years old), 3. anaplastic MB, 4. large cell MB is rare in infants, both of which account for 5-10% of the cases

The histological classification and clinical staging have proven to be less then ideal methods for stratification. Histological subtypes are often quite heterogeneous and exhibit highly variable clinical behavior, with anaplastic subtype typically associated with the worst prognosis, followed by classic and desmoplastic\nodular MB, which correlate with improved overall survival.

MB with extensive nodularity and desmoplastic/nodular MB in infants have a better outcome than the classic MB tumors, while large cell and anaplastic MB behave aggressively. Thus infants with desmoplastic MB should be stratified into a low risk therapeutic group while the large cell MB is rare but points to a poor prognosis that often presents with metastatic disease (Gilbertson and Ellison 2008).

The increasing recognition of MB as a heterogeneous disease, with histological and molecular variants that have distinct biological behavior, affected the disease classification and treatment.

In spite of current aggressive therapies, approximately one third of the patients eventually succumb to the disease due to metastasis. Furthermore the post- treatment squeal, which includes neurological, vascular and long-term neurocognitive impairments, can be devastating for survivors of the disease (Ribi et al., 2005).

It is imperative to gain a better understanding of the molecular alterations and other biological squeal in medulloblastom for future targeted therapies that are more effective and less toxic.

A combination of clinicopathological evaluation and assays based on molecular subgroups of the disease allow stratification of patients into risk groups and more tailored approach to therapy which should prevent the significant adverse effects among survivors.

Studies in the last 5 years have helped to build a consensus on the value and means of using molecular markers in the therapeutic stratification of childhood medulloblastoma (Gilbertson 2004 ; Packer and Vezina 2008 ; Pizer and Clifford 2009).

These studies have revealed the genetic heterogeneity within MB including dysregulation of several signaling pathways. The genetic heterogeneity appears to be the basis for differential response to treatment and give a new impact to the traditional histological subtyping and improve to some extend the accuracy of diagnosis and prognosis and as a consequence the stratification to risk groups (Packer and Vezina 2008).

Although, adult MB is considered different from their childhood counterparts in terms of tumor biology and clinical variables, yet, because of the high incidence of MB in childhood and low incidence in adults most of the studies have been done on the MB of childhood.

Some studies documented differences between childhood and adults tumors with regards to localization, cell of origin, histopathologic features, tumor cell differentiation, and treatment outcome. The adult's MB found to be also genetically distinct from the pediatric MB (Korshunov et al 2010).

Here we focused on the genetic alteration reported so far in MB and their significance in sub-typing, stratification, and medical care.

2. Heritability of medulloblastoma

Neither familial cases of MB, nor MB's cases affected by defined environmental factors have been described so far. Also, no specific chromosomal aberration has been described in more then about 40% of the MB cases. Unlike Ewing sarcoma, where t(11;21) can be found in about 90% of the cases, in MB no main specific gene alteration can be detected. Yet, there is a wide basis to believe that inheritable factors play a significant role in MB pathogenesis and prevalence. Some of the evidence that support this point of view are:

A. **Age of onset**- MB is most prevalent in childhood including about 3% in infancy, mainly medulloblastoma with extensive nodularity, while it is rare in adults. MB is mostly a childhood brain tumor with a peak in 3-9 years age. Inheritable markers are most probably expressed phenotypically at the early ages of life. The younger the patient is, the higher chance that the genetic part is more pronounced, and so in the adults, the latter the age of tumor appearance the higher chance for multi-factorial environmental cause. About 85% of the primary intracranial tumors diagnosed as MB in patients younger then 18 years of age while in adults about 1% of the primary intracranial tumors diagnosed as MB. It is well known that infants are the more vulnerable group with 25-60% rate of cure, while the over all 5-year survival rate in childhood is about 80%. Although, the environmental factors could not be totally excluded, yet the younger age of MB appearance with 35% metastatic, points toward a more pronounced genetic background rather then environmental (Rossi et al 2008, Bar and Stearns 2008).

B. **Severity of the disease**- the most prevalent MB sub-type in infancy is the desmoplastic which is considered the most aggressive sub-type especially when it also appear with metastasis , 35% of the childhood MB are metastatic at presentation. Metastatic phenotype considered as a high risk group with the worst prognosis. Cure rates are lower for infants than for older children. This might point either to the more significant-effective role of the inheritage genetics predisposition in infants then in elderly or adults MB. Also most probably radiotherapy can be particularly more adverse in the immature infant brain (Grill et al 2005; Packer and Vezina 2008; Rutkowski et al., 2009). The main consequence of carniospinal irradiation (CSI) is notably cognitive problems children's IQ can decrease by as much as 30 points in the standard risk group. The high risk group (metastasis, significant post operative residual tumor) remains poor 5-years event free survival (EFS) being 25-40% the worse prognosis is particularly in younger children

Although 5-years overall survival rates have reached 60-80% , survivors often face a variety of long term neurological , neuroendocrine , and social squeal as a result of conventional treatment regimens (surgery, radiotherapy, and chemotherapy (Pizer and Clifford 2009) (Packer and Vezina 2008; Rossi et al 2008, Bar and Stearns 2008). It is imperative to gain a better understanding of the molecular alterations in MB for future targeted therapies that are more effective and less toxic.

C. **Predisposition**- Predisposition to develop MB due to known genetic alterations- some MB cases are associated with known hereditary syndromes such as Gorlin, Turcot and Li-Fraumeni. (Reviewed by Ellison 2010, Northcott, 2011; Onvani 2010) will be discussed in the gene alteration part. All the above points support the suggestion that genetic factors cause predisposition for MB's development.

Most studies on MB have focused on genes that are already known to be involved in the pathogenesis of tumors, such as Wnt, SHH, Notch TP53. The specific genetic pathway/s in MB is/are still unknown.

Studying the different MB's subtypes with the most advanced technologies will significantly contribute to the overall understanding of MB pathogenesis in general and in particular in MB genetic knowledge.

3. Chromosomal aberration and its corroletion to clinicohistopatological classification

Cytogenetics and molecular genetics are two different levels of genetic studies. Both of them are in use for characterization of tumors in general and MB in particular. Nowadays, these tests in combination with other standard methods such immunohistochemistry, significantly improved the diagnosis, prognosis and consequently the treatment modalities and survival of the patients with malignant diseases. Cytogenetics, molecular cytogenetics (FISH, CGH) and molecular genetics are three methods that supplement each other, and their combination leads to the identification of the genes that are involved in tumorigenesis (tumor suppressor genes and oncogenes) and thus can give complete information for prognostic and diagnostic purposes. Although, impressive progress has been achieved in the nano molecular genetics, next generation sequencing, proteomics and transcriptomics, in the last decade, yet, we can not give up the "macro-tests": the old gold standard methods such as cytogenetics and histology. The nano tests are still new and very expensive to implicate to routine work up, they are in a developing stage and the accumulated experience with their use is still limited. There is still missing information regarding the whole range of polymorphism and how to differentiate it from significant changes. Also the exact interactions between all the nano tests (molecular genetics, proteomics and transcriptomics) are only partially understood so far. Moreover the significance and the importance of the immerging field of epigenetics is still not clear. The field of epigenetics is dealing with changes that do not affect the molecular genetics itself but rather the changes in the expression of the gene/s by changing mythlation, acetylation, phosphorilation and ubiquitination (Bernstein et al. 2007; Kouzarides 2007). Its effects include the most delicate interactions of all the living levels, starting from biochemical reaction and the interactions inside the cell compartments, cell to cell, in the organ, in the host and between the host and the environment.

Chromosome analysis of tumor cells plays an important role in the diagnosis, prognosis and follow up of many malignancies. It is a standard of care in hemato-oncology. Culturing solid tumor cells *in vitro* is essential for cytogenetic analysis. The success in getting specific chromosomal aberrations in solid tumors after in vitro culturing is limited because of technical problems such as: an overgrowth of cells from healthy part of the tissue mostly fibroblasts, limited growth of the abnormal tumor cells and low quality of the tumor cell metaphases and also the need for special and well trained cytogeneticists. These are probably the main reasons for the limited and what seems like a non specific chromosomal aberration in medulloblastoma. Only about 40% of the medulloblastomas demonstrate chromosomal aberrations. Presently, advanced technologies such as microarray CGH and next generation sequencing enable us to better evaluate chromosomal aberrations in medulloblastoma. It will take some time for the accumulation of new data regarding chromosomal aberrations using the new methods, mainly because reliable results should be done on a large cohort which include sufficient size group of all MB subtypes.

Copy number abnormalities of chromosome 17 isodicentric, isochromosome of chromosome 17q, loss of 17p, or gain of 17q are the most frequent chromosomal abnormality in medulloblastomas (Mitelman database 2011, Aldosari et al 2002; McCabe et al 2006) it is found in 30-50% of the studied cases (Reardon et al 1997). Isochromosome –isodicentric chromosome 17 is present in approximately one third of the tumors and in some cases is the only chromosomal aberration (Mitelman database 2011; Pfister et al 2009; Ricket and Paulus 2004). It has been observed in 25-30% of childhood MB. In fact there is a loss of 17p and a gain of 17q which is the most common isochromosome in cancer in general (Mitelman database 2011). This might point toward the fact that i(17q) is a general marker of neoplastic process rather then a specific marker of MB. Its role as an indicator for a poor outcome in MB stratification is controversial. The controversial evidence based mainly on the findings of i(17q) also in Wnt pathway subgroup which in consensus considered as a favorable outcome. The question whether to consider copy number abnormality of chromosome 17 as a marker for poor prognosis and to exclude those found to be Wnt pathway, is still in debate (Pan et al 2005; Pfister et al 2009).

Using more sophisticated and advanced techniques such as CGH to profile a panel of 27 primary MB (Reardon et al 1997) revealed frequent loss of 10q, 11, 16q, 17p, and 8p as well as recurrent gains of chromosomes 7, and 17q. These losses and gains were also confirmed by other techniques, such as G-banding, SKY and FISH (Aldosari et al 2002; Avet-Loiseau et al 1999 ; Bayani et al 2000; Eberhart et al 2002; Gilhuis et al 2000). Array CGH of 47 MB (Speicher and Carter 2005) showed gain of 17q, 7, and 1q and loss of 17p, 11p,10q and 8.

There have also been reports, although less frequently of losses on chromosomes 10q, 11, 17p qnd 22 as well as gains on chromosomes 1q, 7 and 7q (Mitelman database 2011; Bayani et al 2000).

SKY analysis of 19 primary MB revealed structural aberrations involving chromosomes 7, 17, 3, 14, 10 and 22.(Bayani et al 2009).

Monosomy 6 is strongly associated with Wnt profile in MB (Clifford et al 2006).

Chromosomal abnormalities including loss of chromosome X in females and loss of chromosome 8, have been found mainly in non SHH/Wnt subgroups.

4. Genetic alterations and its correlation with clinicohistopatological classification

Tumorigenesis is a process in which one of the pathways leading to normal cell development has lost its control and its normal function. In addition, the neovasculization, cell proliferation, differentiation, motility and apoptosis (death) are also altered.

There are two possible categories in tumor specific genetic alteration; one is inheritable or germ cells mutation and the other is acquired alteration. Also there is a difference between general tumorigenesis pathways and tumor specific pathway and general chromosomal aberration and tumor specific chromosomal aberration.

Usually, the tumor specific pathway is a part of the general tumorigenesis pathways but still it is predominant in one specific tumor subgroup, for example RB gene that causes mainly retinoblastoma, WT gene that causes mainly Willm's tumor, both are also causing predisposition to other tumors. Similarly, the acquired gene alteration occurring during the life time, such as BCR/ABL is causing chronic myeloid leukemia and EWSR1-FLI1 is causing Ewing sarcoma. Specific acquired aberration found in addition to the cancer they caused, also in other cancers , there its significance and its prognostic value is different, for instance BCR/ABL points to a favorable prognosis in CML and points to a poor prognosis in acute lymphocytic leukemia (ALL).

Among the life time acquired mutation, one should differentiate between the first event, such as alteration of a gene that causes the disease and has a diagnostic value and those mutations that are considered as the latter (the second or the third) events for example KRAS and TP53 mutation in adenomatose polyposis coli (APC) and MNP1 or FLT1 mutation in acute leukemia. Those gene alterations have mainly prognostic value and may play as a general event seen in other tumors as well.

Unfortunately, neither MB specific chromosomal changes nor MB specific gene were found to be a clear evidence for the possible pathogenesis of MB, neither in MB general nor in one of its subtypes. The understanding of MB pathogenesis is still limited, mainly because most of the MB studies are associated with genes that are already known to be involved in other tumors or syndromes, rather then studying the MB specific gene alterations as the first goal.

Indeed, MB is associated with other (tumor's) syndromes such as Gorlin,Turcot and Li Fraumeni, in which several important developmental signal transduction pathways, including sonic hedgehog (SHH), Wingless (Wnt) and Notch signaling cascades. SHH, Wnt, TP53 and Notch signaling cascades are implicated in the cells migration and localization in the cerebrum, and their proliferation and differentiation. The alterations in these pathways by any component of each signaling pathway may lead to tumorigenesis (Marino 2005; Ingham and Placzek 2006). For example, Gorlin's syndrome characterized by a germ line mutation in the patched homologue 1 (PTCH1) located on 9q22 (Frandon et al 1992) that served as a negative regulator of SHH gene during normal cerebella development. Mutation in PTCH1 gene can cause predisposition to different tumor development including MB with incidence of 5-20% (Friedrich 2007).

Turcot syndrome is characterized by the mutation in the APC a tumor suppressor gene that is predisposed mainly (about 90% during life time) to colon cancer adenomatous polyposis coli (APC), (Hamilton et al 1995) but also predisposed to a lesser extend to other tumors including MB (Huang et al 2000). The APC gene regulates the Wnt signaling pathway.

Recent advances in gene expression profiling techniques have led to the generation of several molecular classification schemes in MB (Thompson et al 2006; Kool et al 2008; Northcott et al 2010 epub).

In general, based on the molecular studies done so far, three main subgroups were defined: SHH, Wnt and non SHH/Wnt pathways which include another 2 subgroups which are less distinct (Thompson et al 2006; Kool et al 2008; Onvani et al 2010; Ellison 2010; Northcott et al 2011). SHH pathway subgroup accounts for 15-25% cases of MB and have a poor prognosis,Wnt pathway subgroup accounts for 15-20% cases of MB and mostly has favorable prognosis, and non SHH/Wnt subgroups account for 60% cases of MB.

According to the Thompson's (2006) classification based on molecular and FISH examination 5 distinct subtypes identified (A to E) including subgroup B in which Wnt pathway and monosomy 6 have been found and subgroup D in which SHH pathway has been found. Kool et al (2008) further corroborated Thompson's classification using CGH and defined 5 subgroups: (A)-Wnt signaling subgroup, (B)-SHH signaling pathway, C and D expression of neural differentiation genes, D and E expression of photoreceptor genes. Subgroups C, D and E are genetically closely related and most often associated with metastatic appearance mainly subgroup E.

SHH pathway MB associated with desmoplastic phenotype (Behesti 2009) and also with large cell and anaplastic MB. They are both reported mainly in infancy and childhood. Metastatic disease at presentation characterizes some SHH pathway mostly large cells and anaplastic MB. Less then half of the SHH pathway MB have PTCH1 mutations or show copy number loss at the PTCH1 locus, 9q22, mutations in SMOH and SUFU are rare thus there must be other undiscovered SHH pathway/s (Thompson et al 2006; Kool et al 2008; Northcott et al 2011).

In contrast Wnt pathway is mostly associated with classic MB (Fattet et al 2009) it has a favorable outcome it tends to be present in childhood in the pre-teen years (6-13 years) but almost do not present in infancy. Most of the children with this tumor survived (Thompson et al 2006). Metastatic disease at presentation is rare in Wnt pathway. There is no report on desmopastic medulloblastoma with Wnt pathway and also large cell and anaplastic MB with Wnt is rare. The APC protein is a regulator of Wnt signaling that function in a complex with other components to regulate several important developmental processes, including proliferation and specification of neural progenitor cells during early cerebellar development (Sillitoe and Joyner 2007). APC function as a tumor suppressor through CTNNB1 (β-catenin) of sporadic cases of MB, a downstream component of the Wnt signaling pathway (Hamilton et al 1995) this account for 15% of the cases. β-catenin by itself also activates transcription of several oncogenes such as MYC and CCND1 resulting in enhanced cell proliferation (Ellison et al 2005).

Only a small part of the Wnt pathway MBs are found to be carrying mutations in CTNNB1 gene-captured by identification of the nuclear activity of β-catenin in the MB. Mutations in APC and AX1N1/2 are rare, thus there are still undiscovered components also in Wnt pathway (Ellison et al 2005; Fattet et al 2009; Norhcott et al 2011).

Most of non SHH/Wnt MBs have a classic pathology and present in infancy and childhood. About half of the large cell and anplastic MBs are non SHH/Wnt. Metastatic disease at presentation also falls into the non SHH\Wnt tumor subgroup.

Other molecular markers beside the above three identified groups is the amplification of MYC family (MYC and MYCN proto-oncogenes), that account for 4-15% of MBs (Rossi et al 2008; McCabe et al 2006). MYCN is an early transcriptional target of the SHH pathway and activation by SHH promotes the expression of the cell cycle proteins cyclinD1 and CyclinD2 leading to GCP proliferation (Behesti amd Marino 2009). A high expression level of MYC is reported to cause progression of MB to an anaplastic phenotype and has been linked to a poor prognosis while even though MYCN shows some association with large cells and anaplastic MB yet it is less established as a marker for an adverse outcome (Aldosari et al 2002; Pfister et al 2009).

Both SHH and Wnt subgroups rarely show copy number abnormalities of chromosome 17, amplification of MYC and MYCN or any other widespread ploidy changes. MB occurred also in 5% of the Li Fraumeni syndrome's patients carrying mutation in the suppressor gene TP53 (Northcott 2009). Other known pathways are involved in the normal cerebellar development found also to be aberrant in some of the MB. For example a disturbance of the RAS-MAP upregulation through downstream components such a MAP2K1,MAP2K2, and MAPK1/3. It is found to be correlated with metastatic behavior (Gilbertson and Clifford 2003). Also, overexpression of the EGF receptor family member ERBB2 is linked to metastatic behavior. A number of proto-oncogenes in MB such as CDK6, PDGFRA, KIT and MYCL1 have been found to be amplified by array CGH. A single copy numbers gains of MET locus on chromosome 7q in 38.5% of the cases in 13 MBs (MacBabe 2006; Tong et al 2004).

The Notch pathway was found to be implicated in MBs pathogenesis in a number of studies. Notch promote granule cell precursor (GCP) proliferation and prevents their differentiation (Behesti and Marino 2009). Increased copy number of Notch2 has been found in 15% of the studied MBs. Also, mutated Hes1 gene that unregulated the Notch pathway have been found in a small study group, although it has been associated with poor prognosis and outcome, its role and implication should be carefully considered and further examined (Fan et al 2004; Thompson et al 2006; Kool et al 2008; Northcott et al 2009).

Due to technology limitations and the availability research strategies most molecular studies of MBs , we are still missing the MB specific molecular markers. Hopefully, MB subtypes specific markers will be discovered by using the advanced technologies which enables us to study MB at different levels: DNA by next generation sequencing, gene expression by transcriptomic and protienomic, epigenomic and miRs.

An accurate classification and the stratification will implicate the medical care. An optimal classification will differentiate between MB in each age interval (infancy, childhood and adult) and between the subgroups in each age.

There is a general consensus that a better understanding of the disease biology should allow us to develop more effective and less harmful treatments of MB.

Northcott et al (2011) generated a class prediction algorithm, an 8-gene classification model which successfully predicted the survival status for 47 out of the 60 patients profiled. The markers of the cerebellar differentiation (β-NAP, NSCLI, TRKC) and component of the extracellular matrix (lysyl hydroxylase[PLOD], collagen TypeVai and elastin) predict favorable prognosis. While genes involved in cell proliferation and metabolism (MYBL2, enolas 1, LDH, HMGI[y], and cytochrome C oxidase) as well as ribosomal protein coding genes predict poor prognosis.

5. MicroRNA (miR) and its corroletion with clinicohistopatological classification

The field on miRNA emerged in the last few years, concentrates on small non coding, single strand RNA molecules that are found to play a regulatory role on gene expression.

Differential microRNA (miR) expression analysis has also contributed to our knowledge on MB pathogenesis. The miRs are the short fragments of endogenous noncoding RNA that play an important role in the developmental processes by regulating gene expression. Target mRNAs are either degraded or translationed by specific miRNAs. Ferretti et al (2008) performed one of the earliest expression profiles on MB. Northcott et al (2009) identified amplification of miR17/92 polycistron proto-oncogen in 6% of pediatric MBs and showed upregulation of miR17/92 expression in a large percentage of primary cases. Similarly, Pierson et al. (2008) demonstrated decreased expression of miR-124a in primary MB as well as in MB cell line. Onvani et al (2010) have reported that miR124a as a negative regulator of CDK6 which are found to be overexpressed in MB (Mendrzyk et al 2005). Additional oncogenic targets, such as miR-30b and miR-30d have also been proposed through miRNA profiling (Lu et al 2009)

Northcott et al (2009) have described subgroup classification based on transcription profile, using mRNA and miRNA examination. They identified 4 distinct subgroups including the well known Wnt and SHH and another two independent subgroup C and D. It has been found that mir17/92, cluster of oncogenic miRNAs, was highly expressed in SHH tumors in association with MYCN expression, while group C was found to be correlated with MYC.

High-resolution SNP array profiling on a group of >200 MB revealed high-level amplification of miR-17/92 on 13q31 (Northcott et al 2009).

It has been found that miR-17/92 and related paralogs (miR-106a/363 and miR-106b/25) were identified as the most highly upregulated miRNAs in MB when compared with normal cerebellum in this analysis. The combination of miR 17/92 amplification and consistent overexpression suggested miR-17/92 as a key player in MB pathogenesis. There is evidence that miR17/92 might cooperate with SHH in MB, as it showed preferential upregulation in SHH subtype.

Recently the role of miRNA in MB has been studied on 14 primary cases using profile of 248 miRNAs showing a general biased downregulation in MB cells as compared to the control cells . A subset of 86 miRNAs which were previously reported to be expressed in neuronal tissues and/or cancer studied in cohort of 34 among them two neuronal candidates miR-9 and miR-125a were chosen for functional analysis. Induction of their expression resulted in the decrease in tumorigenic features: promoted apoptosis, inhibited cell proliferation and impaired anchorage-independent growth. Moreover loss of miR9 and miR125a correlated well with upregulation of truncated trkC which was identified as a target for posttranscriptional repression (Northcott 2009).

In order to discriminate between miRs deregulation in SHH-driven MB from non SHH-cases, 31 MBs studied using a set of 250 miRs. Two groups were defined GLI1-high and GIL1-low. A set of 34 miRs was found with a significant differential expression between the two classes. For functional analysis of the GLI1-high class three candidates (miR-125b, miR-324-5p, and miR-326) exhibiting reduced expression were chosen based on their predicted capacity to target the SHH family members, Smo and Gil1. They were proven to repress Smo mRNA level in the MB cell line (Ferretti et al 2008).

SNPs array profiling of more then 200 MB revealed copy number aberration of multiple unreported regions including high level amplification of miR17/92

Another miRNAome study of 90 MB revealed that four distinct molecular subgroups can be described. These subtypes include the well characterized Wnt and SHH subgroups and another 2 subgroup designated C and D (Northcott et al 2009).
The miR-17/92 was the most highly expressed in SHH-driven MB but also in tumors exhibiting high MYCN (SHH) and MYC (group C,Wnt) expression. MiR-17/92 transcriptional upregulation by N-Myc and Myc and confirming miR-17/92 aberrancy in a large percentage of the MBs (□ about 60%). Based on experiments on mice it was suggested by Northcott et al (2009) that miR 17/92 cooperate with SHH signaling to promote and/or enhance CGNP proliferation.
The miRs studies are still in their initial stage and we are still far from understanding their exact role and how they affect processes in MB pathogenesis.

6. Epigenomic and its corroletion with clinicohistopatological classification

Until recently the thought was that genetic alteration is the main cause of each tumor development and progress. Researchers invest their efforts in finding a tumor specific pattern of genetic alteration. Over the past few years another aspect has arisen which is the deregulation of epigenetics to malignancy (Jones and Baylin 2002;Bernstein et al 2007; Kouzarides 2007; Kongham et al 2008; Esteller 2008).
Epigenetics involves nongenetic DNA modifications that result in changes in gene expression. These changes include gene promoter mythylation on cytocine residues, most frequently of the CpG islands of the promoter, as well as their histone code. These changes are found to be involved in pathogenesis of tumors including MB, through hypermethylation of promoter of tumor suppressor genes and consequently silencing them (Kongham et al 2008).
Fruhwald et al (2001) showed methylation of up to 1% of all CpG island in 17 primary medulloblastoms, it was linked to poor prognosis.
Epigenetics is defined as "mitotically heritable changes in gene expression that are not accompanied by modifications in primary DNA sequence". It is highly correlated with the MB class were ZIC and NSCL1 , encoding transcription factors that are specific for cerebellar granule cells point to the MB arised from cerebellar granule cells.
Anderton et al(2008) have identified tumor –specific methylation of COL1A2 in 77% of the studied primary MBs (46 out of 60) and showed an age-dependent methylation pattern for this gene in desmoplastic tumors, which presented COL1A2 as a potential MB subtype biomarker. Kongkham et al. (2008) identified serin protease inhibitor kuntiz-type2 (SPINT2/HAI-2), an HGF/cMET signaling inhibitor, as a novel tumor suppressor gene that is frequently silenced by promoter hypermethylation in MBs (Kongham et al 2008). Also Waha et al (2007) found promoter hypermethylation-induced reduction of SCG5 expression in primary 16 out of 23 primary cases compared to normal cerebellar controls (Waha 2007), points to its possible role in pathogenesis of MB. Furthermore, promoter hypermethylation-mediated silencing of CASP8, HICI and RASSF1A tumor suppressor genes has also been discovered in more than 30% of MBs by various groups (Lindsey et al 2004).
Pfister et al (2007) showed a striking association between samples classified as either "low methylators" or "high methylators" and patient outcome, where the "high methylators" group exhibited reduced overall survival.
Also the GLI C2H2-type zing-finger protein family member ZIC2 was identified as hypermethylated and thus it has been silenced (Pfister et al 2007).
It has been found that EHMTI function as part of a transcriptional repressor complex that mediates gene silencing by promoting dimethylation of H3K9 (Tachibana et al 2005), a

repressive epigenic modification (Bernstein et al 2007; Kouzarides 2007) in the promoter regions of target genes. An obvious correlation between loss of EHMTI leads to H3K9 hypomethyelation.

Another study using microarray-based differential methylation hybridization (Waha et al 2007) identified hypermethylation of the SCG5 (secretory granule, neuroendocrine protein 1[7B2 protein] gene) in 16 out of 23 (70%) primary MB. Expression of SCG5 found to be downregulated in the MB in comparison with normal cerebral controls. Another gene that found to be down regulated is SPINT2 that was found in 41 out of 56 primary MB. Stable expression of SPINT2 resulted in attenuation of the malignant phenotype: inhibiting cell proliferation, anchorage-independent growth in soft agar and cell motility, of cell lines (Kongham et al 2008). This study suggested that SPINT2 is a suppressor gene. Treatment of MB cell lines suggesting that SCG5 is a suppressor gene (Fruhwald et al 2001) or increased gene with demethylation agent (5-aza-2'deoxycytidine) reduced colony formation expression (Anderton et al 2008; Kongham et al 2008).

The MB epigenomic studies demonstrate that not only the genetic alteration can cause loss of control in a cell and transformation to a malignant cell but also other mechanism can cause malignancy, implicated epigenetic gene silencing as important mechanism of the tumor suppressor gene inactivation in MB.

7. Summary

The reported genetic alterations of MB, either chromosomal or molecular, are so far not specific.The main distinct subgroups are the Wnt and the SHH both account for 30-40% of MB. These pathways are common in many other tumors, suggesting they are not exclusive to MB. There are some other pathways involved in MB pathogenesis that might be more specific to MB. Similarly, the chromosomal aberration i(17q) which is found in about 40% of MBs, as well as in many other tumors including in chronic myelocytic leukemia (CML) can possibly be a secondary chromosomal aberration. Some of the features found in different subtypes but not in an equal distribution, for instance i(17q) were found in 34% ,36%,12% in classic ,large cell and desmoplastic MB respectively and are associate with poor prognosis (Gillbertson & Ellison 2008). Another example NOTCH and PDGF, they both have been found in A and B Kool's subtypes and also subtypes C, D and E share increased expression of neural differentiation genes. Another example is the Wnt-β catenin, found in all subtypes defined in Northcott's classification. This overlapping between the different subtypes, points toward the fact that some of the alterations are not, necessarily, a specific prognostic marker. Studies have been done on a mice model and on cell lines in order to learn more about pathogenesis of MB are important; however the data learned from these experimental systems should be first corroborated with the data learned from human primary MBs, before going to conclusions on the pathogenesis of human MB. This is the reason for focusing in this chapter mainly on the studies done on primary human MBs studies.

Due to the variable results, the exact and specific chromosomal changes in MB which is a crucial event in pathogenesis, is still unknown.

Gilberston and Ellison (2008) wrote in their review: "Genomic-seeing the wood and the trees". The literature is full of studies (over 200 papers) on genetic alteration in MB trying to understand the MB pathogenesis, some of them corroborate with each other. Most of the studies have been done from different research points of view and emphasis, using different technologies. Presently, there are at least 5 different suggestions for classification and stratification of MB: Thompson's (2006), WHO (2007), Kool's (2008), Pefister's (2008) and Northcott's (2011). It is very difficult to combine them to one clear cut classification (Table 1).

***THOMPSON'S (2006) CLASSIFICATION (46)**	**WHO CLASSI-FICATION**	**PROGNOSIS**	**MOLECULAR ALTERATION**	**CHROMO-SOMAL ABERRATION**	**AGE OF ONSET**
A				Gain:17q Loss: 17p	
B	Classic MB	Favorable	Wnt- β catenin↑ CTNNB1-predominant,APC, AXIN!mutation	Monosomy 6	≥3 years
C			SHH PTCH,SUFU mutation	Gain:17q Loss: 17p	
D	Desmoplastic		SHH, PTCH,SUFU mutation		≤3 years
E				Gain:17q Loss: 17p	
***KOOL'S(2008) CLASSIFICATION (52)**	**WHO CLASSI-FICATION**	**PROGNOSIS**	**MOLECULAR ALTERATION**	**CHROMO-SOMAL ABERRATION**	**AGE OF ONSET**
A	classic		Wnt β-catenin mutation NOTCH, PDGF	Monosomy 6	Older children
B	desmoplastic		SHH PTCH1 mutation NOTCH, PDGF	9q loss	Young children years and adults
C	classic	metastases	Neural differentiation genes	17 alteration, loss of X chromosome (females)	children
D	classic	metastases	Neural differentiation genes Photoreceptor genes	17 alteration, loss of X chromosome (females	children
E	classic	metastases	Photoreceptor genes	loss of X chromosome (females	Young children
***PFISTER'S(2009) CLASSIFICATION (80/260)**	**WHO CLASSI-FICATION**	**PROGNOSIS**	**Frequency**		**OS**
MYC/MYCN amplification+10ch.	Large cell/anaplastic	Poor prognosis methastases	6%/4%/10%		13%

aber./ MYC/MYCN amplification +6q-gain+17qgain +10ch.aber.					
6q-gain+10ch.aber.		Poor prognosis	8%		16%
17q-gain/17p-loss/i(17q) +7.5ch.aber.		Poor prognosis	48%/39%/30-48%		56%
6q ,17qbalanced +4ch.aber.					90%
6qdeletion +2ch.aber.		Favorable prognosis	12%		100%
NORTHCOTT'S (2010) CLASSIFICATION (103)*	**WHO CLASSI-FICATION**	**PROGNOSIS**	**MOLECULAR ALTERATION**	**CHROMO-SOMAL ABERRATION**	**AGE OF ONSET**
Wnt			MYC↑ Wnt-β catenin	Monosomy 6	Distributed age median 9-10 years, 3:1 F/M
SHH	Desmoplastic-predominant Anaplastic, large cell		MYCN↑ Wnt-β catenin	Del9q Isochromosome 9p Gain: 3q, 20q, 21q,2 Loss:10q,14	Infants ≤3 years-most common, adults≥16 years
C	Desmoplastic Anaplastic, large cell(23%)	Metastases(46.5 %) Worst prognosis	OTX2↑,FOXG1 B↑, MYC(8q24)↑, Wnt-β catenin Neural development*	Isochromosome (17q) Gain:1q,17q,8 Loss:10q, 5qdistal, 16q,11p ,8p	Childhood peak 3-10 years
D	Desmoplastic Anaplastic, large cell (8%)	Metastases(29.7 %)	OTX2↑,FOXG1 B↑ Wnt-β catenin, Neural development*	Isochromosome (17q) Gain: 17q,8 Loss:11p ,X(females), 8p,8q	Distributed age median 9-10 years

WHO (2007): Classic, desmoplastic, MB with extensive nodularity, anaplastic, Large cell
*For more details see: Louis 2007, Thompson *et al* 2006, Kool *et al* 2008, Pifster *et al* 2009, Northcott *et al* 2010 J. Clin.Oncol., Parenthesis-Year of publication.
** See table 2 in Ellison 2010, Table 2 in Huse and Holland 2010, Table 1-Northcott 2010 J. Clin.Oncol. Parenthesis -Number of samples

Table 1. Medulloblastoma classification according to: WHO- Louis et al 2007, Thompson *et al* 2006, Kool *et al* 2008, Pifster *et al* 2009, Northcott *et al* 2011.

There is also early evidences that epigenetics and miRs might play a role in MB pathogenesis and can be used as a prognostic tool. However , the data regarded to epigenetics and miRs in MB is still limited and uncompleted, as part of the studies done on MB cell line which might point to a candidate involved genes with no assurance for there role in the MB tumor. There are few studies on primary MBs, thus any conclusion from this data is still immature. This emphasized the need for further studying the MB pathogenesis for either specific germ line mutation or other specific level of alteration (transcriptome, proteome, epigenome levels). These should be done as a multi-center study , on a large size of cohort including sufficient number of samples of each MB subtype including adult and childhood MBs. The study should be performed uniformly using different levels of examinations: histologic, cytogenetic, molecular, transcriptome, proteome, epigennetics, and miRs. Hopefully such a study will provide us with more personalized medical care with less adverse side effects.

8. References

Aldosari, N., Bigner, S.H., Burger, P.C., Becker L, Kepner JL, Friedman HS, and McLendon RE.2002. MYCC and MYCN oncogene amplification in medulloblastoma. A fluorescence in situ hybridization study on paraffin sections from the Children's Oncology Group. Arch. Pathol. Lab. Med. 126:549-544.

Anderton, J.A., Lindsey, J.C., Lusher, M.E., Gilbertson, R.J., Bailey. S., Ellison, D.W., and Clifford, S.C. 2008. Global analysis of the medulloblastoma epigenome identifies disease-subgroup-specific inactivationof COLIA2. Neuro Oncol 10:981-994

Avet-Loiseau, H., Venuat, A.M., Terrier-Lacombe, M.J., Lellouch-Tubiana, A., Zerach, M., and Vassal, G. 1999. Comparative genomic hybridization detects many recurrent imbalances in central nervous system primitive neuroectodrmal tumors un children. Brit J Cancer 79:1843-1847

Bar, E.E., and Stearns, D. 2008. New developments in medulloblstoma treatment: the potential of a cyclosporine-lovastatin combination. Expert Opin Invest Drugs 17:185-195

Bayani, J., Zielenska, M., Marrano, P., Kwan Ng, Y., Taylor, M.D., Jay, V., Rutka, J.T., and Squire, J.A.. 2000. Molecular primitive neuroectodermal tumors by using conventional banding, comparative genomic hybridization, and spectral karyotyping. J Neurosurg 2000;93:437-438

Behesti, H., and Marino, S. 2009. Cerebelar granule cells: insights into proliferation, differentiationand role inmedulloblastoma pathogenesis. Int J Biochem Cell Biol 41:435-445

Bernstein, B.E., Meisner, A., and Lander, E.S.. 2007. The mammalian epigenome. Cell 128: 669-681

Brandes, A.A., Franceschi, E., Tosoni, A., Reni, M., Gatta, G., Vencht, C., and Kortmann, R.D. 2009. Adult neuroectodermal tumors pf posterior fossa (medulloblastoma) and of supratentorial sites (stPNET). Crit Rev Oncol Hematol 71:165-179

Clifford, S.C., Lusher, M.E., Lindsey, J.C., Langdon, J.A., Gilbertson, R.J., Straughton, D., and Ellison, D.W. 2006. Wnt/Wingless pathway activation and chromosome 6 loss characterize a distinct molecular sub-group of medulloblastomas associated with a favorable prognosis. Cell Cycle 5:2666-2670

Crawford, J.R., MacDonald, T.J., and Packer, R.J. 2007. Medulloblastoma in childhood; new biological advances. Lancet Neurol 6:1073-1085

Eberhart, C.G., Kratz, J.E., Schuster, A., Goldthwaite, P., Cohen, K.J., Perlman, E.J., and Burger, P.C. 2002 Comparative genomic hybridization detects an increased number of chromosomal alterations in large cell/anaplastic medulloblastomas. Brain Pathol 12:36-44

Ellison, D. 2002. Classifying the medulloblastoma:insight from morphology and molecular genetics. Neuropathol Appl Neurobiol 28:257-282

Ellison, D.W., Onilude, O.E., Lindsey, J.C., Lusher, M.E., Weston, C.L., Taylor, R.E., Pearson, A.D., and Clifford, S.C. 2005. Beta-Catemin status predicts a favorable outcome in childhood medulloblastoma. J Clin Oncol 23:7951-7957

Ellison, D.W. 2010. Childhood medulloblastoma: novel approaches to the classification of a heterogenous disease. Acta Neuropathol 120:305-316

Esteller, M. 2008. Epigenetics in cancer. N Eng J Med 358: 1148-1159

Fattet, S., Haberler, C., Legoix, P., Varlet, P., Lellouch-Tubiana, A., Lair, S., Manie, E., Raquin, M.A., Bours, D., Carpentier, S., Barillot, E., Grill, J., Doz, F., Puget, S., Janoueix-Lerosey, I., and Delattre, O. 2009. Beta-catemin status in paediatric medulloblastoma: correlation of immunohistochemical expression with mutational status, genetic profiles and clinical characteristics. J Pathol 218:86-94

Ferretti, E., De Smaele, E., Miele, E., Laneve, P., Po, A., Pelloni, M., Paganelli, A., Di Marcotulli, L., Caffarelli, E., Screpanti, L., Bozzoni, L., and Gulino, A. 2008. Concerted microRNA control of Hedgehog signalling in cerebellar neuronal progenitor and tumor cells. EMBO J 27:2616-2627

Farndon, P.A., Del Mastro, R.G., Evans, D.G., Kilpatrick, M.W. 1992. Location of gene for Gorlin syndrome. Lancet 339:581-582

Friedrich, R.E. 2007. Diagnosis and treatment of patients with nevoid basal cell carcinoma syndrome (Gorlin-Goltz syndrome-GGS).Anticancer Res 27:1783-1787

Fruhwald, M.C., O'Dorisio, M.S., Dai, Z., Tanner, S.M., Balster, D.A., Gao, X., Wright, F.A., and Plass, C. 2001. Aberrant promoter metylation of previously unidentified target genes is a common abnormality in medulloblastomas-implications for tumor biology and potential clinical utility. Oncogene 16:5033-5042

Gilbertson, R.J. 2004. Medulloblastoma: signalling a change in treatment. Lancet Oncol 5; 209-18

Gilbertson, R.J., and Ellison, D.W. 2008. The origins of medulloblastoma subtypes. Annu Rev Pathol Mech Dis 3;341-365

Gilbertson, R.J., and Clifford, S.C. 2003. PDGFRB is overexpressed in metastatic medulloblastoma. Nat Genet 35:197-198

Grill, J., Saint-Rose, C., Jouvet, A., Gentet, J.C., Lejars, O., Frappaz, D., Doz, F., Rialland, X., Pichon, F., Bertozzi, A.I., Chastagner, P., Couanet, D., Habrand, J.L., Raquin, M.A., Le Deley, M.C., and Kalifa, C. 2005. Treatment of medulloblastoma with postoperative chemotherapy alone: an SFOP prospective trial in young children. Lancet Oncol 6:573-580

Hamilton, S.R., Liu, B., Parsons, R.E. Papadopoulos, N., Jen, J., Powell, S.M., Krush, A.J., Berk, T.,Cohen, Z., Tetu, B. 1995. The molecular basis of Turcot's syndrome. N Eng J Med 332;839-847

Huang, H., Mahler-Araujo, B.M., Sankila, A.,Chimelli L, Yonekawa Y, Kleihues P, Ohgaki H. 2000. APC mutations in sporadic medulloblastomas. Am J Pathol 156:433-437

Ingham, P.W., and Placzek, M. 2006. Orchestrating oncogenesis : variations on a theme by sonic hedgehog. Nat. Rev Genet 7:841-850

Jones, P.A. , and Baylin, S.B. 2007. The epigenomics of cancer. Cell 128:683-692

Kongham, P.N., Northcott, P.A., Ra, Y.S., Nakahara, Y., Mainprize, T.G., Croul, S.E., Smith, C.A., Taylor, M.D., and Rutka, J.T. 2008. An epigenetic genome-wide screem identifies SPINT2 as a novel tumor suppressor gene in pediatric medulloblastoma. Cancer Res 68:9945-9953

Kool, M., Koster, J., Bunt, J., Hasselt, N.E., Lakeman, A., van Sluis, P., Troost, D., Meeteren, N.S., Caron, H.N., Cloos, J., Mrsic, A., Ylstra, B., Grajkowska, W., Hatmann, W., Pietsch, T., Ellison, D., Clifford, S.C., and Versteeg, R. 2008. Integrated genomics identifies five meduloblatoma subtypes with distinct genetic profiles, pathway signatures and clinicopathological features. PLoS One 3:e3088

Korshunov, A., Remke, M., Werft, W., Benner, A., Ryzhova, M., Witt, H., Sturm, D., Wittman, A., Scholter, A., Felsberg, J., Reifenberg, G., Rutkowski, S., Scheurlen, W., Kulozik, A.E., von Deimling, A., Lichter, P., and Pfister, M. Adult and pediatric medulloblastomas are genetically distinct and require different algorithms for molecular risk stratification. J Clin Oncol 2010

Kouzarides, T. 2007. Chromatin modifications and their function. Cell 128:693-705

Lindsey, J.C., Lusher, M.E., Anderton, J.A., Bailey, S., Gilbertson, R.J., Pearson, A.D., and Ellison, D.W. 2004. Identificationof tumour-specific epigenetic events in medulloblastoma development by hypermethylation profiling. 25:661-668

Louis, D.N. 2007 WHO classificationof tumors of the central nervous system. International Agency for Research on Cancer, Lyon.

Lu, Y., Ryan, S.L., Elliott, D., Bingell, G.R., Futreal, P.A., Ellison, D.W. , Bailey, S., Clifford. S.C. 2009. Amplification and overexpression of Hsa-miR-30b, Hsa-miR-30d and KHDRBS3 at 8q24.22-q24.23 in medulloblastoma. PLos One 4, e6159

Marino, S. 2005. Medulloblatoma : developmental mechanisms out of control. Trends Mol. Med 11:17-22

McCabe, M.G., Ichimura, K., Liu. L., Plant, K., Backlund, L.M., Pearson, D.M., and Collins, V.P. 2006. High-resolusion array-based comparative genomic hybridization of medulloblastomas and supratentorial primitive neuroectodermal tumors. J Neuropathol Exp Neurol 65;549-561

Mendrzyk, F., Radlwimmer, B., Joos, S., Kokocinski, F., Benner, A., Stange, D.E., Neben, K., Fiegler, H., Carter, N.P., Reifenberger, G., Korshunov, A., ans Lichter, P. 2005. Genomic and protein expression profiling identifies CDK6 as novel independent prognostic marker in medulloblastoma. J Clin Oncol 23;8853-8862

Mitelman, F., Johansson, B., Mertens, F. (eds) (2011) Mitelman database of chromosome aberrations in cancer. Retrieved from: http://cgap.nci.nih.gov/Chromosomes/Mitelman Database last updated Feb 11, 2011

Northcott, P.A., Nakahara, Y., Wu, X., Feuk, L., Ellison, D.W., Croul, S., Mack, S., Kongkham, P.N., Peacock, J., Dubuc, A., Ra, Y.S., Zilberberg, K., McLeod, J., Scherer, S.W., Sunil Rao, J., Eberhart, C.G., Grajkowska, W., Gillespie, Y., Lach, B., Grundy, R., Pollack, I.F., Hamilton, R.L., Van Meter, T., Carlotti, C.G., Boop, F., Binger, D., Gilbertson, R.J., Rutka, J.T., and Taylor, M.D. 2009. Multiple recurrent genetic events converge on control of histone lysine metylation in medilloblastoma. Nat Genet 41:465-472

Northcott, P.A., Rutka, J.T., Taylor, M.D. 2010. Genomics of medulloblastoma: from Giesma-banding to next-generation sequencing in 20 years. Neurosurg Focus 28: E6

Northcott, P.A., Korshunov, A., WittH, Hielschner, T., Eberhart, C.G., Mack, S., Bouffet, E., Clifford, S.C., Hawkins, C.E., French, P., Rutka, J.T., Pfister, S., and Taylor, M.D. 2011. Medulloblastoma comprises four district molecular variants. J Clin Oncol 29:1408-14

Onvani, S., Etame, A.B., Smith, C.A., and Rutka, J.T. 2010. Genetics of medulloblastoma: clues for novel therapies. Expert Rev Neurother 10:811-823

Packer, R.J., and Vezina, G. 2008. Management of and prognosis with medulloblastoma: therapy at the crossroad. Arch Neurol 65:1419-1424

Padovani, L., Sunyach, M.P., Perol, D., Mercier, C., Alapetite, C., Haie-Meder, C., Hoffstetter, S., Muracciole, X., Kerr, C., Wagner, J.P., Lagrange, J.L., Maire, J.P., Cowen, D., Frappaz, D., and Carrie, C. 2007. Common strategy for adult and pediatric medulloblastoma: A multicenter series of 253 adults. Int J Radiat Oncol Biol Phys 68: 433-440

Pan, E., Pellarin, M., Holmes, E., Smirnov, I., Misra, A., Eberhart, C.G., Burger, P.C., Biegel, J.A., and Feuerstain, B.G. 2005. Isochromosome 17q is a negative prognostic factor in poor-risk childhood medulloblastoma patients. Clin Cancer Res 11:4733-4740

Pfister, S., Remke, M., Benner, A., Mendrzyk, F., Toedt, G., Felsberg, J., Wittmann, A., Devens, F., Gerber, N.U., Joos, S., Kulozik, A., Reifenberger, G., Rutkowsky, S., Wiestler, O.D., Radlwimmer, B., Scheurlen, W., Lichter, P., and Korshunov, A. 2009 Outcome predictionin pediatric medulloblastoma based on DNA cipy-number aberrations of chromosomes 6q and 17q and the MYC and MYCN loci. J Clin Oncol 27:1627-1636

Pierson, J., Hostager, B., Fan, R., and Vubhakar, R. 2008. Regulation of cyclin dependent kinase 6 by microRNA 124 in medulloblastoma. J Neurooncol 90:1-7

Pizer, B.L., and Clifford, S.C. 2009. The potential impact of tumor biology on improved clinical practice for medulloblastoma: progress towards biologically driven clinical trials. Brit J Neurosurg 23:364-375

Polkinghorn, W.R., and Tarbell, N.J. 2007. Medulloblastoma: Tumorigenesis, current clinical paradigm, and effort to improve risk stratification. Nat Clin Pract Oncol 4:295-304

Reardon, D.A., Michlkiewicz, E., Boyett, J.M., Sublett, J.E., Entrekin, R.E., Ragsdale, S.T., Valentine, M.B., Behm, F.G., Li, H., Heideman, R.L., Kun, L.E., Shapiro, D.N., and Look, A.T. 1997. Extensive genomic abnormalities in childhood medulloblastoma by comparative genomic hybridization. Cancer Res 57: 4042-40-47

Ribi, K., Relly, C., Landolt, M.A., Allber, F.D., Boltshauser, E., and Grotzer, M.A. 2005. Outcome of medulloblastoma in children: long-term complications and quality of life. Neuropediatrics 36:357-365

Ricket, C.H., and Paulus, W. 2004. Comparative genomic hybridization in central and peripheral nervous system tumors of childhhod and adolescence. J Neuropathol Exp Neurol 63:399-417

Rossi, A., Caracciolo,V., Russo, G., Reiss, K., and Giordano, A. 2008. Medulloblastoma: frommolecular pathology to therapy. Clin Cancer Res 14:971-976

Rutkowski, S., Gerber, N.U., von Hoff, K., Gnekow, A., Bode, U., Graf, N., Emser, A., Ottensmeiser, H., Deinlein, F., Schlegel, P.G., Kortmann, R.D., Pietsch, T., and Kuehl, J. 2009 Treatment of early childhood medulloblastoma by postoperative chemotherapy and deffered radiotherapy. Neuro Oncol 11:201-210

Sillitoe, R.V., and Joyner, A.L. 2007. Morphology, molecular codes and circuitry produce the three- dimensional complexity of the cerebellum. Annu Rev Cell Dev Biol 23:549-577

Speicher, M.R., and Carter, N.P. 2005. The new cytogenetics: blurring the boundaries with molecular biology. Nat Rev Genet 2005. 6:782-792

Thompson, M.C., Fuller, C., Hogg, T.L., Dalton, J., Finkelstein, D., Lau, C.C., Chintagumpala, M., Adesina, A., Ashley, D.M., Kellies, S.J., Taylor, M.D., Curran, T., Gajjar, A., and Gilbertson, R.J. 2006. Genomics identifies medulloblastoma subgroups that are enriched for specific genetic alteratins. J Clin Oncol 24:1924-1931

Tong, C.Y., Hui, A.B., Yin, X.L. Pang, J.C., Zhu, X.L., Poon, W.S., and Ng, H.K. 2004. Detection of oncogene amplifications in medulloblastomas by comparative genomic hybridization and array-based comparative genomic hybridization. J Neurosurg 100 (2 Supp. Pediatr):187-193

Waha, A., Koch, A., Hartman, W., Milde, U., Felsberg, J., Hubner, A., Mikeska, T., Goodyer, C.G., Sorensen, N., Lindberg, I., Wiestler, O.D., Pietsch, T.,and Waha, A. 2007. SGNE1/7B2 is epigenetically altered and transcriptionally downregulated in human medulloblastomas. Oncogene 26:5662-5668

Part 17

HGF/cMET Signaling Pathway - MBL

30

The Role of HGF/c-Met Pathway Signaling in Human Medulloblastoma

Claudia Faria, Christian Smith and James Rutka
Labatt Brain Tumour Research Centre,
The Hospital for Sick Children, University of Toronto,
Canada

1. Introduction

Medulloblastoma is the most common malignant brain tumor in childhood and represents around 10% of all pediatric cancer deaths. It arises in the cerebellum and originates from aberrant proliferation of neural progenitor cells during development. It has a high tendency to disseminate throughout the central nervous system with as many as 30% of children with metastatic spread at the time of diagnosis. Dissemination is the most important factor associated with poor survival and the leading cause of treatment failure. The current therapies include surgery, radiation and chemotherapy with 5-year survival rates ranging between 50 and 80%. Among long-term survivors, a major concern is the sequelae induced by treatment including endocrinologic, neurocognitive and behavioral dysfunction.

The genetic heterogeneity of medulloblastoma appears to be the basis for differential response to treatment, which leads to the conclusion that current tumor classification systems based solely on histological or clinical criteria are clearly insufficient and limited. Recent studies have identified distinct molecular variants of medulloblastoma that correspond with different clinical presentations, transcriptional profiles, genetic abnormalities and clinical outcomes (Eberhart, 2011; Ellison et al., 2011; Northcott et al., 2010; Pfister et al., 2010). Thus, a better understanding of the molecular biology of this tumor will have significant diagnostic, prognostic and therapeutic value.

Medulloblastoma is associated with dysregulation of the pathways that normally lead to cerebellum development. Over the past few years, different signaling pathways have been shown to play a critical role in medulloblastoma formation and progression. The hepatocyte growth factor (HGF)/c-Met signaling pathway has been implicated in different processes including development and tumorigenesis but only recently has it been demonstrated in medulloblastoma pathogenesis. The receptor tyrosine kinase c-Met is normally activated following engagement with HGF ligand, secreted as a precursor that is proteolytically cleaved in an active form by the serine protease hepatocyte growth factor activator. HGF is a member of the plasminogen-related growth factor family and was originally identified as a growth factor for hepatocytes and as a fibroblast-derived cell motility or scatter factor. The interplay between c-Met and its ligand mediate downstream events that, in the central nervous system, play a critical role in cerebellar granule cell precursors proliferation and survival. Dysregulation of this pathway can promote tumorigenesis through cell migration, invasion and metastasis, angiogenesis and prevention of apoptosis. Met has been found to be overexpressed in a variety of malignancies where its activation can occur by HGF ligation or through ligand independent mechanisms, including mutations and amplifications.

It was shown that medulloblastoma tumor cell lines and surgical tumor samples express HGF and c-Met. Furthermore, overexpression of c-Met is associated with poor clinical outcome. Treatment of medulloblastoma cell lines with HGF induced tumor cell proliferation, anchorage-independent growth and reduced apoptosis in response to chemotherapy. Recently, *Serine protease inhibitor kunitz-type 2* (*SPINT2*), a tumor supressor gene silenced by promoter methylation in medulloblastoma, was identified by our group as a key regulator of HGF/c-Met pathway (Kongkham et al., 2008). Several therapeutic strategies aiming to target and limit the signaling cascade of HGF/c-Met were examined with the c-Met inhibitors being the most promising. Targeting the HGF/c-Met pathway, alone or in combination with standard therapies is likely to improve present treatments in Met-dependent malignancies such as medulloblastoma.

In this chapter we examine the role of the HGF/c-Met pathway in normal cerebellar development and in medulloblastoma formation and progression. We also highlight the most recent advances in targeted therapies to the HGF/c-Met axis in cancer.

2. HGF/c-Met pathway signaling

The HGF/c-Met pathway has been associated with normal development, organ regeneration and cancer. Met is a high affinity tyrosine kinase receptor for hepatocyte growth factor (also known as scatter factor, capable of inducing dissociation and motility). Met is generally expressed in epithelial cells and is activated by HGF produced in surrounding mesenchymal cells or released into the circulation.

During embryogenesis HGF/c-Met signaling is necessary for the development of the placenta, liver, kidney and neuronal tissue but also for the directional migration of skeletal muscle cells (Birchmeier & Gherardi, 1998). In adult tissues, this pathway has been implicated in regeneration and wound healing (Chmielowiec et al., 2007; Huh et al., 2004). Therefore, the HGF/c-Met axis is a key player in cell proliferation, survival and migration and, when dysregulated, can give origin to a variety of cancers.

2.1 Structure of HGF and Met

HGF is a multidomain protein similar to plasminogen, a circulating proenzyme that promotes the lysis of fibrin blood clots in its active form as plasmin. HGF is synthesized as a single-chain inactive precursor and it is converted by serine proteases into an active form with two chains (α and β chain) linked by a disulfide bond. HGF consists of six domains: an amino-terminal hairpin loop domain (HL), four kringle domains (K1-K4) and a serine protease homology (SPH) domain which lacks enzymatic activity (**Figure 1**).

Met, the HGF receptor, is a disulfide-linked heterodimer which results from cleavage of a precursor into an extracellular α chain and a transmembrane β chain. The extracellular region of Met is composed of three domains: the Sema domain (homologous to the Sema domain of the semaphorins and plexins) that includes the entire α chain and part of the β chain; the PSI domain (also present in the plexins, semaphorins and integrins); and four IPT domains (immunoglobulin-like also found in plexins and transcriptional factors). The intracellular region of Met consists of three portions: a juxtamembrane sequence that has the role to downregulate kinase activity upon phosphorylation of Ser975; a catalytic region that activates kinase activity following phosphorylation of Tyr1234 and Tyr1235; and a carboxy-terminal multifunctional docking site that contains two docking tyrosines (Tyr1349 and Tyr1356) essential for downstream signaling (Trusolino et al., 2010).

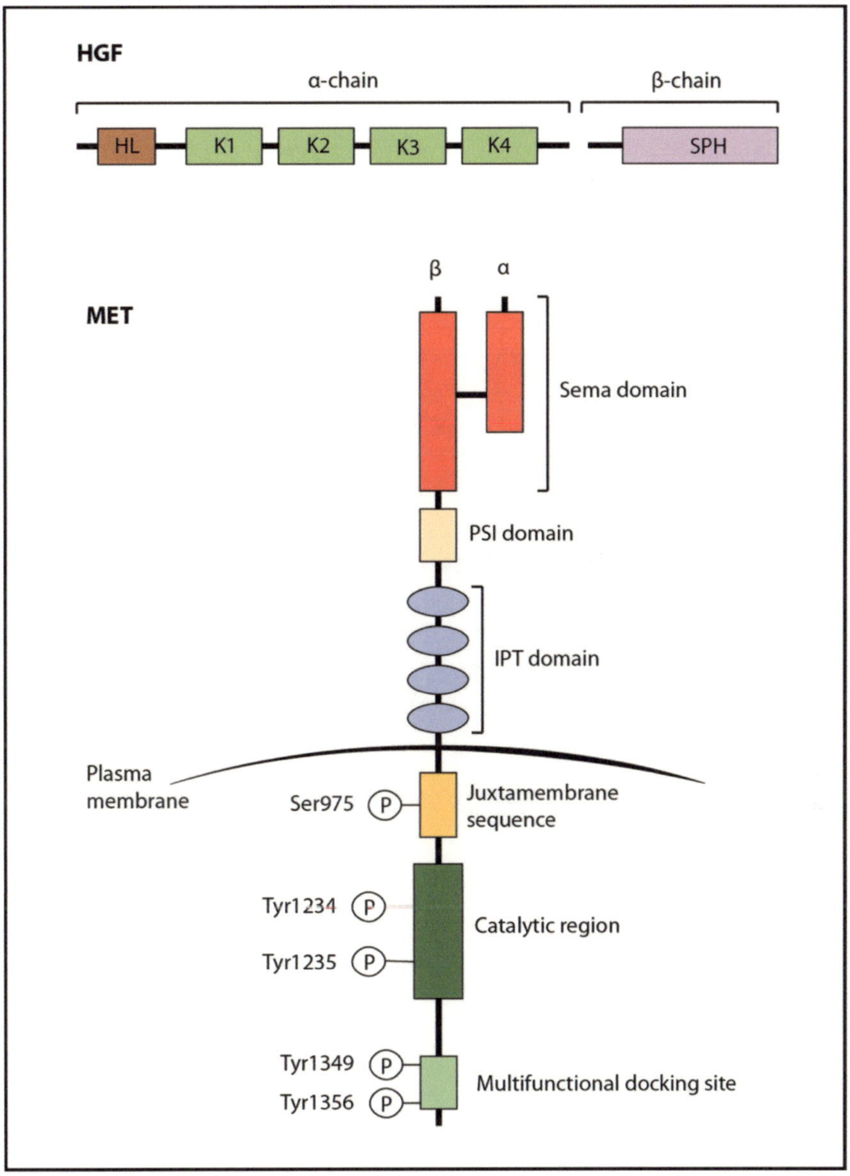

Fig. 1. HGF and Met structures

2.2 Met signal transduction

To activate the Met receptor, the single chain HGF precursor is cleaved into a heterodimeric active form by a protease called HGF activator (HGFA) (Miyazawa et al., 1993). This process is regulated by a protein family of serine protease inhibitors called SPINT1 and SPINT2 (Kawaguchi et al., 1997; Shimomura et al., 1997). Inhibiting the activation of HGF by HGFA, SPINT1 and -2 limit signaling through the HGF/c-Met pathway.

Following HGF binding, the kinase activity of Met is switched on. This process starts with receptor dimerization and *trans*-phosphorylation of two tyrosine residues in the catalytic region (Tyr1234 and Tyr1235) and is followed by phosphorylation of two additional tyrosines in the carboxy-terminal tail (Tyr1349 and Tyr1356). These tyrosines create docking sites for a variety of adaptor proteins and direct kinase substrates including the growth factor receptor-bound protein 2 (Grb2), Grb2-associated adaptor protein (Gab1), son of sevenless (SOS), SRC homology protein tyrosine phosphatase 3 (Shp2), phosphatidylinositol-3-kinase (PI3K) and signal transducer and activator of transcription 3 (STAT3). This leads to the activation of downstream signaling pathways that include the mitogen-activated protein kinase (MAPK), PI3K/AKT and STAT pathways, which mediate Met-dependent cell proliferation, survival, migration and invasion (**Figure 2**).

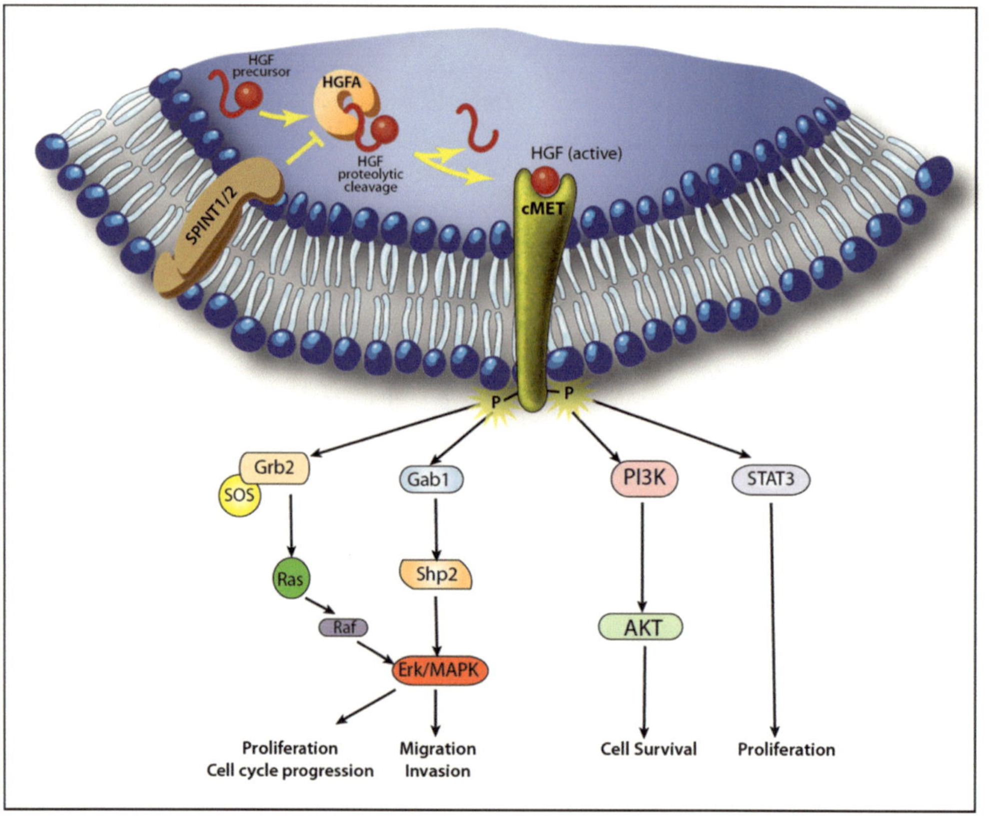

Fig. 2. The HGF/c-Met signaling pathway

The activation of MAPK cascade will sequentially activate different protein kinases whose terminal effectors include extracellular signal-regulated kinases (Erk1 and Erk2), Jun amino-terminal kinases (JNK1, JNK2 and JNK3) and p38. These downstream elements will activate cell cycle regulators leading to cell proliferation and will promote alterations in cytoskeletal functions that control cell migration and invasion. PI3K/AKT activation mediates cell survival and resistance to apoptosis through inactivation of the pro-apoptotic protein BCL-2 antagonist of cell death (BAD) and degradation of the pro-apoptotic protein p53 (Birchmeier et al., 2003). Upon activation of STAT3 by the Met receptor at the plasma membrane, it translocates to the nucleus to operate as a transcription factor regulating the expression of genes implicated in cell proliferation and differentiation (Y. W. Zhang et al., 2002).

Other molecules that interact with the Met receptor include the epidermal growth factor receptor (EGFR), the α6β4 integrin, the semaphoring receptors of the plexin B family and the variant of the hyaluronan receptor CD44 (that links the extracellular matrix and the intracellular cytoskeleton) (Bertotti et al., 2006; Guo et al., 2008; Orian-Rousseau et al., 2002). This crosstalk of Met with different surface proteins highlights the dynamic environment at the plasma membrane and contributes to Met associated biological responses (Lai et al., 2009).

2.3 Regulation of Met signaling

It has been shown that the signaling network around the tyrosine kinase receptor Met is more complex than the known process of recruiting signaling effectors at the plasma membrane and subsequently stimulating intermediates in the cytosol. In fact, this view has been expanded by the finding that Met signals can also originate from endosomal compartments and by a series of other events.

Upon HGF binding, Met is internalized by clathrin-mediated endocytosis and recruited into peripheral early endosomes. This process is mediated by protein kinase Cε (PKCε) that promotes the transfer of active Erk to focal adhesions and, subsequently, the HGF-induced cell migration. From the peripheral endosomes, Met travels along the microtubule network to late perinuclear compartments in a process mediated by PKCα. This juxtanuclear accumulation of Met is a determinant step for activation and nuclear translocation of STAT3 (Kermorgant & Parker, 2005, 2008).

Downregulation of Met signaling involves trafficking and degradation of ligand-activated receptors in the lysosomes. This process is initiated by the association of Met with casitas B-lineage lymphoma (CBL) and endocytic adaptors. Following endocytosis, Met accumulates in multivesicular bodies that later fuse with lysosomes and leads to protein degradation. Met can also undergo sequential proteolytic cleavage at two juxtamembrane sites. The first cleavage occurs in the extracellular domain and is mediated by a disintegrin and metalloprotease (ADAM) originating a 'decoy' fragment that sequesters the ligand and interferes with the receptor's activity. The second cleavage is performed in the intracellular domain, by a γ-secretase and yields a fragment that is destroyed in the proteasome (Hammond et al., 2001)(**Figure 3**).

3. HGF, Met and cancer

The dysregulation of HGF/c-Met signaling has emerged as a key player in several human malignancies, particularly in invasion and metastasis. Human cell lines overexpressing either HGF and/or Met become tumorigenic and metastatic when implanted into nude mice (Rong et al., 1994). Moreover, transgenic mice expressing the receptor or the ligand develop metastatic tumors (Takayama et al., 1997). On the contrary, downregulation of HGF or Met expression in human tumor xenografts decreases tumor growth (Abounader et al., 2002).

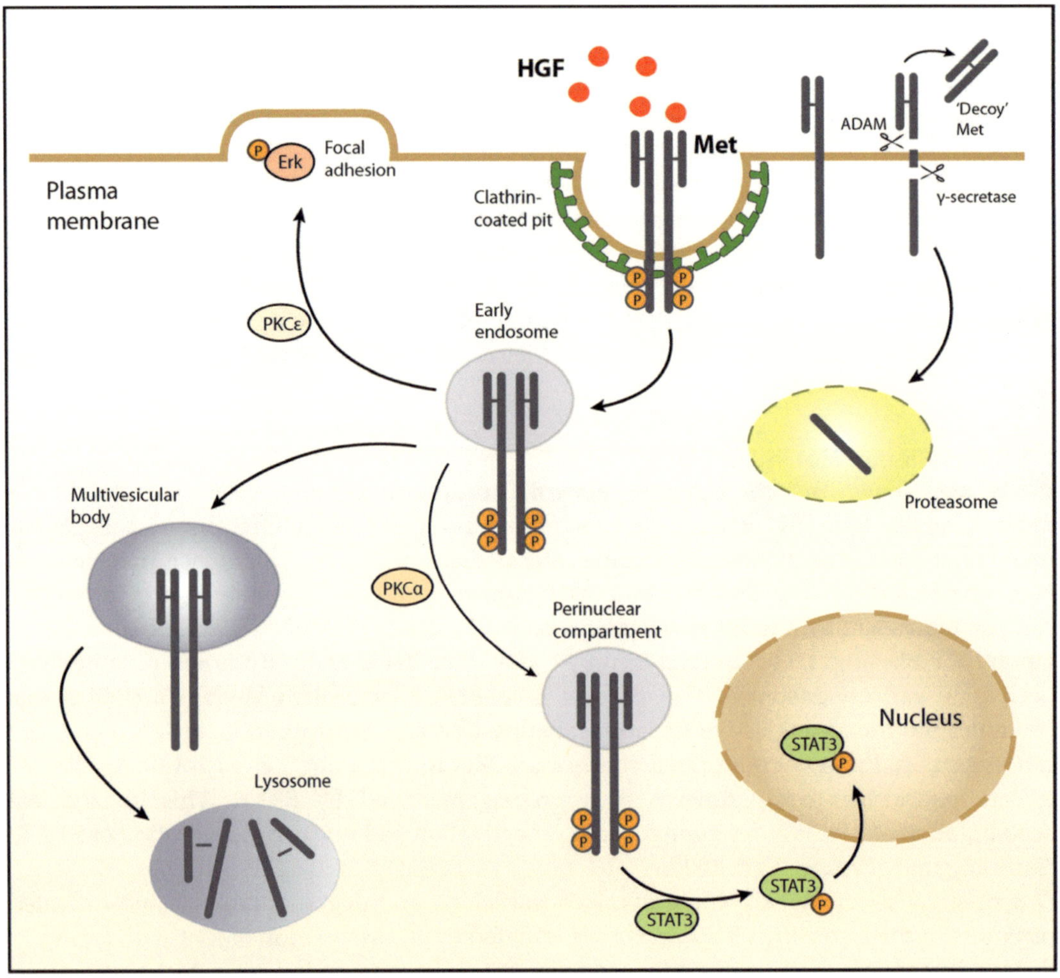

Fig. 3. Mechanisms of Met signaling regulation

There are three biological mechanisms underlying the tumorigenicity of Met: a) the establishment of HGF/c-Met autocrine loops; b) the overexpression of HGF or Met; and c) the presence of activating mutations in the Met receptor (Benvenuti & Comoglio, 2007).

An autocrine mechanism of Met activation is found in some human tumors. For example, osteosarcomas and rabdomyosarcomas are derived from mesenchymal cells which physiologically produce HGF. Glioblastomas and breast carcinomas are derived from ectodermal tissues that normally express Met but not HGF. Experimental models of HGF/c-Met autocrine loops were also able to generate invasive tumors *in vitro* and in transgenic mice (Boccaccio & Comoglio, 2006).

The most frequent mechanism of Met dysregulation found in human tumors is the overexpression of the receptor or its ligand. A large number of studies showed that HGF and Met are expressed in a wide variety of human tumors and in their metastasis. These include carcinomas of the breast, colon, lung, ovary, liver, kidney, upper gastrointestinal tract, pancreas and prostate but also sarcomas, haematopoietic malignancies, melanomas and glioblastomas (Birchmeier et al., 2003).

It has also been shown that high expression levels of Met and its ligand correlate with increased aggressiveness of tumors and patients poor prognosis (Birchmeier et al., 2003). For example, in colorectal cancer patients Met is a powerful prognostic factor for early stage invasion and metastasis (Kammula et al., 2007). Moreover, in a study including 74 clinical samples of low-grade and high-grade gliomas the authors described a correlation of HGF and Met expression levels with tumor grade (Abounader & Laterra, 2005).

The compelling evidence that links Met with human cancer lies in the *MET*-activating mutations found in hereditary renal papillary carcinoma. These mutations were also found in sporadic tumors such as renal carcinoma, gastric cancer, childhood hepatocellular carcinoma and in head and neck squamous cell carcinomas (Boccaccio & Comoglio, 2006; Lai et al., 2009).

The association between cancer and blood coagulation disorders has been known for many years. In fact, approximately 50% of all patients with malignant tumors and up to 90% of those with metastasis have coagulopathies (Wojtukiewicz et al., 2001). Interestingly, Boccaccio *et al.* showed in a mouse model that activation of the oncogene *Met* induced cancer and a thrombohemorrhagic syndrome through transcriptional upregulation of the procoagulation factors plasminogen activator inhibitor type 1 (PAI-1) and cyclooxygenase-2 (COX-2). Upon a first phase characterized by a hypercoagulation state due to Met signaling activation, the mice developed a hemorrhagic diathesis due to exhaustion of the hyperactivated hemostatic system (Boccaccio et al., 2005). At the early step of this process, hypoxia induces transcription of *Met* that, subsequently, activates the transcription of genes involved in hemostasis, such as *PAI-1* and *COX-2*. The activation of the coagulation cascade will lead to fibrin deposition around cells forming an extracellular matrix that will promote angiogenesis and cell migration (Boccaccio & Comoglio, 2005).

HGF/c-Met signaling also has a role in angiogenesis either by direct influence of c-Met activation in vascular endothelial cells, or by regulation of the expression levels of other angiogenic factors in tumor cells. It was previously shown that the HGF/c-Met interaction stimulates proliferation and migration of endothelial cells *in vitro* and induces blood vessel formation *in vivo* (Bussolino et al., 1992). Zhang *et al.* described the "angiogenic switch" in tumor cells upon HGF stimulation by simultaneous upregulation of the proangiogenic vascular endothelial growth factor (VEGF) and downregulation of thrombospondin 1 (TSP-1), an angiogenesis inhibitor (Y. W. Zhang et al., 2003). This process has distinct mediators: while VEGF is modulated by MAPK, PI3K and STAT3, TSP-1 is targeted only by MAPK. An interesting example of this regulation was found in human glioma cells where stimulation with HGF increased the expression levels of VEGF and tumor-associated angiogenesis. The use of HGF and Met inhibitors in experimental tumor models significantly reduced tumor growth and tumor vessel formation (Abounader & Laterra, 2005).

Recently, a new key player of the HGF/c-Met pathway was described. *Metastasis-associated in colon cancer-1* (*MACC1*) was identified by genome-wide expression analysis in primary and metastatic colon carcinomas. Its expression in human tumor samples was found to be an independent prognostic factor for metastasis formation and metastasis-free survival. The experimental studies showed that MACC1 promotes proliferation, invasion and HGF-induced scattering *in vitro* and tumor growth and metastasis in xenograft models (Stein et al., 2009). The authors proposed a positive feedback mechanism where MACC1 acts as a transcriptional regulator of the *Met* gene. The stimulation of the Met receptor with HGF causes the translocation of MACC1 from the cytoplasm into the nucleus. There, MACC1 activates the transcription of the *Met* gene by binding to its promoter (Arlt & Stein, 2009).

The increased amounts of Met receptor will be able to bind more HGF molecules thereby enhancing the pathway signaling and promoting cell proliferation, migration and metastasis.

4. HGF/c-Met signaling in medulloblastoma

4.1 Medulloblastoma overview

Medulloblastoma is the most common malignant childhood brain tumor, comprising 20% of all primary brain tumors in the pediatric population (Crawford et al., 2007). It is an embryonal tumor that arises in the cerebellum from primitive pluripotent precursor cells of the ventricular zone and the external granular layer (Hatten & Roussel, 2011).

The 2007 World Health Organization (WHO) classified medulloblastoma in five variants: classic, desmoplastic, anaplastic, large cell and medulloblastoma with extensive nodularity. Clinical data suggests a favorable prognosis for desmoplastic medulloblastoma and a significant worst outcome for the anaplastic subtype (Gilbertson & Ellison, 2008).

Medulloblastoma formation is strongly associated with dysregulation of the pathways involved in the normal development of the cerebellum. The best characterized pathways in medulloblastoma tumorigenesis are the Sonic hedgehog (Shh), Wingless (Wnt) and Notch pathways (Hatten & Roussel, 2011).

Traditionally, patients are stratified into standard risk and high-risk groups according to age, residual tumor and metastatic disease at diagnosis. High-risk patients include those younger than 3 years of age or having a residual tumor or disseminated disease at diagnosis (Packer et al., 2003). In fact, one third of the patients will have metastasis at the time of diagnosis and two thirds will have leptomeningeal spread by the time of relapse (MacDonald, 2008). Moreover, dissemination is the leading cause of treatment failure and the most powerful factor associated with poor survival (Zeltzer et al., 1999).

Recently, Northcott and co-workers described four molecular subtypes of medulloblastoma using gene expression profiling and some genomic features (Northcott et al., 2010). These medulloblastoma subtypes are distinct with respect to the underlying signaling pathway that is dysregulated and the clinical outcome. The Wnt subgroup includes classic medulloblastomas and has a better prognosis. Most tumors in the Shh subgroup are desmoplastic medulloblastomas and also have good prognosis. The other two subgroups, group C and D, are non-Shh/Wnt, and demonstrate *Myc* overexpression as the main feature of group C, and isochromosome 17q as the main feature of group D. Interestingly, group C patients showed a significantly reduced survival, regardless of their metastatic status.

The treatment for standard risk patients includes surgery, craniospinal irradiation and chemotherapy with reported 5-year overall survival of 80%. For patients with metastatic disease the intensified treatment regimens, including high-dose chemotherapy with autologous stem-cell transplantation and non-conventional radiotherapy, have improved prognosis, with 5-year overall survival rates between 50 and 70% (Gajjar et al., 2006; Sanders et al., 2008). Among survivors, a major concern is the long-term sequelae induced by treatments which include endocrinological, neurocognitive, behavioral, motor and sensitive deficits (Armstrong et al., 2009). Therefore, there is a critical need to identify new molecular targets that improve tumor growth suppression while minimizing the side effects of therapy.

4.2 HGF/c-Met pathway in cerebellar development

During embryonic development, the progenitor cells localized in the ventricular zone of the cerebellum (also called primary germinal zone), along the IVth ventricle, migrate radially to give rise to Purkinje cells, neurons of the cerebellar nuclei and different types of cerebellar interneurons. Simultaneously, the progenitor cells in the rombic lip migrate dorsally to originate the external granule layer (EGL or secondary germinal zone). The peak of proliferation of these cells occurs between postnatal day (P) P5 and P8 in the mouse. Through a tightly regulated mechanism, the progenitor cells in the EGL become postmitotic, differentiate and migrate inwards to give origin to the internal granule layer (IGL), a process that is complete by P20 in the mouse (Marino, 2005).

During the early postnatal period, multiple mitogenic pathways, such as Shh, Wnt and Notch, promote the rapid expansion of progenitor cells in the EGL. It is believed that this vast population of cells includes subgroups of progenitors with distinct genetic properties, that give origin to the different medulloblastoma subtypes (Hatten & Roussel, 2011).

The HGF/c-Met pathway also plays a critical role in cerebellar development. The knockout mice for HGF, Met and SPINT2 are all embryonic lethal (Bladt et al., 1995; Mitchell et al., 2001; Uehara et al., 1995). Comparing the regional expression of HGF and Met in both developing and adult rat brains, Achim and co-workers found expression of HGF in the parietal cortex, striatum and cerebellar deep gray matter in developing but not in adult brain. Abundant expression of Met was also detected in the newborn cortex, thalamus and brainstem (Achim et al., 1997). The analysis of HGF and Met expression in the central nervous system of different mammalian species showed that their neuronal expression is highly conserved during evolution, a sign that they mediate important functions (Jung et al., 1994).

Leraci *et al.* described the expression of Met in the proliferating cells of the external granule layer of the cerebellum and increased proliferation after stimulation of primary cultures of granule cells with HGF. In addition, transgenic mice with partial loss of Met function had a smaller cerebellum with abnormal foliation and balance impairment (Ieraci et al., 2002).

HGF has also been proposed to mediate neurotrophic functions during neurogenesis both in the central and peripheral nervous systems. In fact, it was shown that HGF is a chemoattractant and promotes survival of motor neurons in the embryo. Furthermore, stimulation of sensory and sympathetic neurons with HGF enhances survival, differentiation and axonal growth (Maina & Klein, 1999). Exploring the neuroprotective role of HGF, different groups showed that HGF treatment of primary cerebellar granule neurons prevents apoptotic cell death through activation of the PI3K/AKT pathway signaling (Honda et al., 1995; Hossain et al., 2002; L. Zhang et al., 2000).

To further investigate the influence of aberrant HGF/c-Met pathway signaling on cerebellar development and medulloblastoma initiation and progression, our group genetically engineered a transgenic mouse that expresses a constitutively active mutant of human Met, specifically within the cerebellum. We are in the process of characterizing the cerebellar development in the transgenic line as compared to the wild type, and determine the effects of constitutive Met activation in medulloblastoma pathogenesis.

4.3 HGF/c-Met pathway in medulloblastoma formation

HGF/c-Met signaling has an important role in tumorigenesis and metastatic behavior in several human malignancies but its role in medulloblastoma pathogenesis was only recently described.

Studying a series of 14 human medulloblastoma samples by comparative genomic hybridization Tong *et al.* found amplification of the Met oncogene on chromosome 7q in 38.5% of cases (Tong et al., 2004). A separate group showed a correlation between the expression of HGF and Met in human medulloblastoma samples and patient clinical outcome (Li et al., 2005). When they stimulated medulloblastoma cells with HGF there was an activation of downstream effectors, evidenced by Met, MAPK and AKT phosphorylation. Up-regulation of the pathway was also able to induce cell proliferation, cell cycle progression, anchorage-independent growth and resistance to chemotherapy-induced apoptosis in medulloblastoma cell lines. *In vivo* models overexpressing HGF also had increased tumor growth and invasion (Li et al., 2005). More recently, the same group identified an association between HGF/c-Met signaling and c-Myc in medulloblastoma. They found that HGF induced c-Myc expression both at transcriptional and post-transcriptional levels, leading to cell cycle progression, cell proliferation and increased apoptosis (Li et al., 2008b).

Although the anti-apoptotic functions of HGF/c-Met pathway seem to be predominant, Li *et al.* described enhanced cell death in Daoy cell lines after Met activation. Apoptotic cell death can be induced by two different pathways: the intrinsic mitochondrial pathway and the extrinsic death receptor pathway. In malignant tissues, the tumor necrosis factor-related apoptosis–inducing ligand (TRAIL) has the potential to activate the death receptor pathway upon binding of death receptors DR4 and DR5, which leads to downstream caspase activation and apoptosis (Suliman et al., 2001). Li and co-workers found that increased apoptosis of medulloblastoma cell lines after stimulation with HGF was induced by TRAIL and mediated by DR5 overexpression (Li et al., 2008a). Moreover, the treatment of those cells with a specific c-Met inhibitor (PHA665752) reduced apoptosis indicating that it requires activation of the canonical receptor tyrosine kinase (Li et al., 2008a).

Using an epigenome-wide screening our group identified an inhibitor of HGF/c-Met signaling. SPINT2, a tumor suppressor gene, was downregulated in 73.2% of primary medulloblastoma samples while *Met* was upregulated in 45% of cases. *SPINT2* was silenced by promoter hypermethylation in 34.4% of primary tumor samples (Kongkham et al., 2008). A single nucleotide polymorphism (SNP) array analysis identified hemizygous deletions in the *SPINT2* locus on chromosome 19q13.2 and gains in the *HGF* and *MET* loci on chromosome 7q. The experimental studies using medulloblastoma cells transfected with *SPINT2* showed decreased proliferation, migration and anchorage-independent growth *in vitro* and increased survival times in mouse xenografts (Kongkham et al., 2008). Although *SPINT2* downregulation has already been implicated in other human cancers (Dong et al., 2010; Morris et al., 2005; Parr et al., 2004) this was the first report to establish its role in medulloblastoma pathogenesis.

Binning et al. showed that HGF and Shh cooperate to transform cerebellar neural progenitors in transgenic mice, leading to medulloblastoma initiation and growth (Binning et al., 2008). Furthermore, the treatment of mice bearing Shh+HGF induced tumors with a monoclonal antibody against HGF (L2G7) prolonged survival by increasing apoptosis (Binning et al., 2008). Previous studies had already shown that systemic administration of L2G7 to mouse xenografts of human HGF+/c-Met+ glioblastomas improved survival and reduced tumor growth (Kim et al., 2006).

Knowing that a procoagulant state is often the first manifestation of a malignancy and that it is due to the expression of specific proteins such as tissue factor (TF), Provencal and colleagues analyzed the expression of this protein in human medulloblastoma samples and observed a strong correlation between Met and TF expression levels. Furthermore, the stimulation of Daoy cells with HGF increased the expression of TF and the treatment of those cells with physiological amounts of TF activator (factor VIIa) increased their migratory potential (Provencal et al., 2009). It was hypothesized that the acquisition of a procoagulant phenotype by medulloblastoma favors its dissemination because the enrichment of the tumor environment with fibrin protects the cancer cells from the immune system and forms a matrix for cell migration (Provencal et al., 2009). The same group found that upregulation of TF upon Met pathway activation was associated with increased resistance to the chemotherapeutic drug etoposide (Provencal et al., 2010). This observation suggested that the combination of anticoagulant drugs and chemotherapy could improve the efficacy of chemotherapeutic agents. In fact, this regimen was already tested in metastatic breast cancer with encouraging results (Falanga et al., 1998).

These findings show the importance of the HGF/c-Met pathway signaling in medulloblastoma malignancy. Furthermore, they also provide validation of this pathway as a target for new and promising therapies using small molecular inhibitors and antibodies, some of them already in clinical trials for other cancers.

5. Inhibitors of HGF/c-Met pathway in cancer therapy

The evidence that the HGF/c-Met pathway is involved in the progression and dissemination of several malignancies has generated considerable interest in HGF and Met as major targets in cancer therapy and drug development. Different strategies are being explored and some of them are already being tested in clinical trials. We can consider three main groups of drugs: a) HGF and Met antagonists or competitors; b) Monoclonal antibodies directed against HGF and Met; and c) Small molecule tyrosine kinase inhibitors.

The use of molecular targeted therapies against HGF and Met in medulloblastoma was only recently reported. Our group demonstrated the efficacy of a highly specific small molecular inhibitor (PHA665752) in the treatment of medulloblastoma cell lines by reducing cell proliferation, migration and anchorage-independent growth (Kongkham et al. 2010). Another group used an orally available small molecule inhibitor of Met (SGX523) in medulloblastoma cells and human glioblastoma xenografts. They reported decreased cell proliferation, migration and invasion in the *in vitro* studies and significant reduction of *in vivo* tumor growth (Guessous et al., 2010). The HGF-neutralizing monoclonal antibody, L2G7, was also tested in monotherapy and in combination therapy in genetically engineered mice with medulloblastomas induced by Shh and HGF. The authors reported tumor growth inhibition and increased survival with L2G7 monotherapy (Coon et al., 2010).

Strategies using combined regimens targeting multiple receptor tyrosine kinases are currently under study. This can be achieved in two different ways either by a combination of highly selective agents or by using a single agent that targets multiple specific members of the Met pathway. The use of broad-spectrum agents may have the advantage of reducing drug interactions, but it may also affect other unintended kinases. Stommel *et al.*, studying glioma cell lines, xenografts and human primary glioblastomas, showed simultaneous activation of multiple receptor tyrosine kinases and better responses to combined treatment when compared to monotherapy (Stommel et al., 2007).

We provide a brief summary of the latest advances in HGF/c-Met targeted therapy (**Table 1**).

5.1 HGF and Met antagonists

HGF and Met antagonists or decoys are molecules that bind to the receptor with high affinity without activation of downstream signaling. The activation of Met by HGF involves

Compound	Mechanism of action	Stage of development	References
Biological antagonists			
NK2	Inhibits HGF activity	Preclinical	Montesano et al. 1998; Otsuka et al. 2000
NK4	Inhibits HGF binding to Met	Preclinical	Kuba et al. 2000; Matsumoto et al. 2008; Matsumoto and Nakamura 2008
Uncleaved HGF	Inhibits proteolytic HGF activation	Preclinical	Mazzone et al. 2004
Decoy Met	Inhibits HGF binding and Met dimerization	Preclinical	Michieli et al. 2004
Antibodies			
AMG102 (Amgen)	Anti-HGF (IgG2)	Phase II trial	Burgess et al. 2006; Gordon et al. 2010; Jun et al. 2007
L2G7 (Galaxy Biotech)	Anti-HGF (IgG1)	Preclinical	Coon et al. 2010; Kim et al. 2006; Li et al. 2009
MetMAb (Genentech)	Anti-Met	Phase II trial	Martens et al. 2006
Small molecule inhibitors			
PHA665752 (Pfizer)	Selective inhibitor (Met)	Preclinical	Kongkham et al. 2010; Li et al. 2008a
PF2341066 (Pfizer)	Selective inhibitor (Met and ALK)	Phase II/III	Christensen et al. 2007; Zillhardt et al. 2010; Zou et al. 2007
ARQ197 (ArQule)	Selective inhibitor (Met)	Phase II	Bagai et al. 2010; Munshi et al. 2010
SGX523 (SGX Pharmaceuticals)	Selective inhibitor (Met)	Phase I (discontinued)	Guessous et al. 2010; Y. W. Zhang et al. 2010
XL184 (Exelixis)	Multikinase inhibitor (Met, VEGFR, Ret, Kit, Flt-3, Tie-2)	Phase II/III	http://clinicaltrials.gov
XL880 (Exelixis)	Multikinase inhibitor (Met, VEGFR, PDGFR, Ron, Kit, Flt-3, Tie-2)	Phase II	Qian et al. 2009; http://clinicaltrials.gov
MP470 (Supergen)	Multikinase inhibitor (Met, PDGFR, Ret, Kit, Flt-3)	Phase I	Mahadevan et al. 2007; Qi et al. 2009; Welsh et al. 2009

(VEGFR, vascular endothelial growth factor receptor; Ret, rearranged during transfection; Kit, stem cell factor receptor; Flt-3, FMS-like tyrosine kinase 3; Tie-2, angiopoietin receptor 2; PDGFR, platelet-derived growth factor receptor; Ron, recepteur d'origine nantais)

Table 1. Summary of HGF/c-Met inhibitors.

the dimerization of the receptor upon binding of the two chains of the ligand. HGF has a high affinity site located in the α-chain and a low affinity site in the β-chain, which only becomes accessible after pro-HGF activation (Comoglio et al., 2008). This means that the inactive form of HGF or HGF fragments can interact with Met by binding to the high affinity site but they cannot induce Met signaling because they are unable to promote receptor dimerization.

Examples of HGF competitors are NK2, NK4 and uncleavable HGF. NK2 is a naturally occurring HGF fragment and NK4 is a synthetic truncated form of HGF that contains only the α-chain. This is by far the best studied HGF antagonist and it was shown that it inhibits cell invasion and angiogenesis *in vitro* and in xenografts (Kuba et al., 2000). Uncleavable pro-HGF is an unprocessable form of HGF that competes with active HGF for Met binding and with pro-HGF proteases for HGF proteolytic activation.

Decoy Met is an enzymatically inactive molecule that corresponds to the extracellular domain of the receptor. It interacts with HGF and full-length Met, sequestering the ligand and interfering with the receptor dimerization.

5.2 Monoclonal antibodies directed against HGF and Met

The use of monoclonal antibodies has the following advantages: Specificity against HGF and Met; a relatively longer half-life when compared to other inhibitors; and the potential to induce a host immune response against the tumor cells (Eder et al., 2009).

AMG102 is a fully human IgG2 antibody against HGF that was found to enhance the effects of temozolomide and docetaxel *in vitro* and in xenograft models of gliomas (Jun et al., 2007). A Phase I study used a combination of AMG102 and the antiangiogenic drugs bevacizumab and motesanib in the treatment of patients with advanced solid tumors, showing a stable disease in most patients (Rosen et al., 2008). This molecule has also been tested in Phase II clinical trials for advanced glioblastomas and renal cell carcinomas and a preliminary analysis in glioma patients suggested that AMG102 has limited efficacy as monotherapy (Reardon et al., 2008). Therefore, the most recent clinical trials will use AMG102 in combination therapy (http://clinicaltrials.gov). L2G7 is another anti-HGF antibody that proved to be effective reducing subcutaneous and intracranial glioma xenografts and to increase survival (Kim et al., 2006).

The initial efforts to develop antibodies against Met were unsuccessful because they tended to behave as agonists rather than antagonists, due to its bivalent structure that acts as a natural dimerizing agent. To circumvent this problem a 'one-armed' antibody (OA-5D5; MetMAb), consisting of a monovalent Fab fragment, was developed. It binds to Met with high affinity preventing HGF interaction and subsequent downstream signaling. Martens *et al.* infused MetMAb intratumorally, reporting almost complete inhibition of tumor growth in a glioblastoma mouse model (Martens et al., 2006). Phase II clinical trials using MetMAb in combination with bevacizumav and paclitaxel for metastatic breast cancer and with erlotinib for advanced non-small cell lung cancer have been initiated (http://clinicaltrials.gov).

5.3 Small molecule tyrosine kinase inhibitors

Small molecule inhibitors target the ATP-binding site of the Met receptor, blocking its transphosphorylation. These molecules can also be classified according to their specificity for Met. Highly selective drugs may not be desirable as inhibition of multiple kinases may be more efficient and reduce the development of resistance. On the other hand, off-target inhibition of essential kinases may also be deleterious. With the recent advances in research and the ongoing clinical trials the small molecule inhibitors have emerged as promising drugs (Naran et al., 2009).

PHA665752 is a Met selective inhibitor that was found to be effective in tumor cell lines and xenografts, particularly in a subset of cancers with amplification of the Met gene (Kongkham et al., 2010; Smolen et al., 2006). Due to its low oral bioavailability another drug (PF2341066) with identical structure but more favorable pharmacokinetic properties was designed. PF2341066 selectively targets Met and anaplastic lymphoma kinase (ALK) and was shown to have antitumor cytoreductive activity and antiangiogenic activity in several cancer models (Christensen et al., 2007; Zillhardt et al., 2010; Zou et al., 2007). A Phase II study in non-small-cell lung cancer reported encouraging results with a disease control rate of 87% (Mayor, 2011). The drug is now in Phase III trials. Interestingly, PF2341066 is also being tested in Phase I/II studies in children with recurrent solid tumors, primary central nervous system tumors and anaplastic large cell lymphoma (http://clinicaltrials.gov).

ARQ197 is a highly selective, non-ATP competitive drug with reported clinical activity in several types of solid tumors. A Phase II trial in patients with non-small-cell lung cancer reported improved survival in patients treated with ARQ197 and erlotinib when compared to erlotinib monotherapy (Mayor, 2011).

SGX523 is an orally available ATP-competitive molecule with high selectivity for Met. Although the initial results with *in vitro* and *in vivo* models of medulloblastomas and gliomas looked promising because of its efficacy in reducing tumor growth, the drug was discontinued from a Phase I trial due to renal toxicity (Diamond et al., 2010).

XL184 and XL880 are orally available, non-selective inhibitors, with high binding affinity to both Met and VEGFR and to a lesser extent to other receptor tyrosine kinases such as PDGFR, Ret, Kit, Flt-3 and Tie-2 (Liu et al., 2010). XL184 is being evaluated in a Phase III study in patients with advanced medullary thyroid cancer and in Phase II studies in patients with glioblastoma multiforme and non-small-cell lung cancer that has progressed after previous benefit with erlotinib. XL880 has been tested in Phase II clinical trials in metastatic gastric cancer, papillary renal cell carcinoma and head and neck squamous cell cancer (http://clinicaltrials.gov).

MP470 is a multi-kinase inhibitor, orally available, that was reported to radiosensitize glioblastoma cell lines, through the suppression of RAD51, a DNA repair related protein (Welsh et al., 2009). Additional Phase I clinical studies, currently underway, use MP470 in monotherapy or in combination with standard chemotherapies in patients with metastatic solid tumors and lymphoma (http://clinicaltrials.gov).

6. Conclusion and future directions

The HGF/c-Met signaling pathway plays a significant role in cancer and has emerged recently as a promising target in the treatment of several malignancies. It was shown that HGF and Met are key players in cerebellum development and that their dysregulation is involved in medulloblastoma formation and progression.

Advances in understanding the molecular mechanisms and genetic profiles underlying the different subtypes of medulloblastoma created an urgent need for new and less toxic targeted therapies. HGF/c-Met inhibitors used in the treatment of gliomas *in vitro* and *in vivo* showed efficient reduction in tumor growth and are, therefore, being evaluated in clinical trials. Our preliminary data using a Met selective inhibitor in medulloblastoma cell lines showed that the HGF/c-Met pathway is a novel and promising therapeutic target in this disease.

In the future we will test a panel of available HGF and Met inhibitors using orthotopic xenograft models and our transgenic medulloblastoma mouse model. We hope that the results of our pre-clinical studies will provide the basis for future clinical trials where the HGF and Met inhibitors could synergize with current therapies to increase survival and improve the quality of life of children with brain tumors.

7. Acknowledgment

This work was supported by a grant from the Canadian Cancer Society (grant 2011-700751), and through support from B.r.a.i.n.child, the Wiley Fund and the Laurie Berman Fund for Brain Tumor Research.

CF is a PhD candidate from The Programme for Advanced Medical Education, supported by Fundação Gulbenkian, Fundação Champalimaud, Ministério da Saúde e Fundação para a Ciência e Tecnologia, Portugal.

8. References

Abounader, R. and Laterra, J. (2005), 'Scatter factor/hepatocyte growth factor in brain tumor growth and angiogenesis', *Neuro Oncol,* 7 (4), 436-51.

Abounader, R., et al. (2002), 'In vivo targeting of SF/HGF and c-met expression via U1snRNA/ribozymes inhibits glioma growth and angiogenesis and promotes apoptosis', *FASEB J,* 16 (1), 108-10.

Achim, C. L., et al. (1997), 'Expression of HGF and cMet in the developing and adult brain', *Brain Res Dev Brain Res,* 102 (2), 299-303.

Arlt, F. and Stein, U. (2009), 'Colon cancer metastasis: MACC1 and Met as metastatic pacemakers', *Int J Biochem Cell Biol,* 41 (12), 2356-9.

Armstrong, G. T., et al. (2009), 'Long-term outcomes among adult survivors of childhood central nervous system malignancies in the Childhood Cancer Survivor Study', *J Natl Cancer Inst,* 101 (13), 946-58.

Bagai, R., Fan, W., and Ma, P. C. (2010), 'ARQ-197, an oral small-molecule inhibitor of c-Met for the treatment of solid tumors', *IDrugs,* 13 (6), 404-14.

Benvenuti, S. and Comoglio, P. M. (2007), 'The MET receptor tyrosine kinase in invasion and metastasis', *J Cell Physiol,* 213 (2), 316-25.

Bertotti, A., Comoglio, P. M., and Trusolino, L. (2006), 'Beta4 integrin activates a Shp2-Src signaling pathway that sustains HGF-induced anchorage-independent growth', *J Cell Biol,* 175 (6), 993-1003.

Binning, M. J., et al. (2008), 'Hepatocyte growth factor and sonic Hedgehog expression in cerebellar neural progenitor cells costimulate medulloblastoma initiation and growth', *Cancer Res,* 68 (19), 7838-45.

Birchmeier, C. and Gherardi, E. (1998), 'Developmental roles of HGF/SF and its receptor, the c-Met tyrosine kinase', *Trends Cell Biol,* 8 (10), 404-10.

Birchmeier, C., et al. (2003), 'Met, metastasis, motility and more', *Nat Rev Mol Cell Biol,* 4 (12), 915-25.

Bladt, F., et al. (1995), 'Essential role for the c-met receptor in the migration of myogenic precursor cells into the limb bud', *Nature,* 376 (6543), 768-71.

Boccaccio, C. and Comoglio, P. M. (2005), 'A functional role for hemostasis in early cancer development', *Cancer Res,* 65 (19), 8579-82.

Boccaccio, C. and Comoglio, P. M. (2006), 'Invasive growth: a MET-driven genetic programme for cancer and stem cells', *Nat Rev Cancer,* 6 (8), 637-45.

Boccaccio, C., et al. (2005), 'The MET oncogene drives a genetic programme linking cancer to haemostasis', *Nature,* 434 (7031), 396-400.

Burgess, T., et al. (2006), 'Fully human monoclonal antibodies to hepatocyte growth factor with therapeutic potential against hepatocyte growth factor/c-Met-dependent human tumors', *Cancer Res,* 66 (3), 1721-9.

Bussolino, F., et al. (1992), 'Hepatocyte growth factor is a potent angiogenic factor which stimulates endothelial cell motility and growth', *J Cell Biol,* 119 (3), 629-41.

Chmielowiec, J., et al. (2007), 'c-Met is essential for wound healing in the skin', *J Cell Biol,* 177 (1), 151-62.

Christensen, J. G., et al. (2007), 'Cytoreductive antitumor activity of PF-2341066, a novel inhibitor of anaplastic lymphoma kinase and c-Met, in experimental models of anaplastic large-cell lymphoma', *Mol Cancer Ther,* 6 (12 Pt 1), 3314-22.

Comoglio, P. M., Giordano, S., and Trusolino, L. (2008), 'Drug development of MET inhibitors: targeting oncogene addiction and expedience', *Nat Rev Drug Discov,* 7 (6), 504-16.

Coon, V., et al. (2010), 'Molecular therapy targeting Sonic hedgehog and hepatocyte growth factor signaling in a mouse model of medulloblastoma', *Mol Cancer Ther,* 9 (9), 2627-36.

Crawford, J. R., MacDonald, T. J., and Packer, R. J. (2007), 'Medulloblastoma in childhood: new biological advances', *Lancet Neurol,* 6 (12), 1073-85.

Diamond, S., et al. (2010), 'Species-specific metabolism of SGX523 by aldehyde oxidase and the toxicological implications', *Drug Metab Dispos,* 38 (8), 1277-85.

Dong, W., et al. (2010), 'Epigenetic inactivation and tumor suppressor activity of HAI-2/SPINT2 in gastric cancer', *Int J Cancer,* 127 (7), 1526-34.

Eberhart, C. G. (2011), 'Molecular diagnostics in embryonal brain tumors', *Brain Pathol,* 21 (1), 96-104.

Eder, J. P., et al. (2009), 'Novel therapeutic inhibitors of the c-Met signaling pathway in cancer', *Clin Cancer Res,* 15 (7), 2207-14.

Ellison, D. W., et al. (2011), 'Definition of disease-risk stratification groups in childhood medulloblastoma using combined clinical, pathologic, and molecular variables', *J Clin Oncol,* 29 (11), 1400-7.

Falanga, A., et al. (1998), 'The effect of very-low-dose warfarin on markers of hypercoagulation in metastatic breast cancer: results from a randomized trial', *Thromb Haemost,* 79 (1), 23-7.

Gajjar, A., et al. (2006), 'Risk-adapted craniospinal radiotherapy followed by high-dose chemotherapy and stem-cell rescue in children with newly diagnosed medulloblastoma (St Jude Medulloblastoma-96): long-term results from a prospective, multicentre trial', *Lancet Oncol,* 7 (10), 813-20.

Gilbertson, R. J. and Ellison, D. W. (2008), 'The origins of medulloblastoma subtypes', *Annu Rev Pathol,* 3, 341-65.

Gordon, M. S., et al. (2010), 'Safety, pharmacokinetics, and pharmacodynamics of AMG 102, a fully human hepatocyte growth factor-neutralizing monoclonal antibody, in a first-in-human study of patients with advanced solid tumors', *Clin Cancer Res,* 16 (2), 699-710.

Guessous, F., et al. (2010), 'An orally bioavailable c-Met kinase inhibitor potently inhibits brain tumor malignancy and growth', *Anticancer Agents Med Chem,* 10 (1), 28-35.

Guo, A., et al. (2008), 'Signaling networks assembled by oncogenic EGFR and c-Met', *Proc Natl Acad Sci U S A,* 105 (2), 692-7.

Hammond, D. E., et al. (2001), 'Down-regulation of MET, the receptor for hepatocyte growth factor', *Oncogene,* 20 (22), 2761-70.

Hatten, M. E. and Roussel, M. F. (2011), 'Development and cancer of the cerebellum', *Trends Neurosci,* 34 (3), 134-42.

Honda, S., et al. (1995), 'Localization and functional coupling of HGF and c-Met/HGF receptor in rat brain: implication as neurotrophic factor', *Brain Res Mol Brain Res,* 32 (2), 197-210.

Hossain, M. A., et al. (2002), 'Neuroprotection by scatter factor/hepatocyte growth factor and FGF-1 in cerebellar granule neurons is phosphatidylinositol 3-kinase/akt-dependent and MAPK/CREB-independent', *J Neurochem,* 81 (2), 365-78.

Huh, C. G., et al. (2004), 'Hepatocyte growth factor/c-met signaling pathway is required for efficient liver regeneration and repair', *Proc Natl Acad Sci U S A,* 101 (13), 4477-82.

Ieraci, A., Forni, P. E., and Ponzetto, C. (2002), 'Viable hypomorphic signaling mutant of the Met receptor reveals a role for hepatocyte growth factor in postnatal cerebellar development', *Proc Natl Acad Sci U S A,* 99 (23), 15200-5.

Jun, H. T., et al. (2007), 'AMG 102, a fully human anti-hepatocyte growth factor/scatter factor neutralizing antibody, enhances the efficacy of temozolomide or docetaxel in U-87 MG cells and xenografts', *Clin Cancer Res,* 13 (22 Pt 1), 6735-42.

Jung, W., et al. (1994), 'Expression and functional interaction of hepatocyte growth factor-scatter factor and its receptor c-met in mammalian brain', *J Cell Biol,* 126 (2), 485-94.

Kammula, U. S., et al. (2007), 'Molecular co-expression of the c-Met oncogene and hepatocyte growth factor in primary colon cancer predicts tumor stage and clinical outcome', *Cancer Lett,* 248 (2), 219-28.

Kawaguchi, T., et al. (1997), 'Purification and cloning of hepatocyte growth factor activator inhibitor type 2, a Kunitz-type serine protease inhibitor', *J Biol Chem,* 272 (44), 27558-64.

Kermorgant, S. and Parker, P. J. (2005), 'c-Met signalling: spatio-temporal decisions', *Cell Cycle,* 4 (3), 352-5.

Kermorgant, S. and Parker, P. J. (2008), 'Receptor trafficking controls weak signal delivery: a strategy used by c-Met for STAT3 nuclear accumulation', *J Cell Biol,* 182 (5), 855-63.

Kim, K. J., et al. (2006), 'Systemic anti-hepatocyte growth factor monoclonal antibody therapy induces the regression of intracranial glioma xenografts', *Clin Cancer Res,* 12 (4), 1292-8.

Kongkham, P. N., et al. (2010), 'Inhibition of the MET Receptor Tyrosine Kinase as a Novel Therapeutic Strategy in Medulloblastoma', *Transl Oncol,* 3 (6), 336-43.

Kongkham, P. N., et al. (2008), 'An epigenetic genome-wide screen identifies SPINT2 as a novel tumor suppressor gene in pediatric medulloblastoma', *Cancer Res,* 68 (23), 9945-53.

Kuba, K., et al. (2000), 'HGF/NK4, a four-kringle antagonist of hepatocyte growth factor, is an angiogenesis inhibitor that suppresses tumor growth and metastasis in mice', *Cancer Res,* 60 (23), 6737-43.

Lai, A. Z., Abella, J. V., and Park, M. (2009), 'Crosstalk in Met receptor oncogenesis', *Trends Cell Biol,* 19 (10), 542-51.

Li, Y., et al. (2005), 'The scatter factor/hepatocyte growth factor: c-met pathway in human embryonal central nervous system tumor malignancy', *Cancer Res,* 65 (20), 9355-62.

Li, Y., et al. (2008a), 'Hepatocyte growth factor enhances death receptor-induced apoptosis by up-regulating DR5', *BMC Cancer,* 8, 325.

Li, Y., et al. (2008b), 'Functional and molecular interactions between the HGF/c-Met pathway and c-Myc in large-cell medulloblastoma', *Lab Invest,* 88 (2), 98-111.

Li, Y., et al. (2009), 'Interactions between PTEN and the c-Met pathway in glioblastoma and implications for therapy', *Mol Cancer Ther,* 8 (2), 376-85.

Liu, X., Newton, R. C., and Scherle, P. A. (2010), 'Developing c-MET pathway inhibitors for cancer therapy: progress and challenges', *Trends Mol Med,* 16 (1), 37-45.

MacDonald, T. J. (2008), 'Aggressive infantile embryonal tumors', *J Child Neurol,* 23 (10), 1195-204.

Mahadevan, D., et al. (2007), 'A novel tyrosine kinase switch is a mechanism of imatinib resistance in gastrointestinal stromal tumors', *Oncogene,* 26 (27), 3909-19.

Maina, F. and Klein, R. (1999), 'Hepatocyte growth factor, a versatile signal for developing neurons', *Nat Neurosci,* 2 (3), 213-7.

Marino, S. (2005), 'Medulloblastoma: developmental mechanisms out of control', *Trends Mol Med,* 11 (1), 17-22.

Martens, T., et al. (2006), 'A novel one-armed anti-c-Met antibody inhibits glioblastoma growth in vivo', *Clin Cancer Res,* 12 (20 Pt 1), 6144-52.

Matsumoto, K. and Nakamura, T. (2008), 'NK4 gene therapy targeting HGF-Met and angiogenesis', *Front Biosci,* 13, 1943-51.

Matsumoto, K., Nakamura, T., and Sakai, K. (2008), 'Hepatocyte growth factor and Met in tumor biology and therapeutic approach with NK4', *Proteomics,* 8 (16), 3360-70.

Mayor, S. (2011), 'MET inhibitors: translating from bench to bedside', *Lancet Oncol,* 12 (1), 14.

Mazzone, M., et al. (2004), 'An uncleavable form of pro-scatter factor suppresses tumor growth and dissemination in mice', *J Clin Invest,* 114 (10), 1418-32.

Michieli, P., et al. (2004), 'Targeting the tumor and its microenvironment by a dual-function decoy Met receptor', *Cancer Cell,* 6 (1), 61-73.

Mitchell, K. J., et al. (2001), 'Functional analysis of secreted and transmembrane proteins critical to mouse development', *Nat Genet,* 28 (3), 241-9.

Miyazawa, K., et al. (1993), 'Molecular cloning and sequence analysis of the cDNA for a human serine protease reponsible for activation of hepatocyte growth factor. Structural similarity of the protease precursor to blood coagulation factor XII', *J Biol Chem,* 268 (14), 10024-8.

Montesano, R., et al. (1998), 'Differential effects of hepatocyte growth factor isoforms on epithelial and endothelial tubulogenesis', *Cell Growth Differ,* 9 (5), 355-65.

Morris, M. R., et al. (2005), 'Tumor suppressor activity and epigenetic inactivation of hepatocyte growth factor activator inhibitor type 2/SPINT2 in papillary and clear cell renal cell carcinoma', *Cancer Res,* 65 (11), 4598-606.

Munshi, N., et al. (2010), 'ARQ 197, a novel and selective inhibitor of the human c-Met receptor tyrosine kinase with antitumor activity', *Mol Cancer Ther,* 9 (6), 1544-53.

Naran, S., Zhang, X., and Hughes, S. J. (2009), 'Inhibition of HGF/MET as therapy for malignancy', *Expert Opin Ther Targets,* 13 (5), 569-81.

Northcott, P. A., et al. (2010), 'Medulloblastoma Comprises Four Distinct Molecular Variants', *J Clin Oncol.*

Orian-Rousseau, V., et al. (2002), 'CD44 is required for two consecutive steps in HGF/c-Met signaling', *Genes Dev,* 16 (23), 3074-86.

Otsuka, T., et al. (2000), 'Disassociation of met-mediated biological responses in vivo: the natural hepatocyte growth factor/scatter factor splice variant NK2 antagonizes growth but facilitates metastasis', *Mol Cell Biol,* 20 (6), 2055-65.

Packer, R. J., Rood, B. R., and MacDonald, T. J. (2003), 'Medulloblastoma: present concepts of stratification into risk groups', *Pediatr Neurosurg,* 39 (2), 60-7.

Parr, C., et al. (2004), 'The hepatocyte growth factor regulatory factors in human breast cancer', *Clin Cancer Res,* 10 (1 Pt 1), 202-11.

Pfister, S. M., et al. (2010), 'Molecular diagnostics of CNS embryonal tumors', *Acta Neuropathol,* 120 (5), 553-66.

Provencal, M., et al. (2010), 'Tissue factor mediates the HGF/Met-induced anti-apoptotic pathway in DAOY medulloblastoma cells', *J Neurooncol,* 97 (3), 365-72.

Provencal, M., et al. (2009), 'c-Met activation in medulloblastoma induces tissue factor expression and activity: effects on cell migration', *Carcinogenesis,* 30 (7), 1089-96.

Qi, W., et al. (2009), 'MP470, a novel receptor tyrosine kinase inhibitor, in combination with Erlotinib inhibits the HER family/PI3K/Akt pathway and tumor growth in prostate cancer', *BMC Cancer,* 9, 142.

Qian, F., et al. (2009), 'Inhibition of tumor cell growth, invasion, and metastasis by EXEL-2880 (XL880, GSK1363089), a novel inhibitor of HGF and VEGF receptor tyrosine kinases', *Cancer Res,* 69 (20), 8009-16.

Reardon, D.A., et al (2008), 'Phase II study of AMG 102, a fully human neutralizing antibody against hepatocyte growth factor/scatter factor, in patients with recurrent glioblastoma multiforme.', *J Clin Oncol,* 26 (Abstr 2051).

Rong, S., et al. (1994), 'Invasiveness and metastasis of NIH 3T3 cells induced by Met-hepatocyte growth factor/scatter factor autocrine stimulation', *Proc Natl Acad Sci U S A,* 91 (11), 4731-5.

Rosen, P. J., et al. (2008), 'AMG102, an HGF/SF antagonist, in combination with anti-angiogenesis targeted therapies in adult patients with advanced solid tumors', *J Clin Oncol,* 26 (Abstr 3570).

Sanders, R. P., et al. (2008), 'M1 Medulloblastoma: high risk at any age', *J Neurooncol,* 90 (3), 351-5.

Shimomura, T., et al. (1997), 'Hepatocyte growth factor activator inhibitor, a novel Kunitz-type serine protease inhibitor', *J Biol Chem,* 272 (10), 6370-6.

Smolen, G. A., et al. (2006), 'Amplification of MET may identify a subset of cancers with extreme sensitivity to the selective tyrosine kinase inhibitor PHA-665752', *Proc Natl Acad Sci U S A,* 103 (7), 2316-21.

Stein, U., et al. (2009), 'MACC1, a newly identified key regulator of HGF-MET signaling, predicts colon cancer metastasis', *Nat Med,* 15 (1), 59-67.

Stommel, J. M., et al. (2007), 'Coactivation of receptor tyrosine kinases affects the response of tumor cells to targeted therapies', *Science,* 318 (5848), 287-90.

Suliman, A., et al. (2001), 'Intracellular mechanisms of TRAIL: apoptosis through mitochondrial-dependent and -independent pathways', *Oncogene,* 20 (17), 2122-33.

Takayama, H., et al. (1997), 'Diverse tumorigenesis associated with aberrant development in mice overexpressing hepatocyte growth factor/scatter factor', *Proc Natl Acad Sci U S A,* 94 (2), 701-6.

Tong, C. Y., et al. (2004), 'Detection of oncogene amplifications in medulloblastomas by comparative genomic hybridization and array-based comparative genomic hybridization', *J Neurosurg,* 100 (2 Suppl Pediatrics), 187-93.

Trusolino, L., Bertotti, A., and Comoglio, P. M. (2010), 'MET signalling: principles and functions in development, organ regeneration and cancer', *Nat Rev Mol Cell Biol,* 11 (12), 834-48.

Uehara, Y., et al. (1995), 'Placental defect and embryonic lethality in mice lacking hepatocyte growth factor/scatter factor', *Nature,* 373 (6516), 702-5.

Welsh, J. W., et al. (2009), 'The c-Met receptor tyrosine kinase inhibitor MP470 radiosensitizes glioblastoma cells', *Radiat Oncol,* 4, 69.

Wojtukiewicz, M. Z., et al. (2001), 'The hemostatic system and angiogenesis in malignancy', *Neoplasia,* 3 (5), 371-84.

Zeltzer, P. M., et al. (1999), 'Metastasis stage, adjuvant treatment, and residual tumor are prognostic factors for medulloblastoma in children: conclusions from the Children's Cancer Group 921 randomized phase III study', *J Clin Oncol,* 17 (3), 832-45.

Zhang, L., et al. (2000), 'Hepatocyte growth factor protects cultured rat cerebellar granule neurons from apoptosis via the phosphatidylinositol-3 kinase/Akt pathway', *J Neurosci Res,* 59 (4), 489-96.

Zhang, Y. W., et al. (2002), 'Requirement of Stat3 signaling for HGF/SF-Met mediated tumorigenesis', *Oncogene,* 21 (2), 217-26.

Zhang, Y. W., et al. (2003), 'Hepatocyte growth factor/scatter factor mediates angiogenesis through positive VEGF and negative thrombospondin 1 regulation', *Proc Natl Acad Sci U S A,* 100 (22), 12718-23.

Zhang, Y. W., et al. (2010), 'MET kinase inhibitor SGX523 synergizes with epidermal growth factor receptor inhibitor erlotinib in a hepatocyte growth factor-dependent fashion to suppress carcinoma growth', *Cancer Res,* 70 (17), 6880-90.

Zillhardt, M., Christensen, J. G., and Lengyel, E. (2010), 'An orally available small-molecule inhibitor of c-Met, PF-2341066, reduces tumor burden and metastasis in a preclinical model of ovarian cancer metastasis', *Neoplasia,* 12 (1), 1-10.

Zou, H. Y., et al. (2007), 'An orally available small-molecule inhibitor of c-Met, PF-2341066, exhibits cytoreductive antitumor efficacy through antiproliferative and antiangiogenic mechanisms', *Cancer Res,* 67 (9), 4408-17.

Part 18

The Importance of Redox Regulation of Malignant Cell Survival

31

The Impact of Redox Balance in Brain Tumors

Pinar Atukeren
Istanbul University, Cerrahpasa Medical Faculty, Department of Biochemistry
Turkey

1. Introduction

In a normal cell, there exists a balance between the free radical generation and the antioxidant defense (Devi et al., 2000). It has long been documented that cancer cells are under increased and persistent oxidative stress due to increased reactive oxygen species. Oxidative stress describes the state of a cell whose antioxidant mechanisms can not manage its content of free radicals (Figure 1). As a consequence, cellular constituents are disrupted, and free radical reactions become less controllable since endogenous antioxidants are themselves injured by oxidative insults. Oxidative stress induces a cellular redox imbalance which has been found to be present in various cancer cells compared with normal cells; the redox imbalance thus may be related to oncogenic stimulation (Valko et al., 2006). Increased intrinsic reactive oxygen species (ROS) stress in cancer cells has been speculated to be due to a number of factors such as oncogenic stimulation, increased metabolic activity, and mitochondrial malfunction (Pelicano et al., 2004).The cellular redox state has important effects on the control of cell survival, apoptosis, and expression of tumor suppressor genes. A high cell redox state would encourage tumor formation by creating an enhanced cell proliferative environment. In opposition to this, a high cell redox state would also support increased apoptosis, which would inhibit tumor formation by eliminating partially transformed cells. In addition to ROS, various redox metals, due to their ability to generate free radicals, or non-redox metals, due to their ability to bind to critical thiols, have been implicated in the mechanisms of carcinogenesis. (Leonard et al., 2004; Valko et al., 2005). Cancer cells can generate large amounts of hydrogen peroxide and this, if it occurs in vivo, may contribute to their ability to mutate and damage normal tissues, and, moreover, facilitate tumour growth and invasion (Burdon, 1995). Indeed, it has been suggested that persistent oxidative stress in tumour cells could partly explain some important characteristics of cancer. A wide variety of normal and malignant cell types generate and release superoxide or hydrogen peroxide in vitro either in response to specific cytokine and growth factor stimulus or constitutively in the case of tumour cells (Szatrowski at al., 1991). Tumors of the nervous system are among the most common and pharmacologically intractable neoplastic disorders. Malignant peripheral nervous system tumors include neuroblastoma, the most common extracranial solid tumor. Because of the frequency with which neuroblastoma is metastatic or otherwise surgically incurable at the time of diagnosis, treatment of this tumor often involves chemotherapy. Malignant gliomas comprise the majority of primary brain tumors. (Louis et al., 2002). Of these, glioblastoma multiforme (GBM) is the most common and has the poorest prognosis. It is therefore apparent that a more complete understanding of malignant gliomas and the pathophysiologic mechanisms responsible for tumor growth, invasion, and resistance to therapy is needed. Meningiomas are the most common types of the non gliomatous primary brain tumors, followed by schwannomas.

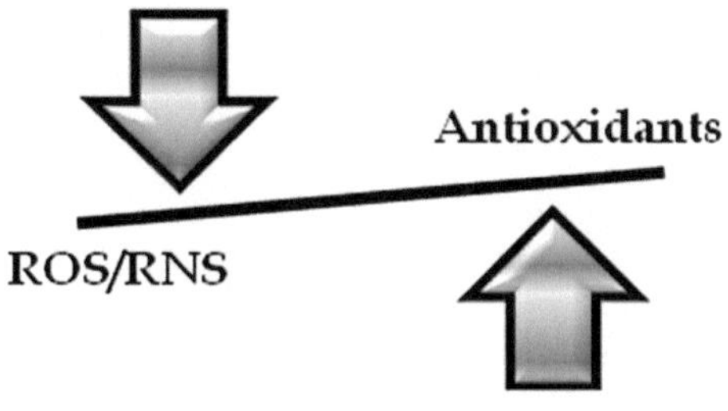

Fig. 1. Oxidative stress balance

2. Oxidative stress and neuronal redox countenance in the brain

Redox balance in neural tissue has an important role in the pathophysiology of neurotoxicity from free radical generation, but also in the pathophysiology of neurotoxicity from free radical generation. The concept of redox status includes both physiological and pathological effects of redox phenomena. ROS are particularly active in the brain and neuronal tissue and aggressive to glial cells and neurons. In-built endogenous antioxidant system plays its decisive role in prevention of any loss due to free radicals. However, imbalanced defense mechanism of antioxidants, overproduction or incorporation of free radicals from environment to living system leads to serious penalty and therefore to neuronal death (Halliwell, 2001). The brain has high content of peroxidizable unsaturated fatty acids, high oxygen consumption per unit weight, high content of iron which is a key in lipid peroxidation and a shortage of antioxidant defense systems (Floyd, 1999) so is more susceptible to oxidative stress compared to other tissues and is unique as a target organ for metastatic growth being surrounded by the blood-brain barrier. The generation of ROS, or free radicals, can exceed the scavenging ability of endogenous antioxidants, resulting in a shift of the redox state of the brain to the oxidative state.

The concentrations of free heavy metals are also tightly controlled in the nervous system by transport proteins such as ferritin (Sies, 1993), thus limiting the non-enzymatic catalysis of hydroxyl radical formation. The nervous system contains some antioxidant enzymes; including Cu/Zn- and Mn dependent superoxide dismutase (SOD), and glutathione peroxidase (GPx) which are expressed in higher quantities than catalase (Shivakumar et al., 1991; Hussain et al., 1995). This spectrum of enzymatic defences suggests that the brain may efficiently metabolize superoxide but may have difficulties in eliminating the hydrogen peroxide produced by the reaction. The accumulation of hydrogen peroxide is of major concern since the brain contains large quantities of iron and copper (Moos, 1995), which may catalyse the formation of the hydroxyl radical and induce lipid peroxidation (Oubidar et al., 1996)(Fig.1). Exogenous antioxidants are nowadays considered a promising therapeutic approach since they could play an important role in preventing and/or minimizing neuronal oxidative damage (Halliwell, 2001; Uttara et al., 2009).

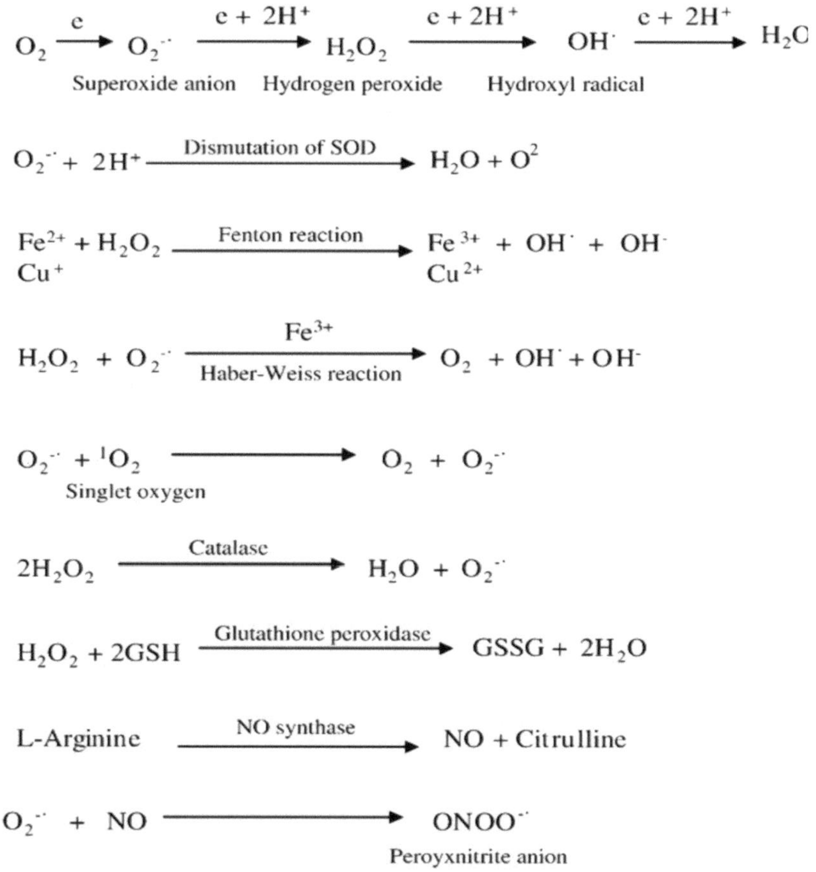

Fig. 2. Reactions of oxygen and nitrogen species

3. Reactive oxygen species (ROS) and reactive nitrogen species (RNS)

Reactive oxygen species (ROS) and reactive nitrogen species (RNS) are products of normal cellular metabolism. The interest in the role of oxygen-free radicals, more generally known as ROS and of RNS in experimental and clinical medicine is consequential (Halliwell, 1999). ROS/RNS are known to play a dual role since they can be either harmful or beneficial (Valko et al., 2004). Utile effects of ROS are having physiological roles in cellular responses to noxa and in the function of a number of cellular signalling systems. The harmful effects of ROS are balanced by the antioxidant action of nonenzymatic antioxidants in addition to antioxidant enzymes (Halliwell, 1996). ROS/RNS are known to act as secondary messengers controlling various normal physiological functions of the organism. In addition, ROS and RNS participate in various redox-regulatory mechanisms of cells in order to protect cells against oxidative stress and maintenance of cellular redox homeostasis. The cumulative production of ROS through either endogenous or exogenous insults is common for many types of cancer cell that are linked with altered redox regulation of cellular signaling pathways. ROS are not only toxicants to the cell, but also second messengers in intracellular signal transduction, and control the action of several signaling pathways. RNS include a series of metabolites which are nitric oxide, nitrite, peroxynitrite with functional implication mainly in vascular stability. Overproduction of reactive nitrogen species is called nitrosative stress (Klatt & Lamas, 2000). This may occur when the generation of reactive nitrogen species in a system exceeds the system's ability to neutralise and eliminate them. Nitrosative stress may lead to nitrosylation reactions that can alter the structure of proteins and so inhibit their normal function and there has been much interest in the roles nitric oxide may play in the pathogenesis of GBM. When ROS/RNS levels exceed a certain threshold, deleterious effects are apparent and became dangerous for cell integrity (Panayiotidis et al., 1999; Barbouti et al., 2002). Oxidative stress can be defined as a deterioration of redox signaling and control (Jones, 2006). Overproduction of reactive oxygen species (ROS) and reactive nitrogen species (RNS), a decreased antioxidant defense system, or both typically results in significant protein oxidation (Hensley et al., 1995; Stadtman & Berlett, 1997), lipid peroxidation (Markesbery & Lovell, 1998; Butterfield & Lauderback, 2002), and DNA/RNA oxidation (Butterfield et al., 2001). Increased formation of ROS and RNS in the cells can contribute to the process of carcinogenesis through either direct genotoxic effects or indirect via modification of signaling pathways that lead to altered expression of numerous genes. Modulations of cell signaling pathways can activate transcriptional factors, like AP-1, NF-jB, HIF-1, and p53 among others (Arrigo, 1999; Bensaad, 2005). These transcriptional factors control the expression of genes the protein products of which participate in complex signal transduction pathways that can lead to cell transformation.The effect of reactive oxygen and nitrogen species is balanced by the antioxidant action of nonenzymatic antioxidants, as well as by antioxidant enzymes. Such antioxidant defences are extremely important as they represent the direct removal of free radicals, thus providing maximal protection for biological sites. As key mediators of cellular oxidative stress and redox state, ROS and RNS also provide plausible platforms for drug design. In fact, the efficacy of a number of established anticancer drugs.

4. Redox status and apoptosis

The intracellular redox state which is directly related to the production of intracellular reactive oxygen species in cancer cells has also been indicated to control the aggressiveness of cancer cells. Cancer development represents a multistage process in which at least three distinct stages which are; initiation, promotion and progression are involved (Klaunig, 2004) and is characterized with increased cell growth and/or decreased capacity for apoptosis. Apoptosis is potentially a protective mechanism against both exogenous carcinogens and inflammatory states and is regulated in part by the cellular redox state. Since apoptosis is caused by elevated levels of free radicals, decreased concentrations of free radicals due to the excessive administration of antioxidants might actually stimulate survival of damaged cells and proliferation into neoplastic state and thus rather promote process of carcinogenesis than interrupt it. Mitochondrial driven apoptosis is most interesting when ROS mediated mechanisms are being considered. Typical features in apoptosis include permeabilization of the mitochondrial membrane in a process associated with ROS generation. Some of the physiological effects of free radicals may be mediated through their influuence on redox sensitive transcription factors (Suzuki et al., 1997) and consequently modulation of gene expression (Cimino et al., 1997). Although care should be taken before concluding that free radicals are intracellular second messengers, there is growing agreement that they act as modulators of cell signaling and messenger systems. Therefore, it seems that the cellular redox status, defined as the balance between intracellular oxidants and antioxidants, is regulated so as to lie within an optimal range for cell survival. The importance of cellular antioxidant capacity as the result of a complex cell program involves enhanced motility and a profound change in energy metabolism so avoiding oxidative damage and escaping excess ROS in the primary tumor site in cancer cells explain why redox signaling pathways are important.

5. Antioxidant defence

Cells have numerous protective mechanisms that maintain the concentrations of ROS within a range compatible with survival. The most efficient enzymatic antioxidants involve superoxide dismutase, catalase and glutathione peroxidase (Mates et al., 1999). Non enzymatic antioxidants involve vitamin C, vitamin E, carotenoids, thiol antioxidants (glutathione, thioredoxin and lipoic acid), natural flavonoids, melatonin and other compounds (McCall & Frei, 1999). Some antioxidants act in a hydrophilic environment, others in a hydrophobic environment, and some act in both environments of the cell. Glutathione (GSH), a thiol-containing tripeptide, is a major antioxidant and a cofactor of glutathione peroxidases (Meister, 1995); it is present in large quantities in the developing nervous system It has been hypothesized that some trophic factors may upregulate neuronal antioxidant capacities (Mattson and Furukawa, 1996). If neuronal death involves an imbalance of the redox status towards oxidation, antioxidants should be protective.

GSH is a major intracellular antioxidant present ubiquitously in the brain in millimolar amounts. GSH detoxifies intracellular H_2O_2 to H_2O and O_2 via oxidation to glutathione disulfide (GSSG) by the enzyme GPx. GSSG is recycled to GSH via glutathione reductase (GR). The GSH/GSSG ratio is critical to maintaining the intracellular redox balance (Smith et al., 1996). A decrease in total GSH levels, or an imbalance in the ratio of reduced to oxidized GSH may cause oxidative stress (Stadtman & Berlett, 1997) and lipid peroxidation (Markesbery & Lovell, 1998). So, the brain is heavily dependent on GSH as a primary endogenous neuroprotectant. It has been reported that elevation of intracellular GSH in tumour cells is associated with mitogenic stimulation (Shaw & Chou, 1986), that GSH controls the onset of tumour-cell proliferation by regulating protein kinase C activity and intracellular pH (Terradez et al., 1993). GSH and its dependent enzymes work in concert with other antioxidants and antioxidant enzymes to protect cells against reactive oxygen intermediates (Sies, 1986). So, it can be said that reduced GSH plays a role in the rescue of cells from apoptosis. GPx and GR decrease and protein oxidation increases in patients with glioblastoma multiforme and transitional meningioma and clear different oxidative status was found in the two kinds of tumors which represent specially one of the most malignant and most benign tumors respectively (Tanriverdi et al., 2007) and it was shown that there is a complex relationship between pro- and anti-apoptotic molecules in glioblastoma multiforme pathogenesis, thus targeting multiple pathways with advanced chemotherapeutic agents or radiotheraupetic regimens following total resections might be helpful in patients with glioblastoma multiforme (Atukeren et al., 2010). So the development of chemopreventive strategies would be desirably based on an association between a particular beneficial effect and a redox condition, as for example, with antioxidant protection against oxidative stress.

6. Mitochondrial redox status

One of the important sources for ROS generation is the mitochondria where some of the oxygen is reduced by single steps of one electron reduction, thus releasing superoxide radical and other ROS (Giorgio et al., 2007). However, it is difficult to detect the occurrence of the superoxide radical in intact mitochondria, most probably in consequence of the presence of high SOD activity therein. Mitochondria have long been known to generate significant quantities of hydrogen peroxide as mitochondrial generation of superoxide to that of hydrogen peroxide is known. Since mitochondria are the major site of free radical generation, they are highly enriched with antioxidants including GSH and enzymes, such as SOD and GPx, which are present on both sides of their membranes in order to minimise oxidative stress in the organelle (Cadenas & Davies, 2000). Superoxide radicals are efficiently detoxified initially to hydrogen peroxide and then to water by Cu/ZnSOD and MnSOD. The redox components of the cell consists of interlinked mitochondrial redox indicators: glutathione (GSH/GSSG), thioredoxin (Trx/TrxR), glutaredoxin (Grx), peroxiredoxins (Prx), systems dependent solely on steady flux of NADPH generated through reduction of $NADP^+$ by NADH by the energetic component of mitochondria (Figure 3). Trx/TrxR system reverses protein disulfide linkages that occur in thiols of oxidized cysteine residues (Holmgren, 1985). Upregulation in the activity of the Trx/TrxR system seen in many tumors is thought to be a result of increased ROS production associated with oncogenic transformation and correlates with resistance to apoptosis and tumor cell proliferation (Baker et al., 1997; Lincoln et al., 2003). Disruption of the cellular redox state via inhibition of TrxR, either in the cytosol or the mitochondria has been shown to increase the ratio of oxidized/reduced Trx, increase ROS, modulate cell signaling, sensitize cancer cell lines to chemotherapeutic agents, and induce cell cycle arrest, senescence and apoptosis of cancer cells (Urig &vBecker, 2006; Mukherjee & Martin, 2008) so decrease in mitochondrial bioenergetic capacity and altered redox status should be

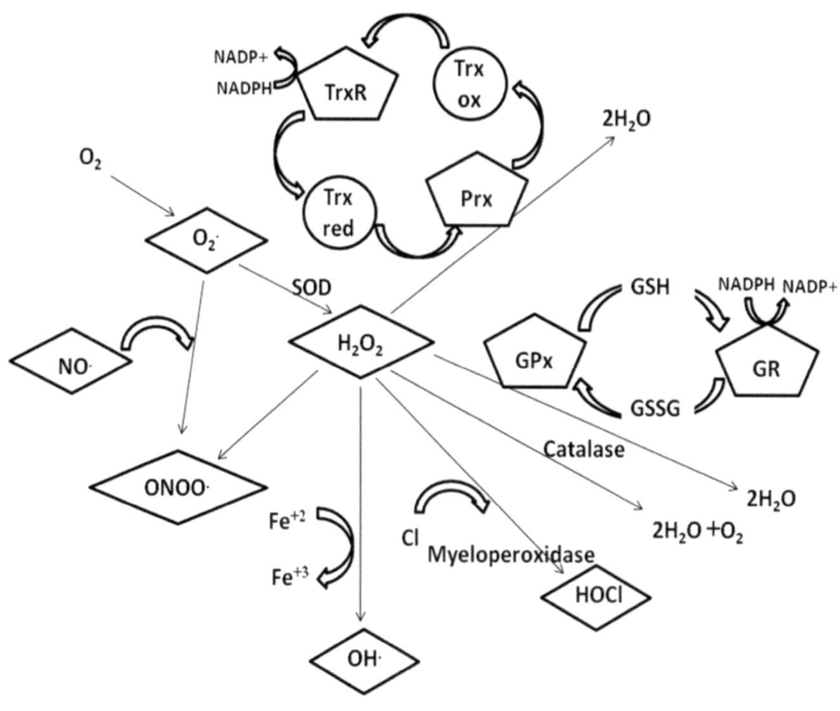

Fig. 3. Redox reactions

viewed as a concerted process. Prx are a family of proteins that function in antioxidant defense and in redox signaling cascades by reaction with peroxides. During their catalytic cycle, oxidized species of Prx are reduced and reactivated by thioredoxin or glutathione (Immenschuh & Baumgart-Vogt, 2005; Winterbourn & Hampton, 2008) and GSH is important for a wide range of cellular redox active proteins and pathways, including glutaredoxin (Grx), glutathione S-transferase (GST), glutathione peroxidase (GPx) and more (Meister & Anderson, 1983; Go et al., 2009).

7. Prospects of antioxidant therapy

Several antioxidant defense mechanisms have evolved to protect cell components from the harmful effects of ROS and RNS. As is known two major groups of endogenous antioxidants are low molecular weight antioxidant compounds such as vitamin C and vitamin E, lipoic acid and ubiquinones and antioxidant enzymes (Gilgun-Sherki et al., 2001). Antioxidant enzymes activity and concentration of nonenzymatic antioxidants in human brain tumours were evaluated and significant increases in all enzyme activities and decreases in GSH and ascorbate levels were observed in brain tumors (Dudek et al., 2004) and consistent differences in the levels of antioxidants in different types of brain tumors were emphasized in different studies (Hanimoglu et al., 2007; Tanriverdi et al., 2007; Tuzgen et al., 2007; Zengin et al., 2009). The relationship between oxidative gene polymorphism and the risk of brain tumors is investigated and it was seen that; the increased risk of glioma and meningioma type brain tumors is related with variants in some antioxidant enzyme genes (Rajaraman et al., 2008) and in a study, tissue expression of MnSOD is suggested to be a prognostic marker for glioblastoma (Park et al., 2009). The importance of daily intake of antioxidants among people with malignant glioma was shown in various studies (Il'yasova et al., 2009; DeLorenze et al., 2010). Recently, exogenous antioxidants are considered a promising therapeutic approach in preventing or minimizing neuronal oxidative damage (Halliwell, 2001; Uttara et al., 2009). Recent interest has been focused on dietary phenolic antioxidants, such as carotenoids, cinnamic acids and flavonoids, as potentially useful agents (Fresco et al., 2006; Uttara et al., 2009). In a study, the effects of flavonoids which are natural polyphenolic antioxidant compounds in brain development, neuroprotection and glial tumor formation are discussed and suggested to develop new therapeutic approaches (Nones et al.; 2010). Curcumin as a polyphenol gets attention in blocking brain tumor formation in a study. The chemopreventive and anticarcinogenic action of curcumin is shown and suggested as this might be due to its ability to inhibit proteins that initiate protective signals (Sudarshana et al., 2009). Also, Gynostemma pentaphyllum extract selectively shifted H_2O_2 concentration in glioma tumor cells to toxic levels due to increased SOD activity so can be suggested for cancer therapy (Schild et al., 2010) and the apoptotic effect of γ-Mangostin in Garcinia mangostana fruit was investigated and it was suggested as a potential in developing an anti brain tumor agent (Chang et al., 2010). In another study, the potential therapeutic effect of resveratrol being a dietary phytochemical antioxidant, is investigated in glioma type brain tumors (Gangliano et al., 2010). Also another study implies the importance of using nutritional antioxidants such as lycopene for their potential therapeutic benefit in the adjuvant management of high-grade gliomas (Puri et al., 2010). So antioxidants are incontestably implicated in brain cancer treatment and they may protect against side effects from conventional therapies, as well as enhance chemotherapy and support anticancer activities. Obviously, antioxidants must be chosen based on their ability to treat a particular redox event or they must act contextually and evolve with the redox conditions to restore balance.

8. Conclusion

Various studies showed that not only oxidants but the redox status as a whole modulates mechanisms regulating neuronal fate. The deleterious effects of high concentrations of antioxidants and the protective actions of sublethal oxidative challenges suggest that neuronal survival depends on the maintenance of an adequate redox status between the two extremes of oxidative and reductive stress, respectively. In addition to its widespread consequences for our understanding of fundamental aspects of neuronal death, the concept of neuronal redox status as opposed to oxidative stress may have clinical implications. Neuronal survival thus seems to be associated with an optimal redox status; an imbalance towards oxidation leads to oxidative stress, whereas high doses of antioxidants may induce a reductive stress. Maintenance of intracellular redox state is critical to cellular homeostasis therefore tumor selectivity in targeting at the cellular and enzymatic levels are of great interest to the rational design of treating compounds. Targeting the mitochondrial apoptotic regulatory machinery is also a promising anticancer approach and in many studies thiol redox platforms were used to discover and develop drugs. Strategies for redox balance analysis rely on different assumption and this approach gives a dynamic idea of what is the general oxidative status in a given condition and evaluation of redox potential of molecules gives idea of what really happened in a period that is a function of half life of a given molecule so this maybe utilized in parallel to gain a more representative picture of a clinical conditioning evolution. Hence, chemotherapeutic outcomes are not compromised, administration of antioxidants capable of maintaining the antioxidant defense system in brain may protect cancer patients from the apparent cognitive rigors of chemotherapy and these redox manipulating compounds could be used in conjunction with existing treatments to beneficial effect. So, it can be said that, as a preliminary approach, to determine optimal doses of antioxidants in order to design treatment protocols respecting the redox homeostasis would be useful.

9. Acknowledgment

I would like to express my gratitude to all those who I am deeply indebted; Prof.Dr.Bekir Kocazeybek, Prof.Dr.Ibrahim Balcioglu, Prof.Dr.Tuncay Altug, Prof.Dr.Ezel Uslu, Ms.Iva Simcic, Mr. Sanju Paul Kadavil, dear friends and my dear family whose encouragement and support helped me to carry on my academic career, complete my work and enlightened my path. I would be honored to dedicate this chapter to women in science all around the world.

10. References

Arrigo, AP. (1999). Gene expression and the thiol redox state, *Free Radic. Biol. Med.*, Vol. 27, pp.936–944

Atukeren, P.; Kemerdere, R.; Kacira, T.; Hanimoglu, H.; Ozlen, F.; Yavuz, B.; Tanriverdi, T.; Gumustas, K. & Canbaz, B. (2010). Expressions of some vital molecules: glioblastoma multiforme versus normal tissues, *Neurol Res.*,Vol.32, No.5, pp. 492-501

Baker, A.; Payne, C., Briehl, M. & Powis, G. (1997). Thioredoxin, a gene found overexpressed in human cancer, inhibits apoptosis in vitro and in vivo, *Cancer Res.*, Vol. 57, pp. 5162-5167

Barbouti, A.; Doulias, PT.; Nousis, L.; Tenopoulou, M. & Galaris D. (2002). DNA damage And apoptosis in hydrogen peroxideexposed Jurkat cells: bolus addition versus continuous generation of $H_{(2)}O_{(2)}$, *Free Radic. Biol. Med.*, Vol. 33, pp. 691-702

Bensaad, K. & Vousden, KH. (2005). Savior and slayer: the two faces of p53, *Nat. Med.*, Vol. 11, pp. 1278-1279

Burdon, RH. (1995). Superoxide and hydrogen peroxide in relation to mammalian cell proliferation, *Free Radic. Biol. Med.*, Vol. 18, pp. 775- 794

Butterfield, DA.; Drake, J.; Pocernich, C. & Castegna, A. (2001). Evidence of oxidative damage in Alzheimer's disease brain: central role for amyloid beta-peptide, *Trends Mol Med.*, Vol. 7, pp. 548-554

Butterfield, DA. & Lauderback CM. (2002). Lipid peroxidation and protein oxidation in Alzheimer's disease brain: potential causes and consequences involving amyloid beta-peptide-associated free radical oxidative stress, *Free Radic Biol Med.*, Vol. 32, pp. 1050-1060

Cadenas, E. & Davies KJA. (2000). Mitochondrial free radical generation, oxidative stress, and aging, *Free Rad. Biol. Med.*, Vol. 29, pp. 222-230

Chang, HF.; Huang, WT.; Chen HJ. & Yang LL. (2010). Apoptotic Effects of γ-Mangostin from the Fruit Hull of Garcinia mangostana on Human Malignant Glioma Cells, *Molecules,* Vol. 7, No. 15(12), pp. 8953-66

Cimino, F.; Esposito, F.; Ammendola, R. & Russo, T. (1997). Gene regulation by reactive oxygen species, *Curr. Topics Cell Regul.*, Vol. 35, pp. 123-148

DeLorenze, GN.; McCoy, L.; Tsai, AL.; Quesenberry, CP Jr.; Rice, T.; Il'yasova, D. & Wrensch M. (2010). Daily intake of antioxidants in relation to survival among adult patients diagnosed with malignant glioma, *BMC Cancer,* Vol.19, pp. 10-215

Devi, GS.; Prasad, MH.; Saraswathi, I.; Raghu, D.;, Rao, DN. & Reddy, PP. (2000). Free radicals antioxidant enzymes and lipid peroxidation in different types of leukemia, *Clin Chim Acta,* Vol. 293, pp. 53-62

Dudek, H.; Farbiszewski, R.; Rydzewska, M.; Michno, T. & Kozłowski A. (2004). Evaluation of antioxidant enzymes activity and concentration of non-enzymatic antioxidants in human brain tumours, *Wiad Lek.*, Vol. 57, No. 1-2, pp. 16-9

Floyd, RA. (1999). Antioxidants, oxidative stress, and degenerative neurological disorders, *Proc Soc Exp Biol Med,* Vol. 222, No. 3, pp. 236- 45

Fresco, P.; Borges, F.; Diniz, C. & Marques, M.P.M. (2006). New insights on the anticancer properties of dietary polyphenols, *Med. Res. Rev.*, Vol. 26, No. 6, pp. 747-66

Gagliano, N; Aldini, G.; Colombo, G.; Rossi, R.; Colombo, R; Gioia, M.; Milzani, A.; & Dalle-Donne, I. (2010). The potential of resveratrol against human gliomas, *Anticancer Drugs.*, Vol.21, No.2, pp. 140-50

Giorgio, M.; Trinei, M.; Migliaccio, E. & Pelicci, PG. (2007). Hydrogen peroxide: a metabolic by-product or a common mediator of ageing signals?, *Nat Rev. Mol. Cell Biol.*, Vol. 8, pp. 722-728

Gilgun-Sherki, Y.; Melamed, E. & Offen, D. (2001). Oxidative stress induced neurodegenerative diseases: the need for antioxidants that penetrate the blood brain barrier, *Neuropharmacology,* Vol. 40, No. 8, pp. 959- 75

Go, YM.; Pohl, J. & Jones, DP. (2009). Quantification of redox conditions in the nucleus, *Methods Mol. Biol.,* Vol. 464, pp. 303–317

Halliwell, B. (1996). Antioxidants in human health and disease, *Ann. Rev. Nutr.*, Vol. 16, pp. 33–50

Halliwell, B. & Gutteridge, JMC. (1999). *Free Radicals in Biology and Medicine,* 3rd ed., Oxford University Press, Oxford, UK

Halliwell, B. (2001). Role of free radicals in the neurodegenerative diseases: therapeutic implications for antioxidant treatment, *Drugs Aging,* Vol. 18, No. 9, pp. 685-716

Hanimoglu, H.; Tanriverdi, T.; Kacira, T.; Sanus, GZ.; Atukeren, P.; Aydin, S.; Tunali, Y.; Gumustas, K. & Kaynar, MY. (2007). Relationship between DNA damage and total antioxidant capacity in patients with transitional meningioma, *Clin Neurol Neurosurg.,* Vol. 109, No. 7, pp. 561-6

Hensley, K.; Hall, N.; Subramaniam, R.; Cole, P.; Harris, M.; Aksenov, M.; Aksenova, M.; Gabbita, SP.; Wu, JF.; Carney, JM. & et al. (1995). Brain regional correspondence between Alzheimer's disease histopathology and biomarkers of protein oxidation, *J. Neurochem.,* Vol. 65, pp. 2146–2156

Holmgren, A. (1985). Thioredoxin, *Annu. Rev. Biochem.,* Vol. 54, pp. 237–271 Hussain, S.; Slikker, Jr W. & Ali, S.F. (1995). Age-related changes in antioxidant enzymes, superoxide dismutase, catalase, glutathione peroxidase and glutathione in different regions of mouse brain, *Int. J. Dev. Neurosci.,* Vol. 13, pp. 811- 817

Il'yasova, D.; Marcello, JE.; McCoy, L.; Rice, T. & Wrensch, M. (2009). Total dietary antioxidant index and survival in patients with glioblastoma multiforme, *Cancer Causes Control,* Vol.20, No. 8, pp. 1255-60 Immenschuh, S. & Baumgart-Vogt, E. (2005). Peroxiredoxins, oxidative stress, and cell proliferation, *Antioxid. Redox Signal.,* Vol. 7, pp. 768–777

Jones, DP. (2006). Redefining oxidative stress, *Antioxid. Redox Signal.,* Vol. 8, pp. 1865–1879 Klatt, P. & - Lamas, S. (2000). Regulation of protein function by S-glutathiolation in response to oxidative and nitrosative stress, *Eur. J. Biochem.,* Vol. 267, pp. 4928–4944

Klaunig, JE. & Kamendulis, LM. (2004). The role of oxidative stress in carcinogenesis, *Annu. Rev. Pharmacol. Toxicol.,* Vol. 44, pp. 239–267

Leonard, S.S., Harris, G.K., & Shi, X. (2004). Metal-induced oxidative stress and signal transduction, *Free Radic. Biol. Med.,* Vol. 37, pp. 1921–1942

Lincoln, D.; Ali Emadi, E.; Tonissen, K. & Clarke, F. (2003). The thioredoxin–thioredoxin reductase system: over-expression in human cancer, *Anticancer Res.,* Vol. 23, pp. 2425–2433

Louis, D.N.; Pomeroy, S.L. & Cairncross, J.G. (2002). Focus on central nervous system neoplasia, *Cancer Cell,* Vol. 1, pp. 125–128

Markesbery, WR. & Lovell, MA. (1998) Four-hydroxynonenal, a product of lipid peroxidation, is increased in the brain in Alzheimer's disease, *Neurobiol Aging,* Vol. 19, pp. 33–36

Mates, JM.; Perez-Gomez, C. & De Castro, IN. (1999). Antioxidant enzymes and human diseases, *Clin. Biochem.,* Vol. 32, pp. 595–603

Mattson, M.P. & Furukawa, K. (1996). Programmed cell life: Anti-apoptotic signaling and therapeutic strategies for neurodegenerative disorders, *Restor. Neurol. Neurosci.,* Vol. 9, pp. 191- 205

McCall, MR. & Frei, B. (1999). Can antioxidant vitamins materially reduce oxidative damage in humans?, *Free Rad. Biol. Med.*, Vol. 26, pp. 1034–1053

Meister, A. & Anderson, ME. (1983). Glutathione, *Annu. Rev. Biochem.*, Vol. 52, pp. 711-760

Meister, A. (1995). Glutathione biosynthesis and its inhibition, *Methods Enzymol.*, Vol. 252, pp. 26-30

Moos, T. (1995). Developmental profile of non-heme iron distribution in the rat brain during ontogenesis, *Dev. Brain Res.*, Vol. 87, pp. 203-213

Mukherjee, A. & Martin, S. (2008). The thioredoxin system: a key target in tumour and endothelial cells, *Br. J. Radiol.* Vol. 81, pp. 57–68

Nones, J.; Stipursky, J.; Costa, SL.; Gomes, FC. (2010). Flavonoids and astrocytes crosstalking: implications for brain development and pathology, *Neurochem. Res.*, Vol. 35, No. 7, pp. 955-66

Oubidar, M.; Boquillon, M.; Marie, C.; Bouvier, C.; Beley, A.; & Bralet, J. (1996). Effect of intracellular iron loading on lipid per- oxidation of brain slices. *Free Radic. Biol. Med.*, Vol. 21, pp. 763-769

Panayiotidis, M.; Tsolas, O. & Galaris, D. (1999). Glucose oxidaseproduced H2O2 induces Ca2+ dependent DNA damage in human peripheral blood lymphocytes, *Free Radic. Biol. Med.*, Vol. 26, pp. 548–556

Park, CK.; Jung, JH.; Moon, MJ.; Kim, YY.; Kim, JH.; Park, SH.; Kim, CY.; Paek, SH.; Kim, DG.; Jung, HW. & Cho, BK. (2009). Tissue expression of manganese superoxide dismutase is a candidate prognostic marker for glioblastoma, *Oncology*, Vol.77, No. 3- 4, pp. 178-81

Pelicano, H.; Carney, D. & Huang P. (2004). ROS stress in cancer cells and therapeutic implications, *Drug Resist Updates*, Vol. 7, pp. 97–110

Puri, T.; Goyal, S.; Julka, PK.; Nair, O.; Sharma, DN & Rath, GK. (2010). Lycopene in treatment of high-grade gliomas: a pilot study, *Neurol India*, Vol. 58, No. 1, pp. 20-23

Purkayastha, S.; Berliner, A.; Shawn Fernando, S.; Ranasinghe, B.; Ray, I.; Tariq, H. & Probal BanerjeE, P. (2009). Curcumin blocks brain tumor formation, *Brain Research*, Vol. 1266, pp. 130-138

Rajaraman, P.; Hutchinson, A.; Rothman, N.; Black, PM.; Fine, HA.; Loeffler, JS.; Selker, RG.; Shapiro, WR.; Linet, MS. & Inskip, PD. (2008). Oxidative response gene polymorphisms and risk of adult brain tumors, *Neuro Oncol.*, Vol. 10, No. 5, pp. 709- 715

Schild, L.; Chen, BH.; Makarov, P.; Kattengell, K.; Heinitz, K. & Keilhoff, G. (2010). Selective induction of apoptosis in glioma tumour cells by a Gynostemma pentaphyllum extract, *Phytomedicine*, Vol. 17, No. 8-9, pp. 589-597

Shaw, JP. & Chou, IN. (1986). Elevation of intracellular glutathione content associated with mitogenic stimulation of quiescent fibroblasts, *J. Cell. Physiol.*, Vol. 129, pp. 193–198

Shivakumar, BR.; Anandatheerthavarada, HK. & Ravindranath, V. (1991). Free radical scavenging systems in developing rat brain. *Int. J. Dev. Neurosci.*, Vol. 9, pp. 181-185

Sies, H. (1986). Biochemistry of oxidative stress, *Angewandte Chem.*, Vol. 25, pp. 1058–1071

Sies, H. (1993). Strategies of antioxidant defense, *Eur. J. Biochem.*, Vol. 215, pp. 213-219

Smith, CV.; Jones, DP.; Guenthner, TM.; Lash, LH. & Lauterburg, BH. (1996). Compartmentation of glutathione: implications for the study of toxicity and disease, *Toxicol. Appl. Pharmacol.*, Vol. 140, pp. 1-12

Stadtman, ER. & Berlett, BS. (1997). Reactive oxygen-mediated protein oxidation in aging and disease, *Chem. Res. Toxicol.*, Vol. 10, pp. 485–494

Suzuki, YJ.; Forman, HJ. & Sevanian, A. (1997). Oxidants as stimulators of signal transduction, *Free Radic. Biol. Med.*, Vol. 22, pp. 269-285

Szatrowski, TP. & Nathan, CF. (1991). Production of large amounts of hydrogen peroxide by human tumor cells, *Cancer Res.*, Vol. 51, pp. 794– 798

Tanriverdi, T.; Hanimoglu, H.; Kacira, T.; Sanus, GZ.; Kemerdere, R.; Atukeren, P.; Gumustas, K, Canbaz, B. & Kaynar, MY. (2007). Glutathione peroxidase, glutathione reductase and protein oxidation in patients with glioblastoma multiforme and transitional meningioma, *J. Cancer Res. Clin. Oncol.*, Vol. 133, pp. 627–633

Terradez, P.; Asensi, M.; Lasso de la Vega, MC.; Puertes, I.; Vin˜a, J.; Estrela, JM. (1993). Depletion of tumour glutathione in vivo by buthionine sulfoximine: modulation by the rate of cellular proliferation and inhibition of cancer growth, *Biochem. J.*, Vol., 292, pp. 477–483

Tuzgen, S.; Hanimoglu, H.; Tanriverdi, T.; Kacira, T.; Sanus, GZ.; Atukeren, P.; Dashti, R.; Gumustas, K.; Canbaz, B. & Kaynar, MY. (2007). Relationship between DNA damage and total antioxidant capacity in patients with glioblastoma multiforme, *Clin Oncol (R Coll Radiol).*, Vol. 19, No. 3, pp. 177-81

Urig, S. & Becker, K. (2006). On the potential of thioredoxin reductase inhibitors for cancervtherapy, *Semin. Cancer Biol.*, Vol. 16, pp. 452–465

Uttara, B.; Singh, A. V.; Zamboni, P.; Mahajan, RT. (2009). Oxidative stress and neurodegenerative diseases: a review of upstream and downstream antioxidant therapeutic options, *Curr.Neuropharmacol.*, Vol. 7, No. 1, pp. 65-74

Valko, M.; Izakovic, M.; Mazur, M.; Rhodes, CJ. & Telser, J. (2004). Role of oxygen radicals in DNA damage and cancer incidence, *Mol. Cell. Biochem.*, Vol. 266, pp. 37–56

Valko, M.; Morris, H. & Cronin, MTD. (2005). Metals, toxicity and oxidative stress, *Curr. Med. Chem.*, Vol. 12, pp. 1161–1208

Valko, M.; Rhodes, C. J.; Moncol, J.; Izakovic, M. &Mazur,M. (2006). Free radicals, metals and antioxidants in oxidative stress-induced cancer, *Chem. Biol. Interact.*, Vol., 160, pp. 1–40

Winterbourn, CC. & Hampton, MB. (2008). Thiol chemistry and specificity in redox signaling, *Free Radic. Biol. Med.*, Vol. 45, pp. 549–561

Zengin. E.; Atukeren, P.; Kokoglu, E.; Gumustas, MK. & Zengin, U. (2009). Alterations in lipid peroxidation and antioxidant status in different types of intracranial tumors within their relative peritumoral tissues, *Clin Neurol Neurosurg.*, Vol. 111, No. 4, pp. 345-51